MATERIA MEDICA OF INDIA AND THEIR THERAPEUTICS

MATERIA MEDICA OF INDIA
AND THEIR
THERAPEUTICS

BY

RUSTOMJEE NASERWANJEE KHORY

AND

NANABHAI NAVROSJI KATRAK

GYAN

Published by

Gyan Publishing House
5, Ansari Road
Daryaganj, New Delhi-110002
Phone: 011-47034999, 9811692060
E-mail: books@gyanbooks.com

Distribution Network
gyanbooks.com
India, USA, Canada, UK, Australia

ISBN: 978-93-6920-084-9 (HB)
First Published, 1903

2nd Impression 2025

Printed at: Gyan Press, Delhi.

MATERIA MEDICA OF INDIA AND THEIR THERAPEUTICS
Author: RUSTOMJEE NASERWANJEE KHORY AND NANABHAI NAVROSJI KATRAK

MATERIA MEDICA OF INDIA

AND THEIR

THERAPEUTICS.

BY

RUSTOMJEE NASERWANJEE KHORY,

Honorary Physician, Sir J. J. Hospital and attached to Bai Motlibai and Sir Dinsha Petit. Hospitals; Member of the Royal College of Physicians, London; Fellow and Licentiate of Medicine of the University of Bombay; Doctor of Medicine (Brux.); Late Syndic and Dean of the Faculty of Medicine, University of Bombay; Late President, Grant College Medical Society; Fellow of the Royal Medical and Chirurgical Society of London; Fellow of the Obstetric Society, London; Justice of the Peace for the City of Bombay; Author of "The Digest of Medicine," "The Principles and Practice of Medicine," "The Bombay Materia Medica and Their Therapeutics"; Examiner in Materia Medica and Therapeutics and in Midwifery and Diseases of Women and Children, University, Bombay;

AND

NANABHAI NAVROSJI KATRAK,

Licentiate of Medicine and Surgery (Bombay), Justice of the Peace for the City of Bombay; Late Chairman of the Standing Committee and Member of the Municipal Corporation of Bombay; Late Secretary and Vice-President of the Grant College Medical Society, Bombay.

BOMBAY:

PRINTED AT THE CAXTON WORKS.

1903.

To

The Right Honourable

LORD REAY, G.C.S.I., G.C.I.E., LL.D., &c.,

Late Governor of Bombay.

In grateful recognition of eminent services rendered to the cause of education in general and medical education in particular, and of many and beneficent medical reforms introduced in the Bombay Presidency, and the sympathetic solicitude evinced for raising the status and position of the local medical profession,

This work has been, by permission, respectfully dedicated.

Organic Drugs from the Vegetable Kingdom.

THE drugs belonging to this kingdom are treated in this work according to the system of natural orders, as this is the most scientific and practical of the various systems made use of in works on botany. At any rate the importance of this system so far as medicine is concerned cannot be questioned. The arrangement and sequence of the various natural orders have been determined after consulting various authors, under the hope that they will be found convenient.

Ranunculaceæ.

Bachanâga, buttercup or crowfoot family.

Ranunculaceæ is derived from Ranunculus, a little frog, as many species grow in moist places where frogs abound.

Habitat.—Cold, damp climates. Mountainous places.

Characters.—Herbs or shrubs with an acrid watery juice ; when applied fresh quickly produce a blister. Leaves alternate or opposite, generally much divided, sometimes entire with dilated and sheathing petioles. Stipules generally absent or united to the base of the petiole. Flowers small yellow, most complete ; sepals, petals and stamens all distinct hypogynous, Corolla 5 with imbricate æstivation, seeds without an aril, embryo minute at the base of homogeneous horny albumen, roots tuberous.

Properties.—The leaves and roots of many species when taken in excess produce symptoms of irritant poisoning. The different parts of the plant at different seasons abound in a volatile acrid principle which possesses local irritant, and in some cases even vesicant properties ; the acrid principle being volatile is dissipated by drying or by infusing it in boiling or even cold water. Some plants contain in addition a narcotic principle. A few plants are simply bitter tonics, alteratives and stimulants. Among the natives the poisonous plants are known as Bish nâga. The word is derived from bish—poison, and nâga—a root, a plant with poisonous root. The non-poisonous plants are known by the name of Nirbishi ; nir—against, and bisha—a poison.

Aconitum Ferox.

Habitat.—Himalaya mountains, Northern India, Nepaul, Cashmere and Sikkim.

Parts used.—The dried tuberous root.

Vernacular.—Arab.—Bish, khanikeel, namir. Beng.—Batsnâb, Bish, Mitha, telia Ati-singiabish. Bomb.—Bachnâb. Cing.—

Vachanâbhi. Duk.—Bachnâg. Guz.—Shingadio-vachnâg. Hind.—Teliyâ-bis, Bishnâb. Kâlâbâchnâg Singya-bis, Mithâ-Zahar, Bish, Bikh. Malay.—Vatsa-nâbhi. Mar.—Wuchnâk. Punj.—Moura-bikh. Pers.—Bishnâg. Sans.—Vatsanâbhâ, Visham, Shringi-bish. Tam.—Visha-navi, Vasha-nâbhi. Tel.—Ati-vassa, Vasanabhi.

Teliya means greased or oiled, to preserve them from the action of the air. Vatsa-nabhâ means navel of children, as the root resembles in appearance the navel of children. Shringe-bish from shingia or shingdân, which means a horn, and bish a poison. The smooth and tapering root of aconite resembles in appearance a goat's horn.

Characters.—The tuber is heavy, horny, fusiform or conical, generally wrinkled, dark or yellowish brown externally, and shining black within ; in shape it resembles a deer's horn. It is from 2 to 4 inches long and about an inch wide at the crown or base ; it breaks with a resinous fracture and could be reduced to a coarse powder ; the smell is very disagreeable, resembling that of cat's urine, the taste acrid and stimulating ; a portion of it when chewed causes a tingling sensation and numbness on the tongue, the sensation remaining unabated for a long time. Dose of the root 1 to 2 grains.

Constituents.—A crystalline alkaloid called napelline or pseudo aconitine, similar to aconitine (one pound yielding one drachm). It has a transparent vitreous appearance, soluble in boiling water, less soluble in ether, chloroform and alcohol. Is weaker than Aconitine. A valuable hypnotic. Dose, ¼ to ½ gr. A good substitute for opium and chloral.

Preparations.—(1) Liniment. (2) Tincture 1 in 8 of alcohol. Dose, 2 to 5 ms.

Actions and uses.—Aconitum ferox is diaphoretic, diuretic, antipyretic and anodyne. It is more diuretic and less antipyretic than A. napellus. The tincture is antiphlogistic and useful in nasal catarrh ; also in tonsillitis, sore throat, coryza, neuralgia and acute gout. The liniment is used for chilblains.

Aconitum Heterophyllum.

Habitat.—India, Himalaya.

Parts used.—The dried tuberous roots.

Vernacular.—Duk.—Ativish, Ataicha, Atvikâ, Vajje-Turki. Guz.—Atavakhâ-ni-kali, Atvasek. Hind.—Atis, Patis-Batis. Mar.—Ativish. Pers.—Vajje-Turki. Tam.—Ati vadayam. Tel.—Ati-vasa.

Ativisha—meaning counteracting poison.

Characters.—Two varieties, grey and white. White tubers are young, plump, of a pale ash colour, ovoid and half an inch to an inch long. External surface wrinkled and marked with scars of rootlets. At the broad end there are 2 or 3 scale-like rings, the remains of fallen scaly leaf buds. Grey tubers are longer and shrivelled ; both break with a resinous fracture, their interior is white, taste very bitter. Dose of the powder as a tonic, 5 to 15 grs. As an anthelmintic, 3 to 5 grs. As an antiperiodic, 20 to 30 grs.

Constituents.—An intensely bitter alkaloid—Atisine, Aconitic acid, Tannic acid, Pectous substance, abundant starch, fat, a mixture of oleic, palmitic-stearic glycerides, vegetable mucilage, cane-sugar and ash, 2 p.c.

Preparation—Tincture (1 in 8). Dose 10 to 60 ms. Bâlâgolia given to infants for restlessness and to keep them quiet. It contains 3 narcotics namely, Cannabis, Opium, and Dhatura, and the remainder 28 bitters and aromatics.

Devdâr yâdi kvâth.—Decoction.

Ativish, Shiâjirûn, Râto Dhamaso Gokharu, each one part, fry the mass and add Sunth, Kaephal, Nagarmoth, Kariatun, Kadu, Dhânâ, Himaj, Gajapipli, Dhamâso, Ringani, Galo, Kakdasingi, of each one part make a decoction (1 in 20). Dose, 4 to 12 drs. used during convalescence from fever, acute diseases, parturition, &c.

Actions and uses.—Bitter, stomachic, aphrodisiac, tonic, and antiperiodic, given during convalescence from such debilitating diseases as fevers, acute inflammatory affections, &c., used also in cough, dyspepsia and in diarrhœa depending thereupon, in which case it is given in combination with aromatics, bitters, and astringents such as Tinospora, Bonduc-nuts, Holarrhena, &c. It has been given as an antiperiodic in malarial fevers with some success, but is much inferior to quinine. Combined with vâvading it is given to expel worms.

Aconitum Lycoctonum.

Habitat.—Europe, N. Asia, Himalaya.

Part used.—The tubers.

Vernacular.—Arab.—Khanik-el-zeb. Hind.—Bika.

Constituents.—It contains two alkaloids : Lycoctonine, soluble in ether, but sparingly so in water ; and acolyctine, soluble in water, but insoluble in ether.

Aconitum Napellus, B. P.

Aconite—meaning a rock, as the root grows upon steep rocks.

Napellus—meaning a little turnip, the shape of the root being like that of the turnip.

Habitat.—Europe, Himalaya, Alps, North America.

Parts used.—The tuberous root, Aconiti Radix, B. P., and Aconiti Folia.

Vernacular.—Eng.—Wolf's-bane, Monk's-hood, mousebane, Indian Aconite, Nepaul Aconite. Arab.—Khanik-el-nemer. Beng.—Dudhia bikha. Guz.—Nagapuri Bachanaga, Dudhio Vachanaga, Hind.—Dudhia bikha, Kota bikha, Batsnab-bish, Mahoor. Panj.—Telia Kachang. Bomb.—Bachnab, Tel Vasanabha. Can.—Vasanabhi.

Khanik-el-zeib and Khanik-el-nemir. Khanik, the slayer, and Zeib, a wolf. Nemir, a panther. It means slayer of wolf and panther. Aconite was used to destroy wild beasts.

Visham, visha, a name common to any poison.

Characters.—Flowers deep blue, helmet shaped. Leaves in segment, wedge-shaped and deeply cut, and when chewed giving a sensation of tingling on the tongue and lips. Root of a brown colour, tuberous, horny, irregular and roughly wrinkled, conical, 2 to 3 inches long and one inch in thickness at the crown, the lower portion tapering and marked with a few scars and fragments of rootlets; on the top are the remains of leaflets. The root bark is thick and enclosing a seven-rayed star-shaped pith, which is whitish and starchy. The cut surface is yellowish white and resinous and made up of wedges. It is without any marked odour, the taste is somewhat sweetish at first, then becomes acrid and radish-like; when chewed it leaves a tingling sensation on the tongue for a long time. Dose, $\frac{1}{2}$ to 2 grs.

Constituents.—The chief active principle is the alkaloid aconitine in the proportion of ·03 p.c. Pseudo aconitine or napelline or Veratroyl Aconine, Pseudo aconine, and Aconella, which resembles narcotine, also Picraconitine, aconitic acid, resin, fat, and sugar.

Pseudo aconitine or Veratroyl Aconine or Napellina or Napelline is weaker than aconitine. It is more soluble in hot water and less soluble in ether and chloroform.

Aconitina, B. P., aconitine, aconitia is identical with benzoyl aconine. To obtain it mix the alcoholic extract with hot water, remove the oil and resin, cool and filter, then precipitate with ammonia, exhaust the precipitate with ether, distil and dry. Met with in colourless hexagonal, or rhombic prisms, or white amorphous solid of alkaline reaction. With acids it forms salts. It is readily soluble in alcohol or chloroform, less so in ether, nearly insoluble in cold water (1 in 150), in hot water (1 in 50), and in petroleum spirit; melts at a temperature of 375° F. A drop of even a very weak solution causes a tingling sensation on the tongue. $\frac{1}{100}$ gr. of aconitine is equivalent to about 1 grain of aconite root Dose, $\frac{1}{240}$ to $\frac{1}{80}$ grain. The salts of aconitine, namely hydrochloride and hydrobromide are both crystalline.

Preparation.—Of the leaves, Extractum aconiti. Extract of aconite. Dose, $\frac{1}{6}$ to $\frac{1}{2}$ grain. Of the root, Extractum aconiti fluidum, each drop contains one grain of the powdered root. Dose, $\frac{1}{2}$ to 2 ms.

Tinctura aconiti, B. P. (1 in 20). Dose, 5 to 15 ms., if frequently repeated 2 to 5 ms.

Linimentum aconiti, B. P. (2 in 3).

St. Jacob's Oil.—It probably contains aconite liniment, ether, alcohol, turpentine, red colouring matter and water. According to another formula it contains turpentine, aconite liniment, carbolic acid, alcohol, ether, capsicum and origanum.

Preparation.—Of aconitina. Unguentum aconitinæ, aconitine ointment, B. P., contains aconitine (2 p. c.)

Injectio aconitinæ hypodermica, contains 1 grain in 240 ms. Dose, 1 to 2 ms.

Oleatum aconitinæ, oleate of aconitine. Contains 2 p.c. of aconitine in oleic acid for external use.

Anodyne amyl colloid. It contains aconitine, veratrine, and hydride of amyl dissolved in collodion. A good application in neuralgia &c.

Bachnag Powder. To prepare it, soak small pieces of the root in milk for several hours, dry and powder. Dose, $\frac{1}{8}$ to $\frac{1}{2}$ gr.

Physiological action.—Aconite is sedative, anodyne, mydriatic and poisonous. It depresses circulation and respiration. It is a powerful depressant of the sensory nerve ends of nervous and of muscular apparatus of the heart, respiration and the spinal nervous system. It does not affect the cerebrum. At first it stimulates the vagus centre in the medulla, and lowers the heart-beat, the respiration, and arterial tension. This is soon followed by cardiac depression and paralysis of the vasomotor centre. As a sedative upon the nerve ends in small quantity it produces a little tingling and then numbness as on the tongue and lips. It also produces diaphoresis and diuresis. It acts upon the stomach and intestines, producing increased secretion. It causes constriction in the fauces, and produces nausea, vomiting and more or less salivation.

In toxic doses there is loss of sight and hearing, with dilated, sometimes contracted pupils, cold clammy sweats, great numbness, lowering of the body heat, loss of motion, sensation and impairment of reflexes, ending in convulsions, syncope and death; consciousness is generally retained to the last. Locally it is a powerful sedative, paralysing the sensory nerves around painful areas and producing numbness.

Therapeutics.—As a powerful antiphlogistic, its chief use is in the early stages of acute cararrhal or sthenic fevers, acute catarrhal inflammation and vascular excitement. In inflammation of serous membranes as acute pleurisy, in pericarditis, in orchitis, in acute peritonitis, and in acute rheumatism, if given early, it is very useful.

It should not be given in asthenic patients, in weak, fatty, or dilated heart, in continued fevers, in gastro-intestinal irritation and pulmonary inflammation. As a powerful vascular and cardiac sedative, it is given in cardiac hypertrophy without any organic lesion, and in nervous palpitation. It is also given in scarlet fever, measles, erysipelas, acute catarrh, acute bronchial affections, in coryza, tonsillitis, exophthalmic goitre, and asthma; also in croup, either spasmodic or inflammatory. Given with Dover's powder, it is very useful in breaking up a cold or an attack of influenza. It is a popular remedy with singers. They take it occasionally to clear their voice. It is very beneficial if given in local congestive neuralgia, as facial neuralgia or those affecting the branches of the fifth nerve; in diarrhœa or dysentery or in suppressed menstruation following a chill or exposure to cold and in congestive dysmenorrhoa. Given in gonorrhœa it prevents chordee. In cases requiring the passage of a catheter, tincture of aconite in drop doses prevents the chill following the cathetrism. Aconitine in $\frac{1}{240}$ grain doses is used hypodermically in acute inflammations, accompanied with high fever. As a local anodyne the liniment is applied to relieve the pain and itching in herpes zoster, pruritis and chilblain ; in neuralgia and chronic rheumatism. Aconitine ointment is a powerful local sedative and used locally in facial neuralgia, also in orchitis and painful affections of the joints. In odontalgia the tincture may be rubbed on the gums. It should not be used on an abraded surface. Aconitine ointment is very efficient in trigeminal neuralgia.

Aconitum Palmatum.

Habitat.—Himalaya, Mishmi.

Parts used.—The tubers.

Vernacular.—Bomb.—Bikhma, Vakhama ; Guz.—Vakhamo ; Hind.—Bishama.

Characters.—Tuber generally branched, colour light brown, hard and horny and breaking with a short starchy fracture. Externally the surface is longitudinally furrowed. Internally compact, shining and yellowish. Taste intensely bitter, but not acrid. Smell somewhat pungent and aromatic. Dose, 5 to 10 grs.

Constituents.—An alkaloid identical with atisine, starch, &c.

Preparation.—Infusion (1 in 20). Dose, 1 to 4 drs.

Actions and uses.—Stomachic, bitter, antiperiodic and anthelmintic; used in fevers, dyspepsia and diarrhœa. It has been also tried in cholera.

Adonis Vernalis.

False hellebore or the pheasant's eye.

Habitat.—Southern Europe and Asia.

Parts used.—The leaves and stalks.

Characters.—A perennial herb of a wild growth. Dose 3 to 6 grs.

Constituents.—The active principle is a bitter hygroscopic glucoside, called adonidin, aconitic acid,—adonido quercitrin, adonidic acid and sugar (adonido-dulcite).

Adonidinum-adonidin. A canary-yellow powder of intensely bitter taste and neutral reaction. It is soluble in water, ether and alcohol. Dose $\frac{1}{20}$ to $\frac{1}{8}$ gr.

Preparations.—Extractum adonidis liquidum. Dose, 1 to 2 ms. Tinctura adonidis. Tincture of adonis (1 in 8). Dose, 10 to 30 ms. Infusum adonidis. Infusion of adonis (1 in 40). Dose, 1 to 4 drs.

Physiological actions.—Fresh plant is acrid, irritant and vesicant; dry plant is cardiac stimulant, tonic and diuretic, similar in action to digitalis. It acts more promptly, slowing the heart beats, increasing the force, and raising the blood pressure in the arteries. It is rapidly eliminated in the urine. It is not cumulative and can be given for a long time without danger. In large or poisonous doses it at first excites the heart and then causes paralysis of the cardiac motor nerves. Adonidin is more energetic than degitoxin. It is also a cardiac sedative like belladonna.

Therapeutics.—As a diuretic it is used to remove œdema or dropsy due to diseases of the heart, chiefly the dilated heart with mitral regurgitation. It slows the respiration, relieves throbbing headache, perspiration and dyspnœa. In epilepsy it may be given with potassium bromide.

Anemone Pulsatilla.

A. pratensis (pulsatilla nigri-cans.) A. patens (pulsatilla vulgaris.) Pasque flower. Wind flower. Meadow anemone.

Anemone, from anemos the wind, wind flower, the herb grows in windy places.

Pulsatilla, from pulsere, to beat or strike, it pulsates from the wind striking or beating against the tree.

Pratensis, from pratum, a meadow or belonging to meadow; its place of growth.

Habitat.—England, Siberia, Temperate and Alpine Himalaya.

Parts used.—The flowering herb.

Vernacular.—Pers.—Shakaykel-naaman.

Characters.—Stems simple and erect, with large terminal flowers, Flowers bell-shaped, violet or purple. Fruits achenes, numerous. Root, dark-brown, oblique. Leaves silky and villous. All parts covered with soft silky hairs. Without any odour and of an acrid taste. Dose, 2 to 10 grs.

Constituents.—An acrid yellow oil, anemonal, which is converted in the presence of water into anemonin or pulsatilla camphor; the chief active principle anemonic acid; and acrid anemone camphor. Anemonin, anemoninum or pulsatilla camphor is obtained from various species of anemone. Distil the herb with water, and evaporate the distillate. It resembles camphor and is neutral white, friable, crystals or needles without odour, of an exceedingly acrid taste, soluble in chloroform and hot alcohol and sparingly so in ether and water; on the addition of alkalies it is converted into anemoninic acid, a crystalline insoluble powder; dissolves in alkalies with a yellow colour. Dose, $\frac{1}{6}$ to $\frac{1}{2}$ gr. in pill.

Preparation.—Extractum pulsatillæ liquidum. Dose, 1 to 5 ms.

Tinctura pulsatilla (1 in 10). Dose, 2 to 10 ms. Infusion (1 in 40). Dose, 1 to 4 drs.

Physiological action.—Diuretic, general stimulant, antispasmodic sedative, mydriatic, expectorant, galactagogue and emmenagogue; in toxic doses irritant. When chewed it increases the secretion of saliva. It lowers the heart, and arterial tension, reduces the respiration and the body heat. In large doses it causes nausea, vomiting and diarrhœa, and in toxic doses paralysis with stupor followed by convulsions and death. Locally it causes numbness, tingling, skin inflammation and eruptions.

Therapeutics.—The root is mixed with milk and given internally. Pulsatilla is now particularly used in functional uterine derangements as leucorrhœa, amenorrhœa, dysmenorrhœa, and other painful affections of the pelvic organs; also in rheumatism, gout, nervous headache, orchitis and epididymitis, in both of which it relieves inflammation and also the pain. As an antispasmodic it is used in coryza, rhinitis, bronchitis, asthma, whooping cough, and hysteria; as a gastric sedative it is given in dyspepsia, gastritis, flatulence, &c. Anemonin is used in asthma, bronchitis, whooping cough, &c.

Locally, 1 of tincture to 10 of water is used as an injection for leucorrhœa; mixed with walnut husk, it is used for dyeing the hair black. It is applied to scaly skin diseases and to unhealthy ulcers, syphilitic sores &c.

Cimicifuga Racemosa, B. P.

Syn—Actæa Racemosa, Bugbane, black snake root, black cohosh, rattle root.

Cimicifuga, that which drives away bugs, in allusion to the use of one variety to drive away bugs.

Habitat.—Rich woodlands, Cashmere, Temperate Himalaya, United States.

Parts used.—The dried rhizome with the attached rootlets. Cimicifugæ—Rhizoma-Cimicifuga syn. Actææ Racemosæ Radix, B. P.

Characters.—Rhizome 2 to 6 inches long and ½ inch to 1 inch in diameter, horizontal, thick, hard and covered with cup-shaped scars; the roots are brittle, especially near the rhizome; on section they form 3 to 5 wedge-shaped woody bundles, separated by medullary rays, colour brownish-black, odour slight, taste bitter and nauseous like that of opium.

Constituents.—Resins (3½ p. c.), fat, starch, gum, tannic and gallic acids, sugar, volatile oil (when fresh), and an acrid crystallizable neutral principle known as cimicifugin. Of the two resins, one is soluble in alcohol, but not in ether, and the other soluble in ether and alcohol as well.

Cimicifugin. To obtain it act upon the rhizomes with alcohol, precipitate the solution with acetate of lead, remove the lead with sulphuretted hydrogen and evaporate.

Characters.—A powder of a yellowish-brown colour, soluble in alcohol and chloroform, slightly so in ether and water. Dose, ½ to 2 grs.

Preparation.—Extractum cimicifugæ liquidum, B. P. Dose, 5 to 30 ms. Extractum cimicifugæ. Dose, 1 to 4 grs. Tinctura cimicifugæ, Tincture of Actæa Racemosa, B. P. (1 in 10). Dose, 30 to 60 ms.

Physiological action.—The root is alterative, stomachic, emmenagogue, aphrodisiac, diuretic, diaphoretic, and antispasmodic. Its action on the heart, circulation, and the nervous system is similar to that of digitalis. On the unstriped muscular fibres its action resembles that of ergot. In small doses it is a gastric stimulant. It increases the activity of the generative organs and the menstrual flow, also stimulates the bronchial mucous membranes and the kidneys. In large doses it slows the heart, but increases its force, also raises the arterial tension. In toxic doses it acts as an irritant, dilates the pupils, produces dimness of sight, headache, nervous tremor, violent delirium, giddiness, nausea, vomiting, and depression of pulse.

Therapeutics.—It has been given in chronic muscular rheumatism, lumbago, torticollis, intercostal neuralgia, sciatica, pleurodynia, and headache due to fatigue. As a stomachic tonic it is given in dyspepsia due to alcoholism, and as a nervine tonic in delirium tremens, hysteria, ovarian neuralgic pains, chorea and impotence or seminal discharges ; as an ecbolic it increases the flow of menses. It is also useful in menorrhagia and metrorrhagia, subinvolution of the uterus, and in irritable womb affections, &c. As an expectorant it is of benefit in acute and chronic bronchitis and phthisis. In puerperal mania or puerperal peritonitis, also in puerperal hypochondriasis, its good effects are well marked. Cimicifugin is given to excite the contraction of the uterus to check or allay after-pains of delivery.

Actæa spicata, or baneberry (Eng.), possesses properties similar to cimicifuga racemosa.

Clematis Triloba.

Habitat.—Mountains of Western India.

Parts used.—The leaves.

Vernacular.—Guz.—Rânjâi. Hind.—Rânjâi. Mar.—Morvel. Sans.—Laghu-karani.

Laghu-karani.—Laghu, small or light, and karani, ear, in allusion to the shape of the leaves.

Characters.—A climber, young branches tomentose and silky, leaves on longish petioles, simple or alternately divided, elliptical, or ovate and lanceolate, flowers large and white.

Preparation.—Infusion (1 in 20). Dose, 1 to 2 ozs.

Actions and uses.—Alterative and sedative, used like sarsaparilla in blood diseases, such as syphilis, chronic fevers and scrofula. It is also given in leprosy. The juice of the leaves, combined with that of the leaves of holarrhena antidysenterica, is dropped into the eye for the relief of pain in staphyloma.

Coptis Teeta.

C. trifoliata—Coptis or mishmi teeta.

Habitat.—Assam, China, Thibet, Mishmee Mountains.

Parts used.—The dried rhizome.

Vernacular.—Arab.—Urûk, Màhâmirân Assam.—Mishmee, Teeta ; Chin.—Sou-lene or Chynlen, Honglane ; Cing.—Pita-karo-. sana. Eng.—Goden thread root. Guz.—Haladio Vachnâg. Hind. Bomb.—Mishmitita and Maha-miran.

Urak, a kind of turmeric ; Mismi means bitter.

Characters.—Two varieties—superior rhizome, creeping, golden yellow, thick as a cane and marked with spinous projections where the rootlets have been broken off. Jointed, nuckle-like at the upper end; knotty, perfectly dry and brittle. Inferior rhizome, as thick as a goose-quill, rootlets thin and wiry, breaks with a short fracture, centre spongy, taste intensely bitter, without any odour. The root, when chewed, tinges the saliva yellow. Dose, 15 to 60 grs.

Constituents.—Berberine, 8½ p.c., a colourless alkaloid coptine and resin.

Berberine, a yellow, bitter crystalline alkaloid, also found in Hydrastis, calumba root, berberry and Thalictrum foliolum.

Preparation.—Tinctura coptidis (1 in 10). Dose, 30 to 60 ms. Infusum coptidis (1 in 20). Dose, 1 to 2 fld. ozs.

Actions and uses.—Bitter, stomachic tonic, antiperiodic and alterative; also local stimulant. As a tonic its influence in restoring appetite and increasing the digestive power is very marked. Largely used, in native practice, in dyspepsia and in convalescence from acute diseases. It has a gentle action on the bowels. In ague and other fevers it may be given both during and after the paroxysms. Under its use patients recover from acute diseases manifestly improved in strength. As an alterative it is used in enlarged liver and spleen. Especially used in jaundice. Locally it stimulates the mucous membranes, and is used as a gargle in sore throat and ulcers in the mouth. It is also used, combined with Berberis asiatica, in conjunctivitis and as a snuff in coryza.

Delphinium Denudatum.

Habitat.—Sirmoor, Lahore, Punjab.

Parts used.—Tubers and seeds.

Vernacular.—Greek—Saturyno. Arab—Zhadvar, antila. Bom.—Jadwar Nirbishi. Pers.—Mâh-pârvin, Mafarfin. Sans.—Jadavàr.

Jadwar.—The great purifier of blood or antidote. Mah-parwin.—Moon and Pleiades, the plant blossoms in summer when the Pleiades rise.

Nirbishi, Nir opposed to and Bisi belonging to Bis or poison, that is, it is opposed to, or an antidote to, poison.

Characters.—Tubers small, blackish-brown, irregularly ovoid, wrinkled, somewhat conical, seldom more than an inch long and ½ inch in diameter, having a few horn-like projections at the top, the remains of rootlets. Cut surface, softish, of a dark-brown colour and homogeneous, unctuous to the touch, taste bitter, odour fruity.

Constituents.—Some species contain delphinine and staphisagrine. Both soluble in alcohol, staphisagrine is insoluble in ether in which delphinine is soluble.

Preparation.—Decoction (1 in 10). Dose, 2 to 4 drs.

Actions and uses.—Alterative, stomachic tonic, and anodyne. As a tonic it is used during convalescence from fevers; as an alterative in syphilis and rheumatism. The root is chewed to relieve toothache. Delphine resembles aconitine, and is antidotal against muscarine and digitaline. Staphisagrine acts like curare and paralyses the motor nerves.

Remarks.—According to Persian medical works Jadwâr is found growing together with Bish (A. ferox), to which and to snake poison Jadwâr is considered an antidote.

Delphinium Brunonianum.

Vernacular.—Samp-phali (Hind).

Habitat.—Punjab, Himalaya.

Characters.—The root has a strong scent of musk.

Actions and uses.—The juice is used to destroy ticks in animals.

Delphinium Cœruleum.

Vernacular.—Dakhan-ghu, a Punjab plant, used to kill maggots.

Caltha palustris.—The marsh marigold found in marshes in the Western Himalaya. The root is poisonous.

Delphinium Zalil.

Habitat.—Khorasan and Badghis.

Parts used.—The herb.

Vernacular. — Arab. — Zireer. Hind — Astruck Trayamâna. Burm.—Pai. Bomb.—Trâya-mân, Gul-Jalil. Guz.—Trayaman. Mah.—Trayaman. Pers.—Zalel, Asfrak. Punj.—Asbarga-yafiz-Gâfiz. Sans — Trâya matika, Bolâ deva, Balâ-bhadra, Arjaka, Mangalyarha.

Characters.—Herb light-brown or yellow, placed in water it tinges it bright yellow; stems angular and furrowed, a span high and generally torn lengthwise; flowers pubescent, perfect, ribbed, yellow like those of Asfara-bârri and surrounded by pointed follicles. Taste bitter and somewhat aromatic; odour honey-like.

Constituents.—A dark-reddish acid resin; two neutral principles (white and yellow), tannin, and two bitter alkaloids, somewhat similar to delphinine and berberine, ash, 17·8 p.c.

Preparation.—Ash and decoction (1 in 20). Doze—2 to 6 drs.

Actions and uses.—A bitter tonic, alterative, anodyne, diuretic and parasiticide. As a tonic it is used in fevers and dyspepsia; as an alterative and diuretic in enlargement of the abdominal viscera, as liver and spleen, in jaundice and dropsy. Locally, mixed with lime-juice, the ash is used in parasitic affections of the skin, as scabies, itch, &c. With barley meal a poultice of it is used in inflammatory swellings.

Remarks.—Sometimes the rhizomes of valeriana hardwickii are sold by native druggists for this drug.

Delphinium Staphisagria, B. P.

Staphisagria means wild dried grape. The fruits are in clusters and resemble wild grapes.

Delphinium, a dolphin.—The shape of unopened flowers is like that of a dolphin's head.

Habitat.—Mediterranean Coast, France, Italy, Levant, Asia Minor.

Parts used.—The seeds. Staphisagriæ Semina, B.P.—Semen Pedicularis, stavesacre seeds.

Characters.—An annual or biennial plant. Flowers in racemes. They are bluish or purple, the seeds are irregularly triangular or obscurely quadrangular, arched or straight, blackish brown, becoming dull, greyish brown by keeping. Testa brownish grey, wrinkled and deeply pitted with reticulated ridges. The interior of the seeds is soft, whitish, and contains oily albumen, enclosing a small embryo. The taste is nauseous, bitter and acrid, without any odour. Dose of the powder, 1 to 2 grs.

Constituents.—Seeds contain several alkaloids—delphinine, delphinoidin, delphisine, and staphisagrine. It also contains resin, fatty matters, a bitter principle, volatile oil, and fixed oil 25 p. c., malic acid, proteids, mucilage. The fatty oil could be extracted by ether.

Delphinine, Delphinina, Delphia.

Characters.—An amorphous, brownish white or yellowish crystals.

Manufacture.—Obtained by boiling the decoction of the seeds with magnesia, treating the precipitate with alcohol and evaporating. It is insoluble in water, soluble in alcohol, ether, dilute acids and chloroform. Dose $\frac{1}{4}$ to $\frac{1}{2}$ gr.

Staphisagrine.—An amorphous yellow alkaloid of a bitter acrid taste. Insoluble in ether, soluble in chloroform and alcohol.

Preparation.—Of the seed; unguentum staphisagriæ, ointment of staphisagria, stavesacre ointment, B. P. (4 in. 23). Oleum staphisagriæ. Tincture (10 p. c.) Dose, 5 to 10 ms.

Preparation of Delphinine.—Ointment (20 grs. to 1 oz.)

Physiological action.—The seeds are parasiticide (owing their property to the fixed oil), violent emetic, diuretic and cathartic. The alkaloid delphinine, which is a local irritant, produces tingling, burning, and inflammation of the skin. It is a heart poison, and, like aconitine and veratrine, it depresses the heart and respiration. In large doses it leads to paralysis of the spinal cord and asphyxia. Internally it has to be used very guardedly.

Therapeutic uses.—The powdered seeds are used, as an ointment, to destroy scabies, pediculi, vermin, lice, &c.; as a liniment for rheumatism, neuralgia, &c.

Delphinine is given internally in dropsy, rheumatism, spasmodic asthma and neuralgia ; externally the ointment or an alcoholic solution is applied over the painful nerve areas, in neuralgia, toothache and earache. Delphinine and staphisagrine are antidotes to muscarine and digitalin poisoning.

Helleborus Niger, Helleborus Officinalis. Black Hellebore.

Habitat.—South Europe, Germany, Nepaul Mountains.

Part used.—The dried rootlets and rhizome.

Vernacular.—Arab—Khartik Kuerbeck Kharbec-ul-aswad. Bomb. —Kutki. Duk.—Kutki. Eng.—Hellebore. Guz.—Kuddu. Hind.—Kutki, Kuddu. Mar.—Bâla-kadu. Pers.—Khârbek-e-hindi. Tam.—Kataka-rohini. Sans.—Kataka-rohani, Katuruni. Singh.—Calurana.

Characters.—Roots black, and hence the name. As met with in the bazaar it is of two different colours, each having a different name, the red known as Kadu and black, Kali Kutaki. In both the rhizome is knotty, in short broken pieces 1 to 3 inches long, in size resembling a goose quill. Externally smooth and of a brownish white colour, slightly shrivelled and marked with scars of fallen rootlets. Very fragile, light soft, and can be compressed between the fingers. On section the cut surface appears as if made up of layers or scales. Has a white broken ring between the centre and the external surface ; odour heavy, resembling that of majith or tobacco. Taste somewhat acrid and very bitter. The colour is brownish dark. In size somewhat thicker. Externally each piece is covered over with numerous (from 3 to 4) longitudinally nerved scales, or marks of leaflets.

Dose, powdered rhizome as a tonic, 10 to 30 grs.; as a purgative, $\frac{1}{2}$ to 1 dr.

Constituents.—Helleborine, Helleborein—both crystalline and poisonous, resin, fat, &c.

Helleborine.—Insoluble in water, but soluble in alcohol and chloroform.

Helleborein.—It is crystalline, very soluble in water, slighty so in alcohol and insoluble in ether. Dose, $\frac{1}{16}$ to $\frac{1}{10}$. gr. Used as 1 p.c. solution.

Preparation.—Fluid extract of black hellebore. Dose, 3 to 20 ms.

Extract of black hellebore. Dose, 1 to 4 grs., cautiously.

Physiological action.—In small dose it is a bitter tonic, stomachic, also antiperiodic. In large doses a drastic hydragogue, cathartic and an emmenagogue. In toxic doses a violent, gastro-intestinal irritant, giving rise to vomiting, purging, vertigo, cramps and convulsions, often ending in death. As a purgative it resembles colocynth. Helleborin is an active poison ; when applied to the tongue it causes, like aconite, tingling sensation. Internally as a narcotic it causes paralysis of motion and sensation, congestion of the brain and spinal cord, dilated pupils, and death.

Helleborein is an irritant of the mucous membranes of the eyes, nose, stomach, intestines, giving rise to conjunctivitis, sneezing, salivation, nausea, vomiting and purging. In small doses, like digitalis, it acts as a cardiac tonic, but slows the frequency of the pulse. In large doses it quickens the pulse, ultimately paralysing the heart. The respiration is at first increased, then slowed, and at last becomes laborious, there is increased activity of the kidneys and uterus. In toxic doses there is gradual paralysis, followed by convulsions, and death.

Therapeutics.—Hellebore is given in acute cerebral affections, fevers, dyspepsia and in jaundice; the natives give it in combination with holarrhena antidysenterica seeds in amenorrhœa, melancholia, mania, insanity, worms, dropsies, skin diseases. Helleborein, as a substitute for digitalis, is hypodermically injected or given internally in smaller doses in diseases of the heart. As a local anæsthetic it is more powerful than cocaine ; 3 to 4 drops of 1 p. c. solution of helleborein causes complete anæsthesia of the cornea; on the addition of a little erythrophlœin, the anæsthetic effect lasts for a very long time.

Helleborus Fœtidus.—Bear's foot. Decoction or syrup of leaves used for asthma, hysteria, hypochondriasis. Dose 5 to 20 grs.

Helleborus Viridis is the green hellebore. The root is used like the root of H. Niger.

Hepatica Triloba.—Liver wort.

Habitat.—North America, Europe.

Part used.—The leaves.

Characters.—Leaves reniform, 3-lobed, 2 inches long. Dose, ½ to 2 drs.

Constituents.—Tannin, mucilage.

Preparation.—Decoction (1 in 20). Dose, 1 to 2 ozs. Infusion (1 in 20). Dose, 1 to 2 ozs.

Actions and uses.—Demulcent, tonic deobstruent ; given in liver disorders and in respiratory diseases, such as phthisis, bronchitis, &c.

Hydrastis Canadensis, B.P.

Golden seal, eye balm, orange root, yellow paint, ohio curcuma.

Hydrastis.—So called because its active properties are found in the watery juice, or because it grows in marshy or watery places.

Golden seal.—In allusion to the yellow rhizome, once used as a yellow paint and dye.

Habitat.—North America, Canada, &c.

Parts used.—The dried rhizome and rootlets. Hydrastis Rhizoma Hydrastis Rhizome, B. P.

Characters.—Rhizome, yellowish brown, tortuous, 2 inches long and ¼ of an inch thick, longitudinally wrinkled and breaking with a short resinous fracture; bark thick and reddish-yellow, with medullary rays, pith large, of a greenish-yellow colour, exhibiting a ring of 10 bright yellow wood bundles; roots thin and brittle; taste bitter and odour slight. Dose, 5 to 30 grs.

Constituents.—Hydrastine, berberine, xanthopuccine, canadine, starch, sugar, resin, and a fluorescent compound.

Hydrastina. Hydrastine.—To obtain it, add hydrochloric acid and water to the powdered root. Filter and remove the precipitate of berberine, and add ammonia to the filtrate, To purify hydrastine add alcohol, filter through charcoal and crystallize. It occurs in the root to the extent of 1·5 p.c.

Characters.—In white crystals, resembling strychnine in appearance, very sparingly soluble in water, soluble in alcohol, ether and chloroform. Taste very bitter; combined with acids it forms salts; on dry distillation, it is converted into trimethylamine and meconin. Dose, ¼ to 1 gr. From hydrastine is prepared an oxidation product, hydrastinine.

To obtain hydrastinine, oxidize hydrastine with binoxide of manganese and sulphuric acid. Hydrastinine hydrochloride, the salt generally used, occurs as light yellow crystals deliquescent, of bitter taste, soluble in water (1 in 1) and alcohol (1 in 3). Dose, ½ to 1 grain; in a 10 p.c. solution it is used as an injection hypodermically for uterine hæmorrhages.

Berberine.—Occurs as yellow crystals, soluble in alcohol and water, and insoluble in ether. Canadine.—In white needles; Canadine sulphate is soluble in water and alcohol. Xanthopuccine.—In yellow crystals. It unites with acids to form salts. It is probably impure berberine.

Preparation of Hydrastis.—Extractum hydrastis liquidum, B. P.—Liquid extract of hydrastis. Dose, 5 to 15 ms.

Hydrastin.—A dry extractive. It is obtained by evaporating extractum hydrastis liquidum. It consists chiefly of hydrochloride of berberine. It should not be confounded with the crystalline alkaloid—Hydrastine. It is of a bright yellow colour. Dose 2 to 6 grs.

Tinctura Hydrastis, B.P. Tincture of Hydrastis (1 in 10). Dose, ½ to 1 drm.

Physiological action.—Alterative aperient, antiperiodic, diuretic and antiseptic. In small doses it is a bitter and stomachic tonic. It has a stimulating action on the mucous membrane of the stomach and intestines. It promotes appetite, increases gastro-intestinal secretions, and stimulates the flow of bile. It is a good deobstruent to the glandular system. It causes uterine contractions If long continued, it deranges digestion and leads to constipation. It is a poison to the protoplasm and arrests the movements of the white corpuscles. Hydrastine is similar in action to quinine. It produces effects on the nervous system and causes ringing in the ears.

Hydrastinine is utero vaso constrictor, antispasmodic and cardiac stimulant.

Therapeutics.—As a stomachic tonic it is used in atonic dyspepsia gastro-intestinal catarrh, jaundice, in catarrh of the bladder, uterus, vagina, &c., and in chronic alcoholism. It stimulates the liver in habitual constipation. In menorrhagia and other uterine hæmorrhages, it is given in preference to ergot and iron, also used in hæmoptysis and night sweats of phthisis.

Hydrastine, the alkaloid, and hydrastin, the dry extractive, are both used as antiperiodics like quinine, in chronic malaria and in intermittent fevers. As alteratives they are given internally in all forms of catarrh, chiefly of the stomach, duodenum, bile-ducts, bladder, uterus, vagina, &c. As cholagogue it is given in constipation and in sluggish liver. Externally as an injection, the solution of the extract (1 in 50), or the infusion of hydrastis (1 in 50) is used in chronic gonorrhœa, leucorrhœa, gleet, and in chronic nasal catarrh. The solution is also applied to syphilitic sores in the mouth, throat, &c., to rectal fissures and fistula, to anal prolapse, hæmorrhoids, cracks and fissures of the nipples, abrasions, erosion and ulceration of the os and cervix. As an ointment (1 in 25) it is used in eczema. It is also used as a local antiseptic dressing for unhealthy wounds and cancerous ulcers.

Hydrastinine hydrochloride is used hypodermically in menstrual irregularities a few days before the expected time. Combined with ergot and cannabis it has been used in uterine hæmorrhages, such as congestive dysmenrrhœa, menorrhagia and metrorrhagia, also in metritis, endometritis, pyosalpingitis, &c.; also to induce abortion. Given also in epilepsy, hydrophobia, strychnine poisoning, with good results. Externally applied in acne and hyperidrosis.

Nigella Sativa—N. Indica.

Habitat.—The Mediterranean countries. Cultivated in India.

Parts used.—The seeds. Mugrela seeds.

Vernacular.—Arab.—Kamûne-asvad, Hubba tussoudâ. Beng.—Kâl-Zira. Bomb.—Kelanji. Bur.—Satmung-net. Can.—Karé-jirágè. Cing.—Kaluduru. Duk.—Kalanji. Eng.—Small fennel flowers.

Egypt—Habes-souda. Guz.—Kalijiri. Hind.—Kalajira, mugrila. Malyal.—Karum-chirakam. Mar.—Kalajire. Pers.—Siyah-berang, shunez. Sans.—Krishna-jiraka, Karavi, Sushavi. Tam.—Karin-shiragum. Tel.—Nalla-jilakara. Singh.—Kaloo-dooroo.

Characters.—It is probably the black cumin of the Bible. The seeds resemble coarse gunpowder and are triangular, the umbilical end smaller than the other. Surface, black, wrinkled and marked by irregular depressions. Testa rough. Internally the seeds contain a white oily kernel of a strong aromatic odour, resembling lemons, sassafras or cubebs. The taste is oily at first, after a time it resembles that of garlic. Dose, 4 to 8 grs.

Constituents.—The seeds contain a fixed oil 37.5 and volatile oil 1.5, albumen 8.25, mucilage 2, albumen 1.8, organic acids 0·9, metarabin 1.4, melanthin, resembling helleborin, 1.4, ash 4·5, moisture 7.4, sugar glucose 2.5 and arabic acid 3.2, &c.

Preparation.—Medicated oil (oleum mugrelæ) Tincture (1 in 8). Dose, 30 to 60 ms. Decoction mugrela (1 in 20). Dose, 4 to 8 fluid drs.

Actions and uses.—Anthelmintic, diuretic, galactagogue, emmenagogue and carminative. It as an aromatic adjunct to purgative and bitter remedies. A decoction of the seeds just after delivery is given to stimulate the uterus to contraction and to increase the secretion of the milk ; also in worms. As a carminative and stomachic with plumbago-root, it is given in dyspepsia, loss of appetite, diarrhœa and intermittent fevers. As an emmenagogue it is used in amenerrhœa and in dysmenorrhœa. In large doses it causes abortion. Locally it is largely used brayed in water to remove painful swellings of hands and feet.

Remarks.—The seeds are scattered between woollen shawls and clothes as a protection against insects.

Pæonia Officinalis.

Habitat.—Temperate Himalaya and Europe.

Parts used.—The tubers.

Vernacular.—Pers. and Arab.—Fawania Aod-el-Salib. Bomb.—Ud salap. Eng.—Peony rose, officinal Peony. Hind.—Ud salap.

Ude salam is a corruption of Aod-el-salib, meaning wood of the cross." The wood on section shows two lines crossing each other like a cross. Aod-el-salib is also the name of Peony corallina or male peony, the roots of which is turnip shaped.

Pæon, the physician of the gods.

Characters.—Tubers irregular, flattened, turnip shaped, one to two inches in length and from ½ an inch to 1 inch in thickness. Hard, heavy, and conical ; external surface or epidermis brownish, shrivelled, tough, and fibrous or rugous, with numerous fissures radiating from the centre. At the top is a hard conical point, the remains of a stem.

2

When cut, the tuber is starchy and presents a bluish surface, resembling catechu or chobchini, and consists of 2 or 3 rings. Smell peculiar, acrid, and resembles that of ipecacuanha. Taste slightly acrid and nauseous. Dose, 3 to 10 grs.

Constituents.—Tuber contains malates, oxalates and phosphates, a little tannin, sugar, starch and a volatile oil.

Actions and uses.—Acrid, alterative, antispasmodic, and emmenagogue. As an antispasmodic it is used in uterine obstructions, biliary, intestinal and renal colic, hysteria, epilepsy, palpitation of the heart, asthma and convulsive affections. It is, however, in great repute as an emmenagogue in dysmenorrhœa and amenorrhœa, to stimulate the secretion of menses. As an alterative, it is used in syphilis, torpor of the liver and ascites. In large doses it is poisonous, causing giddiness, vomiting, &c.

Remarks.—The peasantry of Europe, even nowadays, put a garland of these seeds round the necks of children during dentition, or a bag containing pieces of the root is suspended from the neck, under the superstitious belief that it wards off convulsions.

Pænia Emodi.

Habitat.—Panjab.

Part used.—The tuber.

Vernacular.—Mamekh.

Actions and uses.—Similar to those of Pæonia officinalis.

Ranunculus bulbosus. Crowfoot.

Habitat.—Europe, North America.

Parts used.—The herb and corm.

Characters.—The plant is hairy, 6 to 18 inches high. The bulb at the stem base. Dose—$\frac{1}{2}$ to 1 drs.

Constituents.—A volatile oil, anemonine, and anemonic acid.

Preparation.—Decoction, infusion (1 in 20). Dose, 1 to 2 ozs.

Actions and uses.—Irritant, diuretic and narcotic. Locally applied to the chest in bronchitis. Also in rheumatism, sciatica, neuralgia, &c.

Thalictrum Foliolosum.

Habitat.—Temperate Himalaya, Khosia Hills, Sutlej Valleys, Kamaon Mountains.

Parts used.—The root.

Vernacular.—Bomb.—Piaranga, Mimeeree. Eng.—Gold thread, Meadow rue, Poorman's rhubarb. Hind.—Shuprak Mamiran, Pilijari. Punj.—Bur-moti, Gurbiani. Sans.—Pitaka. Pilijari—pili, yellow, and jari, jar, a root. The root is yellow.

Characters.—The root, often mistaken for Coptis Teeta. It is creeping and of yellow colour, as thick as a goose quill; surface slightly contorted, knotty, and covered with scales, the remains of rootlets. Cut surface is resinous, of a deep yellow colour and hollow in the centre. Light yellow rings arranged in wedges, found between the hollow and the external portion. Taste bitter, odour resembling that of Fel bovinum. Dose—5 to 10 grs.

Constituents.—Berberine and a yellow bitter extractive.

Preparation.—Tincture (1 in 8). Dose, 20 to 30 ms. Liquid extract. Dose, 5 to 20 ms., and snuff.

Actions and uses.—Aperient, bitter tonic and febrifuge, used in atonic dyspepsia, jaundice and flatulence, in the interval of intermittent fever and during convalescence from fevers and acute diseases, as an aperient, it acts gently on the bowels, a good substitute for rhubarb. The snuff is used in coryza. It is a febrifuge of some power.

Magnoliaceæ.

The magnolia or Bâdiana family.

Trees or shrubs, leaves alternate, beautiful leathery and stipulate. Flowers sweet and fragrant, white or red, and distinct, handsome with large sepals and petals in two or more rows. Fruits cone-like, stellate or capsular, with numerous carpels, one-celled, dry or succulent, dehiscent or indehiscent and distinct or somewhat coherent; seeds solitary or several, albumen fleshy and homogeneous.

Habitat.—Temperate climates, Tropics, Hindustan, Japan, China.

Properties.—Plants in this order are remarkable for their bitter, tonic, astringent, and aromatic properties; they contain an essential oil, a bitter principle and sometimes tannic acid.

Drimys Winteri or Wintera Aromatica.

Habitat—South America.

Part used.—The bark.

Vernacular.—Eng.—Winter's Bark.

Characters.—Bark in quills or curves, in thickness 2 to 4 lines. Colour greyish brown, with granular fracture; odour similar to that of canella or cinnamon, often substituted for cinnamon and sometimes called Winter's cinnamon. Canella bark has been termed spurious Winter's bark. Dose, 10 to 30 grs.

Constituents.—Winterene—a volatile oil, Resin 10 p.c.; tannin 9 p.c.

Preparation.—Tincture (1 in 10). Dose, ½ to 1 dr. Infusion (1 in 20). Dose, 4 to 12 drs.

Actions and uses.—Tonic, aromatic, and stimulant; given for colic, flatulence, scurvy, &c.

Illicium Verum, B. P.

Illicium, meaning allurement, *i.e.*, from its odour and attractive appearance. Verum, verus, true, genuine, or real type.

Habitat.—Cochin China.

Parts used.—The fruit and oil, oleum anisi, oil of anise, B. P.

Vernacular.—Arab.—Raziyanaje, Badiani Khatai. Bomb.—Badian. Burm.—Nanat-paen. Duk.—Anas-phala. Eng.—Star-anise, Chinese anise, aniseed. Hind.—Anasphil. Pers.—Badia-ni-Khatai. Tam.—Anashápu. Tel.—Marati-mogga.

Star anise.—The manner in which they grow is peculiar, the pods being in small clusters joined together at one end and diverging in 8 rays.

Characters.—A shrub ; Fruit pedunculate, of an iron-brown colour, formed of 8 carpels arranged like stars. Each carpel oval, with a broad base, compressed on both walls, and having a boat-like prominence at the top, woody, wrinkled and hard to the touch. The cavity reddish-brown and glossy, opening by a slit at its upper margin ; seed, one in each carpel, smooth, shining, ovato oval, ribbed only on one side and glossy, of a brown or chestnut colour and oily ; taste of the seeds like that of anisum, sweet, aromatic, acrid at first, then astringent and, lastly, bitter. Taste of carpel like that of kabab chini. Dose 5 to 30 grs. It contains integuments or capsules, 78 p. c., and seeds 22 p.c.

Constituents.—Star anise contains volatile oil, 4 to 5 p.c. Saponin, proto catechuic acid, shikimic acid, resin, mucilage, cane-sugar and ash, 2 p.c. The volatile oil is chemically identical with the oil distilled from the fruits of pimpenella anisum and is obtained by distillation with water.

Oleum anisi, B. P., a clear colourless or pale-yellow liquid, of fruity odour and mildly aromatic sweet taste, becomes red on exposure to air, the colour resembles that of ol. fœniculi, composed of 2 parts, $\frac{1}{5}$ being a liquid anethol or anese camphor isomeric with oil of turpentine and $\frac{4}{5}$ solid anethol with small amount of terpene, safrol, anisic acid, &c. Dose $\frac{1}{2}$ to 3 ms.

Preparation.—Infusion (1 in. 20). Dose, 1 to 2 ozs.

Actions and uses.—Stimulant carminative, anodyne, and diuretic. Internally an infusion of the fruits is of great service in flatulent colic, spasmodic affections of the intestinal canal ; also in infantile retention of urine. The powdered capsules are stimulant and carminative. For oil see Pimpinella anisum. An inferior variety is occasionally sold by Mahomadan or Bohree druggists as true Badiana. The fruits are abortive, with hardly any odour, narrow, and have 13 carpels instead of eight. The colour is darker, reddish-brown and they are much wrinkled on the under surface. The ends of the carpels are more turned up than in the true variety. The taste is feebly aromatic and slightly bitter and astringent. It contains only a bitter principle and tannin.

Illicium Religiosum.

Habitat.—Cultivated round Buddhist temples in China and Japan.

Part used.—The fruit.

Vernacular.—Shikimi.

Characters.—Fruit similar to Star-anise, having 8 carpels, thin, more woody, shrivelled wrinkled, and end in a curved beak, odour clove-like and faint ; taste unpleasant.

Constituents.—It contains a liquid volatile oil, Protocatechuic acid, Shikiminic acid, Sikimipicrin, shikimin (poisonous). The volatile oil of the leaves contains saffrol, eugenol, shikimol and liquid anethol.

Actions and uses.—The fruits have poisonous properties causing vomiting, dilated pupils, epileptiform convulsions and even cyanosis.

Illicium floridanum and I. parviflorum have fruits with 13 and 8 carpels respectively. Bark is substituted for cascarilla.

Liriodendron Tulipifera.

Habitat.—United States, China.

Parts used.—The bark.

Vernacular.—Eng.—Tulip-tree.

Characters.—Bark in quills or curved pieces, a line or two in thickness, colour purplish-brown, fissured and covered with thin ridges. Inner surface smooth and whitish. Taste astringent. Dose, ½ to 1 drachm.

Constituents.—Volatile oil, resins, liriodendrin, tulipiferine, tannin.

Preparation.—Infusion (1 in 20). Dose, 4 to 8 drs. Decoction (1 in 20). Dose, 4 to 8 drs. ; fluid extract, 20 to 40 ms.

Action and uses.—Bitter tonic, given in dyspepsia, intermittent fever, also in chronic rheumatism.

Magnolia Glauca.

Swamp sassafras, beaver tree, sweet bay.

Habitat.—United States.

Part used.—The bark.

Characters.—The bark in thin quills or curved pieces ; colour orange brown, externally fissured and warty. Taste astringent, bitter; used as a powder. Dose, ½ to 1 dr.

Constituents.—Volatile oil, resin, tannin and a crystalline principle magnolin which is insoluble in water, but soluble in ether and alcohol.

Preparation.—Infusion (1 in 20). Decoction (1 in 20). Dose, 1 to 2 fl. ozs.

Actions and uses.—Tonic, aromatic, bitter, antiperiodic, diaphoretic, alterative. Resembling cinchona, and given in fevers, malaria, gout, chronic rheumatism, catarrhs. In fever it arrests the paroxysms.

Michelia Champaca—M. Nilagirica, Hill Champa.

Habitat.—India, Nilgiris, temperate Himalaya. It is cultivated for the sake of its yellow sweet-scented tulip-like flowers, which are offered to the Hindu deities.

Parts used.—The bark, leaves and flowers.

Vernacular.—Burm.—Sa-ga. Eng.—Golden or yellow champa. Beng.—Champaka. Can.—Sumpagahy. Cing.—Sappu (M. Nilagirica). Guz.—Rae champa. Hind.—Champa. Duk.—Champa. Mar.—Pivala Champa. Malyal.—Bongas jampacca. Sans.—Piti. champaka suvarna, champaka-pushpam. Tam.—Shempang shembugha. Tel.—Champa Kamu R. Dipapushpa, (lamp flower), from depa, bright, shining; and pushpa, flowers. The flowers are shining and bright.

Characters.—M. Champaca, leaves fall off during the cold season, when the tree is full of flowers. Bark light-brown externally, and can easily be removed from the wood by mere scratching; inner surface reddish brown; mottled with longitudinal green stripes and irregular pale yellow dots or scars; taste somewhat bitter and very acrid; odour faint. M. Nilagirica. Bark light-brown, also brittle and covered with lichens and mosses, of bitter taste and odour. Dose of the bark, ½ to 1 dr.

Constituents.—M. Champaca. The bark contains a volatile oil, fixed oil, resin, tannin, mucilage, starch and sugar. M. Nilagirica contains a volatile and fixed oil, acrid resin, tannin, sugar, starch, calcium oxalate &c.

Preparation.—Infusion (1 in 20). Dose, ½ to 1 ounce. Decoction (1 in 20). Dose, ½ to 1 ounce.

Actions and uses.—Deobstruent alterative, bitter, stomachic, emmenagogue and demulcent. The leaves are applied to indolent swellings; the bark is febrifuge and alterative and used as a substitute for guaiacum in chronic rheumatism. The root is an emmenagogue; it is used in disordered menstruation to increase the flow, and as an aromatic bitter during convalescence from fevers. The infusion of flowers is demulcent and diuretic and given in gonorrhœa to relieve scalding. Flowers beaten up with sweet-oil are applied to the nose in fœtid nasal discharges. The oil of the seeds is rubbed over the abdomen to relieve flatulence.

Anonaceæ.

The custard-apple or Sitáphala order.

Trees or shrubs with powerful aromatic taste and smell. Leaves alternate, simple and exstipulate. Flowers usually green or brown; fruit dry, or succulent; carpels distinct or united, so as to form a fleshy mass. Seeds one or more, albumen ruminated, anatropal.

Properties.—Generally aromatic and fragrant, in all their parts. The order furnishes some edible fruits. Varieties Anona squamosa, Custard-apple, Sweetsop, Sitaphal; Anona muricata, Soursop; A. reticutala, Ramphal, Bullock-heart.

Anona Squamosa.

Habitat—Western India ; cultivated in India and America.

Parts used.—The leaves, root and seeds.

Vernacular.—Arab.—Shurifa. Beng.—Luna, meba. Burm.—Amesa, auza. Cing.—Atta. Eng.—Custard apple, sweet sop. Duk.—Sitaphal. Hind.—Sitaphal. Malay.—Buwah-nona, shri-kaya. Mar.—Sitaphal. Pers.—Shurifah. Sans.—Ganda gutea. Tam.—Sitapallam. Tel.—Sitapundu. Maleal.—Ata-chika.

Characters.—The root is dark-brown, bark scabrous. Seeds dark brown and polished with bi-lateral ridges, one end umbilicated, or with a ring and a central pit, the interior contains ruminate albumen of a brownish colour ; taste acrid and oily; odour nauseous, leaves lanceolate, smooth, glaucous, of a dark-green colour and of a pungent and offensive odour. Dose, 5 to 10 grs.

Constituents.—Oil and resins. The seeds, leaves and immature fruit contain an acrid principle.

Preparation.—Ointment.

Actions and uses.—Insecticide. The seeds and leaves are poisonous to insect life. The crushed leaves are applied to the nostrils in hysteria; and mixed with salt and made into a poultice are applied to sores infested with maggots; an ointment of pounded seeds is used externally in guinea worm, and for removing lice from the hair; also applied to abscesses to hasten maturation. The natives apply to the os well-pounded seeds to procure abortion. The root is used as a drastic purgative and given in melancholia. The drug requires to be used with caution.

Bocagea Dalzellii and Guatteria Laurifolia.

Habitat.—Concan, Travancore.

Part used.—Leaves.

Vernacular.—Mar.—Sageri, Kochrik, Harkin-jal.

Characters.—Leaves polished, narrow, oblong, acute or obtuse, 5 to 9 inches long and 1 to 2 inches broad, coriaceous, serrated, the base acute or rounded, taste pungent and bitter. Flowers white, carpels smooth, globose, contain 2 mature seeds.

Constituents.—Tannin and gallic acid. A crystalline body, related to sinigrin of mustard seed.

Actions and uses.—Leaves are used as fomentation in rheumatism.

Menispermaceæ.

The Gulavela, Moon-seed, or cocculus family.

Menispermaceæ, from mene, the moon, and sperm, a seed, the fruit being kidney or moon (crescent) shaped.

General characters.—Shrub, climbing, trailing or woody. Leaves simple, entire, exstipulate, alternate. Flowers rarely unisexual, generally diœcious, petals shorter than sepals, stamens distinct, sometimes monadelphous, imperfectly developed or wanting, seeds solitary, moon or kidney-shaped fruits, small carpels, distinct, some species contain a narcotic and a bitter principle, mucilage or starch and a yellow colouring matter.

Habitat.—Tropics.

Properties.—Generally they are bitter tonics, and antiperiodic. One species, kâkamari, contains an excess of narcotic principle in its seeds.

Anamirta Paniculata, B.P.

A. cocculus. Menispermum cocculus. Cocculus Indicus.

Cocculus is a diminutive of coccum—a berry. Indian berry. Paniculata, having Panicles or flowers.

Habitat.—East India, Ceylon, Malayan Islands, East Indies, Malabar, Assam, Concan Islands, Travancore, Bengal.

Parts used.—A neutral principle obtained from the fruits. Picrotoxinum, Picrotoxin, B. P.

Vernacular.—Eng.—Levant nut, Indian berry, fish berry. Burm.—Hong. Arab.—Khanak-ul-kalb. Beng.—Bakain-ka-phal Kâka mâri. Bomb.—Karvatzad. Can.—Kâka mâri. Cing.—Tittaval. Duk. —Kaka mari. Guz.—Kôk phala, jermai. Maleal.—Gaarla-phalla, Polla. Hind.—Kakmari. Malay.—Tuba bidji, Pallak-kaya. Mar.—Karwi, Pers.—Zeheri mahi. Punj.—Neti mala. Tam.—Kakka-calli-maram. Tel.—Kakichampa. Sans.—Kâka-phala. Zeheri mahi, from Zeher a poison, and mahi, a fish. The seeds, when given to fishes, are intoxicating and poisonous.

Characters.—A climbing shrub. Berries in a long bunch, when dry, larger in size than a pea or a small grape, kidney-shaped wrinkled, and of a dark-brown purple colour, surface rough, highly tubercled or wrinkled, and marked with a circular scar at the hilum; seed oily and yellow; kernel brown, resinous and oily; taste acrid and bitter; smell rancid and oily. Dose, 1 to 2 grains.

Constituents.—The berries or seed-kernels contain picrotoxin, an active, neutral, non-nitrogenous crystalline principle; anamirtin or cocculin, and a fixed oil in large quantities. The pericarp or shell contains an alkaloid menispermin united with cocculinic acid; para menispermin, a neutral crystalline principle; hypopicro-toxic acid; also resin, fat and gum.

Picrotoxin, picrotoxinum, from picros bitter, and toxikon, poison. It has properties of a bitter poison. To obtain it triturate aqueous extract of seeds with magnesia, exhaust in hot alcohol, evaporate and purify; seeds contain from ½ to 1 p. c. of picrotoxin.

Characters.—Neutral, colourless, shining, prismatic crystals, without any odour, and of a very bitter taste; soluble in cold water (1 in 330), in boiling water (1 in 35), in cold alcohol (1 in 13), in boiling alcohol (1 in 3), freely soluble in glacial acetic acid, in solution of potash, in olive oil or lard (1 in 500), and in glycerine (1 in 60). It does not form salts. Dose internally, $\frac{1}{100}$ to $\frac{1}{25}$ grain.

Preparation of Picrotoxin.—Liquor picrotoxini aceticus, about 2 grains to 1 fluid ounce. Dose, 2 to 8 minims. Pigmentum picrotoxini (1 grain in 1 drachm) contains picrotoxin, acetic acid, castor oil and eucalyptus. Pilula picrotoxini, $\frac{1}{60}$ grain of picrotoxin with milk, sugar and glycerine of tragacanth to make one pill—unguentum picrotoxini, 10 grains to 1 ounce. Injectio picrotoxini hypodermica, 1 in 360 of water. Dose, 3 to 6 minims, equal to $\frac{1}{60}$ of a grain.

Preparations of the berries.—Extractum cocculi fluidum; fluid extract of cocculus. Dose, 1 to 3 minims. Unguentum cocculi—ointment of cocculus (80 grains to 1 ounce). Decoctum cocculi—decoction of cocculus (1 to 20). Dose, 1 to 2 fluid drachms. Tinctura cocculi,—tincture of cocculus (1 to 8). Dose, 2 to 15 minims.

Physiological action.—Insecticide, nervine sedative, cerebro-spinal excitant, and intoxicant. Used in Europe to adulterate beer, and in India to increase intoxicating effects of country liquors, also to intoxicate or poison fish and to stupefy wild cattle for capture. As a cerebro-spinal excitant its action simulates those of belladonna and nux vomica, and gives rise to the symptoms resembling those of the epileptiform convulsions. It is a powerful stimulant of the secretions of the skin, saliva, intestines, of all the motor and inhibitory centres in the medulla, especially of the respiratory centres and also of the vagus. At first it stimulates the heart and respiration; after a time the heart becomes slower, and there is stoppage of the action of the diaphragm. In large doses it causes muscular twitchings, in co-ordination, spasms of the flexors, of a tonic alternating with clonic, or of a choreaic character, stupor, epileptiform convulsions, trembling, exalted reflexes followed by insensibility, coma and death.

Therapeutics.—As an insecticide, the tincture is used as a wash to destroy pediculi which may infest the body. The ointment is used in certain parasitic affections of the skin, such as prurigo, itch and ring-worms of the scalp, care being taken to avoid the application over an abraded skin. The natives use the juice of the leaves with that of the root of gloriosa superba to kill guinea-worm. In India the seeds are given internally, like belladonna and nux vomica, to stimulate the secretions of the skin, saliva, intestines.

Picrotoxin is a nervine tonic; and it is used in chronic paralysis and in paralysis of the sphinctor ani and of the sphinctor vesicæ; in epilepsy when the attacks are nocturnal, in other spasmodic diseases, and in chorea. It is a valuable remedy in $\frac{1}{120}$ of a grain in nightsweats of phthisis. Also given in flatulent colic, and in dysmenorrhœa (given two days before the term), in leucorrhoea with mucopurulent discharge (accompanied with lumbar pain); in vomiting, with headache and in giddiness. It is an antidote to morphine, chloral, and chloroform poisoning. A dose of one $\frac{1}{20}$ grain is equivalent to 30 grains of chloral.

Chondrodendron Tomentosum, B. P. Pareira Brava.

Chondrodendron—chondros, a cartilage or grain, and dendron, a tree, in allusion to the grain-like or cartilaginous warty protuberances on the bark.

Tomentosum, meaning woolly.—The under side of the leaves being grey and hairy.

Habitat.—Brazil, Peru, West Indies.

Parts Used.—The root. Pareiræ radix, Pareira Root, B.P.

Characters.—Climbing woody plant ; leaves very large ; fruits grape-like, root cylindrical, twisted, from ¾ of an inch to 4 inches in diameter and from 4 inches to 4 feet in length, covered with a thin blackish-brown bark, with longitudinal furrows and transverse ridges and fissures ; internally yellowish-brown or grey, with well-marked concentric or eccentric zones and radiating rays, without odour and of a bitter taste. Dose of the powdered root, 30 to 60 grs.

Constituents.—Pelosine or cissampeline, an alkaloid, said to be identical with berberine ; Tannin, some resin, bitter yellow matter, starch and ash 4 p.c.

Pelosine or cissampeline.—Boil the root in water, add sulphuric. acid, precipitate with potassium carbonate, purify by dissolving in solution of sulphuric acid ; finally treat with charcoal. Characters.—Amorphous, insoluble in water, sparingly soluble in ether and carbon sulphide, freely soluble in chloroform,acetone, benzol and alcohol

Preparation.—Extractum pareiræ liquidum, B. P.—liquid extract of Pareira. Dose, ½ to 2 fluid drs. Decoction pareiræ—Decoction of Pareira (1 in 20). Dose, 1 to 2 ozs.

Physiological actions.—Laxative, diuretic and bitter tonic, similar to uva ursi and chimaphila. Its chief action is, however, on the mucous membrane of the urinary organs, which it stimulates.

Therapeutics.—It is given in painful micturition due to catarrh of the bladder, ureters or the kidneys or to the presence of gravel. In dropsy, and in chronic cystitis it increases the flow of urine. In suppurative kidneys, in gonorrhœa, gleet and leucorrhœa, it diminishes the unhealthy discharges. As a tonic it is used like any vegetable bitter, and like calumba given during convalescence from fevers. In poisonous bites the leaves are applied externally.

Cissampelos Pareira.

Parts used.—The root.

Habitat.—West Indies, common in hedges. Singapore, Ceylon.

Vernacular.—Beng.—Agnad-akanadi. Cing.—Veni—Wâela. Eng.—Velvel leaf. Guz.—Karandhis. Hind.—Dukh nirbishi, Harjori. Mar.—Paharvel. Punj.—Tikri, Katori. Sans.—Amboshta, Akanadi, Patha, Venivel, Pahadamula, Vanatiktika. Sind.—Tikri, Katori. Tam.—Ponmootootai. Tel.—Pata.

Venivel means a braided creeper, so called in allusion to the large, roundish bracts of the female flowers, resembling plaited hairs of children and women

Characters.—It is a tall, woody creeper, root-bark of a dark-brown colour, rough, crooked, with prominences, stem tortuous, knotty and seldom branched; bark soft, light and slightly furrowed. On section the root-bark is waxy and presents a radiating menispermal ring of a whitish-grey colour; the ring is similar to that found in calumba. The taste is sweetish, aromatic at first, then becomes intensely bitter; smell aromatic. Dose 30 to 60 grs.

Constituents—Cissampeline or Pelosine, $\frac{1}{2}$ p.c. in the root. It is identical with bebeerine.

Preparation—Decoction (1 in 20). Dose, 1 to 2 ozs.

Actions and uses.—Bitter tonic, diuretic and antilithic. Given in chronic cystitis, fever, and in diarrhœa, The powdered root is dusted over ulcers with benefit.

Cocculus Leæba.

Habitat.—Punjab, Sindh and Carnatic, Arabia, Persia, Afghanistan.

Part used.—The shrub.

Vernacular.—Punjab—Ullar-bellar, Parvati.

Characters.—Scandant shrub.

Actions and uses.—Bitter toinc; similar to those of Tinospora cordifolia.

Cocculus Villosus.

Habitat.—Tropical India.

Parts used.—The roots and leaves.

Vernacular.—Beng.—Huyer, Haer. Can.—Dagadi. Guz.—Patala Galori. Hind.—Farid-buti, Dier, Jamte-ki-bel. Mar.—Vasanvel, Tana. Sans.—Jal-Jamni, Vasa-dani, Patalagarudi, Vasana-valli. Tam.—Kattuk-kodi. Tel.—Chipura-tige, Katle-tige. Duk.—Jamti-ka-gratta.

Vasanvalli, from vas, fragrance, giving a fragrant perfume.

Jal—Jamni,—Jala, water and Jam, Jamvoun, to coagulate, in allusion to the property of the juice of the leaves of forming a coagulum or jelly.

Farid buti, in allusion to the legend of Shaik Farid having sustained his life upon the water rendered thick and mucilaginous by shaking the leaves of this plant. According to some, Pedalum murex (Gokharu) is the plant which they name Farid-buti.

Characters.—A widely distributed climbing plant, root very crooked, twining round on itself and giving off few fibrous rootlets; surface smooth, colour light-brown, odour peculiar and taste bitter and disagreeable; leaves on old branches, thick, succulent, oblong or ovate, cordate, orbicular or sagitate, obtuse, and more or less downy. Dose, 1 to 1½ drm.

Constituents.—Resin, alkaloid and an acid. Resin is yellowish-green and soft; odour fragrant, of that of tolu balsam. Soluble in benzine.

Preparation.—The mucilage of leaves and decoction of root (1 in 10). Dose, 1 to 2 ounces.

Action and uses.—Alterative and demulcent. The juice of the leaves coagulates in water into a green jelly, which is applied externally as a cooling application in prurigo eczema, impetigo, &c. Sweetened with sugar it is given in gonorrhoea to soothe the smarting and scalding. The root is an alterative, and mixed with pepper and milk is used by the natives for the same purposes as sarsaparilla. With bonduc nut (sagorgota) it is a favourite remedy in dyspepsia and colic in children. Experience has shown that the use of the root as an alterative, laxative and sudorific is beneficial in chronic rheumatism and syphilitic cachexia.

Coscinium Fenestratum.

Hibitat.—Ceylon. Western Peninsula.

Part used.—The stem.

Vernacular.—Eng.—Tree turmeric, False calumba. Bomb.—Jhar-ki-haldi. Can.—Doda mara-darasina. Cing.—Venivel. Duk.—Huldi-ka-jhar. Hind.—Jhar-ki Haldi. Malyal.—Mara Manjjal. Mar.—Jhade-halede. Sans.—Daru-haridrakam. Tam.—Mara-munjil. Tel.—Mani-pasupu.

Characters.—Stem cylindrical and woody, bark pale and corky, wood of a greenish-yellow colour; on section porous, with medullary rays and no concentric rings. Taste bitter. Dose, ½ to 1 drachm.

Constituents.—Berberine.

Preparation.—Infusion (1 in 20). Dose, 4 to 12 drs. Tincture (1 in 10). Dose, ½ to 1 dr.

Actions and uses.—A bitter stomachic and tonic, used in fevers during convalescence; like calumba, it is found very useful. The natives apply a paste of it to the head as a cooling application.

Jateorhiza Columba, B. P.—Cocculus Palmata.

Jateorhiza, meaning healing root; palmata, the palm of the hand The leaves are palmately lobed. Calumba, from Colombo in Ceylon, the original habitat of the plant.

Habitat.—Mozambique Forests, East India Islands, Ohio.

Parts used.—The dried root Calumbæ Radix, Calumba Root, B. P.

Vernacular.—Arab.—Sakel hamam. Bomb.—Kalamb-kachri Cing.—Kalumbu. Duk.—Kalamb-ki-jer. Eng.—Calumba root; Columbo. Guz.—Kalumbo. Hind Kalamb-ki jer. Pers.—Bikle. Kalambah. Tam.—Kalamba-ver. Tel.—Kalamba veru.

Sak-el-hamam, means dove's foot, from the resemblance of the hairy ovaries and three parted stigmas to the leg and foot of a dove.

Characters.—The fresh roots are fleshy and fusiform, cut in transverse slices or circular discs. The dry root is met with in flat, circular or oval, transverse slices, about 1 to 2 inches in diameter, and from 3 to 6 lines in thickness. Each slice is very light-brown externally and yellow internally. It is corky looking and shrunken in the centre. The most central portion is formed of tubular corky fibres. External to it is another layer, which is also corky and made up of flat or tape-like fibres cut transversely. This portion is surrounded by another outermost layer, which is nearly flat, of a yellow colour, and hard, and to which the bark is firmly adherent. Each slice breaks very readily and with a short mealy fracture. The taste is very bitter, aromatic and mucilaginous. The odour resembles that of azadarach; the root is often more or less worm-eaten. Dose, 5 to 30 grs.

Constituents.—A non-nitrogenous, crystalline, neutral, bitter principle, calumbin; an alkaloid, berberine; calumbic acid, starch 35 p.c., mucilage and ash 6 p.c.

Calumbin.—Exhaust the root with alcohol or ether; evaporate and crystallize. In white crystals, slightly soluble in water, of a bitter taste.

Calumbic acid is found in combination with berberine. It is obtained by adding hydrochloric acid to the extract of calumba, and treated with lime water.

Characters.—White crystalline flakes; sparingly soluble in cold water, alcohol and ether.

Preparations of the root.—Infusum calumbæ, B. P. (1 in 20). Dose, ½ to 1 oz. Liquor calumbæ concentratus, B.P. (1 in 2). Dose, ½ to 1 dr. Tinctura calumbæ, B. P. Tincture of calumba (1 in 10). Dose, ½ to 1 dr.

Extractum calumbæ fluidum. Fluid extract of calumba. Dose 5 to 30 ms.

Physiological action.—A non-irritant bitter, without astringency, a good stomachic tonic like quassia, and gentian. It is a stimulant of the mucous membranes of the mouth, salivary glands, œsophagus, stomach and intestines, and increases their secretion. It increases appetite and digestion, and thus promotes the constructive tissue changes. If in large doses and long continued, it produces catarrh of the stomach and intestines and interferes with digestion.

Therapeutics.—As a tonic it is generally given in hectic fever and during convalescence from acute and chronic fevers and other diseases. In atonic dyspepsia, with loss of appetite and deficient secretions of the stomach and intestines, in diarrhœa, cholera, in vomiting, and in flatulence, the infusion is given with benefit. A nice vehicle for administering acids, alkalies, aromatics and cathartics. Externally the natives use the powder of the root as an antiseptic on ulcers and wounds.

Remarks.—It is one of the few bitter tonics which do not contain tannic or gallic acid, hence can be combined with iron salts.

Menispermum Canadense and M. Fenestratum.

Syn.—Canadian moon-seed, Texas or yellow parilla, vine maple.

Habitat.—Eastern United States.

Parts used.—The rhizome and rootlets.

Characters.—A woody climbing plant, stems round and striated, rhizome thick, yellowish-brown, knotty and wrinkled externally.—Roots brittle, break with a tough fracture, yellow within. Bark thick and porous, without any odour, and of a bitter taste. Dose 10 to 30 grains.

Constituents.—Berberine, Menispine—s tarch, resin and tannin. Menispine is a white powder, soluble in alcohol and ether.

Preparation.—Extractum menispermi fluidum—fluid extract of menispermum. Dose, 30 to 60 ms. Menispermino—a dry extractive. Dose, 1 to 5 grs.

Actions and uses.—Stomachic, bitter tonic, alterative and diuretic ; used for the same purposes as calumba. A good substitute for sarsaparilla in scrofulous conditions, gout and rheumatism and in gravel affections. It stimulates the intestinal glands, but not the liver ; and is given in dyspepsia, general debility, &c.

Stephania Hernandifolia.

Habitat.—Nepal, Singapore, Ceylon.

Part used.—Stems.

Vernacular.—Beng—Agnad-akanadi. Sans.—Vanatiktika.

Characters.—Striated stems.

Actions and uses.—Similar to those of Cissampelos pareira.

Tinospora Cordifolia. T. Crispa. Cocculus Cordifolius.

Habitat.—Konkan, forests of Tropical India ; Konkan, Western Coast of India.

Parts used.—The stem and fecula (starchy extract Gulancha).

Vernacular.—Arab.—Gilo. Beng.—Gadancha. Bomb.—Gulavela Gilo, Giroli. Burm. Singo-mone. Can.—Amrita-balli. Cing.—Rasakinda. Duk.—Gulbel, Gulwail. Goa.—Amritvel. Guz.—Gado, gulvel. Hind.—Guluncha, Gulbel, Giloe. Maleal.—Amrita, chitramruta. Malay.—Citamerdu. Mar.—Gulwail Gharol. Pers.—Gulbel. Panj.—ak-Gillo, Gularich. Sans.—Somavalli, Amurta, Guduchi, Pittaghni, Bhishak-pryia, Nirjara, Chinnaruha. Tam.—Shendilkodi. Tel.—Tippa-tinge,

Starchy extract (Fecula).—Beng.—Palo, Sat-i-gilœ. Bomb.—Galo satta. Duk.—Gulancha, satva. Sikkim.—Gurjo. Hind.—Giloe-ka-sat. Pers.—Salte gilo. Tel.—Tuppa sattu.

Pittaghni—pit means bile, and agne, fire or destroying ; bile destroying.

Bishak pryia, dear to physicians ; Nirjara, not perishing,

Chin narhua means growing when cut. The stem, when placed upon a bush in the open air, will retain its vitality throughout the hot season and put forth leaves and roots during the rains.

Characters.—Climbing shrub. Those spreading on trees of Mangifera Indica and Azadirachta Indica are used for medicinal purposes. Fresh bark is papery ; dry bark is externally of a dull-brown colour, inner portion green and succulent and easily separable from the wood ; wood, of a light white colour and presents wedges separated by depressed radiating menispermal medullary rays ; taste very bitter and mucilaginous.

Constituents.—The root and stem contains starchy extract, bitter principle and a trace of berberine.

Preparation.—Infusion of Gulancha (1 in 10). Dose 1 to 2 ozs. Tincture of Gulancha (1 in 8). Dose, ½ to 2 drs. Starchy extract or fecula Dose, 10 to 20 grs. The extract is prepared by powdering the stem and washing out the starch with water and drying the sediment. Pieces of various shapes and sizes, of a pure white colour ; taste bitter and mucilaginous, and it adheres to the tongue like Vansa Lochana.

Actions and uses.—Fresh stem is more efficacious than the dry and is a good substitute for calumba. It is a stomachic bitter tonic, alterative, aphrodisiac, antiperiodic and demulcent, given in dyspepsia and in debility caused by repeated attacks of fever. Like Peruvian barks it is a good febrifuge ; used in enlarged spleen. As an alterative given in secondary syphilis, rheumatism, leprosy, skin diseases, such as impetigo, and in jaundice. As a diuretic and demulcent it is given in dysuria, in scanty high-coloured urine due to catarrh of the bladder. The juice of the stem, combined with pâkhanbhed and honey, is given in gonorrhæa. The fecula is nutritious, largely used in native practice in cold, fevers, and seminal weakness, also in urinary affections.

Remarks.—Herbalists sell the stems of cocculus malabaricus for gulavela, but the stem of cocculus malabaricus is hard, thick, less fleshy and not so efficacious as gulavela.

A wreath, known as kamlâ-in-mâlá or jaundice wreath, and made of the fresh stem, each piece about an inch long and tied in the middle in loose knots with a piece of thread, and being placed an inch apart from one another, is put round the neck of jaundiced patients, under a common belief among the credulous natives that the wreath has the property of lessening the force of jaundice, and that its good effects are manifested by the wreath in increasing in length in proportion as the force of jaundice diminishes. This is a mere delusion. The increase in the length of the wreath is due to the drying up of the stems by lapse of time and to the narrowing of the knots of the thread over the stems.

Tiliacora racemosa.

Habitat.—Tropical India, Ceylon.

Part used.—The shrub.

Characters.—A climbing shrub.

Vernacular.—Tel.—Mushadi. Beng.—Tiliakora. Hind.—Bagor Mushadi.

Actions and uses.—Bitter and stomachic, used like other bitters. Among the natives it passes for a remedy for snake-bite.

Berberidaceæ.

The daruhalada or barberry family.

Shrubs or herbs, leaves alternate, compound, usually exstipulate, stem generally free from hairs, but often spiny; stamens hypogynous; equal to petals in number; anthers two-celled, each opening by a valve from the bottom to the top. Fruit baccate or dry and capsular. Seeds with minute embryo, albumen, fleshy and horny.

Habitat.—Temperate parts of Europe, America and Asia and mountains of North India.

Properties.—Acid, bitter and astringent; acid properties are due to the presence of oxalic acid.

Berberis Aquifolium.

Habitat.—Pacific Slope of the United States, Western United States.

Part used.—The root.

Vernacular.—American barberry. Holly-leaved barberry, mountain grape, Oregon grape.

Characters.—Root, 1 to 2 feet or more in length and about one-fourth in breadth, extremely hard and tough; colour, bright golden yellow, cortical portion thin and papyraceous, dull-greenish or brownish-yellow. Intense, but pleasant bitter taste. Dose, 10 to 30 grs.

Constituents.—It contains an alkaloid berberina or berberine, also a peculiar resinous matter.

Preparation of the root.—Liquid extract. Dose, 10 to 30 ms. Tincturæ (1 to 10). Dose, 10 to 40 ms.

Physiological action.—In small doses, bitter tonic, stomachic astringent and antiperiodic; in large doses cathartic and diuretic, producing watery motions accompanied with pain.

Therapeutics.—Used in malarial intermittent, remittent and typhoid fevers, diarrhœa, and dyspepsia; as an alterative and tonic it is given in scrofulous and cancerous affections and in secondary or tertiary syphilitic diseases, in syphilitic cachexia and in chronic scaly or squamous eruptions, more particularly in psoriasis and pityriasis; also useful after a long mercurial course to eliminate mercury from the system. As a cathartic and diuretic it increases the secretions and thus relieves hepatic congestion and frees intestinal secretions ; hence, in habitual constipation, it is combined with cascara sagrada. In pain, soreness and burning sensation along the urinary or biliary tracts, with a tendency to gall-stone or urinary calculi, it is a very useful remedy. As a glandular stimulant it is given in chronic tonsilitis and in enlargements of the prostate.

Berberis Aristata.

Berberis Lycium, raisin barberry, Indian Lycium (ophthalmic barberry), B. Asiatica and B. Canadensis or B. Vulgaris (European variety).

Habitat.—Mountainous parts in North India, Nepaul, Nilgiri, mountains of Ceylon. Various species of barberry occur on the Nilgiri mountains.

Parts used.—The stem, wood and root-bark (Berberis cortex), fruit or dry berries, and extract.

Vernacular.—The root-bark. Arab.—Dar-hald. Bomb.—Dar-halad. Hind.—Dar-halad, Dar-chob. Daru-haridra (the wood). Pers. —Dar-hald, Dar-chob. Eng.—Indian Barberry, Nepaul barberry, yellow wood, turmeric wood. Sans.—Daru haridra. Tam.—Mulla-bubla, Puttar.

The extract. Arab.—Huzazi-Hindi. Bomb.—Rusot, Raswanti. Hind.—Rusot, Raswat. Sind.—Raswal. Pers.—Fil-zahrah.

The fruit or berries. Arab.—Ambar-baris. Bomb.—Zarishk. Duk.—Zarish. Hind.—Zarishk chitra. Hydrabad—Vilayati amali. Pers.—Zarishk.

Rasot, Rasuth—Ras, juice, and uthna to boil ; Raswanti—Rasa, a juice, and vanti, a pulp; Daruhalad—Daru, wood, and halad, turmeric. The wood is yellow. This term is also applied to the yellow root or wood of curcuma aromatica, curcuma longa and coccinium fenestratum.

Characters.—The stem is met with in circular pieces, each from 1 to 2 or 4 inches long, and about 1 to 2 inches in diameter ; very bitter and of an astringent taste. The root-bark is smooth and brittle and of a dull grey or yellow colour ; on section the stem presents a central ring with numerous radiating wedge-like projections, made up of fibrous cells ; between these projections is a spongy substance perforated by small holes. The fruits are larger than English barberries, shrivelled, much compressed, often oval and of a bright-red colour ; most of them abortive, but a few contain oblong seeds ; they resemble raisins ; they are met with in black, moist, sticky masses. Taste very acid and astringent, owing to the presence of tartaric, oxalic and malic acids ; most of them are abortive. The extract rusota is a dark brown, lumpy mass of a bitter, astringent taste, and of the consistence of opium. Dose of the root-bark, 20 to 30 grs.

Constituents.—The root and wood contain in great abundance a yellow alkaloid berberine or berberina, oxyacanthine, fat, resin, tannin, also berbamine and another alkaloid. The fruit contains malic and citric acids and tannin.

Berberine, Berberina.—A bitter, orange-yellow, acicular crystals, soluble in hot water and alchol, insoluble in ether. With acids forms salts ; with chloroform, ether and alcohol forms crystalline compounds. Dose, 1 to 5 grs. Berberine is also contained in the root of calumba, coptis teeta, hydrastis, podophyllum, menispermum, xanthoxylum, &c.

Preparation.—Decoction of the root (1 in 20). Dose, 1 to 2 ozs. Infusion of the stem (1 in 20). Dose, 1 to 2 ozs. Tincture of the cortex (1 in 4). Dose as a tonic, ½ to 2 drs; as an antiperiodic, 4 to 6 drs. Syrup or preserves of fruit ; liquid extract not miscible with water. Dose, ½ to 2 drs.

Rusot, an impure watery extract prepared from powdered stem or wood, by exhaustion with water, filtration and admixture with cow's milk and final evaporation. It is readily soluble in water, partly so in rectified spirit, forming a yellow solution.

Actions and uses.—The bark and stem—Tonic, diaphoretic, stomachic, antiperiodic, and a gentle but certain aperient, used in malarial fevers, diarrhœa, dyspepsia, dysentery, ague, during convalescence from fevers and acute diseases. As an alterative, it is used in bilious complaints, torpid liver, dropsy and jaundice. With gypsum, it is given in metrorrhagia. The berries are cooling and acid, and used as refrigerant in febrile diseases, diarrhœa, &c. The extract (Rusot) is an anodyne, tonic and febrifuge, internally used like the bark. Externally, rusot, mixed with alum, rock salt, chebulic myrabolams and opium, is applied round the orbit in painful affections of the eye, as in black eye, &c. Mixed with honey, it is applied to ulcers in the mouth. It is also applied to relieve pain of cancer and of neuralgia. Berberine.—The alkaloid is given internally in malaria, dyspepsia, diarrhœa, sickness of pregnancy, &c. Berberine carbonate, berberine hydrochlorate, berberine phosphate and berberine sulphate, are used in malarial affections, amenorrhœa, enlargement of spleen, anorexia, vomiting of pregnancy and intestinal catarrh.

Caulophyllum Thalictroides.

Vernacular.—Blue cohosh, papoose or squaw root, blueberry, blue or yellow ginsing.

Habitat.—Rich woodlands, Canada, Northern United States.

Parts used.—The rhizome and rootlets.

Characters.—Rhizomes are horizontal, 4 inches long, ¼ of an inch thick, knotty on the upper surface with stem-scars and branches; externally greyish-brown, inside whitish and tough. Rootlets many and matted, without any odour, and of a sweetish and acrid taste. Dose 15 to 20 grs.

Constituents.—A resin-caulophyllin, 12 p.c. saponin or leontin, a glucoside, tannin, wax and an alkaloid-caulophylline. The alkaloid is colourless, tasteless and without any odour. Caulophyllin.—To obtain it, exhaust the root with alcohol, pour the alcoholic extract into water. It is a brown resinoid powder. Dose, 1 to 4 grs., in pill with glycerine of tragacanth.

Preparation.—Tinctura caulophyllinæ, Tincture of caulophyllum (1 in 4). Dose, 1 to 4 drs. Extractum caulophyllinæ liquidum—Liquid extract of caulophyllum. Dose, ½ to 1 dr. Liquor caulophyllin et pulsatillæ co. Dose, ½ to dr. Infusion and decoction (1 in 10) Dose, 2 to 4 drs.

Physiological action.—Caulophyllin is stimulant, tonic, demulcent, diuretic, emmenagogue and antispasmodic; also parturient; it causes intermittent contraction of the gravid uterus.

Therapeutics.—Used in deficient labour pains, in menstrual derangements, as spasmodic dysmenorrhœa. It checks muscular contraction in cases of threatened abortion, and also relieves spasmodic after-pains. It is given in atony of the uterus, in prolapsus uteri, and in sub-involution. Combined with pulsatilla it is found useful in acute rheumatism, leucorrhœa, vaginitis, urethritis and in hysteria. Saponin is a sternutatory.

Podophyllum Emodi.

Habitat.—Interior range of Himalaya, Cashmere, Shikim Hazara, &c.

Parts used.—The rhizome, roots, fruits, and the resin.

Vernacular.—Hind.—Papra or papri, Bhavan-bakra or Bakra, Chimyaka. Sans.—Parpata, vakra.

Characters.—Rhizomes similar to those of podophyllum peltatum except that the rhizome of P. Emodi is cylindrical, more crowded above with tuberosities and stem scars, the under surface covered with many depressed oval or circular roots. Dose, 5 to 15 grs.

Constituents.—Resin, 10 to 12 p. c., sugar, fat, gum, &c., the resin is in much greater quantity than in podophyllum peltatum.

Preparation.—Tincture (1 in 30). Dose, 5 to 20 ms; resin-podophyllin, ⅛ to 1 gr.

Actions and uses.—Cholagogue, alterative, bitter tonic, given as a sure purge, with slight griping in torpid liver. Uses similar to those of podophyllum peltatum.

Podophyllum Peltatum, B. P.

Podophyllum.—Podos foot, and phyllon, "leaf." The leaf is 5 to 7 partite, which resembles the foot of aquatic ducks or domestic fowls.

Peltatum.—Pelta, a light shield. The leaf petioles are attached to the middle of lamina like a shield.

Habitat.—United States. Rich woods of Canada.

Part used.—The rhizome and rootlets. Podophylli Rhizoma, Podophyllum Root, B. P., the resin; Podophylli Resina, Podophyllum Resin, B. P.

Vernacular.—Eng.—The American May-apple, wild mandrake or vegetable mercury, so called, as it is a powerful biliary purgative.

Characters.—A perennial herb, stem pale green, with a white flower at its summit. The root is dark reddish-brown, smooth or slightly wrinkled, in nearly cylindrical pieces, which are knotty, each knot is marked on its upper surface by a circular depressed scar; on the under surface are numerous brittle, brownish rootlets. It breaks with a short starchy fracture; on section it is white or pale-yellow or brown. It has a characteristic odour and a bitter acrid taste. Dose, powdered root, 5 to 20 grs.

Constituents.—Resin podophyllin 4 to 5 p.c.; an alkaloid berberine, Podophyllo quercetin, starch, gum, fat, and sugar. Podophyllum Resine, podophylli Resina, B.P., is obtained from the root when a concentrated tincture is precipitated by acidulated water. It is an amorphous powder of a herby odour, acrid bitter taste; colour varies from pale-yellow to deep orange-brown, soluble in alcohol, alkaline liquids, and partly so in ether. Dose, ¼ to 1 gr. It is an ingredient of various cathartic pills. The active portion of the resin consists of podophyllotoxin, which contains 70 to 80 p.c. of the cathartic principle, and is made up of picropodophyllin held in solution by picropodophyllic acid. There is also another inactive acid—podophyllic acid. Picropodophyllin is obtained by treating podophyllotoxin with an alkali. It is a neutral, crystalline, bitter mass of a white colour, soluble in chloroform, acetone, sparingly soluble in ether, benzin, hot water and weak alcohol. Podophyllic acid—an inactive resin acid, soluble in alcohol. Podophyllo quercetin is the colouring matter—occurs in yellow needles, soluble in alcohol, sparingly so in chloroform and insoluble in water. The Indian plant yields 10 to 12 p.c. of podophyllin resin and 56 p.c. of podophyllotoxin, whereas the American species yields 5 p.c. of resin and 40 p.c. of podophyllotoxin.

Preparation.—Tinctura podophylli, B.P. (1 of the resin in 30 ms.) Dose, 5 to 15 ms. Pilula podophyllin composita. Podophyllin ¼ gr., aloes 1 gr., capsicum ½ gr., belladonna extract ¼ gr., glycerin tragacanth q.s. to make one pill. Pilula podophyllin et quininæ—Quinine sulphate 1 gr., podophyllin $\frac{1}{12}$ gr., milk sugar $\frac{1}{12}$ gr., extract of belladonna $\frac{1}{6}$ gr., aloes $\frac{1}{6}$ gr. Make one pill. Extractum podophylli fluidum—fluid extract of podophyllin. Dose, 3 to 20 ms. Tinctura podophyllin ammoniata made with aromatic spirit of ammonia (1 in 50). Dose, 2 to 6 ms. Pilula podophyllin, ¼ of a grain of resin triturated with milk sugar, acacia, in one pill. Pilula podophylli cum belladonnæ et strychninæ, otherwise known as Tonic liver pills—contains: Podophyllin ¼ grain, extract belladonna ¼ grain, strychnine $\frac{1}{80}$ grain in one pill. Pilulæ podophylli et pepsinia—Digestive granules, ¼ of a grain in each; Liquor podophylli cum belladonna et strychnina. Dose, 1 dr. Liquor podophylli et pepsinæ. Dose, 1 dr.

Actions and uses.—Podophyllin is an active cholagogue and cathartic. In small doses it is given in sick headache, in dyspepsia with deficient bile in the stools, in habitual constipation due to torpid liver and in bilious vomiting. It is generally combined with henbane, belladonna or cannabis to counteract its griping effects. In dropsy, rheumatism, syphilis, it is generally given along with other purgatives as jalap, colocynth, &c., or combined with cream of tartar and calomel. As a derivative it is given in catarrhal or malarial jaundice. In large doses it acts as a gastric irritant. The root may be given as an alterative.

Nymphæaceæ.

The water lily family ; aquatic herbs ; leaves cordate and floating ; flowers solitary ; Thalamus, large, fleshy, forming a disc-like expansion, more or less surrounding the ovary ; carpels numerous, united, forming one compound ovary ; fruit indehiscent, many-celled ; seeds numerous ; embryo minute.

Habitat.—Northern temperate regions and tropics.

Properties.—Bitter and astringent ; rhizomes and seeds of many species contain starch.

Nymphæa Alba.

N. Versicolor, Poini. N. Odorata, sweet-scented water lily (Eng.)

Habitat.—Bengal, Ajmir, Pastkur Lake.

Parts used.—The flowers and seeds.

Vernacular.—Beng.—Buro Sundli. Bomb.—Poini. The seeds kumabija.

Characters.—The flowers are smaller than those of kamala, and of variegated colours. The seeds are very small and tubercled. Dose, 10 to 30 grs.

Preparation.—Syrup of flowers. Dose, 1 to 2 drachms.

Actions and uses.—Demulcent, astringent and refrigerant, and used in dysentery in combination with sugar ; other properties are similar to those of N. speciosum, for which it is often substituted.

Euryale Ferox.

Nymphæa stellata.

Habitat.—Calcutta, North India.

Parts used.—The seeds.

Vernacular.—Beng.—Makana. Bomb.—Makhana. Hind.—Makana. Kash.—Jawur. Chin.—Kien-shih, ki-tu. Tel.—Nallani padmam.

Characters.—The fruit, large orange or pear-shaped, indehiscent, interior white, hard, starchy, contains 8 to 15 round black seeds of the size of peas and full of flour. The seeds are farinaceous, and when fried, roasted or rather baked, they are known as Dhani.

Actions and uses.—Dhani is invigorating and used as an article of food ; also as an astringent, nutritive, and tonic, used in seminal discharges, In Bombay makana is imported from Mathura and Benares.

Nelumbiaceæ.

The water bean family.

Aquatic plants, creeping in the horizontal direction, attached to the earth by numerous fibres ; leaves, peltate, floating on the surface of water and are mucilaginous ; flowers large and showy, thalamus very large, flattened at the top, excavated, presenting numerous cavities, each containing a single carpel ; fruit nut-like, half buried in the cavity ; Seeds solitary, without albumen, embryo large ; plumule well developed.

Habitat.—Northern temperate and tropical regions, stagnant waters.

Properties.—Fruit of all species are edible ; rhizomes, starchy, astringent and bitter.

Nymphæa Edulis. N. Esculanta.

Castalia Edulis.

Habitat.—India.

Parts used.—The roots and flowers.

Vernacular.—Arab.—Nilu-far. Beng.—Choto Sundhi, Kanval. Bur.—Kiyan-nu. Can.—Nyadale-huvu. Cing.—Nalun. Duk.—Alli-phul, Chhota-kanval. Eng.—Edible lotus, pond lily. Guz.—Kanval. Hind.—Chhota-kanval. Malyal.—Allit-tamara, Anpala. Mar.—Kamula. Pers.—Nilufar. Sans.—Kamala. Tam.—Ambal, Allitamarai. Tel.—Kotika, Kalharomu.

Characters.—Aquatic plant, leaves oval, entire, downy underneath, margin slightly waved, petioles attached to the margin, flowers white, seeds numerous. The root, very bitter and astringent. Dose 10 to 30 grs.

Constituents.—The root contains gallic and tannic acids, starch, gum, &c.

Syrup. Dose, 1 to 2 drs. Decoction (1 in 20). Dose, 1 to 2 ozs.

Actions and uses.—Demulcent, diuretic and nutrient. Other characters same as those of Nelumbium speciosum. The roots are used as an article of diet.

Nelumbium Speciosum.

Nymphæa Lotus. N. Pubescens.

Habitat.—India, Persia, China, Thibet, Japan, Ceylon.

Parts used.—The flowers, filaments and anthers.

Vernacular.—Eng.—Egyptian lotus, Egyptian or Pythagorian bean. Arab.—Nilufar. Assam.—Kyrob. Beng.—Burrshaluk, Komol, Padma. Bur.—Kyah-phyn. Cing.—Juda-tebolu. Duk.—Kung-evelka. Hind.—Kamala, Koi-podoma, Kanbal-kukri. Malyal.—Tamara. Pers.—Nilofer (the seeds). Sind.—Pabban, Kooni, Guz.—Nilofara, the seeds, kamar kakali. Goa.—Seveka. Can.—Nyadale-huvu. Tam.—Tamaray-Ambal. Tel.—Tella kaluva, Alli-kolung. Mar.—Kamal. Sans.—Padma, Kamala, Pundarik, Kakonada, Indwara.

Characters.—An aquatic herb, leaves floating, peltate and roundish, upper surface green, under surface bluish; flowers, when fresh, are large, white and showy. The dry flowers have a brown colour, sepals 4 or 5, the petals numerous, and in several whorls, filaments petaloid, seeds (Kamala kakari) solitary, without albumen. The structure of the seed receptacle has been compared to a wasp's nest, or a pomegranate, cut in half; in shape oval. Externally smooth and brownish or greyish-black; surface covered with numerous minute whitish dots, testa horny, cotyledons white and starchy and covered with a thin almond-coloured membrane, embryo green. Dose, powdered seeds, 10 to 30 grs.

Constituents.—The rhizome and seeds contain resins, glucose, metarabin, tannin, fat and an alkaloid, similar to nupharine, identical with that obtained from nuphar luteum.

Preparation.—Syrup of flowers. Dried flowers 2 ounces, sugar 1 ounce, and water 5 fluid ounces. Dose, 1 to 3 drs. Compound decoction of flowers and filaments with liquorice (1 in 10). Dose, 4 to 12 drs.

Actions and uses.—The seeds are demulcent and nutritive; the filaments and flowers are cooling, astringent, bitter and expectorant. Syrup of flowers is used in coughs, to check hæmorrhage from bleeding piles, in sanguineous fluxes from the bowels, and in menorrhagia. The lotus flowers and fresh leaves with sandalwood or emblic myrobalans are used as a cooling application to the forehead in cephalalgia, to the skin in erysipelas and to other external inflammations. A cooling bed sheet made of kamala is used for fever patients with high fever. The seeds, with those of Euryale ferox (Makhana), are used as an article of diet. The starch contained in the rhizome, when collected, constitutes a sort of arrowroot known to Chinese as Ghaanfeen. The powder of the seeds, Kamarkakri, is known by the name of Bhesabola. These two products come from Shanghai, and are largely used by native women as a demulcent in leucorrhœa. Bhesabola should not be mistaken for Bhosabola, which is a variety of Hirabol.

Papaveraceæ.

The Afima or Poppy family.

Papaver is derived from papa, pap, or thick milk, in allusion to its use for children, to nourish and cause sleep.

General Characters.—Herbs or shrubs, usually with a milky white, yellow or blood coloured, acrid and narcotic juice; leaves alternate, more or less divided, peduncles long, one-flowered; flowers white, pink, yellow, rose or red coloured, also showy, regular and symmetrical; sepals 2 or 3. Fruit one-celled, either pod-shaped with two parietal placentas or capsular, with several placentas, dehiscing by valves or pores, seeds numerous, albuminous, with minute embryo near the base of fleshy albumen; seeds contain a bland, nutritive fixed oil. Taste bland and wholesome.

Properties.—Many plants are narcotic, some are acrid and poisonous, a few emetic, and others cathartic.

Argemone Mexicana.

Habitat.—West Indies, all over India.

Parts used.—The milky juice of the fresh plant and a fixed oil of the fresh seeds.

Vernacular.—Beng.—Buro Shyala-kanta. Burm.—Matnal,Khyao. Can.—Bolurakkisa, Datturi. Duk.—Bharamdandi, Pila-dhatura. Eng.—Mexican poppy, yellow thistle, gamboge thistle. Guz.—Pilat Dhatura. Hind.—Bharbhand, Shiyal-kanda, Satyanasa, Faringi-Dhotra, Pivola-Dhotra. Malyal.—Brahma-danti. Mar.—Daruri. Spanish.—Figo del inferno. Sans.—Himavatel Bramha danda. Tam.—Birama-dandu, Kurukkam-chedi. Tel.—Bramha-dandi-chettu.

Remarks.—Daruri. The word Daru means gunpowder, the seeds resemble the grains of gunpowder.

Pivala Dhotra—Pivala, yellow, and Dhotra, corruption of dhatura. The flowers and leaves of dhotra are yellow, and resemble flowers and leaves of Dhatura.

Kante Dhotra—the herb is prickly or full of kantas or prickles.

Figo del inferno, "The fig of hell," on account of its strong prickles.

Faringi Dhotra—The plant having been first introduced into India by Firingis (Portuguese).

Characters.—The yellow milky juice resembles gamboge; leaves thick, glaucous, of a greenish colour and marked with whitish veins on the posterior surface; the mid rib and the veins are here and there studded with prickly thistles, which are also found on the borders of the leaves; flowers bright yellow, capsules oblong, oval, about 1 to 1½ inch long and five partite; convex portions covered with prickles; the depressions are free; seeds many, round and of a dark-brown colour, corrugated and tubercled with a thick white band and resemble *Kuma bija*. On section they are resinous and oily; oil, pale-yellow, clear, and of a nauseous odour, but without any disagreeable taste. Dose of the oil, 20 to 60 ms.

Constituents.—The leaves and capsules contain morphia, the seeds contain an oil 36 p.c. carbohydrates and albumen 49 p.c., moisture 9 p.c., and ash 6 p.c., The ash contains alkaline phosphates and sulphates.

Actions and uses.—The juice is alterative and used in syphilis, leprosy and gonorrhœa along with the juice of aristolochia bracteata. The seeds are narcotico-acrid. The oil and extract from the seeds are laxative and sedative, combining the action of castor-oil and cannabis Indica. The oil is used in cholera, dropsy, painful colic. As substitute for ipecacuanha, the seeds are given in dysentery and other intestinal affections. Locally the juice or the oil is used as a soothing application to indolent ulcers, herpetic eruptions, leucoderma, syphilitic ulcers and warts. It relieves strangury caused by blisters. Fresh root is applied to scorpion bites.

Chelidonium Majus.

Great or garden celandine, Tetter wort.

Habitat.—Europe, North America, waste lands and rocky places. Chelidonium. It is derived from chelidon, a swallow, as it flowers at the coming of, and dries up at the departure of, the swallows.

Part used.—The whole plant.

Characters.—Perennial herb; leaves pinnate; flowers yield saffron-yellow milky juice ; root reddish-brown, branching, several headed ; fruit a capsule, two-valved ; seeds numerous ; odour unpleasant; taste acrid. Dose, 10 to 40 grs.; fresh juice, 5 to 20 ms.

Constituents.—Chelerythrine, sanguinarine ; chelidonine, protopine, chelidoxanthin (a yellow crystalline substance), chelidonic (jervic or malic) acid, chelidoninic acid, gum, and chlorophyll.

Chelerythrine.—To obtain it, shake the extract with ether. The solution contains chelerythrine, leaving behind chelidonine.

Chelidonine—Digest the extract in hydrochloric acid and precipitate with ammonia.

Chelidoxanthin, a bitter neutral principle, occurs in yellow needles.

Preparation.—Fluid extract. Dose, 10 to 30 ms. ; Extract—Dose, 10 grs. ; Infusion (1 in 40). Dose, 1 to 2 ozs.; Expressed juice, 5 to 20 ms.

Actions and uses.—Drastic cathartic, expectorant, diuretic and diaphoretic. In over doses poisonous ; given in jaundice, liver diseases, whooping cough, dropsy, scrofula, intermittent fever and phthisis. Externally as an irritant it is used for warts, opacity of cornea, corns, urticaria, itching, &c.

Glaucium luteum (Hornpoppy) and **Glaucium corniculatum.**—Both contain alkaloids similar to those in chelidonium majus.

Eschscholtzia Californica.—Chamisso.

Syn.—California poppy.

Habitat.—California.

Part employed.—The whole plant.

Characters.—An herbaceous, glabrous, glaucescent plant ; leaves alternate, petiolated and multified, with linear lobes and no stipules ; flowers supported on long peduncles, terminal, regular and hermaphrodite. The receptacle is a hollow cone, upper border bears a calyx, coralla, perigynous golden-yellow, sepals two valvate united throughout their entire length, but detached at the base in the form of a funnel. Fruit dehiscent, linear, oblong, dry and capsular, traversed longitudinally by ten projecting ribs extending as far as the base into two rigid valves, bearing the seed at the edges ; seeds contain an albuminous, fleshy matter enveloping the embryo.

Constituents.—It contains morphine and a glucoside.

Preparation.—Fluid extract of the plant 15 to 30 ms.

Actions and uses.—Soporific, the same as that of morphine. It does not cause any bad taste nor does it cause any dryness in the mouth, nausea, vomiting, difficulty during urination, &c. ; given in headache.

Meconopsis Wallichii, M. Aculeata, M. Nepalensis.

Habitat.—Temperate Himalaya.

Part used.—The plant.

Vernacular—Hind. Guddikum, Gudia. Eng.—Prickly poppy. Panj.—Kanta.

Characters.—A large herbaceous plant, flowers blue, purple, and showy root tapering, 6 inches long and bifurcated 1½ inch in breadth. Smooth below and scaly at the upper part from the scar remains of leaves ; between the scales are stiff yellow bristles. It is brown externally, and white, soft and spongy within, containing a large central pith ; odour somewhat musky.

Constituents.—Manganese and ash 12.7 p.c.; a yellow viscid extract containing crystalline matter.

Actions and uses.—Narcotic. Possess very poisonous properties.

Papaver Rhœas, B. P.

Habitat.—Europe.

Parts used.—The fresh petals. Rhœados Petala, Redpoppy petals, B. P.

Vernacular.—Eng.—Common red poppy or corn poppy. Bom.—Janglidrika. Arab.—Nabatul-khash, khashul-ahmar. Beng.—Lal-poshta. Bur.—Hin-bin-ami. Can.—Kempu khasa-khasi-gida. Duk.—Lal-khaskhas. Guz.—Lal-khas-khas, Lala. Hind.—Gullala, jangli mudrika, Malyal.—Chovanna. Mar.—Tambada-khasa-khasa. Pers.—Kohnare surk-khas-khas-i-mansur. Sans.—Rakla-postu Mudrika. Tam.—Shivappugacha. Tel.—Erra-posta-kaya-chetta.

Kaskhas-i-mansur,—because it sheds its petals very quickly.

Mudrika, Mudra (a seal or mark) stamped with the mudra or seal, which resembles the capsule in shape. This is in allusion to the stigma of the capsules of lala used by the Hindus, after bathing, as a mark or Tilaka impressed upon the middle of their forehead. The stigma resembles in shape mudra, a seal or a chakra.

Characters.—Flowers large, of a reddish colour, and resemble those of opium, fresh petals of a bright scarlet colour mainly used for their colouring matter, odour characteristic and very unpleasant; taste bitter; capsules smaller than those of poppy, globular, 2 inches broad, smooth and having a lustrous surface and entire margin; odour heavy, like that of poppy.

Constituents.—Milky juice, containing a red crystallizable colouring matter, and an alkaloid called rhœadine.

Rhœadine is tasteless, non-poisonous, insoluble in water, alcohol, ether, chloroform, benzol or liquor ammonia ; soluble in weak acids.

Preparation.—Syrupus rhœados, B. P. (1 in 4·5). Dose, ½ to 1 dr.

Actions and uses.—The petals are slighty expectorant, other properties are similar to those of poppy capsules, but much milder ; syrup is used as a colouring agent.

Papaver Somniferum, B. P. The Opium or Garden Poppy.

Habitat.—Asia Minor, Persia, China, Africa, Italy, Greece, England, United States and India.

Parts used.—The nearly ripe and dried capsules—Papaveris capsulæ, Poppy capsules B.P., petals, seeds and the inspissated juice, Opium B.P.

Somniferum.—To bring sleep. This drug causes sleep.

Vernacular.—Arab.—Bazrul-khas-khas. Beng.—Poshto. Burm.—Bhin-si. Eng.—Maw seeds (black), white poppy. Malay.—Banga-pion. Pers.—Tukhme-koonar, Khas-khas. Sans.—Chosa, Postu-bijam. Tam.—Gasa-gasalu. Tel.—Kasa kasa. Mar. Guz. Duk. Hind.—Koknar, post, Khas-khas. Malayal.—Khas-khas-karu. Can.—Khas-khasi.

The vernacular names for the tree, capsules and seeds of poppy are made up by affixing the vernacular for the tree, capsules and seeds to the vernacular for the poppy.

Seeds.—Two varieties, P. Somniferum, or poppy with black seeds ; and P. Album, or poppy with white seeds.

Characters.—P. Somniferum is an annual plant, with thick branching yellow root, stem 2 to 4 inches high, leaves thick, smooth and glaucous, 6 to 10 inches long; sessile, oval, tapering at the base, toothed and green, with prominent veins, and white midrib. Flowers large, terminal, silver-grey; sepals 2 green, petals 4, yellow or violet; fruit a capsule, globular, 1 to 3 inches wide, flat at the top, the bottom glaucous. The pericarp is pale brown externally and marked with dark spots. It has a bitter taste. Unripe capsule is marked in 3 or 4 places with 3 or 4 longitudinal incisions, from which the juice or opium is obtained, the incisions being limited to the middle third of the capsules, avoiding the inner capsular diaphragm, as, otherwise, the juice would escape into the central cavities of the capsules. Each capsule has a very small, thick stalk at the bottom, with a large radiating sessile stellate stigma at the top, which distinguishes them from colocynth or bael fruits. Seeds numerous, reniform, very small, reticulated, whitish-grey or greyish-black, taste sweet and oily. Black seed poppy (maw seed) has purple or red flowers, capsules smaller and rounder, seeds black. White seed poppy has white flowers and white seeds.

Contituents.—Capsules and seeds contain a large percentage of a bland fixed oil, used as food and for burning in lamps. The oil is of a pale golden colour, dries easily, and of an agreeable odour ; partially soluble in cold alcohol (1 in 25) and in boiling alcohol (1 in 6), and used like olive oil. Dose, ½ to 1 dr.

Preparation.—Of the capsules (deprived of the seeds). Syrupus papaveris (1 in 3). Dose, ½ to 1 fluid dr. Of the capsules, including seeds—Decoction papaveris (1 in 10). Extractum papaveris. Dose, 2 to 5 grs.

Actions and uses.—The unripe capsules are active medicinal agents, but their narcotic effects are less powerful and less certain than those of opium. They are given for the relief of cough and to check diarrhœa in infants. Locally the capsules are used as anodyne fomentations, and also as emollients. Their poultice is applied to bruised, inflamed, excoriated and swollen parts, to tender and irritable ulcers, and to the eyes in ophthalmia. Seeds are demulcent and nutritive, also mild astringent; mixed with sugarcandy and cardamoms they are given in diarrhœa and dysentery. Decoction is used externally to sprains, contusions, bruises, &c.

Opium, B. P.

Opium, the juice, obtained by incision from the capsules, inspissated by spontaneous evaporation.

Vernacular.—Arab.—Afim, Afyun, Labnul, Ahi-phen. Beng.—Aphim, Aphin. Bom.—Aphim, appoo. Burm.—Bein, Bhain. Can.—Aphimu. Chin—Ofu-yung, Opien. Cing.—Abim. Eng.—Opium. Duk.—Afim. Greek.—Opion. Guz.—Chasa, Aphion. Hind.—Afyun. Malyal.—Kasha-kasha, Karuppa. Mar.—Aphin. Pers.—Mahanul Tiryake. Shir-i-khuskhus. Sans.—Aphina, Apay-num, Chasa, Aphim. Tam.—Casha-pal, Apini. Tel.—Gasha-gashala-palu.

The Arabs converted opion, from Greek opos, into Afiun, opos meaning sap or juice of plants.

Ahi-phena—Ahi, a snake, and Phena, the foam, from the belief that afima was not a vegetable product, but a produce obtained from the foam of snakes. Tiriyake, the juice which Rustam obtained from Kaikaos to give to Sohrab. It is said to have contained opium in its composition.

Characters.—Fresh opium is homogeneous, milky and of the consistence of gum. On keeping it for some time it becomes dry, of a brown colour, and hard, oily and dark. Opium is found in irregular lumps or globular cakes covered with agglutinated mass of poppy leaves, or with the capsules of a species of rumex; each cake weighs on the average about 2 lbs. and upwards. A fresh cake is plastic, somewhat moist, coarsely granular externally, internally smooth and of a reddish-brown colour. The taste is bitter, and it has a strong characteristic narcotic odour. Dry cake contains from 13 to 15 p.c. of morphine. Fresh cake yields about 9 p.c. Dose, ½ to 2 grs.

Adulterations.—Sand, stones, litharge, charcoal, camel's dung, tragacanth, molasses, acacia leaves and stems, poppy capsules, also the juice of opuntia dellenia, and calatropis gigantea, the extract of tobacco plant, dhatura, hemp; gum and resinous matter from figs called lassa; resin from shorea robusta, pulp of tamarind and bael fruit, gum and the seeds of hygrophilla spinosa; starchy substances as linseed, poppy-seed, &c.

Varieties.—Turkey, Asia Minor, and Smyrna opium yields from 10 to 13 p.c. of morphine; Constantinople from 10 to 13 p.c.; Egyptian from 6 to 7 p.c.; East Indian (Malwa and Garden Patna) from 5 to 7 p.c.; Persian 8 to 10 p.c., and European varieties, such as English, French, 14 to 23 p.c.

In the British Pharmacopœia any variety of opium, containing not less than 7·5 p.c. of anhydrous morphine when dry is directed to be used in the preparations of tincture of opium and extract of opium; for other preparations it has been directed that opium when dried and powdered should contain not less than 9½ p.c. and not more than 10½ p.c. of anhydrous morphine. In the case of opium of a higher strength it is directed to bring it to the required strength by diluting it with another specimen of opium containing between 7·5 p.c. and 10 p.c. of morphine or with milk-sugar.

Constituents.—Opium contains a large number of alkaloids, organic acids, and neutral substances.

The most prominent alkaloids are morphine; narcotine 2 to 8 p.c.; codeine 0·2 to 0·7 p.c.; thebaine or paramorphine 0·15 to 1 p.c.; pseudomorphine 0·2 p.c.; papaverine 1 p. c.; narceine 0·2 to ·7 p.c. The organic acids are meconic acid 4 p.c.; lactic acid 1·25 p c., which exists in combination with the alkaloids. Bitter neutral principles, as meconin 0·3 p.c., meconosin and porphyroxine. Opium also contains resins, a trace of volatile oil, glucose, sugar, gum, pectin, caoutchouc, wax, fat, colouring matter, odorous principles, and ash 6 p. c.

Morphina, B.P.—Morphine—Morphia.

Occurs as a white amorphous powder, or shining, transparent acicular prisms, without any odour, and of a bitter taste, insoluble in water and ether, soluble in hot alcohol (1 in 36), soluble in oleic acid and fixed oils. Dose, $\frac{1}{10}$ to $\frac{1}{3}$ gr.; $\frac{1}{4}$ of a grain of morphine is equal to 1 grain of opium used in chemical testing.

Preparation.—Oleatum Morphinæ, a local sedative, 1 in 60 to 1 in 10.

Morphinæ hydrochloridum, B. P., morphine hydrochloride.—In acicular prisms of a silky lustre or a white crystalline amorphous powder of a bitter taste and neutral reaction, soluble in cold water (1 in 24), in alcohol (1 in 50), boiling water (1 in 1). Dose, $\frac{1}{8}$ to $\frac{1}{2}$ gr.; one grain is equal to 9½ grains of crude opium, 8 grains of powdered opium, 4⅗ grain of extract of opium, and 117 minims of tincture of opium.

Preparations.—Of morphine hydrochloride, B. P.—Liquor morphinæ hydrochloridi, B. P. (1 gr. in 110 ms.) Dose, 10 to 60 ms.; Suppositoria morphinæ, B. P. ¼ grain of morphine hydrochloride in each; Suppositoria morphinæ cum sapone (½ grain each); Tinctura chloroformi et morphinæ composita, B. P. (1 gr. of morphine hydrochloride in 110 ms.) Chloroform 1½ fluid ounces, morphine hydrochloride 87½ grains, diluted hydrocyanic acid 1 fluid ounce, tincture of capsicum ½ fluid ounce, tincture of Indian hemp 2 fluid ounces, oil of peppermint 14 minims, glycerine 5 fluid ounces, alcohol 90 p.c. to make one pint. Dose, 5 to 15 ms. Trochiscus morphinæ, B. P. in $\frac{1}{36}$ grain in each ; Trochiscus morphinæ et ipecacuanhæ, B. P., $\frac{1}{36}$ grain in each, with $\frac{1}{12}$ of a grain of ipecacuanha.

Morphinæ Acetas, B. P., Morphine Acetate.—To obtain it, neutralize morphine with acetic acid.

Characters.—A white crystalline or amorphous powder of a bitter taste, acetous odour, and of a neutral reaction; loses acetic acid on exposure to the air, soluble in water (1 in $2\frac{1}{2}$), in alcohol (1 in 100). It spoils by keeping. Dose, $\frac{1}{8}$ to $\frac{1}{2}$ gr.

Preparations.—Liquor morphinæ acetatis, B. P. (1 gr. in 110 ms.) Dose, 10 to 60 ms. Injectio morphinæ acetatis hypodermica (1 gr. in 6 ms.) Dose, 1 to 2 ms. Injectio morphinæ et atropinæ hypodermica —Injectio morphinæ acetas 3 drachms, atropine sulphate 1 grain. Dose 1 to 3 minims. (3 ms. contain $\frac{1}{2}$ grain morphine acetate and $\frac{1}{80}$ grain of atropine.) Atropine, although antagonistic to morphine, increases the sedative action and counteracts disagreeable effects of morphine as headache and constipation.

Morphinæ Hydrobromidum, a white amorphous powder, soluble in water. Dose, $\frac{1}{8}$ to $\frac{1}{2}$ gr. ; Morphinæ Lactas, a white crystalline salt, soluble in water (1 in. 8). Dose, $\frac{1}{8}$ to $\frac{1}{2}$ gr.

Morphinæ Meconas.—White needles, soluble in water (1 in 34). Less disagreeable in its effects than other opium salts. Dose, $\frac{1}{8}$ to $\frac{1}{2}$ gr. Used as hypodermic tablets. Liquor morphinæ bimeconatis (1.25 p.c.) about the same strength as tincture of opium. Dose, 5 to 40 ms.

Nepenthe.—An alcoholic solution of morphine meconate in sherry-wine=strength of tincture of opium.

Morphinæ Sulphas, Morphine sulphate.—In white acicular crystals, without any odour, taste bitter and of a neutral reaction, soluble in water (1 in 21), contains 80 p.c. of morphine. Dose, $\frac{1}{8}$ to $\frac{1}{2}$ gr. Liquor morphinæ sulphatis (1 p.c.) Dose, 10 to 60 ms.

Morphinæ tartras, B. P., Morphine tartrate—prepared by the combination of morphine and tartaric acid in molecular proportions. White crystalline powder or tufts of acicular crystals, soluble in cold water (1 in 11), almost insoluble in alcohol. Dose, $\frac{1}{8}$ to $\frac{1}{2}$ gr., Injectio morphinæ hypodermica, B. P. 1 gr. in 22 ms. Dose, 2 to 5 ms. Liquor morphinæ tartratis, B. P. (1 in 110). Dose, 10 to 60 ms. Winslow's soothing syrup.—Morphine, essence of anise, and syrup of tolu. Each ounce contains morphine $\frac{1}{8}$ grain.

Morphinæ Phthalas.—In glassy scales, soluble in water (1 in 5) for hypodermic injection. Dose, $\frac{1}{8}$ to $\frac{1}{2}$ gr.

Apomorphinæ Hydrochloridum, B. P.—Apomorphine hydrochloride, Apomorphine hydrochlorate.

Manufacture.—Heat morphine or codeine hydrochloride with hydrochloric acid without access of air, dissolve in water; to the solution add sodium carbonate; treat the precipitate thus formed with ether and add little hydrochloric acid.

Characters.—Small greyish, white shining crystals of a bitter taste and without any odour. It has a neutral or faintly acid reaction. It is soluble in water (1 in 50), more readily so in alcohol, is insoluble in ether and chloroform. The solution becomes green by exposure to the air. Dose, $\frac{1}{20}$ to $\frac{1}{10}$ of a grain hypodermically; by the mouth, $\frac{1}{10}$ to $\frac{1}{4}$ of grain. Mistura apromorphinæ et terebeni, $\frac{1}{10}$ grain in 1 ounce. Dose, 1 oz. Syrupus apomorphinæ hydrochloridi, $\frac{1}{4}$ grain in 1 ounce. Dose, $\frac{1}{2}$ to 1 dr. Injectio apomorphinæ hypodermica, B. P. 1 grain in 110 minims. Dose, 5 to 10 ms.

Papine, an active principle of opium; an anodyne without any narcotic or convulsive elements. A safe opiate for children, free from its bad after effects, as nausea, vomiting, constipation, &c. Dose, adults 1 dr.; children, 1 year or under, 2 ms.

Codeina, B. P. Codeine, Codea, Methylmorphine.

Treat morphine with caustic soda and chloride or iodide of methyl (·3 or ·5 p.c. in opium).

Characters.—Frequently contaminated with other alkaloids; colourless, or yellowish white, octohedral crystals or rhombic prisms, translucent, without odour; taste bitter, alkaline reaction, soluble in water (1 in 80), boiling water (1 in 17); readily soluble in alcohol, chloroform, dilute acids and in excess of ammonia water, soluble in ether (1 in 30). Dose, $\frac{1}{4}$ to 2 grs.

Codeinæ phosphas, B.P., Codeine phosphate.—The phosphate of the alkaloid obtained from opium or morphine.

Characters.—White crystals of a slight bitter taste, soluble in water (1 in 4), much less soluble in alcohol; suitable for hypodermic injection (1 grain in 6 minims). Does not cause any local irritation; contains 70 p.c. of the alkaloid. Dose, $\frac{1}{4}$ to 2 grs. Syrupus codeinæ, B. P., one fluid drachm contains $\frac{1}{4}$ grain of codeine phosphate. Dose, $\frac{1}{2}$ to 2 drs.

Hypodermic tablets contain $\frac{1}{4}$ gr. of codeine in each; Codeine and glycerine jelly. Dose, 1 dr.; Lozenzes $\frac{1}{3}$ gr. each; Pastils $\frac{1}{4}$ gr. each for cough; Pilula codeinæ composita. Codeine $\frac{1}{4}$ gr.; Extract of nux vomica $\frac{1}{2}$ gr.; Extract of lettuce $\frac{1}{4}$ gr.; make a pill—for diabetes. Apocodeine, prepared from codeine.—An amorphous powder, soluble in water; hydrochloride of codeine acts as an emetic; used hypodermically. Dose, $\frac{1}{10}$ to 1 gr.

Narceina.

Narceine difficult to obtain in a pure state.

Characters.—Occurs as white silky acicular crystals, neutral, taste slightly bitter: readily soluble in boiling water, in water (1 in 400), very soluble in alcohol, and insoluble in ether. Dose, $\frac{1}{8}$ to $\frac{1}{2}$ gr.

Preparation.—Sodium narceine salicylate, otherwise known as antispasmin. A white powder, soluble in water; contains 50 p.c. of narceine. Dose, $\frac{1}{2}$ to 1 gr.

Acidum Meconicum.

Meconic acid 4 p. c. in opium. To obtain it, add chloride of calcium to infusion of opium, the precipitate of calcium meconate is washed with hot water and treated with hydrochloric acid ; meconic acid is deposited. Pearly scales, sparingly soluble in water, readily so in alcohol.

Narcotina. Narcotine.

Characters.—Brilliant white, inodorous, neutral crystalline prisms contained in opium (2 to 8 p. c.), insoluble in water or potash solution, soluble in chloroform (1 in 3), alcohol (1 in 100), and ether (1 in 125), freely soluble in benzol. Dose 1 to 3 grains. As an antiperiodic it has been used in India for ague. Narcotinæ hydrochloride, Narcotine hydrochloride. Dose, 2 to 10 grs.

Cotarnine Hydrochloride (stypticin.)—A salt of Cotarnine, a base obtained from narcotine. Occurs as yellow crystals soluble in water and alcohol. Dose, $\frac{1}{4}$ to $\frac{1}{2}$ gr.

Papaverina. Papaverine.

Characters.—Delicate, colourless crystals or prisms, does not form salts with acids. Insoluble in water, slightly so in alcohol and ether. Dose, $\frac{1}{12}$ to $\frac{1}{3}$ grain.

Preparations of Opium.

Acetum opii.—Black drop—vinegar of opium; opium 10 p. c. macerate with nutmeg 3, sugar 20, dilute acetic acid, to make 100. Dose, 5 to 20 ms.

Denarcotized opium, Deodorized opium, Opium deodoratum; it contains morphine 14 p. c. To obtain it, add ether to opium to remove the constituents, which are soluble in ether, as narcotine and odorous principles which leave bad after effects. Mix the dry residue with milk-sugar. Dose, $\frac{1}{2}$ to 2 grs.

Extractum opii, B. P., extract of opium; standardized to contain 20 p. c. of morphine. Dose, $\frac{1}{4}$ to 1 gr.

Extractum opii liquidum, B. P., contains $\frac{3}{4}$ grain of morphine in 110 minims. Dose, 5 to 30 ms.

Emplastrum opii, B. P., opium plaster (1 in 10), contains opium and resin plaster.

Emplastrum cephalicum, contains extract of opium 6, Burgundy pitch 18, lead plaster 76.

Linimentum opii, B. P., contains equal parts of tinctura opii and linimentum saponis.

Pilula saponis composita, B. P. (20 p. c. of opium), contains opium 1, hard soap 3 and syrup of glucose 1. Dose, 2 to 4 grs.

Pilula plumbi cum opio, B. P., contains $12\frac{1}{2}$ p. c. of opium—opium 1, acetate of lead 6, and syrup of glucose 0.7. Dose, 2 to 4 grs.

Pilula ipecacuanhæ cum scilla, B. P.; pill of ipecacuanha with squill, contains 5 p. c. of opium and 5 p. c. of ipecacuanha—Dover's powder 3, squill 1, and ammoniacum 1. Dose, 4 to 8 grs.

Pulvis opii compositus, B. P., contains 10 p. c. of opium—opium 3, black pepper 4, ginger 10, carraway fruit 12, tragacanth powder 1. Dose, 2 to 10 grs.

Pulvis cretæ aromaticus cum opio, B. P. ($2\frac{1}{2}$ p. c. of opium), contains aromatic powder of chalk 39 and opium 1. Dose 10 to 40 grs.

Pulvis ipecacuanhæ compositus, B. P., Pulvis ipecacuanha et-opii., Dover's powder (1 in 10) contains ipecacuanha 1, opium powder 1, and potassium sulphate 8. Dose 5 to 15 grs.

Pulvis kino compositus, B. P. (5 p. c. of opium), contains kino 75, opium 5, and cinnamon bark 20. Dose 5 to 20 grs.

Suppositoria plumbi composita, B. P., contains 1 grain of opium, 3 grains of acetate of lead in each, made in oil of Theobroma.

Tinctura opii, B. P., Tincture of opium (laudanum), 1 grain of opium in 15 minims. Dose 5 to 15 ms.

Tinctura camphoræ composita, B. P.—Camphorated tincture of opium—compound tincture of camphor.—Paregoric elixir—$\frac{1}{4}$ grain of opium in 60 minims; contains tincture of opium 60·9, benzoic acid 4·6, camphor 3·4, oil of anise 3·1, diluted alcohol to make 1,000. Dose $\frac{1}{2}$ to 1 dr.; for children, 5 to 20 ms.

Tinctura opii ammoniata, B. P., ammoniated tincture of opium (5 grains of opium in one fluid ounce)—contains tincture of opium 3 ozs., benzoic acid 3 drs., oil of anise 1 dr., solution of ammonia 4 ozs., and alcohol to make 20 ozs. Dose 30 to 60 ms.

Vinum opii—Wine of opium (22 grs. of ext. op. in 1 oz.) Dose 10 to 40 ms.

Unguentum gallæ cum opio.—B. P., Gall and opium ointment contains $7\frac{1}{2}$ p. c. of opium.

Bala goli—A native preparation, extensively used, contains opium and other narcotics, aromatics and bitters.

Trochisci glycerrhizæ et opii, Troches of glycyrrhiza and opium—contains ext. glycyrrhizæ, opium powder, oil of anise and sugar, (opium $\frac{1}{13}$ gr. in each).

Squibb's diarrhœa mixture contains: Tinct. opii 1, spt. camphoræ 1, capsici 1, chloroform $\frac{1}{2}$, alcohol to make 5. Dose for children, 1 to 10 ms.; for adults, $\frac{1}{2}$ to 1 dr.

Liquor opii sedativus—sedative solution of opium (Battley's sedative) resembles Ext. opii. liq. B. P.

Physiological action.—It depends upon the combined effects of the various alkaloids and other principles obtained from it. Opium in medicinal doses at first stimulates the brain, heart and respiration; this effect is soon followed by general depression. Generally opium is analgesic, hypnotic, antispasmodic, diaphoretic, narcotic and cerebral depressant. Its chief action is on the cerebro-spinal system and through the nerves it acts upon all the organs of the body. It affects the ganglia at the base of the brain, giving rise to contracted pupils, vomiting, and slow respiration. Under its use the grey matter of the cord is first stimulated, and there are increased reflexes. This is soon followed by depression, as evidenced by the lowering of perception and sensation. The cutaneous vessels are dilated at first, as shown by a sense of heat felt on the external ear, itching and rose-coloured skin eruptions. This is followed by pallor and coldness of the limbs and fingers. The generative organs are stimulated. In medicinal doses, taken for some time, it affects all the secretions except milk and sweat, which are increased. It causes dryness of the mouth and throat, lessens the secretion of the stomach and thus impairs appetite. The secretion of bile is also diminished and constipation results. The action of the heart is increased, and there is increased arterial tension. The cerebral functions are at first exhilarated, the ideas flow rapidly, and there is a sort of mild intoxication. This is soon followed by drowsiness and sound sleep, often disturbed by dreams, and often followed, on waking, by headache, constipation, indigestion and depression of spirits. If any pain be present it is relieved, but a larger dose will be necessary on subsequent occasions. In full doses the cerebral symptoms are accentuated, but the stimulation is of short duration. The after-effects become more marked. The mouth becomes very dry, digestion is impaired, there is nausea, vomiting and profuse sweat. The heart is depressed, the circulation lowered, the oxidation is interfered with, and there is loss of body heat. The pupils are contracted, there is intense itching of the nose with retention of urine. The cerebral depression is soon followed by headache, vertigo, slow and laborious respiration. In poisonous doses, sterterous breathing and coma supervene, followed by feeble pulse, cold clammy perspiration, contracted pupils followed by dilation as the end approaches, cyanosis of the face and fingers, followed by abolished reflexes, deep coma, paralysis of respiratory centres, and death.

Therapeutic uses.—Opium is given to relieve severe pain from any cause, except in cerebritis and to allay any irritation. As an antispasmodic it is extensively used. It allays irritation and produces sleep in insomnia, sciatica, neuralgia, lumbago, cancer, intestinal, renal, or hepatic colic, calculi, &c. ; also in tetanus, in morbid states of the abdominal viscera, as gastritis, gastrodynia, in hernia and in diseases of the urino-genital system. To check excessive secretion it is largely used in diarrhœa, dysentery, nervous and sympathetic vomiting, and in excessive expectoration ; also in diabetes, ptyalism and lecorrhœa, &c. In diabetes and polyuria, codeine is invariably preferred. As a support to the general system it is given in low fevers, in low states of the system accompanied by tremors, in low muttering delirium, and in surgical cases to promote the healing of wounds and ulcers. In high fevers it is combined with mercury, aconite, camphor, antimony, &c. As a narcotic it is used in all inflammatory conditions, acute and chronic, except in those of the respiratory tract and in albuminuria, where its administration has led to deaths by coma or by apnœa. In peritonitis it is highly beneficial. As a sudorific, combined with ipecacuanha and camphor, it is given to promote diaphoresis in fevers, harassing cough and in coryza. In India it is largely used by *chundoolees* for its aphrodisiac effects. As a hæmostatic it is useful to check hæmorrhages, chiefly from the uterine fibroids and cancer, combined with other hæmostatics. As a soporific, in spite of all its defects, it is the drug most extensively used as being certain in its effects. Opium is given to quiet the nervous system ; hence it checks or controls the reactionary fevers. In threatened abortion its use is extremely beneficial. Externally it has a sedative action upon the cutaneous nerves, and as anodyne poultices it is largely used to relieve pain. It forms an important ingredient in all anodyne applications used in gout, rheumatism, and ophthalmia. It is also used as plaster, suppository, and as a paint in painful piles, ulcers, &c. For hypodermic purposes its alkaloids alone are used.

Bala goli is given to children in wakefulness, diarrhœa, colic and general irritability, but its use as a rule should be deprecated, as disastrous consequences sometimes result from its use. Young children are more susceptible to opium than adults, and women more so than men. Some have idiosyncrasy for it, and cannot tolerate even the smallest dose. In persons taking opium medicinally or for the first time, the exhilarating effects are of short duration, and they often pass into a state of drowsiness; but with habitual opium-eaters the exhilarating symptoms are of longer duration. The coma of opium narcosis can be diagnosed from that due to alcohol, and apoplexy. In opium poisoning pupils are contracted. In alcohol they are dilated. In apoplexy they are contracted unequally.

Morphine hydrochloride is an anodyne, hypnotic and narcotic. The soporific effect of opium as a whole is mostly due to this alkaloid; it is four times as strong as the crude opium. It produces less vascular and arterial excitement, less headache, less vertigo, less subsequent depression and less constipation. It allays nervous irritability, diminishes pain, induces sleep, arrests secretions, except that of the skin, which it promotes. Full effects are speedily induced by its hypodermic injection. It is given in cardiac dyspnœa, in rheumatism, gout and in puerperal convulsions; also in aortic stenosis and in paroxysms of angina pectoris. In large doses it is a narcotic poison.

Morphine Acetas is given in diabetes like codeine, and like it controls the formation of sugar.

Apomorphine Hydrochloride.—In small doses it is a valuable expectorant; in large doses a safe, certain and quick emetic when given hypodermically and also when taken by the mouth; vomiting is generally followed by sleep. It is useful in cases of irritant and narcotic poisoning, alcoholic intoxication, impaction of foreign bodies in the air passages, &c. Although a derivative of morphine, it can be used in cases of poisoning by morphine salts. As an expectorant, combined with morphine, it is used in hacking cough, bronchial asthma and in phthisis. It relieves hiccough, spasms of chorea, epilepsy, &c. In catarrh of the larynx and of bronchi and in capillary bronchitis it is given with salicylate of ammonia with good result.

Codeine is a respiratory sedative and hypnotic, It is not a very active alkaloid, its soporific effects being feeble, while tetanic effects being altogether absent. Its chief value depends upon its power of lessening the quantity of sugar in the urine in diabetes. It is given in various affections of the heart, as a palliative for cough in phthisis and for the relief of abdominal pains, in nervous insomnia, and in cases where sleep is prevented by the pain of rheumatism or cancer or by distressing cough. In ovarian neuralgia, codeine in ½ grain doses three times a day is given with good results. As a gastro-intestinal sedative, it lessens irritability of the stomach and intestines, hence useful in nausea, vomiting (from any cause), diarrhœa, gastrodynia, &c.

Paramorphine or thebaine is a powerful spinal excitant and tetanizer, resembling strychnine in action.

Narcotine.—Hypnotic, tonic, and antiperiodic, only next to quinine. Used in ague, in general debility due to prolonged lactation, and during convalescence from acute diseases. Also given in headache, constipation, &c.

Papaverine is narcotic and convulsant. It is free from the ill effects of opium, as headache, giddiness, &c. It contracts the pupils.

Narceine is hypnotic, but is without the bad after-effects of morphine.

Treak Farook.—A native preparation containing opium. It occurs as an oily, unctuous semifluid, of a darkish blue or brownish dark colour. The taste is sweet. The odour is sweet and resembles that of liquorice. Used as a tonic, stimulant and antispasmodic, in myxœdema beriberi, anasarca, rheumatism, vomiting, diarrhœa, tetanus, seminal debility, &c. It is also given in the collapse stage of cholera and in poisoning by venomous animals.

Sanguinaria Canadensis.

Indian (red) paint, Blood-root, Red Puccoon.

Sanguinaria, from sanguis, blood. The plant, when incised, emits blood-like juice.

Habitat.—United States, North America, Canada.

Part used.—The rhizome.

Characters.—A perennial plant ; flower white, single on an erect stalk ; petals tinged with rose or purple ; rhizome 2 inches long, $\frac{2}{5}$ of an inch thick, cylindrical, somewhat branched and wrinkled, colour reddish brown ; on section whitish internally, with numerous small reddish resin cells ; bark thin ; odour faint ; taste bitter and acrid. Dose, 1 to 3 grs. ; as an emetic, 10 to 30 grs.

Constituents.—Sanguinarine, chelerythrine. protopine, homochelidonine, citric and malic acids, resin, starch, gum, albumen, sugar, and ash, 8 p. c.

Sanguinarine, an alkaloid is the active principle of the plant.

To obtain it, infuse the root in hot water and add acetic or dilute hydrochloric acid to the hot solution and precipitate the solution with ammonia. Boil the residue with charcoal and evaporate. It is a white powder, of a coffee-brown colour ; taste acrid ; soluble in alcohol, ether, benzene. Dose, $\frac{1}{12}$ to $\frac{1}{8}$ gr. ; as an emetic $\frac{1}{2}$ gr.

Chelerythrine.—To obtain it, pass hydrochloric acid gas through the ethereal tincture, dry the precipitated hydrochlorate, and dissolve it into hot water, filter and add liquor ammoniæ.

A lemon-coloured salt. Also found in chelidonium majus.

Protopine gives, with sulphuric acid, deep purple colour. It is also found in papaver somniferum and chelidonium majus.

Preparations—Extractum sanguinariæ fluidum ; fluid extract of sanguinaria. Dose—2 to 5 ms. ; as expectorant and stimulant.

Tinctura sanguinariæ, tincture of sanguinaria, (1 in 8). Dose, as an expectorant, 5 to 60 ms. ; as an emetic, 1 to 2 drs.

Acetum sanguinarinæ. Dose—10 to 30 ms.

Sanguinarinæ nitras. Dose—$\frac{1}{20}$ gr.

Sanguinarinæ sulphas. Dose—$\frac{1}{30}$ gr.

Physiological action—Locally it is a feeble escharotic. Internally emetic, stimulant tonic, alterative, narcotic, sternuatatory, emmenagogue and expectorant. In small doses it stimulates the stomach and increases the circulation. In large doses it depresses the pulse and causes nausea. In full doses it depresses the heart and respiration and produces salivation, sneezing, vomiting, purging and great prostration. In excessive or toxic doses it is a violent irritant ; at first it stimulates the heart and increases the arterial tension, then it depresses the heart, lowers the arterial tension and finally paralyses the heart ; it also lowers the reflexes ; pupils are dilated, there are active vomiting, diarrhœa, burning in the stomach, faintness, vertigo, dim vision, cold sweats, great thirst and paralysis of the heart and respiration, followed by collapse and death.

Therapeutics.—It is used in pneumonia, rheumatism, chronic nasal catarrh, croup, bronchitis, whooping cough and in throat affections; also in atony of the stomach and in torpid liver, jaundice and duodenal catarrh. Given as an aphrodisiac in spermatorrhœa, as an emmenagogue in amenorrhœa due to anæmia, and in syphilis. When inhaled it causes violent sneezing. Externally it is applied to indolent ulcers, nasal polypi, warts, chancres, and also over fungous granulations and scaly eruptions

Violaceæ. The Banaphasha or Violet Family.

Herbs or shrubs, leaves simple, stipulate, with involute vernation, alternate or opposite ; flowers blue, pink or white, handsome, irregular ; fruit one-celled, capsular, three-valved, dehiscent, loculicidal ; seeds numerous ; embryo straight ; albumen fleshy.

Habitat.—Europe, Siberia, America, Africa and Malacca.

Properties.—Some species have a delicate fragrance, some contain an emetic principle known as emetine or violine ; a few are mucilaginous, others are reputed to be anodyne ; some are purgative.

Viola Tricolor.

Pansy.

Viola Pedata.—Blue violet.

Habitat.—North America, Europe.

Parts used.—The flowering herb and rhizome.

Characters.—The flowering herb is from 4 to 12 inches high and angular; leaves round and cordate ; flowers yellow, white, blue or purplish. Taste bitter. Dose, 10 to 60 grs.

Constituents.—An active principle, Violin allied to emetine Salicylic acid, resin, &c.

Preparation.—Decoction (1 in 20). Dose, 1 to 2 ozs.

Actions and uses.—Mucilaginous, expectorant, emollient and laxative. Violine is emeto-cathartic. Poultice of the herb in milk is used in impetigo, also in eczema of the face and head. Given internally in constitutional syphilis, scrofula and bronchitis.

Viola Odorata.

Habitat.—Temperate climates, Europe, North America.

Parts used.—The flowering herb.

Vernacular.—Arab.—Banaphasa, Behussej. Beng.—Bonosa. Duk. —Banaphashaka. Eng.—March violet, sweet violet. Guz.—Banaphasha. Hind.—Bagabanoshsa. Mar.—Baga-banosa. Pers.—Bag-i-Banaphasha. Tam.—Vayilettu.

Bagh-i-Banaphasha—Bâg, garden, and Banafsha, violet. Kashamiri Banaphasha is the name given to the whole plant, and the Pul-i- Banaphasha, to the flowers only.

Characters—A dry herb, colour brownish, without any stem, consists of leaves and sometimes flowers, variegated, yellow, white, blue or purplish, with long filiform stalks. Roots dry, thready, fibrous, pale yellow, knotty, slender, some as thick as a quill, and slightly furrowed. Leaves cordate at the base, reniform or heart-shaped and dentate at the upper part. Flowers purple, violet, blue or pink and irregular. Carpels three nerved and brown. Corolla, with a long, narrow tapering spur, which extends beyond the calyx. Smell sweet, nauseous, and resembling that of ipecacuanha. Taste nauseous, bitter and mucilaginous. Dose—15 to 60 grs.

Constituents.—The flowers contain a colouring matter, a volatile oil, three acids, viz, violenic and salicylic acids and another red acid, and an emetic principle called violin, identical with emetine; viola quercitrin allied to rutin (mandelin), sugar, &c.

Preparations.—Infusion of the root (1 in 10). Dose, 1 to 2 ozs. Decoction (1 in 10). Dose, 1 to 2 ozs. Syrup of flowers (1 in 6). Dose, 2 to 4 drs.

Actions and uses.—The root is nauseating and diaphoretic, somewhat similar to ipecacuanha, given in fevers. The petals, especially of the purple flowers, are diuretic, refrigerant and expectorant, also laxative, given along with other aperients as tamarind, myrobalans, &c., in coughs, nephritis, with scalding and scanty urine, fevers, syphilis scrofula, skin diseases, chronic diarrhœa and dysentery.

Ionidium Suffruticosum, Viola Suffruticosa.

Habitat.—Tropical parts of Asia and Australia.

Parts used.—Root and leaves.

Vernacular—Beng.—Nunbora. Burm.—Keoki-bin. Duk.—Ruttonpuruss Ruttanpuras. Hind.—Ratanpurs. Mar.—Ratanpurs.

Mal.—Oorela tamara. Sans.—Padma charini, charati. Tam.—Urela tamara. Tel.—Purusha ratnam Nela Kobbari.

Characters.—Roots yellowish white, tapering downwards, 3 to 4 inches in length and covered with a corky bark ; leaves small, lanceolate, subsessile and alternate ; taste of the plant mucilaginous. Dose—20 to 60 grs.

Constituents—The root contains an alkaloid, soluble in ether and alcohol, forming salts with mineral and vegetable acids ; Quercitrine, another colouring matter, soluble in water, but insoluble in alcohol; mucilage ; acid resin, and oxalates.

Preparation.—Infusion or decoction (1 in 10). Dose, 2 to 6 drs. Liniment and electuary.

Actions and uses.—Tonic, demulcent and diuretic, used in gonorrhœa, general debility and in affections of the urinary organs; externally, with some mild oil, it is used as a cooling application for the head.

Ionidium Parviflorum.—In South America it is used as a specific in elephantiasis. It is there known as "Cuchunchulli de Cuença."

Bixaceæ.

Bixineæ or Flacourtiaceæ. The Kesar or chaulmogara family, shrubs or small trees, leaves alternate, exstipulate, leathery and often dotted ; fruit dehiscent or indehiscent, with a thin pulp in the centre ; pulp differently coloured ; seeds numerous, and often covered with withered pulp ; albumen fleshy and oily.

Habitat.—Hottest parts of E. and W. Indies and Africa.

Properties.—Many species, are feebly bitter, stomachic and astringent. The fruits of some are edible and wholesome. The bark of one variety is emetic.

Hydnocarpus Anthelmintica, False Chaulmugra.

Habitat.—China.

Part used.—Seeds.

Vernacular.—Chinese Lukrabo or Ta-Fung-Tsze, Dai-Phong-tu.

Characters.—The seed is about half the length of chaulmugra seed, but of equal diameter. The shell thicker and harder and marked with raised ridges. The seeds, after extraction of the oil, are used as vermifuge.

Actions and uses.—Used in leprosy, lepra, itch, pityriasis, psoriasis, syphilis, cracks on hands, &c.

Hydnocarpus Wrightiana. H. Inebrians.

Habitat.—Western Peninsula, Concan.

Parts used.—The seeds and oil.

Vernacular.—Cing.—Rata kekuna, makulu. Duk.—Jangli-Badam. Eng.—Jungle almond. Hind.—Jangli-Badam. Mar.—Kowtee. Maleal.—Moratti, Tamna. Mar.—Kadu-kavatha, Kowtee. Tam.—Maravattay. Tel.—Niradi-Vittulu.

Characters.—Fruit globose and of the size of an apple ; rind rough, occasionally tubercled and of a brown colour ; seeds numerous, obtusely angular, of a dark-brown colour and embedded in a scanty white pulp, which is firmly adherent to the testa ; albumen oily, white when fresh, and dark-brown in the dry seeds. On expression the seeds yield an oil of a pale sherry colour ; odour resembles that of chaulmogra.

Constituents.—The seeds contain about 44 p. c. of the fixed oil, which also contains some gynocardic acid. Does not give any crystalline or fatty deposit on long keeping.

Preparations.—Infusion (1 in 20). Dose, 1 to 2 ozs. Oil. Dose—10 to 30 ms. Paste containing Hydnocarpus Wrightiana 2, Jatropha Curcas-oil 2, Sulphur 4, Camphor 1, Lime-juice 20 ; used for rubbing on scaly eruptions.

Actions and uses.—The oil is used as a substitute for chaulmogra oil. It is an alterative, stimulant and parasiticide. The seeds, like chaulmogra, are used externally in obstinate skin diseases, such as scabies, lichen and prurigo. An infusion of seeds is used as a wash or injection in gonorrhœa, or into the vagina in fœtid discharges after delivery. The oil, with lime-water, is used as a liniment for scurf on the head, and, like chaulmogra, in the treatment of leprosy and for rheumatic joints. With alkaline ashes it is used in certain parts of India as a stimulant dressing for phagedenic ulcers, foul sores, and to remove maggots. By some authors this species is regarded as belonging to the natural order Pangiaceæ allied to Papayaceæ.

Gynocardia Odorata. Syn Hydnocarpus Odoratus.

Habitat.—Rangoon Forests, Malayan Peninsula, Sikkim and Khassia Hill.

Parts used.—The seeds and oil from the seeds.

Vernacular.—Burm.—Talien-noe. Chin.—Tafung-tsze. Hind.—Chaulmogra, Petarkura. Pers.—Chaulmogra. Lepcha.—Tuk-Hung.

Characters.—The fruits grow upon the stem and main branches, and are globular, each contains 3 or 4 seeds ; seeds rough-skinned, hard, about 1 inch in diameter, many, ovoid, irregular, more or less angular and round or flattened ; testa thin, smooth and brittle ; albumen plenty. When expressed yield 30 to 50 p. c. of the oil.

Constituents.—Oleum Gynocardiæ, Chaulmogra oil.—It is a fixed oil, very bulky, of a sherry wine or brownish colour. The odour is nauseous and peculiar. Dose, 2 to 15 ms. The oil deposits on keeping crystalline fat, and contains palmitic acid 60 p. c., and therefore solid in cold climates. It contains Gynocardic acid 11 p. c., the active ingredient; cocinic acid 2·5 p. c., and hypogœic acid 4 p. c. Both of the latter acids are found either combined with glycerides as fats or in a free state. Gynocardic acid is a fatty acid, crystallizes in yellowish flakes, and has an an acrid burning taste. Dose, ½ to 2 grs.

Preparations.—Of the oil, pearls or pills, and unguentum gynocardiæ (1 in 4).

Actions and uses.—The seeds and oil are alterative and tonic, used to improve the state of the blood as in leprosy, phthisis, skin diseases, &c. By some the oil is regarded as a specific in leprosy, and, no doubt, in some cases it has very beneficial effects. It is also used in scrofula, secondary syphilis, phthisis and rheumatism with stiff joints, both externally as an inunction or ointment, and internally with mucilage, or as capsules or pearls. Gynocardic acid ointment, 15 to 25 grains to an ounce of vaseline is used in herpes, tinea, leprosy and other skin affections. It should be given after meals in milk or with cod-liver oil.

Flacourtia Cataphracta.

Habitat.—India, Assam, Nepaul, Behar.

Parts used.—The fruit, leaves and bark.

Vernacular.—Arab.—Zarnab. Bomb.—Joggam. Can.—Talisapatri. Cing.—Talispatturu. Duk.—Tajpat. Barmi. Eng.—Many spined Flaucortia. Beng. and Hind.—Talispatri, Barahmi, Paniala, panijala. Mar.—Tambat. Sans.—Talisha, Prachinamalaka. Tam.—Panijala, Talishapatri. Tel.—Talisapatri. Port.—Joggam.

Characters.—Leaves oblong or lanceolate, long, annulate, glabrous, crenato-serrate; petiole short. Leaves and shoots resemble rhubarb in flavour; fruit of the size of a plum, indehiscent, purple, containing 5 to 6 seeds; seeds obovoid; endocarp hard; testa coriaceous, taste acid. An oil is extracted from the seeds. Dose of the leaves—20 to 60 grains.

Preparation.—Infusion of the bark (1 in 10). Dose, 4 to 12 drs.

Actions and uses.—The bark is refrigerant and astringent, used in fevers to allay thirst, correct foul taste and prevent nausea and biliousness. Leaves and young shoots are stomachic, and given in diarrhœa, dysentery and even in consumption. Infusion of the bark is used in hoarseness of the voice. The fruit is edible.

Cochlospermum Gossypium, Bombax Gossypium.

Habitat.—Behar, Orissa, Deccan, Garwal and Bundelkhand.

Parts used.—The gum (Indian Tragacanth).

Vernacular.—Arab.—Kaserae-hindi Kather, Samaghul-qatade-hindi. Cing.—Ella-imbul. Eng.—Golden silk-cotton tree, yellow-flowered cotton tree. Duk. and Hind.—Pili Kapas, Katera-gond (the gum). Mar.—Kathalio gunda. Maleal.—Shima-punji, Tachema-pungee. Pers.—Katerae-hindi, Kathera. Tam.—Tanaku maram. Tel.—Konda-gogu chettu.

Characters.—Large trees, bearing large golden-yellow flowers appearing in spring when the tree is destitute of leaves; Fruit capsular, of the size of lemons, containing within them cotton; seeds kidney-shaped; testa hard. The gum, known as kateera, is obtained from the trunk of the tree. It is greyish white in colour, translucent, in large white or yellowish, irregular or twisted vermicular pieces or tears, with a tendency to split up readily into flat scales; when moistened it swells into transparent jelly; taste mucilaginous; a good substitute for tragacanth.

Preparation.—Lozenges and mucilage.

Actions and uses.—The gum is demulcent and astringent, used in cough, hoarse throat and scalding in the urine; mixed with curd or whey it is largely used in diarrhœa and dysentery. Experience has verified its good results in the cases of the last-named diseases.

Remarks.—In Bombay the gum of sterculia urens, known as karâi gunda, is sold for katira gunda.

Bixa Orellana, B. Indica. Annatto Bush.

Habitat.—America; cultivated in India.

Parts used.—The pulp and seeds.

Vernacular.—Eng.—Annatto bush, arnotto. Brazilian—Uracuara. Beng.—Nutkaner, Latkan. Burm.—Thidew. Can.—Kuppa Manhala. Cing.—Kaha-gaha. Duk.—Kisti. Hind.—Capurji, Latkan. Malay.—Kasumba-kling. Maleal.—Kurungu-munga. Mar.—Sendri, Kisree. Tam.—Kuragu-manjal. Tel.—Jafra chettu.

Characters.—The plant does not thrive without plenty of sun. The pulp covering the seeds is of a deep red colour, from this the colouring matter, known as arnotta or annatto, is made The annatto exists in cakes of a black colour, becoming red-brown on exposure to air. It has a peculiar odour and a disagreeable bitter taste. The seeds are triangular, compressed on two sides and chanelled lengthwise. On one side the top is obtusely mucronate; the kernel is white and oily. Dose of the seeds, 5 to 20 grs.

Constituents.—A colouring matter, called bixin, obtained from minute red leaflets, soluble in alcohol, concentrated sulphuric acid and ether. Insoluble in water.

Preparation.—Powder of seeds and pulp. Dose, 5 to 10 grs.

Actions and uses.—The root and seeds are febrifuge, astringent and slightly purgative, used in dysentery and in diseases of the kidneys; as a stomachic tonic they are given in convalescence from fevers and in general debility. Its principal use is as a dyeing agent and used to colour butter, cheese, chocolate, &c.

Capparidaceæ.

The Hurahura, or caper family.

Herbs, shrubs or rarely trees; leaves simple or lobed, alternate, generally exstipulate, rarely spiny with stipulate appendages; flowers yellow, white or purple; fruit dehiscent and pod-shaped or indehiscent and baccate; seeds one or many, usually reniform and without albumen, cotyledons leafy.

Habitat.—Chiefly tropical, may be found in temperate climates.

Properties.—Similar to those of cruciferæ, *i.e.*, pungent, stomachic, stimulant and antiscorbutic. Some are aperient, diuretic and anthelmintic, and some are poisonous, owing to the acrid principle being large in quantity.

Gynandropsis Pentaphylla, Cleome Pentaphylla.

Habitat.—India and all tropical countries.

Parts used.—The plant and seeds.

Vernacular.—Eng.—The five-leaved cleome. Beng.—Kamal, Katkoduku, Shada-hurburija. Bomb.—Kanphuti. Cing.—Waila. Duk.—Hulhul. Hind.—Karaila, Hulhul. Maleal.—Kara-vella, Tai-vala. Mar.—Tilavana, Mabli. Sans.—Surjavarta, Arkapushpika. Sind.—Beghara. Tam.—Nai-kaduga, Nai-vella. Tel.—Vaminta.

Characters.—A five-leaved cleome, a weed; flowers whitish or purple; seeds black, small, numerous and kidney-shaped, resembling those of cleome viscosa, and having a faint flavour of mustard; leaves 5 foliolate, and leaflets obovate. The whole plant is viscid and covered with glandular hairs; odour peculiar, like that of asafetida. Dose of the powdered seeds, 15 to 25 grs.

Constituents.—The plant contains a fixed oil; seeds, when crushed, develop an acrid volatile oil, similar in properties to mustard oil, also a resin.

Preparation.—Decoction (1 in 20). Dose, 1 to 2 ozs.; medicated oil.

Actions and uses.—Seeds are antispasmodic, sudorific, and carminative, used in fevers, bilious affections and infantile convulsions. Bruised leaves rubefacient and even vesicant, applied to the boils and buboes to promote suppuration. The juice of the leaves, beaten with salt, is used as drops in earache. The whole plant, boiled in sweet oil, is used in leprosy. As an antispasmodic it is given in hysteria. The seeds are used as a substitute for mustard seeds.

Cratæva Religiosa, Capparis Trifoliata, C. Roxsburghii.

Religiosa—The leaves being used for religious purposes.

Habitat.—Malabar, Canara, Tropical Africa.

Parts used.—The leaves and bark.

Vernacular.—Eng.—Holy garlic pear, three-leaved caper. Burm.—Ka-dat. Duk.—Burmi-ki-jhar. Beng.—Barun, Tiktoshak. Can.—Nirvala, Bilapatri. Cing.—Bilapatra. Guj.—Vaivaruna. Hind.—Bilasi, Varvunna. Malyal.—Vilva-patrani. Mar.—Koomla, Haravarana, Kurwan Vayavarana. Sans.—Koom Varuna Ashamarighana (the leaves), Belpatra, Tapia. Tam.—Mavilinga-maram. Tel.—Vivapatri, Usik manu. Panj.—Barna.

Ashamarighana—Ashamari, means gravel or stone, and Ghân, to kill or to remove. This is in allusion to the use of the drug as lithontriptic in urinary diseases, renal calculi, &c.

Bela-patra, which means like the leaves of Bela. The leaves in both are three-foliolate.

Characters.—The tree is planted around tombs and temples in India; root-bark soft, when fresh of a dirty white colour, outer surface wrinkled and here and there marked with fissures of a dirty brown colour, internally white, soft and fragile; odour heating, nauseous and disagreeable ; taste bitter and pungent. Leaves three-foliolated, leaflets lanceolate, fine-pointed and smooth, upper surface dark green, under surface of a light colour. When bruised the leaves have a disagreeable smell like that of hellebore ; taste bitter and pungent. Dose, 5 to 20 grs.

Constituents.—The bark contains a principle similar to saponin.

Preparations.—Varuna ashes ; Decoction of the root-bark (1 in 10). Dose, 1 to 2 ozs. Infusion of the leaves (1 in 10). Dose, 1 to 2 ozs. Compound decoction.—C. Religiosa, tribulus terrestris, ginger, carbonate of potash, honey and water. Dose, 1 oz. A compound powder, known as Varunadya-churna, contains ashes, bark powder of C. Religiosa and potassium carbonate. Varunadyaguda, a confection contains bark, treacle and a number of aromatics and diuretic substances.

Actions and uses.—Stomachic tonic, laxative and lithontriptic. Given to promote appetite and to increase the secretion of bile. As a diuretic the root-bark is used in dropsy and urinary disorders, in calculous affections, combined with tribulus terrestris. As an alterative the compound powder is given in ascites, calculus, in chronic enlargements of glands, as liver, spleen, and in affections of the bladder and uterus. Fresh leaves and roots, mixed with cocoanut juice and ghee, is given in rheumatism, also as food to reduce corpulence. A paste of the leaves is applied to soles of the feet to relieve swelling and burning sensation. The leaf is smoked in caries of the bones of the nose.

Cleome Viscosa. C. Icosandra, Polanisia Viscosa. P. Icosandra, Sticky Cleome (Eng.)

Habitat.—Tropical India and other warm countries.

Parts used.—The seeds and plant.

Vernacular.—Beng.—Hurhurya. Can.—Hucha-sasavi. Duk.—Chowri-ajawana. Eng.—Dog mustard, sticky cleome. Hind.—Hurhura, Halhul. Malyal.—Kat Kuddaghoo. Mar.—Hulahul, Kanphuti, Pivala Tilavana. Port.—Bredo mamma. Sans.—Adity-a-bhakta, Arka Kanta. Tam.—Naaveli. Tamool.—Nahi Kuddaghoo. Tel.—Kukka-vaminta.

Nahi-kuddaghoo.—Dog mustard.

Kan-phuti, from kan, ear, and phuti to tear or burst ; the juice is a popular remedy for purulent discharges from the ear.

Characters.—An annual viscous weed, from one to two feet high, stem furrowed and studded with glandular capitate hairs ; leaves digitate on long petioles, channelled and of a reddish colour ; leaflets three to five, obovate, finely serrated at the margin. The leaves have a pungent flavour. Flowers yellow and axillary, capsules long, striated and hairy; seeds of the size of mustard seeds, small, many, reticulated, black and reniform, compressed and netted with a white scar near the hilum ; taste, on chewing the seeds, hot, and mucilaginous like Mullabija. The fresh plant, when crushed, gives out a volatile oil like that of garlic or mustard. Dose, 10 to 30 grs.

Preparation.—Infusion (1 in 10). Dose, ½ to 1 oz.

Actions and uses.—Carminative, pungent, anthelmintic and antiseptic ; seeds are used in round worms, to expel flatus in children, also in fever and diarrhœa. The juice of leaves is rubefacient like mustard ; mixed with salt it is dropped into the ear in otorrhœa. An infusion of the seeds is used for unhealthy ulcers and to kill maggots..

Capparis Spinosa.

Habitat.—Afghanistan, West Asia, Deccan, Gujerat.

Parts used.—The bark of the root.

Vernacular.—Eng.—Caper plant. Syrian—Kabur. Turkish—Kabariet. Arab.—Kiabara. Pers.—Kabar-Karak (fruit). Sans.—Kakadani-karira (fruit). Hind.—Karu, Karer (the oil). Duk.—Karya (the oil).

Characters.—The bark is like half quills, outer surface smooth, slightly fissured and greyish brown, within brown and resinous ; taste slightly bitter and pungent. Dose, 10 to 30 grs.

Constituents.—The bark contains a neutral bitter principle of a sharp irritating taste, resembling senegin. The flower buds contain capric acid and a glucoside which yield, on boiling with sulphuric acid, isodulcite and a colouring matter similar to quercetin ; also some gelatinous substance. The fresh plant contains a volatile oil, having properties of garlic oil.

Preparation.—Infusion (1 in 10). Dose, ½ to 1 oz.

Actions and uses.—Similar to that of senega ; alterative, antiscorbutic, stimulant, expectorant and diuretic. The root-bark is used in palsy, gout, rheumatism, cough and dropsy. Locally the powder is applied to malignant sores, also to boils and swellings. The juice of fresh plant, like cleome juice, is dropped into the ear to kill worms ; a fair sustitute for senega.

Capparis Zeylanica. C. Acuminata.

Vernacular.—Beng.—Kalukera. Tel.—Paliki. Mar.—Waghauli. Hind.—Govindphal. Tam.—Authinidi-kai. Used as refrigerant and cooling.

C. Aphylla. Eng.—Thorny caper bush. Hind.—Ardanda. Sans.—Hiunkara. Tam.—Katallikai. Tel.—Adonda, arudonda. These are used as counter-irritants. The fruits are used as a picl

Cadaba Indica. C. Farinosa.

Habitat.—Western India.

Vernacular.—Eng.—Indian Cadaba. Tam.—Velivi. Tel.—Ada morinika, Chekonadi, Chimurudu. The root is reputed as aperient and anthelmintic.

C. Trifoliata.

Habitat.—Carnatic, Ceylon.

Parts used.—Leaves and flower-buds.

Vernacular.—Tam.—Viluthee, Maunthak-kooroonthu.

Characters.—Cadaba Trifoliata—leaves palmate, three-foliate, leaflets oblong, lanceolate and 2 inches long.

C. Indica—leaves simple, ovate, oblong, acute and mucronate, from 1 to 1½ inches long. C. Farinosa—leaves hoary, ovate or oblong, obtuse and about 1 inch long. Dose of the leaves, 2 to 4 drs.

Constituents.—Leaves contain a bitter alkaloid, soluble in ether and alcohol and two organic acids—one resembling cathartic acid. Also nitrates and carbonates of lime. The ash contains alkaline chlorides, sulphates and carbonates.

Preparation.—Decoction of leaves (1 in 10) Dose, 2 to 4 ozs.

Actions and uses.—Stimulant, antiscorbutic and aperient. Decoction of leaves of C. Indica is used as anthelmintic in round worms. The juice of C. Trifoliata is given in dyspepsia in children. Leaves are used as purgative, emmenagogue and antiphlogistic, combined with myrobalans and ginger, or with senna and Epsom salt. In amenorrhæa and dysmenorrhœa a decoction of the leaves, combined with castor-oil and turmeric, is found useful. It is also given in syphilis, scrofula and rheumatism. Externally the leaves are used as varalians with the leaves of odina wodier to relieve rheumatic pains, and as a poultice to boils to promote suppuration. The leaves are used by the natives in preparing medicated oils.

Cruciferæ or Brassicaceæ.

Mustard (Rai) turnip and cabbage family.

Cruciferæ, from crux, a cross in allusion to the Maltese cross like arrangement of the four petals.

General Characters.—Herbs or, rarely shrubs, leaves alternate and exstipulate. Flowers cruciform, yellow, white or pink, rarely purple; and generally a mixture of these colours. Stamens tetradynamous, Inflorescence in racemes or corymbose. Racemes opposite the leaves or terminal and ebracteated. Fruit a siliqua or silicula. Seeds many, each seed superior, generally stalked and pendulous. All plants have a pungent bitter and acrid juice. The seeds are acrid and contain a fixed and volatile oil. The plants contain starch, sugar, iodine and sulphur.

Habitat.—They are met with in temperate, frigid and tropical climates.

Properties.—Many are nutritive, some pungent acrid, others antiscorbutic ; some used as ordinary vegetables.

Sisymbrium Irio.

Habitat.—North India, Persia and Europe.

Part used.—The seeds.

Vernacular.—Eng.—Hedge mustard, London rocket. Bom.—Khakshi. Arab.—Khubab. Fars.—Shafterak. Hind.—Khub-kalan, Khaksi. Mar.—Rantikhi. Mezenderan.—Shalumbi. Pers.—Khakshi. Tabriz —Surdan. Turkistan— Shiwaran.

Khuba-kalan—Khuba means good and Kalan Kallo or Maror (Guz.) means beauty. This drug is used by women to increase their beauty and promote fat.

Characters.—The seeds resemble those of asâlio, but are smaller and of a yellowish red colour. They are small, oblong or oval, and marked with a groove. When placed in water they become coated with a transparent mucilage ; taste is mucilaginous and oily, not so pungent as asâlio and has a hot flavour like that of mustard. Dose of the powdered seed—15 to 45 grs.

Actions and uses.—Expectorant, stimulant and antiscorbutic. An ingredient in many tonic confections used by the natives ; given in coughs, asthma, hoarseness, and to promote expectoration. Native women use it under the belief that they thereby fatten the body. Externally they are used as poultice over boils and inflammatory swellings.

Raphanus Sativus.

Garden radish. R. Caudatus. Raphanus Raphanistrum—wild radish.

Habitat.—Gujerat, Punjab.

Parts used.—The plant, root.

Vernacular.—Eng.—Long-podded radish, Garden radish. Bom. —Mulo, Muro. Arab.—Bazr-el-Fujl. Beng.—Mula, Muli. Burm.—Moula or Moula. Can.—Mullangi. Duk.—Mulli. Hind.—Mula, Muro. Pers.—Turb. Sans.—Mulaka. Tam., Tel.—Mullangi.

Characters.—Root tapering, seldom branched, of a white colour and a pungent taste ; leaves long and generally lyrate, petiole broadly channelled ; taste somewhat pungent ; seeds resemble those of sarasun, but are larger and of a reddish brown colour ; testa very minutely reticulated. On trituration the roots and seeds yield, with water, a fixed oil.

Constituents.—Seeds and root contain a fixed oil, a sulphuretted volatile oil, resembling mustard-seed oil. The oil is colourless and has the taste of radishes. It contains sulphur and phosphoric acid.

Preparation.—Juice of leaves. Dose, ½ to 1 dr. ; infusion of seeds (1 in 10). Dose, 1 to 6 drs.

Actions and uses.—The seeds and leaves are diuretic, laxative and lithontriptic. The root is used as an edible vegetable. All parts of the plant are used in urinary diseases and in cases of gravel.

Lepidium Sativum.

Habitat.—North of Asia, Persia, cultivated in all countries.

Part used.—The seeds.

Vernacular.—Arab.—Hab-el-rashad, Half. Beng.—Aliveri. Bom.—Ahaliva, Asalia. Burm.—Samah-ni, Samung-ni. Duk.—Halim. Guz.—Assalia. Hind.—Tara-tezak, Halim, Chansar, Chandrika. Eng.—

Common garden cress. Mar.—Ahaliva. Pers.—Turrah-tezak. Sans.—Chandrasura. Tam.—Alivirai. Tel.—Adiyali, Adala Vitala.

Characters.—The seeds resemble in size those of Khubakalan, but are larger. They are of a reddish colour, oblong, somewhat angular and curved slightly on one side, surface rugous. Near the point of attachment there is a white scar, from which a small channel extends to $\frac{1}{3}$ the length of the seeds. They are without odour, but of a pungent and mucilaginous taste. Doses—as alterative, 5 to 15 grs.; as aperient, 20 to 40 grs.

Constituents.—A volatile, aromatic oil and a fatty oil.

Preparation.—Infusion cold (1 in 10). Dose, 4 to 6 drs.

Actions and uses.—Aperient, alterative, tonic, aphrodisiac and carminative. A cold infusion is used to relieve hiccough. As an alterative the seeds are used in chronic enlargements of the liver and spleen. As a restorative tonic they form an ingredient in aphrodisiac confection or rabree, and are given in seminal debility and leucorrhœa. As a carminative they are given as an adjunct to purgatives. The bruised seeds, mixed with lime-juice, are used as application for the relief of local inflammatory and rheumatic pains. Taken alone they act as aperient.

Lepidium Iberis.

Habitat.—Persia.

Part used.—The seeds.

Vernacular.—Arab.—Bazr-el-khum-khum, Bazr-el-hawah, Kasisas. Eng.—Pepper grass, Pepper wort. Hind.—Towdri, Todari. Ispahan—Kaduma. Kirman—Mardarakht. Pers.—Tondripha-Towdri. Tabriz.—Darina.

Characters.—The drug consists of white, yellow or black seeds, with some portion of rhomboid-shaped pods. In shape the seeds resemble lentils, but are smaller. They are yellowish red, ovate, flat or roundish, convex on both surfaces, and have a membranous white ring springing from the hilum. The ring spreads on both sides and separates the surfaces. A small groove extends from the hilum and disappears about the middle of both the surfaces. The taste is mucilaginous, slightly pungent, and resembles that of asâlio ; that of the cotyledons, burning. When soaked in water the seeds become thickly coated with mucilage. Dose, 20 to 60 grs.

Constituents.—An amorphous bitter principle.—Lepidin, a sulphuretted volatile oil and gum.

Preparations.—Confection and tea.

Actions and uses.—The seeds are diuretic, carminative, sudorific and stimulant. The confection is given in dropsy, bronchitis, fevers and with pepper in atonic dyspepsia, accompanied with flatus Externally the seeds are used as a rubefacient in rheumatism.

Helianthemum Canadense.—Frost wort.

Habitat.—North America.

Part used.—The herb.

Characters.—The herb, perennial, 6 to 15 inches high, hairy; leaves, long and woolly beneath; flowers broad, yellow; calyx pubescent; taste bitter and astringent. Dose, 5 to 30 grs.

Constituents.—A bitter glucoside and tannin 11 p. c. Used as infusion, decoction, extract.

Actions and uses.—Tonic, astringent and alterative; in large doses emetic; given in scrofula, syphilis, diarrhœa; as a gargle in sore throat.

Capsella Bursa Pastoris.—Shepherd's purse.

Habitat.—Europe and widely naturalized.

Part employed.—The herb. Dose, 20 to 60 grs.

Preparations.—Fluid extract. Dose, $\frac{1}{4}$ to 1 fl. dr.; Tincture (1 in 8), 1 to 4 fl. drs.

Actions and uses.—Diuretic, hæmostatic, stimulant and tonic, recommended in all forms of kidney affections, in chronic diarrhœa, dropsy of the abdomen, &c.

Cochlearia Armoracia, B. P., Armoracia Rusticana, Nasturtium Armoracia.

Habitat.—Europe, cultivated in Britain.

Parts used.—The fresh root. Armoraciæ Radix—Horseradish root, B. P.

Vernacular.—Eng.—Common horseradish. Hind.—Muli.

Characters.—Root nearly cylindrical and marked with leaf-scars at the crown, about half an inch to an inch in breadth and one foot long, yellowish externally and whitish internally; has a characteristic pungent odour and pungent taste when scraped, cut or bruised. Dose, 10 to 30 grs.

Constituents.—A volatile oil, identical with oil of mustard, and resin. The oil is dissipated by drying.

Preparation.—Spiritus armoraciæ compositus, B. P.—Horseradish 5 ounces, dried bitter orange peel 5 ounces, bruised nutmeg 55 grains, alcohol 25 ounces, and distilled water 25 ounces; distilled to 2 pints. Dose, 1 to 2 drs.

Actions and uses.—Stimulant, masticatory and diuretic; externally rubefacient, irritant and vesicant; used in atonic dyspepsia, rheumatism, dropsy and hoarseness of voice. Locally used for the same purposes as mustard in the form of liniment or cataplasm. Its action is due to the volatile oil, and hence should be used fresh.

Remarks.—Sometimes aconite or monkshood is sold for horseradish, which it resembles; accidents have occurred.

5

Cheiranthus Cheiri.

Habitat.—Northern India.

Part used.—The seeds.

Vernacular.—Eng.—The wallflower. Hind.—Tcdri surkh. Panj.—Lahori subu.

Characters.—Seeds small, linear, acute and reddish. They contain myrosine and an oil like that found in Raphanus sativus. Dose, 10 to 30 grs.

Actions and uses.—Emmenagogue and deobstruent; used in paralysis, uterine disorders and disordered liver, also for enlarged glands.

Brassica (Sinapis).

Varieties.—B. Alba, B. P., B. Nigra, B. P. Syn.—Sinapis Alba and Sinapis Nigra.

Habitat.—Asia, South of Europe, United States.

Parts used.—The seeds, sinapis albæ Semina B. P., Sinapis Nigræ Semina B. P., powder of the mixed seeds. Sinapis. Mustard B. P. and a volatile oil, oleum Sinapis volatile B. P.

Brassica—cabbage; the fruit resembles cabbage.

Mustard—mustum ardens, burning must, in allusion to the seeds, which were once pounded with must or vinegar; also in allusion to its burning and pungent taste.

Vernacular.—Arab.—Khardal. Beng.—Rai. Burm.—Moung-ngyin kung ziyen. Can.—Sasave. Cing.—Rata-aba, Ganaba. Duk.—Rayan. Eng.—Mustard. Guz.—Rayi. Hind.—Rayi. Malay.—Savi Sasavi. Mar.—Mohari. Pers.—Sipandan, Sarshaf Sans.—Rajika, Tuverica. Sarshapaha, Asuri. Tam.—Kadagu. Tel.—Avalu.

Characters.—White mustard—flowers yellow and in racemes, pods ribbed with a long ensiform beak; fruit a siliqua $1\frac{1}{2}$ inch long, sword-shaped and four to six seeded; seeds $\frac{1}{12}$ of an inch thick and globular, with circular hilum; testa yellowish, finely pitted and hard; embryo oily; two cotyledons, one folded over the other. It is without odour when entire or powdered, almost inodorous when triturated with water. Taste pungent, but less acrid than that of the black variety. Black mustard—flowers small, yellow, on peduncles at the end of the branches; pods smooth, erect, and with a short beak. The fruit $\frac{3}{4}$ of an inch long, oblong, globular and tapering, 3 to 7 seeded; seeds smaller than those of the white variety ($\frac{1}{25}$ inch in diameter); testa hard, minutely pitted and reddish brown or dark. It is without any odour when entire or powdered, but, when triturated with water, the odour becomes pungent and penetrating. The taste is smarting, pungent and acrid. Dose, 15 to 60 grs.

Constituents.—Sinapis Alba contains a bland fixed oil, 20 to 25 p.c., a crystalline substance Sinalbin; Sinapine sulpho-cyanide, Lecithin, mucilage (only in testa); Myrosin, a ferment; proteids, ash 4 p. c. The ash consists of potassium phosphate, magnesium phosphate and calcium phosphate. Sinalbin and myrosin, acting on each other in the presence of water, produce sugar, sinapine sulphate and sulpho-cyanide of acrinyl, a rubefacient principle, similar to that found in the volatile oil of black mustard. Black mustard contains myrosin and sinigrin (potassium myronate), 0·5 p. c. Myrosin and sinigrin, when acted upon by water, form sulphocyanide of allyl, which is the volatile oil of mustard. It also contains fixed oil 25 p. c. sinapine sulphocyanide, lecithin mucilage, proteids and ash 4 p.c.

The fixed oil, obtained by expression is a yellowish green, non-drying fluid of a slight odour and bland mild taste. It solidifies on cooling. It contains glycerides of oleic, stearic and erucic or brassic acids. It is used as a diet in certain parts of India.

Sinalbin, only found in the white variety, in pearly crystals, or colourless prisms, soluble in water, sparingly so in alcohol.

Volatile oil of mustard B. P.—A yellowish limpid liquid, highly refractive, of a pungent and acrid odour and taste. It contains chiefly sulpho-cyanide of allyl, with traces of carbon sulphide.

Preparations.—Charta sinapis B.P. or mustard paper. Linimentum sinapis, B. P.—volatile oil of mustard, 1½ fluid drachm ; camphor, 2 drachms ; castor-oil 5 fluid drachms, and alcohol, 4 fluid ounces.

Physiological actions.—Flour of mustard is nervine, stimulant, emetic and diuretic ; externally rubefacient, counter irritant and vesicant. In small doses it promotes digestion and removes flatus ; in large doses it is a stimulating and sure emetic in over-feeding, indigestion and in narcotic poisoning, when given with hot water. It is an irritant to the skin. Its chief use, however, is as an external remedy to relieve local pain, to stimulate the viscera and to act as a counter-irritant. The volatile oil, in the form of charta or plaster, acts as a stimulant and vesicant to whatever part it is applied. Its application causes redness, heat and severe burning pain. If applied for a long time it causes vesication by setting up local inflammation. It is extensively used as a household remedy to rouse patients from syncope, low states of the system and from unconsciousness. As a counter-irritant it is largely used in all internal inflammations.

Therapeutic uses.—It is applied to remove muscular, neuralgic, and rheumatic pains, in colic, gastralgia, in inflammation of the air passages of the lung, pleura, pericardium, &c. The volatile oil is highly irritant. Taken internally it produces gastro-enteritis. The liniment is applied as a rubefacient and also as a vesicant to swollen joints. As a derivative, mustard foot-baths or hip-baths are largely used in fevers, uterine derangements, especially amenorrhœa and dysmenorrhœa ; in headache, cerebral congestion, in cardiac and in chest pains, &c. The fixed oil is applied to promote the growth of hair. The powder is often mixed with wheat flour to weaken its irritant effects

Brassica Juncea.

Sinapis Juncea, Sinapis Ramosa, Brassica Ramosa.

Habitat.—India, South Russia.

Parts used.—The seeds.

Vernacular.—Burm.—Moung-ngyin. Can.—Lasane. Cing.—Garraba, Rataaba. Eng.—Indian mustard, Russian sarepta mustard. Hind.—Sursun. Malyal.—Kadiya. Mar.—Mohare. Pers.—Saurshuf. Sans. —Rajika Tuvarica. Sind.—Suraibij.

Characters.—Seeds oblong, light, reddish brown, clean and bright, closely resembling those of sinapis nigra, but larger.

Actions and uses.—similar to those of sinapis nigra, for which it is a good substitute. If previously deprived of its fixed oil, its activity is increased. If kept for a long time, it loses its pungency.

Brassica Campestris.

Habitat.—Europe and Russian Asia.

Parts used.—Root and seeds.

Vernacular.— Eng.—Swedish turnip Can.—Sasave. Guz.—Sarasava. Hind.—Surson. Mar.—Sherus. Pers.—Sarshuf.

Other varieties also produce edible roots and seeds and resemble black mustard in property, and probably in constituents.

Brassica Napus—Cultivated rape-seed or cole seed. The seeds are black, but larger than mustard seeds, finely pitted and slightly acrid. A large quantity of bland fixed oil is expressed from the seeds known as turnip seed oil. The cake, left after expression of the oil, is known as oil-cake.

Brassica Rutabaga—seeds small and contain a pungent oil.
Brassica Chinensis yields. Shanghai oil.

Brassica Rapa—Rape or colza. The turnip.

Vernacular.—Hind. —Sarsun, sursr, surras, Duk.—Rayan. Arab. —Luft. Beng.—Shalgam, Gonghi, Sarsho. Burm.—Mung-la-do-waing. Eng.—Rape or colza. Guz.—Sursul. Pers.—Gouglu. Sans.—Asuri shershape. Sind.—Gohheu.

Asuri.—Means Sorceress. Village witches were detected by means of this oil. The oil was dropped into cups filled with water, each cup bearing the name of the suspected woman. If the oil takes the form of a woman in any of the cups, the person whose name is on the cup is declared to be a witch.

Characters.—The seeds are blue-black and pitted, larger than mustard or turnip seeds. They are slightly acrid. They yield a bland oil known as rapeseed oil. This oil—Sursun tel, is largely used in India as an emollient and rubbed over the whole body in leucoderma, paralysis and rheumatism. It keeps the skin soft and clean, and is believed to promote the growth of hair and to remove lice and scurf. The natives use the oil as an article of diet.

Anastatica Hierochuntina.

Habitat.—Deserts of Syria, Palestine, Arabia.

Part used.—The dried herb.

Vernacular.—Arab.—Kaphe-Miryana, Kaphe-Ayesha. Hind.—Garbha phula. Eng.—Mary's flower, Rose of Jericho. Pers.—Panja-i-Mariam. Guz.—Garbhaphul.

Garbha phula—Garbha, a womb, and phula a flower. The opening of the plant when put in water, and its closing in again when dry, is symbolical of the opening of the womb in childbirth and the closing of it after delivery. In Palestine, it is termed Kaf Maryan, Mary's flower, in allusion to the tradition that the plant blossomed on the Christmas eve to salute the birth of the Redeemer and paid homage to his resurrection by remaining expanded till Easter. Kaphe Ayesha, so called by the Mohamedans, in allusion to the tradition that the plant expanded at the birth of Ayesha, who was the favourite wife of the Prophet and mother of the faithful.

Characters.—Dry herb of brownish white colour and of the shape of a fig. The stem is short and woody and branched in a corymbose manner. The branches when fresh spread out straight upon the ground, but after withering, the hygrometric stems curve inward so as to form a round ball ; in this state they are blown out by the winds from place to place. Hence they are supposed to be the Gurgal, rolling things or wheel of Isaiah. The root is thin and occupies the same place as the stalk of a fig. Each branch is studded with numerous small capsules which are white and hairy. In shape the whole herb resembles a water goblet The top of it is formed of two marginal concave wings, between which a curved prickle-like process projects. It possesses a curious hygrometrical property, *viz.* when placed in water it spreads flat by absorbing it. This property is preserved for years

Preparation.—Cold infusion (1 in 10). Dose, 2 to 6 drs.

Actions and uses.—The cold infusion is given in difficult labour in which the effects seem to be more mental than physiological.

Fumariaceæ.

The Fumitory order.

Herbs smooth, with brittle stems and a watery juice; leaves multiple, exstipulate, often with tendrils, alternate much divided ; flowers irregular, unsymmetrical, in pink, red, yellow, or white inflorescence, and racemose ; fruits small, pod-like, dehiscent or indehiscent, one or two seeded and succulent ; seeds shining and crested ; albumen fleshy.

Habitat.—India, Japan, Persia, and in temperate climates.

Properties.—All plants possess bitter, acrid, astringent, emmenagogue and aperient properties.

Fumaria Officinalis.

Habitat.—Persia. Nepaul, Bombay.

Part used.—The plant.

Fumaria.—From fumus, fume or smoke. The plant irritates the eyes like smoke.

Vernacular.—Arab.—Shahteraj, Baklat-ul-malik. Bomb.—Pitapapra. Chin.—Tsze-hwa-ti-ting. Eng.—Common fumitory. Hind.—

Pitapapra. Pers.—Shahturuz. Sans.—Kshetera parapati, yavana paipata Beng.—Shatera Pitpapra.

Characters.—The drug is of a greyish yellow colour and resembles in appeara nce trayamana. It consists of broken leaves, stems, capsules, flowers and seeds; leaves greenish,thick and narrow; stems greyish yellow, one to two inches long, furrowed and rather quadrangular ; capsules very small, gryish green, tubercled, slightly compressed and with a transverse ridge scar to the apex; flowers irregular, unsymmetrical and either violet coloured or white; seeds very small and consist of fleshy albumen; taste bitter, acrid and astringent, odour acrid and disagreeable.

Constituents.—Fumaric acid, and fumarine,—a crystalline organic base.

Fumaric acid is isomeric with maleic acid. It may be obtained by de-hydration of malic acid ; it exists ready formed in several plants, namely, Corydalis bulbosa, Glaucium flavum, Lichen Islandicus, It is also found among the products of the oxidation of protein compounds by nitro-hydrochloric acid.

Fumarine exists in irregular 6-sided crystals or monoclinic prisms. Insoluble in alcohol, chloroform, benzol, bisulphide of carbon and amyl alcohol; sparingly soluble in water and soluble in ether.

Preparation.—Decoction (1 in 10). Dose, 1 to 2 ozs.

Actions and uses.—Diuretic, diaphoretic, tonic, alterative, anthelmintic, and aperient ; useful in syphilis, scrofula, constipation and dyspepsia, due to torpor of the liver or intestines. It is allied in its properties to taraxacum. With black pepper it is given in ague and jaundice ; also given to purify the blood in skin diseases.

Remarks.—What is sold under the name of Ghati-pita-papado is an acanthaceous plant often substituted for Pita-papado. The true Pita-papado is sold in the bazaar under the Persian name Shahtira.

Corydalis Cava. C. Tuberosa.

Syn.—Hollow-rooted fumitory.

Habitat.—United States.

Part used.— The root (tuber).

Constituents.—Corydaline, corycavine and other bases.

Preparation.—Powdered root (tuber), 10 to 40 grains. Fluid extract. Dose—10 to 40 ms. Dry extract Dose 1 to 5 grs.

Actions and uses.—Alterative, antisyphilitic, antiperiodic, tonic, diuretic and resolvent. It seldom disagrees with the stomach, and may be employed as a tonic in irritable condition of that organ. It is especially given in scrofula, syphilis, cutaneous affections, urinary diseases and debility.

Corydalis Govaniana.

Habitat.—Western Himalaya.

Part used.—Yellow juice.

Actions and uses.—Alterative ; given in scrofula, skin diseases &c.

Polygalaceæ.

Milk wort family.

Polygalaceæ from poly, much, and gala, milk ; it is believed to increase the milk in female animals.

Shrubs, or herbs. Leaves alternate or opposite, simple and exstipulate. Flowers irregular, unsymmetrical and apparently papilionaceous (wings being formed by the calyx). Fruit indehiscent, loculicidal and occasionally winged ; seeds pendulous, smooth or hairy, with a caruncula next the hilum ; albumen copious and fleshy.

Habitat.—Found everywhere.

Properties.—Bitter and acrid ; roots milky, and used as tonic, febrifuge and stimulant ; some are emetic, purgative, diuretic, diaphoretic and expectorant. Some have edible fruits, and others contain a saponaceous principle.

Krameria Triandra B. P.—Peruvian Rhatany, Krameria Argentea B. P. Para Rhatany.

Habitat.—Peru, South America, New Granada, Bolivia and Para.

Part used.—The dried root. Krameriæ Radix—Krameria root—Rhatany root B. P.

Characters.—Shrubs. Root in cylindrical pieces. Para Rhatany—bark smooth, thick, of a purplish brown colour, marked with deep transverse fissures or cracks. Internally rough and scaly. Wood pale and of a reddish brown colour and firmly adherent to the bark, fracture short and splintery. Taste astringent and tinges the saliva yellow. Dose, 10 to 60 grs. Peruvian Rhatany—bark dark, reddish brown, easily separable from the yellowish wood, thinner, astringent. in taste, and tinges the saliva red. Dose, 10 to 60 grs.

Constituents.—The bark contains krameric acid, Tannin 40 p.c., Rhatanic red, starch, sugar, gum, wax and calcium oxalate.

Rhatanic red or ratanhia red.

Manufacture.—Boil kramero tannic acid with diluted sulphuric acid ; when it splits up into glucose and the colouring principle, which is similar to that found in horsechestnut and tomentilla. With potash it is converted into protocatechuic acid and phloroglucin.

Preparation.—Liquor Krameriæ Concentratus B. P. (1 in 2.) Dose, ½ to 1 dr. Extractum Krameriæ B. P.—Extract of Krameria. Extract of Rhatany. Dose, 5 to 15 grs. Infusum Krameriæ (1 in 20). Dose, ½ to 1 oz. Trochiscus Krameriæ B.P.—Rhatany lozenges (1 grain of extract in each.) Trochiscus Krameriæ et Cocainæ B. P. (Extract 1 grain and Cocaine $\frac{1}{20}$ grain in each.) Tinctura Krameriæ B. P.—Tincture of Rhatany (1 in 5). Dose, ½ to 1 dr.

Actions and uses.—A powerful astringent, alterative and tonic ; used in chronic diarrhœa and dysentery ; also to check passive hœmorrhages as menorrhagia, leucorrhœa and gleet. In incontinence of urine it is also beneficial. Externally, as gargle or lozenges, it is given in sore throat ; as an injection or enema, for fissure of the anus, leucorrhœa, and as a wash in cracked nipples. It is also used as dentifrice. Locally it is applied to spongy gums. As an alterative it is given in rheumatism, syphilis and scrofula. It is also used as an application for the bites of venomous reptiles.

Polygala Crotalarioides.—In India the root is used as an expectorant.

P. Tenuifolia, a Chinese plant, the root of which in contorted quilled pieces, is used in cough; the leaves are given in spermatorrhœa.

Polygala Chinensis. *Habitat.*—Pasture lands throughout India.

Vernacular.—Arab.—Lubanat. Hind.—Maradu. Mar.—Negli. Pers.—Furfur.

Polygala Alba.—White or false senega.—The root contains polygalic acid 3 p. c. Used as infusion and tincture.

P. Polygama.—P. Rubella.—Bitter polygala, the root and herb contains a bitter principle similar to senegin, and is used as a diaphoretic, laxative and tonic in bronchial catarrh &c.

Polygala Senega B. P.

Habitat.—Woods, rocky soil, United States, Honan, Shensi.

Part used.—The dried root, Senegæ Redix—Senega Root B. P.

Sengh.—Snake root, milk wort, mountain flax.

Senega.—The term is derived from Seneca, an American Indian tribe who used it for snake-bite.

Characters.—Indigenous perennial plant. Flowers small and white and at the summit of the stem ; root 4 or 5 inches long, slender and of a yellowish brown colour, enlarged at the top into a knotty crown, contorted and often curved, longitudinally wrinkled, breaking with a short fracture ; cortex horny, translucent, free from starch grains, and enclosing a white or yellowish porous wood ; taste at first somewhat sweet, and afterwards acrid ; odour distinctive. Dose—3 to 20 grs.

Adulterations.—Ginsing root, cypripedium root, Gentian root, and Cynanchum Vincetoxicum root ; but they all differ in odour and taste.

Constituents.—A neutral glucoside called Senegin, 2 to 5 p. c., probably identical with saponin ; Polygalic acid, a volatile oil, a fixed oil, 8 to 9 p.c. ; tannin, gum, resin, sugar 7 p.c. ; pectin, malates, and yellow colouring matter.

Senegin.—To obtain it exhaust the root with alcohol, concentrate and precipitate with ether. A white amorphous powder, without any odour, freely soluble in alcohol and cold water, forming a soapy emulsion with boiling water ; with hydrochloric acid it is decomposed into glucose and sapogenin.

Polygalic acid, sparingly soluble in alcohol, insoluble in ether and chloroform.

Fixed oil.—Obtained from the root by ether—contains virginic acid, to which the aroma is due. Volatile oil contains valerianic ether and methyl salicylate.

Preparations.—Infusum Senegæ B. P. (1 in 20). Dose, ½ to 1 oz. Liquor Senegæ Concentratus B. P. (1 in 2). Dose, ½ to 1 dr. Tinctura Senegæ B.P. (1 in 5). Dose, ½ to 1 dr. Extractum Senegæ fluidum—Fluid extract of senega. Dose, 10 to 20 ms.

Syrupus senegæ contains fluid extract of senega 20, ammonia water 5, and sugar 10. Dose, 1 to 2 drs. Syrupus scillæ compositus—compound syrup of squill—8 p. c. Dose, 20 to 30 ms.

Physiological action.—Stimulating expectorant, emmenagogue, diuretic and diaphoretic. In large doses gastro-intestinal and throat irritant, producing cough, increased salivation, sneezing and nasal catarrh. In small doses it removes the tightness and feeling of oppression from the chest. Senegin has a stimulating action on the mucous membranes, especially of the pulmonary tract. It is a powerful depressant of the heart and of the muscular and nervous systems. It is eliminated by the kidneys, skin and bronchial mucous membrane, which it stimulates and irritates.

Therapeutics.—As a stimulating expectorant it is largely used alone or in combination with ammonium carbonate in chronic bronchitis, pneumonia, asthma, croup and whooping cough ; it relieves the cough and promotes expectoration. It is not of much use if the bronchial mucus expectoration is tough and scanty; as a diaphoretic and diuretic, it is sometimes employed in anasarca and dropsy due to albuminuria ; as an emmenagogue it is used with benefit in amenorrhœa.

Sapindacæ.—The Aritha or Soap Wort Family.

Sapindacæ from sapo, soap, and Ind, " Indian," Indian soap. The fruit is saponaceous and contains a vegetable principle named saponine.

Large trees or twining shrubs, and rarely climbing herbs; leaves generally compound, rarely simple, alternate or opposite, often dotted and with or without stipules. Flowers unsymmetrical, generally polygamous ; ovary, generally two to three-celled. Fruit capsular or fleshy and indehiscent, some sweet are with an acid flavour ; seeds exalbuminous, superior arillate. Most prominent property of this family is the presence of a saponaceous principle.

Habitat.—Tropics.

The plants are astringent, aromatic, diuretic, diaphoretic and aperient. Some species are poisonous.

Schleichera Trijuga.

Habitat.—Burma, Ceylon, S. India, Himalayas.

Parts used.—The bark and oil.

Vernacular.—Eng.—Ceylon oak. Hind.—Kosimb. Tam.—Pu-maram. Tel.—May Rahatangah. Mal.—Puvam. Can.—Sagade, Chakota.

Characters.—Fruit a drupe of the size of a nutmeg ; the husk is grey, fragile, covered with soft, blunt prickles; seeds 1 to 3, oblong, smooth, truncated at the base and surrounded with pulpy arilla ; taste acid ; bark thick, with a soft, outer corky layer ; inner bark firm, hard and breaks with a short fracture ; colour pale red ; taste astringent.

Constituents.—The bark contains tannin and ash.

Actions and uses.—The pulpy arilla is sub-acid. The bark is astringent, and mixed with oil, it is applied to cure itch and other skin eruptions ; the oil under the name of Macassar oil is used as a stimulant application to the scalp to promote the growth of the hair.

Sapindus Trifoliatus. S. Rubiginosus.

Habitat.—South India, Ceylon, Bengal.

Part used.—The pulp of the fruit.

Vernacular.—Arab.—Finduk-i-hindi, Bandak-e-hindi. Beng.—Buro-ritha. Bur.—Miavenen-suc-khe-si. Can.—Kukate-kayi, Thaly marathu, artala. Cing.—Penela. Duk.—Rithah. Eng.—Indian filbert, Soapnut tree, soap berry. Guz.—Aritha. Hind.—Ringin, Dodan, Ritha. Malay.—Punnan-kotta. Mar.—Ritha, Areeta Ringin. Pers.—Ratah. Sans.—Phenila, Arishta. Tam.—Pannan-kottai, Puvandi. Tel.—Kunkudu-kayalu.

Characters.—Berries dry, generally three, united together, or separate ; skin thin, shrivelled and of the colour of raisins ; when ripe soft and of a greenish colour. In shape somewhat resembling a kidney. When united together, points of attachment are marked by a heart-shaped scar ; pulp translucent ; berry one-seeded ; seed round, smooth, black and shining ; testa hard and bony ; kernel yellowish brown and oily ; smell of the berry like that of burnt sugar, and that of the pulp resembling that of Khajura ; taste sweet at first, afterwards becoming bitter. Dose of the pulp, 2 to 6 grs.

Constituents.—Saponin 11·5 p.c. Glucose and pectin. The thick cotyledons contain white fat 30 p.c. It saponifies readily.

Actions and uses.—Expectorant, emetic, anthelmintic and purgative. Externally stimulant and irritant ; used in asthma, colic, worms, and as a purge combined with scammony. Externally applied to the mucous membrane of the nose to rouse patients from insensibility in hysteria, epilepsy, hemicrania and melancholia ; also applied to scrofulous and other glandular swellings and to bites of venomous reptiles ; used also to destroy pediculi and to wash and cleanse the hairs of the head. Pessaries made of the kernel of the seeds are used in amenorrhœa and after childbirth to stimulate the uterus to a healthy contraction.

Remarks.—It resembles sikakai. The fruit pulp is said to be fifty times more powerful in cleaning linen than soap. Berries of S. Saponaria, S. Rurak, S. Emarginatus, S. Detergens are all used for the purposes of soap-making owing to the presence of Saponin. S. Mukorassi is the soap-nut of Northern India, and is called Dodan in the Punjab.

Paullinia Sorbilis—Guarana—Brazilian Cocoa.

Habitat.—N. and W. Brazil.

Part used.—Guarana, a dried paste of crushed seeds deprived of aril and moulded into cylinders and dried by sun or fire.

Characters.—A climbing plant; fruit of the size of grape or hazel nut, ovoid, pyriform, 6-ribbed, seeds resembling hazel nut seeds, 2 or 3 filling the fruit. Arillus white; taste bitter ands astringent. Guarana is made by slightly roasting and powdering the dried seeds and then made into a stiff paste or dough with water; with this paste broken seeds are also mingled and made into cylindrical rolls or elliptical cakes or sticks. The paste is dark-brown or of a fawn-yellow colour; odour slight, resembling chocolate; taste bitter and astringent, partly soluble in water and alcohol. Dose, 10 to 60 grs.

Constituents.—Contains a bitter crystalline principle; guaranine 3.5 to 6.5 p. c., identical with caffeine or theine. Tannin—Paullini tannic acid 26 p. c., resin, greenish fixed oil, fat, albumen, starch, gum and saponin, ash 2·5. p.c.

Guaranine.—Powder the paste. Boil it with litharge and water. Filter the solution, pass sulphuretted hydrogen through the solution to precipitate lead; evaporate and crystallize. Dose, 1 to 5 grs.

Paullini tannic acid precipitates ferric salts, gelatin, gold and silver salts.

Preparations.—Extractum guaranæ fluidum—fluid extract of guarana, not miscible with water. Dose, 10 to 60 grs. Tinctura guaranæ (1 in 4). Dose, ½ to 1 dr. Syrup. Dose, 2 to 4 drs. Elixir Guaranæ—a tincture of guarana treated with magnesia to liberate the alkaloid, and flavoured. Dose, ½ to 2 drs. Elixir Erythroxyli et Guarano contains coca and Guarana 7½ grains each in one fluid drachm. Dose, 1 to 2 drs.

Physiological actions.—Nervine stimulant, tonic and astringent. It affects both the sensory and motor nerves, but more so the sensory nerves. It causes hyperæsthesia and also convulsions. Its action on the heart and respiration is to stimulate them at first and then to depress them. It produces restlessnses, and quick perception, slows the pulse, impairs digestion and causes irritation of the bladder. It is given chiefly in relieving neuralgic affections, such as hemicrania, sick headache occurring during menstruation or after a debauch. As a tonic it is given in diarrhœa and phthisis; also in convalescence from acute diseases, &c. Guaranine may be employed in the same way as caffeine.

Dodonæa Viscosa. D. Augustifolia.

Habitat.—Throughout India, Neilgherries, and Punjab.

Part used.—The leaves.

Vernacular.—Can.—Bandarika. Hind.—Sanatta, Banmendru. Eng.—Jamaica-switch sorrel. Mar.—Jakhmi, Bandari.

Characters.—Leaves green, more or less viscid, containing shining yellowish resin ; taste sour and astringent.

Constituents.—Gum, acid resins 27·3. Albumen, Tannin. Of the two resins one is insoluble in ether ; both are soluble in chloroform, alcohol, liquid ammonia and in fixed alkalies.

Preparation.—Tincture (1 in 10). Dose, 15 to 30 ms.

Actions and uses.—Alterative, laxative, febrifuge and tonic, given in rheumatism, gout and fevers. The leaves make excellent poultice and varalians and retain heat for a long time when applied to painful swellings and rheumatic joints.

Æsculus Indica.—Himalayan horse-chestnut, made into a paste and applied to rheumatic joints ; the seeds are used as food.

Acer pictum and acer cæsium.—The knots in the stems are, like Quassia, made into cups and used for drinking water in rheumatism.

Cardiospermum Halicacabum.

Habitat.—India.

Part used.—The herb.

Vernacular.—Eng. Heart's pea. Arab.—Taftaf, Habb-el-Kulkul. Beng.—Nayaphataki, Lotaphatakari, (seeds). Burm.—Mala mai. Can.—Kanakaia. Cing.—Jyotish-muttee. Duk.—Shib-Jub. Guz.—Karodio. Hind.—Kanaphata. Mal.—Ulinja. Mar.—Kanphuti, Shib-jal. Sans.—Karnasphota, Paravata-padi, Jyantisha mati. Tam.—Modda-coatan. Tel.—Budha-kakara, Nella Gulisi-tenda, Vekkudutige.

Paravata-padi. Pigeon's foot. Karansphota-karan, an ear, and sphota, or phota a crack. It is used for the cure of crack in the ear.

Characters.—A climbing plant, leaves glabrous, biternate ; leaflets oblong, coarsely cut and serrated; root white and fibrous, of a disagreeable odour and of an acrid, nauseous and bitter taste.

Constituents.—Saponin.

Preparation.—Decoction of the root (1 in 10). Dose, 4 to 10 drs. A compound powder containing leaves of C. Halicacabum, carbonate of potash, root of acorus calamus, root-bark of Terminalia Bellerica in equal parts ; mix, make powder. Dose, 1 drachm in amenorrhœa.

Actions and uses.—Diuretic, laxative, stomachic, alterative and rubefacient, given in rheumatism, nervous diseases, piles, chronic bronchitis and phthisis ; also in amenorrhœa. The leaves fried are also applied to the pubes to increase the menstrual flow in amenorrhœa; the eaves, besmeared with castor-oil, are applied over rheumatic pains, swellings and tumours of various kinds. The juice of the plant is dropped into the ear in earache and discharge from the meatus.

Hypericaceæ.

The St. John's wort family. Herbs, shrubs or trees. Leaves opposite, rarely alternate, exstipulate, simple dotted and bordered with black glands; flowers regular; sepals 4 or 5, unequal, united at the base, unbricated; petals hypogynous; stamens numerous; fruit capsular; seeds minute, numerous and exalbuminous.

Habitat.—Both temperate and hot regions.

Properties.—They contain resinous yellow juice, which is purgative; some are tonic, astringent and diuretic.

Hypericum Perforatum.

Habitat.—Hilly parts of India.

Part used.—The juice.

Vernacular.—Arab.—Hyufarikun. Pers.—Dadi, Jao-i-Jadu.

Jao-i-Jadu means magic barley.

Constituents.—A volatile oil, hypericum-red—a blood-red resin, having the odour of chamomile.

Actions and uses.—Nervine tonic, and astringent, given in hypochondriasis; also used as an anthelmintic emmenagogue and diuretic. The juice was used as an application to wounds.

Guttiferæ or Clusiaceæ.

The Kokama or Mangosteen family. Guttiferæ—from gutta, a drop, and ferre to bear. Plants yield gum, or resinous juice in drops.

General characters.—Trees or shrubs, sometimes parasitical, with resinous juice; leaves entire, simple, coriaceous, opposite and exstipulate. Flowers perfect, sometimes unisexual; stamens monadelphous, distinct, of a fragrant odour. Fruits globular, dehiscent or indehiscent, edible, of delicious flavour and astringent taste; seeds solitary or numerous, frequently arillate, oily and without albumen.

Habitat.—Tropical parts, specially S. America and Africa.

Property.—Many contain a yellow gum resin, of an acrid and purgative character, and some contain edible fruits.

Ochrocarpus Longifolius.

Habitat.—Western Peninsula.

Part used.—The dried flower buds.

Vernacular.—Bomb.—Tambra Nagakesara. Eng.—Cobra's saffron. Guz.—Rati Naga-kesara, Gor iundi (the fruit). Hind.—Nagesura. Mar.—Tambra Naga-kesara, Punnag, Suringi. Pers.—Nara-Mushka Sans.—Naga kesara, Punnaga.

Naga kesara—Naga, a cobra, and kesara, saffron. Cobras are said to be fond of these blossoms on account of their fragrance. The true Naga-kesara is Mesua Ferrea.

Characters.—Flower buds resemble kababchini in size and form; and are of a cinnamon colour; some are hermaphrodite; others male only. On opening the male bud a group of anthers, adherent to one another and forming a small ball, is seen. The colour of the anthers is deeper than that of the calyx. In the hermaphrodite variety, on removing the anthers, is seen the ovary with a large stigma. The seed, is large as an acorn, exudes a viscid, gummy fluid when cut. The smell is aromatic and taste acrid. Dose, 1 to 2 grs.

Actions and uses.—The flower-buds are used as fragrant adjuncts to decoctions and medicated oils. They are stimulant, aromatic, stomachic, bitter and astringent; used, like taja, elachi, tamalapatra, in great thirst, irritability of the stomach and excessive perspiration, and also given in dysentery with benefit. A paste of it is used to fill up the cavities of caried teeth to relieve toothache.

Mesua Ferrea: M. Roxburgha, M. Coromandalina.

Habitat.—Bengal, Himalaya and Andamans.

Parts used.—The flower-buds, root, bark and oil.

Vernacular.—Beng.—Nag-kesar; Burm.—Ken-gan Gungan. Can.—Naga-ampagi .Eng.—Iron wood tree. Hind.—Nagesar, Nagkasar. Malyal.—Beluta, Champagum-veila. Mar.—Nag-champa. Sans.—Kesaramu, Nagasara, Naga-kesaram, Kangal, Kanna. Tam.—Irul-maram, Nagashappu, Shirunagappu. Tel.—Chikati-manu Nag-kesaram.

Characters.—Flower buds are large and white; sepals thick, membranous and orbicular; petals spreading; anthers large and golden-yellow; fruit ovoid, conical shaped and chestnut like in size, the base surrounded by the persistent sepals; seeds 1 to 4, dark-brown; testa smooth round the base of the young fruits. Dose, 1 to 2 grs.

Constituents—The fruit contains an oleo resin and an essential oil. The seeds contain a fixed oil. The hard pericarp contains tannin. The resin is in tears; it sinks in water. It is partially dissolved in rectified spirit, amyl alcohol and ether, but wholly in benzol. The essential oil is very fragrant, of a pale yellow colour and of the odour of flowers. and resembles chian turpentine.

Preparations.—Syrup (1 in 10). Dose, ½ to 1 dr. Ointment and oil. Decoction of root (1 in 10). Dose, 2 to 4 drs.

Actions and uses.—The dried blossoms, root, and bark are bitter, aromatic and sudorific. Unripe fruits are aromatic, acrid and purgative. Flower-buds are used in dysentery. The oil is used as an application for rheumatic joints; an ointment of the powder of blossoms, with butter, is applied to bleeding piles and for burning sensation of the feet.

Garcinia Xanthochymus. Xanthochymus Pictorius.

Habitat.—Eastern Bengal, Eastern Himalayas, Western Peninsula.

Part used.—The fruit.

Vernacular.—Beng—Outh or osht. Assam.—Tepor. Burm.—Matun. Hind.—Dampel. Tel.—Iswara-mamadi. Tam.—Tamalamu, chitaka.

Characters.—A yellow fruit, very acrid, of the size of a small apple.

Preparation.—Compound syrup, contains, in addition to osht, rock salt, pepper, ginger, cumin-seeds and sugar.

Actions and uses.—Same as those of G. Indica.

Garcina Mangostana.

Habitat.—Malacca, Malayan Peninsula, Singapore, India, Archipelago.

Parts used.—The rind of the fruit and pulp.

Vernacular.—Beng.—Mangusatan. Bomb.—Mungeestun. Burm.—Men-gû-young, Zalai Mango-si. Chin.—Shan-chulukwo. Eng.—Mangostine. Hind.—Mangustan. Malay.—Manggusta.

Characters.—Fruit, a drupe as large as a small apple. When fresh the outer skin is soft, fibrous, and of a red colour; pulp is snow-white, enveloping the seeds; flavour very grateful and delicate; dry fruit is globular and of a dark-brown colour, with a radiating flat or compressed six-parted stigma at the top, with a four-parted hard and thick adherent calyx at the bottom. When cut the interior is hollow and occasionally contains a small quantity of dark coloured dried pulp. The rind is corky-looking and sprinkled with a yellow colouring matter. The odour is somewhat aromatic. The taste is acidulous and astringent. Dose, 10 to 30 grs.

Constituents.—The rind contains mangostin, resin and tannin.

Mangostin. To obtain it, boil the rind in water ; to remove tannin, exhaust by boiling alcohol, and evaporate. The resulting product is mangostin and resin. To precipitate the resin re-dissolve in alcohol and water.

It occurs in small yellow scales, without any taste, neutral reaction, insoluble in water, but readily soluble in alcohol and ether; also in hot dilute acids. Concentrated nitric acid converts it into oxalic acid. With alkalies it forms yellow solutions.

Preparations.—Extract. Dose, 3 to 10 grs. Tincture of the rind (1 in 10). Dose, ½ to 1 dr. Syrup of the pulp (1 in 5). Dose, ½ to 1 dr.

Actions and uses.—The rind is a powerful astringent and a good substitute for Indian bael, and is used, in intestinal catarrh, advanced cases of dysentery and chronic diarrhœa ; also in leucorrhœa, gonorrhœa and chronic diarrhœa of children. Locally the solution of pulp is used as an astringent gargle in tonsilitis, and as a local application in prolapsus ani and vaginæ.

Garcina Indica and G. Purpurea.

Habitat.—Western Peninsula, Amboyna.

Parts used.—The concrete oil, fruit, seeds and bark.

Vernacular.—Eng.—The fruit, Red mango. Bomb.—Amsul, kokuma. Goa.—Brindao. Mar.—Ratambi—Bhirand. The concrete oil. Eng.—Kokuma butter. Guz.—Brindao is a corruption of Bhirand, Kokumbela, kokamanu-ghee. Mar.—Birandela, Kokumchatela.

Characters.—The concrete oil is extracted from the poundel seeds by boiling, and then moulded into oval-shaped balls, when it is known as kokuma butter. It resembles in appearance country soap (kapparavanji-sabu). It is hard, of a dirty white colour, dry, easily pulverisable and unctuous to the touch. The fruit is globular in size, and resembles an orange. It is of a yellow colour and contains an acid pulp and several seeds. The seeds are black, reniform, wrinkled and compressed laterally, and resemble *amali* seeds in size, and contain a fixed oil. Each seed has a 4-parted wing-like calyx, with a short stalk at its base. Kokama or amsul is the pulp of the fruit cleared of the seeds and dried in the sun and slightly salted. It is of a black colour and an oval shape. The epidermis is wrinkled. At the base of kokama the calyx and the remainder of the stalk are often seen. The smell and taste are acid.

Constituents.—The concrete oil boiled with soda yields hard soap. which is decomposed by sulphuric acid, leaving fatty acids as stearic acid, myristic acid and oleic acid. The seeds contain fat 30 p.c. The fruit contains cellulose, an extractive and insoluble residue.

Preparation.—Syrup of the juice (1 in 5). Dose, ½ to 1 teaspoonful. Decoction of the bark (1 in 10). Dose, 4 to 6 drs.

Actions and uses.—Cooling. demulcent, emollient and antiscorbutic. It is used in the form of syrup in irritation of bowels, leading to diarrhœa and dysentery and as a refrigerant in fevers. In scurvy it is used in place of lemon-juice. The oil—kokum butter—is an excellent emollient application to cracks and fissures of the lips, hands and feet, and over the nipples and to excoriations in other places. Used by the natives as an ointment base combined with lard, and as suppositories and pessaries, and no doubt is a good substitute for oil of theobroma and for simple ointment. It keeps well in Indian climates. The bark and leaves are astringent and used as a decoction in dysentery.

Garcinia Hanburii, B.P.

G. Morell var. Pedicellata, G. Pictoria, Hebradendron Cambogioides.

Habitat.—Camboja, Bengal, Assam, S. India, Cochin China, Siam.

Part used.—Gum resin Cambogia, B. P., Gutta Gamba, Gamboge.

Vernacular.—Eng.—Gamboge. Arab.—Rubbe-Revand, Gotagauba. Beng.—Tamal. Bur.—Tanoto asi, Sanato-pin. Can.—Jarigehulimara Tamal (juice). Cing.—Gokatu, Melliyani, Kana-Goraha. Duk.—Ussarehe-Rewand. Guz.—Revinchini Khatai. Hind.—Gota-ganba, Tamal. Mar.—Rewanchini, Tamal. Pers.—Gotaganba, Ussarehe-i-rewand. Sans.—Tapinja, Tapiccha, The, Tamala, the juice. Tam.—Ireval, Karakapuli. Tel.—Revalchini-pal.

Tamala.—A pigment for making sectarial mark on the forehead. Ussarh-i-rewand.—An extract of rhubarb (Rheum palmatum). Both are similar in colour and properties.

Characters.—Siam gamboge is the true gamboge of commerce. A yellow juice which exudes in drops from leaves or ducts of the middle bark or branchlets when broken or from wounds in the trunk. The gum resin when hardened is called Rawanchni Khatai, and the juice when in a fluid state Ravanchinio-siro. The gum resin is brittle and of a deep orange colour. It is met with in two different varieties. The cake or lump or coarse gamboge. It is the gum resin collected on the leaves of the tree or in cocoanut-shells and then transferred into large flat earthen vessels, in which it is exposed to the air for some time, and before it hardens completely, it is moulded into cakes. The cakes or amorphous masses are of earthy fracture, their external surface is brownish yellow and marked with blue spots, due to the mixture of foreign bodies with the resin. In this state it is known as Revanchini khatai or Gamathi-rhubarb, so called on account of its being moulded into the shape and size of true rhubarb, and of being similar to it in taste and odour. The cylindrical, pipe or roll gamboge is superior ; and hence officinal ; its surface is longitudinally striated from the impressions of the bamboo reeds into which the liquid juice is poured ; is met with in round, solid or hollow and striated pieces, which break with a smooth glistening conchoidal fracture ; the fractured surface is dull smooth and of a uniform reddish yellow colour. When powdered it is bright and yellow ; rubbed with water it forms a yellow emulsion. The taste is acrid. It has no odour. Dose, ½ to 2 grs.

Constituents.—Gum resin contains gum 25 p.c., resin or gambogic acid 70 p.c., on which its activity chiefly depends, wax and ash 1 p.c. The resin is soluble in alcohol and ether. In it resides the colouring matter and medicinal properties.

Preparation.—Pilula cambogiæ composita, B.P., contains Gamboge, Barbados aloes, compound cinnamon powder, each 1 oz., hard soap 2 ozs., and syrup of glucose 1 oz. (1 in 6). Dose, 4 to 8 grs. Compound powder contains gamboge 3 drs., powdered rock-salt 3 drs., galangal and ginger each 2 drs. Dose, 10 to 40 grs. Pil. Catharticæ Co. contains Ext. Colocynth Co. 3 grs., calomel 1 gr., Ext. jalap 1 gr., Gamboge ¼ gr. for one pill. Dose, 1 to 2 pills.

Physiological actions.—The gum resin is an efficient and active hydragogue and drastic purgative, and anthelmintic In large doses it acts as an acrid poison, causes gastro-enteritis and even death. In small and repeated doses it is a cathartic, accompanied with nausea and vomiting, colicy pain, and watery stools. The powder is sternutatory.

Therapeutic uses.—Seldom given alone; generally in combination with pârâkajali, rock-salt and galangal, or with calomel, jalap, and cream of tartar. Given to relieve torpor of the liver due to malaria, and in dysentery in very small doses, (gr. $\frac{1}{16}$) at short intervals. It should never be given in irritable condition of the stomach and bowels, nor in cases where there is a tendency to abortion or to uterine hæmorrhage. A paste of it, combined with zedoary, is used as an application to sprains, bruises, and swollen parts. The natives use it locally with cashew-nut as an application for the removal of piles.

Calophyllum Wightianum.

Habitat.—Canara, Travancore.

Part used.—The gum.

Vernacular.—Tam.—Sirra Punnai. Malay.—Sira Punnai. Can. —Babbe.

Characters.—Large translucent, irregular lumps; colour yellow, of horny texture, and brittle; without any odour; the taste is soapy. Mixed with water it softens, and disintegrates into granular matter and oil globules. The water dissolves a portion of it and becomes viscid.

Calophyllum Tomentosum.

Habitat.—Western Peninsula, Ceylon.

Parts used.—The gum.

Vernacular.—Mar.—Pannai.

Characters.—Black and opaque; taste feebly astringent; soluble in cold water.

Calophyllum Inophyllum. Balsamaria Inophyllnm.

Alexandrian laurel, sweet scented calophyllum.

Calophyllum, Kalos beautiful and Phullon a leaf.

Habitat.—Tranvancore, Ceylon, Andamans.

Parts used.—The bitter oil from the seeds and resin.

Vernacular.—Bomb.—Undi, undel. Burm.—Phung-nyet. Can.—Wuma mara. Cing.—S. Domba-gass. Malyal.—Punna. Mar.—Undi. Sans.—Punnaga, Kesova. Tam.—Punnaigam. Tel.—Pannegachettu. Ceylon—Domba oil. Duk.—Surfan. Beng.—Sultana-champa. Eng.—Laurel nut oil.

Characters.—Fruit dry, ovoid or round and greenish yellow; skin brown or black and much wrinkled; nut hard, woody and white; seeds oily consisting of two hemispherical cotyledons closely united; the kernel contains 60 p. c of oil. The oil is obtained from the seeds by expression, and is known as bitter oil or oil of Weandee. It is yellow-green, bitter and aromatic.

Constituents.—A resinous substance and oil. The resin is soft, of a parsley odour, and resembles myrrh. It melts easily and dissolves readily in alcohol. Does not yield umbelliferone by dry distillation.

Preparations.—Liniment and paste. The paste is made by mixing together pounded seeds of undi, seeds of cashew-nut, borax and gamboge.

Actions and uses.—Only used externally. The oil is rubefacient and irritant; mixed with hydnocarpus oil it is used for rheumatic joints, swollen glands, &c.; also in certain skin diseases as scabies and exanthematous eruptions. A paste of the seeds is used to hasten maturation of enlarged glands, abscesses, and boils. The pounded bark is used as an application for swelled testicles.

Schima Wallichii.

Habitat.—Eastern Himalaya, Nepaul, Assam, Burmah.

Part used.— The bark.

Vernacular.—Hind.—Makriya Chilauni.

Chilauni.—Means that which causes itch.

Characters.—The bark, with its liber cells like glistening needles, resembles cowhage. The bark is thick and smooth; external surface irregular, marked with fissures and exfoliations; colour brown.

Constituents.—The parenchyma contains starch and a red colouring matter. Dose of the powdered bark, 1 to 3 grs.

Actions and uses.—A mechanical irritant and vermicide; given in tapeworms. To be followed by castor-oil.

Ternstrœmiaceæ or Camelliaceæ.

The Tea or Camellia family.

Trees or shrubs; leaves four, leathery, alternate stipulate, sometimes dotted. Flowers regular, showy, rarely polgyamous; sepals 5 to 7, coriaceous; petals 5 to 9, imbricated; stamens, hypogynous. Fruit capsular, dehiscent; seeds few, arillate; albumen scanty.

Habitat.—South America, North America, China, East Indies.

Properties.—Stimulant and astringent.

Camellia Theifera. B.P.

Camelea Thea. The teaplant.

Habitat.—England, India, China, Upper Assam, Japan, Ceylon.

Parts used.—The leaves and the alkaloid. (Theine or caffeina, B.P.)

Vernacular.—Eng.—China tea plant. Ind.—Cha, Chai. Mal.—Bluch tea. Pers.—Chaba Chai Kosh.

There are three varieties of this genus.—Thea Bohea and Thea viridis, natives of China and Thea Assamica, which furnishes Assam tea. These are not distinct species but varieties of one termed Thea sinensis. At one time Thea Bohea was supposed to be the source of black tea and that green tea was obtained from Thea Viridis.

Characters.—Leaves 1 to 3 inches long, petiolate, acute at both ends, irregularly serrate, of a peculiar odour and bitter, astringent taste. They are often scented with orange, rose, jasmine and sweet scented olive. Green tea consists of the leaves, quickly dried after gathering. Black tea—the leaves are dried some time after they are gathered, or after they have undergone some kind of fermentation by which they change from green to black. Green tea is often artificially coloured black by a mixture of prussian blue and gypsum, or of gypsum and indigo and a little turmeric. The aroma in tea is due to the volatile oil separated during the process of drying by heat. Dose, a teaspoonful.

Constituents.—Manufactured tea contains a peculiar volatile oil, tannic and gallic acids; quercetin so called boheic acid; theine an alkaloid identical with caffeine; also the alkaloids xanthine and theophylline (dimethylxanthine). The volatile oil is most abundant in green tea. Xanthine is also found in muscles along with creatine, as products of muscular waste. Theophylline is similar in character to theobromine. It forms salts with hydrochloric or nitric acid, with platinum and gold chloride and a double salt with mercuric chloride. It occurs in acicular crystals soluble in warm water. Theine is obtained from coffee, cocoa seeds, guarana, paraguay tea, kola nuts, &c. It occurs in the form of beautiful silky prisms. Soluble in water, Dose, 3 to 5 grains; hypodermically, $\frac{1}{4}$ to 1 grain for the relief of neuralgic pains.

Preparation.—Infusion. Dose, 2 to 6 oz.

Physiological actions.—Tea is a refreshing and stimulating beverage, soothing, analgesic and sudorific. When indulged in to excess it affects the heart, the vaso-motor centre and motor nerves and also the stomach, giving rise to nausea, vomiting, flatulent dyspepsia, tremulousness of the limbs, pallor of the face, feeble pulse, supra-orbital headache, hallucinations and nightmare. It diminishes the waste of the body, and is therefore indirectly nutritive. It increases the assimilation of nitrogenous and hydro-carbon food.

Therapeutics—Given as a household drink. Among the natives an infusion of tea with trikatu is used as a carminative and diaphoretic in fevers, dyspepsia, in mental overwork, &c. Its tannin combines with the gelatine of the food, and hence its excess leads to dyspepsia and also to constipation. Its use should be avoided in hysteria, insomnia, in those suffering from cardiac valvular disease. Theine is a nervine stimulant and is very beneficial in headache, neuralgia, nervous depression. It is often combined with benzoate of sodium, which increases its solubility. Like curare, it causes muscular contractility when brought in contact with it. Compared with coffee its action upon the excretions is to diminish the elimination of carbonic acid, and also of urea, uric acid and waters.

Dipteraceæ—Dipterocarpeæ.

The Sumatra camphor or the Garajan family.

Large trees with resinous juice; leaves feather-veined, involute and alternate; calyx tubular, ultimately enlarged into wing-like expansion; fruits dehiscent or indehiscent, one-seeded; seed solitary and ex-albuminous.

Habitat.—Tropical parts of the East Indies, Java.

Properties.—These plants contain an oleo-resin, to which they owe their properties.

Dipterocarpus Turbinatus, D. Incanus, D. Alatus.

Habitat.—Chittagong, Pegu, Burma, Tenasserim.

Part used.—The oleo resin (balsam).

Vernacular.—Eng.—Wood-oil tree. Beng.—Batisal Shweta-jaryan. Bomb.—Garajana-tela. Burm.—Kanyin. Cing.—Hora-gaha. Eng.—Wood-oil tree, Gurjun balsam. Hind.—Jayan-ka-tel. Garajana-ka-tela. Mar.—Duhun-el-garjan. Tam.—Yennar.

Characters.—The trunk exudes or yields on incision the oleo resin or balsam, which when fresh, is an opaque grey fluid, which soon separates into two layers; the upper one viscid, transparent liquid of a dark-brown colour, and lighter than water; the lower one thick and of consistence of dirty white sediment; taste bitter aromatic, and the odour resembles that of copaiba. It is soluble in pure benzol, chloroform, bisulphide of carbon and essential oils. Partially soluble in methylic, ethylic and amylic alcohols, ether, acetic acid, carbolic acid or caustic potash. Dose, ½ to 2 drs.

Constituents.—The balsam contains an essential volatile oil of a pale straw colour; also dry semi-transparent resin; and a crystallizable acid—Garjanic acid; and volatile matters.

Preparation.—Emulsion (1 to 4 of extract of malt). Dose, ½ to 2 drs. Liniment (1 in 1 of lime water.)

Physiological action.—Alterative and stimulant. It has a stimulant action upon the mucous membranes, especially that of the urinary tract, and is excreted by the kidneys. Like copaiba, it forms glycuronic acid in the system which appears in the urine; with nitric acid it forms a pecipitate of gurjanic acid, which is mistaken for albumen. The precipitate, however, disappears when heated. The glycuronic acid renders the urine antiseptic and prevents the development of bacteria.

Therapeutics.—Given in leprosy, both internally and externally; also in gonorrhœa, menorrhagia, gleet and various other affections of the urinary organs and in skin diseases; also used in cough with purulent expectoration like copaiba, for which it forms a good substitute.

Vateria Indica. V. Malabarica. Chloroxylon dupada.

Hābitat.—Western Peninsula.

Parts used.—The resin and fat.

Vernacular.—Eng.—White dammer Indian copal, Piney tallow tree. Can.—Dupamara. Cing.—Halgass. Hind.—Safed Dammar. Maleal.—Payani Kunlurukaru. Tam.—Vellay-Kungilium, Dupada. Tel.—Dupadamaru, Tella.—Damaru.

Characters.—The resin, which is light greenish or amber coloured, exudes from the tree. It burns with a steady light and gives off pleasant smell. The seeds yield an oil known as Piney tallow of Canara.

Constituents.—The seeds contain solid fat 49·2 p. c., which resembles the solid fats of Garcinia and Bassia. It is a greenish yellow, bleaches rapidly on exposure to light, and has a peculiar balsamic odour. It contains oleic and other fatty acids.

Actions and uses.—The tallow is emollient and stimulant, used locally for chronic rheumatic joints; its chief use is, however, as a general ointment base but more especially in the preparation of nitrate of mercury and other ointments. The resin is used as an incense.

Shorea Robusta.

Habitat.—Central India, Western Bengal.

Part used.—The resin.

Vernacular.—Arab.—Qanqahar. Beng.—Dhuna, Rala. Bomb.—Sala, Rala (the resin). Can.—Guggala. Cing.—Dummala. Hind.—Dhuna, Dhona, Rala, Damar, Rosina. Eng.—The saul tree. Malyal.—Kungiliyam. Duk.—Rala. Mar.—Rala, Guggilu, Dhuna Pers.—Loalemonatehari. Sans.—Asva-karana, Sâl Guggilam, Konshi-kaha. Tam.—Kungiliyam. Tel.—Guggilamu.

Asva-karana, Asva, a horse, and karana, an ear, in allusion to the leaves resembling in shape the horse's ear.

Characters.—Resin obtained from the tree is a deposit between the bark and the wood. It occurs in irregularly cylindrical pieces marked with longitudinal striæ on its surface. Sometimes the pieces are colourless, the colour often varying from dark brown to pale amber or yellow, and red. It is very brittle, and consists of small granules, which can easily be reduced to a fine powder. Generally tasteless, but sometimes the taste resembles nearly that of turpentine. Its powder is easily fusible. When thrown into the flame of a candle it soon takes fire and gives out thick volumes of fragrant smoke or a big blaze. Dose, 10 to 30 grs.

Preparations.—Ointment (1 in 3), and plaster (1 in 2).

Actions and uses.—Stimulant and demulcent. The natives use it for fumigating sick rooms. Externally, as plaster or ointment, it acts as a stimulant. A paste of it mixed with brandy and white of eggs is a very useful and soothing application for the relief of lumbago and other rheumatic pains. The natives use the powder of Rala as an astringent application to the relaxed uvula; it has also been tried in dysentery with some good results.

Dryobalanops Camphora, D. Aromatica. Shorea Camphorifera.

Habitat.—Sumatra, Borneo.

Part used.—Camphor having a different odour from that of ordinary camphor and being less volatile.

Vernacular.—Eng.—Borneo camphor, Borneol or camphyl alcohol. Bomb., Hind.—Baras Kapura, Bhimsani Kapura, Kafur. Sans.—Pakva and Apukva Kapur.

Characters.—It occurs in small pieces, resembling those of ordinary camphor, but is harder and heavier, and sinks in water. It is also less volatile and has a somewhat different odour, the odour resembling that of common camphor, with the additional smell of patchouli or ambergris. It is converted into ordinary camphor by the addition of nitric acid. It may be prepared from ordinary camphor by heating it with potash. Besides camphor, the tree yields a liquid known as camphor oil or Borneene, which is isomeric with oil of turpentine. It must not be confounded with the ordinary camphor oil, which drains out of crude laurel camphor. The odour resembles that of cajuput, camphor and cardamoms combined. The high price of this camphor prohibits its use as ordinary camphor.

Preparation.—A compound powder called by the Jains Vasakshepa (Sans.), or Kabir (Abir), which contains sandalwood, Borneo camphor, saffron and musk. Dose, ½ to 2 grs.

Actions and uses.—Stimulant, antispasmodic, aphrodisiac. As a stimulant application it is used in conjunctivitis.

Tiliaceæ.

The lime tree, Linden or the Bahuphali family.

Trees, shrubs, or rarely herbs; leaves stipulate, simple, lobed and alternate; flowers generally yellow; sepals distinct or coherent, valvate in æstivation and deciduous; fruits samaroid and many-celled, dry or pulpy; seeds solitary or numerous; albumen fleshy; embryo erect.

Habitat.—Chiefly found in the tropics, a few being found in the northern parts of the world.

Properties.—Allied to those of Malvaceæ; they are mucilaginous, emollient and demulcent; some bear edible fruits; many yield useful fibres for manufacturing purposes, and valuable timber.

Corchorus Olitorius.—C. Trilocularis.

Habitat.—Asia, Africa, Peninsula, Bengal, Punjab.

Parts used.—The seeds and leaves.

Vernacular.—Beng.—Banpat Kooshta, Bhangipat. Bomb.—Rajajira seeds, Isband. Burm.—Phetwun. Chin.—Dimoa. Eng.—Jew's mallow, jute. Guz.—Rajajira. Hind.—Pat, the plant Baphalli. Malay.—Ramitsjua. Mar.—Kurru Chuntz. Sans.—Nadika, Peta, Putta. Tam.—Perinta. Tel.—Parinta Kura.

Characters.—Seeds similar in shape to those of Bhauphali, but smaller, angular, darker, harder and extremely bitter; leaves oblong; capsules, trilocular. Dose of the seeds, 30 to 90 grs.

Preparation.—Infusion of leaves (1 in 10). Dose, 1 to 2 oz.

Actions and uses.—The leaves and seeds are bitter, mucilaginous and demulcent. The infusion of the leaves is given in fevers and in congested liver. The plant, reduced to ashes, is used as an alterative in congestion of the liver and dyspepsia.

Grewia Tiliæfolia, G. Arborea, G. Elastica.

Habitat.—Western India, Ceylon, Burma.

Part used.—The bark.

Vernacular.—Beng.—Dhamani. Can.—Butaleas, Thadsal. Hind.—Dhaman. Mar.—Dhaman. Sans.–Dharmana. Tam.—Thada. Tel.—Charachi.

Characters.—Leaves hoary beneath, cordate, dentate; flowers yellow; berries of an acid flavour; bark thick, white internally and grey externally; tuber papery, peeling off, leaving a rough green surface beneath; very mucilaginous and sweetish to the taste.

Preparation.—Infusion (1 in 10). Dose, 1 to 2 oz.

Actions and uses.—Demulcent, given in dysentery.

Grewia Asiatica.

Habitat.—Ceylon, Burma.

Parts used.—Fruit and bark.

Vernacular.—Beng.—Shukri. Cing.—Dowaniya. Hind.—Phalsa. Mar.—Phals. Sans.—Parusha-Phala-Traya. Tel.—Putiki.

Characters.—Fruits acid, colour dark brown; kernel hard.

Preparation.—Infusion (1 in 10). Dose, ½ to 1 oz.

Actions ana uses.—Cooling and refrigerant; the bark is demulcent, and given in fever and dysentery.

Grewia Scabrophylla.

Habitat.—West Indies.

Parts used.—Leaves, stem and fruit.

Vernacular.—Mar.—Khat-khate.

Characters.—Leaves scabrous.

Actions and uses.—Mucilaginous; used as a substitute for althæa.

Corchorus Humilis, C. Fascicularis, C. Antichorus.

Habitat.—Tropical India, Bengal, Africa.

Parts used.—The whole plant.

Vernacular.—Poona.—Mogarmithi, Beng.—Jangli-pat, Bilnalita. Bomb.—Bhaphali. Duk.—Magar Mithi. Hind.—Hirankhari.

Herankhari—Haran, deer, and khari, a hoof, from its resemblance to deer's hoof.

Characters.—Small prostrate weed; root woody; branches several, small, slender and spreading out from the root; leaves oblong, serrated, small, wrinkled, thick, mucilaginous and of a greenish dark colour; flowers small, yellow, in the axils of leaves and in bunches of two or three; capsules about ½ to 1 inch in length and hairy externally; each capsule composed of three carpels, containing many small, angular, dark-red coloured seeds; seeds very bitter.

Preparation.—Infusion (1 in 10). Dose, 1 to 2 ozs.

Actions and uses.—The plant is mucilaginous, somewhat astringent and nervine tonic. It is a common ingredient in aphrodisiac confections. It is used in gonorrhœa, seminal debility and urinary diseases.

Remarks.—Bhaphali. This name should not be mistaken for Bhaphali, the Marathi name for Peucedanum grande, an umbiliferous plant. In peucedanum grande, the whole plant, including leaves, capsules, &c., are diminutive; not so in corchorus fascicularis.

Frankeniaceæ.—The Frankenia or sea heath order.

Herbs or shrubs; leaves opposite, exstipulate; flowers sessile; calyx tubular and persistent; petals 4 or 5, hypogynous; stamens distinct; ovary superior, one-celled; fruit capsular, dehiscent; seeds numerous, minute; embryo straight in the middle of albumen.

Habitat.—South Europe, North Africa.

Properties.—Mucilaginous, aromatic.

Frankenia Grandifolia, Yerba Reunia.—Flax Herb.

Habitat.—California, South of Europe.

Parts used.—The herb.

Characters.—The herb is mucilaginous and slightly aromatic.

Constituents.—It contains a peculiar astringent principle and a large amount of sodium chloride.

Preparation.—Fluid extract. Dose, 10 to 20 ms., chiefly used as an injection or as a gargle, much diluted.

Action and uses.—Generally used as an injection in catarrhal affections of the nares and the genito-urinary tract. In vaginal leucorrhœa the injection is said to be peculiarly beneficial.

Caryophyllaceæ.

The pink or clove wort, or the zaharasa family.

Herbs erect, low or prostrate; stems smaller at the joints; leaves opposite, entire, exstipulate and connate at the base; flowers hermaphrodite or rarely unisexual, white or pink coloured; fruits one-celled, rarely more; seeds numerous and small; embryo curved round albumen; albumen mealy.

Habitat.—Temperate and cold climates.

Properties.—Most of them have no important medicinal properties some are galactagogue and others alterative.

Dianthus Anatolicus.

Habitat.—Thibet, Armenia.

Part used.—The plant.

Vernacular.—Hind.—Kanturiyun. Pers.—Kanturiyun.

Characters.—Plant densely tufted ; stalk short, woody and branched ; stems slender, with one or more flowers ; leaves rigid, slender, with thick midrib and margin.

Constituents.—Contains a little saponin.

Preparation.—Decoction (1 in 10). Dose, 1 to 2 fluid ozs.

Actions and uses.—Similar in property to common centaury (Erythrœa centaurium). Also stomachic and tonic like gentian.

Polycarpæa Corymbosa.—A small plant.

Habitat.—India.

Part used.—The plant.

Vernacular.—Tam.—Nilaisedachi.

Actions and uses.—Used internally and externally for the bites of venomous insects and reptiles.

Saponaria Vaccaria—Gypsophila Vaccaria.

Habitat.—India, Central Europe.

Part used.—The root.

Saponaria, soapy, that is, its mucilaginous juice forms a lather with water.

Vernacular.—Arab.—El-sabuniyeh. Beng.—Sabusie. Eng.—Perfoliate soap wort. Hind.—Sabuni. Romans.—Struthium, Radicula.

Characters.—The entire plant is bitter and of a saline taste; roots long, of the size of a quill, cylindrical and branching ; bark thick, easily separable, reddish externally and white within.

Constituents.—Saponin—is obtained by exhausting the powdered root with boiling alcohol ; on cooling saponin is deposited as a white amorphous friable substance, without any odour, having an acrid taste ; soluble in weak alcohol ; insoluble in water, forming an emulsion ; heated with an acid and boiled, the solution is converted into Sapogenin, which, on evaporation, gives needle-shaped crystals. Saponin is also found in Gypsophila struthium, saponaria officinalis, illicium anisatum, caulophyllum, senega, quillaja, &c.

Preparation.—Infusion (1 in 20). Dose, ½ to 1 oz.

Actions and uses.—Alterative, stimulant, purgative, diuretic and sternutatory. It stimulates the mucous membranes, and may be used in cough, chronic bronchitis, pleurisy, asthma, &c. It is also used in liver diseases, jaundice, syphilis, gout and chronic skin diseases.

Malvaceæ.

The Bhinda or Mallow family. Malvaceæ.—Derived from Malva, mallow or soft, the plants having soft and downy leaves and emollient properties.

Characters.—Herbs, shrubs or trees, often with hairs; leaves alternate, stipulate, downy, palmate; flowers showy, regular and axillary, surrounded by an involucre of variegated colours; fruits indehiscent or dehiscent, capsular or baccate; carpels one, two or many-seeded; seeds reniform or ovate and hairy, generally without albumen; embryo curved, cotyledons, twisted like chrysalis.

Habitat.—Temperate climate, tropics.

Properties.—Demulcent and mucilaginous; from the liber of many species, tough fibres are obtained. The hairs covering the seeds constitute cotton.

Abelmochus Esculentus.—Hebiscus Esculentus.

Habitat.—East Indies.

Parts used.—The immature capsules and ripe seeds or unripe fruit.

Vernacular.—East Indies—Ochro, Gombo, Bandikai. Arab.—Bamiya. Beng.—Ramturai, Dhenrus. Bomb.—Bhinda. Burm.—Ba-lu-wa, yung-ma-da. Can.—Bendekayi. Cing.—Bandaka. Duk.—Bhendi. Eng.—Edible Hibiscus, Okro, Gombo. Guz.—Bhindu. Hind.—Bhendi, Ramturai. Maleal.—Ventak Kaya, Venda. Mar.—Bhenda. Pers.—Bamiya. Sans.—Darwika, Teridisha, Bhinda. Tam.—Vendaik-kay; Tel.—Benda-kaya.

Ramaturai (the fruit) resembles in shape Turai, the fruit of Luffa acutangula (Palwal). The fruit also resembles in shape the früit of Trichosanthes dioica.

Characters.—Fresh immature capsules are from 2 to 6 inches long, broad at the base and tapering at the apex, furrowed and somewhat hairy, particularly at the ridges, abounding in copious bland and viscid mucilage, each capsule consisting of from 6 to 9 valves or cells, containing a single row of smooth, white, round seeds, turning black when ripe and dry.

Constituents.—Fresh capsules contain pectin, starch, mucilage and ashes, rich in salts of potash, lime and magnesia. The ripe seeds contain phosphoric acid.

Preparation.—Decoction (1 in 10). Dose, 1 to 2 ozs.

Actions and uses.—Emollient, demulcent, diuretic, cooling and aphrodisiac, given in irritation of the throat, catarrh of the bladder, dysuria and gonorrhœa.

Abutilon Indicum.

A. Asiaticum, Sida Indica, Sida Mauritiana, Sida populifolia.

Habitat.—Tropical India, Ceylon, waste grounds.

Parts used.—The bark, leaves and seeds.

Vernacular.—Arab.—Masht-el-ghoul. Beng.—Gungi-potari, Balbij. Bomb.—Chakra-bhenda, Madami-pitari (the seeds). Burm.—Thama Khai-ok. Can.—Shri-mudrigida. Cing.—Anoda-gaha. Duk.—Kangoi, Dabbe Gunji.' Eng.—Country mallow. Goa.—Tubocuty. Guz.—Kangoyi Kapata, Daboli. Hind.—Kali Kanghi, Anter-vela. Maleal.—Petaka-putti, Oram. Pers.—Darakhte-shanah. Mar.—Petari, Madmi Chakra-bhenda. Panj.—Ali, Khiratipala, Pataka, Limbal. Tam.—Payruntuthi. Tel.—Tutti, Tutturu-benda, Nagu-benda.

Characters.—Bark thin, long, tough and fibrous, also striped, externally cinnamon-coloured, covered with a silky, hoary tomentum, internally white ; taste bitter and astringent ; leaves roundish, cordate, acuminate, serrated, velvety on both sides, of a pale green colour and mucilaginous; seeds reniform; testa dull brown and hairy; in size resembling Elachi dana. On section yellowish white within ; taste mucilaginous and pea-like. Two varieties of seeds are met with—(1) tomentose and hoary, Bulabija of the shops, and (2) with purple stems called Kalo Kanghi.

Constituents.—The leaves contain mucilage, tannin, organic acid and traces of asparagin and ash containing alkaline sulphates, chlorides, magnesium phosphate and calcium carbonate.

Preparation—Decoction of the seeds and bark (1 in 10). Dose, 1 to 2 oz., and mucilage of bruised leaves.

Actions and uses.—Seeds demulcent ; the bark diuretic and cooling, used, like althæa, in gonorrhœa strangury, &c.

Althæa Officinalis.

The mallow. Marsh mallow.

Habitat.—Temperate climates, Europe, Western and Northern Asia; salt marshes, New York.

Part used.—The flowers, leaves, roots and carpels.

Mortification root, sweet weed, Wymote, Marsh mallow.

Vernacular.—Pers. and Hind.—Gul-Khairu (flowers). Persian.—Tukhm-i-Khitimi (carpels) ; Risha-i-Khinni (the root).

Characters.—Flowers from 1 to 2 inches long with three different colours—yellowish at the base, green in the middle, and pink or violet at the top ; calyx five partite, thick and covered with whitish hairs ; petals five and bearded at the base and on their inner surface. In the centre of the flower is a conical-five-angled projection, the stamenal column and pistil ; root hairy, of a whitish colour, both externally and internally, cylindrical and somewhat tapering, breaking with a short granular fracture ; parenchyma is filled with starch, and contains also scattered cells of calcium oxalate crystals. The root has a faint, peculiar, aromatic odour and a sweet mucilaginous taste; carpels of a dark-brown colour, reniform and hairy, with a groove on its back, having two surfaces jointed together at the hilum by a notch. A portion of it near the hilum is convex and reticulated. Beyond this the surface is studded with hairs. Near the margin the surface is marked with fan-like ridges. It encloses one seed. The taste is mucilaginous. Dose of the root, ½ to 1 dr.

Constituents.—Dry root contains an organic principle, althein or asparagin 2 p.c.; mucilage called bassorin or althæa 25 p.c.; Pectous matter or pectin 10 p.c.; fixed oil, sugar 8 p.c.; fatty oil, starch, 35 p.c.; ash 5 p.c. Tannin only in the outer bark, containing phosphates. Mucilage is precipitated by neutral acetate of lead, and hence differs from gum arabic. It differs from cellulose, as althæa does not turn blue by iodine when moistened with sulphuric acid, and is not soluble in ammoniacal solution of oxide of copper.

Bassorin can be obtained from asparagus, liquorice, belladonna roots and sweet almonds.

Asparagin occurs as hard, transparent, colourless crystals; soluble in cold water (1 in 50); insoluble in alcohol and ether. An aqueous solution of it dissolves in yellow oxide of mercury, hence recommended as a vehicle for hypodermic injection of yellow oxide of mercury. Dose—1 to 2 grs.

Althæa root is a constituent of Massa Hydrargyri (25 p.c). Dose, 1 to 15 grs.

Preparations.—Decoction of the root (1 in 10,) used as an emollient, enema, poultices and ointment. Infusum althæa contain carpels and flowers (1 in 20). Dose, 1 to 2 ozs. Syrupus althæa, syrup of marsh mallow. Contains althæa, alcohol, glycerine and sugar. Dose *ad libitum.*

Actions and uses.—The different parts of the plant are mucilaginous, emollient and demulcent. Althæa acts mechanically; it forms a soothing covering over the inflamed parts and protects them from friction. The root is given internally in inflammation of the lungs, intestines and bladder. It forms an useful ingredient of various cough mixtures, pectoral syrups, &c. Mixed with sweet oil, the leaves and flowers are applied as poultices and fomentations to burns and to parts bitten by venomous animals. As a demulcent the decoction is used as an enema in irritable and inflamed state of the vagina and rectum. Althein is a good diuretic and given in cystitis, in irritable cough due to congestion of the pharynx, in ascitis, in anasarca due to Bright's disease, and in gout.

In pharmacy the powdered root, being very absorbent, is used to harden pills, electuaries, &c.

Gossypium Barbadense, B.P.—Gossypium Herbaceum. G. Arboreum. G. Indicum—G. Stocksii and other Species.

Habitat.—Hot countries, Asia, Africa, Egypt, America.

Parts used.—Root bark, cotton seed-oil, and the hairy covering of the seed, Gossypium, cotton, cotton wool, B. P.

Vernacular.—Arab.—Kuttun, Nabut-ul-gutu, Shagratul-gutu. Beng.—Karpas, Rui, Shuter-gucht. Burm.—Wabin, Gim. Can.—Hatti-gida. Concani.—Denkapus (sacred cotton). Cing.—Kapu.

Duk.—Rui-kapas. Eng.—Cotton. Guz.—Ru-vona (hairy covering), kapasia (seeds). Hind.—Rui, Binola. Malyal.—Pamtai. Mar.—Kapasi, kapas. Pers.—Pambah. Sans.—Karapasaha, Karpasi. Tam.—Punji, Van-paruti. Tel.—Patti-chettu, Karpasamu.

Characters.—Herb from 2 to 6 feet high; leaves long petioled, palmate, 3 to 5 lobed, and of a green or darkish green colour; flowers yellow, capsular, 3 to 4 celled, opening by many valves, acute, oblong or ovate, and containing numerous seeds; seeds oblong or ovate, pointed at one end and covered with silvery white hairs; hairs or covering of seeds, or purified cotton, is not easily separable; testa hard and of a blackish colour. On section the seeds are oily; the bark of the washed root (G. radicis cortex,) in thin flexible bands or quills, of a brownish yellow colour, externally slightly ridged and marked with black dots or transverse lines; the inner surface is whitish and of a silky lustre, tough and fibrous; fibres, separating into papery layers; no odour; taste slightly pungent and astringent. Dose of the root 30 to 60 grs.

Gossypium.—Hairs of the seeds freed from other impurities and deprived of fatty matter. They are pure white, soft, fine filaments, hollow, spirally twisted and slightly thick at edges. They are without any odour or taste.

Oil of the seed—Oleum Gossypii Seminis (cotton-seed oil.) The fixed oil is obtained by cracking off testa, grinding kernels and expressing and purifying. Its amount varies from 10 to 30 p.c. It is often substituted for olive oil, brazil or para-nut oil, and for beech oil or oil from Fagus sylvetica; It is sometimes used in the preparation of camphor and ammonia liniments.

Constituents.—The root-bark contains starch, chromogene 28 p.c.; fixed oil, resin, glucose, tannin, starch and ash 6 p.c. Chromogene, a yellow substance, becoming red and resinous by age; soluble in alcohol (1 in 14), chloroform (1 in 15), ether (1 in 23), and benzol (1 in 22). The oil, oleum gossypii seminis—cotton-seed oil, as expressed from the seeds, is of a yellow colour, highly viscous, without any odour, of bland taste and neutral reaction; soluble in ether, but slightly soluble in alcohol. It contains oleine, and a green feeble yellow colouring matter.

The hairs contain cellulose inorganic matter, fixed oil, albuminoids lignin, &c.

Preparation.—of the bark. Decoctum Gossypii (1 in 5). Dose, 1 to 2 ozs.; used as an emmenagogue. As a parturient, it is superior to ergot. Extractum gossypii radicis fluidum—fluid extract of cotton root bark; macerate the bark with glycerine and alcohol and percolate. It is not miscible with water. Dose—10 to 60 ms. Of the hairs, purified cotton, absorbent cotton or cotton wool. To prepare it, add alkalies to cotton to remove greasiness, adherent impurities and moisture; then add solution of chlorinald lime and hydrochloric acid. Cotton is insoluble in ordinary solvents, but soluble in solutions of ammonium sulphate of copper. Under the microscope these hairs are found to be hollow and twisted bands spirally striate and slightly thickened at the edges. Absorbent cotton, which is now the official cotton or cotton wool, B. P., is used in the preparation of pyroxylin or gun cotton. Cotton gauze or cotton wool tissue consists of a thin sheet of absorbent cotton wool between two layers of gauze. Medicated cotton is cotton wool medicated with the following, viz, alum, arnica, benzoic acid, camphor, chrysophanic acid, cubebs, carbolic acid, salicylic acid, boracic acid, krameria, opium, resorcin and tannic acid.

Artificial Sponges.—Absorbent cotton formed into balls and covered with antiseptic gauze. Also made of absorbent cotton covering a glass capsule filled with an antiseptic as eucalyptus, carbolic acid, thymol, &c., to be broken by pressure.

Pyroxylinum.—B. P. Pyroxylin ; soluble gun cotton ; colloxylin—collodion cotton. It is prepared by the action of sulphuric and nitric acids and water on cotton, by macerating, washing, draining and drying ; chiefly used in the preparation of collodium, collodion B. P.

Collodion—to prepare it dissolve pyroxylin 1 in a mixture of ether 36 and alcohol 12. It is a syrupy colourless liquid of an ethereal odour, is highly inflammable, and dries quickly on exposure to air, leaving a thin transparent film, which contracts rapidly on drying. It is insoluble in water or alcohol.

Camphoid, a substitute for collodion. It is a solution (1 in 40) of pyroxylin. It contains pyroxylin 1, camphor and absolute alcohol 20 each. Used as a vehicle for the application to the skin of such drugs as iodoform, phenol, salicylic acid, resorcin, chrysophanic acid and ichthyol.

Hæmostatic collodion.—To obtain it, mix together collodion 100, carbolic acid 10, and tannic acid 5, or acid benzoic 5.

Styptic collodion.—To prepare it, take absolute alcohol 10, benzoin 1, and dissolve. To the solution add tannic acid 10, ether 40, and gun cotton 1.

Collodium Flexile, B. P., elastic collodion, flexible collodion. To prepare it, mix thoroughly collodion 12 with Canada turpentine ½, and castor-oil ¼. Flexible collodion is used in the preparation of collodium cantharidatum or collodium vesicans.

Collodium Vesicans, B. P.—Blistering collodion, cantharidal collodion. To prepare it, take blistering fluid 20 and pyroxylin ½, and mix.

Collodium novum, a new kind of collodion —To obtain it, mix and make a solution of mastiche 3, Balsam of Peru 1, narcotine 1, and chloroform 5.

Anodyne colloid ; syn.—Amyl colloid. To obtain it, take amyl hydride 1 ounce, aconitine 1 grain, veratrine 6 grains, collodion 2 ounces ; very often half the quantity of amyl hydride is replaced by alcohol (absolute) or by amylic alcohol.

Celloidin—it is pyroxylin purified by solution in alcohol and ether. Photoxylin—Dinitrocellulose—prepared by nitrating wood wool ; dissolved in a mixture of alcohol and ether, it resembles collodion ; used to form artificial aural tympana.

Carbolic collodion : 20 grains carbolic acid to 1 ounce of styptic colloid; used for toothache. Collodium cum oleo crotonis 1 in 7, used as a counter-irritant. Collodium callosum.—A mixture of flexible collodion 60 with extract of Indian hemp 1 and salicylic acid 8, used as an application for corns, warts, and lupus. Collodium cum iodoformo (1 to 12), for venereal sores. Collodium ichthyol (7 to 1). Collodium iodi, iodine 1 to flexible collodion 15. Collodium Peruvianum—Balsam of Peru 1 to collodion 9. Collodium Salicylicum—Salicylic acid 1, flexible collodion 5. Collodium Salicylicum cum zinci chlorido.—Zinc chloride 1, salicylic acid 2, collodion 15. Collodium Salicylicum et lacticum—salicylic and lactic acids, each 10, collodion 80. Collodium Salol, Salol collodion.—Ether 4, salol 4, collodion 30; For acute rheumatism. Crystallin.—A combination of ether and methyl alcohol, a good substitute for collodium.

Actions and uses.—A syrup of cotton flowers is given in hypochondriasis; their poultice is applied to burns and scalds. The carpels are astringent. An unripe capsule, with opium and nutmeg inserted into its interior, incinerated and reduced to powder, is used in dysentery. Decoction of the root-bark is used as abortifacient, emmenagogue and oxytocic, it increases labour pains during delivery, and is given in amenorrhœa, dysmenorrhœa, uterine hæmorrhages and to procure abortion. The seeds, made into tea, are mucilaginous, and used in dysentery and diarrhœa. They are demulcent, laxative, aphrodisiac, expectorant and galactagogue. The juice of the leaves is used in scanty lactation. Pounded cotton seeds mixed with ginger, is applied to orchitic swelling. The leaves, with oil, are applied to gouty joints. The fibres are protective, and used to cover up wounds, on which they act mechanically by keeping off dirt and germs. Burnt cotton is applied round dropsical and paralyzed limbs, swollen legs, rheumatic and gouty joints, and in children to the chest in bronchitis and pneumonia to preserve heat and moisture and also to act as a sort of fomentation.

Absorbent cotton is a good absorbent of water, and used for excluding air from injured surfaces and to allay pain, as in burns, scalds, erysipelas, and articular rheumatism. Soaked in antiseptic solutions, it is applied directly to wounds and ulcers, to absorb the discharges. Among the natives burnt cotton is used to stop blood as well as to cure ulcers. Sometimes spider's web is used as a substitute for cotton. Pyroxylin is highly inflammable and explosive. Collodion is inflammable, and when applied, there is rapid evaporation of its ether; and it leaves a thin film of pyroxylin on the surface. It is used as a protective application over wounds, burns, ulcers, slight cuts, cracks and fissures, over inflamed surfaces, as in erysipelas, in skin diseases, chapped nipples, &c. Styptic collodion is an hæmostatic and protective. It contains tannin, and is therefore used to stop bleeding from leech bites; as an antiseptic it is used for cuts and wounds and for arresting hæmorrhages. Flexible collodion is used in drawing edges of a wound together, bringing pressure on buboes, boils, carbuncles, &c. In acute orchitis the chord and scrotum are coated with it with benefit.

Vesicant collodion is a more convenient form of applying liquor epispasicus, the advantage being that it does not spread to the surrounding parts. It is used in neuralgia, lumbago and muscular pains.

Oleum gossypium seminis, like olive oil, is demulcent, and used as a lubricant in preparing various liniments. Collodium novum is an antiseptic and used to relieve pain in neuralgia, and acute or chronic rheumatism.

Hibiscus Abelmoschus. A. Moschatus (Bamia Moschata).

Habitat.—Tropical countries.

Part used.—The seeds.

Vernacular.—Arab.—Hub-ul-Mishk Kabbamisk. Burm.—Ba-lu-wa-ki. Beng.—Mushak-danah, Kasturi-dana. Bomb.—Mishka-dana. Cing.—Kapu-kinaissa. Duk.—Musek, Kalakasturi bhendi-ke-bing. Eng.—Musk-mallow. Guz.—Mushak-dana. Hind.—Mushak-danah. Pers.—Mushk-danah. Malyal.—Katta-kasturi. Mar.—Bhenda-che-bij. Sans.—Tata Kasaturika. Tam.—Kattuk-kasturi. Tel.—Kasturi-benda. East and West Indies.—Ochro, Gombo, Bandikai.

Abelmoschus is a corruption of Hub-ul-mishk.

Kabbamisk, a grain of musk.

Tata Kasaturika.—Tata, creeping, and Kasturika, musk-plant, in allusion to this musk-smelling plant rising above the ground at first and then bending upon itself like a creeper. The seeds of Ramturai are often passed off for Mishka dana, being similar in shape and size.

Characters.—Seeds aromatic, resembling Bhenda-seeds in size. They are of a brown colour, irregularly kidney-shaped, their surface marked with concentric rings, pointed at one end. Odour musky but not perceptible unless well bruised.

Constituents.—Gum, albumen, fixed oil, a solid crystalline matter, odorous principle and resin. The fixed oil is a greenish yellow fluid, which solidifies on exposure to the air. The solid crystalline matter is white, pearly, of a pleasant taste, and soluble in ether. The odorous matter is a light green fluid, of the strong smell of musk. It is not volatile.

Actions and uses.—Stimulant, carminative, cooling and demulcent, given in gonorrhœa, catarrh of the bladder and hoarseness of voice. The seeds are stomachic and used after being mixed with coffee. Powdered seeds steeped in alcohol are used as an application for the bites of serpents.

Remarks.—Abelmoschus esculentus, hibiscus esculentus. Eng.—Okro. Guz.—Bhinda. Egyp.—Bamia. The capsules are held in esteem as a vegetable.

Hibiscus Cannabinus.

Habitat.—Western India, Tropics.

Parts used.—Flowers and seeds.

Vernacular.—Arab.—Hab-el-zalim. Beng.—Mesta-pat, Nalki. Can.—Punday, Pundrika. Chin.—Hiang-ma. Duk.—Ambari. Eng.—The fibres, brown Indian hemp, Dukhani hemp, hemp cuved hibisleas.

Hind.—Patsan, Sunnee. Mar.—Ambari. Panj.—Sankokla-patsan. Pers.—Hab-el-zalim. Tam.—Palungo, Relacha. Tel.—Gongukuru. Sind.—Sujjado.

Characters.—The plant has white flowers with purple stamens; pods prickly, seeds like cardamoms, with a black skin and white kernel. The fibres are known under the name of sunnie or sunn hemp. True sunn is derived from crotolaria juncea, or Dukhani hemp. The seeds yield an edible fixed oil. Dose of the seeds, 5 to 15 grs.

Actions and uses.—The juice of the flowers, with sugar and black pepper, is used as a remedy in biliousness and fevers. The seeds are fattening, tonic, and aphrodisiac, being an ingredient in aphrodisiac confections.

Remarks.—Hab-el-zalim is also an Arabic name for artichoke seeds, as well as for the fruit of Habzelia œthiopica (monkey-pepper.)

Hibiscus Rosa Sinensis.

Habitat.—India, Konkan.

Parts used.—The roots and flowers.

Vernacular.—Arab.—Anghar-e-hindi. Beng.—Orphul, Joba, Uru, Juva. Bomb.—Jasund, Jasus. Burm.—Khounyan. Can.—Dasvalada huvn. Chin.—Chukin. Duk.—Jasut Gudhel. Eng.—Shoeflower. Guz.—Jasutnu-phul. Hind.—Jasun, Juva. Malyal.—Shempariti, Kambangsaptu. Madras.—Shappathupu. Mar.—Jasavanda. Pers.—Angharac Hindi. Sans.—Jaba or Japa-pushpam. Tam.—Sapatta-cherri. Tel.—Dasana-japa-pushpam.

Jasovanda is also a name given to Jonesia-asoka, for which this should not be mistaken.

Shoe-flower. The petals are used by the Chinese to blacken their eyebrows and to blacken their shoe leather.

Characters.—A common garden shrub. Leaves ovate, cordate, closely serrate, acuminate and of a green or darkish green colour; flowers large, of a red colour, mucilaginous and fleshy; roots long, tapering, of a whitish colour and mucilaginous in taste. There are several varieties, some with single white or yellow flowers, others with double red flowers. The root of the white flower variety is mostly preferred and used in medicine.

Preparation.—Infusion (1 in 10). Dose, 1 to 2 ozs., and mucilage,

Actions and uses.—The petals are demulcent, and emollient. As a refrigerant drink its infusion is given in fevers, as a demulcent in cough and cystitis; combined with milk, sugar and cumin, it is given in gonorrhœa. In menorrhagia, combined with lotus root and the bark of eriodendron anfractuosum, it is of benefit.

Hibiscus Sabdariffa.

Habitat.—Tropics.

Part used.—The fleshy red calyx.

Vernacular.—Beng.—Lal-mesta. Burm.—Thambau-khyenboung. Can.—Pundi-soppu. Eng.—Red sorrel, Roselle. Duk.—Lal-ambara. Hind.—Patwa. Mar.—Lal-ambari. Tam.—Pulychay-kire, Shemay-kashli-kire. Tel.—Yaragogu, Panj Patwa.

Characters.—The fleshy red calyx, when dried, is used as a fruit and as an article of diet like tamarind.

Constituents.—Potash, tartaric and malic acids, watery extract, cellulose, &c. Dose, 15 to 25 grs.

Preparation.—Jelly and syrup. 1 to 2 drs.

Actions and uses.—Demulcent and cooling, used as a cooling drink in biliousness, fevers and cough. It is sometimes combined with common salt, pepper, molasses and asafetida.

Malva Sylvestris—M. Rotundifolia—M. Vulgaris.

Habitat.—Temperate climates.

Part used.—The fruit.

Vernacular.—Arab.—Khubazi, Anjil. Bomb.—Khubazi, Towdri (the seeds). Eng.—Common mallow, marsh mallow. Pers.—Kitmi-i-Kuchak, Nan-i-Kulagh. The seed Towdri.

Characters.—Fruit of a light brown colour; carpels from 10 to 12, reniform, very beautifully reticulated, and closely arranged on the axis, giving the whole fruit the form of an artificially made thread button ; in the centre or at its top there is a conical projection, which is the remnant of styles, and at the base a leathery calyx with or without a small pedicle adherent to the fruit. The taste is mucilaginous, and resembles that of Gul-i-khitmi.

Constituents.—Mucilage and a bitter extractive.

Preparation.—Decoction and infusion (1 in 20). Dose, 1 to 2 ozs.

Actions and uses.—Mucilaginous, demulcent and cooling, used in coughs and other irritable conditions of the mucous membranes of the throat and pulmonary tract, in inflammation of the bladder and in hæmorrhoids ; other properties are similar to those of althæa.

Pavonia Odorata.

Habitat.—N.-W. Provinces, Sind, W. Peninsula, Burma and Ceylon.

Part used.—The root.

Vernacular.—Beng.—Bala. Can.—Balarakkasi-gida. Hind.—Sugandhe-bala. Mar.—Kala Vala. Pers.—Bulla Hrivera. Sans.—Bulla Hrivera. Tam.—Peramutiepu. Tel.—Erra-kati, Chitli-benda.

Characters.—Root 7 to 8 inches long, twisted, giving off numerous thin fibres, having a delicate musky odour ; bark light brown, and smooth; wood hard and yellowish ; plant covered with sticky hairs ; flowers pink ; seeds brown, and oily ; odour delightful.

Preparations.—Infusion (1 in 10). Dose, 1 to 2 ozs. Compound decoction, known as Shadanga Paniya. It contains the roots of Pavonia odorata, andropogon muricatus, cyperus rotundus, or Cyperus pertenius, and red sandalwoods; herbs of oldenlandia herbacea, and dry ginger, each 1 drachm make decoction; used in fevers as a cooling and stomachic acid drink. Dose, 1 to 2 ozs.

Actions and uses.—Demulcent, carminative, stimulant, diaphoretic and diuretic; used in flatulent dyspepsia, hysteria, nervous headache and in low state of the system; also in fevers, gout, rheumatism and cough.

Sida Cordifolia.

S. Acuta, S. Retusa, S. Rhombifolia, S. Carpinifolia, S. Spinosa.

Habitat.—The tropics, Australia, Bengal.

Parts used.—The roots and leaves.

Vernacular.—Arab.—Hulbahe-barri. Australia—Queensland hemp, jelly leaf, Beng.—Barjala, Bijband, Chuka, Hamaz, Kowar, Sirivadi, Babila. Cing.—Katekan, Babila Sirivadi. Guz.—Balu-Jangli-methi. Hind.—Bariara, Gulsakari, Kharenti, simak (seeds). Malyal.—Cheru, paruva. Mar.—Chikana-pata, Tupa Karia, Tukati. Pers.—Shanbalide-barri, Shamlite-dashti. Sans.—Bala, Bala-Baty alaka, Pat. Tam.—Malai-tangi, Pilambasi, Visha-badi. Tel.—Chitia Mutti, Subadevi.

Jelly leaf. The leaves being mucilaginous. Chiknapata—chikna, means mucilaginous, and pat, a leaf. Bala is the general name for plants of this genus. There are five such balas, viz., Bala, Maha bala, Atibala, Naga bala, and Rajabala.

Characters.—Roots woody, hard and fibrous; taste sweetish, and resembling common liquorice root; bark light, yellowish brown; leaves cordate, rhomboid or lanceolate, tomentose or more or less dentate, highly mucilaginous.

Constituents.—The root contains asparagin and gelatine.

Preparation.—Infusion of root (1 in 10). Dose, 1 to 2 ozs.

Actions and uses.—The roots are cooling, astringent, bitter tonic, febrifuge, demulcent and diuretic. Given with ginger in fevers and urinary diseases; also in rheumatism. As a demulcent the juice is given in gonorrhœa, leucorrhœa and chronic diarrhœa. The root of S. carpinifolia is locally used by the Hindoos as a paste, with sparrow's dung, to burst boils. The leaves of S. cordifolia are made into varalians and applied to the eyes in ophthalmia.

Thespesia Populnea. Hibiscus Populnea.

Habitat.—Bengal and Ceylon.

Parts used.—The leaves, bark, fruit and seeds.

Vernacular.—Eng.—Portia-tree, Tulip tree. Beng.—Poresh. Bomb.—Bhindi. Can.—Kandarola-mara, Pooarasoo. Cing.—Gansuri, Suria-gass. Duk.—Paras-pippal. Guz.—Parasa-pipalo. Hind.—Paras-pipal, Pahari-pipal. Mar.—Bhendi, Parasa. Malyal.—Puvva-rasha. Sans.—Parisa, Gargha, Bhanda, Supara Shavaka. Tam.—Puvarasa maram. Tel.—Gangaravi.

Characters.—Leaves thick, cordate, broad, acuminate, with long petioles, darkish green above and pale beneath ; flowers large, yellow, and bell-shaped; fruit a capsule of the size of a common lemon, oblong, depressed and coriaceous, when dry of a darkish brown colour ; fresh fruits abound in a viscid yellow juice, which is highly glutinous, and resembles gamboge ; the seeds contain a dark red oil, known as huile-amère.

Constituents.—The heart wood contains a garnet-red resin insoluble in water, soluble in alcohol, chloroform and alkalies; sparingly soluble in benzol and in ether.

Preparation.—Juice of leaves; decoction of the bark (1 in 10). Dose, 1 to 2 ounces.

Actions and uses.—Alterative and stimulant ; the decoction is given internally in scabies and other skin diseases. Externally the juice of leaves is applied in scabies, psoriasis, &c.; varalians of leaves are applied to rheumatic and painful swollen joints.

Sterculiaceæ.—The silk-cotton, or Murada Singa family.

Sterculiaceæ, from stercus, " excrement," in allusion to the fœtid odour of flowers or fruits of some of the species.

Characters.—Trees or shrubs, Leaves alternate, simple or compound ; flowers white, red or yellow, regular or irregular, perfect or abortive and unisexual ; petals sometimes absent ; stamens united by their filaments into a column, indefinite ; anthers, 2-celled, extrose; fruits a number of follicles or capsular, rarely baccate ; seeds with fleshy and oily albumen ; embryo straight or curved.

Habitat.—Tropics and temperate climates.

Properties similar to those of malvaceæ, generally mucilaginous, demulcent and emollient ; some are considered emetic, diuretic and purgative.

Abroma Augusta.

Habitat.—India.

Parts used.—The root and sap of the bark.

Vernacular.—Beng.—Ulat-Kambal. Bomb.—Olak Tambol. Eng.—Devil's cotton.

Characters.—Small tree or shrub ; leaves ovate, oblong and serrulate, under-side tomentose or scabrous ; flowers dark-purple and drooping ; fruit dry, 5-celled, capsular, with 5 truncated wings, dehiscent when ripe, each cell containing numerous black seeds ; roots with thick, brown, fibrous bark, exuding, when cut, a thick gummy substance. Dose of the root, 30 to 60 grs. The sap, 10 to 30 grs.

Constituents.—The root-bark contains gum, wax, a non-crystalline extractive matter and ash 11·64 p.c., but no manganese.

Actions and uses.—The root and the sap are uterine tonic and emmenagogue ; with black pepper given in congestive and neuralgic dysmenorrhœa and amenorrhœa, either given a week before or during menstruation. It is a very valuable substitute for hydrastis, viburnum, and pulsatilla.

Adansonia Digitata—The Baobab tree.

Habitat.—Cultivated in India.

Parts used.—The pulp of the fruit, bark and leaves.

Vernacular.—Arab.—Habhabu, Bahobab. Burm.—Bila-magisi. Duk.—Gorikha-amali, khatyan. Eng.—Monkey bread, Ethiopian sour gourd. Guz.—Chora Amala, Gorakha Chincha, Sumpura (the fruit). Hind.—Rookha, Hathi-khatiyan, Gorak-amli, Mar.—Churi Chintza, Gorakh-chinch. Tam.—Papara pulia maram. Anai-puliya. Senegal—El-omarah, oufa. The fruits El-Kongles.

Gorukha chinch.—Gorukha, the name of a Hindoo monk of old, and chinch, tamarind. In allusion to the old monk, who is said to have taught his disciples under this tree. The fruits, when dried (shells), are used as water pots by the monks.

Hathi Khatiyan—Hathi, elephant, and Katiyan, fibre. It means elephant's flax, in allusion to the great strength of the fibre prepared from its bark.

Characters.—Tree with trunk of an enormous size ; fruit, bottle or cucumber-shaped ; shell hard, woody, light and covered with dull green felt-like yellowish down or brown hairs. The interior of the fruit consists of a soft, corky substance, tough and fibrous in structure and a sub-acid pulp, of a brownish red colour. It consists of mucilage, which is firmly adherent to and surrounds the seed. The seeds are enclosed in a horny shell ; they are kidney-shaped, rough externally, of a rusty red colour, acid flavour and sour taste. The bark yields a white semi-fluid gum, which is colourless, tasteless and insoluble in water. It contains calcium oxalate and resin.

Constituents.—The pulp contains phlobaphenes, mucilage and gum, glucose, tartrate and acetate of potash, and other salts, &c. The pericarp contains phlobaphene, albuminoids, gum, colouring matter, carbonate of potash and soda, &c. The leaves contain wax, glucose, salts, gum and albuminoids. The bark contains wax, tannin, gum, albuminoids, carbonate and chloride of sodium and potassium and a glucoside adansonin antagonistic to strophanthus.

Preparation.—Decoction of bark (1 in 10). Dose, 1 to 2 ozs.

Actions and uses.—The pulp of the fruit is astringent and demulcent, given in dyspepsia, diarrhœa, dysentery, cough and other pulmonary affections. The bark is demulcent and aperient and given for similar purposes. As a refrigerant (acid drink), like tamarind, the pulp is used in fevers. The leaves are used as varalians in painful swellings. The dry powder of the leaves, called Lallo, is used to check excessive perspiration. Dose, 5 to 15 grs.

Bombax Malabaricum—B. Heptaphyllum.

Habitat.—India, tropical.

Parts used.—The gum and root.

Vernacular.—Beng.—Rakto-semul. Bomb.—Musta-semul (the gum), Supari-ka-phul. Burm.—Lapan-La-i. Can.—Mullu, Burraul-mara, Macharas. Cing.—Kattu-Imbal. Duk.—Sopari-ka-phul, Kanton-ka-Khatyan. Eng.—Red silk-cotton tree. Guz.—Shemalo (the gum), Mocharas. Hind.—Ragat-semul, Mocharas, Supari-ka-phul. Mar.—Sairi. Malyal.—Mulu-elavu. Panj.—Sum. Sans.—Mocha, Kanta-kadruma, Shemalo, Solmali-mocharas. Duk.—Semal, Kantonka Khatyan. Tam.—Illavam. Tel.—Buruga-manu, Mocharas (gum).

Kanta-kudruma, means a tree with hard conical prickles. Sopari-ka-phul—Mocharas a name given to the gum, is from sopari—areca catechu, in allusion to the fact that children masticate the blunt thorns of B. Malabaricum.

Characters.—Tree large, remarkable for its height, and covered with hard conical prickles, deciduous when in flowers ; flowers large, red, bright, with a green cup-shaped calyx, followed by egg-shaped green capsules ; seeds numerous, of a black colour, and covered by long silky hairs, or a quantity of fine cotton ; this cotton is not used like ordinary cotton on account of smoothness and want of adhesion between fibres.

Mocharas is not a normal juice, but the product of diseased action, which consists in the proliferation of the cells of the bark ; the gum only exudes from the bark, which has been so injured by decay or by insects. On incisions into the diseased bark, a number of small cavities are seen, which contain a jelly-like substance, some granular matter and starch. Thus in appearance Mocharas resembles galls more than gum ; when first exuded it is in whitish fungous pieces, which gradually turn red, and finally mahogany-like. In some pieces holes made by insects are distinctly seen, the galls thus resembling kakada-singa. It is very brittle, the fractured surface being resinous-looking and red. The taste astringent, and resembles chikani sopari. The root is as large as a carrot ; bark dark-brown externally and reddish within, fibrous, tough and studded with a soft spongy substance. The taste is feebly astringent, and gummy or mucilaginous. Dose of the gum, 10 to 40 grs.

Constituents.—The seeds yield 25 p.c. of a sweet non-drying oil, of a light yellowish brown colour which contains crystalline, insoluble fatty acids 92·8 p.c. The cake of the seeds contains nitrogenous compounds, fat, extractive matter, woody fibre and ash.

Preparation.—Decoction of root (1 in 20). Dose, 1 to 2 ozs.

Actions and uses.—The root is astringent, alterative, demulcent and restorative, used in diarrhœa, dysentery and menorrhagia ; also in high-coloured urine with copious deposit. As an alterative and restorative, the natives use a pakh (confection) in tuberculosis of the lungs and other wasting diseases. The gum is used as an astringent and demulcent for the same purposes, but more especially in dysentery, menorrhagia and in diarrhœa of children. Native women use it largely after delivery to stop menses during lactation. It is a chief ingredient in various restorative, expectorant and aphrodisiac confections. Found to be a valuable substitute for gum kino, red gum, &c.

Eriodendron Anfractuosum.

Habitat.—Asia and Africa.

Parts used.—The root and gum.

Vernacular.—Beng.—Shwet Shimool. Burm.—Tembo-le-bin. Can.—Buramara. Cing.—Imbul, Pulim. Duk.—Khatyan. Eng.—White silk cotton tree. Hind.—Hattian, Safed-semul, Tulaper. Guz.—Dholo-shemlo. Maleal.—Paniala, Mullila-pula. Mar.—Shamieula, Pandhra Saur. Sans.—Sveta-shelmah. Tam.—Elavum-maram. Tel.—Buruga-chettu.

Characters.—The tree yields a dark coloured opaque gum, insoluble in water. This plant is sometimes preferred to the red silk variety.

Constituents.—Albuminoids, fat, non-nitrogenous extractive. The ash contains potash and phosphoric acid.

Preparation.—Decoction of root (1 in 10). Dose, 2 to 4 drs. Gum.—Dose, 10 to 90 grs.

Actions and uses.—The young roots and fruits are demulcent and astringent, and used in diarrhœa, dysentery and menorrhagia. The gum (Hattian-ka-gond) is used in bowel complaints.

Helicteres Isora.

Habitat.—Central and Western India, Western Peninsula, Ceylon.

Parts used.—The fruit and root-bark.

Vernacular.—Beng.—Atmorha. Bomb.—Murada Siaga. Duk.—Dhamni Kavuna. Eng.—East Indian screw plant. Cing.—Leeviya gaha. Guz.—Mriga Shing. Hind.—Kupaise, Joa-ka-phal, Marorphali. Mar.—Varkati, Dhamani, Maedasingi. Sans.—Avurtuni Mrigashinga. Tel.—Sayamali. Tam.—Valambirikai. Pers.—Pechak, Burkisht Hisht bar.

Mriga Shinga, mruga,-deer, and shenga, a horn, deer's horn, from the twisted form of the carpels.

Characters.—The tree resembles common hazel tree; fruit covered with a yellowish brown tomentum, thickest at the base. The stalk is long and club-shaped; carpels five, slender, angular and extending from the stalk. Each carpel is of a greenish brown colour, and twined round the other, giving the whole fruit the shape of a corkscrew, and opening longitudinally in front; seeds many, in a single row, black rhomboid, highly polished, taste mucilaginous and slightly bitter; root-bark dark brown and studded with round tubercles. Dose of the powdered fruit, 5 to 15 grs.

Preparation.—Liniment from powdered fruit. Decoction of root (1 in 10). Dose, ½ to 1 oz.

Actions and uses.—Demulcent and mildly astringent. Powdered fruit is given with other drugs to stop griping in the bowels and flatulence in children. The root-bark is given in diabetes. The root may be substituted for that of althæa. The Hindus use the powder of the root with castor-oil as an application inside the ears in offensive sores and discharges.

Pentapetes Phœnicea.

Habitat.—The hotter parts of India.

Part used.—The capsules.

Vernacular.—Hind.—Dopahariya. Beng.—Katcula, Bandhuli. Mar.—Tambri-dufari. Tam.—Naga-pu. Sans.—Bandhuka, Bandhu-jiva, Arka Vallubha Pushparakta.

Bhandhujiva, living in association or groups. Arka Vallabha, beloved of the sun. Pushparakta, red flowered.

Characters.—Plant found in wet places during the monsoon. Fruit capsular; capsules mucilaginous, sub-globose, bristly, 5-celled, 5-valved; calyx inferior, 5-partite, bristly; cell containing 8 to 12 seeds, arranged in vertical rows.

Actions and uses.—Demulcent, given in coughs and scalding in the urine.

Pterospermum Suberifolium.

Habitat.—India. Godaveri forests, Ginji Hills.

Part used.—Flowers.

Vernacular.—Cing.—Welaug gas. Tam.—Teddi maram. Tel—Nolika-chettu. Hind.—Muchkand. Sans.—Much-kunda.

Much Kunda muchu—mungo, means mucus, and kund, a sweet smelling flower.

Characters.—Flowers white, fragrant. They render water gelatinous.

Actions and uses.—The flowers are used externally, as a paste in hemi-crania.

Pterospermum Acerifolium.

Habitat.—India, Assam.

Parts used.—Flowers, bark and leaf.

Vernacular.—Sans.—Karnikara. Hind.—Kamar-Kath-champa. Beng.—Kanak-champa. Sikkim—Hathepaila. Nagee. Burm.—Toung-jihet-woon.

Preparation.—Bhasm (ash).

Actions and uses.—The white tomentum from the under surface of the leaf is used as a hæmostatic to stop bleeding. The Bhasm, mixed with kamala, is used as an application in suppurating small-pox.

Sterculia Acuminata—Kola Acuminata.

Female Kola.—Gongo nuts, kola nuts, guru nuts.

Habitat.—Tropical forests of West Indies, Africa, Soudan, Senegambia, Angola.

Parts used.—The seed or nut.

Characters.—Tree handsome and large; flowers yellow, with 5 follicles, each containing one seed. Seeds, one inch long, and flattened testa, brownish with blackish spots; odour nutmeg like; taste aromatic. The green canals are present in the pith and bark. Dose, powdered nuts, 15 to 20 grains.

Constituents.—Caffeine, in much larger proportion than in any member of the group except guarana. Theobromine and a glucoside—kolanin, which splits up in the presence of a ferment into free caffeine and glucose; also starch, sugar, gum, proteids, fat, volatile oil, and tannic acid. Kolanin is decomposed by saliva and gastric juice.

Preparations.—Tincture (1 in 5). Dose, ½ to 1 drm. Extract. Dose, 3 to 10 grains. Fluid extract. Dose, 10 to 30 minims. Kola Wine. Dose, 1 to 2 ounces. Neo Kola is a coloured powder from kola nuts, flavoured with vanilla and used as a beverage. Kolatina, paste of Kola nuts. Dose, 1 to 2 drs.

Physiological Action.—Kola is a nervine stimulant, tonic and astringent. The fresh nuts are used as food and as aphrodisiac. This latter property is due to their containing essential oil which is absent in the dry nuts. It is eaten to ward off fatigue and depression, to support the strength, to allay inordinate appetite, to assuage thirst, to promote digestion, and render those using it cheerful in spirits and capable of prolonged fatigue in the same manner as coca leaves.

Therapeutics.—Like guarana and coca it is used in gastric catarrh dyspepsia of alcoholism, sea sickness and syphilis. It counteracts the intoxicating influence of alcohol, and the depressing effects of tobacco. It is employed in cardiac and nervous asthma. It contains tannin, and hence given in chronic diarrhœa and in gastro-intestinal irritation. As an aphrodisiac kola is used to allay the sense of exhaustion, and thus stimulate the sexual appetite. In dipsomania, wasting diseases, neurasthenia, and cephalalgia where caffeine is indicated, it is of benefit. It is a valuable adjunct to the administration of mercury and iodides, and a good substitute for tea or coffee. Kolanin is a tonic and stimulant given for neurasthenia and migraine.

Remarks.—The preparations of Kola should be taken at or between meals.

Sterculia Fœtida.

Habitat.—Concan, Malabar, Ceylon.

Parts used.—The leaves, fruit and bark.

Vernacular.—Eng.—Hell's Incense, Wild almond. Hind.—Jangli badam. Mah.—Narakha Uda, Narkya Uda. Tam.—Pinari maram, Kudrap dukhu.

Kudrap-dukku—resemblance of its large follicle to the testicle of a horse.

Characters.—Leaves compound, peltate, leaflets 7 to 9, oblong lanceolate, acuminate; wood of a light brown colour, soft and fibrous; the odour resembles that of human ordure, and hence the name. carpels oblong, many seeded; seeds elliptical, an inch long and covered with a hard brown shell which is velvety within, covered by a felt like skin, and enclosing an oily white kernel. The skin softens in water like bassorin. Flowers panicled, brownish red at the base, and of a stercoraceous odour.

Constituents.—The kernel contains fixed oil, 40 p.c., and starch. The oil is thick, pale yellow, bland and non-drying, depositing crystalline solid fats, and fatty acids, consisting of oleic, and small quantity of lauric acids.

Actions and uses.—The fruit is demulcent and astringent, and used in gonorrhœa. The leaves and bark are aperient, diaphoretic, diuretic, and used in dropsy, rheumatism &c. The seeds are used for eating.

Sterculia Urens.

Habitat.—Throughout India, Ceylon.

Part used.—The gum.

Vernacular.—Beng.—Buli. Can.—Penari. Hind.—Bâli, gûlû, kûlû, karai, kalru, kur katila, katira. Guz.—Karai. Mar.—Pandrûk, kâvali, kundūl. Sans.—Balika. Tel—Kalvi, Thabsû. Tam.—Valley putali.

Characters.—Often confounded with cochlospermum gossypium. The seeds yield an oil containing much stearin. A gum exudes from young branches, from panicled inflorescence and from petioles of leaves; also from large canals in the pith and bark, where it is contained in the tissues. It is a soft solid mass, soluble in cold water, forming a milky solution.

Constituents.—Mucic acid, obtained by treating gum with nitric acid, and ash 4 p.c.

Actions and uses.—The gum is used for making native sweetmeats; the mucilage has no adhesive power. Its uses are similar to those of Tragacanth.

Sterculia Scaphigera.

Vernacular.—Chinese—Ta-hai-tsze, Boatam-paijang.

Characters.—The fruit contains large quantity of gum. The fruit is elongated, ovoid and terminates at the lower extremity by a large oblique cicatrix; externally dark brown, deeply wrinkled; pericarp like thin epidermis, containing dark resinous looking pulp and 2 cotyledons covered by a thin fragile shell. On maceration, the pericarp swells, forming a large gelationous mass.

Constituents.—The pericarp contains a green oil, bassorin, a brown astringent matter and mucilage; the nucleus contains cellular tissue, fatty matter, bitter extractive and starch.

Actions and uses.—Similar to those of Tragacanth.

Byttneriaceæ.

The chocolate family. Trees, shrubs, or under shrubs, sometimes climbing. Leaves simple, alternate; calyx valvate, corolla absent, stamens hypogynous, definite; filaments united; anthers 2-celled introse. Confounded with sterculiaceæ, malvaceæ, and Tiliaceæ.

Habitat.—Tropical plants.

Properties.—Mucilaginous. Some species bear edible fruits.

Theobroma Cacao, B. P.

Theobroma. Theos, a god; and Broma, food—food for the Gods, in allusion to its delicious qualities.

Habitat.—South America, Brazil, Mexico, West Indies, Tropics.

Parts used.—A concrete oil expressed from the seeds, oleum theobromatis, B. P., cacao butter or oil of Theobroma.

Characters.—Fruit large, fusiform, with ten shallow furrows and with blunt ridges covered with tubercles, single or 2 or 3 together. Pericarp or shell thick, tough and 5-celled. Seeds many, closely packed in tears, size that of an almond; they are angular and pressed against one another and immersed in the pulp, which is copious, sweet and buttery. From the pulp is prepared a beverage or a distilled spirit. 100 parts of seeds contain 12 parts of shells or thin husks which envelope the seeds and 88 parts of kernels. In the seed is found theobromine, resembling caffeine. Cocoa, otherwise known as rock cocoa, consists of the seeds with husks roasted, deprived of the oil, ground in a mill mixed with flour of rice, barley and sugar, and put up in a powdered form. Chocolate contains cocoa mixed with sugar, cloves, sassafras nuts, vanilla, and arnatto as a colouring agent, made into a paste and cast into moulds, or pressed in cakes. The aroma in chocolate is due to the aromatic principle which develops when the leaves are roasted.

Chocolate is often adulterated with starch, barley, rice flour, lard &c. Both cocoa and chocolate are used in the preparation of agreeable beverages. The beverages often disagree, as they contain fatty and oily substances.

Constituents.—The seeds contain about 50 p.c. of a concrete fat or a fixed oil, which is known as butter of cocao or oleum theobromatis; starch 16 p.c.; an alkaloid theobromine 2 to 4 p.c.; caffeine and proteids 18 p.c.; sugar, colouring matter and ash 3 to 4 p.c. Butter of cocao, oil of theobroma. To obtain it, warm or dry the seeds or bury them in a heap for a few days in a box, and then dry; next press them through rollers and extract the oil. The oil may also be extracted by expression, by decoction or by solution in chloroform or ether.

Characters.—A yellowish white solid concrete mass, breaking with a smooth fracture, and has the faint odour of cocoa; the taste is bland and agreeable; it has a neutral reaction. It is soluble in alcohol, ether and oil of turpentine and insoluble in water. The oil contains stearine, and a little oleine laurin, arachin, resin, and glycerides of formic and butyric acids. Dose, ½ to 1 dr.

Theobromine—Demethylxanthine is an alkaloid forming salt (closely allied to caffein). To obtain it, exhaust the kernels with hot water, add acetate of lead and filter the precipitate; then remove lead by sulphuretted hydrogen, treat the residue with alcohol and evaporate. It may be synthetically obtained from xanthine, a substance nearly related to uric acid. A crystalline white powder of a bitter taste; sparingly soluble in alcohol, chloroform, water and ether. Dose, 1 to 5 grs.

Preparations of the oil.—Emulsion; suppositories; Ceratum theobromine or red salve; to prepare which melt together, cocoa butter 35, white wax 35, oil of almonds 30, carmine, oil of rose and ammonia water.

Preparations of Theobromine.—Diuretin—a combination with sodium salicylate. Uropherine, a combination of theobromine with lithium salicylate or with lithium benzoate. Iodo theobromine, a combination of sodium salicylate and sodium iodide with theobromine.

Actions and uses.—The concrete oil is nutrient, emollient and demulcent, generally used as an excipient for suppositories, pessaries, ointments &c.; used externally for abrasions and inflamed surfaces. The alkaloid theobromine and its salts are diuretic and nervine stimulant, generally given with nitro-glycerine, menthol, cocaine, apomorphine, caffein, &c. Cocoa is used as a nutritious beverage like tea and coffee, but is less stimulant than the latter. As a diuretic and stimulant it is used in Bright's disease.

Tamaricaceæ.

Tamaricaceæ—The Padvasa or Tamarisk family.

Shrubs or herbs.—Leaves alternate, entire scale-like; flowers small, racemose, spiked; fruits dehiscent and one-celled; seeds numerous comose, and without albumen; embryo straight.

Habitat.—Northern Hemisphere and Mediterranean basin.

Property.—The bark of some of these plants is astringent, bitter and tonic. Some species, as Tamarix Mannifera, contain a saccharine substance known as Mount Sinai Manna, supposed to be an exudation produced in consequence of punctures of species of coccus insects which infest this plant. The ashes of some species contain large quantities of sulphate of soda.

Tamarix Gallica—T. Indica. T. Orientalis. T. Articulata.

Habitat.—Sind, Panjab, Asia, Africa, Europe.

Parts used.—The galls and sugary exudation or manna. The galls are called the Tamar fruits in Persian works.

Vernacular.—Arab.—Asl, Tarfa-Jaz, Mazaj (exudation) gazanjebin. Beng.—Jhav. Bomb.—Mayun (galls). Duk.—Jhav, Ferash. Eng.—Tamarisk. Guz.—Jhav, Hind.—Jhav, Padvas, Ferash. Panj.—Pharwan, Pilchi, Rukh. Pers.—Darakhte zamarisk (manna), Gaz. Sans.—Jhavuka, Shor-gaz. Tam.—Shavukku. Tel.—Shiri-Saru Manu.

Burree mai.—The galls on T. Gallica are smaller than those of Majuphala or true galls. These are of a dirty brown colour, roundish or ovate, irregularly shaped or angled and knotty. They are of various sizes. Sometimes 2 or 3 are united together; some of them present a slender (stalk-like) woody portion at their base; surface tubercled and also wrinkled; the cut surface brownish red; the cavity sometimes containing the insect (coccus manniparus) or a resinous-looking exudation, which is nothing more than excrementitious matter.

Choti mai.—The galls on T. articaluta. The galls are of a darkish brown colour and knotty, resembling a pea in size. They are smaller than those of Burree mai. The shape is globular, not angled. The surface is resinous-looking, round, knotty, of the size of a pea and of yellowish brown colour, of a slight balsamic smell.

The manna occurs in small grains, which are white at first, but have a tendency to liquefy and form a yellow fluid-like honey. The taste is astringent at first, but after a time becomes glutinous. Manna is produced upon tamarisk willow, or oak, in consequence of the puncture of an insect (coccus manniparus). Dose of manna, 1 to 8 drs. Dose of the galls, 5 to 15 grs.

Constituents.—Manna; a thick yellow syrupy liquid containing cane-sugar, glucose, levulose, dextrin and water. Galls contain tannin 50 p. c.

Preparations.—Decoction of galls (1 in 10). Dose, $\frac{1}{2}$ to 4 drs, Tincture (1 in 8). Dose, $\frac{1}{2}$ to 1 dr. Ointment (1 in 5). Compound ointment with opium (14 in 1 of opium).

Actions and uses.—Galls are astringent, used in chronic discharges and watery fluxes, as leucorrhœa, diarrhœa and dysentery; also in hæmorrhagic diathesis. Locally used as pessaries. The manna is a mild aperient and expectorant, and forms an ingredient in aperient and cough mixtures. These galls are as effective as, or rather superior to, the true galls.

Erythroxylaceæ.

General characters.—Tree or shrubs often climbing; leaves usually opposite or whorled, rarely alternate, stipulate and furnished with peltate hairs; flowers perfect or polygamous, arising from imbricated scale-like bracts; calyx persistent without glands; petals with two parallel membranous plates at their base; stigma capitate; fruits drupaceous, woody nut or samaroid; seeds solitary; ovules sessile and anatropal; embryo straight.

Habitat.—Brazil, West Indies.

Properties.—Some are tonic, others purgative, and others stimulant and sedative. The wood of some is used for dyes.

Erythroxylum Coca, B. P.

Habitat.—Peru, Bolivia, Tea districts of India, Ceylon, Java, South America.

Parts used.—The dried leaves of Erythroxylum coca, and other varieties. Cocæ Folia, Coca leaves, B. P., and an alkaloid—Cocaina, B. P.

Erythroxylum—from erythros red and xylon, wood. The wood has a red colour.

Characters.—A small shrub; leaves small, thin, with short petioles 1½ to 3 inches long and 1 to 1½ inches broad, obovate, entire, glabrous, obtuse or emarginate, both sides reticulate, midrib prominent and with a curved line running on each side from base to apex; colour brownish green; odour tea-like; taste slightly bitter and aromatic; on chewing it benumbs the lips and tongue. Should not be confounded with cocao, the leaves of Theobroma cacao. Dose of the leaves, ½ to 2 drs.

Constituents.—Coco leaves contain hygrine, truxil cocaine (truxilline or cocamine); cocaine (a crystalline alkaloid). Benzoyl ecgonine (a derivative of cocaine); aromatic oil, coca tannic acid, coca wax, cinnamylcocaine, &c. In the Java leaves is found an alkaloid tropococaine, a compound of benzoic acid and a base.

Hygrine.—A volatile liquid alkaloid; colour yellow; taste burning; odour that of trimethylamine.

Ecgonine is obtained by heating cocaine with hydrochloric acid, when cocaine will split up into methylic alcohol, benzoic acid and ecgonine.

Cocaina, B. P., Benzoyl-methyl-ecgonine.

To obtain Cocaine treat coca leaves with alcohol and acidulate with sulphuric acid; treat the precipitate or the colouring matter with lime. The aqueous solution contains cocaine sulphate; to this add potassium carbonate, then agitate it with ether and alcohol and decolorize with animal charcoal, evaporate and crystallize. The leaves contain more cocaine than other parts, and a small quantity of other alkaloids. India and Java leaves contain less cocaine and more of the other alkaloids. It occurs in colourless monoclinic prisms, of a bitter taste, followed by sensation of tingling and numbness on the tongue. It has an anæsthetic action on all mucous membranes. It has decided basic properties, combining with acids to form salts. It is almost insoluble in water, insoluble in glycerine, soluble in alcohol (1 in 10), ether (1 in 4), chloroform (1 in $\frac{1}{2}$), castor-oil, olive-oil and other fixed oils (1 in 12), oil of turpentine (1 in 14), benzol, toluol and amylic alcohol (1 in 3), petroleum spirit (1 in 80). Hot water decomposes it, forming an acid solution which contains benzoylecgonine, ecgonine and cocaine benzoate. Cocaine solution kept for a time becomes mouldy and covered with fungi. To avoid this, it is recommended to add boric acid, perchloride of mercury, salicylic acid, camphor, chloroform, thymol, &c. Dose, $\frac{1}{20}$ to $\frac{1}{2}$ gr. in pills or tablets. As pure cocaine is soluble in fats and oils, it is always used externally as local anæsthetic combined with fatty substances.

Preparations.—Ceratum cocainæ (1 in 30) of petroleum; used for burns, pruritis, scalds, urticaria, &c. Bougies of cocaine contains $\frac{1}{2}$ grain with cocao butter, used in urethritis. *Obstetric cones* or suppositories of cocaine. These contain cocaine with boracic acid and butter of cocao. *Collodium cocainæ* contains 2 p.c. of cocaine with flexible collodion. It allays itching *Emplastrum cocainæ*—1 in 50, of lead plaster used for sciatica, neuralgia, corns, bruises, &c. *Cocainæ oleas*—Cocaine oleate contains oleic acid with 5 p.c. of the alkaloid. *Vaselinum Cocainæ* contains cocaine 1 p.c. *Tabellæ cocainæ*—Cocaine tablet $\frac{1}{20}$ grain in each with chocolate, given in sea sickness and in sickness of pregnancy; also in chloroform or alcoholic vomiting.

Salts of cocaine. *Cocainæ citras.*—Hygroscopic crystals, used by dentists. Dose, $\frac{1}{20}$ to $\frac{1}{2}$ gr. *Cocainæ hydrobromidum.* Dose, $\frac{1}{20}$ to $\frac{1}{2}$ gr. *Cocainæ hydroiodidum*—Colourless crystals, slightly soluble in water. Dose, $\frac{1}{20}$ to $\frac{1}{2}$ gr. *Cocainæ hydrochloridum* B. P. cocaine hydrochlorate, cocaine muriate, cocaine hydrochloride. To obtain it, acidulate the extract of coca leaves with sulphuric acid, neutralize with lime and filter. To the filtrate add hydrcohloric acid and recrystallize. It occurs in colourless crystals or white crystalline powder, has a neutral reaction; taste bitter, producing a tingling sensation on the tongue followed by numbness. Applied to the eye, it dilates the pupil. Soluble in cold water (1 in $\frac{1}{2}$), alcohol (1 in 4), in glycerine (1 in 4). Insoluble in olive oil and almost insoluble in ether. Dose, $\frac{1}{5}$ to $\frac{1}{2}$ gr.

Cocaine and chloroform anæsthesia. It consists in the use of chloroform inhalation and at the same time hyodermically injecting cocaine as in operations on the eye and throat. *Lamellæ cocainæ*, B. P., contains $\frac{1}{50}$ grain of cocaine hydrochloride. *Hypodermic tablets*, $\frac{1}{10}$ gr. to $\frac{1}{6}$ gr. in each. *Pilula cocainæ hydrochloridi*, $\frac{1}{5}$ gr. in each with milk-sugar. *Trochisci cocainæ hydrochloridi*, $\frac{1}{12}$ gr. in each. *Injectio cocainæ hypodermica*, B. P., 11 minims contain 1 grain of cocaine hydrochloride, known also as *Liquor cocaine hydrochloratis*, contains about 10 p.c. of the salt mixed with half a grain of salicylic acid to make 6 drachms of the liquor. Dose, 2 to 5 ms. *Pastillus cocainæ hydrochloridi.*—Each contains $\frac{1}{10}$ grain of the salt. *Trochiscus krameriæ et cocainæ*, B.P., contains extract of krameria 1 gr. and cocaine hydrochloride $\frac{1}{20}$ of a gr. in each. Used to allay irritation of the throat. *Cocaine lactas*—A white thick honey-like mass, easily soluble in water; used locally along with the treatment of tuberculous cystitis with lactic acid. *Cocainæ nitras*—Cocaine nitrate. Large colourless crystals, freely soluble in water. Dose, $\frac{1}{20}$ to $\frac{1}{2}$ gr. for hypodermic injection (1 in 50). *Cocainæ salicylas*, cocaine salicylate, minute, snow-white crystals, deliquescent. Used hypodermically in spasmodic asthma. Dose, $\frac{1}{20}$ to $\frac{1}{2}$ gr. *Cocainæ sulphas*. Dose, $\frac{1}{20}$ to $\frac{1}{2}$ gr. *Cocainæ phenas*—Cocaine carbolate, a combination of cocaine and carbolic acid. Honey-like fluid, soluble in alcohol; used as solution 1 p.c. Dose, $\frac{1}{20}$ to $\frac{1}{4}$ gr. in pill. Given internally in catarrh of the stomach. Locally the solution is applied to caried tooth to relieve the pain.

Preparations of coco leaves.

Extractum cocæ liquidum, B.P.—Liquid extract of coca. Syn.—Extractum erythroxyli fluidum. It is not miscible with water unless free from wax. Dose, $\frac{1}{2}$ to 1 dr. *Elixir cocæ*.—1 in 6 of simple elixir. Dose, 1 to 4 drs. *Elixir erythroxyli et Guaranæ*—Each fluid drachm contains $7\frac{1}{2}$ grains of coca and guarana each. Dose, 1 to 2 drs. *Extractum cocæ* (solid). In pills or pastils (4 of leaves to 1 of spirit). Dose, 2 to 15 grs. *Infusum cocæ* (1 in 50). Dose, $\frac{1}{2}$ to 2 ozs. *Tinctura cocæ* (1 in 5). Dose, 1 to 2 fluid drs. *Vinum cocæ* 1 in 8 of sherry. Stimulant, checks vomiting caused by irritable stomach and relieves the pain of gastralgia. Dose, $\frac{1}{4}$ to $\frac{1}{2}$ oz. *Pastillus cocæ extracti* $2\frac{1}{2}$ grs. of the extract in each. Used in aphonia due to relaxed vocal cords.

Physiological actions.—Coca leaves and their preparations are remarkable for their food-replacing properties. They are stimulant, muscular and nervine tonic, diuretic, diaphoretic, and narcotic. Locally anæsthetic and nervine sedative. Coca is anoalgous to tea or coffee, but is more sustaining. In small doses it is an aromatic bitter tonic. It stimulates the stomach, the nervous system, kidneys, respiration and the heart and raises the arterial tension; as a stimulant to the brain it increases its blood-supply, produces wakefulness, also appeases fatigue, hunger and thirst and increases muscular strength and power of endurance. It checks the process of tissue waste and also lessens the quantity of urea. As a diuretic it increases the flow of urine, and also stimulates the intestinal peristalsis. Locally it acts on a limited area. When applied or hypodermically injected its effect on the mucous membrane and the skin is to cause profound anæsthesia. On the tongue it destroys its taste and its sensibility. On the eye it causes dilatation of the pupil, paralysis of accommodation and sometimes ptosis. It resembles in its general action atropine. In both the effects on the heart, respiration, blood, pupils, salivary glands, skin and intestines are alike.

Cocainism, or a cocaine habit, is marked by loss of appetite, loss of sleep, feebleness of mind and body, emaciation, general marasmus, ascites, fetid breath, hallucinations, debasing habits, selfishness, great depravity and insanity.

Therapeutics.—The liquid extract of coca leaves is given in sea sickness, vomiting of pregnancy, in pains due to ulcer of the stomach, gastric indigestion and in hæmorrhage from the bowels. The leaves are smoked to relieve asthma, hay fever and sore throat. The extract is given internally in melancholia, epilepsy, insanity, diabetes, spermatorrhœa, &c. In excessive doses coca is injurious like opium or fermented liquors. In moderate doses it counteracts the injurious effects of tobacco and alcohol. Coca wine is an agreeable stomachic stimulant. It checks gastric irritation and vomiting, and relieves the pain of gastralgia. It relieves hoarseness of voice in singers and speakers; and is also given in seminal debility. In diabetes it has been tried in place of codea. It steadies the nerves of excitable persons. Its leaves may be smoked as cigars. Cocaine hydrochloride is used as a paint or as an hypodermic injection to benumb the pains of inflamed parts; also applied to deaden the sensibility of healthy parts, as the eye, ear, nose, urethra, uterus, &c. In coryza a 4 p. c. solution is applied to the nostrils. In gonorrhœa 2 p.c. solution is injected into the urethra. It is sometimes used as an injection into the back in hydrophobia, tetanus, incontinence of urine, lead colic, sciatica, lumbago, in ophthalmic surgery and also in minor operations. Locally the solution or the oleate is applied to burns, painful ulcers, fissures of anus, hæmorrhoids, &c. As vaginal pessaries it is used in various forms of retarded parturition where the expulsive pains are absent or deficient. Its infusion is likewise used as an application to the throat or as an injection into the bladder before lithotrity or into the urethra before the passage of sounds or catheters, and to the gums for teeth extraction. To have a marked effect it should reach the terminal filaments of sensory nerves. In moles and warts 6 grains to a drachm of glycerine should be used locally before the application of nitric acid. The oleate of cocaine is a good application in pruritis ani or vaginæ and in skin diseases attended with itching.

Erythroxylon Monogynum. E. Indicum.

Habitat.—Western Peninsula, Ceylon, Cuddapah District.

Parts used.—The wood bark and leaves.

Vernacular.—Can.—Adavi, goranti. Eng.—Red cedar, bastard sandal or cedar. Tam.—Tevadarum, Devdarune.

Cedar in allusion to the wood being fragrant like cedar.

Characters.—Shrub. Bark pale and resinous; leaves cuneate, obovate; wood fragrant.

Constituents.—No cocaine, but the leaves contain a bitter and tonic alkaloid which may have sustaining property.

Preparations.—Infusion of leaves (1 in 20). Dose, ½ to 1 oz. Decoction of the bark (1 in 10). Dose, ½ to 1 oz.

Actions and uses.—Leaves are refrigerant, bitter tonic and nutrient, possessing properties similar to those of coca. The bark is also a tonic; the leaves are eaten during famine times in India.

Cedrelaceæ.

The mahogany or Toon tree, or Rohana chhala family. It is composed of large trees; leaves alternate, pinnate, exstipulate and entire; flowers generally numerous; fruits capsular, dehiscent.

Habitat.—Tropical parts of America and India.

The properties of this order are aromatic, tonic, astringent, febrifuge and fragrant. Many are valuable timber trees.

Cedrela Toona.

Habitat.—Peninsula and Bengal.

Parts used.—The bark, gum and flowers.

Vernacular.—Bombay.—Kooruk. Beng.—Toon. Burm.—Thit-ka-du. Can.—Sauolamara Tanda. Eng.—Indian mahogany, or white cedar, or toon tree. Hind.—Toona. Malyal.—Arana maram. Mar.—Kooruk. Sans.—Tunna-Nandevreksha. Tam.—Wunjooli maram. Tel.—Nandi.

Characters.—Bark smooth and grey; flowers small, yellow and sweet scented like honey; gum transparent, in stalactiform masses, colour yellow, surface polished. It first swells and then dissolves in water, forming a thick gelatinous mucilage; seeds numerous, imbricated and winged.

Constituents.—Resin, extractive matter, gum, &c.

Preparation.—Decoction (1 in 10). Dose, 1 to 2 ozs.

Actions and uses.—Fruit and bark astringent, but not bitter. With bonduc nut as a tonic and antiperiodic it is given in fevers, rheumatism and dysentery; flowers are emmenagogue, and given in disordered menstruation; the wood is used in making surgical instruments; it must not be mistaken for thuja, which is incorrectly called white cedar.

Chloroxylon Swietenia.

Habitat.—Ceylon, Western Peninsula.

Part used.—The bark.

Vernacular.—Eng.—Satin wood. Cing.—Buruta. Hind.—Rakata Rohidi, Ragatrora. Mar.—Haladarava, Bhiree. Tam.—Mududa Vummaai, Kodavah. Tel.—Biluda-parasham.

Characters.—The tuber of the bark is dark-brown and very rough from the presence of elliptical corky lentils, which are loosely attached. When separated they leave a smooth pale surface within. It yields a kind of gum, dark reddish brown or amber coloured, which is allied to gum-arabic, is insoluble in water, swells and becomes a whitish jelly. The wood is the satin wood of India used in making stethoscopes.

Constituents.—The bark contains tannin.

Preparation.—Decoction (1 in 20). Dose, ½ to 1 oz.

Actions and uses.—Astringent and anodyne, used for sprains, contusions and for painful joints.

Soymida Febrifuga, Swietenia Febrifuga, S. Rubra.

Habitat.—India, Ceylon.

Parts used.—The bark.

Vernacular.—Eng.—Bastard cedar, redwood tree. Beng.—Rohana. Hind.—Rohana, Rohitaka. Sans.—Patranga. Can.—Swamy. Mur.—Rohine Rheyu. Tam.—Shem. Tel.—Sunu, Sonuda.

Characters.—Bark in tubular quills, about an inch in diameter. Externally of a brown colour, smooth, with numerous cracks and covered with small warty growths, which, when they fall off, leave brown rings; taste bitter and astrrngent. Dose, 10 to 20 grs.

Constituents.—It contains a bitter principle, colourless resinous matter, starch and tannic and gallic acids.

Preparation.—Decoction (1 in 20). Dose, ½ to 1 oz. Tincture (1 in 8). Dose, ½ to 1 dr.

Actions and uses.—Bitter tonic, astringent and antiperiodic, like Peruvian bark; in large doses it leads to vertigo and stupor; given in intermittent fevers, dysentery, general debility and diarrhœa. As an injection or a wash, its decoction is used in leucorrhœa, gonorrhœa and as a gargle in sore throat.

Canellaceæ.

The canella order. Leaves alternate; anthers longitudinal and dehiscent; absence of disk, presence of a style; seeds albuminous; flowers unsymmetrical; albumen horny.

Habitat.—West Indies and America.

Properties.— Aromatic, stimulant and tonic.

Canella Alba.

Laurel-leaved canella, wild cinnamon.

Habitat.—West Indies.

Part used.—The bark canellæ cortex—canella bark. Spurious winter's bark.

Characters.—Flowers white and aromatic; fruit (berries) blackish; bark whitish, in quills, 6 to 24 inches long, grey coloured. The corky layer is orange-red and marked with scars; inside striated with resin cells; the odour between that of cloves and cinnamon; taste bitter and biting. Dose, 15 to 30 grs.

Constituents.—Volatile oil, resin, bitter principle, starch, mannite sugar; the oil is sometimes substituted for oil of cloves.

Preparation.—Powder.

Actions and uses.—Aromatic, tonic and stimulant; given in gout, rheumatism, secondary syphilis, menorrhagia, amenorrhœa, and gastric debility; generally given with aloes.

Meliaceæ.

The bead tree, nima or margosa family.

Trees or shrubs ; leaves exstipulate, alternate, pinnate, or simple, generally oblique and serrated ; flowers small and very fragrant ; fruits baccate, capsular or drupaceous ; seeds few, arillate, exalbuminous.

Habitat.—Tropics.

Properties.—The plants of this order are remarkable for their bitter, tonic and astringent properties ; some are powerful purgatives ; some bear edible fruits ; some species are poisonous.

Aglaia Roxburghiana.

Habitat.—Western India, Ceylon.

Part used.—The seeds.

Vernacular.—Can.—Totilla-kayi. Hind.—Priangu. Sans.—Priyanga, Syama, Kantalva, Nandini.

Characters.—Fruit subglobose or pilose, 1 to 2-celled and 1 to 2-seeded ; buff-coloured when fresh, brown and wrinkled when dry ; shell thin, with an aril, pink and fleshy ; seeds flat, irregular and slightly convex, ½ inch in diameter ; odour aromatic and astringent.

Constituents.—Quercitannic acid and ash.

Preparation.—Infusion (1 in 20). Dose, 1 to 2 ozs.

Actions and uses.—Refrigerant and astringent ; used in fevers, diarrhœa and liver affections ; as an alterative it is given in leprosy.

Carapa moluccensis, Granatum littoreum. A tree of the muddy sea coasts of India and Ceylon. The Malays use the bark, which is bitter and astringent, in colic, diarrhœa and other abdominal diseases.

Amoora Rohituka, Andersonia Rohituka, Meleacea Wightiana.

Habitat.—Assam, Oudh, Western Peninsula.

Part used.—The bark.

Vernacular.—Assam.—Amora-amari. Beng.—Tiktaraj. Burm.—Chayau-ka-yo. Can.—Muttala gida. Cing.—Hingul-gas. Hind.—Harrin-hara, Sohaga. Maleal.—Chemmara Mar.—Rohituka Sans.—Rohituka, Rohini, Rohera, Plihagna, Plihashatru. Tam.—Shem-maram. Tel.—Chawa-manu, Rohitaka.

Pliha-ghna, spleen destroyer ; Pliha-shatru, enemy to spleen.

Characters.—Fruit dull-yellow or reddish, 3-celled, containing 3 seeds ; seeds chestnut-coloured, enclosed in thick fleshy arilla ; bark blackish brown, externally covered with very rough elliptical warty projections and minute fissures ; substance of the bark deep, reddish brown and of a striated short fracture. Fresh bark soft and can easily be cut. Taste very astringent.

Constituents.—Two yellow resins, starch, colouring matter, tannin and salts ; both resins are soluble in ether, but one is insoluble in alcohol and alkaline solutions the other is soluble in both these liquids, and is of an acid nature.

Preparation.—Decoction (1 in 10). Dose, ½ to 1 oz.

Actions and uses.—Alterative, astringent and tonic, given in enlarged glands, as liver and spleen, in corpulence and in general debility.

Melia Azedarach, M. Bukayun, M. Sempervires.

Habitat.—North of India, Bengal, Mysore, Bombay, China, United States.

Parts used.—The root-bark, gum, leaves, flowers, fruit and oil of the seeds.

Vernacular—Arab.—Mab-ul-dan (the seed). Beng.—Maha nimb, Ghora nim. Burm.—Simbo Karva. Can.—Bavena Betta-da. Cing.—Luna-middella. Duk.—Gora nimb. Eng.—Persian lilac, Pride of China, Evergreen bead tree. Guz.—Bakayan. Hind.—Bakayan, Maha nimb. Malayal.—Malai vempu. Mar.—Goru-nima, Dongracha lim. Panj.—Drek. Pers.—Darakat-i-azad, Tak. Sans.—Hemadruma Parvat nimba, Arishta. Tam,—Male Vembu. Tel.—Vepa manu, Nimbarun. Tabrishtan.—Takhak. Shiraz—Taghak.

Characters.—The root-bark, when fresh is curved or quilled, thick spongy and warty; externally of a dark-brown colour, with irregular ridges ; internally brown or covered with white striæ ; taste astringent, also bitter and nauseous. The bark yields a gum,which is in large tears, the surface cracked and fissured, the pieces are vermiform, colour pale yellow or amber. It is soluble in water, forming a pale-coloured mucilage ; leaves bi-pinnate ; leaflets obliquely ovate, lanceolate, acute, serrated and glabrous ; flowers small, purple, lilac-coloured, sweet-scented and fragrant ; fruit a drupe when dry, oblong or elliptical, colour reddish, dark brown or yellow of the size of cherries ; epidermis, shining and wrinkled ; pulp poisonous, glutinous to the touch and of a disagreeable smell; nut hard, of a yellowish brown colour, 5-celled, each cell containing a seed enclosed in a dark coloured testa ; seed of the shape and size of a wheat grain, oblong, compressed at the upper part and slightly pointed, generally of a pale brown colour; cotyledon greyish white and oily; on crushing the seed the odour is very acid and disagreeable. Dose of the root, 15 to 60 grs.

Constituents.—Noncrystalline resinous substance—the active principle, sugar, tannin, &c.

Preparation.—Decoction of the fresh bark (1 in 10). Dose, ½ to 1 oz.

Actions and uses.—In small doses, the bark is a bitter tonic, astringent, antiperiodic, anthelmintic, given to children in round worms, and to adults in fever and indigestion ; leaves and flowers are alterative and diuretic. The juice of the leaves is used in fevers, dyspepsia, general debility, jaundice, worms, scrofula, boils, leprosy, &c. Externally the flowers and leaves are discutients ; as a poultice they are made warm and applied to the head in nervous headaches. A poultice of the flowers is said to kill lice and to cure eruptions of the scalp ; a paste of the leaves is applied hot to unhealthy ulcers, to indolent scrofulous glands and to pustular eruptions. The drug is a narcotic poison in large doses, producing giddiness, dimness of sight, mental confusion, stupor, dilated pupils and stertor. It also acts as a gastro-intestinal irritant, producing vomiting and purging.

Azadirachta Indica. Melia Azadirachta.

Habitat.—Himalaya, Persia.

Parts used.—The root-bark, fruit, flowers, leaves, gum and oil of seeds.

Vernacular.—Ceylon—Kohomba. Duk., Beng.—Nim. Burm.—Kamakha, Them-bauma. Can.—Bevinamara, Isa-bevu. Cing.—Telko-homba. Chin.—Lientaze, Ku-lien-taze. Eng.—Ash-leaved bead tree, morgosa, Indian lilac. Guz.—Limbado. Hind.—Nim. Maleal —Weppa, Aria Bepon. Mar.—Limba. Pers.—Azaddarakhti-Hindi. Sans.—Nimba. Tam.—Vembu, Vepa Veypam. Tel.—Yeppa Nimbarnu.

Characters.—Bark coarsely fibrous ; externally rough, fissured and of a rusty grey colour ; internally yellow and foliaceous, readily separated into thin layers ; taste bitter and astringent. The petioles are thickened at the base, slender, round and about a foot in length; surface of a brownish colour and longitudinally furrowed, taste bitter ; flowers small, darkish brown when dry and tubular ; leaves pinnate ; leaflets oblique, dentate, lanceolate and smooth on both surfaces, taste very bitter; fruit when ripe is purple, one-celled, one-seeded, fleshy within, with a hard, woody shell containing an oily bitter kernel, greenish white with a brown testa ; dried fruit resembling small raisin, dark, oval and slightly oblong; surface wrinkled; pulp adherent to the stone; seeds of a brownish white colour, angular and pointed at the top, surface reticulated and fibrous ; epicarp very brittle and containing one or two almond coloured kernels, which are oily and nauseously bitter ; the expressed oil from the seeds contains a large amount of sulphur; the colour is pale yellow, odour garlic-like, taste very bitter. It coagulates at a low temperature without losing its transparency. The gum is yellowish, in vermiform pieces.

Constituents.—The seeds contain a resinous oil known as margosa or neem oil. The bark contains a neutral resinous bitter principle, Margosine, non-crystalline and without alkaloidal properties, catechin, gum, sugar and tannin.

Margosine is obtained by exhausting the bark with alcohol, and precipitating the solution with water. The precipitate is next purified by solution of benzene, carbon sulphide, ether and alcohol.

Resinous oil, Margosa or neem oil. The recently expressed oil from the seeds, when exposed for some time, deposits a white sediment (an alcoholic bitter extract). It is easily soluble in ether, chloroform, carbon bisulphide, benzole, &c. When repeatedly agitated with alcohol it loses its bitterness and its alliaceous odour. It consists of fixed fatty acids, probably oleic, stearic and lauric acids, also butyric and valeric acids. Dose, 2 to 5 ms.

The cake, left after expression of the oil, contains another neutral principle; insoluble in ether or alkaline solution but solouble in chloroform.

Preparations.—Tinctura Azadirachtæ (1 in 8).—Dose, ½ to 1 dr. *Decoctum Azadirachtæ* of the root-bark and fruit (1 in 5). Dose, 1 to 2 ozs. as an antiperiodic.

Punch-nimb-churnu.—A compound powder of five parts of the tree. These are—leaves, bark, root, flowers and fruit—all pounded together and used. Dose, 5 to 20 grs.

Actions and uses.—The bark and leaf stalks are astringent bitter tonic and antiperiodic, and used in intermittent and paroxysmal fevers and for general debility and convalescence after febrile and other diseases. The leaves are discutient. and local stimulant and used as varalians or poultices to disperse indolent glands and swellings. The young trees yield a kind of sweet juice (toddy) which, when fermented, is used as stomachic and anthelmintic and is given in worms and jaundice. The pulp is applied to boils, pustular eruptions, opens sores and bruised joints. The compound powder *pancha nimba churun* is tonic, and given in convalescence after fever. The fruit is a purgative, anthelmintic and alterative. The oil of the seeds is bitter, anthelmintic and stimulant, given in leprosy, intestinal worms, piles and urinary diseases. The gum is used by lying-in women as a uterine stimulant. The seeds are used for killing pediculi, and the powdered kernel for washing the hair and as a remedy for mange in dogs. The oil, mixed with other oils, is applied to skin diseases, suppurating scrofulous glands, and leprous ulcers. It is rubbed on the skin in rheumatic affections and to the head in headache. The oil contains sulphur, and therefore, with alkalies, it is used in skin diseases.

Remarks.—The Nimba is one of the pancha-tikta, or five bitters.

Melia Dubia, M. Superba, M. Composita, M. Robusta.

Habitat.—E. and W. Peninsula, Ceylon.

Part used.—The pulp of the fruit.

Vernacular.—Bomb.—Kodu-khajura. Can.—Kad-bevu Ara-bevu. Cing.—Lunu-midella. Guz.—Lembarro, Kadukbajur. Hind.—Dinkarling. Mar.—Nimbarra. Sans.—Arangaka. Tam.—Mallay Vemboo.

Kadukhajur means bitter khajur (dates). Kalakhajur is black dates. The fruits resemble dates.

Characters.—Tree smaller than Melia-azadirach ; fruit, when dry, resembling a date in size, shape and colour ; epidermis, dark-brown and deeply wrinkled, also rugous ; apex blunt and studded with small tubercles, with a stalk and a five partite calyx at the base. Pulp firmly adherent to a large and very hard stone, it is sticky and of a brownish red colour, swelling when soaked in water ; taste of the pulp bitter and nauseous ; seed covered with a dark-brown polished testa ; kernel very oily and of sweet taste. Dose of the pulp, 30 to 60 grs.

Constituents.—A glucoside, a fatty oil, wax, malic acid, glucose, mucilage and pectin. The glucoside, is a crystalline bitter principle, of a slightly acid reaction, soluble in alcohol, ether and water.

Actions and uses.—Bitter carminative and anthelmintic, given in colic and other bowel complaints, and also in worms. Locally an ointment made of the juice of fresh fruit, with sulphur and curd heated together, is used for scabies and wounds affected with maggots.

Naregamia Alata.

The Goanese ipecacuanha.

Habitat.—Western Peninsula, India.

Parts used.—The stem and roots.

Vernacular.—Can.—Nela-Narigu, Nalakanu-gida. Goa.—Trifolio, Avacari. Mah.—Kapur Bhendi. Malay—Nela naregam. Mar.—Pittve. Pittpapra, Pittmari, Tinapana.

Avacari (Goa), a corruption of the word ocari, which means emesis. The root is used as an emetic.

Characters.—Stem dirty green, bark firmly adherent, slender, sparingly branched and rising from the root-stalks ; root-stalks knotty, contracted and warty; tubers mealy; powder light-brown ; odour like that of valerian, pungent and aromatic ; taste slightly bitter and nauseous. Dose, 5 to 10 grs.

Constituents.—It contains an alkaloid—Naregamine, an oxidizable fixed oil, wax, sugar, resin and alcoholic extract (containing asparagin), gum, starch, pectin, albuminous and colouring matters and ash 10 p.c.

Naregamine.—To obtain it, agitate the extract with dilute sulphuric acid. It is an amorphous, slightly coloured residue. It forms salts with sulphuric, nitric and hydrochloric acids. The solution is precipitate by tannin, potassio mercuric iodide, and iodine.

Preparations.—Tincture (1 in 8). Dose, $\frac{1}{2}$ to 1 dr. Liquid extract of a golden brown colour. Dose, 45 to 75 ms. Decoction (1 in 10). Dose, $\frac{1}{2}$ to 1 to oz.

Actions and uses.—Diaphoretic, emetic, expectorant, and stimulant to the mucous membranes ; given in dysentery with success. It is also given in rheumatism and biliousness. It is a fair substitute for ipecacuanha.

Sycacarpus Rusbyi.

Habitat.—South America.

Part used.—The bark.

Characters.—The odour of the bark is slight, but peculiar, and the taste unpleasant, not bitter, and slightly nauseous.

Constituents.—Oxalate of lime in large monoclinic crystals. Gutta-percha, a resinous secretion, a yellowish-white, amorphous, sometimes slightly granular substance; caoutchouc; and an active principle.

Preparation.—Fluid extract. Dose, 5 to 30 ms. Tincture (1 in 10). Dose, ½ to 1 dr.

Actions and uses.—At first stimulant, expectorant like apomorphine, carbonate of ammonia, and strychnine and then sedative; given in acute bronchitis and in chronic pulmonary cases accompanied with viscid secretion, or when the cough is dry and harsh.

Walsura Piscidia, Trichilia Trifoliata, T. Emetica.

Habitat.—Travancore, Ceylon, Malabar.

Parts used.—The bark and nut.

Vernacular.—Arab.—Jauz-el-kai, Rukeh. Burm.—Joe-boe. Tam.—Walsura. Tel.—Walurasi.

Jauzel-Kai means an emetic nut.

Characters.—Bark ¼ inch thick, brown, irregularly and longitudinally fissured, separated in flakes. The liber is cinnamon coloured, hard and compact; taste bitter and astringent.

Constituents.—Saponin, a resin of a light brown colour and tannin.

Preparations.—Ointment of the powdered nut.

Actions and uses.—The bark is stimulant, expectorant, emmenagogue and violent emetic. The nut is used as a hair-wash to kill lice. The ointment is used to cure itch. The bark is used to poison fish.

Remarks.—The fruit of Randia dumetorum is often used as a substitute for emetic nut.

Aurantiaceæ.—The orange family.

Aurantiacæ—aurum (gold), from the yellow colour of the fruit.

Characters.—Trees or shrubs. Leaves alternate, exstipulate, dotted, and with the blade articulated to the winged petiole; flowers regular, fragrant; calyx short, urn shaped, 3 to 5-toothed; petals or sepals equal in number; stamens equal, or some multiple of them; disk hypogynous and annular; fruit indehiscent; seeds solitary or numerous, ex-albuminous; cotyledons thick and fleshy.

Habitat.—Chiefly natives of East Indies, cultivated throughout the warmer regions of the globe.

Properties.—The plants have receptacles containing an essential oil, which renders them fragrant; used in perfumery and for flavouring purposes. The volatile oil is found in leaves, petals and rinds of fruits. The rind contains also a bitter principle. The pulp is acid and saccharine.

Citrus Aurantium, var. Bigaradia, B. P.

C. Vulgaris.—The bitter orange.

Aurantium, from aurum, gold. From the colour of the fruit.

Orange, from Arabic naranj.

Habitat.—North India, Circars, Aurangabad, West Indies, United States, Spain.

Parts used.—The fresh outer part of the pericarp—Aurantii Cortex Recens B. P. The dried outer part of the pericarp—Aurantii Cortex Seccatus B. P., orange flower. B. P. And the volatile oil distilled from fresh flowers.

Vernacular.—Arab.—Naranj. Beng.—Kumla-neebu, Narangi. Burm.—Lieng-mau, Sung-zen. Chin.—Kan, Kiuh. Can.—Kittale. Cing.—Narang-ka. Duk.—Narangi. Eng.—C. aurantium, the sweet or Portugal orange and Citrus vulgaris, the bitter orange or Caracoa orange. Hind.—Narangi, Kamlaneeboo, Indian Cintra. Malay.—Simao, Jeruk-manis. Maleal.—Madra, Narranji. Mar.—Naringa. Pers.—Narang. Portuguese—Porto-gallatto. Sans.—Swadu-naringa, Nagranga, Jambira, Karuna-nembu. Tam.—Kitchili Kolinjy. Tel.—Kitchidi, Kittali, Narangamu.

Cintra is the name of the mountain valley near Lisbon.

Characters.—A small tree, with beautiful foliage ; spines axillary, solitary, young shoots glabrous ; leaves oval, elongated, acute, sometimes slightly toothed ; petioles more or less dilated and winged ; flowers fragrant, large and white ; fruit nourishing, roundish or ovoid, usually depressed, red or yellow, terminated by a small knob ; cells 9 to 12, many seeded; rind convex, containing vesicles of oil ; colour deep orange-red externally, rough and glandular; inner surface covered with small amount of spongy portion ; pulp sweet. Epidermis glandular and rough, inner layer spongy, of a fragrant pleasant odour and bitter aromatic taste. Dried rind in thin strips or bands. Dose of the rind, 15 to 30 grs.

Constituents.—The rind of the fruit contains a volatile oil, isomeric with oil of turpentine ; gum resin, a fixed oil, hesperidin, a bitter crystalline principle, tannin, ash 4-5 p.c. The flowers and rind of the fresh fruit contain a volatile oil called oil of neroli ; a fragrant yellowish liquid of a bitter aromatic taste ; soluble in alcohol (1 to 1). It gives the peculiar odour to eau-de-cologne or to Spiritus odoratus. Dose, 1 to 3 ms. The leaves and young unripe fruit contain a volatile oil called the oil of orange leaf or neroli petit grain, or essence de petit grain. This oil contains Limonene 20 p.c., Nerolol 30 p.c., Nerolyl acetate 40 p.c., Geraniol 3 p.c.

Preparations.—Of the rind, *Infusum aurantii*, B. P. (1 in 20). Dose, ½ to 1 oz. *Extractum aurantii amari fluidum.*—Fluid extract of bitter orange peel. Dose, ½ to 1 dr. *Infusum aurantii compositum*, B. P.—Dried orange peel ½ ounce, fresh lemon peel ¼ ounce, cloves 55 grains, water 1 pint. Dose, ½ to 1 oz. *Syrupus aromaticus*, B. P., Tinctura aurantii 5 oz., aqua cinnamomi 5 ozs., syrup 10 ozs. Dose, ½ to 1 dr. *Syrupus aurantii floris* B. P. (1 of orange flower water in 9).

Dose, $\frac{1}{2}$ to 1 dr. *Syrupus aurantii* (1 of tincture in 8). Dose, $\frac{1}{2}$ to 1 dr. *Tinctura aurantii*, B. P.—Tincture of orange peel (1 in 4). Dose, 30 to 60 ms. *Elixir aromaticum.*—Aromatic elixir contains compound spirit of orange, precipitated calcium phosphate, syrup, alcohol and water. Dose, 1 to 3 drs. *Vinum aurantii*, B. P. (10 p.c. of alcohol). Dose, 60 to 120 ms. Aqua aurantii floris, B. P. Dose, 1 to 2 ozs.

Orange peel is also an ingredient in the preparation of tinctura gentianæ composita. Dose, 1 to 4 drs. Tinctura cinchonæ composita. Dose, 1 to 4 drs.

Actions and uses.—Aromatic bitter, stomachic, carminative and stimulant of the nervous system. These properties are due to the volatile oil it contains. Its preparations are valuable additions to bitter infusions used in dyspepsia and flatulence, but they are used mostly as adjunct to other stomachics as a flavouring agent. It is invaluable in scurvy. The oil, in large doses, produces violent colic and even convulsions.

Citrus Medica, var. Limonum, B. P.

Habitat.—North India, Mediterranean, foot of Himalaya; cultivated in Southern Europe.

Parts used.—Juice—Succus Limonis, B. P., and the fresh outer part of the pericarp, Limonis cortex, B. P., and volatile oil, oleum Limonis, B. P.

Vernacular.—Arab.—Lemu Qalambak. Beng.—Karna-nebu. Bur.—Kigi-samyasi. Can.—Dodda-nimbe. Cing.—Lokka-dehi. Eng. —True lemons. Guz.—Motu-limbu. Hind.—Korina-neboo. Malyal. —Valya-cheru narauna. Mar.—Thora-limbu. Pers.—Kalanbak. Sans, —Limpaka, Maha-Jambira, Nimbuka, Vijapura, Madhukarkatika. Tam.—Periya-elumihcham. Tel.—Pedda-ninuna-pandu.

Characters.—A straggling bush or tree, more tender than the orange tree, having many angular branches ; colour of the bark grey, that of branches green, and that of twigs reddish ; leaves spiny, evergreen, ovate, acute and serrate ; flowers sweet scented ; colour from white to purplish pink ; fruit ovoid, berry with nipple-shaped extremity, the rind—Limonis Cortex is smooth and marked with punctations over the oil glands ; pulp acid and yellowish. The natives use in medicine two varieties—Godaria Limbu thick-rinded ; the Kagaji limbu has a thin rind. In shape both are globular, their size varying from walnut to that of a small orange; colour also varies from shades of green to yellow ; their interior is juicy. The juice succus limonis, lemon juice is acid ; each lemon yields from 6 to 8 drs. It is contained in conglomerated cells separated in different layers or carpels. On the margin of each layer one or two seeds are attached ; seeds smaller than those of orange ; rind or the peel is in narrow thin bands, adherent to their spongy white inner layer. It has a deep yellow colour and is glandular, odour fragrant, taste bitter aromatic. The fragrancy is due to the presence of the volatile oil in the rind.

Citrus Medica, var. Citron.

Habitat.—Foot of the Himalaya, Peninsula.

Parts used.—The rind, juice and oil.

Vernacular.—Arab.—Utraj. Beng.—Honsa nebu Begpura. Bomb.—Mahalung. Bur.—Sh-Onsakhava. Can.—Mada-lada-hannu.—Eng.—Citron. Guz.—Turanj, Bijorun. Hind.—Mahalung Leemoo. Maleal—Narauna. Pers.—Duk-Turanj Limoo. Sans.—Phala-pural karuna Mahalunga. Tam.—Nartlamlpazham. Tel.—Mahipala, Bijalpura.

Characters.—The fruit is pineapple shaped, large and oblong; peel pale yellow, rough, from the presence of oil-glands, inner surface having only a small quantity of white spongy portion. The juice contains 7 to 9 p. c. of citric acid and is a slightly turbid yellowish liquid.

Constituents.—Lemon juice contains citric acid 7 to 10 p.c., phosphoric and malic acids ; also citrates of potassium and other bases; sugar, mucilage and ash. Dose, 4 to 6 drs. Lemon peel contains a volatile oil, hesperidin, a bitter crystalline glucoside, chiefly in the white of the rind ; and ash 4 p.c. Hesperidin, a bitter principle 5 to 8 p. c. in yellow crystals, sparingly soluble in boiling water and ether, readily soluble in hot acetic acid, also in alkaline solutions. Volatile oil. Oleum limonis, B. P., is obtained by expression from fresh lemon peel, and is isomeric with oil of turpentine. It is a pale-yellow limpid liquid of a fragrant odour and aromatic bitter taste, soluble in alcohol (1 in 3). It contains citrene or limonene 76 p. c., citrol 7-8 p.c., cymene and citronellal. Dose, ½ to 3 ms.

Preparations.—Spiritus limonis, spirit of lemon ; used for flavouring purposes. Spiritus ammoniæ aromaticus, B. P. Spiritus aurantii compositus. Acidum Citricum—Citric acid—obtained from the juice of the lemon or the lime, by adding chalk to form calcium citrate and by decomposing by sulphuric acid. It occurs in colourless rhombic crystals, soluble in water. The solution of 17 grs. in 4 drs. of water is equal to 4 drs. of lime juice; or sufficient to neutralize potassium bicarbonate 25 grs. or sodium bicarbonate 20 grs., or Ammonium carbonate 15 grs. Dose, 10 to 30 grs. Tinctura limonis, B.P. (1 in 4). Dose, 30 to 60 ms. Syrupus limonis, B.P. Lemon peel 1 ounce, lemon juice 25 ounces, sugar 38 ounces, alcohol q. s. to weigh 4 pounds and one ounce. Dose, ½ to 1 dr.

Actions and uses.—The juice, rind of the fruits and volatile oil are used in medicine. The peel is bitter tonic and stomachic, used for flavouring tinctures and infusions. It is also stimulant and carminative, given in indigestion, flatulence, and as a corrective to purgatives. It is also extensively used to disguise the taste of medicines such as quinine, &c. The lemon juice is refrigerant, cooling and antiscorbutic, analogous to orange juice, but it contains more citric acid and less syrup, and hence called acid of lemons. The juice taken internally enters the blood as alkaline citrates, potassium salts and phosphoric acid. The citrates are partly oxidized into carbonic acid and water. The potassium salts and phosphoric acid act upon the red corpuscles. They precipitate uric acid and thus promote the formation of calculi. If long continued, the juice or citric acid impairs digestion and impoverishes the blood. It is supposed to dissolve organic matters in the system; hence used in the treatment of atheroma. Fresh juice is useful in scurvy. It is an ingredient in many refrigerant and diuretic effervescing drinks, used in allaying febrile heat and thirst, in subduing restlessness, promoting the action of the skin and kidneys. It is given in inflammatory affections and in dyspepsia with vomiting. Its power of conveying alkalies into the blood renders it useful in acute rheumatic affections, sciatica, lumbago, &c., also given in obesity in large quantities with good results. It is often used with potassium bicarbonate and honey by the natives as a gargle in diphtheria and sore throat. Externally it relieves itching if applied in pruritis of the vulva, scrotum, is applied in sun-burn, and to check post partem hæmorrhage. The essential oil is a stimulating liniment for the relief of rheumatic pains. The juice of baked lemon is used in bilious affections and to stop diarrhœa.

Seville or Bigardi orange comes from Spain, Madura, China and India. Mandarin (citrus levensis) comes from South of Europe ; the latter is very small in size, flattened at both ends and has a very thin rind.

Citrus Bergamia, C. Limetta.

Habitat.—Italy, Sicily, France, Jamaica, Indian Peninsula, Bengal.

Part used.—The soluble oil from the rind of the fresh fruit.

Vernacular.—Arab.—Limu, Limu Hamiz. Beng.—Niboo. Burm.—Than-ba-ya, Shouk. Chin.—Tan-pu-lo. Can.—Nimbe-hanun. Cing.—Dehi. Duk.—Limboo. Eng.—Acid lime, Bergamotto lime, Adam's-apple, common sour lime. Guz.—Nimbu. Hind.—Neemboo. Mar.—Zimbu. Malay.—Eroomitchee-narakam cheru-narama. Pers.—Limue-rtush. Sans.—Nimbooka, Jambira-phalam. Tam.—Elumich, Elimicham. Tel.—Gaja-nimma, Jambira-nimma.

Characters.—A small tree, resembling in characters lemon, orange, &c. Flowers small, of a delicious peculiar odour ; fruit paler coloured than lemon, pyriform or globose, and smooth; rind with receptacles for oil; pulp greenish, aromatic and of an acid taste.

Constituents.—The rind of the fresh fruit contains a volatile oil, hesperidin and ash. The volatile oil, Oil of Bergamot is obtained from unripe greenish but full-grown fruits by expression and distillation of the outer rind. It is a greenish thick liquid, faintly acid, of a peculiar fragrant odour and aromatic bitter taste ; soluble in alcohol, liquor potassæ and glacial acetic acid. It contains several hydrocarbons, such as Citrene, Bergaptene or Bergamot camphor ; Linalool and linalool acetate (or bergamiol), upon which its value chiefly depends. It is an ingredient of spiritus odoratus.

Actions and uses.—Stimulant and aromatic. The natives use the juice as refrigerant, antiscorbutic and antiseptic in dyspepsia, fevers, and vomiting. The oil is chiefly used externally as a perfume in the manufacture of toilet articles.

Rutaceæ.

The rue family.

Trees, shrubs, or rarely herbs. Leaves alternate or opposite, exstipulate, simple or pinnated and dotted; flowers regular or irregular and perfect; calyx and corolla with a quaternary or quinary distribution of their parts; ovary sessile or elevated on a gynophore; fruits capsular, carpels united or distinct; seeds solitary or in pairs, radicle superior.

Habitat.—South of temperate zone; cultivated in the East.

Properties.—Antispasmodic, febrifuge, diuretic and tonic.

Ægle Marmelos.

Cratæva marmelos, Feronia pellucida.

Habitat.—Malabar, Coromandel, dry forests in India.

Parts used.—The fruit (pulp).

Vernacular.—Arab.—Sapharajale-hindi, Shul. Beng.—Shriphal, Bela. Bomb.—Shriphal. Burm.—Oosheet. Can.—Bila-patri-hannu. Cing.—Bellika. Duk.—Belphal. Eng.—Bael, Bengal Quince. Guz.—Bilinu-phal. Hind.—Shriphal, Bela. Malay.—Tanghai. Mar.—Bela. Pers.—Saphara-jale-hindi. Maleal.—Kuvelam. Sans.—Bilva-phalam, Mahura. Tam.—Vilva-maram. Tel.—Maradu-pandu, Malu-remu-chettu.

Shriphal is derived from Shri—the goddess of abundance, and phal, a fruit. It is an emblem of increase and fertility. The tree is sacred to the goddess of riches, and is cultivated everywhere in Hindu gardens. Shriphal is also the name given to cocoanut, in allusion to the fruit possessing an abundance of good properties.

Characters.—Fruit of various shapes and sizes, oval, oblong, elliptical, roundish. Small ones of the size of a hen's egg, large ones being as big as cocoanuts. Rind very hard, woody, nearly smooth, becoming stony when dry and of a lightish yellow, cherry-red or brown colour; surface tubercled and dotted; pulp of a brownish red colour, firm, and having 12 or more stony carpels, and in the cavities between the carpels and surrounding the seeds is a tenaceous transparent gluten-like or a gummy resinous substance in angular fragments, of a reddish brown colour, which becomes hard on drying, but continues transparent. It is insoluble in water. The carpel contains seeds, which are hairy, one or more in each carpel; odour (of the pulp) aromatic and agreeable; taste astringent and resembling that of jambu; leaves pinnate or ternate, leaflets oblong, broad, lanceolate and crenulate; green or dark green in colour, smooth, shining and thick, and of an aromatic smell and taste; root-bark thin, of a light pink colour and somewhat astringent. Dose of the pulp, 15 to 30 grs.

Constituents.—The pulp contains mucilage, pectin, sugar, tannin, a volatile oil, bitter principle, and ash 2 p.c. The wood ash contains potassium and sodium compounds, phosphates of lime and iron, calcium carbonate, magnesium carbonate, silica, sand, &c. The fresh leaves, on distillation, yield an oil of a yellowish green colour and neutral reaction, of an aromatic odour and bitter taste ; soluble in alcohol and miscible with carbon bisulphide.

Preparations.—Extractum belæ liquidum. Dose, 1 to 2 drs. Decoction (1 in 5). Dose, ½ to 1 oz.

Actions and uses.—The ripe fruit is nutritious, delicious, aromatic, alterative, and laxative. It is given with sugarcandy to prevent the growth of piles and to remove habitual constipation. A decoction of unripe or half ripe fruits, or unripe fruit baked for 6 hours is astringent, digestive and stomachic, and is given in diarrhœa and dysentery. When taken in excess it often causes flatulence. Syrup of ripe fruits is used in dyspepsia. The root-bark is refrigerant, and is given in fevers, asthma with palpitation of the heart. In native practice a poultice of the leaves is applied to the head in the delirium of fever, and to the chest in acute bronchitis. The decoction of the leaves is given in asthma. A marmalade of bael fruit is a household remedy for diarrhœa and dysentery.

Remarks.—The root is one of the ingredients of the decoction of *dasa mula*, or the ten roots.

Atalantia Monophylla.

Limonia Monophylla, Trichilia Spinosa.

Habitat.—Western Peninsula, Ceylon, Malabar Coast, Ghauts, Bombay Presidency, Mahableshwar, Coromandel.

Part used.—The oil.

Vernacular.—Eng.—Wild lime. Can.—Katunimbe. Maleal. —Malvaregam. Mar.—Makhur-limbu. Tam.—Katelle-nucha. Tel. —Konda-nimma.

Characters.—Leaves fragrant like those of orange ; berry globular, yellow, divided into 4 cells by membranous septa ; pulp like that of lime, but scanty, each cell containing one seed ; rind, of a faint odour of orange peel and full of oil cells ; oil is aromatic and of a dark green colour.

Preparation.—Decoction of the leaves.

Actions and uses.—The oil is only used externally as a stimulant in rheumatic joints, paralytic limbs, &c. The root is antispasmodic and stimulant. Decoction of the leaves is applied in itch.

Barosma Betulina, B. P.

B. Crenulata. B. Serratifolia.

Habitat.—South Africa, Cape Colony.

Part used.—The dried leaves. Buchu folia, B. P. Buchu leaves.

Barosma, from baros, heavy, and osme, smell or odour. The odour of the leaves is heavy and powerful. Betulina, from Betu, birch, the leaves resemble those of birch tree. Crenulata, from crena, a notch, the leaves are crenulate or notched.

Characters.—Shrub. B. Betulina leaves $\frac{1}{2}$ to $\frac{3}{4}$ inch long, of a dull yellowish green colour, rhomboid, ovate, rigid, and cartilaginous when moist; surface glabrous, somewhat warty, margin denticulate, apex blunt and recurved; oil glands visible near the margin; odour and taste strong and characteristic. Dose of the leaves, 15 to 30 grs.

Constituents.—Volatile oil, resin, lignin, bitter extractive principle, (rutin, or barosmin) gum and salts.

Volatile oil, obtained by the distillation of the leaves is the active principle and contains a body of a peculiar, penetrating, peppermint-like odour; on cooling it separates barosma camphor or diosphenol, a steoropten occurring in white needle-like crystals.

Preparations.—Infusum Buchu B. P.—Infusion of Buchu (1 in 20). Dose, $\frac{1}{2}$ to 1 oz. Extractum buchu fluidum, fluid extract of buchu. Dose, 10 to 60 ms. Tinctura Buchu, B. P.—Tincture of Buchu (1 in 5). Dose, $\frac{1}{2}$ to 1 dr.

Physiological action.—Diuretic, diaphoretic, and stimulant. In small doses it causes a sense of heat in the stomach, increases appetite, stimulates the heart beat, and increases the action of the skin by causing slight diaphoresis. It is eliminated by the kidneys, the urine becomes darker and of a strong aromatic odour, leaving a brownish deposit. In large doses it is a gastro-intestinal and renal irritant, producing vomiting, purging and strangury.

Therapeutics.—Given in gravel, chronic pyelitis, chronic bronchitis, catarrh of the bladder and in urethritis; also in diseased prostate, in lithiasis, and in retention or incontinence of urine. In atonic dyspepsia, chronic rheumatism it is generally combined with alkalies.

Feronia Elephantum, Anisiphalins Rumphii, Cratæva Vallanga.

Habitat.—India, Gujerat, Bengal, Travancore.

Parts used.—The leaves, ripe and unripe fruit and gum.

Vernacular.—Arab.—Kabit. Beng.—Kat-bel. Burm.—H'man. Can.—Bilvalitha, Kavita Vriksea. Cing.—Dewul. Duk.—Kavit. Eng.—Elephant apple or wood apple, London—Amrad (gum). Guz.—Kavit Kotha, Ghate-gund (gum). Hind.—Bhuin-koit, Katbel, Kawit. Malyal.—Vilampozham. Mar.—Kavitha. Pers.—Kabit. Portuguese.—Balong. Sans.—Bhu-kabid-thazi, Kupitha, Kapiprya, Dadhiphala. Tam.—Vela Villa Vila, Vellanga. Tel.—Kapihamu Nola, Puli.

Elephant apple or wood apple. The pericarp of the fruit is hard like wood or elephant skin.

Kapitha, the apple on which monkeys dwell. Kapipriya, that which is dear to monkeys. Dadhiphala, Dadhi or Dahi means, coagulated milk, and Phal, the fruit. The taste of the fruit resembles that of coagulated milk.

Characters.—Leaves with from 5 to 7 leaflets, pinnate, cuneate or obovate, crenate at the top, pellucid and dotted. When crushed they smell like fennel, *varialee*; fruit light grey or dirty white in colour, globose and covered with a scurfy epidermis; rind dull green, woody, granular and very fragile; pulp of a pale greyish pink colour; seeds numerous, oblong, compressed, thick and fleshy; smell aromatic; taste somewhat acid and astringent. The gum, *ghati gund*, is semitransparent, and in roundish tears or irregular masses, colourless, or of a yellow or brownish red colour. With water it is readily soluble without residue, and forms a thick, tasteless, viscid mucilage like that of Bavala gund (gum acacia), the major portion is different from gum-arabic, and contains abundant crystals of mucic acid. Dose of the pulp, 15 to 25 grs.

Constituents.—The pulp contains a large quantity of citric acid with potash, lime and iron. The leaves yield an essential oil similar to that obtained from bael leaves.

Preparation.—Fluid extract. Dose, ½ to 1 dr. medicated oil. Puncha Kapittha. Composed of the five allied products, viz. flowers. bark, fruit, leaves and root, made into a medicated oil and applied to the whole body in fevers. Compound powder. Kapith Ashtaka—Kapith—Elephant apple. Ashtaka, eight. A compound preparation of eight drugs, which are highly astringent. These contain Kapith or Koth (the pulp) 8, Sakar 6, Dalimba-chhal 4, Amali-chhal 3, Bela-phal 3, Dhauri-phul 4, Naga-kesar 1, Taj 4. Mix and make a powder. To this add Ajamod 3, Pipali 3, Miri 4, Jirun 4, Dhana 4, Pipali-mula 3, Valo 2, Sanchal 2, Elachi 4, Tamala-patra 2, Chitrk 1, Sunth 2. Mix and make a powder. Astringent carminative and stomachic. Dose, 1 to 2 drs. Used in chronic dysentery and diarrhœa.

Actions and uses.—The young leaves are stomachic, lithontriptic, and carminative, used in dyspepsia and diarrhœa; also used in lessening red sand from the urine. The unripe fruit is astringent, and, like bael, is used in diarrhœa and dysentery. The ripe fruit is refreshing, anti-scorbutic, digestive and tonic, the syrup is used in salivation, sore throat and in strengthening the gums. The gum is a good substitute for gum-arabic, the mucilage is more viscid than that of gum-arabic, and is used with honey in diarrhœa, dysentery, and to relieve tenesmus of the bowels. The pulp or the powdered rind is used as a local application for bites of venomous insects.

Limonia Acidissima, L. Crenulata.

Habitat.—Himalaya, Coromandel, Malabar, Assam, W. Peninsula Hurdwar.

Parts used.—The fruit, leaves and root.

Vernacular.—Hind.—Beli. Mar.—Naibel. Malyal.—Jerukat narigam. Tel.—Torelaga.

Naibel.—Nai, Navi, barber. Barber's bael fruit, used by barbers in Java instead of soap.

Characters.—Shrub, with pinnate leaves, with 2 or 3 pairs of leaflets ; leaflets oblong, crenated ; with solitary spines, and winged petioles ; flowers corymbose, corymb umbelliform, small, white and fragrant ; root yellow, bitter and aromatic, fruit small, globular, of the size of a nutmeg or pea or grape, 'yellowish, but red when perfectly ripe ; structure similar to that of the lime ; pulp flesh-coloured, highly acid and somewhat bitter and aromatic ; cells four ; seeds three.

Preparation.—Infusion of leaves and decoction of root (1 in 10). Dose, 1 to 2 ozs.

Actions and uses.—The leaves are antispasmodic, given in epilepsy. The root is purgative and antispasmodic, given in colicy pains ; the dried fruit is a tonic and is given in fever and dyspepsia associated with flatus.

Remarks.—The fruit is considered by the Arabs as a prophylactic against small-pox, malignant fever and plague.

Murraya Exotica. Chelsia paniculata.

Habitat.—Himalaya, Ceylon, Bengal, China.

Parts used.—Flowers and leaves.

Vernacular.—Beng.—Kamini. Burm.—Thanat-kha, May-kay. Cing.—Attaireya-gass. Eng.—Honey-bush, Cosmetic-box, China-box. Hind.—Bibzar, Koonti. Konkan.—Kamoun, Murchole. Mar.—Kounti. Tel.—Noga-golunga.

Honey-bush.—The fragrance of its white flowers is like that of honey.

Characters.—An ornamental shrub with beautiful dark-green pinnate leaves. Leaflets coriaceous, flowers white and sweet-smelling, resembling in taste and odour Murraya kœnigii.

Constituents.—Flowers contain a glucoside named Murrayin.

Preparation.—Infusion (1 in 10). Dose, ½ to 1 ozs.

Actions and uses.—Tonic and stomachic, like Murraya kœnigii and used similarly.

Murraya (Bergera) Kœnigii.

Habitat.—Himalaya, Bengal, Ceylon, W. Peninsula.

Parts used.—The leaves, root and bark.

Vernacular.—Beng.—Barsunga Karia-phalee. Burm.—Pindo-sin. Can.—Karibevu. Cing.—Kara-pinchee-gass. Duk.—Karya-pak. Eng.—Curry-leaf tree. Guz.—Gora-nimb. Hind.—Katnim, Karripak, Kudia-nim. Malayal.—Karu-veppa. Panj.—Ganda-nimb. Mar.—Harhunimb, Jhirang, Jirani. Maleal.—Barsanga. Sans.—Krishna-nimbu, Saurabhi-nimba. Tam.—Karu-vembu. Tel.—Nalyal Karivepa.

Saurabhi nimb.—Sorab, soram, fragrant smell, The neem is fragrant. Joran, Jirana, to digest. The plant is digestive.

Characters.—Leaves pinnate with numerous leaflets, alternate, unequally oblique and serrated, upper surface dark green and dotted, under surface of a light colour ; odour powerful ; taste pungent, bitter and acidulous; root spreading, with numerous suckers; bark soft and thick, odour agreeable; taste like that of fresh ginger.

Constituents.—The leaves contain a volatile oil resembling the oil of Ægle Marmelos; a resin; and a crystalline principle named kœnigin (glucoside).

Preparation.—Infusion (1 in 10). Dose, 1 to 2 ozs.

Actions and uses.—Tonic, stomachic, and febrifuge, given with bitters in dyspepsia, loss of appetite, and in general debility; also in dysentery and to stop vomiting. The bark and root are local stimulants and used as application to wounds by venomous animals.

Peganum Harmala.

Habitat.—N. W. India, Western Deccan.

Part used.—The seeds.

Vernacular.—Eng.—Syrian Rue. Arab.—Harmal. Beng.—Isband. Bomb.—Haramaro, Ispanda. Duk.—Ispand, Harmaro. Hind.—Islamlahori, Ispand. Pers.—Isband, Sipand. Tam.—Vanai-virai. Tel.—Shima, Garante, Vittulu.

Characters.—The drug consists of seeds mixed with a few pedicles and portions of capsules; seeds are of a dull greyish brown colour, several, irregularly angular, curved on one side. Each covered with a rough tomentum, easily separable from the testa by scratching; odour strong, heavy and disagreeable, resembling that of cannabis or govarni-sing; taste resinous, persistent and bitter.

Constituents.—A resin of a narcotic odour and two alkaloids viz., Harmaline and Harmine; Harmaline when treated with hydrochloric acid, yields Hermatol, in orange-red crystals sparingly soluble in water; Harmine may be obtained by oxidizing harmaline with nitric acid; It occurs as colourless crystals, insoluble in water; very little soluble in alcohol and ether. Fuming hydrochloric acid converts it into harmal. When oxidized by means of chromic acid, it yields herminic acid—silky tufts.

Preparations.—Decoction (1 in 20). Dose, ½ to 1 oz. Tincture (1 in 8). Dose, 30 to 60 ms.

Actions and uses.—Stimulant of the sexual organs, alterative, also emmenagogue like ergot, savine and sitap used internally in amenorrhœa and as a fumigatory in palsy, and lumbago; it increases the flow of milk and menses.

Remarks.—Native midwives use it for procuring abortion. Mendi seeds are often substituted for Ispanda; both are alike in form and colour.

Paramygnya Monophylla.

Habitat.—Sikkim, Himalaya, Bhutan, Ceylon.

Parts used.—Fruits and root,

Vernacular.—Mar.—Karru-wagete.

Characters.— The root-bark is brown and scabrous; taste bitter; fruits resemble those of capparis zeylanica. The bark contains large crystals of oxalate of lime.

Actions and uses.—Diuretic and alterative.

Luvunga Scandens.

Habitat.—Himalaya, Bengal.

Part used.—The fruit or berry.

Vernacular.—Sans.—Kakkola. Beng.—(the oil) Kakala.

Characters.—Berries glandular, papillose, of a terebenthinate odour and taste. Contain 1 to 4 dark-green oily seeds; testa membranous.

Preparation.—Perfumed medicinal oil (kakkolaka). Hair oil.

Ruta Graveolens—var. Angustifolia.

Habitat.— Cultivated in the East, South Europe.

Parts used.—The plant, fresh leaves and oil.

Vernacular.—Arab.—Sudaba. Bomb.—Satapa. Can.—Nagadali-sappu. Cing.—Aruda. Duk.—Saaf. Eng.—Peganon of Scripture, Garden rue, Herb of grace. Guz.—Scradab, Sitapa. Hind.—Satari Amda. Mar.—Sudab. Malay.—Sadab. Pers.—Sudap. Sans.—Somalata, Brahmu Sadapata. Tam.—Arvada. Tel.—Arudu.

Characters.—Herb, perennial, about 2 or 3 feet high, glaucous-green, smooth or tubercled; leaves long, petioled; leaflets small, dotted, linear, oblong or obovate and very minutely crenate; under surface pale, upper surface glaucous green or dark-green; flowers yellow; fruit capsule obtuse, shortly pedicelled 4 or 5 lobed; corymbs spreading, bracts lanceolate; sepals triangular, acute; petals ciliate; seeds black, many; odour peculiar and resembling somewhat that of Tulasi; taste pungent, nauseous and slightly bitter. Dose, powdered leaves, 5 to 20 grs.

Constituents.—An essential volatile oil (Oleum Rutæ), and Rutin—a bitter, yellow glucoside. The oil is a viscid fluid of a greenish yellow colour and neutral reaction, solidifies in crystalline laminæ resembling those of anise oil. The chief volatile constituents are methyl-nonyl ketone. The ketone was formerly regarded as capric or rutic aldehyde. It also contains lauric aldehyde and a hydrocarbon, analogous to oil of turpentine and borneol. Dose, 1 to 3 ms.

Preparations.—Decoction (1 in 10). Dose, 1 to 2 ozs., and essential oil.

Physiological actions.—Locally an active irritant. In small doses tonic, digestive, and aphrodisiac, causes heat in the throat, nausea, eructations, and flatulence. It irritates the skin, kidneys and bronchi, and increases their secretions. It stmulates the heart, increases the frequency of its action and diminishes its tension. It also leads to hyperæmia of the uterus and ovaries, and increases the menstrual flow. It is promptly diffused, and may be found in the urine, sweat and breath. In large doses it sets up gastro-enteritis, with violent vomiting, purging, bloody urine and dysuria. In poisonous doses it is a narcotic and irritant poison, causing great prostration, convulsions, suppression of urine, often giving rise to abortion.

Therapeutics.—It is a most powerful aphrodisiac. The juice or the decoction of fresh leaves is used as an anthelmintic in children, and as an injection (rectal) against thread-worms. The oil is stimulant, carminative and antispasmodic, given with aromatics in colic, hysteria, epilepsy, and flatulence; as an emmenagogue in amenorrhœa, Externally the oil is applied to the chest in chronic bronchitis, to glandular enlargements, to rheumatic painful parts and to scaly eruptions. Locally it produces inflammation and vesication. The natives give it extensively to increase the flow of urine and menses. The varalians of the leaves and oil are used in tympanitis.

Ampelidaceæ or Vitaceæ.

The vine family. Climbing shrubs—juice watery; joints swollen and separate from each other ; leaves simple or compound, alternate above and opposite below ; flowers regular, green, small and stalked ; fruit succulent, 2-celled ; seeds erect, few—2 in each cell ; testa bony ; albumen hard.

Habitat.—Warm regions, Caspian ; cultivated in the South of Europe.

Properties.—Leaves, stems and unripe fruits are juicy, the juice being acid, owing to the presence of tartaric acid and acid potassium bitartrate. Ripe fruits are also juicy, but sweet owing to the formation of glucose or grape-sugar.

Leea Macrophylla.

Habitat.—Hotter parts of India.

Part used.—Tuberous root.

Vernacular.—Beng.—Tolsu mudriya. Burm.—Kya-bet-gyee. Mar.—Dinda. Sans.—Dholsa Mudra, Dholusa-mudrika.

Characters.—Herbaceous plant; leaves large; flowers small, and white, stems straight and pointed; root woody, porous and tough, of a deep red colour and very bulky; bark dark-brown, scabrous and striated. Internally the bark is deep-red. The odour is astringent and agreeable. The tubers are mucilaginous.

Preparations.—Poultice of the root and paste.

Actions and uses.—Local stimulant. The root is applied over guineaworm and to obstinate chronic sores to promote their healing. A paste of it is applied in ringworm.

Leea Sambucina. L. Staphylea. Staphylea Indica.

Habitat.—Hotter parts of India, Burmah.

Parts used.—The roots and leaves.

Vernacular.—Beng.—Kurkur-Jihwa. Burm.—Ka-let. Goa.—Diono. Hind.—Kurkurgihwa. Mar.—Karkani. Portuguese.—Ratanhia. Tel.—Ankadoo.

Characters.—Stems shrubby with straight branches; leaves pinnate; leaflets stalked; flowers greenish white; fruit the size of a small cherry; root porous, woody and tough; bark scabrous, of a dark-brown colour, taste astringent and odour agreeable.

Preparations.—Decoction (1 in 10). Dose, ½ to 1 oz.

Actions and uses.—Stomachic, tonic and astringent, used in diarrhœa, dysentery, colic; also used to relieve thirst during fever. Externally it is used for ringworm. Roasted leaves are applied to the head in vertigo. The juice of fresh leaves is digestive, and given in diarrhœa and chronic dysentery.

Vitis.—Different species of vitis are remarkable for their containing tannin; hence useful as astringents. Some of them are acrid, owing to their containing needle-shaped crystals of oxalate of lime, which cause mechanical irritation; hence used to promote suppuration of boils. The dried tubers and stems are not acrid. In them the oxalate crystals mat together and thus become blunt. They contain large quantities of potash and lime salts, and are therefore used as diuretic and antacid in urinary diseases.

Vitis Araneosus.

Vernacular.—Hind.—Kamraj, Chamar-Musli. Mar.—Bendri, Bendervel, Ghorvel.

Ghoravela, from ghora, a horse, and vel, vine. The young shoots and leaves are given to horses as a cooling medicine. The root is used as astringent in diarrhœa.

Vitis Carnosa.—V. Cordata, Cissus Carnosa; found in the hedges and forests in Bengal.

Vernacular.—Beng.—Amallata. Eng.—Fleshy wild wine. Guz.—Khatumbro. Hind.—Kassar Amal-bel. Mah.—Odi, Ambat-vel. Tel.—Mandula-mari-tigae, Kani-apa-tige.

Actions and uses.—The root is remarkably acrid; used as an application to boils.

Vitis Indica. Vitis Rugosa.

Habitat.—Western Peninsula India, Deccan, Tennaserim.

Parts used.—The leaves and tubers.

Vernacular.—Eng.—Indian wild vine. Hind.—Amdhuka. Beng.—Amdhiaka, Amoluka. Duk.—Jangali Draksha. Maleal.—Shembravulli. Mar.—Randraksh, Kole-Jan.

Characters.—Climbing plant, slightly hairy ; stem striated, rather contorted especially at the joints, and smooth; leaves trifoliate, smooth and succulent; leaflets lateral, obliquely cordate, acuminate, oblong and serrated on the top ; tubers 1 to 2 feet long, tapering at both ends, brown externally, having wart-like protuberances arranged in circular rings, internally red and juicy. The leaves are rich in salts of potash and lime ; fresh leaves are acrid owing to the irritation caused by the presence of needles of oxalate of lime ; berries black when ripe, full of purple juice, taste acrid, somewhat sweet and mucilaginous.

Preparation.—Decoction of tubers (1 in 10). Dose, ½ to 1 oz.

Actions and uses.—Antiscorbutic, alterative and stimulant; used in syphilis, scrofula, scurvy, general weakness, chronic skin diseases, &c.

Vitis Pedata.

Vernacular.—Beng.—Goali-lata. Mar.—Gorpadvel. Sans.—Godhapadi or Iguano's foot.

Godhapadi, Godha,—the reptile, lizard, and padi-pedis foot, from the fancied resemblance of the leaves to the foot of the reptile Galoli.

Actions and uses.—The leaves are astringent. The decoction is used to check uterine and other fluxes.

Vitus Quadrangularis—Cissus Quadrangularis.

Habitat.—India, Arabia.

Parts used.—The dried stalk, leaves and juice.

Vernacular.—Beng.—Harajora, Hasjora. Burm.—Shazavu-lese. Can.—Mangaruli. Duk.—Maller. Guz.—Hadashankar, Chodhari. Hind.—Nallar, Harsankar. Malay.—Jungilam-parinda. Mar.—Hera Shankar, Hada Jodi, Chodhari-kandavel. Sans.—Ashti-sandhna, Vagra-valli. Tam.—Piranda-kodi. Tel.—Nalla-ratiga.

Hara Shankar.—Hara or Hada, a bone, and Sankar, a chain, in allusion to the jointed stems like a chain of bones.

Asthi Sandhana—Asthi, bone, and Sandhana, to join or to heal, in allusion to the stem having a resemblance to the articulations of bones, from this it is supposed to be useful in healing or reducing fractures and dislocations.

Characters.—Stem obtusely quadrangular, smooth, greenish, generally dichotomously branched, nodes jointed ; leaves thick, entire or three-lobed ; juice acrid. Dose of the powder, 20 to 40 grs.

Preparation.—Decoction (1 in 5). Dose, ½ to 1 oz.

Actions and uses.—Alterative and stimulant, given in dyspepsia, loss of appetite and scurvy ; also in irregular menstruation. The juice is given mixed with gopi chandan, ghee and sugar. Paste of the fresh stem is astringent, and locally applied to dislocations, sores and fractured limbs ; juice of the stem is dropped into the ear in otorrhœa and into the nose to check epistaxis.

Vitis Setosa—Cissus Setosa—C. Cordata.

Habitat.—Peninsula.

Vernacular.—Hind.—Harmal, Haljar. Mah.—Khaj-golicha-vel. Tam.—Puli naravi. Tel.—Bara-butsali.

Actions and uses.—The leaves are very acrid; roasted and oiled they are applied to indolent tumours to promote suppuration, and to painful swelling to assist in the extraction of guinea-worms.

Shamraj and Bhojraj are short pieces of stems of the two species of Vitis, and used as an astringent in gonorrhœa.

Vitis Vinifera.

Habitat.—Himalayas ; cultivated in Europe, &c.

Parts used.—Grapes and raisins, or dried grapes without stones.

Vernacular.—Arab.—Kerm. Beng.—Angur, Drakhya. Burm.—Sabisi, Sabya-si. Bomb.—Drakhsha, Kishamisha. Can.—Drakshi-hannu. Cing.—Mudra-palam. Duk.—Angura Daka. Eng.—Grapes, Grape vine, the vine. Guz.—Draksha. Hind.—Angura, Dakha, Kishamisha, Monakha (raisins) Malyal.—Munteri. Mar.—Draksha. Pers.—Angura, Gureb (the juice). Sans.—Draksha phalama, Mridoica. Tam.—Diraksha-pazham, Dirippa Zham. Tel.—Gostini-pondu.

Characters.—Berries succulent, of an ovoid form, often globose ; ovary, 2-celled, ovules two in each. There are two varieties—Kali draksh and Kishamish. The former is black in colour and large. Kishamisha is small, brownish red or pale yellowish brown. The fruit, not being articulated with the rachis or the rachis with the branch, remains attached to the plant and withers on it. The dry fruits are called raisins. In large and old raisins the pulp is found crystallized in nodular masses. Varieties of raisins.—Sultanas, muscatels and currants. Muscatels are raisins dried in the sun, Sultanas are remarkable for the absence of seeds. Currants, corruption of Corinth, where they were originally grown, are a very small variety of raisins.

Constituents.—The pulp contains grape sugar, cream of tartar, gum and malic acid. The seeds contain a bland fixed oil and tannic acid ; skin of the fruit contains tannic acid.

Preparations.—Juice, ashes of the wood, and Asava or wine "Draksha arishta." Used in the preparation of fermented liquors, vinegar, &c.

Draksha arishta—a spirituous preparation (Medicinal Wine). Make a decoction of Raisins 20, and water 60. To the filtrate add treacle, cinnamon, cardamom, Folia malabarica, flowers of mesua ferrea—Fruit of Aglaia Roxburghiana—Black pepper, long pepper, and seeds of embelia ribes each 2 parts. The whole is then set aside for a fortnight and allowed to ferment. Dose 1 to 4 drachms. As a stimulant given in congh, consumption and enlarged glands.

Actions and uses.—Skin and stones from the grapes should be removed before use. Raisins are refrigerant, demulcent, cooling, and also aperient, generally used to sweeten medicinal preparations and given to relieve thirst in fever, and inflammatory affections and in constipation. The leaves are astringent, and used in diarrhœa. The ashes of the wood are used as prophylactic against stone and in uric acid diathesis. The natives apply the paste of the ashes to swellings of testicles and to piles. Black raisin is generally used as an ingredient in purgative mixtures. Kishamish is used also as an ingredient of several confections.

Pittosporaceæ.—The Pittosporum family.

Characters.—Trees or shrub. Leaves simple, alternate and exstipulate; flowers regular; sepals and petals hypogynous; stamens 5; ovary superior; fruit baccate or loculicidal capsule; seeds numerous; embryo minute; albumen fleshy.

Habitat.—Australia, Africa.

Properties.—Resinous properties. Some bear edible fruits.

Pittosporum Floribundum, P. Ceylonicum. Celastrus Verticillatus, Senacia Nepalensis.

Habitat.—Himalayas, Western Ghauts, Peninsula.

Part used.—The bark.

Vernacular.—Mar.—Vekhali Vishari. Hind.—Vel-kali, Vehyente. Cing.—Katteya-goss.

Vikhari means specific for poison.

Characters.—Bark in quills; external surface grey and marked by warty prominences forming circular rings; inner surface smooth of ight-brown colour; odour aromatic, resembling carraways; taste very bitter. Dose, as a febrifuge, 5 to 10 grs.

Constituents.—A bitter glucoside—Pittosporin, and an aromatic oleo resin.

Preparation.—Decoction (1 in 10). Dose, ½ to 1 oz.

Actions and uses.—Bitter, aromatic, febrifuge and expectorant. In large doses narcotic; used in fevers and in chronic bronchitis with good results. It is used by the natives as an antidote against snake poison.

Xanthoxylaceæ.

The prickly ash family. Trees or shrubs; resembling in their characters Rutaceæ. Differing from it in having polygamous flowers. Fruits sometimes baccate and indehiscent. In rutaceæ universally capsular. Seeds always albuminous in xanthoxylaceæ. In rutaceæ some are albuminous while others are exalbuminous.

Habitat.—Temperate climates and tropics, especially America.

Properties.—Pungent, aromatic and bitter, stimulant, febrifuge, tonic, sudorific, sialogogue and emmenagogue.

Toddalia Aculeata, T. Rubricaulis. Scopalia Aculeata, T. Asiatica, T. Nitida, Paulinia Asiatica.

Habitat.—Himalaya, Ceylon, W. Peninsula, Coromandel Coast.

Parts used.—The root-bark and fruit (berries).

Vernacular.—Cing.—Kudu-miris. Duk.—Jangli kali mirachi. Eng.—Lopez root. Hind.—Jangli kali mirch, Dahan. Mal.—Kaka Toddali, Mulakatani. Mar.—Limri. Sans.—Kanchan, Dahan. Tam.—Kaka-toddali, Mirla-karan-maram. Tel.—Konda-kashinda, Varra-kasimi.

Kanchana (Sanskrit word) means golden—the orange colour of the fruit. Dahan means burning, in allusion to the burning taste or pungency of berries.

Characters.—Stem and branches prickly ; fruit of the size of a pea, orange coloured, highly pungent. When ripe, dried berries are dark-brown or black and of the odour of citron; root small, white, woody and cylindrical ; bark soft, yellow, with a corky external layer, wrinkled longitudinally, and containing cells filled with oleo-resin ; taste hot and peppery.

Constituents.—The bark contains a resin, essential oil, and a bitter principle. The oil is limpid, of a green colour ; odour that of citron and of a bitter aromatic taste.

Preparations.—Infusion (1 in 20). Dose, ½ to 1 oz. Tincture (1 in 10). Dose, ½ to 1 dr. Liniment of the root.

Actions and uses.—Berries pungent, like black pepper. The bark bitter stomachic, carminative, tonic and antiperiodic. The bark is given in hill and jungle fever. The whole plant is febrifuge, carminative, tonic and stimulant. Internally the root is given in general debility and during convalescence from fever and other chronic diseases. Under the name of Lopez root, it had once some reputation for diarrhœa in Europe. The liniment is used in rheumatism.

Xanthoxylon Rhetsa, X. Alatum. X. Budrunga. X. Acanthopodium. X. Hamiltonianum. X. Oxyphyllum.

Habitat.—W. Peninsula, Tropical Himalaya, Assam, Colombo.

Parts used.—The carpels and bark.

Vernacular.—Burm.—Toung-than. Arab.—Faghireh. Beng.—Tambul. Can.—Jimmi-mara. Cing.—Kattoo-keenagaso. Chinese-Hwatseau, Tsm-tsian. Eng.—Japanese pepper or Indian prickly-ash, pepperwort. Hind.—Nepali-dhanyia, Tejphala, Durmur, Budrang. Malyal.—Mulila. Mar.—Tisal Trephal, Chirphal. Pers.—Kababeh, Kushadeh. Sans.—Tumburu (carpels). Tam.—Rhetsa-maram. Tel.—Rhetsa-maram, Tisal chira phola kokali.

Tumburu, means coriander. It has the peculiar flavour of coriander and is similar in size and shape. Hwa-tseau—pepper flower. Faghireh—open-mouthed, the dried carpels adhering at one end and open at the other. Kababeh Kushadeh—open-mouthed cubebs. Rhetsa-maram (Tel.) means a council tree. The hill people held their council or panchayet under this tree to settle their disputes. Prickly ash. The bark is prickly. The aromatic, pungent property is confined to the pericarp.

Characters.—The tree is armed with prickles ; fruits dehiscent, small and oval ($\frac{1}{4}$ of an inch in diameter), resembling malkagani; surface wrinkled and pitted ; colour brownish, dark externally and brown within. It has a small woody stalk at its base and is bifid from the top down to more than half its length. Seeds black, very hard and shining, resembling pepper ; odour lemon-like and oily ; taste acidulous ; bark in irregular flat pieces of various sizes, externally brownish, consisting of several layers of a brownish red colour, corky and spongy. Dose of the seeds, 10 to 20 grs.

Constituents.—The bark contains a bitter crystalline principle, identical with berberine ; a volatile oil, and resin. The carpels contain a volatile oil, resin, a yellow acid principle and a crystalline solid body, xanthoxylin, consisting of carbon, oxygen and hydrogen, but devoid of nitrogen. Xanthoxylin is isomeric with oil of turpentine. It is a stearopten, a pale, viscid non-drying oil ; a pure hydrocarbon, to which its aroma is due.

Preparations.—Infusion of bark and decoction (1 in 10). Dose, 1 to 2 ozs.

Actions and uses.—Stimulant, aromatic, carminative, and alterative. The seeds are used like pepper as condiment. As a stimulant they are given in dyspepsia, diarrhœa. The bark is tonic and aromatic; the seeds are used as an ingredient in guraku (tobacco for the hukka), and given in atonic dyspepsia, fevers, rheumatism. Sometimes the essential oil is used as stimulant, especially in cholera.

Xanthoxylon Fraxineum.

X. Americanum, X. Carolinianum, X. Clava Herculis, Toothache shrub (Eng.) ; Prickly-ash.

Habitat.—N. America, United States, Canada.

Parts used.—The bark and berries.

Clava Herculis—Clava, club ; in allusion to the resemblance of the strong cone-like warts on the bark to the club of Herculis.

Characters.—X. Americanum—prickly shrub, bark in curved or quilled fragments, outer surface brownish grey, with whitish patches and minute black dots, faintly furrowed, with some brown, glossy, straight two-edged spines, linear at the base, inner surface whitish, smooth, without any odour ; taste aromatic, but soon becoming bitterish and pungent. Dose, powdered bark, 5 to 30 grs. Powdered berries, 10 to 40 grs.

X. Fraxineum—Shrub covered with sharp scattered prickles; leaves imparipinnate ; leaflets ovate, downy. Bark with prickles protruding through the corky cones ; branches covered with large prickles. X.

Clava Herculis, or southern bark, very thick, with conical projections and stout brown spines.

Constituents.—Two resins.—A bitter principle, probably identical with berberine ; a volatile oil, tannin, a fixed oil, colouring matter, gum, sugar and ash, 12 p. c.

Preparations.—Extractum Xanthoxyli Fluidum. Dose, ½ to 1 dr. Decoctum Xanthoxyli (1 in 20). Dose, 1 to 2 ozs.

Physiological action.—Alterative, diffusible stimulant, aromatic, bitter, carminative, sialogogue, emmenagogue, sudorific and masticatory. In the mouth it causes tingling sensation. It increases the secretions of the salivary glands, liver, stomach, intestines and pancreas. It stimulates the heart, increases the arterial tension. As an alterative its action is similar to that of mezerion, guaiacum, stillingia, &c.

Therapeutics.—Indicated in rheumatism, scrofula, syphilis. jaundice due to catarrh of the bile ducts, indigestion, intestinal colic, general debility and dropsy; also in low forms of fevers, diphtheria, hæmorrhage from the stomach, bowels or urinary organs. Locally it is applied to old and indolent ulcers, and used as masticatory in toothache, and hence the name toothache shrub. In pharyngitis gargle of the decoction is useful.

Xanthoxylon piperitum, Fagara pipenta, Chin-iva-chu-ya grows in India and China; a powerful aromatic, used in place of ginger and pepper. The active principle resides in the bark, leaves and pericarp. A poultice made of its bruised leaves and rice-flour is used in sore throat ; mixed with camphor the powdered leaves are applied to porrigo decalvans.

Simarubaceæ.

The Maharukha or Quassia family.

Shrubs or large trees, leaves without glands or dots, alternate, compound or simple, sometimes exstipulate ; flowers regular, axillary or terminal ; disk conspicuous ; ovary stalked, 4 or 5-lobed, 4 or 5-celled fruit indehiscent one seeded and drupaceous ; carpels 4 or 5.

Habitat.—Tropical parts of India, America and Africa.

Properties.—A bitter principle, characteristic of this order; many are tonic and febrifuge.

Ailanthus Excelsa.

Habitat.—Baroda, Broach, Coimbatore, Ceylon, Ghauts, Behar.

Parts used.—The bark and leaves.

Vernacular.—Bomb.—Maharukh. Can.—Dodda-mari. Guz.—Mahto Araduso ; Hind.—Mahanib, Arna. Maleal.—Peru-mara. Mar.—Maruk. Pers.—Samaga. Sans.—Arala. Tam.—Peru-maram. Tel.—Pedda-manu Peyyapa.

Characters.—This tree resembles the prickly ash. The bark is of an ash colour. Externally very thick and rough and marked by numerous ridges; internally yellow or white and fibrous, taste aromatic, pleasant, but bitter ; leaves tomentose when young, old leaves glabrous, long and abruptly pinnated ; taste bitter ; leaflets from 10 to 14, in pairs and coarsely toothed at the base. Dose, 15 to 60 grs.

Constituents.—The bark contains an acid principle, ailantic acid. It is wax-like, reddish brown and very bitter ; very easily soluble in water, less so in alcohol and ether, and insoluble in chloroform and benzol.

Preparations.—Infusion of the bark (1 in 20). Dose, 1 to 2 ozs.

Actions and uses.—Bitter, stomachic, tonic, febrifuge and astringent. An infusion of the bark is given with curd in atonic dyspepsia, diarrhœa and fever. As a tonic it is given in general debility and anorexia; generally combined with other vegetable bitters. The juice of the fresh bark is given with cocoanut milk and aromatics in general debility in women—chiefly after child-birth—to stop after-pains. The infusion of the bark is used as rectal enema to destroy ascarides.

Remarks.—It is a good substitute for Kuda Chhala.

Ailanthus Glandulosa.

Habitat.—China, South Europe, France, United States.

Part used.—The bark.

Vernacular.—Chin.—Chau-chu, Chua-chu.

Characters.—The tree, called the tree of heaven—forms the food of the silk-producing insect, Bombyx Cynthia. The bark is thick externally and rough internally ; the colour is pale-yellow and of a fibrous texture. Dose, 5 to 30 grs.

Constituents.—Volatile oil and an oleo resin.

Preparations.—Tinctura ailanthus, tincture of ailanthus (1 in 10). Dose, 10 to 60 ms. Inhalation of the oil. Dose, 5 to 10 ms. Extractum ailanthus fluidum.—Fluid extract of ailanthus. Dose, 15 to 30 ms. Decoctum ailanthus (1 in 25). Dose, 4 to 8 drs.

Physiological actions.—The properties are similar to those of tobacco. They depend on the presence of oleo resin. It is a decided nauseant, drastic cathartic and vermifuge. The volatile oil is antispasmodic and nauseant. It causes vertigo, dull headache, pain in the back, weakness, numbness in the limbs, cold and clammy skin, impairment of mobility, depression of the heart, cerebrum and of the spinal cord, leading to small and weak pulse, slow and laborious respiration, &c.

Therapeutics.—Used as an inhalation in palpitation of the heart, spasmodic asthma and hiccough. As an anthelmintic the decoction of the fresh bark (1 to 20) or the oleo resin in drachm doses is given against tape worms. It is also given in scarlatina with dark eruptions and delirium.

Ailanthus Malabaricus.

Habitat.—Western Ghauts of the Indian Peninsula, Ceylon.

Parts used.—The bark and resinous juice.

Vernacular.—Sans.—Sarala. Can.—Doop, Baga dhup, Hem-mara (resin). Malyal.—Peru-maratoli Mattip-pal. Mar.—Ood. Cing.—Walbelingas, Kumbalu. Tam.—Peru-maram. Tel.—Muttipal. Travancore—Mutti-pal.

Sarala is regarded as a substitute for pine resin (pinus longifolia).

Characters.—Bark rough, very thick and studded with bright garnet-looking resinous grains; taste pleasant and slightly bitter; the bark yields a fragrant resinous juice, dark-brown or grey, of the consistence of thick treacle, known as Mutti-pal.

Constituents.—Commercial resin contains 77 p. c. of pure resin, and the rest impurities. Resin is soluble in alcohol, and, on evaporation, leaves a very viscous, transparent, light-brown liquid.

Preparation.—Infusion (1 in 10). Dose, $\frac{1}{2}$ to 1 oz.

Actions and uses.—Bark bitter, tonic and febrifuge, given in dyspepsia and fever. The resin is demulcent, and mixed with milk it is given in dysentery and bronchitis. The resin is also used for incense, as, when burnt, it gives out fragrance.

Balanites Roxburghii, B. Indica, B. Egyptica.

Habitat.—Drier parts of India and Egypt.

Part used.—The fruit pulp.

Vernacular.—Africa—Saum. Arab.—Haleluz. Beng.—Hingana-bita, Hinggo. Guz.—Hingoria. Hind.—Hinggo Hingan, bet. Mar.—Hingana. Malyal.—Nanchunta. Sans.—Ingudi Vrikshaha, Ingua, Tapastam-munipadapa, Gauri-tvac. Egypt—desert date (ripe), Egyptian myrobolan, (unripe). Tam.—Nanjundan. Tel.—Gari-chettu, Ringri.

Gauritvac is derived from Gauri, goddess of abundance, and twac, "worship." Gurus (Hindu priests) prepare an oil from the seeds and use it in the ceremony of initiating a Hindu.

Characters.—A small thorny tree, leaves bifoliate; flowers, greenish white; fruit wrinkled and tuberculated on the surface, of a pale yellow or brownish yellow colour, of the shape of bijorun or egg or lime, oblong and slightly compressed at the base, where a short woody stalk is attached. The surface is marked with five longitudinal grooves; rind very thin and highly brittle, containing within it a soapy pulp or mesocarp, which is unctuous and oily when touched, and adherent to the woody shell; the nut is fibrous, of a pale white colour, and contains one large seed; seed homogeneous, oily, resinous and of a dirty grey colour, and having a disagreeable odour; pulp exceedingly bitter and of an offensive greasy smell. Dose of the pulp, 2 to 20 grs.

The shell is filled with gunpowder and is used in India for fireworks.

Constituents.—The bark yields a principle allied to saponin. From the seeds is extracted the oil known as Zachun oil or Zaitun oil of Africa. The oil resembles that of Arachis hypogœa ; it congeals at zero. It contains fatty acids. It is a slow drying oil, and becomes white when exposed to the sunlight. The pulp contains an organic acid, saponin, mucilage and sugar.

Actions and uses.—Leaves acrid, purgative, anthelmintic and expectorant, used in worms in children, cough and irritation of the throat. It is a good emulsifier. In action it resembles senega. The oil expressed from the seeds is applied to burns and excoriations, and also to freckles.

Cascara Amarga, Picramnia Antidesma.

Honduras Bark, Picramnia Bark.

Habitat.—Mexico, West Indies.

Part used.—The bark.

Characters.—Bark from five to six inches in length, firm and heavy, of a brownish grey colour, outer layer striated and longitudinally fissured ; inner bark of the trunk is from one quarter to three-eighths of an inch in thickness. In taste the bark, when chewed, imparts a moderate degree of bitterness with a slightly yellow saliva.

Preparations.—Extractum cascara amarga liquidum. Dose, 30 to 60 ms. The dry extract. Dose, 3 to 5 grs.

Actions and uses.—A powerful tonic, alterative, diuretic and antisyphilitic, used in syphilis, rheumatism and chronic skin diseases, as eczema, psoriasis &c., also in chronic hepatic disorders and chronic nasal catarrh. The use of tobacco and alcohol seems to counteract its usefulness.

Picræna Excelsa, B. P.

Picræna, from Pikros, bitter. The plant is extremely bitter.

Excelsa, from ex out, and celsus, beyond meaning surpassing in bitterness.

Quassia or Quassy, the name of a negro who first used this bark as a remedy against malignant fever.

Habitat.—Jamaica, Guiana. West Indian Islands. Surinam.

Part used.—The bark. The wood of the trunk and branches, Quassiæ Lignum—Quassia wood, B. P.

Vernacular.—Beng.—Bharangi (the bark). Hind.—Kashshing. Jamaica.—Bitter ash or bitter wood.

Characters.—Bark brownish grey, smooth and wrinkled ; wood yellowish white, thick, dense, tough, hard, and porous, used as chips or raspings; the taste is intensely and purely bitter. It is without any odour ; on longitudinal section the wood exhibiting elongated cells containing crystals of calcium oxalate. Dose, 20 to 60 grs. Wood is made into cups and sold as bitter cups or quassia cups.

Constituents.—A bitter principle, picrasmin or quassin ; an alkaloid, resin, mucilage and pectin.

Picrasmin or quassin is obtained by adding soda to the Quassia infusion, precipitating with tannin, decomposing the precipitate with oxide of lead or lime and dissolving with alcohol. Occurs in crystals, very bitter, soluble in hot alcohol, chloroform ; sparingly so in cold water, soluble in alkaline or acid solutions.

Preparations.—Liquor quassiæ concentratus, B. P. (1 in 10). Dose, ½ to 1 dr. ; Infusum quassiæ, infusion of quassia, B P. (1 in 100). Dose, ½ to 1 oz. ; Tinctura quassiæ, tincture of quassia, B. P. (1 in 10). Dose, ½ to 1 dr. ; Extractum quassiæ, extract of quassia. Dose, 1 to 3 grs.

Actions and uses.—A pure bitter, febrifuge and anthelmintic, chiefly used in atonic dyspepsia, with pain after eating, in vomiting, in regurgitation of food, in atonic diarrhœa, and in loss of appetite ; as an anthelmintic, an enema made of its infusion is used against threadworms. In convalescence from intermittent fever with bilious vomiting, in atonic gout and in dropsy from debility, it has been much employed combined with sodium bicarbonate. It contains no tannin ; hence it can be combined with persalts of iron without producing black colour.

Picrasma Quassioides—Brucea Quassioides.

Habitat.—Sub-tropical Himalaya, South China.

Parts used.—The wood and bark.

Vernacular.—Hind.—Kashshing. Beng.—Bharangi.

Characters.—Wood, in pieces, covered with a dark-brown bark, having a netted surface and marked with transverse scars of a light yellow colour with a central pith.

Constituents.—The bark contains resinous deposits and crystals of oxalate of lime. The wood contains a crystallizable principle, probably quassin, a bitter resin-like principle, a non-crystallizable resinous body and an alkaloid.

Preparations.—Infusion (1 in 40). Dose, ½ to 1 oz. Tincture (1 in 10). Dose, ½ to 1 dr.

Actions and uses.—The bark is bitter tonic, less bitter than true quassia, and used for the same purposes. As a parasiticide the wood is used to kill insects. As a febrifuge it is given in fevers.

Remarks.—Bharangi is also the name of the roots and stems of Clerodendron serratum.

Samadera Indica—S. Pentapetala.

Habitat.—Western Peninsula, Ceylon.

Part used.—The bark.

Vernacular.—Sans.—Lokhandi. Cing.—Somadasa-gass. Eng.—Niepa bark. Mal.—Karinghota. Tam.—Niepa.

Characters.—A tree, very high; leaves large, alternate, and oblong ; fruit a drupe-oval and compressed, one seeded, colour brown, surface smooth or reticulated and coriaceous. The wood is yellow and bitter like quassia wood. The bark is in quills, externally minutely fissured; colour dark-brown, with light-coloured patches here and there; suber exfoliated. It has a short fibrous fracture.

Constituents.—A bitter oil from the seeds. The oil contains olein palmitin, stearin; and a bitter principle, samaderin, yellowish, soluble in water and alcohol.

Preparation—Decoction (1 in 10). ½ to 1 oz.

Actions and uses.—The decoction of the bark and wood is given with myrobolans in fever. The oil is a good application in rheumatism. The bark is a good substitute for quassia.

Simaba Cedron.

Habitat.—Central and South America.

Part used.—The seeds.

Characters.—Flowers hermaphrodite; fruit pear-shaped, of the size of hen's egg; other characters similar to those of simaruba.

Constituents.—An active principle—Cedrine.

Preparation.—Fluid extract. Dose, 1 to 10 ms. Powdered seeds. Dose, 1 to 10 grs.

Actions and uses.—Tonic, stomachic and antiperiodic, much valued as a remedy for the bites of serpents and insects. It is taken internally and also applied to the wound. As an antiperiodic it is given in intermittent fevers and in neuralgia. It is also given in dyspepsia and colic of the intestines.

Zygophyllaceæ.

The Dhamaso, Guaicum or Bean caper family. Zygophillaceæ, yoke-leaf. The leaves are bifoliate, yoked and in pairs.

Herbs, shrubs, or rarely trees. Leaves stipulate, opposite, usually imparipinnate or rarely simple, dotless; flowers perfect, regular and symmetrical, bearing a fleshy disk, white, red or yellow; sepals 5, glandless; filaments 8 or 10, having small scales; ovary lobed, 4 or 5-celled, surrounded by glands; ovules 2, filiform; albumen little or none; fruit capsular, dehiscent or separating into cocci, with winged expansions; seeds albuminous; cotyledons foliaceous.

Habitat.—Beyond the tropics.

Properties.—Some of the plants are resinous and possess stimulant and alterative properties; others are diaphoretics and anthelmintics. Some have hard and durable wood.

Fagonia Arabica. F. Brugnieri. F. Cretica.

Habitat.—N. W. India, Sind, Panjab, W. Peninsula, Egypt.

Part used.—The plant.

Vernacular.—Bomb.—Dhamasa. Guz.—Dhamasa. Dhamaso. Him. —Spalaghzai. Hind.—Ustar-khar, Damahan, Damahar. Mah.—Dhamasa. Pers.—Bad-aurd. Sans.—Dusparsha. Sind.—Dramahui.

Dusparsha.—The term is derived from Du or Duha, which signifies painful or frightful, and Sparsha, to touch. The plant is prickly or thorny, and hence painful to the touch. Bad-aurd means carried by the wind.

Characters.—Plant prickly and of a greyish brown colour. The drug consists of stems, leaves and thorns, all in broken pieces. The stem is slender and of a greyish colour, surface marked with longitudinal furrows; bark tough. On section the wood is soft, light, and brittle; stem is hollow in the centre and containing a white pith; leaves linear, oblong and narrowed, specially at the base, thick and succulent when fresh; their margin is curved backwards, colour greyish, dark; surface wrinkled; thorns conical, longitudinally furrowed and a little below the apex, jointed, and of a reddish colour; taste bitterish and astringent; odour somewhat aromatic.

Preparations.—Infusion and decoction (1 in 10). Dose, 1 to 2 ozs.

Actions and uses.—Local sedative. Stimulant, febrifuge, bitter and alterative. Its poultice is used to promote suppuration of abscesses; an infusion of it is used as a gargle in sore mouth. Steam inhalation is useful in fevers. As a bath it is used in irritability of the skin, with intense scratching.

Guaiacum Officinale, B. P.—G. Sanctum, B. P.

Sanctum, sanctus, consecrated, used as incense in worship.

Habitat.—West Indies, South America.

Parts used.—The heart wood, Guaiaci Lignum, B.P., Lignum vitæ and the resin of the wood Guaiaci Resina, or Guaiac, B. P.

Lignum Vitæ means the wood of life, because of its durability like Rock-wood.

Characters.—Wood hard, of a brown or greenish brown colour, heavier than water, resinous, with irregular concentric rings surrounded by yellow albumen; when heated or boiled in salt water, or burning it in a fire, it emits a balsamic resin, whose odour is feebly aromatic and taste slightly acrid and disagreeable. The resin is in irregular masses or globular tears, very brittle, of a greenish brown colour; when broken it has a glassy lustre within. Almost insoluble in water, soluble in alcohol and ether, chloroform and alkaline fluids. Dose of the resin, 5 to 15 grs. It should not be given with mineral acids and sweet spirit of nitre.

Constituents.—The wood contains resin 20 to 25 p. c., yellow colouring matter, watery extract 3 to 4 p. c., and ash 1 p. c. The resin consists of guaiacic acid, resembling benzoic acid, guaiaretic acid 10 p. c., guaiaconic acid 70 p. c., beta resin 10 p. c., gum and guaiac yellow. The guaiac yields by dry or destructive distillation

Guaiacene, of the odour of bitter almonds ; and Guaiacol, a colourless aromatic oil ; Pyroguaiacin (in green scales) ; creosol, which resembles guaiacol. It also contains yellow colouring matter, gum &c.

Preparations of guaiacium resin. Mistura guaiaci, B. P. (1 in 40). Dose, ½ to 1 oz. Tinctura guaiaci ammoniata, B. P. (20 p. c.) contains Guaiacum resin 4 ozs., oil of nutmeg 30 ms., oil of lemon 20 ms., strong solution of ammonia 1½ ozs.; alcohol to make a pint. Dose, ½ to 1 dr. in mucilage or syrup. Trochischus Guaiaci Resinæ, B. P. (3 grs. in each). Extractum Guaiaci Fluidum—Fluid extract of guaiacum. Dose, 10 to 20 ms. Of the wood, Liquor sarsæ compositus concentratus, B. P. (1 in 10). Dose, 2 to 8 drs.

Physiological action.—Diaphoretic, alterative, stimulant, expectorant, antirheumatic and antisyphilitic. In large doses laxative. Taken internally it acts as a local stimulant, producing acrid sensation in the throat, salivation, warmth in the epigastrim, increase of the gastric juice, bile and intestinal secretions. If long continued it acts as a gastro-intestinal irritant, leading to nausea, vomiting, purging and severe headache. It enters the blood and is excreted by the liver, bronchi, skin and kidneys.

Therapeutics.—It is used in the treatment of chronic gout, chronic rheumatism, sciatica, lumbago, scrofula, syphilis, amenorrhœa and neuralgic dysmenorrhœa. A special remedy in tonsilitis, given in ½ dr. doses of the tincture, as an emulsion with yolk of egg to abort the disease, or to cure inflammation.

Tribulus terrestris, T. Zeylanicus, T. Lanuginosus.

Habitat.—India and other warm countries.

Parts used.—The fruit and root.

Vernacular.—Chin.—Peh-tsih-li. Eng.—Woolly caltrops. Arab.—Khasak-us-saghir. Beng.—Ghokhuri. Burm.—Sule-anen. Can.—Negalu-gida. Cin.—Niranche, Sembu, Niringhi. Duk.—Ghokru. Guz.—Mitha Gokharu. Hind.—Chhota Gokhru. Maleal.—Neringil. Mar.—Lohan Ghokaru. Panj.—Bhukhri, Bakhra-kokullak. Pers.—Gokhru-khurd, Khare-khasaka, Hasak Shagkir. Sans.—Trikantaka, Ikshugandha, Vanasrangata, Gokshura, Gokshuraka. Tam.—Kokullah-neringi. Tel.—Chiri Palleru.

Gokshura, derived from Go-gao, a cow and Ksura, a divided hoof, in allusion to the cloven shaped appearance of the carpels or cocci of the fruit, which, like a cloven hoof, adhere together in pairs. Ikshugandha means aroma of the plant.

Characters.—Fruits roundish, somewhat compressed, five-cornered, and covered with prickles or thorns, of a lightish yellow colour, and of the size of a marble. At the base is a furrowed club-shaped stalk ; carpels, five. Each carpel has four strong prickles, two on each side ; seeds several, oily, enclosed in hard stony cells, taste astringent and agreeable, odour aromatic ; the root when fresh is slender, fibrous, about 4 or 5 inches long, cylindrical and of a light brown colour. Dose, 5 to 20 grs.

Constituents.—The extract of the powdered fruits contains an alkaloid, a resin, probably the source of the aroma, fat and mineral matter, 14 p.c.

Preparations.—Confection. Dose, 1 to 2 drs. Infusion and decoction (1 in 10). Dose, 1 to 2 ozs.

Actions and uses.—Alterative, diuretic, demulcent, and aphrodisiac. An infusion is used to relieve painful micturition, to increase the flow of urine, and as a vehicle for diuretic medicines in dysuria, gonorrhœa, urinary disorders, and for the relief of nocturnal emissions, incontinence of urine and impotence ; its action closely resembles that of buchu and uva ursi. It is generally given with hyoscyamus and opium.

Remarks.—The root is one of the ten drugs which go to form a compound decoction known as Dasamula dakvatha.

Varieties.—Mitha (sweet), and Kadava (bitter) Gokharu. Mitha Gokharu, or true Gokharu of old writers, is also known as Chhota or Bethha Gokharu. The Kadava Gokharu, otherwise known as Motha or Ubha Gokharu, is the fruit of Pedalium Murex. Like true Gokharu, its fruits are provided with thorns or prickles, but its carpels have no resemblance to cow's hoof. Kadva Gokharu is bitter and mucilaginous, while the true Gokharu is astringent and alterative.

Tribulus Alatus.

Habitat.—Grown in Sindh, Punjab, Beloochistan.

Vernacular.—Eng.—Winged caltrops. Punjab.—Hasak. Sind.—Nindo trikund, Latak.

Characters.—Fruit pyramidal, broadly winged, cocci and 2-seeded; spines confluent. The fruit has some aperient properties.

Linaceæ.

The Alasi or Flax family.

Linaceæ, from Linum, flax or linen thread.

Herbs, or rarely shrubs. Leaves alternate, opposite or rarely verticillate, entire and exstipulate ; flowers hypogynous, regular, very showy ; calyx imbricated ; ovary 3 to 5 celled ; fruit capsular, many celled ; seeds two in each cell, with little or no albumen, embryo straight.

Habitat.—Temperate climates.

Properties.—Mucilaginous, demulcent and sedative. A few of them are stimulant, bitter tonic and purgative. The seeds contain mucilage and an oil, and hence they are demulcent and emollient. The plants are remarkable for the tenacity of their liber-fibres.

Linum Usitatissimum, B.P.

Linum, a thread. Eng.—linen, that is, its fabric. Usitatissimum, usitatus, most useful, common or familiar.

Habitat.—Common in most temperate countries, Central Asia, Egypt, South of Europe.

Parts used.—The dried ripe seeds. Linum. Linseed B. P. ; Linum contusum—crushed linseed B. P., and the oil, oleum lini B. P. expressed from them.

Vernacular.—Arab.—Bazen, Dhonul-kattau. Beng.—Tesi-Mosina. Bomb.—Alashi. Burm.—Humatoze. Can.—Aloshi-yaune. Chin.—Hu-ma-tsze. Eng.—Flax-seed, Linseed or Lintseed. Hind.—Suf Ulsi, Tisi. Mar.—Alshi javas. Maleal.—Bidgierammi. Malyal.—Cheru-chana Vittiute-eima. Pers.—Tukhm-i-Katau, Tukhame-zaghira. Sans.—Atasi. Tam.—Alishi-verai-yenney. Tel.—Allivi-tullu.

Characters.—A cultivated annual plant ; seeds small, flat, ovoid, with an acute edge, and an oblique blunt point at one end, of a brownish red colour, shining on the surface and white within; the seed coat contains mucilage, the surface is studded with fine pits or depressions, with a ridge just below the apex, having the hilum in the hollow. Seed nuclei or cotyledons are two, large and oily, and contained within the external covering, within which is a thin mucous envelope. The flax seed or linseed oil cake is the cake left after the expression of the oil. It contains nitrogen and a little oil and ash 6 p.c. The whole linseed, when powdered or ground, is known as linseed meal. It yields about 25 p.c. of the fixed oil.

Constituents.—The seed-nucleus contains a fixed oil 30 to 35 p.c.; the epithelium contains mucilage 15 p.c., proteid 25 p.c., amygdalin, resin, wax, sugar and ash 3 to 5 p.c. The ash contains phosphates, sulphates and chlorides of potassium, calcium, and magnesium.

Oleum Lini B.P.—Oil of flax seed, linseed oil. To obtain it, the seeds, when fresh, are expressed, without the use of heat or dried with heat, and then crushed and pressed. It is a yellowish, oily, limpid liquid without any colour. It has a neutral reaction, a peculiar odour and bland taste. It becomes thick or solidifies when at a very low temperature. It is soluble in ether (1 in 3), chloroform and oil of turpentine and absolute alcohol (1 in 10). Consists chiefly of the glyceride of linoleic acid ; heated with oxide of lead it dries up into a transparent varnish. known as Linoxyn. By saponification it yields glycerin and fatty acids. namely linoleic, oleic, palmitic and myristic acids. On exposure to the air the linoleic acid has a great affinity for oxygen, becomes resinoid and converted into oxylinoleic acid, making it a drying oil. Linoleic acid is also found on drying poppy seed oil, which is also a drying oil. Dose. ½ to 2 ozs.

Mucilage.—It contains in the dry state mineral substances 10 p. c., which, when removed, the linseed mucilage is allied to althæa mucilage. On mixing with boiling nitric acid the mucilage yields mucic acid.

Preparations of the oil.—Emulsion; Linimentum calcis B.P (50 p.c.), known as lime liniment, carron oil liniment. For external use for burns ; Sapo mollis—soft soap—Potassium oleate. To obtain it, mix linseed oil 400, potassa 90, alcohol 40 and water, apply heat till the mixture becomes soluble. It is a soft unctuous mass ; colour brownish yellow, soluble in hot water (1 in 5), alcohol (1 in 2). The officinal soft soap is made with olive oil.

Preparations of the seed.—Decoctum lini (1 in 30), infusum lini, linseed tea (1 in 30) ad libitum.

Physiological action.—Demulcent, expectorant, diuretic and emollient. In large doses it is laxative. In small doses it stimulates the kidneys. It is oxidized in the system and excreted as a resinoid body in the urine. Its infusion is given in inflammation of the mucous membranes of the respiratory, digestive and urinary organs ; also in vesical and renal irritation.

Therapeutics.—As it contains a mucilaginous principle and a little oil it is given with honey in coughs and catarrh. As a demulcent and diuretic it is given in renal colic, cystitis, vesical irritation, strangury, vesical catarrh and calculi. Fumigation with the smoke of linseed-oil is used for colds in the head and hysteria. The decoction, owing to the oil it contains, is useful for enema. Ground meal is chiefly used for poultices applied to enlarged glands, boils, gouty and rheumatic swellings, to the chest in pneumonia, &c. The oil is laxative and given in piles. Locally made into an emulsion with lime water it is a valuable non-oil irritant application in burns and scalds. Linimentum calcis or carron liniment, is so called from having been first very extensively used in the Carron iron foundry. The oil is often added to purgative enemata instead of the castor-oil. Liber fibres are cooling to the body and lessen perspiration, and hence used as an article of dress. Lint or ghanu kaparun and tow are prepared from fibres and used in surgery. Linum catharticum or purging flax possesses purgative properties. Bird lime, a brown turpentine-like substance, is the residue left on burning the linseed oil.

Oxalidaceæ.

The amboti or wood sorrel family. Herbs rarely shrubs or trees, generally with an acid juice. Leaves non-glandular, punctate, rarely opposite, alternate, usually compound or occasionally simple and with or without stipules ; flowers yellow or pink coloured, regular and symmetrical ; fruits capsular, three to five-celled, generally angular, occasionally drupaceous ; carpels distinct and indehiscent ; seeds few, with fleshy albumen.

Habitat.—Tropics and temperate regions ; most abundant at the Cape of Good Hope and tropical America.

Properties.—The plants generally possess refrigerant properties and are remarkable for their juice.

Averrhoa Bilimbi.

Habitat.—Cultivated in hotter parts of India on account of their acid fruits ; and Burmah.

Part used.—Fruit.

Vernacular.—Beng.—Blimbi. Bomb.—Anvulla. Bur.—Kalazoun-ya-si. Cing.—Bilin. Eng.—Bilimbi cucumber. Guz.—Bilambdi. Duk.—Bilambu. Sans., Hind.—Kamaranga. Malay.—

Blimbing-tasi. Maleal.—Wilumpi, Kari-chakka. Tam.—Pulich-chakkay. Tel.—Pulusu-kayalu. Portuguese—Bilimbinos.

Averrhoa Carambola.

Vernacular.—Beng.—Kamaranga, kamarak. Burm.—Zoungyah. Chin.—Wu-lien-taze. Can.—Kamarak. Duk.—Khamrag. Eng.—Chinese gooseberry. Guz.—Kamarak. Hind.—Kamaranga, Kamrak. Malay.—Blim-bing-manis karmal.—Maleal.—Tamaratonga. Portuguese—Carambola. Tam.—Tamarttam-maram. Tel.—Tamarta-kaya.

Characters.—A. Bilimbi, fruits yellowish, smooth, fleshy, green, five-lobed, rounded, of the size of a small mango, hence the English name cucumber tree ; unripe fruit is intensely acid ; ripe fruit acid-sweet. A. Carambola.—Fruits sweet and sour, yellow, with five acute angles and a yellowish, thin, smooth rind, the size of a hen's egg.

Constituents.—They contain a watery pulp, which contains much acid potassium oxalate.

Preparations.—Syrup (1 in 10). Dose, 1 to 2 drs. ; and conserve of the fruits. Dose, ½ to 1 dr.

Actions and uses.—Antiscorbutic. Fruits are used as an acid vegetable and for preserve. The syrup is used as a cooling medicine in fevers. The juice is used to remove iron moulds or stains. The leaves are a good substitute for sorrel.

Biophytum Sensitivum—Oxalis Sensitiva.

Habitat.—Tropical India, Java, Asia, Africa, Moluccas.

Part used.—The plant.

Vernacular.—Beng.—Bunmaranga. Guz.—Zarer. Hind.—Lajalu, Lak-chana. Maleal.—Toda-wadi. Mar.—Lagri.

Characters.—Plant 6 to 10 inches long; leaves resembling those of Bhui amala ; flowers small, greenish brown and in umbels, coming out of the axils of leaves, smell resembling that of bhanga or of decaying grass ; taste at first acidous, mucilaginous and astringent, becoming, after a time, bitter ; seeds red and shining.

Preparations.—Infusion and decoction of the root (1 in 20). Dose, 4 to 12 drs.

Actions and uses.—Acid, refrigerant and cholagogue ; used in fever and torpid liver ; mixed with gingelly oil it is given in gonorrhœa and in lithic acid diathesis. It is a constant ingredient in various alterative decoctions. Mixed with butter, the powdered seeds are applied to wounds and abscesses.

Oxalis Corniculata, O. Monadelpha, O. Pusilla.

Habitat.—Asia, Europe, India, Malay Islands.

Parts used.—The plant and fresh juice.

Vernacular.—Arab.—Hemenbab, Hemba, Homad-mad. Beng.—Chuka-tiputti, Amrulsak, Omlote. Bomb.—Amboti, Bhin-surpati, Amrulsak. Can.—Pullam-purachi-sappu. Duk.—Ambuti. Eng.—Indian sorrel, horned-wood-sorrel. Hind.—Amboti, Amrul-chuka, Khatta-metha, Set-patti. Malyal.—Puliyarai. Sans.—Shuk-lika, Chuk-rika, Chaugeri Shata-ambusta, Amlika, Shata, Danta. Tam.—Puli-yari kiray. Tel.—Pulla-chinta. Siam.—Amla-lonika.

Amla-lonika is derived from am, acid, and lonika, like loni or purslane.

Characters.—Leaves slender, prostrate and hairy, on long petioles, divided into three segments, each obcordate and finely fringed with white hairs or ciliated at the margins ; upper surface glabrous, lower hairy ; flowers yellow ; capsule very hairy, conical and furrowed ; seeds many, transversely ribbed ; taste very acid and astringent.

Constituents.—It contains acid potassium oxalate.

Preparations.—Fresh juice. Dose, ½ to 1 dr. Decoction of leaves (1 in 10). Dose, 1 to 2 ozs.

Actions and uses.—Cooling, refrigerant, appetizing and astringent; given in mild cases of dysentery, prolapse of the rectum and vagina, and as a stomachic, in fever and biliousness. The fresh juice is given as an antidote to poisoning by dhatura.

Geraniaceæ.

The crane's bill family.

Geranos, a crane, from the resemblance of the elongated beak of the seed or capsule to a crane's bill.

Herbs or shrubs, with articulate swollen joints ; leaves simple, opposite or alternate, with membranous stipules ; flowers symmetrical and showy ; sepals 5 imbricate ; petals 5, twisted, in æstivation ; fruit, 5 carpels attached by means of their styles to an elongated axis or carpophore, from which they separate (when ripe) from below upwards by the curling up of the styles ; seed one in each carpel, ex-albuminous; embryo convoluted.

Habitat.—The Cape of Good Hope.

Properties.—Astringent, resinous and aromatic.

Geranium Maculatum.

Habitat.—North America.

Part used.—Rhizome.

Syn.—Crane's bill, Alum root, American kino, Astringent root, American Tormentilla, crow foot, dove foot.

Maculatum—macula, spotted. Leaves acquire white spots by age. Alum root, because it contains tannic and gallic acids or being a good substitute for kino and catechu.

Geranium Nepalense—G. Oscillatum. Found in Himalaya, Nilgiris, Ceylon. The rhizome is used in medicine, and is known as Bhanda Rewil (Hind.); and used in diseases of the kidneys.

Geranium Robertianum.—Robert herb.—grows in Europe, Himalaya. Ther rhizome is used as astringent and diuretic in hæmorrhages and gravel.

Geranium Moscatum, Erodium Moschatum, stoik's bill. A good diaphoretic.

Erodium cicutarium.—A good diuretic given in dropsy.

Geranium Wallichianum.

Habitat.—Temperate Himalayas, Afghanistan, Kuram Valley.

Part used.—Rhizome.

Vernacular.—Afghan.—Mamiran. Arab.—Ibrat-ur-raai: Ibrat ur-raai means shepherd's needle.

Characters.—Indigenous perennial plant. The rhizome is horizontal, cylindrical, two to three inches long, half an inch or less thick, tuberculated longitudinally, wrinkled and dark brown; the bark is thin; wood wedges yellowish, forming a circle near the cambium line; medullary rays broad, central pith large; rootlets thin and fragile; taste pleasant and astringent; no odour. Dose, powdered rhizome, 20 to 40 grs.

Constituents.—Tannin 12 to 27 p. c. Gallic acid, red colouring matter, starch, pectin, sugar.

Preparations.—Extractum Geranii Fluidum.—Fluid extract of geranium. Dose, 10 to 40 ms. Dried extract, otherwise called Geranin. Dose, 1 to 5 grs. Tincture (1 in 10). Dose, 20 to 40 ms. Decoction (1 in 20). Dose, ½ to 1 oz.

Actions and uses.—Powerful and efficient astringent like tannic acid. As a tonic it is given with hydrastine in chronic diarrhœa and dysentery, passive hæmorrhages, in relaxed condition of the mucous membranes, as gonorrhœa, gleet, leucorrhœa, diabetes, cholera, &c. Locally used as a gargle in sore throat and in ulceration of the mouth; as an injection to relaxed vagina, uvula, rectum, &c.

Celastraceæ.

The Malakangani or spindle tree family.

General characters.—Shrubs or small trees; leaves simple, generally alternate, and rarely opposite; stipules small and deciduous; flowers small, regular, perfect and rarely unisexual; stamens opposite the sepals; fruits 2, 3 to 5-celled, drupaceous and indehiscent or capsular; seeds ascending, arillate; disk large, flat, surrounding the ovary and albuminous.

Habitat.—Warmer parts of Asia. India.

Properties.—Seeds contain an acrid principle; the seeds of some contain an oil of a stimulating nature.

Celastrus Paniculatus, C. Montana, C. Rothiana, C. Senegalensis, C. Nutans, Scutia paniculata.

Habitat.—Hilly districts, Himalaya and Ceylon.

Parts used.—The seeds and the oil.

Vernacular.—Bomb.—Malakanguni. Eng.—(the oil) oleum nigrum, Staff tree. Guz.—Malakaguni. Hind.—Malakangani. Mar.—Kanguni. Sans.—Vanhiruchi, Katumbhi, Jyotish-mati. Tam.—Ati-parich-cham, Malkang-uni. Tel.—Mala-erikata, Bavungi, Gundu Mida, Valuluvai Danti-chettu.

Jyotish-mati, meaning light possessing. In allusion to their supposed property of stimulating intellectual powers and sharpening memory.

Characters.—Fruit resembling tirphal in size, three-celled and globose. In form resembling the open-mouthed fruits of kapus. Fruit with a small stalk at the base, surface rugous and of a faint yellow colour ; seeds hard, angular, and somewhat pointed at one end. In form and size similar to draksha bija colour brownish red, surface wrinkled and covered with a kind of brownish powdery substance ; kernel oily and almond-like ; taste biting and hot ; embryo green, situated in the middle of the kernel ; oil of a deep reddish-yellow colour, becoming, when kept for a time, thick like honey. Dose, 3 to 10 grs.

Constituents.—The seeds contain an oil, a bitter resinous principle, tannin and ash 5 p. c. The oil is obtained from the seeds by exhaustion with ether. It is a thick, reddish, bitter oil, of an aromatic odour. Oleum nigrum—an empyreumatic black oil—is obtained by the destructive distillation of the seeds of C. paniculatus, to which Loban, lavang, jaiphal, and javantri are often added. Dose, 5 to 15 ms.

The bitter resinous principle resembles glucosidal resin. It is extracted from the seeds with proof spirit or ether, or by shaking the oil with alcohol. It is insoluble in cold and boiling water.

Preparations.—Decoction of seeds (1 to 10). Dose, ½ to 1 ozs.

Pomatum.—1 in 8 of butter known as Magz sudhi or brain polisher, so named under the belief that it promotes the intelligence of pundits and learned men who use it as an application for the head.

Actions and uses.—The seeds are alterative, stimulant and nervine tonic, combined with aromatics and given in rheumatism, gout, paralysis and leprosy. The oil is used as pomade and also as rubefacient for relieving rheumatic pains of a malarious character and in paralysis. Oleum nigrum has been tried in berberi with some benefit.

Elæodendron Glaucum, E. Paniculatum, E. Roxburghii, Neerij Dichotoma.

Habitat.—India, Ceylon, Darjeeling.

Parts used.—The bark and leaves.

Vernacular.—Can.—Tamrooj. Hind.—Bakra, Chauri. Jamrasi Mar.—Bhut-pal, Tamrooj. Punj.—Marandu, Jamoa. Tam.—Karkava, Irkuli. Tel.—Nerija-Neradi.

Bhut-pal—Bhut, a demon, and pal, palo the plant. The leaves are used to remove the Bhut or demon of which women are supposed to become possessed in hysteria.

Characters.—Leaves opposite, short petioled, acutely oblong or obtusely serrate, both surfaces polished, upper surface shining ; root-bark compact and brittle, in small fragments of a dull reddish colour, and covered by a scabrous suber, which is yellowish externally and brick-red internally ; bark and leaves bitter and astringent to taste.

Constituents.—The bark contains an alkaloid, 2 resins, tannin 8 p.c., glucose 5 p.c. and ash 18 p.c. The ash contains calcium carbonate and calcium oxalate. The alkaloid is separated by lime and chloroform. It gives a purplish colour with sulphuric acid, and yellow with nitric acid. With acids, it forms salts, which are soluble in water.

Resins.—One is soluble in ether and amylic alcohol ; the other in rectified spirit.

Actions and uses.—Astringent, stimulant and deobstruent. The dried leaves are used as a fumigatory in hysteria ; also as a sternutatory to relieve headache. The bark rubbed with water is used to remove any sort of swelling, and used as a deobstruent in enlargement of glands. The natives use it as a remedy for snake-bites. Both the leaves and bark are astringent like matico.

Euonymus Atropurpureus B.P., Euonymus Crenulatus, E. Pendulus, E. Tingens, E. Europœus, E. Americanus.

Bitter ash, Peg wood, Indian arrow wood, prick wood, burning bush, strawberry tree.

Habitat.—Western Peninsula, Himalaya, Nilgiri, shady places.

Part used.—The bark of the root—wahoo bark.

Vernacular. Hind.—Barphali, Sikhi, Rạngchul, Guli, Papar, Çhopra, Kunku Kesari.

Characters.—Ornamental shrub ; branches slightly quadrangular ; flowers dark-purple, in cymes ; fruit capsular, smooth, 4-lobed.

The dried bark in quill or curved pieces, outer surface covered with a thin scaly suber, which is soft, corky and friable, colour ash-grey, with dark ridges or patches ; inner surface smooth, pale, tawny and white. It breaks with a short fracture ; odour is faint and characteristic ; taste mucilaginous bitter and acrid. Dose, $\frac{1}{2}$ to 1 dr.

E. Crenulata bark is almost white. The inner portion of the bark of E. Tingens is also white and the arillus yellow.

Constituents.—The bark contains tannin, sugar, but no alkaloid. An amorphous bitter principle, euonymin ; atropurpurin identical with dulcite ; resins, asparagin ; euonic acid, fixed oil, albumen, wax, starch and ash 14 p.c.

Euonymin.—To obtain it add chloroform to the dried extract or the tincture, shake the solution and evaporate ; then add to the residue ether or alcohol and acetate of lead. Dissolve the precipitate by sulphuretted hydrogen and evaporate. It is soluble in water, alcohol and ether. Dose, ½ to 2 grs.

Resin.—Amorphous, of a greenish colour, without any taste, insoluble in water, and soluble in ether. Atropurpurin.—A glucoside, identical with dulcite.

Preparations.—Extractum euonymi. Dose, 1 to 5 grs. Extractum euonymi siccum, B. P. Euonymin. Dose, 1 to 2 grs. Extractum euonymi liquidum, not miscible with water. Dose, to 1 dr. Tinctura euonymi.—Tincture of enonymi (1 in 5). Dose, 10 to 40 ms.

Compound Pills.—Enonymin, gr. i ; Extract of Henbane, gr. 1 ; Extract of Rhubarb, gr. 1; Extract of Nux vomica, gr. ¼ ; Aloin, gr. ¼ ; Make one pill—as a cholagogue, Liquid preparations containing enonymin with pepsine, cascara sagrada and bismuth are used in proprietary medicines.

Actions and uses.—Euonymus is cholagogue, hepatic stimulant, diuretic, antiperiodic, antiparasitic, and tonic. The action is similar to that of podophyllin. As a cathartic it is similar to rhubarb, but only weaker. It is generally associated with aloes, jalap, rhubarb, or colocynth. It increases the flow of bile and promotes other secretions. In over-doses it is a gastro-intestinal irritant. *Therapeutics.*—A good remedy for torpid liver, bilious diarrhœa, habitual constipation, dropsy, pulmonary affection and pediculi. With pepsin it is a valuable hepatic and digestive agent ; hence given in indigestion, flatulence. The fruit of E. Europeus is used to destroy lice.

Remarks.—The inner bark of E. tingens is used to make sectarial marks on the forehead by the Hindus. The vernacular name, Kunkun, has reference to the colour of the arillus, Kunku being the red powder used to make a mark on the forehead of the Hindus. E. Europeus is the common spindle tree ; the wood is used to make spindles.

Rhamnaceæ.

The Boedi, buckthorn, Christ's thorn family.

General Characters.—Shrubs or small trees. Leaves spiny, simple, alternate or rarely opposite ; flowers small, perfect ; stamens perygynous ; petals involute, sepals valvate ; fruits dry, capsular fleshy and indehiscent ; seed erect, one in each cell ; albumen fleshy.

Habitat.—Universal.

Properties.—Some plants have acrid and purgative properties. A few are used in the preparation of dyeing materials. The bark in some of the species is highly astringent. In others it is bitter, tonic and febrifuge.

Rhamnus Frangula.

Alder buckthorn, black alder, dog wood, Persian berries.

Habitat.—Europe, Holland.

Part used.—The bark.

Characters.—Bark from the trunk and branches; in small quills, smooth, of a purplish or of a greyish brown or black colour, with white lenticles; outer layer corky, with many whitish elongated transverse markings; inner layer brownish yellow and fibrous. When chewed it colours the saliva yellow; taste pleasant, sweetish bitter, no odour. Gives red colour to lime water, yellow colour to cold water, and brown to hot water.

Constituents.—A glucoside—frangulin or rhamnoxanthin, emodin, isœmodin, resin, tannin, ash 5 p. c. Frangulin, a glucoside. To obtain it, macerate the bark in solution of carbon bisulphide, evaporate, add alcohol and again evaporate. Occurs in crystals, of a lemon yellow colour, without any odour or taste; insoluble in water, sparingly soluble in alcohol or ether; identical with cathartin. With hydrochloric acid it splits up into glucose and frangulic acid. Emodin.—Trioxymethyl anthraquinone, a reddish crystalline principle, a decomposition product of frangulin. Isœmodin or frangulic acid, is a bitter laxative.

Preparations.—Extractum Rhamni Frangulæ. Dose, 15 to 60 grs. Extractum Rhamni Frangulæ liquidum—Fluid extract of frangulæ. Dose, 1 to 4 drs. Trochisci Rhamni Frangulæ, otherwise known as aperient fruit lozenges. Syrupus Rhamni Frangulæ. Dose, 1 to 4 drs. Decoction (1 in 40). Dose, 1 to 2 ozs. Ointment (1 to 8 of lard).

Physiological action.—The bark is purgative; when fresh it is a violent gastro-intestinal irritant, producing vomiting, purging and much pain. Dried bark is not irritant; a safe purgative, alterative, tonic and diuretic.

Therapeutics.—Given in dropsy, in constipation of pregnancy, also in chronic cutaneous affections, in rheumatism and in secondary syphilis. Ointment is used for itch and parasitic affections. Frangulin is identical with cathartin (the active principle of senna).

Remarks.—Emodin is also found in rhubarb root.

Rhamnus Purshianus, B. P.

Habitat.—Pacific Coast of the United States, California.

Part used.—The dried bark. Cascara sagrada or Rhamni Purshiani cortex or sacred bark, B. P. chittem bark, Bearberry Persiana or Purchiana bark.

Characters.—A small tree. The bark in curved quills or nearly flat pieces, thick, brownish or greyish white externally, and whitish within, easily separable, marked with spots of adherent lichen, without any odour and of bitter taste. Dose of the powdered bark, 3 to 15 grs.

Constituents.—Neutral, bitter, crystalline, yellow principle, resembling frangulin; three resins:—Emodin, tannin, oxalic and malic acids, and a white crystalline sublimate.

Preparations.—Extractum Cascaræ Sagradæ liquidum. Extractum Rhamni Purshiani liquidum, B. P.—Liquid extract of cascara sagrada. Dose, ½ to 1 dr. Extractum cascaræ sagradæ, B. P. Dose, 2 to 8 grs. Syrupus cascaræ aromaticus, B. P. Dose, ½ to 2 drs. Elixir cascara sagrada contains liquid extract of cascara 8, tincture of orange 2, alcohol 1, cinnamon water 3, syrup 6. Dose, ½ to 2 drs. Cascara cordial contains cascara sagrada, Berberis aquifolium root, coriander seeds gr. 15, Angelica root gr. 2, oil of anise gtt. 10, oil of orange gtt. 10, oil of cassia gtt. 2, extract liquorice grs. 12, sugar 5 drs. Given in constipation, dyspepsia, hæmorrhoids, and as an excipient for nauseous drugs. Dose, ½ to. 1 dr. Cascara capsules ½ dr. of liquid extract in each or 3 grs. of solid extract. Some contain, in addition, Euonymin. 1 gr. in each. Dose, 1 to 2. Cascara lozenges contain chocolate with 2 grs. of solid extract in each. Pilula Cascaræ Composita.—Extract of cascara 1½, Extract of nux vomica ⅛, alcoholic extract of belladonna ⅛, milk-sugar 1, in one pill; a nice aperient; Syrupus Cascara Sagrada—Liquid extract of cascara 4 ozs., liquid extract of liquorice 3 ozs., carminative tincture 2 drs., syrup 20 ozs. Dose, 1 to 4 drs. Tinctura laxativa contains liquid extract of cascara sagrada 2, aromatic spirit of ammonia 2, spirit of chloroform 2, tincture of belladonna 1, tincture of nux vomica 1, miscible with water. Dose, 20 to 60 ms., used as a laxative. Liquor cascara aromaticus contains aromatics, alcohol and saccharine. Dose, 1 to 3 drs., used as an adjuvant to constipating drugs.

Actions and uses.—The dried bark is purgative, tonic, and febrifuge. In large doses cathartic. It improves the appetite and digestion. It promotes the gastric, hepatic and pancreatic secretions, produces large, soft, and painless evacuations. Useful in chronic constipation due to torpor of the liver in catarrhal jaundice, and atony of the stomach and intestines; after its disuse the bowels act naturally. It acts best on an empty stomach and in a concentrated form. Purgative action is due to the resins, and the tonic effects to the bitter principle. Given as a tonic and laxative in habitual constipation, associated with hæmorrhoids, dyspepsia, &c. It sometimes cures gout or rheumatism where salicylate of soda has failed.

Rhamnus Wightii, R. Catharticus.

Habitat.—Western Peninsula, Ceylon, Nilgiris

Parts used.—The bark and berries.

Vernacular.—Eng.—Buckthorn. Bomb.—Rukta Rohida. Guz. —Rakta Rohido. Mal.—Rakta Rohida. Mar.—Ragatrora.

Characters.—Bark in thick hard pieces ; colour brownish red. The texture tough and fibrous, bark from the young wood fragile and soft; taste highly astringent ; berries black, size of a pea, 3 to 4 seeded; taste bitter and acrid. Dose, ½ to 2 drs.

Constituents.—A crystalline principle ; resins, tannin, a bitter principle, malic and cathartic acids, sugar, starch, albuminous matter, salts and ash. The ash contains silica, alumina, lime, iron, magnesia, &c.

Preparations.—Fluid extract. Dose, ½ to 2 drs. Decoction (1 in 10). Dose, ½ to 1 oz. Syrup. Dose, 2 to 4 drs.

Actions and uses.—Astringent, tonic and deobstruent, given in relaxed condition of the system like cinchona bark, Combined with Boedi chhala, it is given in bloody fluxes ; locally it is applied to swollen glands and tumours.

Remarks.—The name Raktarohida properly belongs to Amoora Rohituka, order Meliaceæ. This name is popularly applied to several astringent drugs.

Zizyphus Jujuba. Z. Trinervia. Rhamnus Jujuba.

Habitat.—South of Asia.

Parts used.—The bark, leaves and lac.

Vernacular.—Arab.—Zruf, Ussli Suddir, Sidra Nabig, Unabe Hindi. Beng.—Kul, Budri. Burm.—Hyi-bin, Hzee zugi. Can.—Elonji-mara, Gub-mara. Cing.—Maha-debara, Duk.—Ber-chuni. Eng.—Jujube tree. Guz.—Boedi, Bora, Goud. Hind.—Ber, Boer. Maleal.—Elantha Perintodali. Malay.—Bidara. Mar.—Bora. Pers.—Kumara. Sans.—Wadari or Badari, Dir, Parni, Vanokoli. Tam.—Ellendi. Tel.—Regu-pandu.

Characters.—Bark scabrous, externally (like Babul chhal) darkish brown and deeply and longitudinally fissured. Internally pinkish or reddish, very tough and fibrous, taste highly astringent, odour rather disagreeable ; leaves one to two inches long, short petioled, alternate, three-toothed, oblong, obtuse, glabrous above and tomentose beneath, margins serrated, thick, coriacious and very mucilaginous when bruised. Dose, ½ to 1 dr.

Constituents.—The bark and leaves contain tannin and a crystallizable principle, ziziphic acid and sugar.

Preparations.—Paste of leaves ; infusion of leaves (1 in 10). Dose, ½ to 1 oz., and decoction of the bark (1 in 10). Dose, ½ to 1 oz.

Actions and uses.—The bark is astringent, used in leucorrhœa, diarrhœa and hæmorrhagic fluxes, generally combined with Talabija. The paste of the leaves, with those of Ficus glomerata, is used locally for scorpion bites ; and as a poultice to promote suppuration of boils. With catechu the leaves are given as cooling and refrigerant. The root is used in fevers.

Remarks.—A kind of lac known as Bhuri lak or Bora lak, is found as excrescence upon the branches. It is an ingredient in the preparation known as Lakha shadi tela.

Zizyphus Vulgaris.

Habitat.—India, Persia, China.

Part used.—The dried fruit.

Vernacular.—Arab.—Unnab. Bomb.—Unnab-khorasani. Eng.—Jujube. Hind.—Fetni, Pitni. Pers.—Unnab, Sinjid-i-jilani. Sutlej.—Amlai.

Characters.—Fruit dry, oblong and of a red colour, in size resembling small nutmeg or dried date; surface smooth, shining and wrinkled and presenting a small cup-shaped depression at its base, in the centre of which a small stalk is attached; pulp greyish yellow, spongy, unctuous and lumpy to the touch. In the centre of the fruit is a small stone, which is pointed on both sides and adherent to the pulp; taste sweet, sub-acid and moderately astringent like that of fresh apple. A fine gum lac is obtained from this tree.

Constituents.—The fruit contains mucilage and sugar; the bark and leaves contain tannin; the wood contains a crystallizable acid (ziziphic acid), tannin and sugar.

Preparation.—Decoction of the bark (1 in 20). Dose, $\frac{1}{2}$ to 1 oz.

Actions and uses.—Similar to those of dried raisins or prunes. The fruit is aperient, demulcent, expectorant and tonic; used in habitual constipation, rheumatism and chronic skin diseases. It is a chief and constant ingredient in pectoral syrups and confections. The leaves, when chewed, are said to destroy the sense of taste of disagreeable medicines. The decoction of the bark is used externally as an astringent wash to wounds and ulcers.

Ventilago Madraspatana. Funis Viminalis.

Habitat.—Ceylon, Burma, and Southern India.

Part used.—The root-bark.

Vernacular.—Beng.—Ruktupita. Can.—Popli-chukai. Mar.—Khandvel, Lokhandi. Sans.—Rakta-valli. Tam.—Vambadam. Tel.—Surugundu, Erra-chiratali.

Raktavalli.—Red creeper.

Characters.—A climbing shrub; root $\frac{1}{2}$ to 1 inch in diameter, rough and scaly; colour reddish, of a metallic lustre.

Preparation.—Medicated oil. The powdered bark, with gingelly oil.

Actions and uses.—Parasiticide. The oil is used locally for itch and other skin eruptions.

Anacardiaceæ.

The Bhilamo or Cashew (Kaju) family.

Anacardiaceæ, from ana, alike or according to, and cardia, the heart, in allusion to the fruit, which is heart-shaped.

General characters.—Trees or shrubs abounding in resinous gummy, acrid milky and sometines poisonous juice, which becomes black on drying; leaves alternate, exstipulate, simple or compound and dotless; flowers regular, often small and unisexual; fruit indehiscent drupe or nut-like; seeds edible, without albumen.

Properties.—Many plants contain a milky juice of a resinous, gummy and acrid character. In some the juice is poisonous. In pistachio nut the seeds are solitary, without albumen. Seeds of some species are used as food. The juice of Kaju and Bhilama is acrid, corrosive and of a black colour. The mango (Amba) of India is a luscious fruit. Some plants yield turpentine. Many furnish varnishes and dyes.

Anacardium Occidentale. Acajuba Occidentalis. Cassuvium Pomiferum.

Habitat.—An American plant, cultivated on sea-coasts of India, Tropics. Imported from Goa.

Parts used.—Seeds or kernels (almond fruits). Bark, tar, and spirit distilled from the fermented juice of the torus.

Vernacular.—Amboyna.—Boa frangi. Beng.—Kaju Hidjii badam. Bur.—The-ho-thayat. Can.—Gerapoppu. Cing.—Kaju-atta. Duk.—Kajuki-Jutli. Eng.—Cashew-nut. Guz.—Kaju. Hind.—Kaju, Hijli-badam. Mar.—Kaju. Maleal.—Parunki-mavah, Keppal Cherum. Malay.—Jambu-monat. Pers.—Badam-i-Pharangi. Sans.—Bijara-sala. Tam.—Kala-mavah, Kothai-mundiri. Tel.—Jedi-mamedi, Mamedi-vittu.

Boa frangi—Portuguese fruit.

Characters.—Flowers sweet smelling, pea-shaped, yellow or red; peduncle or torus, enlarged and fleshy, containing a sweet and astringent juice and used as edible fruit each peduncle having at its end a small kidney-shaped nut (kaju). The nut is an inch long, flattened on both sides, smooth and shining; the pericarp contains quantities of acrid, caustic and vesicating oily liquid. The acridity is destroyed by roasting the nut, when it becomes edible, as an article of food and as an ingredient in chocolate; hence, when ground up with cocoa, the nuts make a good chocolate. The tarry, acrid, oily fluid is obtained by heating the pericarp. From the fermented juice expressed from the torus or thalamus, a kind of spirit is distilled. The spirit has a peculiar flavour due to the volatile, aromatic principle contained in the rind of the torus. It is similar to the fermented cedar, but is superior to rum or arrack. A kind of astringent gum is exuded from the trunk, which is a fair substitute for gum-arabic. The gum occurs in reddish, yellow or brown stalactiform masses; with water it forms glairy, turbid mucilage. The tar is obtained from the pericarp by roasting the fruit.

Constituents.—The tar contains anacardic acid 90 p.c. and cardol 10 p.c., to the latter the blistering property is due. The kernel contains a sweet, bland, pale yellow oil, similar to olive oil, that from the mesocarp is thick, brown and viscid. It becomes darker when exposed to the air, and is soluble in alcohol and ether. The wood contains catechin.

Anacardic Acid.—The pericarps are exhausted with ether and distilled. The solution contains anacardic acid and cardol; the residue is next washed with water to free it from tannin. It is then dissolved in alcohol. To the solution is next added oxide of lead, which precipitates insoluble lead salts of anacardic acid. The acid thus obtained occurs as white crystalline mass without any odour. On heating it is decomposed, producing colourless fluid oil of the odour of rancid fat when burned. Cardol.—To obtain it, the alcoholic solution of the pericarp, after removing anacardic acid, is next distilled ; to the distillate add acetate of lead and sulphuric acid. The precipitate contains cardol as a yellow oily liquid, insoluble in water, soluble in alcohol and ether.

Preparations.—Infusion of bark (1 in 20). Dose, ½ to 1 oz. Tinctura anacardii (1 in 10) of the pericarp. Dose, 2 to 10 minims ; used as a vermifuge. Unguentum anacardii.—Blistering ointment (1 of the tar in 10 of vaseline).

Actions and uses.—The tar is a powerful irritant, a good, rapid and safe vesicant and a blistering agent. It gives rise to a dark-coloured stain and an eczematous inflammation of the skin, producing copious flow of serum. It is used in tuberculous leprosy, ringworm, corns, obstinate ulcers, piles, &c. The oil being insoluble in the fluid of the alimentary canal, 3 or 4 drops of it can be swallowed with impunity. It is also used to preserve wood from the attack of insects. The tincture is used as a vermifuge. The bark is given in diabetes insipidus. The spirit is a powerful diuretic and soporific, given to promote secretion of urine. It is also used as an application for rheumatism. Cardol is eliminated with the urine and fæces.

Buchanania Latifolia, Chirongia Sapida, Spondias Elliptica.

Habitat.—Hotter parts of India, Jumna, Ajmir, Panjab.

Part used.—The seeds.

Vernacular.—Burm.—Thitsai, Lambò. Beng.—Chironji, Piyala. Can.—Murkalu, Noas Kool. Guz.—Charoli, Pia-Tal. Hind.—Piyal, Charoli. Mar.—Charoli, Panj. Mal.—Mura, munga, peru. Panj.—Chirauli. Sans.—Poyala, Chara, Tapasa-priya. Tam.—Mowda, Aima. Tel.—Chara-mamidi.

Tapasa-priya—dear to hermits.

Characters.—Fruit sub-globose, drupe, slightly compressed, ½ inch in diameter, colour deep purple ; stone hard, 2 valved ; kernels laterally compressed, brown, or mottled dark brown, ¼ inch in length and ¼ in breadth ; cotyledons oily ; flavour agreeable and nutty.

Constituents.—Albuminoids 28 p.c., mucilage 2·5 p.c., oil 58 p.c., and fibre and ash 3·5 p.c. The expressed oil is straw coloured, of a sweet taste and limpid. It congeals into a white semi-solid mass at a low temperature.

Preparation.—Emulsion, which contains almonds, dates without stone, seeds of cucumber and sessamum, made into a paste, in milk or water. Dose, 2 to 4 drs.

Actions and uses.—Demulcent, nutritive and expectorant, given in cough and in general debility. The oil is used as an application for baldness.

Mangifera, Indica, M. Montana, M. Domestica.

Habitat.—East Indies and other tropical countries.

Parts used.—The kernel, gum, resin, fruit, leaves, flowers, bark, &c.

Vernacular.—Arab.—Maghzak Ambaj. Beng.—Ama, Amgachh. Bomb.—Amba. Burm.—Siyapin, That-yat. Can.—Mavena. Chin.—Mang-wo. Cing.—Amba-attamba. Duk.—Am. Eng.—Mango tree, Guz.—Amba, Keri, Ambosi (dried raw decorticated fruit). Hind.—Am, Amba-kaper, Ambosi Amchur Am khusk (dried fruit). Mar.—Amachura, Amba. Maly.—Mushchi. Pers.—Darakhte Ambah. San.—Ammara-chutu, Sahakara, Prajapati, Makau-lamu. Tam.—Manga-maram. Tel.—Mamidi-chettu.

Characters.—Fruit juicy, drupe of various shapes and sizes of several varieties, differing very much in flavour ; stone compressed and fibrous. The kernel is large and covered with a papery testa; cotyledons two, plano-convex, lobed and often unequal, bitter and astringent ; gum resin found in pieces exuding from the fruit at the time of flowering and just before ripening ; generally found deposited upon tender portions of the plant ; leaves long, lanceolate, stiff and of a darkish green colour ; young leaves very delicate and of a pale or pale reddish colour, of an astringent taste and an acidulous aromatic smell ; bark dark-brown and longitudinally fissured, inner part of a light, white, pale yellowish or reddish colour, of an agreeable aroma and an astringent taste. A kind of spirit is prepared from the mango. It is used for the same purpose as whisky. It gives about 60 p. c. of alcohol. Dose of the kernel, 10 to 30 grs.

Constituents.—The dried unripe peeled fruit contains water 21 p.c., watery extract 61·5 p.c., cellulose 5 p. c., insoluble ash 1·5, soluble ash 1·9 The soluble ash contains alkalies as potash ½, tartaric and citric acids 7, and malic acid 12·6. The ripe fruit contains yellow colouring matter, chlorophyll product, soluble in ether, bisulphide of carbon and benzol, less readily soluble in alcohol. The bark contains tannin. The kernel contains gallic acid and tannin, fat, sugar, gum and ash.

Preparation.—Fluid extract of the bark. Dose, 5 to 15 ms.

Physiological action.—The bark is astringent and tonic. The ripe fruit is invigorating, refreshing and nutrient, also somewhat laxative. The unripe fruit is acid, astringent and antiscorbutic. Ambosi is a valuable antiscorbutic owing to its containing citric acid. The ashes of the leaves are applied to burns and scalds. Tender leaves, dried and made into a powder, are used in diabetes. The kernel is astringent and anthelmintic. Amba-no-chick, or the gum resin, mixed with lime juice, is used locally in scabies. The bark is astringent, anthelmintic and used in nasal catarrh and for lumbrici. As an astringent it is given in diarrhœa, also to check hæmorrhages from the nose, stomach, intestines, uterus, and lungs. It also checks profuse muco-purulent discharges as leucorrhœa, gonorrhœa, &c.

Odina Wodier.

Habitat.—Hotter parts of India.

Parts used.—The bark and gum.

Vernacular.—Beng.—Jival. Bomb.—Shimpti. Burm.—Hnaubai Nabhay. Can.—Shimtee Poonu. Cing.—Hick-gass. Duk.—Besharam Kashmal. Guz.—Shembat, Jingna-gund (gum). Hind.—Shimpti. Kimul.—Moye-chhala. Mal.—Uthi. Malyal.—Udi maram. Mar.—Mageer, moye. Sans.—Aja Shringi, Jiyal, Jingini Netra-ushadhi. Tam.—Oaday maram, anicarra. Tel.—Oddi-manu Gampina.

Aja Shringi.—Goat's horn; Netra-ushadhi, Netra eyes, and aoshad medicine. It is a collyrium for the eyes.

Characters.—Gum in large tears or stalactiform masses of a yellowish tinge or amber colour, very brittle and friable or in angular pieces, each piece marked with fissures ; taste disgreeable and mucilaginous, one half of it soluble in water,-the remaining forming a slimy or glairy and turbid mucilage on account of the oil it contains ; the bark externally is ash-coloured, scabrous, fissured, fibrous and soft ; internally the fibres are covered with a reddish powdery substance ; taste slightly astringent.

Constituents.—The bark contains tannin and ash, the ash contains considerable quantity of potassium, carbonate, and hence deliquescent.

Preparation.—Decoction of bark (1 in 10). Dose, ½ to 1 oz.

Actions and uses.—Astringent, used as a gargle for the mouth; also as a lotion for skin eruptions. The bark mixed with Morgosa oil (Neem oil) is said to be a very useful application for chronic ulcers. The gum beaten up with brandy is used as an application to sprains and bruises. The gum is given internally in asthma and as a cordial to women during lactation.

Pistacia Integerrima, Rhus Kakrasingi, Rhus Succedanea.

Habitat.—Sub-Alpine Himalaya, Punjab.

Part used.—The galls.

Vernacular.—Beng.—Kakara Sringi. Can.—Dushtapu-chattu. Duk.—Kakada-singi. Eng.—Zebra wood tree. Guz.—Kakara-singi, Sumak (the fruit). Hind.—Kakar-singi. Mah.—Kakada-shingi. Sans.—Kara-kata-sringi. Tel.—Kakara-shingi. Tam.—Kakkata-shingi.

Characters.—Galls large, hollow, horn-like and curved, rough, pale greenish grey externally, single or sometimes lobed. They vary in size and shape, some of them resembling bivalve shells, others obovate or obcordate, generally purse-like, cylindrical and tapering at either end. Near the neck or at the attached end is the midrib of the leaf, upon which the gall has been formed ; it appears to have split into two. Between the halves is a small hole, which is the passage for the insect ; surface smooth and here and there wrinkled, furrowed and marked with tubercles. It is brittle, and breaks with a crackling noise. Internal surface of the sac has bright yellow colour like that of dried blood ; odour slightly aciduous ; taste strongly astringent, bitter and similar to that of Himaja. Dose of the powder, 10 to 30 grs.

Constituents.—Tannin.

Preparations.—Decoction (1 in 10). Dose, ½ to 1 oz.

Actions and uses.—Astringent, tonic and stimulant, generally given with demulcents and aromatics in cough, bronchitis, phthisis, asthma, difficulty of breathing, and as a tonic in fevers and want of appetite. It allays thirst, difficulty of breathing and to check vomiting. As an astringent it is largely used in diarrhœa, dysentery, piles, &c. A paste of them is applied in psoriasis.

Pistacia Lentiscus.

Habitat.—South of Europe, Asia Minor, Calcutta, Levant, Island of Scio.

Parts used.—The bud, bark, leaves, fruit and a concrete resinous exudation (mastiche).

Vernacular.—Arab.—Uluk-bagh-dame, Kinnak, Rumi-mastaka (resin). Guz., Beng.—Rumi-mastaki. Eng.—Gum Mastiche. Hind.—Rumimostike, Kundar-rumi. Mar.—Rumi-mastaki. Pers.—Kinnah, Kinnoli. Tam.—Irumi-malait-taki. Tel.—Rumaroha Ramu.

Characters.—True mastiche obtained from the stem by incision is rarely met with in the Indian market. It occurs as small, oval, smooth, yellowish white tears, brittle, being usually covered with its own dust, resembling gum resin, friable, of a vitreous fracture, softening in the mouth and becoming ductile when chewed, shining and transparent ; larger tears of an inferior variety are found mixed with bark and earthy matter; taste slightly terebinthinous; odour agreeable, flavour weak and balsamic ; it melts at moderate heat and exhales a sweet odour. Insoluble in water, soluble about 80 p.c. in alcohol, leaving a substance resembling caoutchouc, which isdissolved by ether. It gives its name to the process of mastication, being largely chewed in the East. Isasa or sveta kundola, is sometimes passed off as true mastiche. Dose of the powder, 20 to 60 grs.

Constituents.—A trace of volatile oil, two resins, Alpha resin or mastichic acid 90 p. c., and Beta resin or mastichine 10 p. c., also an ethereal oil. Mastichic acid is soluble in alcohol. Mastichine resembles copal, is insoluble in cold but soluble in hot alcohol and soluble in ether.

Actions and uses.—It is a mild stimulant and diuretic, used in catarrhs of the respiratory and urinary passages ; as an aphrodisiac combined with salep it is given in genital debility ; also used as a masticatory. It is used by dentists for filling cavities in caried teeth. When kept in the mouth it perfumes the breath. The paste is applied to the chest in catarrh, bronchitis or to relieve local pain.

Pistacia Vera, Pistacia Khinjuk, Pistacia Cabulica, P. Pushtu.

Habitat.—N.-W. India, Beloochistan, Sind, Syria, Persia, Afghanistan.

Parts used.—The fruit, galls, husks and oleo-resin.

Vernacular.—Pers.—Darakht-i-Pistah ; the oleo resin, Saker. (kundrune Talkh). Baluchi.—Kabuli mastaki, Bombay—Mastic. Beng.—Pistan. Bomb. the nuts—Pistan. Eng.—Pistachio nuts. Arab.—Fustuk. Guz.—Pistam. Hind.—Pistan. Ind.—Pisteh. Pers.—The outer husk, Posti-pista ; (the galls), Gul-i-Pisteh Buzgunj.

Gul-i-pisteh means flowers of pista. The term is applied to the galls of P. Khinjak and P. Cabulica, natives of Scinde, from their supposed resemblance to the flowers.

Characters.—The fruit is of the size of an olive ; husk reddish ; taste astringent, and odour terebinthinate ; within the fruit is a woody shell or nut of a brownish white colour, with hard, horny and polished texture and ovoid shape ; the kernel or almond is of a pale greenish colour and covered with a thin brownish red and brittle skin, which can easily be removed by scratching. It contains much oil, the taste is sweet and balsamic, flavour agreeable and resinous. Gall is a small, ovoid, fig shaped, spherical excrescence, of a brownish red colour, about half an inch long and half an inch in diameter at the apex, having a hole at the base communicating with a hollow cavity within, thus resembling a small fig bud. At one end of the gall is a scar, the remains of a fallen leaf. The walls are thin, brittle and translucent ; taste acidulous and astringent ; odour terebinthinous ; oleo resin is similar in appearance, characters and properties to true mastiche, but more opaque and less clean. Dose of the fruit, 1 to 2 drs. ; of the galls, 10 to 30 grs.

Constituents.—Galls and husks contain tannic acid 45 p.c., gallic acid, resin or oleo resin 7 p.c., to which the odour is due. Kernel contains an aromatic oil, which soon becomes rancid. Galls are soluble in water 65 p.c., in spirit 75 p.c., and in ether 31 p.c.

Preparation.—Confection. Dose, 1 to 2 drs.

Actions and uses.—The kernel is nutrient, demulcent and restorative. The galls are astringent and demulcent, used in diarrhœa, dysentery and in excessive expectoration.

Pistacia Terebinthus, Terebinthus Vulgaris, P. Atlantica, P. Palestina.

Habitat.—Europe, South of France, Algeria, Asia, Mediterranean Basin, Africa, Island of Scio or Chio, and Cyprus.

Parts used.—The concrete oil ; liquid oleo-resinous exudation ; (terebinthina chia) and galls.

Vernacular.—Arab.—(The oil) Butum, Ilak-el Ambat, Katinge-rumi (Galls), Hab-ul Khizra. Afghan.—Khinjak. Hind.—(Oleo resin) Cabuli Mistaki. Eng.—Chian turpentine, Cypress turpentine, East Indian mastich. Pers.—Zunghari, Sukhur. Baluch—Gwan.

Characters.—The oleo-resin is a thick tenacious, greenish yellow liquid, becomes hard by keeping, loses its volatile oil, and becomes a concrete, soft, translucent mass or tears, with a fennel, citron or jasmine-like terebinthinate odour and faintly bitter, mastiche-like, agreeable taste. It is free from the bitterness and acridity of turpentine. Galls are small sacs found on the margin of the leaves, single, or three or four combined, of a pink colour, terebinthinate odour and astringent taste; used as an emulsion. Dose of the oleo-resin, 5 to 15 grs., and of the galls. Dose, 3 to 10 grs.

Constituents.—Volatile oil, resin, mastichic acid, and masticin.

Preparation.—Mistura Terebinthinæ chiæ, contains 30 grains in 1 ounce, emulsified with tragacanth and acacia.

Pilula Terebinthinæ chiæ contains chian turpentine 3, and sublimed sulphur 2 in each. Dose, 1 to 2 pills.

Pilula Terebinthinæ et zinci contains chian turpentine 4, zinc sulphatis 1. Dose, 1 to 3 pills.

Actions and uses.—Similar to those of Rumi mastachi. Its chief use is, however, as a remedy for cancer of the female pelvic organs. It is said to cause disappearance of the cancerous infiltration. Galls are astringent.

Rhus Aromatica, R. Acuminata.

Fragrant sumach, sweet sumach.

Habitat.—United States, Cashmere Valley.

Part used.—The root bark.

Characters.—Shrub, 2 to 6 feet high, stems straight, branching at the top; flowers yellow, in spikes; fruit in clusters, red and acid; when broken the odour is very strong and fragrant; root-bark contains a volatile oil. Dose, 10 to 30 grs.

Constituents.—The root-bark contains several resins, calcium and potassium salts, malates, tannin, a volatile oil, fat, mucilage, &c.

Preparations.—Tincture (1 in 5). Dose, 5 to 30 ms.; fluid extract, not miscible with water. Dose, 5 to 30 minims; solid extract, 1 to 5 grs.

Actions and uses.—Pungent, aromatic, astringent, tonic, diuretic and stimulant, exerting its influence principally on the urinary organs. Used in diabetes, cystitis, hæmaturia, albuminuria; in nocturnal incontinence of urine in children; in hysterical eneuresis in adults; in involuntary painful micturition, where the urine is loaded with mucus and pus or as is found in old persons due to loss of tone in the bladder to retain the urine; also given in night sweats, in hæmorrhage from the kidneys, bladder or uterus and in other passive discharges, as leucorrhœa, atonic diarrhœa, dysentery, &c.

Rhus Coriaria.

Habitat.—Persia, Syria, Asia Minor, Mediterranean Basin.

Parts used.—The fruit, leaves and bark.

Vernacular.—Arab.—Sumaka, Tumtum. Eng.—Blue-leaved Sumach, Star-leaved Sumach. Hind.—Tratraka. Panj.—Talri. Pers.—Sumaka Mahi.

Characters.—Fruit a drupe, small, flat, of the size of Guvara-bija or lentil, hairy and of a reddish colour, surface smooth, shining and pitted here and there ; calyx small and of a brown colour ; epidermis fragile, so that the seed escapes readily; seed greyish brown, very hard, flat, reniform, and resembling a pea, having a white scar at the centre; leaves about a foot long and pinnate, with 5 to 7 hairy leaflets; elliptical, woolly and serrate. Dose, 20 to 30 grs.

Constituents.—The leaves contain a colouring matter, and tannin. The fruit contains bimalate of lime.

Preparations.—Decoction (1 in 10). Dose, ½ to 1 oz. Paste of leaves ; gargle ; liquid extract, dose ½ to 1 dr. Infusion (1 in 10). Dose, ½ to 1 oz.

Actions and uses.—A good substitute for Rhus aromatica, refrigerant and astringent, used in scurvy, diarrhœa, dysentery, and to check bilious vomiting ; in catarrh of the stomach and bowels, indigestion, cholera, in hæmatemesis and in hæmoptysis ; also used in leucorrhœa. It strengthens the gums. Locally the paste is applied over the pubes to check diuresis ; mixed with charcoal powder it is applied to unhealthy sores and in piles A gargle is used in catarrhal affections of the pharynx and in ulcers of the mouth. The bark is a powerful astringent. The liquid extract prepared by boiling the leaves, bark and fruit is given to check diarrhœa. Poultices of the leaves are used as applications to the abdomen in the diarrhœa of children.

Remarks.—The leaves are used as a substitute for gall nuts in the production of grey colours for dyeing and tanning leathers.

Rhus Glabra.—Smooth sumach.

Habitat.—America, California.

Parts used.—The fruit, leaves and bark.

Characters.—Bark smooth, greyish red, covered with scattered warts (galls) ; fruit a drupe in clusters, of small crimson berries, sub-globular, densely hairy ; seeds roundish or oblong and smooth. Without any odour and of an acidulous taste Dose, ½ to 1 dr.

Constituents.—The fruit contains acid calcium and potassium malates, tannin 6 p. c. and colouring matter. The seeds contain a fixed oil ; galls contain tannin 60 to 70 p.c

Preparations.—Infusion and decoction (1 in 20). Dose, 1 to 2 ozs. Fluid extract, not miscible with water. Dose, 1 to 2 drs. ; gargle.

Actions and uses.—Astringent, refrigerant, diuretic, and antiseptic, given in catarrh of the stomach and bowels, in dysentery, gonorrhœa, &c. ; also as a diuretic and refrigerant in fever and diabetes. In catarrh of the throat, in pharyngitis and other mouth affections it is used as a gargle. The infusion is used as a wash for ulcers, wounds, &c.

Rhus Toxicodendron.

Trailing sumach, poison ivy.

Habitat.—Canada, United States.

Part used.—The fresh leaves.

Characters.—Shrub, erect, leaves long, petiolate, trifoliate; lateral leaflets sessile, long, obliquely ovate, pointed, terminal at the base, wedge shaped or rounded ; leaflets entire, downy, glabrous and notched; dried leaves papery, brittle, without any odour ; taste astringent and acrid ; applied to the skin they set up erysipelatous inflammation. On incision the plant yields an acrid poisonous juice, which turns black by exposure to the air. Dose of the powdered leaves, 1 to 4 grs.

Constituents.—A poisonous principle—Toxicodendric acid, tannin, fixed oil, mucilage, and wax.

Toxicodendric acid.—To obtain it bruise the leaves with slaked lime, macerate with water, add sulphuric acid and distil. The distillate is an acid, which is a colourless solution, highly volatile ; almost absent in dried leaves. The poisonous principle is also found in Rhus pumila and Rhus diversiloba and Rhus venenata (swamp sumach). The last is most poisonous.

Preparation.—Tinctura Rhois Toxicodendri.—Tincture of Rhus toxicodendron (1 in 2). Dose, 2 to 5 ms. Emplastrum Rhois Toxicodendri.

Physiological action.—A cutaneous irritant ; locally applied, it causes redness and swelling of the affected part, with itching and vesicular eruptions. It is also an irritant of the mucous membranes, causing conjunctivitis, redness and tumefaction of the mouth and throat, great thirst, nausea, vomiting often choking pain, worse at night, diarrhœa, with bloody stools and diureris. In favourable cases desquamation of the epidermis follows, lasting some time. It is given internally in chronic eczema, in vesicular erysipelas, in typhoid fever, and even in rheumatism. In affections of the fibrous tissue, in erythema, herpes and pemphigus and in nocturnal rheumatic pains, the administration of Rhus is attended with benefit. In paralysis, due to rheumatic diathesis or to exposure to cold and wet, it is useful. As a local application it is used as a lotion in sprains, superficial burns, bites and stings of insects.

Semicarpus Anacardium.

Anacardium Latifolium, A. Officinarum—Marking-nut tree (Eng.)

Habitat.—Hotter parts of India, Ceylon, Burmah.

Parts used.—The fruit or nut and oil.

Vernacular.—Arab.—Baladar (nut), Hab-al-kalb, Hatul-phahama, Inkar-diya. Beng.—Bhela, Bhelava. Burm.—Khi-si chailem khyd. Can.—Ghera-mara Giru Duk.—Bhilawan. Eng.—Marking-nut. Guz.—Arushu Bhilamu. Hind.—Bhela, Bhilava. Mar.—Bhilama, Bilba, Bibnava. Malyal.—Kanpura Cherun-kuru. Mal.—Sambiri, Thembari. Pers.—Biladuro. Sans.—Bhallataka, Arshoghani, Bhellatike Bijama, Arush-kara. Sing.—Kiri Badulla. Tam.—Shayug cottay, Sheran-kottai. Tel.—Bhallatamu-jodi, Chettu Tumnaoda Mamedi.

Arush-kara means causing sores.

Arshagani—Arsha or Harasha (Guz). piles and gni, to destroy. Bhilamo is a destroyer of piles, and hence the name. Marking-nut is so called as the nuts are used extensively for marking linen. It is also used in the preparation of a black varnish.

Characters.—Fruit, a nut resting upon a receptacle, the whole resembling in shape the heart of an animal. Nut obliquely cordate, flattened on both sides, smooth, shining and wrinkled; colour black, epidermis minutely pitted with a small broad stalk at its base where the receptacle is attached; pericarp in two layers, the inner one hard and the outer one leathery; between these layers are cells which contain a black resinous, viscid, acrid juice or vesicating oil, which is known as marking ink. The oil can be obtained by boiling the whole nut without depriving it of its pericarp. The nut is prepared for internal use by first boiling it and then washing with cold water. Dose of the oil, ½ to 2 ms.

Constituents.—The almonds contain a small quantity of sweet oil; the pericarp contains a vesicating oil 32 p.c., soluble in ether, which blackens on exposure to the air. It resembles the oil obtained from Anacardium occidentale.

Preparation.—Paste, containing juice of marking-nut 1, plumbago zeylanica 1, baliospermum montanum 1, Euphorbia neriifolia 1, Asclepias gigantea 1, sulphate of iron 1, molasses 1, mix. Used as an application to scrofulous glands of the neck.

Actions and uses.—The black thick juice of Bhilamo, is chiefly used as a stimulant; locally caustic and vesicant. As a local stimulant it is applied for the relief of rheumatic pains, leprous affections, inflammation of bones and joints, bruises and sprains. When applied over the skin it causes intense pain and swelling, its thin epidermis causes deep bluish coloured vesicles and intractable sore. The mark does not disappear for many months or even for life. The pain of the application is best relieved by salines internally and lead lotion externally; the whole fruit or the seed is edible, like that of the cashew. It is boiled and then washed with cold water before use. The oil obtained from it, mixed with butter or oil, is used by the natives as stimulant, narcotic, digestive, alterative and nervine tonic, and given in dyspepsia, worms, nervous debility, asthma and epilepsy. As an alterative it is given in scrofula, venereal diseases and leprosy, and to relieve asthmatic attacks. Sometimes the fruit is heated in the flame of a lamp and the oil allowed to drop in milk. This is given in cough due to relaxed uvula and palate. Its internal use requires great caution. It is used locally to procure abortion. The vapour of the burning pericarp is applied to cold swelling and to cure piles. The mature receptacle is fleshy and sweetish-sour; boiled and eaten with cocoanut and charonji as an aphrodisiac.

Remarks.—The natives mix Bilama in the preparation of mercurial compounds under the belief that it counteracts the dangerous effect of mercury, namely, salivation.

Spondias Mangifera.

Habitat.—Throughout India.

Parts used.—The fruit, bark and gum.

Vernacular.—Beng.—Amrai. Burm.—Gue-bin. Can.—Amatemara, Pundi. Duk.—Janglitam. Eng.—Wild mango, Hog plum-tree. Hind.—Ambra, Amra, Maryam Kaiphar. Malyal.—Ampazham. Mar.—Ambada. Pers.—Darakhte Maryam. Sans.—Amrataka, Amrat, Adhvaga-bhogya, Pitta-Vriksha. Tam.—Mare-man-chedi. Tel.—Pita-vruk shamu, Toura-manudi.

Adhvaga-bhogya means travellers' delight.

Pittavriksha.—Bile tree. The bark is used to lessen biliousness.

Characters.—Fruit a drupe of the size of a pullet's egg, oval, fleshy, yellow when ripe; gum smooth, shining, reddish brown or yellowish, in stalactiform pieces, resembling tragacanth; with water it forms transparent jelly, or incompletely soluble mucilage. Dose of the bark, 10 to 30 grs.

Preparation.—Decoction (1 in 10). Dose, $\frac{1}{2}$ to 1 oz. Extract, 5 to 15 grs.

Actions and uses.—The pulp is astringent, stomachic and acid, and used in dyspepsia. The bark and gum astringent and demulcent, and used in dysentery.

Burseracæ or Amyridacæ.

Myrrh (Hirabola) and frankincense family.

General characters.—Trees or shrubs, leaves compound, frequently dotted; flowers small, perfect and rarely unisexual; disk and stamens perigynous; ovary sessile, superior, from 1 to 5-celled; ovules in pairs; fruit dry, 1 to 5-celled; seeds ex-albuminous, superior. The plants secrete a fragrant gum resin or a resinous juice and turpentine.

Habitat.—Tropical regions of America, Africa and India.

Properties.—Some plants are bitter purgative and anthelmintic; others are tonic, stimulants and antispasmodic.

Balsamodendrons.

Trees of this family yield a gum resin similar in characters and properties to that obtained from the trees of the Boswellian family. The same remarks apply to the arrangement and classification of the plants of this order as in the case of Boswellia.

Commiphora (Balsamodendron) Opobalsamum, Balsamum Gileadense.

Habitat.—Arabia.

Parts used.—The balsam or oleo-resin, known as Balm of Gilead or Balm of Mecca, fruit and wood.

Vernacular.—Arab.—Akulla Balasân, Habel-Balasana, Dhonulbalsan. Bomb.—Roghan-i-Balsan, the wood Ud-i-Balasana. Duk.—

Balasan katela. Eng.—Balm of Gelead. Mecca—gum balsam tree, Indian bdellium. Egypt.—Belasan. Hind.—Roghan-i-Balsan. Ind.—Dohnula Balashana; oleo resin, Roghane-bulsan.

Characters.—The balsam is collected by making deep incision through the bark down to the wood. Another method is to extract it by boiling the leaves and wood in water. A greenish turbid balsam, resembles copaiba in colour and consistence. The genuine oleo-resin is greenish turbid fluid, sinks in water. It burns like naphtha without injuring the wood. Cotton dipped in it can be washed quite clean in water. Its odour is similar to that of chini-kababa or oil of rosemary. The taste is acrid, aromatic and bitter. When rubbed on the palm of the hand it loses its essential oil and becomes sticky. Hence, if kept for some time, it becomes yellow and sticky. The fruit is ovate, oblong or obovate, elevated on a very small stalk and with a ring-like calyx at the base; surface wrinkled and of a reddish brown colour. There is a small projecting style at the top, from which four longitudinal ridges spread downwards and extend to the calyx; pericarp is brittle; seed one, resinous looking; oily and of a brown colour, taste balsamic, odour resembling that of turpentine; wood of a pinkish colour and heavy, met with in pieces; covered with layers of papery bark; bark yellow, tubercled; odour fragrant; taste oily. Dose of the balsam, 3 to 15 ms.

Constituents.—The balsam contains a volatile oil 30 p.c., hard resin 64 p.c., soft resin 4 p.c., and bitter principles 0·4 p.c.

The volatile oil is mobile, without any colour and of a fragrant odour, soluble in alcohol and ether; sulphuric or nitric acid gives it a deep red colour and on the addition of water it is precipitated as a resin.

Resin is honey yellow, transparent and brittle, dissolves with difficulty in alcohol and ether, dissolves readily by heat; also soluble in oils. Soft resin is brown, very glutinous and without any odour or taste.

Preparation.—Decoction of wood and fruits (1 in 20). Dose, 4 to 8 drs. balsam and oil.

Actions and uses.—The fruit is carminative, stomachic, expectorant, and stimulant, given in combination with gum acacia, in chronic coughs, diarrhœa and dysentery. A paste of it is locally applied to indolent sores and on recent cuts or bleeding wounds. The balsam is astringent and demulcent, given in profuse mucous discharges from urino-genital organs as gonorrhœa, gleet, leucorrhœa and chronic catarrh in old persons. The wood has properties similar to those of the fruit.

Balsamodendron Playfairii.

Habitat.—Arabia, N. Africa.

Part used.—Gum resin.

Vernacular.—Somalis—Hattai. Muscat—Dukh. Arab.—Dijj.

Characters.—The gum resin resembles myrrh. It occurs in irregular pieces of wax-like appearance, cracked in all directions, externally yellowish brown or liver-coloured and incrusted on one side with reddish sand ; inodorous and of a bitter acrid taste. Agitated with water it forms an emulsion, frothy and milky. Dose, 5 to 15 grs.

Preparation.—Plaster.

Actions and uses.—Similar to those of other balsams, used as plaster for the chest and limbs in rheumatic pain. Also as a stimulating application to wounds, in coughs and as a suppository for piles. Internally it is used as demulcent and expectorant.

Balsamodendron Myrrha, B. P., Commiphora Myrrha.

Habitat.—Arabia, Somali Country, Africa, Socotra, Yamen.

Part used.—The gum resin from the stem. Myrrha—myrrh, B.P.

Vernacular.—Arab.—Mukala, Murr, Habak, Hadee (Bdellium, perfumed). Beng.—Bola, Bomb.—Bysabole, Bhensabole, Mhaisagaggul (Indian Bdellium). Can.—Bola. Cing.—Gauda-rasa, Bolam. Duk. —Bol. Eng.—Myrrh, Bole. Guz.—Bol. Hind.—Bal. Mar.—Hirabola, Balata, Bola. Mahomedans—Batareh. Pers.—Bola. Sans. —Vola Minaharma, Gandha Rosaha, Rasaghandhaba, Saindhava, Samudra gugul. Tam.—Vellaip-paam. Tel.—Balimtra-polam.

Bhensa means a buffalo, and Bola myrrh. It is called buffalo myrrh, because it is given to buffaloes to increase the flow of milk.

Sindhava Gugula or Samudra Gugula means resin coming from beyond the sea.

Characters.—Low bush or small tree. Trunk very large, branches many, knotty, irregular and at right angles, terminating in sharp spines ; leaves trifoliate and long, leaflets sessile, obovate ; fruit long and pyriform. Gum resin is found in the bark and pith and may exude spontaneously as a juice. It is soft, oily, yellowish at first, then becomes roundish, irregular tears or hard masses of a brownish or reddish brown colour, waxy looking ; odour balsamic ; taste bitter, acrid and aromatic. With water it gives a brownish yellow emulsion. With nitric acid a purple colour, Dose, 5 to 30 grs.

Varieties.—Turkish is the best. The Arabian, is called by the Arabs "Mur" and by Somalis Hirabul or Mul-mul. The Indian myrrh is called Bissabol or Bhesabol. It is very impure. Meenahurma, another variety. It is of a yellowish white colour, very opaque, like ammoniacum and of a bitter taste. It is used to extract guineaworms. It acts by poisoning the animal and making it loosen its hold upon the tissues.

Constituents.—A volatile oil, also called myrrhenol or myrrhol, an oxygenated etherial volatile oil 2 p.c., resin myrrhin, 25 to 40 p. c., which by fusion becomes converted into myrrhic acid, gum 40 to 60 p.c., bitter principle—a glucoside, salts as calcium phosphate, and carbonate, &c.

The volatile oil, obtained on distillation from myrrh, is neutral in reaction, and of the odour of myrrh. It is a pale yellow coloured thick viscid liquid, identical in formula with thymol and carvol.

The resin, called myrrhin, which by fusion becomes converted into myrrhic acid, is soluble in alcohol, chloroform and ether. Fused with potash it gives protocatechuic acid and pyrocatechin. The bitter principle, obtained by exhausting the resin with warm water, is an amorphous, brittle, brown substance, sparingly soluble in water, of an intensely bitter taste. It is a glucoside.

The gum is soluble in water. It is adhesive, making a stable paste. It is partially precipitated by acetate of lead, and hence differs from gum-arabic.

Preparation.—Pilula aloes et myrrhæ, B.P. (2 in 9). Dose, 4 to 8 grs. Tinctura myrrhæ, B.P. Tincture of myrrh (1 in 5). Dose, ½ to 1 dr. Decoctum aloes compositum, B.P. Dose, ½ to 2 ozs. Pilula rhei composita, B.P. Dose, 4 to 8 grs. Mistura ferri composita, B.P. Dose, ½ to 1 oz.

Physiological action.—Disinfectant, antispasmodic, emmenagogue, expectorant and tonic. Externally astringent and stimulant. In small doses as a gastric stimulant it promotes appetite and digestion. In large doses it is a gastro-intestinal irritant and causes nausea, vomiting and diarrhœa. It quickens the cardiac action, diminishes bronchial secretions, stimulates the uterus, and is a good emmenagogue.

Therapeutics.—Given in fevers, epilepsy, generally combined with iron and bitters; mixed with molasses it is given for anæmia, amenorrhœa and bronchial catarrh, and to native women, for 11 days after confinement, for involution of the uterus. As stimulant to mucous membranes it diminishes excessive secretion from mucous surfaces of the pharynx, bronchi, vagina, uterus, and bladder, hence it is largely used as expectorant in chronic bronchitis and phthisis; also in leucorrhœa; as an antispasmodic, combined with tonics, it is given in hysteria, asthma, epilepsy. As a tonic it is given in flatulence, constipation, and atonic dyspepsia. In diphtheria the tincture of myrrh, combined with glycerine, is given internally every one or two hours with benefit. It prevents the hair falling off. Locally as a stimulant to the mucous membrane of the mouth, it is used as a gargle for spongy gums, relaxed throat, aphthæ and sore mouth; also as a dentifrice in tooth-powder; as a stimulant and disinfectant its fumes are applied on sores and foul ulcers. Dissolved in asses' or women's milk it is dropped into the eye in purulent ophthalmia.

Boswellia.

The gum resin—olibanum or frankincense, is derived from species of this genus. These are found in Eastern Africa, Socotra, Arabia, and several species of this family yield olibanum more or less similar in characters and properties. From the similarity of the vernacular names of the gum resin from boswellia trees to the names of that obtained from Balsamodendrons, some confusion has arisen, but it is of no practical importance, because all have similar, if not identical, properties, and are used for nearly the same purposes. Attempts will be made here to keep the matter, as far as possible, clear of ambiguity. They will all be described under three heads

Boswellia Glabra.

A gum resin from Somali Country in Africa, Arabia.

Vernacular.—Arab.—Luban, Kundar. Burm.—Bringi-loban. Duk.—Farangi aud. Eng.—Indian frankincense. Malyal.—Koonthre-Kuni. Pers.—Kundur. Tam.—Kungli, Parangi Shambirani. Tel.—Gugulu, Parangi Shambrani.

Boswellia Thurifera, B. Serrata, Canarum Hirsutum.

Deccan, Konkan jungles, Belgaum, Ajmir, East India.

Vernacular. — Arab. — Zuchir, Guj Kundur, Yakar. Bombay Market.—Laban Meyeti, Pandhri Esesh, Pandhri Loban, Dhup. Beng. — Kundro, Salai-gund. Cing.—Kundrikam. Duk. — Luban Kundur. Eng. — Olibanum. Guz. — Gujar-gugar. Hind. — Gugal, Awul, Kundur, Dupsalai Sukha, Bizoza, Chandel-ghar, Ganda Biroza. Indian.—Guggul. Mahometan.—Mukul. Malyal.— Kundurukkan. Sans. — Kundurya-salaki-neryasan. Tel.—Kunduruk Kam-pishin, Anduga pisunni.

Boswellia Carterii, B. Floribunda, Boswellia Papyrifera.

The gum resin from Abyssinia.

Vernacular.—Arab.—Bastaja, Kishar, Kundur, Koshfa. Bomb.—Esesh-Visech. Eng.—Frankincense, African or Arabian olibanum, frankincense tree. Guz.—Isasa. Hind.—Seta Kundura, Selagonda. Mah.—Visesha. Sans.—Kundari or Sveta Kunduru.

Characters.—Olibanum. According to the native classification there are several kinds. *Kundura zakara*, male frankincense, is in reddish white or deep yellow and circular tears. *Kundura Unsa*, female frankincense, is yellowish white, translucent or in pale tears. *Madahraja Kundur*, artificial spherical tears made by shaking the moist exudation in a basket. *Kishar Kundur* or *Dhupa* (India Bazaar) or Kashfa-resin, in flat and scaly pieces, obtained from the bark of the tree, which is coated with the exudation or scurf, known as Dhupa. The exudation in powder is known as Dukok Kundura or dust of olibanum. Dhupa (Guz.) is used in the Indian temples as an incense. *Visesha*, olibanum, the gum resin obtained by making incisions in the bark when the gum is exuded resembles Babula gunda or Kera gunda; has the colour and consistence of Canada-balsam. It occurs in large, clean, detached, yellowish tears or flat pieces, globular or pear-shaped, and often translucent. Papery bark is sometimes found adherent to flat pieces, colour whitish, pale yellow or brown, and unctuous to the touch ; before the flame of a lamp it burns very readily and is reduced to a black mass; does not emit much smoke; odour rather disagreeable, balsamic and terebinthinate; it softens in the mouth; soluble in ether and spirit of wine; taste slightly pungent and bitter and terebinthinate; kept for a time in water, it turns into a milk-white opaque and sticky mass, a soft whitish pulp, and then rubbed into a mortar, it forms an emulsion. Gandha Biroza, which is fragrant and transparent, is prepared from the gum resin as soft ductile pieces of a greenish or white colour, similar in appearance to Venice turpentine. Dose, 10 to 30 grs.

Constituents.—Olibanum contains volatile oil 4 to 7 p. c., mostly (olibene) resin, 56 to 75 p. c., gum 30 p. c., a bitter principle and ash 3 p. c.

Preparation.—Olibanum ointment—olibanum, sesamum oil and white wax, equal parts, melted together. Lepa or paste. Emulsion, plaster or fumigation.

Actions and uses.—Properties similar to those of the products of pines and firs as Burgundy pitch, &c.; stimulant, expectorant, demulcent, emmenagogue and discutient. As a discutient Visesha, or Gunda-biroza is applied to indolent swellings, buboes, &c.; as stimulant expectorant, chiefly used in chronic pulmonary affections, in bronchitis, bronchorrhœa and chronic laryngitis, pharyngitis, &c. As a demulcent it is used in bloody fluxes; an oil distilled from Gunda-biroza is given in gonorrhœa. Native women take it to increase menstruation. As fumigation it is much used in bronchitis and fevers. Its lepa or ointment is a useful stimulant application for sprains, bruises, dislocations, carbuncles, boils and ulcers.

Canarium Commune, Bursera Paniculata.

Balsamodendron Zeylanicum.

Habitat.—Penang, Moluccas, Mauritius, Ceylon, Southern India, Manilla.

Part used.—The concrete oleo resin, which exudes by excision—Elemi.

Vernacular.—Eng.—Java Almond. Elemi tree, East Indian Elemi. Hind.—Jangli badam. Malay.—Kanari.

Characters.—Bark yields a concrete resin in conical tears or large pieces hanging from the trunk and branches. At first it is a limpid, oily liquid, white and sticky or soft and yellowish, but soon becomes thick, wax-like and yellow. It readily softens when heated, and has the odour of fennel and lemon or terebinthinate; taste bitter, and pungent. Kernels or almonds are three-angled; seeds similar to those of Pistacia terebinthus. They yield a bland oil and some solid fat of an agreeable sweet taste, and smell of turpentine.

Constituents.—Volatile oil 10 p. c. and resin (brein) 60 p.c., resin (amyrin) 25 p. c., bryoidin, breidin, and elemic acid.

Preparation.—Unguentum elemi (1 in 5); emulsion of nuts or seeds, and oil. Dose of the emulsion, 4 to 8 drs.

Actions and uses.— Demulcent, stimulant and expectorant, given in gonorrhœa, gleet, and leucorrhœa. The emulsion of the kernels is used as a substitute for Mistura amygdala. The ointment is used as a stimulant application to ulcers and chronic skin diseases.

Canarium Bengalense, Darjeeling Gokal Dhup, a native of Sylhet. Resin exudes from fissures or wounds in the bark. It is clear amber-coloured and soft; after a time becomes hard and brittle; resembles copal.

Gardenia cancamum is a gum resin obtained from a Gardenia. It is fragrant like myrrh, and used for fumigation. Medicinally it is given in corpulence and to reduce spleen; also used as an emmenagogue. It is locally applied to cure toothache.

Canarium Strictum.

Habitat.—Western Peninsula, Tinavelly, Malabar, Philippine Islands.

Part used.—Resin.

Vernacular.—Beng.—Kâla-damar, Manda dup, Gugal, Dup. Duk.—Kala dammar. Eng.—Black dammer. Guz.—Kalo-domar. Hind.—Kala dammar. Maleal.—Canari, Thelli-mara. Tam.—Karrapu-damar, Kongalam-maram. Tel.—Nalla-rajan.

Characters.—Dammar, an oleo resin, exudes from incisions or is obtained by lighting fire at the base of the tree till the bark has become charred, when the resin begins to exude in large stalactitic mass, of a shining colour when viewed *en masse*; it is deep red-brown when held between the eye and the light; odour strong, terebinthinate and resembling fennel and lemons, taste bitter and pungent. Insoluble in cold, partially soluble in boiling alcohol on the addition of camphor. Its powder is readily soluble in oil of turpentine. When burnt it emits a more resinous smell and burns with more smoke than white dammar. It is chiefly used in the manufacture of bottling wax, varnishes, &c.; a good substitute for Burgundy pitch.

Constituents.—It contains volatile oil and resin. Used as plaster and ointment.

Actions and uses.—Stimulant to the skin; used as an ointment in chronic skin diseases, as psoriasis, ptyriasis, &c.

Remarks.—Vateria Indica is the white dammer tree.

Commiphora Mukal, C. Africana.

Balsamodendron Mukul, B. Agallocha, B. Pubscence, B. Roxburghii.

Habitat.—Indigenous in Sind; W. Himalaya, Central India.

Part used.—The gum resin.

Vernacular.—Resin: Arab.—Moql, Aflatunum Kundur. Beng.—Goobdee, Gugala. Bomb.—Athaisa gugula. Can.—Guggala. Cing.—Gugula, Rata Dummula. Duk.—Gugula. Eng.—East Indian myrrh, Indian and African Bdellium. Salaitree. Guz.—Gugala. Hind.—Gugal, Gubdee, Mukul Athaisa Gugala, Salai-gogil. Mar.—Guggula. Pers.—Bae-ja hudan, Muql. Sans.—Guggalaha-sallake, Drava-Sihla-i-Guggula. Tam.—Gukkul, Kukkulu. Tel.—Maisakshi, Googula.

Characters.—Gugal occurs as yellowish, viscid, brown tears, or in fragrant pieces, mixed with hairs, stems, pieces of bark, &c.; colour brownish dark or golden yellow. Each piece is translucent. It hardens very slowly, and resembles Gulakanda. It is more oily than Hirabola and burns very readily. With water it forms a milky emulsion. The odour is that of olibanum, or terebinthinate, but fainter. The taste is bitter. Mhaisa Gugal is in vermiform pieces and thick, colour lighter and greenish pieces with papery bark attached to them.

Constituents.—Volatile oil, gum resin, bitter principle.

Preparation.—Unguentum gugalæ (1 in 8), tinctura gugalæ (1 in 5). Dose, ½ to 1 dr. Compound pill, known as Yogaraja Gugala, contains Gugala 25, Triphala 15, Suntha, Pipali, Chavaka, Pipali-mula, Chitraka, Hinga, Ajamoda, Sirasa, Jirun, Shahjirun Ranuka-bija, Indra-java, Pahada-mula, Baberang, Kutaki, Atisha, Bharingi, Vekhanda, of each 1, Moravela 2, mix and make a pill mass. Dose, 3 to 5 grs. To be given in decoction of Gorakhamundi (Sphœranthus Indicus). Used as an alterative in syphilis, chronic gonorrhœa, piles, fistulæ, scrofulous skin diseases, chronic rheumatism, consumption and leprosy. Kanchanara Gugala contains Gugala 12, Kanchana-chhala 10, Triphala 2, Trikatu 1, Vayavarana 1, Elachi, Taja, Tamala-patra, each ½, Madha q. s. Mix and make a paste or a pill mass. Dose, 4 to 6 grs. To be given in decoction of Triphâl, or infusion of Khera-chhala. Used as an alterative in enlarged glands in the neck, chronic rheumatism, dropsy, gleet, &c.

Actions and uses.—Alterative, demulcent, stimulant, tonic, antispasmodic and emmenagogue, often combined with aromatics and given in rheumatism, scrofulous affections, and nervous diseases; locally the ointment is used as a stimulant to indolent ulcers, to painful joints, combined with sulphur, catechu and borax.

Remarks.—It is confounded with salaigond obtained from Boswellia Glabra and B. Serrata.

Garuga Pinnata.

Habitat.—India, Madras and Bengal.

Parts used.—The fruit and juice.

Vernacular.—Beng.—Toom. Burm.—Khyong-youk. Hind.—Ghogar, Kharpat. Mar.—Kanghur, Kuruk, Kusar. Panj.—Kharpat. Tam.—Kavi-vembu maram. Tel.—Garuga-chettu, Kalu-gudu.

Characters.—Fruit greenish yellow, of the size of gooseberry. The juice from the leaves gummy and resinous, greenish yellow and translucent, generally in small mamiliform masses.

Constituents.—Gum resin contains 76-5 p.c. of gum, 13·9 of resin, 9-5 of moisture, including volatile oil. The gum is precipitated by ferric salts, and is similar to that of myrrh; resin is neutral, soluble in ether.

Preparation.—Elixir containing the juice of Garuga Pinnata, Adhaloda vesica, Vitex trifolia, mixed with honey.

Actions and uses.—The fruit is eaten and is cooling and stomachic. The juice is expectorant, given in asthma and coughs. Dose of the juice, 1 to 2 drs.

Leguminosæ or Fabaceæ.

The Aghathia, pulse, and Babula family.

Legumen, from legere, to gather. That which may be easily gathered by the hand and not cut.

Trees, herbs or shrubs; leaves petioled, alternate, usually stipulate, simple or variously compound; flowers of various colours, often papilionaceous or globose; fruit sometimes a tomentum and rarely a drupe, usually a legume; hence the name of the order; seeds arillate, one or more sometimes attached to the upper or ventral suture. The albumen is absent or present. The cotyledons are leafy or fleshy.

Properties.—Numerous species are greyish coloured and most graceful plants. Generally this order is poisonous; a few are used as nutritious food by men or animals. In them the poisonous properties are replaced by sugar or starch. The gum exuded by most plants is generally demulcent. The leaves are aperient, and some are used as dyes; the wood is used as timber.

Abrus Precatorius. A. Minor. A. Pauciflorus.

Habitat.—Indigenous in India, wild in tropical countries, West Indies.

Parts used.—The seeds, root and leaves.

Vernacular.—Arab.—Ain-eddik. Beng.—Kunchgula, Gunjachi. Burm.—Khyen-rwœ, Yove-si. Can.—Gul-ganji. Cing.—Olinda. Duk.—Gumchi. Eng.—Bead seed tree, Abrus, Jamaica wild liquorice, Indian or country liquorice, Jumble beads, American seeds, Jequirity, prayer-beads. Guz.—Lal-chanothi. Hind.—Gunch-rutti. Malay.—Dan-sot-ga. Malyal.—Kunni-kuru. Mar.—Gunzha. Pers.—Khak-shi, Chasma-khuros. Sans.—Gunja, Kaka-chinchi-bajama. Tam. Gundumani. Tel.—Guruvenda, Yashti Madhu.

Ain-ed-dik, cock's eye. The seeds resemble cock's eye.

Characters.—Leaves 2 or 3 inches long; leaflets many, small, linear and oval; taste sweet; root woody, hard, much branched and of an acrid odour and taste; seeds albuminous, small, globose, of a brilliant scarlet colour, with a black (scar) patch on the hilum. Three varieties: red, white and black; red seeds bright scarlet, polished, as large as peas and egg-shaped, having black spot containing a white scar at one end, which indicates the place where they were attached to the pods; white seeds (which are used medicinally) larger than those of the red variety, ivory-white, very hard and highly polished, having a scale-like attachment at the hilum. The black seeds are never used medicinally; odour of the seeds disagreeable.

Constituents.—The seeds contain some fixed oil, arabic acid, two proteid poisons, called a-phyt-albuminose and paraglobulin, closely allied to principles found in snake venom, like ricin and to proteids contained in papaw juice. The root, leaves and branches contain sugar, and glycyrrhizic acid.

Preparations.—Medicated oil, "Gunjtel."—Boil together Til-tel 4, and the juice of Bhangro 14, and add Gunj 2 (1 in 10). Infusum Abri.—Infusion of Jequirity (1 of the seeds in 12½), for external application.

Actions and uses.—The seeds are harmless when eaten, but poisonous when a paste of them is applied to open wounds. Applied to the eyes they set up inflammation, œdema of the lids and ulceration of the cornea. The face and neck become swollen and the maxillary glands enlarged.

Internally the seeds are demulcent, expectorant like liquorice; used in cough, and gonorrhœa. The fresh leaves are chewed with cubebs and sugar to relieve hoarseness of voice as in sore throat and aphthæ in the mouth. In spermatorrhœa with bloody discharges, the white abrus leaves and henna leaves triturated with the powder of the root of holostemma rheedii with cumin seeds and sugar are given internally. With chitraka mula the paste of the leaves is applied in skin diseases as leucoderma, and also recommended as a cure for baldness over the scalp. The infusion of the seeds should be used fresh, as in a short time it decomposes and swarms with bacteria. Boric acid may be added to prevent decomposition. It is used as application for the eyes for the cure of pannus and old granular lids. Its use should be followed by weak solution of alum or borax. When applied to the inner surface it produces artificial purulent ophthalmia, varying in intensity with the frequency of the applications. It is also used for the cure of lupus and unhealthy ulcers. The paste of the seed (1 in 4) is used as a rubefacient in sciatica, stiff shoulders and paralysis; the oil is used in removing scurf of the scalp, in prurigo, in exuberant granulations and proliferating cell growths. The dried roots are made use of in the same manner as the liquorice root. Being sweet like liquorice root, it is called liquorice by the Indians.

The Lal Gunza is used by jewellers and goldsmiths as Ratti weights, to weigh gold, diamonds and pearls. In some parts of India the natives use the paste of the seeds to kill bullocks to obtain a supply of hides. They prepare small spikes of the paste of powdered seeds by drying the paste in the sun and use them after the manner of a driver's goad. The spikes are called sui (needles) or suitari (awls).

Acacia Senegal, B. P. Acacia Arabica. Mimosa Arabica.

Habitat.—India, Arabia, Abyssinia, Africa.

Parts used.—The bark extract and leaves, gummy exudation from the stem and branches. Acaciæ Gummi, gum acacia, B. P.

Vernacular.—Arab.—Amghantan Akakia (extract), Mughilan, Sanghi arabi (gum). Beng.—Babular. Bomb.—Kalo-bavala, Maswai-gund, Maklai gond (gum). Burm.—Nan-lung-kyen. Cing.—Andere,

Can.—Kare golbale mara. Duk.—Kali-kikar. Eng.—Indian gum tree, Babul bark. Guz.—Kalo, Bavala-kikar, Oomravate-gund (gum). Hind.—Kikar, Babul. Mar.—Babli, Tamra-gond. Malyal.—Karuvelakam. Pers.—Kharo, Mughilan. Sans.—Kala-babal. Senegal.—Red gum. Tam.—Karu-vel. Tel.—Nalla-umona.

Bark fissured, scabrous, tough and woody; colour dark-red externally and pale-red within. Whole bark can be easily separated into layers; taste astringent. *Gum*, an exudation from stem and branches, a result of the transformation of cell contents under the bark where the gum remains in pouches, obtained by making incisions into the bark; occurs in irregular or broken tears, of pale yellow or deep reddish brown colour, of various sizes, agglutinated or stalactiform masses and angular fragments or pieces. Thick pieces opaque, thin ones transparent; each tear about ½ an inch to an inch in diameter; gum brittle, breaks with a glassy iridescent fracture; taste bland and mucilaginous, without odour, entirely soluble in water and insoluble in alcohol.

Makai or Maklai gund is brought from Aden, is of the best quality, colourless, in large round tears or twisted, or in vermicular pieces, of a white-yellow or reddish colour, allied to gum senegal. Maswai gund is of inferior quality, heavy, hard, fissured and in angular pieces, shining, yellowish red or straw-coloured or brownish yellow or black with a tinge of white, of agreeable odour and mucilaginous and astringent taste, soluble in water, forming a sticky solution. It is free from fungus. Seeds in a single row along the whole length of the pod; on both the margins of the pod and between each seed there is a constriction. Pod about 4 to 5 or 6 inches long, compressed and of a grey, glaucous colour, containing the pulp (Akakia), in which are embedded several seeds. Akakia (extract) is yellowish white mass, resembling lardaceous pus. When dry, of a bottle-green or dammer colour, heavy, hard and easily pulverizable, having the smell of Rajama. It sticks between the fingers. Generally prepared from the juice of *karaz*, the fruit of A. Nilotica and A. Vera. The juice is left to thicken in the pods, which are steeped in water for the purpose, and then pressed and dried in the sun. Dose of the gum *ad libitum* of the extract, 2 to 5 grs.

Constituents.—Gum contains arabic acid, combined with calcium magnesium and potassium; also small quantity of malic acid, sugar, moisture 14 p.c., ash 3-4 p.c.

Preparation.—Mucilago acaciæ B. P. Mucilage of gum acacia (2 in 3). Decoction of bark (1 in 10). Dose, 1 to 2 ozs. Poultice of leaves. Mistura glycerrhizæ composita. Dose, 1 to 4 drs. Pulvis cretæ compositus; Trochisci cubebæ; Trochisci glycerrhizæ et opii.

Actions and uses.—The bark is astringent and tonic, a substitute for oak bark. The decoction is used as a gargle in sore throat, in copious salivation, and as a wash for ulcers; externally applied it allays irritation of excoriations of sores and ulcers by forming a coating. The gum is used as food for diabetic patients, as it is not convertible into sugar. In pharmacy it is used to suspend heavy insoluble powders in mixtures and in making pills. Akakia is astringent, styptic and tonic. A paste of it, with the white of an egg, is applied to burns and scalds and to relaxed condition of the mucous membrane, and as a collyrium for the eyes in conjunctivitis. It is also used to arrest hæmorrhages. Powdered bark with gingelly oil is used externally in cancerous affections. Pods are given in cough. Leaves are local stimulant; poultices of bruised tender leaves are applied to ulcers with sanious discharges. The gum is also demulcent emollient and nutritive and used for irritated condition of the mucous membranes, as in cough, sore throat, catarrh of the stomach and intestines, as diarrhœa, dysentery, leucorrhœa, cystitis, urethritis, &c.; also in irritant poisons.

Acacia Catechu. A. Wallichiana. A. Polyacantha. Mimosa Catechu.

Habitat.—India, Cutch, Ceylon, Malabar, Bengal and Pegu.

Parts used.—The bark, extract prepared from the wood, catechu nigrum, gum, and khairsala.

Acacia.—From Akakia, a thorn, *i.e.* a tree studded with thorns. Catechu, from cuth, "Kaitha," an Indian name for extract or the juice.

Vernacular.—Beng.—Khair (wood). Bomb.—Khera-sara. Burm.—Shia-dza, Sha-shi, Shazibin (wood). Can.—Cuth-kagli (wood). Cing.—Kiheri, Khadir (wood). Duk.—Kath. Eng.—Red catechu, black China catechu. Guz.—Katho, Kheriogund. Hind.—Khera-sara, Kath. Mar.—Khadir, Khair. Malay.—Kachu, Gambia,. Kadaram. Panj.—Kwarech. Sans.—Khadira-sara, Mekashaha, Khadi-ramu (wood). Tam.—Wodalai, Kashketti. Tel.—Khadi-ramu.

Characters.—Bark rough, of a dark-brown colour externally, smooth and reddish within. It resembles Bavala chhala. In some specimens the bark is smooth, of a yellowish colour, rather thin, external surface here and there denuded of its epidermis; taste highly astringent. Catechu—an extract prepared by removing sap, wood and bark—make a decoction of these, strain and finally evaporate to the consistence of jaggary and pour into clay moulds. Divide into squares by string and dry in the sun. Similar product is obtained by boiling water from the unripe pods or twigs.

Khair-sala or Khairsar is a natural catechu, obtained from cavities in the wood of acacia catechu. It is of a pale brownish colour, and an astringent taste. It occurs in small irregular fragments mixed with chips of reddish wood. It is found by persons who split the wood. It has a sweetish but feeble astringent taste. It is also found in the wood of callophyllum tomentosum. Gum Kerio-gunda is of a light yellow or white colour, and resembles the commercial inferior gum. It is met with in spheroidal tears or agglutinated masses. The tears are brittle and porous. It occurs in minute needle-shaped crystals, and does not dissolve in cold water, and forms thick pale-coloured mucilage.

Commercial catechu is often adulterated with fragments of leaves, mats, cloths, ferrous carbonate; or artificially prepared by roasting powdered mahogany, walnut and other coloured woods and then boiling and evaporating the decoction. Dose, 5 to 15 grs. of catechu.

Constituents.—Catechu tannic acid 35 p. c., catechuic acid or catechin, catechu red, gum, quercetin and ash.

Catechu Tannic Acid.—Mix catechu with cold water and evaporate the solution. It is a dark, reddish brown powder oxidising in the air and insoluble in ether.

Catechin or catechuic acid—make a hot solution of catechu, strain and allow to settle. Another method:—Dissolve catechu in dilute alcohol, shake the solution with ether, evaporate and crystallize. Occurs as white needles or crystals ; taste sweetish ; soluble in ether. On heating it is converted into catechu tannic acid. On dry distillation it yields pyrocatechin or catechol, phenol and acetic acid. Fused with potash it gives phloroglucin and proto-catechuic acid.

Preparation.—Infusion (1 in 30). Dose, 1 to 2 fl. ozs. *Kathbal.*—A combination of catechu and myrrh. *Kathlan.*—A confection containing khairsal, rose buds and sugar. *Tinctura catechu* composita nigrum (1 in 5). Dose, ½ to 1 fl. dr. *Pulvis catechu compositus* (4 in 10). Dose, 10 to 40 grs. Catechu ointment (1 in 8). *Trochisci catechu*, 1 gr. in each.

Actions and uses.—Powerful astringent stronger than kino, antiperiodic and digestive. Its action is due to the tannic acid it contains. It is a powerful astringent to the mucous membranes, given in dyspepsia attended with pyrosis, and also in diarrhœa in children, in dysentery, intermittent fever and scurvy ; as a gargle in hoarseness of voice and sore throat. Locally as a dusting powder to hypertrophied relaxed tonsils, ulcerated and spongy gums ; as a gargle in salivation and as an injection in leucorrhœa and to control passive hæmorrhages. The ointment is used in chancres, sore or cracked nipples and eczematous eruptions on the skin ; also leprous indurated ulcers. Its powder is used as a snuff in epistaxis. Kher-sal is a stimulant, expectorant and astringent, given to promote expectoration and to check internal hæmorrhages as hæmoptysis ; also in diarrhœa and dysentery. Kathbal is a tonic and galactogogue, and given as a tonic to women after confinement. Kathalan is used by parturient women after delivery.

Varieties.—The black catechu, Khadira, is in circular flat cakes or round balls, of a dark-brown or reddish colour, with a shining fracture and of a granular appearance. When in irregular masses or square cakes it is known as Box catechu. It is hard and brittle. The granules resemble those of Hira-dakhana. The taste is highly astringent. It sticks to the tongue. It is used for industrial purposes. The pale or pinkish brown catechu, Papri khar, prepared from nuts of areca catechu, used as a masticatory for chewing with betel-leaf. In preparing this, instead of evaporating the decoction till it solidifies, the inspissation is stopped at a certain point and the liquor allowed to cool. It is next allowed to coagulate and crystallize over twigs and leaves thrown into the pots for the purpose. It occurs in irregular quadrangular fragments of a porous earthy appearance, with a laminated texture, easily broken and of a light pinkish brown colour. It is less astringent and less sticky than the black catechu. *Chinai Kath* or *pale catechu.* The extract from the leaves and young shoots of uncaria gambier, prepared at Malacca, Singapore and Penang. There are two varieties, known as true and false. The true Chinai Katha or Gambier catechu is imported from China, and is an earthy-looking substance, of a light brown colour, consisting of cubes, more or less agglutinated. They are dark, reddish brown externally and of a pale cinnamon hue within and porous, friable, and marked with ridge. The taste is bitter and earthy, also slightly astringent, becoming subsequently sweetish. It has no odour. The false variety is not imported from China. It is disc-like or resembling lozenges of a pale white colour, and chiefly composed of Mulatani Mati flavoured with catechu water. Vadino Katho.—Like Chinai Kath, is met with in two forms, true and false. Both occur in irregular lumps of about an inch in diameter. The true form is dark-brown above and pale within. The false is pale or pinkish above and earthy within. Chaki-no-katho.—It occurs in quadrangular squares, of a reddish or pale brown colour above and pale white within; the taste resembles that of clay.

Acacia Concinna.

A. Rugata, Mímosa Saponaria, M. Concinna.

Habitat.—India, Burmah, Nepaul, Assam.

Part used.—The pods.

Vernacular.—Beng.—Banritha. Bom.—Sikekai. Burm.—Ken Chon-se. Can.—Shige-Kayi. Duk.—Sikekai. Eng.—Soap acacia. Hind.—Aila, Rassaul. Malyal.—Chinik-kaya. Mar.—Shika, Telashenga. Sans.—Saptala, Charmakasa. Tam.—Shika. Tel.—Shikaya, Gogu.

Charmakasa.—The word is derived from charma, the skin, and kasa to injure. It means, skin-injurer. The pods have numerous thornlike projections, which injure the skin when handled roughly.

Characters.—Pods or legumes, long and flat, colour darkish or brownish red, surface rugous and highly wrinkled, from 4 to 5 inches in length, and about 1 to 1½ inches in breadth, each pod is bi-valved; valves much wrinkled, marked by a transverse depression on both surfaces and much contracted between the seeds; odour aciduous; taste astringent, sourish and nauseous, and resembling that of kokama or soap-nut "Aritha;" seeds numerous, separate, shining, dark coloured, small and oval.

Constituents.—Pods, freed from seeds, contain saponin 11·2, malic acid 12·75, resin 1, glucose 13·9, gum and colouring matter 21·5, crude fibre 22, and ash 3·75.

Preparations.—Mucilage; infusion (1 in 20). Dose, 1 to 1½ oz.

Actions and uses.—Pods are used by native women as a detergent and a wash for the head. As an expectorant and cholagogue the infusion is given in torpid liver, jaundice and other biliary complaints. It is used by the natives as an adjunct to other purgative medicines. It does not cause griping in the bowels as senna.

A. Farnesiana.

A. Indica, Mimosa Indica, M. Farnesiana.

Habitat.—Panjab, Sind, Assam, Bengal.

Parts used.—The bark, gum and extract.

Vernacular.—Beng.—Guh-babul. Burm.—Nauloon-mien, Can.—Jalli. Duk.—Ghu-kikar. Guz.—Gu-baval. Hind.—Ghu-babul, Iri-babul. Malay.—Pyvelam. Mar.—Iri-babul. Panj.—Vialayeti Kikar. Sind.—Baver. Tam.—Vaday-vulli maram, Kampa-tumma. Tel.—Naga-tumma.

Ghu-baval, Ghu-kikar.—Ghu, means human ordure. The fresh bark, wood and gum having the smell of ordure.

Characters.—The plant contains yellow sweet-scented flowers. The bark exudes a large quantity of gum. The gum is met with in spheroidal tears or in stalactiform masses, of a pale-yellow or dark-reddish brown colour. With water it partially dissolves, forming a gelatinous mucilage.

Preparations.—Decoction of bark (1 in 20). Dose, 4 to 8 drs., and mucilage.

Actions and uses.—Gum is demulcent and emollient; other properties similar to those of A. Arabica. The bark is astringent. Dose, of the powdered gum, 10 to 30 grs.

Acacia Modesta, Amritsar or Binhori gund, similar to Acacia Arabica or Acacia Farnesiana—occurs in small tears, angular fragments or vermiform pieces, marked with transverse lines. The colour is yellow or it is translucent. With water it forms a soluble mucilage of a pale colour.

Acacia Pennata.

Habitat.—India.

Parts used.—Bark and leaf juice.

Vernacular.—Can.—Arar. Hind.—Biswul. Mar.—Shemb.

Characters.—Scandant shrub, numerous prickles; leaflets 30 in pairs, narrow, linear, glabrous; bark in strips, 3 feet long.

Constituents.—Tannin 8·8 p.c.

Preparation.—Decoction of bark (1 in 10). Dose, 2 to 4 drs. Juice of leaves. Dose, a teaspoonful.

Actions and uses.—Leaf juice and bark are astringent and alterative. The juice is given with milk in diarrhœa with green stools in children. In bleeding from spongy gums, the leaves, with cumin and sugar, are chewed. In dysuria the pulp of leaves, with cow's milk, cumin and sugar, is given with benefit.

Agati Grandiflora.

Æschymomene Coccinea, Sesbania Grandiflora.

Habitat.—Western India.

Parts used.—The bark, flowers, leaves and gum.

Vernacular.—Beng.—Bak. Can.—Agashi. Duk.—Agasthi. Guz.—Agosthia. Hind.—Basna. Mar.—Agashta. Sans.—Sthula-pushpa, Vranari Vaka, Agasti. Tam.—Agatli. Tel.—Avisi.

Characters.—Leaves pinnate, oblong ; taste slightly acrid and astringent ; flowers large and fleshy, of a white pale-pink or purplish colour, and acidulous bitterish taste ; bark fissured longitudinally and of a greyish brown colour externally; gum in tears, adhering to the bark, of a dark-brown colour and resembling Damula Akhavena, for which it is a good substitute. It merely softens in cold water ; is insoluble in boiling water and also in alcohol, but soluble in dilute alkalies.

Constituents.—The bark contains tannin and gum.

Preparation.—Decoction (1 in 20). Dose, 4 to 8 grs.

Actions and uses.—The bark is tonic and astringent, given in debility, dyspepsia, diarrhœa, &c. The juice of the leaves is poured into the nose in nasal catarrh with headache ; poultice of leaves is a popular remedy for bruises and sores. The root is given with honey in catarrh of the respiratory passages.

Albizzia Lebbek. A. Odoratissima. A. Latifolia. A. Serissa. Acacia Speciosa. Mimosa Sarissa.

Habitat.—Throughout India, Travancore, Coimbatore.

Parts used.—The seeds, bark, leaves and flowers.

Vernaculars.—Beng.—Sirish. Burm.—Seet, Tseek-the. Can.—Sirasala, Bengha. Duk.—Sirish. Eng.—Sirisas tree. Guz.—Siris. Hind.—Siriss Bussa Kapitana, Bismar. Jabelpore—Sarin. Mar.—Sirisha, Chichva. Malay.—Chichva, Viln vake. Sans—Serisha, shuka-priya, Muridu-pushpa. Tam.—Kattuvagai. Tel.—Peddadu cherram.

Shuka-priya—dear to parrots. Mridupushpa—having soft flowers.

Characters.—Seeds oblong, flat, smooth, of a reddish brown colour, very hard, like those of Cassia Fistula, but smaller in size, resembling Turanj-bin. Both surfaces marked by a depression in the middle, the depression is limited by a distinct, narrow, oblong, broken ring; testa very hard; cotyledons yellow; smell of the cotyledon disagreeable; taste bitterish sweet; flowers large, globular yellowish white on short pedicles. The bark is yellowish brown ; suber in large flakes, much pitted and fissured, on separating the suber a red surface is exposed. The bark is hard and gritty, externally red and white within, taste acidulous and astringent; leaves bipinnate, in 4 pairs, obtuse, oval, glabrous and unequal. From the trunk a kind of gum, Kurunas-seras-gond, is produced. It occurs in stalactiform masses; colour light to deep reddish brown, translucent and with a smooth and polished surface ; very little soluble in water ; the mucilage swells into a gelatinous mass. Dose of the seed, 5 to 10 grs.; of the bark, 10 to 20 grs.

Albizzia Porcera.—The gum, is in granular or warty masses or in tears or vermiform pieces, colour reddish brown, transparent and polished ; water completely dissolves it, and the mucilage is thick and gelatinous.

Albizzia Stipulata produces gum, which is tough and dark-coloured ; water dissolves very little of it. It swells into a cartilage-like mass.

Albizzia Odoratissimus.—The gum is in large transparent tears and superficially fissured. The colour is like that of amber, very little soluble in water ; it swells into a tough colourless mass.

Constituents.—Bark contains tannin, resin 7.5 p.c., and ash 9 p.c.

Preparation.—Decoction of bark (1 to 10). Dose, 2 to 8 drs. anjana.

Actions and uses.—The seeds are astringent, tonic, and used in diarrhœa and in seminal debility. Leaves are used as poultices over boils, skin eruptions and swelling. The powdered bark is used as anjana in eye diseases. A decoction of the bark is used as a gargle in sore mouth. Internally it is a tonic and alterative.

Alhagi Maurorum, Hedysarum Alhagi. A. Camelorum.

Habitat.—Khorasan, Concan, N. W. Provinces.

Parts used.—The plant, juice and manna.

Vernacular.—Eng.—Camelthorn. Arab.—Unani Farakeyun or Athariyun, Shonkul-Jamal, Algoul. Beng.—Javasha. Guz.—Algaul, Javaso, Turaujlein (manna). Hind.—Juvansa. Pers.—Khare Shutar, Ushtar-khar. Sans.—Dura-labha, Yavosa (manna). Tel.—Giri-karmika.

Khare Shutar, camel's thorn. Duralabha—Dur, distant, and alabha, difficult to lay hold of. The plant is found in the wide desert of Persia, Syria, Egypt.

Characters.—The plant with hard spines, leaves oblong, obtuse, coriacious and of a reddish brown colour ; an oil is obtained from the leaves ; the pod is constricted ; flowers reddish, flower-stalks thorny. Manna or sugary exudation in lump or in small whitish and saccharine granular powder mixed with thorns, pods and leaves ; colour dirty-white, smell sugary ; taste sweet, afterwards slightly acrid and bitter.

Constituents.—Manna contains mannite and cane-sugar.

Preparations.—Decoction (1 in 10), Dose, ½ to 1 oz., fresh juice. Manna. Dose, 15 to 40 grs. Extract obtained by evaporating the decoction. It is called yavasakara, and is of a bitter sweet taste.

Actions and uses.—The plant is laxative, diuretic and expectorant. The manna and the extract is laxative, cholagogue, aphrodisiac and demulcent ; given in coughs. The fresh juice is diuretic, and given, in combination with aromatics, in the suppression of urine ; also used in opacities of the cornea, and snuffed up the nose in migraine. A poultice of the plant or its fumigation is used in the cure of piles. The plant is smoked with black dhatura, tobacco and bishops-weed seeds in asthma.

Andira Araroba, B. P.

Habitat.—Brazil.

Part used.—A powdery deposit in cavities in the trunk. Araroba Goa powder, crude chrysarobin B. P. is obtained by cutting down the tree and scraping the powder from the clefts. The powder is rough, tawny-coloured and bitter.

Constituents.—Goa powder contains chrysarobin about 80 p.c., gum 7 p.c., resin 2 p.c., bitter extractive 7 p.c., woody fibre 5 p.c., ash 0·5 p.c.

Chrysarobinum, B. P. commonly, but erroneously, called chrysophanic acid, obtained from crude araroba by extracting it with hot chloroform or hot benzene, evaporating to dryness and powdering. It is a crystalline, yellow or pale orange or ochre coloured powder, becoming brown or dark on exposure to the air. It is without any odour or taste, entirely soluble in hot benzol, hot alcohol, hot chloroform, ether, solution of alkalies, sulphuric acid, hot oil of turpentine ; partially so in petroleum spirit, amylic alcohol, collodion, and various hydrocarbons. soluble in water 7 p.c., benzene 80 p. c.

Preparations.—Unguentum chrysarobini, B. P. (1 in 25), chrysarobin ointment. *Pigmentum Crysarobini* (1 in 10 of liquor *Gutta Percha* or collodion).

Oxidized Crysarobine.—Obtained by the action of sodium peroxide on chrysarobin suspended in boiling water ; used in eczema of the face, genitals, &c., where chrysarobin is contra-indicated.

Plaster Mulls $\frac{1}{10}$ to $\frac{1}{2}$ gr. in every square inch. The Goa powder should be mixed with lime juice or vinegar.

Physiological actions.—Parasiticide. It is a gastro-intestinal irritant, producing large watery bilious stools and vomiting. It irritates the skin and sets up dermititis and follicular inflammation. *Therapeutics.*—As a parasiticide the ointment is used in superficial skin diseases of vegetable origin, as ringworm, herpes, circinatus, cloasma and intertrigo ; also in dhobie's itch, psoriasis and in hæmorrhoids ;

Remarks.—Chrysarobin is incorrectly termed crysophanic acid. It discolours the skin and nails dark yellow ; but the stain can be removed by benzene and by chlorinated lime or by potash solution.

Arachis Hypagæa.

Habitat.—India, Africa.

Parts used.—The seeds and oil (oleum arachis).

Vernacular.—Eng.—Ground-nut, pea-nut, monkey-nut. Beng.—Chini-badam. Burm.—Nubi. Can.—Nilagale, Nelakadali. Cing.—Rata Khaju. Duk.—Bhui Sing. Guz.—Chinia badam, Bhui chana, (the oil) Mithun tela. Hind.—Bhui Sing, Mung-phali, Gor tel. Malay.—Nelak Katala. Mar.—Bhoi-chane. Bhui Sing. Sindh.—Bhui Mung. Tam.—Verk Kadalai. Tel.—Varu Shanaga Kaya.

Chinai Badam.—Being first introduced from China. Gortel, Mithun-tel—Gor, mithun, sweet ; tel, oil.

Characters.—The fruit when mature is a pale yellow, wrinkled and oblong, pod often contracted in the middle and containing 2 or 3 seeds of the size of hazelnut ; seeds brownish red ; testa papery ; kernel white and sweet ; cotyledons plano-convex and more pointed at one end than at the other. The seeds when pressed yield an oil known as Arachis oil, which is used as a substitute for olive oil. The oil is limpid, clear, of a pale yellow colour, of an agreeable odour and olive-oil like taste. It is a non-drying oil. The nuts yielding from 40 to 50 p.c. of the oil.

Constituents.—The oil contains glycerides of palmitin and olein, hypogæic and arachidic acids. The seeds contain, besides the oil, nitrogenous substances, starch, phosphoric acid, potash, magnesia, &c.

Actions and uses.—The seeds are eaten like nuts ; the oil is a good substitute for olive oil ; used as demulcent and emollient in burns, scalds, cracks and fissures ; also used for soap making.

Astragalus Sarcocolla.

Habitat.—Persia, Western Asia.

Part used.—A gummy exudation.

Sarcocolla, from sarkos, flesh, and kolla, a glue, from the colour of the gum being like that of the flesh.

Vernacular.—Arab.—Gujara, Anzeruta Kohl-kirmani. Jahudaneh. Ispahan—Kunjad, Agardhak. Bomb.—Gugara. Eng.—Sarcocolla. Hind.—Gujara. Ind.—Lai. Lat.—Sarcocolla. Pers.—Runjudeb, Guzhad. Kohl-Farsi, Persian collyrium. Shiraj.—Kunderu.

Characters.—The gum is highly adhesive, like powdered frankincense, of a colour va ying from deep red to yellowish white, becoming grey when powdered ; met with in agglomerated friable grains, which are opaque or semi-transparent, without any odour and of a bitter-sweet taste. When heated it swells and emits a heavy smell of burnt sugar. Dose, 5 to 20 grs.

Constituents.—Sarcocolline 65, gum 4·5, gelatinous matter 3·5, woody matter 27. Sarcocolline is soluble in 40 of cold and 20 of boiling water.

Preparation.—Compound dusting powder, contains Gujar, white-lead, each one part and starch 6 parts.

Plaster or lep.—Lepa (a native plaster) contains various stimulant gum resins, anodyne and adhesive ingredients, namely : Gujar 9, jadwar 1, aloes 16, alum 8, isas 8, medalakdi 4, Singa puri dammar 4, frankincense 7, amba halad 7, gamboge 12. To be mixed intimately in Mohvra spirit; used by the bone-setters as plaster for fracture, dislocation, subluxation, contusions, sprains, &c.

Actions and uses.—Styptic, anthelmintic and alterative, used as dusting powder in wounds and ulcers. It is non-irritant. The compound powder is used to check purulent discharges from the eyes. Roasted with onions, its juice is dropped into the ear in otorrhœa and earache. It is internally given to children as an anthelmintic and aperient, and also as an alterative to adults in rheumatism. It acts best when combined with trikatu and nishota.

Astragalus Gummifer, B. P.

Habitat.—Asia Minor and Persia.

Part used.—A gummy exudation obtained by incision from the stem. Tragacantha B. P.

Astragalus, from osteon, bone; and gala, milk. The milky exudation soon becoming horny or bony, or from the seeds being squeezed into the shape of vertebræ. Tragacanth, from Tragos, a goat; and acantha, a thorn—plant, thorny, like goat's head. Hedges made of this plant resist the onslaughts of the goat.

Characters.—Semi-transparent flakes, or contorted bands, difficult to powder, without any odour or taste, insoluble in alcohol or ether, sparingly soluble in cold water, swelling into a thick gelatinous mucilage. It also contains a little starch. Dose, 5 to 30 grs.

Constituents.—Tragacanthin 30 p. c., calcium compound of gummic acid 50 p. c., starch, cell fragments, moisture 14 p. c., ash 3 p. c. containing calcium carbonate.

Preparation.—Glycerinum tragacanthæ B. P. (1 in 5), a translucent, homogeneous jelly. Mucilago Tragacanthæ, B. P., mucilage of tragacanth (6 grains to 1 ounce). Dose, 1 to 2 ozs. Pulvis Tragacanthæ Compositus, B. P., tragacanth, gum acacia and starch, each one part, sugar three parts. Dose, 20 to 60 grs.

Actions and uses.—Tragacanth is demulcent and nutritious, like other gums, but mostly used to suspend resin, heavy powders, and oils in emulsions and mixtures. In large doses it is a vehicle for agents used in gargles. It is given in diarrhœa and dysentery; also for gargles in pharyngitis.

Astragalus Heratensis. A. Strobilifero.

Habitat.—Persia.

Parts used.—Gummy exudation; country tragacanth or gum Katira.

Vernacular.—Arab —Miswak-elabbas, Samagul-kasad, Kathira. Hind.—Katera-gond. Pers.—Katera, Zalzada, Gabina. Tam.—Bodam-pishin. Tel.—Bodam Bunka.

Characters.—It is similar to English tragacanth. Katera-gund is not s.mply the dried juice of the plant, but is produced by metamorphosis of the cell membranes. The stems, when cut transversely, exhibit tough, concentric annual layers, which tear lengthwise into filaments. These enclose a central column containing hard translucent gum-like mass. The gum consists of different layers, spirally twisted, or of tear-like masses or of broad bands, made up of several strata. When in the shape of leaf it is known as flake tragacanth or leaf gum. The superior quality is white and more translucent. It is chiefly imported from Persia. The vermiform tragacanth, also called vermicelli gum, is in string-like pieces. It is very hard, tough, difficult to powder. Inodorous and tasteless. With water it forms a jelly-like mucilage. Dose, 20 to 60 grs.

Constituents.—Contains an insoluble gum or bassorine, a soluble gum, a little starch and ash.

Bassorin is an isomer of starch. It forms sugar when bolied with dilute acids and mucic acid when heated with nitric acid.

Soluble gum. The gum is different to arabin, being rendered turbid by acetate of lead and jelly-like with alcohol.

Preparation.—Mucilage and a compound powder.

Actions and uses.—Demulcent and emollient, used in diarrhœa and dysentery, in which it is generally given in curd (Dahi); other properties similar to those of official tragacanth.

Baptisia Tinctoria.

Wild or false indigo.

Habitat.—North America.

Part used.—The root, bark or the whole plant.

Characters.—Plant 2 to 3 feet high, smooth, succulent, glaucous; flowers yellow, branches knotty, odour disagreeable. When bruised, taste bitter, acrid and nauseous. Dose, 3 to 10 grs.

Constituents.—Baptisine, acrid and poisonous. Baptisin, a bitter glucoside. Baptin a purgative glucoside, a brownish powder, soluble in alcohol.

Preparation.—Infusion and decoction; Extractum Baptisiæ liquidum. Dose, 3 to 10 ms. Baptisin. Dose, 1 to 5 grs. Tinctura Baptisiæ (1 in 10). Dose, 5 to 30 ms.

Actions and uses.—In small doses alterative, stimulant, emmenagogue, tonic, antiseptic and mild laxative. In large doses a powerful emetic and cathartic, leading to gastro-intestinal irritation and inflammation. Given in amenorrhœa, hepatic disorders, scrofula, diphtheria, scarlatina, and dysentery; in continued fever or in the early stage of typhoid fever; cataplasm, or the decoction is used locally in obstinate ulcers and gangrenous sores. Baptisin in small doses is tonic and astringent. In large doses purgative. Given in dysentery.

Bauhinia Variegata. B. Purpurescens. B. Candida.

Habitat.—India.

Parts used.—The bark, buds and gum.

Vernacular.—Can.—Shempag, Kauchivala. Hind.—Kuchnar, Kuvidara, Sona-kauraj. Mar.—Kanchana (the gum Sem or Semla). Malay.—Chovana-numdari. Sans.—Kuvidara. Tam.—Segapu-Menthari. Beng.—Kanchan, Bedal. Burm.—Mahahlœgœ-ni.

Characters.—Bark of the trunk scabrous and tubercled, darkish brown externally and tough, fibrous and reddish internally. On the branches the bark is smooth, of an ash colour externally, and very tough and green or white within ; taste feebly astringent, resembling that of babula bark. The gum (semla gum) is in irregular broken pieces, of amber colour. It sparingly dissolves in water, but soon swells forming a mucilage, which is turbid, milky or jelly-like, containing starch or other insoluble substances.

Constituents.—The bark contains tannin.

Preparation.—Decoction (1 in 10). Dose, 4 to 8 drs,

Actions and uses.—The bark and buds are alterative and astringent. The decoction of the bark is given in leprosy, scrofula, skin diseases and ulcers. In scrofulous enlargements of the cervical glands, the bark, with suntha and rice-water, is given as an emulsion, or in combination with Boswellia serrata, myrobalans, and a number of aromatics. A gargle of the bark with pomegranate flowers and akakia is used in sore throat and salivation. A decoction of the buds is given in menorrhagia, hæmorrhoids and bleeding from the mucous surfaces. A decoction of the buds is given in cough, bleeding piles, hæmaturia and menorrhagia.

Bauhinia Racemosa. B. Parviflora. Piliostigma Racemosa.

Habitat.—Konkan, Mysore, Bengal, Assam.

Parts used.—The bark, leaves and dry extract.

Vernacular.—Beng.—Bauraj. Burm.—Bivai-gin, Hpa-lan. Cing. —Myla. Hind.—Mawil-Ghila, Malu. Mar.—Apta, Patwa. Panj.—Murta. Sans.—Vannaraj, Apta. Tam.—Atcha maram. Tel.—Patwa, Adavi Avisa.

Characters.—A climber; leaves cordate at the base, glabrous above and pubescent below. Leaflets roundish or broadly ovate ; flowers in elegant festoons ; bark reddish brown ; gum in purplish red fragments resembling kino in appearance and properties ; soluble in water and partially so in spirit.

Constituents.—The gum contains tannin and glucose. Dose, 5 to 15 grs.

Preparation.—Decoction of bark (1 in 10). Dose, 2 to 8 drs.

Actions and uses.—Astringent, given in chronic dysentery and diarrhœa.

Bauhinia Tomentosa.—Yellow bauhinia.

Habitat.—Ceylon, Malabar.

Parts used.—The leaves, bark, seeds and flowers.

Vernacular.—Burm.—Ma-ha-hlœ-ga-wa. Can.— Shempage. Cing.—Petan. Eng.—Wild ebony. Malyal.—Kanchana. Sans.—Usa-maduga. Tam.—Kat-ati. Triviat-putram,

Kat-ati.—Kat, dark-coloured, and ati, wood. The wood is strong and black, like ebony.

Characters.—Flowers large and sulphur-coloured ; leaves ovate or roundish at the base, under surface villous ; leaflets oval and obtuse; peduncles 2 flowered ; calyx spathaceous, 5 toothed ; petals oval ; legumes flat and lanceolote ; seeds 5 or more.

Constituents.—Tannin.

Preparation.—Decoction (1 in 10). Dose, 2 to 8 drs.

Actions and uses.—Astringent ; given in chronic diarrhœa and dysentery ; the decoction of the bark and seeds is given as a tonic in hepatic congestion. Bruised bark is applied to tumours and wounds.

Butea Frondosa. B. Superba. Erythrina Monosperma.

Habitat.—Plains of India.

Parts used.—The leaves, flowers, seeds and gum.

Vernacular—Beng.—Palasha-kinaka, Kamarkas. Burm.—Ponk-uway. Can.—Muttaga mara, Chhiul-mootr. Cing.—Kaliya. Duk.—Palasaka, Chinai-gond, Kinya-gond (gum), Palas-papado (seeds). Eng.—Bastard teak, Bengal kino (gum). Guz.—Palas-papdo (seeds), Khakro, Chinia-gond. Hind.—Dhak, Palas, Kamarka (gum). Malyal.—Murukha monum. Mar.—Palasha-kakra. Panj.—Chuchra. Pers.—Palah. Sans.—Palasha, Lakshataru Kinsuka. Tam.—Murukkam, Palas muram. Tel.— Maduga, Kimshuka. The flowers.—Guz.—Palas phul. Hind.—Kesurina phul (flowers).

Lakshataru.—The lac tree. The branches contain lac in large quantities.

Characters.—Leaves ternate, from 9 to 12 inches long, leathery, shining above, and hairy below ; flowers large and irregular, fresh ones of a beautiful, deep yellowish-red colour, and shaded with silver-coloured down, when dry becoming paler in colour ; seeds flat, each about 2 inches long and about 1½ inches in breadth, in shape resembling shell lac ; surface shining, colour of dried blood or reddish ; testa very thin and containing a yellowish brown-coloured leafy cotyledon ; taste somewhat acrid. The inspissated juice obtained from the stem by incision constitutes Bengal kino. Gum when pure, is either translucent and in tears, or in smal , flat or irregular fragments of a brilliant ruby-red colour, softening between the teeth, and highly astringent. Generally mixed with numerous small pieces of corky bark, of a light grey colour; not freely soluble in water and alcohol.

Constituents.—The gum contains kino, tannic and gallic acids 50 p. c., mucilage and ash 2 p. c.; on dry distillation it yields pyrocatechin. The seeds contain a tasteless oil of a yellow colour ; wax, or fat 18 p. c., albuminoid, gum, glucose, organic acids, metarabic acid and phlobaphene, cellulose, ash 5 p. c.

Preparation —Of the gum, compound powder containing 5 p. c. of opium. Dose, 5 to 20 grs. Tincture (1 in 10). Dose, ½ to 2 drs. Of the leaves and flowers, decoction (1 in 10). Dose, 1 to 2 fld. ozs. Infusion of flowers (1 in 10). Dose, 1 to 2 fld. ozs. Decoction of the seeds (1 in 10). Dose, 1 to 2 ozs. Paste.—Take the roots of butea superba, nyctanthes and woodfordia floribunda, the seeds of cassia tora and vernonia anthelmintica, the stem and juice of trichosanthes palmata. Make a paste in water and apply in bites and stings of animals.

Actions and uses.—Leaves astringent and alterative, used in diarrhœa, pyrosis, sweating of phthisis, diabetes, menorrhagia, worms and colic. A hot poultice made of leaves is used to disperse boils and pimples. The decoction is used as an injection into the rectum in diarrhœa, dysentery, and into the vagina in leucorrhœa ; also used as a gargle in sore throat and ulcers of the mouth. The seeds are aperient and anthelmintic, used with success in tape-worms and round-worms. A decoction of seeds and infusion of flowers is used with nitre as a diuretic in dysuria and in retention of urine. Externally the seeds are irritant, and used with lime juice in dhobie's itch, ringworm, indolent ulcers, and fistula. Gum.—A powerful astringent and a good substitute for kino, and may be used for all the purposes for which kino is used. The natives use this gum, combined with rocksalt and other astringents, in pterygium and opacities of the cornea. Flowers are also astringent and diuretic. Varalians of flowers are applied to the pubes in dysuria and retention of urine and to promote menses.

Cassia Absus. Senna Absus.

Habitat.—W. Himalaya, Ceylon.

Part used.—The seeds.

Vernacular.—Arab.—Tash Mezaj, Kushnu Zunk, Habek Sudan. Cing.—Kalu-Kallu, Bu-tora. Duk.—Cha-kuta. Guz.—Chinol. Hind.—Chakasu (seeds). Egypt.—Allakalis. Malyal.—Karin-killa. Mar.—Chamada, Kan-kuti, Chime. Pers.—Chesmak, Chast-migah. Tam.—Karunkanum-kattukkol, Avarai-pattai. Tel.—Chukuddi-pal. Sans.—Chaksu.

Chakasu is a corruption of the Sanskrit word chakshu, which means an eye.

Kalu-Kallu means black horse-gram. The seeds are black and bear resemblance to horse-gram.

Characters.—Seeds black, flat and highly polished, in size resembling big-sized bugs, shape obliquely ovate and flat on both surfaces ; testa horny, tough and thick ; cotyledons yellow ; taste bitter. Dose, 10 to 30 grs.

Constituents.—The seeds contain a trace of manganese, extractive matter, resin and ash.

Preparation.—Powder. Confection. Dose, ½ to 1 dr.

Actions and uses.—Seeds very bitter, aromatic and mucilaginous. As an aphrodisiac they form one of the ingredients of methino-ladu and vakerio-ladu. The seeds, when baked and reduced to powder, are applied under the eyelids in purulent ophthalmia.

Cassia Alata. C. Bracteata. C. Herpitica. Senna Alata.

Habitat.—Travancore ; cultivated in India.

Part used.—The leaves.

Vernacular.—Beng.—Dadmurdan, Dadmari. Burm.—Sim-bo-maiza-li. Can.—Shime-agase. Cing.—Attora. Duk.—Velaiti-agali. Eng.—Ringworm shrub, winged cassia. Hind.—Daomurdan. Malay.—Shima-akatti. Sans.—Divipagustia-Dadrughua. Tam.—Simai-agatti. Tel.—Sima-avisi.

Characters.—Handsome shrub ; flowers in racemes and yellow ; leaves 2 feet long, petiole triangular ; leaflets 8 to 14 pairs, obovate, oblong, obtuse, mucronate and glabrous ; legumes long and enlarged sideways ; taste like senna, but less nauseous.

Preparation.—Extract of leaves. Dose, 1 to 4 grs. Tincture (1 in 5). Dose, ½ to 2 drs.

Actions and uses.—Aperient, general tonic and parasiticide, used like senna ; extract of leaves is a good substitute for extract of colocynth. Externally the juice of the leaves, with or without lime juice, is applied to ringworm and to poisoned bites. Internally given in venereal diseases.

Cassia Acutifolia, B. P. Alexandrian Senna. C. Angustifolia, B. P.

Indian or Tinnevelly senna, C. Officinalis, C. Lanceolata, C. Oborata, Jungle senna, C. Elongate, Mecca or Bombay senna.

Habitat.—Africa, India.

Part used.—The leaves.

Vernacular.—Arab—Pero-sana-e-Hindi. Beng.—Shon-pat. Duk.—Nat-ki-sanapat. Eng.—Senna. Hind., Guz.—Sona-mukhi. Tam.—Nela-ponna. Tel.—Nela Tangedu.

Leaves of Solenostemma argel, Tephrosia appollinea, and coriaria myrtifolia, are often substituted for senna leaves.

Acutifolia—Acutus, sharp; and folium, leaf. Leaves sharp-pointed.

Angustifolia—Angustus, narrow; and folium, leaf. Leaves narrow.

Characters.—Alexandrian senna. Leaflets pale greyish green, thin and brittle, size ¾ to 1¼ inch in length, mostly lanceolate, acute, entire, unequal at the base, surface finely pubescent, veins distinct ; epidermis hairy, odour characteristic, nauseous and faint ; taste mucilaginous and somewhat unpleasant, nauseous. Senna Indica or Tinnevelly senna, one to two inches in length, lanceolate and acute, unequal at the base, thin, entire, yellowish green, and smooth above, somewhat duller beneath, glabrous or pubescent; taste and odour nauseous. Senna pods or legumes 7 to 8 lines broad at the base, style prominent on its upper edge ; seeds obovate, cuneate and compressed. Dose of the powdered leaves ½ to 2 drs.

Constituents.—The fruit contains *cathartic acid*, but no resin or oil. The leaflets contain an active principle *cathartin*—a combination of cathartic acid with one or two earthy bases. Also sennapicrin ; a peculiar unfermentable sugar—*cathartomannit* or senna sugar or sennit, a trace of volatile oil ; *sennacrol* ; colouring matter allied to chrysarobin—chrysophan, phæoretin ; mucilage, vegetable salts and ash 10 p. c.

Cathartic acid.—An amorphous glucoside. To obtain it, precipitate concentrated infusion with alcohol. Dissolve the precipitate in water, add hydrochloric acid to separate the albumen, purify and filter and precipitate the filtrate with ether. It is formed of carbon, hydrogen, oxygen, nitrogen and sulphur ; a brown powder, soluble in water and quite insoluble in spirit. Decomposed into glucose and cathartogenic acid by mineral acids. Does not possess nauseous or griping properties. Dose, 4 to 8 grs.

Senna picrin.—Bitter principle (glucoside), insoluble in ether.

Sennacrol—Acrid resinous principle (glucoside), soluble in ether, causes griping. The nauseating and griping properties of senna leaves are due to the presence of this resin and of an oil which have no purgative properties.

Cathartomannit.—To the concentrated infusion of leaves, add alcohol and precipitate. Dilute the residue with water, add oxide of lead and evaporate and crystallize. Colourless, rhombic crystals, mostly spheroidal, with curved sides, of a sweet taste, soluble in water (1 in 2), alcohol (1 in 450), ether (1 in 10).

Preparation.—Of the leaves, *Liquor sennæ concentratus*, B. P. (1 in 1), concentrated solution of senna. Dose, ½ to 1 dr. *Confectio Sennæ*, B. P., Electuarium Lenitivum, contains senna eaves 7 ozs. coriander fruit 3 ozs., figs 12 ozs., tamarind 9 ozs., cassia pulp 9 ozs., prunes 6 ozs., extract of liquorice 1 oz., sugar 30 ozs., water sufficient to make 75 ozs. in weight. Dose, 1 to 2 drs. (1 in 11) *Infusum Sennæ* B. P. (1 in 10). Dose, ½ to 1 oz. *Mistura sennæ compositus*, B. P.—Black draught—magnesium sulphate 5 ozs. liquid extract of liquorice 1 oz., compound tincture of cardamoms 2 fld. ozs., aromatic spirit of ammonia 1 fld. oz., infusion of senna to make 1 pint. Dose, 1 to 2 ozs. (1 in 10). *Syrupus sennæ* B. P. (1 in 2), contains senna 40 oz. oil, of coriander 10 ms., alcohol 40 ms., sugar 50 oz., alcohol (20 p.c.) 70 oz. Dose, ½ to 2 drs. *Tinctura sennæ composita*, B. P. (1 in 5). Dose, ½ to 1 dr. *Pulvis Glycerrhizæ compositus*—B. P. compound liquorice powder, contains senna (1 in 6). Dose, 60 to 120 grs. *Elixir sennæ.*—Dose, 1 to 3 drs. In this the cathartic acid is preserved in its full activity, and the nauseating and griping properties are obviated. *Extractum sennæ fluidum*, fluid extract of senna. Prepared by maceration and pressure and flavoured with aromatics. In it the cathartic acid is unoxidised and resin left behind. Dose, 2 drs. *Extractum Sennæ Fluidum Deodoratum.* Exhaust senna with alcohol to remove the resin and oil, dry the solution and exhaust the dried mass with water to dissolve cathartic acid. Dose, 1 to 2 drs. *Preparation.*—Of the legumes. *Extractum sennæ leguminum liquidum.*—Contains cathartic acid, but no resin or oil. Dose, ½ to 1 dr. for children. The Arabians prefer the pods as a sure and safe purgative as they do not gripe. They contain more cathartic acid than the leaflets, and no resin and no volatile oil.

Physiological action.—Efficient and safe cathartic, acting on the small intestines, and producing copious yellow stools with griping and flatulence, generally given combined with carminatives to lessen griping. In small doses it is non-irritant, acts on the intestines, increasing peristalsis and secretions. It does not cause constipation as its after-effects. Given in large doses it is a gastro-intestinal irritant, sets up nausea, vomiting and purging with great flatulence and severe tenesmus. In women it increases the menstrual flow. It often causes purging in children when suckling mothers take it Some people have an idiosyncrasy for senna, and even the smell of the drug causes nausea, vomiting or purging. It is a very safe cathartic when prompt evacuation of the bowels is required.

Therapeutics.—It is given in constipation, determination of blood to the head, biliousness, gout, hæmorrhoids, fissures in the rectum, fevers and rheumatism. It produces soft and easy motions. It should not be given alone, as it causes nausea, griping, flatulence and depression of the pulse. It is a stimulant of the abdominal and pelvic viscera, and as such acts on the small intestines and increases peristalsis and their secretion. It is less powerful than scammony and gamboge, more irritating and stronger in its purgative effects than salines and rhubarb. Unlike rhubarb, it is devoid of tonic properties. It should not be given in inflammatory conditions of the alimentary canal, if there is tendency to intestinal hæmorrhage, in hæmorrhoids, menorrhagia, threatening abortion and prolapse of the uterus or of the rectum. The natives take the leaves with betel leaves, coriander, tamarind manna, fennel, Epsom or Rochelle salts as a corrective and aromatic.

Cassia Auriculata, Senna Auriculata.

Auriculata.—In allusion to the shape of the seeds resembling the auricles of the heart.

Habitat.—Ceylon, Madras, Dekkan, Western Peninsula.

Parts used.—The bark, leaves and seeds.

Vernacular.—Can.—Tangayree, Avara Taravada. Cing.—Ranawora. Duk.—Tarvar, Aval. Eng.—Mature tea tree. Guz.—Avala. Hind.—Tarwar-aval Dantvan (sticks). Malyal.—Ponna-viram, Avar. Mar.—Taravada. Sans.—Mayhari, Talopodo. Tam.—Avarai. Tel.—Tangadu Avar-gidda.

Datavan, from dant, tooth, and van, stick—native tooth sticks, are made of the stems or wood of this plant, which are as thick as the little finger.

Characters.—Bark in pieces or quills, folded like pancakes, in size, colour and form resembling cinnamon. Each piece 2 to 3 or 4 inches long. External surface dark-brown and slightly tubercled. Internally of a reddish colour, surface rugous, very bittle; taste astringent and sweetish; leaves pinnate; leaflets oblong, about an inch long and from 3 to 4 lines in breadth, short petioled, upper suface of the leaves smooth, under surface hairy; colour dark-brown when dry; flowers yellow; legumes compressed and straight, thus differing from those of mendhi avala, which are curved like sheep's horn; seeds heart-shaped, small, flat, obtusely pointed at one extremity, and of a dark-brown colour, without taste or odour.

Constituents.—The bark contains tannin 25 p.c. and ash 5 p.c.

Preparation.—Infusion of leaves (1 in 20). Dose, 4 drs. to 2 ozs. Compound syrup contains the flowers mixed with mocharas and sarsaparilla. Dose, 2 to 4 drs. Decoction of root (1 in 20). Dose, 2 to 8 drs.

Actions and uses.—The bark is tonic and astringent; the powder of the seeds is blown into the eyes in ophthalmia. The infusion is used as a cooling drink in fevers. A powder made with all parts of the plant is given in diabetes and chyloserous urine, and also used by Gujarati women to check excessive menstrual flow. A compound syrup is given for nocturnal emissions.

Cassia Fistula B. P. Catharticarpus Fistula.

Habitat.—Asia, America, Egypt, W. Indies, Africa.

Parts used.—The fruit, the pulp surrounding the seeds—Cassiæ pulpa, B. P.

Vernacular.— Arab.— Katha-el-hinde, Asl-e-Kheyar-sambar. Beng.—Sondhali, Honalu. Burm.—Gnoogyee Nusi. Cing.—Ahilla. Can.—Kakke-kaye, Kunare. Duk.—Girmalah-amaltas. Eng.—Purging cassia, Indian laburnum (pulp), drumstick, pudding pipe. Guz.—Garmalu. Hind.—Amaltas, Bhawa. Kathel Mal.—Konnan. Malay.—Mentus. Mar.—Bhava Baya. Pers.—Khiya-chambar. Sans.—Aragbudha, Suvarnuka. Tam.—Rajataru or Nripadruma Mambala-konnai. Tel.—Suvarnamu Kayalu.

Khiyar Chambare—chambara, a necklace, in allusion to the structure of the pods, which resembles "a necklace." Katha-el-Hind means Indian cucumber, the pods having some resemblance, in shape, to fresh and young cucumber.

Asal-i-Khiyara Chambara.—Asal means honey. The pulp of Khiyara Chambara tastes like honey. Suvarnaka, from suvern-gold in allusion to the golden-yellow flowers. Rajataru—Raj means royal; and taru, a tree, the tree being uncommonly beautiful when in flowers.

Characters.—Pod cylindrical, of a dark-brown colour, about 2 feet in length and 1 to 1½ inch in diameter; stalk short, but woody, blunt end or the apex is contracted into a point; within the pod are numerous cells, arranged one upon the other transversely ; each cell is thin, membranous, flat on both surfaces, and contains a seed, which is oval, flat, and of a reddish brown colour and surrounded by pulp which is soft, glutinous and of a dark colour, in smell and taste resembling Khajura. It becomes mouldy and sour by keeping.

Constituents.—The pulp consists of sugar 60 p. c., mucilage, astringent matter, gluten, colouring matter pectin, calcium oxalate and ash.

Preparations.—Confectio sennæ, B. P. Dose, 1 to 2 drs. Decoction (1 in 10). Dose, 1 to 2 ozs. Compound decoction—known as Aragbadhadi—contains cassia pulp, picorrhiza kurroa, chebulic myrobalans, long pepper-root, and cyperus rotundus. Used as a cathartic. Dose, 4 to 6 drs.

Actions and uses.—Laxative—pulp seldom used alone, as it causes colic, griping and flatulence. Used as an adjunct to other purgatives. When given for a long time it tinges the urine dark-brown. The pulp is employed to adulterate essence of coffee. The seeds are emetic.

Therapeutics.—The bark and leaves, mixed with oil, are applied to pustules. The root is a strong purgative. The pulp recommended to persons of dyspeptic habits. Dose of the pulp as a laxative, 30 to 80 grs.

Cassia Obovata. C. Æthiopica. C. Obtusa.

Habitat.—Punjab, Sindh, W. Peninsula. Mysore, Egypt, Arabia Senegal, Jamaica

Part used.—The herb.

Vernacular.—Arab.—Senna-baladi. Burm.—Puve-kam-yoe. Can.—Nela-varike. Cing.—Sena-kela, Nilavari. Eng.—Italian senna, jungle senna, Jamaica senna, Tripoli senna. Guz.—Mendhi-avala, Surti-sunamukhi, Bhui Taravara. Hind.—Bhui Taravara. Mar.—Mulkacha Shona-makhi. Malayal.—Nila-vaka. Tam.—Nila-vagai.

Senna baladi.—Wild senna. The plant is said to grow in wild places. Mendhi-avala.—Mendhi, a sheep ; and avala (C. Auriculata), a name of the plant, in allusion to the shape of the pods resembling the horns of a sheep.

Characters.—The drug consists of pieces of stems, flowers, pods, and leaves; stems slender, hairy, and of a greenish brown colour ; pods curved, resembling the horn of sheep (Mendhi) ; leaves pinnate ; leaflets from 4 to 6 pairs, obovate, glabrous above and dark beneath ; colour darkish green ; taste and odour of the leaves resembling those of sonamukhi.

Preparation.—Infusion (1 in 20). Dose, 2 to 6 drs.

Actions and uses.—Leaves purgative ; other actions and uses similar to those of senna. The whole plant is used locally as an application in pityriasis, psoriasis, &c.

Cassia Occidentalis. Senna Occidentalis. C. Sophera.

Habitat.—India.

Parts used.—The leaves and seeds.

Vernacular.—Eng.—Negro coffee, round-podded cassia. Beng.—Kala-kasunda. Bomb.—Kasonda, Hikala. Burm.—Mezali. Can.—Dodda-tagase. Cing.—Peni-tara, Uru tora. Duk.—Kasundi, Gajarsag. Guz.—Kasundi. Hind.—Kasa-murda, Brihat-chitra-kasundi, Gajar sag. Mar.—Ronta-kola, Hikalabija. Malyal.—Peya-vera, Ponnam Takara. Sans.—Kasa marda, Sourna May harie. Tam.—Ponna verai, Naltam Gokarai. Tel.—Nuti Kosinda, Kush-mardha.

Kasa Marda, Kasa, Khaus, meaning cough, and marda, destroyer. Destroyer of Cough.

Characters.—An herbaceous plant or a small shrub, 3 to 5 feet high, leaves pinnate; leaflets in 3 to 5 pairs, obliquely oblong or lanceolate, finely pointed, green, glabrous above and pale beneath. On bruising the leaves the smell is very fœtid ; taste pungent and very acrid ; root tapering, fibrous, of a brownish white colour and very bitter ; smell aromatic, musk-like ; legumes linear, turgid or glabrous and many-seeded ; seeds horizontal with cellular partitions. Dose of the seeds, 4 to 10 grs. in children ; of the leaves, 1 to 2 drs.

Constituents.—The root contains a resinous substance ; a bitter, non-alkaloid principle. Leaves contain cathartin, colouring matter and salts. The seeds contain tannin, sugar, gum, starch, cellulose, chrysophanic acid, calcium sulphate and phosphate and fatty matter (olein and margarin), malic acid, sodium chloride, magnesium sulphate, iron, silica, &c.

Preparation.—Infusion of root (1 in 20). Dose, 4 to 8 drs. Decoction of whole plant (1 in 10). Dose, 2 to 6 drs.

Actions and uses.—The whole plant is purgative, alterative and expectorant, given in hysteria, and whooping cough. The seeds are purgative and given to children with cow's or human milk in convulsions. The root is antiperiodic, and given in fevers and neuralgia. The whole plant is used in cutaneous maladies, as ringworm, scabies, pityriasis and psoriasis ; also as an application over boils and carbuncles.

Cassia Tora, C. Tagara, C. Fœtida, C. Obtusifolia, Senna Tora.

Habitat.—India.

Parts used.—The leaves and seeds.

Vernacular.—Sans.—Prabhunatha, Chakramarda, Dradrugna, Arab.—Kul-kul, Sanji, Saboyah, Aines-saratin. Beng.—Takola, Chakondia. Burm.—Dan-ky-wai. Can.—Takkarike. Cing. –Tora. Duk.—Tarotah. Guz.—Kowaria. Hind.—Chakaund, Panwar, Dadmardan. Malyal.—Takara. Mar.—Tankli, Tarota. Sans.—Chakra marda, Prapunata, Prapunada, Uranaksha. Mahometan—Sanjasoboyah. Pers.—Kulkul-sanji. Tam.—Takaruni, Ushit Tagaria. Tel.—Tantepu chettu.

Chakra-marda—Chakra, a ring or wheel, Murda to destroy. Destroying ringworm, and Aines-saratin, crab's eyes.

Characters.—The leaves generally close at night time. They are in three pairs, the uppermost pair being largest and longest; leaflets obovate and obtuse; taste mucilaginous and nauseous; seeds greyish brown or darkish. They are of various shapes, some cylindrical and pointed at one end, others roundish or ovate, others again rhomboid, in size resembling methi, but somewhat larger; surface tubercled and marked with yellowish or greenish yellow narrow stripes, the stripes occupying the upper and lower surfaces of the seed.

Constituents.—The seeds contain a glucosidal substance similar to emodin which agrees with crysophanic acid in most of its properties. The leaves contain a principle similar to cathartin and a red colouring matter as in senna leaves; also mineral matters.

Preparation.—Decoction (1 in 10). Dose, 4 to 12 fld. drs. Paste contains Cassia tora 6 parts, psoralia corylifolia 4 parts, and carrot seeds 2 parts. To be soaked for 8 days and then locally applied in itch.

Actions and uses.—It has a great reputation as an alterative in all kinds of skin diseases accompanied with induration, as leprosy, cheloid, psoriasis, &c. The juice of the leaves is applied to relieve cutaneous inflammation caused by bhilamo. The seeds, mixed with karanja-tela (pongamia glabra), are used locally as an application for ringworm. With sour milk it is used externally in eczema. A paste of the root with lime juice is used for ringworm, also for buboes in plague. The decoction of the leaves is aperient and given to children during teething. Locally they are used as a poultice over boils to hasten suppuration.

Remarks.—Lately the seeds have been used as a substitute for coffee.

Cæsalpinia Bonducella.

Syn.—Bonducella Guilandina.

Habitat.—India, tropical parts of Asia and Africa.

Parts used.—The kernel of the seeds, oil and leaves.

Vernacular.—Arab.—Akit-makit, Bonduk-i-Hindi. Beng.—Nata, Koranja, Jhagra-gula. Bomb.—Sagura-ghota. Gajaga-kakachia. Can.—Gajaga-kayi. Cing.—Kumburu-atta. Duk.—Gajga. Eng.—Bonduc-nut, Nicker tree. Guz.—Sagara-gota, Gajga-atchka, Kakachia. Hind.—Kat-karanj, Kat-kaleja, Karaijo Sagargota. Malay.—Kalan-chick-kuru. Mar.—Gajra, Sagara-gota. Pers.—Khaya-i-Iblis. Sans.—Kubarakshi-phalam, Keti-aranja. Tam.—Kazhar-shikkay. Tel.—Gach-chakaya.

Khaya-i-Iblis—Khaya means testicle, and Iblis the devil. It means the devil's testicle, from the resemblance of the seeds in shape and appearance to human testicles. Bonduc.—The Arabic word Bondaka, or the Persian Funduk, means a ball of earth or a filbert.

Characters.—Seeds globular, very smooth, shining and of a dull grey colour; shell thick and bony; surface traversed by minute brownish coloured stripes, cotyledon, or the kernel dull white, wrinkled and hard; taste bitter and rather mucilaginous; leaves large, pinnate and prickly; leaflets small, glabrous and of a dark-green colour. The oil is obtained by expression of seeds.

Constituents.—The kernels contain a non-alkaloidal bitter principle, guilandina. The cotyledons of the seeds contain a fixed oil 25, bitter principle or resin 2, sugar 6, salts 3, albuminoid matter 20, starch 35, and tannin. Bitter principle.—A white bitter powder without acridity, entirely soluble in essential and fatty acids, in alcohol, acetone, chloroform and glacial acetic acid; very little soluble in ether, bisulphide of carbon; almost insoluble in petroleum and water.

Preparation.—Pulvis Bonducellæ compositus. Compound powder containing bonduc 2 parts, black pepper 1 part, and pipli 1 part. Dose, 5 to 20 grs.

Actions and uses.—The kernels are bitter tonic, antiperiodic and anthelmintic. The juice of fresh leaves is febrifuge and used in chronic fevers. The seeds, powdered and mixed with black pepper as are febrifuge and alterative tonic and are given in general debility to check hæmorrhages, and in quotidian, tertian, quartan fevers. As an anthelmintic the kernels, mixed with leaves and flowers of butea frondosa and with flowering tops of Artemisia maritima are given for intestinal worms. The fixed oil is emollient and used as an embrocation and to remove freckles from the face and to stop the discharges from the ear; sagaragota, with powdered cloves, is given to relieve the pain of colic and vomiting.

Remarks.—The seeds are worn as necklaces by pregnant women under the belief that it prevents abortion.

The soap-nut (Sapindus triphatus) is also known by the name of Bunduk-i-hindi, with which bonducella should not be confounded.

Cæsalpinia Coriaria. Poinciana Coriaria.

Syn.—American sumach—Divi-divi or Libi-dibi (Eng.)

Habitat.—Himalaya.

Parts used.—The legumes.

Vernacular.—Duk.—Amriqka Sumaq. Pers.—Shumage-amriqah Tam.—Shumak.

Characters.—Dried pods oblong, compressed, somewhat obtuse, curved laterally; externally of a dark-brown colour. Underneath the outer skin of the pods and between it and the inner layer is an astringent matter, an impure tannin of a light yellow colour. Dose, 30 to 60 grs.

Constituents.—Pods contain 60 p. c. of tannin, starch, gum and woody fibre.

Preparation.—Decoction (1 in 40) as injection.

Actions and uses.—The powder is antiperiodic, and given in intermittent fevers. The decoction of the legumes is astringent, and used as an injection in bleeding piles and for prolapsus ani in children.

Cæsalpinia Digyna.

Habitat.—Himalaya, Ceylon.

Parts used.—The root.

Vernacular.—Vakeri-mula.

Characters.—The root is tuberous.

Preparation.—Infusion (1 in 10). Dose, 2 to 8 drs.

Actions and uses.—Alterative and astringent, given with milk, cumin, sugar and ghee, in diarrhœa and other chronic fluxes; also in phthisis and scrofulous affections.

Cæsalpinia Sappan.

Habitat.—E. and W. Peninsula.

Part used.—The wood.

Vernacular.—Arab.—Bukam. Beng.—Bokom. Duk., Guz. Hind., Mar., Bomb.—Patanga. Burm.—Tainniy. Cing.—Patangi. Eng.—Sappan wood. Bookum or Bukhum wood, Brazil wood. Malyal.—Chappannam. Pers.—Bakam. Sans.—Patong. Tam.—Vartangi, Vattekku. Tel.—Okanu katta, Patang, Bakaup chekka. Can.—Patanga-chekke.

Characters.—The wood hard, heavy, of a light reddish colour, here and there sprinkled with a reddish resinous substance; taste oily and acrid; odour acrid; often used as logwood.

Constituents.—Red colouring matter—sappan red or brazillin, gallic and tannic acids. Sappan red occurs in colourless rhombohedron or monoclinic prisms. It resembles hæmatoxylin, and, like it, is soluble in ether, alcohol and water; contains carbon 67·11 p.c., hydrogen 5·43 p.c., and oxygen 27·46 p.c.

Gulala or red powder contains patanga and phataki, mixed with tavakhir (arrowroot), cheap aniline dyes are now used instead. The dry powder of Gulal is used by the Hindus during the Holi festival and in other religious ceremonies. It is also used by a sect of Hindus for teka mark on their forehead.

Actions and uses.—Astringent, given in intestinal and pulmonary hæmorrhages and in menorrhagia; also in diarrhœa and dysentery. A decoction of it is a good substitute for logwood, and used for the same purposes as Rakta-chandana. Gulala is used as a dusting powder in otorrhœa.

Cicer Arietinum.

Habitat.—Warm climates, India.

Parts used.—Seeds, acidulous water or acid exudation.

Vernacular.—Arab.—Humuq. Beng.—Chana, But-kale, Batoola. Bomb.—Harabara-chana. Burm.—Ku-lo-pan. Can.—Kadali. Duk.—Harbarah. Eng.—The Bengal gram, common chick-pea, parched gram (the pulse). Guz.—Chaya, Channa, Chuna-no-Khato (acidulated water). Hind.—Chana, Buroarmani. Italian—Cece. Mar.—Herbera,

Chana. Panj.—Nakhud. Pers.—Chola. Sans.—Chana-kamal, Chennaka. Tam.—Kadalai. Tel.—Sana-galoo-chanaka.

Spurious chanano khato is merely sulphuric acid diluted and tinged with kirmaja.

Characters.—An annual small plant; leaves pinnate; stems covered with glandular hairs, containing oxalic acid and acid oxalates. With the dew these exude and hang in drops, ultimately forming crystals; leaflets small and hairy, of a greenish grey colour and of an acidulous taste; seeds or pulse gibbous, mucronate, of a yellowish or reddish brown colour; testa brittle, containing yellow cotyledons. Chana-no-Khato or the vinegar is an acid liquid of a dull, dirty colour—an exudation from the hairs, stem, leaves and other parts of the plant. The vinegar is collected by spreading white cloth upon the plant during the season of dew, when the exudation becomes mixed with the dew and is taken up by the cloth and finally wrung out in a vessel. The acidulated water, when evaporated, is known as Chana-no-Khara, which is a white powder, which exists in fine needle-shaped crystals and has an acidulous taste.

Constituents.—The fluid contains water holding in solution oxalic, acetic and perhaps malic acids. The husked seeds or the pulse contains water 11·5, albuminoids 21, starch 59, phosphoric acid 1, oil 4, ash 2, fibre 1, &c. Nitrogen per ounce is 14 grains.

Actions and uses.—The vinegar is an acid liquid similar to that found in Kamarakha, bilambi, &c. It is used as stomachic, refrigerant and laxative in dyspepsia and to promote digestion and to remove flatulence and costiveness. The juice of leaves possesses similar properties; medicated vapour baths, prepared by adding the plant to boiling water, are used to relieve dysmenorrhœa. A poultice of the leaves is applied to sprained and dislocated limbs. The seeds are astringent, and given in dysentery. Chana is the most favourite pulse with the natives. It is taken raw or parched, in green or ripe state.

Clitoria Ternatea.

Habitat.—India, Ceylon.

Parts used.—The root and seeds.

Vernacular.—Arab.—Buzrula, Mazariynne-hindi. Beng.—Kalizer, Shavet-upurajita, Vish-mi-karanti. Burm.—Oung-maiphyoo. Can.—Karnike. Cing.—Nil-katarodu. Duk.—Gokarna, Phiki-kijar Ghutti. Eng.—Winged-leaved Clitoria. Guz.—Garani. Hind.—Gokarana, Aprajita. Mar.—Kajali, Gokarana. Maleal.—Kaka-valli. Pers.—Nabate-bikhe-hayat. Mazeriyun-i-Hindi (Indian mezereon). Sans.—Nilagheria, Aparjita, Ashphota, Vishnu Karanta Gokarna. Tam.—Kakkanan-kodi. Tel.— Tella-Dintana.

Characters.—Root white, tapering, branched and fleshy; taste acrid and bitter; root-bark soft and thick; seeds generally black or greyish brown, minutely mottled green and black, oblong, round or nearly reniform, with a white scar at one margin, slightly compressed near the edges. The ends of some seeds are smooth as if cut off by a knife; testa brittle, containing two cotyledons, which are full of granular starch, thus resembling sena-bij; taste oily, acrid, bitter and disagreeable.

Constituents.—The root-bark contains starch, tannin and resins. The seeds contain a fixed oil, a bitter resin, which is the active principle, tannic acid, glucose a light-brown resin, and ash 6 p. c.

Preparation.—Infusion (1 in 8). Dose, 1 to 2 ozs. Alcoholic extract. Dose, 5 to 10 grs. A compound powder containing clitorea seed 1, acid tartrate of potassium 2, ginger 1. Dose, ½ to 1 dr.

Actions and uses.—The root is demulcent, diuretic and laxative, and is given in fever, croup, chronic bronchitis, ascites, dropsy, and enlargements of the abdominal viscera. As a demulcent the infusion is used to relieve irritation of the bladder and urethra, and also given in bronchitis. The juice of fresh root is blown up the nostrils in hemicrania. The extract is a brisk purgative—a good substitute for kala-danah, gulbas bija and jalap.

Copaifera Lansdorfii, B. P. C. Officinalis.

Habitat.—Brazil, Amazon Valley.

Part used.—The oleo-resin obtained from the trunk—Copaiba, Copaiva, B.P.

Characters.—The exudation is thick, brown and viscid, generally translucent, of a characteristic aromatic odour and bitter acrid taste. Entirely soluble in absolute alcohol, ether, chloroform, benzene, fixed and volatile oils, in petroleum spirit (1 in 4); insoluble in water. Dose, 30 to 60 ms. It is erroneously named balsam; it does not contain cinnamic or benzoic acid.

Constituents.—Volatile oil, bitter principle and resin. The resin contains capaivic acid. The volatile oil—Oleum copaibæ, B. P., oil of copaiba. To obtain it, distil the exudation with water or steam. A colourless or pale-yellow oily liquid, with the aromatic, bitter, nauseous taste and odour of copaiba; soluble in absolute alcohol (1 in 1). Dose, 5 to 20 ms. Resin copaiba.—A residue left after distilling off the volatile oil from copaiba. A yellowish body, brittle, of acid reaction. Soluble in amylic alcohol, and benzol. It contains copaivic acid, which is crystallizable, and a trace of viscid resin. Dose, 15 to 20 grs.

Preparations.—Mistura copaibæ composita—compound copaiba mixture. Copaibæ 1, spiritus ætheris nistrosi 1, Liq. potassæ ¼; mix and stir. Then add Tinct. lavandulæ Co. 1, syrup 2, water 8. Dose, 1 dr. Emulsion, pills, capsules, electuary.

Physiological action.—Laxative, expectorant, diuretic, and stimulant of the genito-urinary organs. Taken into the stomach it causes heat, acid eructations, loss of appetite, heaviness and diarrhœa. The urine is increased in quantity and loaded with solid constituents. In large doses it irritates the skin, stomach, intestines and kidneys. It causes gastric catarrh and nephritis. The urine becomes scanty, containing albumen casts and even blood, with pain in the loins; on the skin it produces itching and even eruptions, as psoriasis, urticaria, &c. The oil and resin are soon absorbed into the blood. They are eliminated by the excretions and may be found in the urine, breath, milk and perspiration.

Therapeutics.—As a diuretic it is given in ascites, not depending upon albuminuria. Chiefly used in gonorrhœa after the acute symptoms have abated, in acute and chronic bronchitis with excessive expectoration and in hæmorrhoids. In cystitis in the female it may be injected into the bladder. In chronic skin diseases, as psoriasis and urticaria, it is used with great benefit. The volatile oil is good for throat affections, while the oleo-resin is used for diuretic purposes.

Crotalaria Juncea, C. Bengalensis, C. Fenestrata, C. Tenuifolia.

Habitat.—Throughout the plains of India.

Parts used.—The seeds, leaves and fibres.

Vernacular. — Beng.—Shon-pat, Ghoresun. Mastan-pat. Bomb.—Maesta-pat, Taag-ambharee. Burm.—Paisan. Can.—Pundinaru, Shana-bina. Cing.—Kesma. Duk.—Janab. Eng.—Sun or Bengal hemp. Guz.—Sun. Hind.—Sann, shunum. Mar.—Taga, Sonalla, Sans. Malay—Jenapa-vera, Pulivanji. Tam.—Wakkoo-gana-pam, Shanambo.

Sun is often confounded with sunnee, a fibre obtained from Hibiscus cannabinus.

Characters.—Seeds compressed, markedly reniform, of a light or greyish brown colour; surface shining, glabrous and slightly tubercled; cotyledons hard, bony and yellowish red; taste and smell like that of phaseolus mungo.

Constituents.—The leaves contain abundance of mucilage, a little solid fat, and a resin soluble in ether.

Preparation.—Infusion (1 in 10). Dose, 1 to 2 ounces.

Actions and uses.—Refrigerant, demulcent and emmenagogue, used in fevers and in skin diseases, such as impetigo, and psoriasis. As an emmenagogue it is used to increase the flow of menses; sometimes they cause abortion. Dose of the seeds, 10 to 30 grs.

Remarks.—This plant furnishes a coarse fibre called Sana, Taaga, or Bengal hemp. It is used for making oakum and surgical tow.

Cylista Scariosa.

Habitat.—Concan, Orissa, Deccan.

Part used.—The roots.

Vernacular.—Concan—Ranghevad.

Ran-gevad. Ran, wild; and Ghevadas a kind of Dolichos-lablab. It resembles Dolichos.

Characters.—Root tapering, woody, upper portion 2 inches in diameter, dark brown and covered here and there with circular light-brown scars; on section, the central portion is pithy, surrounded by medullary rays of a light colour; the woody tissue is porous and red; taste astringent and bitterish.

Constituents.—Tannin, starch, and soft yellow resin but no alkaloid.

Preparation.—Decoction of the root (1 in 10). Dose, 4 to 8 drs.

Actions and uses.—Astringent, given in dysentery and leucorrhœa. Applied externally to reduce swellings.

Dalbergia Sympathetica. D. Volubilis.

Habitat.—W. Peninsula.

Part used.—The plant.

Vernacular.—Goa.—Titabli. Mar.—Pentgul, D. Volubilis, Alei.

Characters.—A scandent shrub, stems covered with thick, large, blunt thorns; leaves pinnate; leaflets obtuse, silky beneath; flowers axillary, in cymes; calyx, silky; corolla yellowish white, pod one-seeded and obtuse.

Preparation.—Infusion of leaves (1 in 20). Dose, 2 to 8 drs, Decoction of root (1 in 20). Dose, 2 to 8 drs.

Actions and uses.—The leaves are alterative, and used in syphilis and rheumatism. The bark is stimulant and used locally to remove pimples. The juice of the leaves is used in aphthæ as a gargle in sore throat. The root is demulcent. Internally the juice or decoction of the root is given with cumin seeds in gonorrhœa.

Derris Uliginosa.

Habitat.—E. Himalaya, Ceylon, W. Peninsula.

Part used.—The Bark.

Vernacular.—Beng.—Panlata. Mar.—Kajarvel, Kirtana.

Kirtana.—Worm creeper. It is a poison to worms and their larvæ creeping in the fields.

Characters.—The bark dark-brown and scabrous, thickly studded with corky warts. Taste astringent and acrid.

Constituents.—The bark contains a neutral crystalline principle, wax, two resins, two colouring matters, an alkaloid, an acrid glucoside, allied to saponin, gum, and mineral matter 8 p.c.

Preparation.—Decoction (1 in 20). Dose, 2 to 8 drs.; a medicated oil.

Actions and uses.—Alterative and insecticide; the bark is used as a fish poison and also as a poison to kill worms and insects which infest leaves and flowers; as an alterative, it is given in rheumatism, chronic paralysis and dysmenorrhœa combined with asafetida, garlic, plumbago root and used externally in rheumatism.

Desmodium Gangeticum.

Habitat.—India, Burma, Ceylon.

Parts used.—The root and bark.

Vernacular.—Beng.—Salaparni. Guz.—Salavan. Hind.—Sarivan. Mar.—Salparni, Daye. Sans.—Daye, Shalparni.

Shalparni.—Having leaves like the Shal (Shorea robusta.)

Characters.—Plant sub-erect ; stems angular, from 3 to 4 feet high, and largely covered at the top with short grey hairs ; leaves oblong, from 3 to 6 inches, long, rounded at the base and narrowed towards the point; flowers pale and purple; legumes 6 to 8, jointed and compressed; joints small, rather roundish or kidney-shaped, and covered with minute hooked hairs ; fresh root of a light white colour ; taste of the root-bark astringent ; odour slightly aromatic.

Constituents.—The root contains extractives, resin, oil, an alkaloid, ash 6 p.c. containing a trace of manganese.

Preparation.—Decoction (1 in 10). Dose, 2 to 6 drs. Compound decoction. Dasamula de Kvatha.—Dasa, ten ; mula, the root ; and quath, a decoction. A decoction of ten plants. Containing: Salavan 1, Pithvan 1, Bhui-ringani 1, Dorali-mula 1, Chotta Gakhoru 1, Bela 1, Tetu mula 1, Shevana 1, Patola 1, Takla 1. The first five plants are known as minor plants, called Hrasva pancha-mula or Laghu pancha-mula. The last five are called Vrihat pancha-mula or the five major plants. Dose, 1 to 2 ozs.

Actions and uses.—Febrifuge, alterative and tonic. Given in fever, derangements of the bile, during convalescence from chronic fevers ; also in remittent and puerperal fevers, inflammatory diseases of the lungs, and in diseases of the brain; also in catarrhal affections, vomiting, cough, asthma and dysentery.

Ormocarpum Sennoides.

Habitat.—Western Peninsula, Ceylon.

Vernacular.—Can.—Kadunugge. Tam.—Katmorunga. Tel.—Adavimunaga.

Characters.—A low shrub, young shoots and flowering parts are hairy and of a pale yellow colour, and covered with glutinous secretion. Leaves pinnate, alternate, oblong and obtuse ; flowers 3 to 6, yellow ; racemes short and axillary ; pods jointed, pendulous, muricated and glutinous.

Preparation.—Decoction of the root (1 in 10). Dose, 4 to 6 drs. Liniment.

Actions and uses.—Tonic and stimulant. The liniment is used in paralysis and lumbago.

Desmodium Triflorum. D. Heterophyllum. Hedysarum Triflorum.

Habitat.—Bengal and Peninsula India.

Part used.—The plant.

Vernacular.—Beng.—Kulalaia. Hind.—Kadalaya. Mar.—Ranmethi. Tam.—Serupullady. Tel.—Moonoodoo-moordoo.

Characters.—Stems procumbent ; leaves trifoliate ; leaflets obovate or obcordate, pubescent or hairy ; peduncles axillary, solitary, 1 to 3 flowered ; legumes hispidly pubescent, 3 to 6-jointed ; joints truncated ; flowers, small and blue.

Preparation.—Decoction (1 in 10). Dose, 2 to 8 drs.

Actions and uses.—The leaves with milk are used as galactagogue. and as carminative they are used in diarrhœa and convulsions in children. The fresh plant bruised is applied to indolent ulcers.

Dolichos Biflorus.

Habitat.—India.

Part used.—The seeds.

Vernacular.—Beng.—Kulthi, Kultho-kulle. Can.—Hurali. Eng.—Madras horse-gram. Guz., Hind.—Kulthi. Mal.—Muthera, Mædiri. Sans.—Kalutha, Culutu ; Mar.—Kulitha, Kultha. Tam.—Kollu. Tel.—Walawalli, Ulava.

Characters.—Two varieties—red and white. The seeds are of different colours, varying from light red to dark red and black. Those which are light red are mottled green or dark. In size they resemble chaksu, are highly polished and shining, having a white scar about the middle of the margin ; testa very thin and brittle ; cotyledons whitish.

Constituents.—Albuminoids, starch, oil, ash and phosphoric acid.

Preparation.—Decoction (1 in 10). Dose, 4 to 8 drs.

Actions and uses.—Astringent, diuretic and tonic. The decoction is used in urinary diseases and menstrual derangements. Parturient women use it to promote lochia ; also given to check profuse leucorrhœa and menstrual fluxes. Like Ankola powder, a powder of these seeds is applied to the skin to check cold sweats.

Entada Scandens, Acacia Scandens, Mimosa Entada.

Habitat.—Tropics.

Part used.—The seeds.

Vernacular.—Bomb.—Gardul. Beng.—Gila-gach. Cing.—Pus wael. Duk.—Gradul. Guz.—Suvali-amli. Hind.—Garabi. Mar.—Garambi, Gartdul. Maleal.—Parin-kaka-vulli. Panj.—Kastori-kaman. Tel.—Gila-tiga. Sikkim Pangra. Lepcha, Takdokhyen.

Characters.—Legumes several feet long and 4 to 5 inches broad, surrounded with thick, firm, polished, entire rim ; joints 10 to 30, one-seeded, ligneous, swelled in the centre and transversely furrowed ; seeds very large, each about 2 inches in diameter, flat or compressed, and roundish or heart-shaped ; surface very shining, smooth and of a dark-red colour, having a blackish scar at the hilum ; testa of a reddish colour and thick ; cotyledons two, like that of Bhui-singa ; taste slightly bitterish ; a drop of water placed on it becomes milky owing to the escape of oil globules and granular matter.

Constituents.—Contains a viscid, turbid oil 7 p.c., and a little saponin.

Actions and uses.—Irritant and emetic. A paste of them is applied to relieve inflammatory glandular swellings in the axilla, known to the natives as Kakha Bilari. It is applied to swollen hands and feet in cases of general debility with marked relief. The seeds are used as soap to wash the hair.

Erythrophlœum Guinense, E. Judiciale.

Habitat.—Central and Western Africa.

Part used.—The bark.

Vernacular.- Eng.—Casca bark, doom bark, sassy bark, ordeal bark.

Characters.—The bark has an astringent, acrid, bitter taste, and when powdered excites violent and persistent sneezing.

Constituents.—An active glucosidal principle, called Erythrophlœine.

Erythrophlœinæ Hydrochloridum—yellowish white granular, crystals, soluble in water. The solution has an acrid, bitter taste. Dose, $\frac{1}{40}$ to $\frac{1}{24}$ gr.

Preparation.—Tinctura Erythrophlœi, (1 in 10). Dose, 5 to 10 ms

Physiological actions.—Cardiac tonic, sedative, hydragogue and diuretic. In large doses emetic and narcotic, producing nausea, vomiting, intense headache, narcosis and death. Erythrophlœinæ hydrochloridum combines the actions of Digitalin and Picrotoxin. It strengthens and slows the heart's action, contracts the arterioles and increases the secretion of urine. It is not cumulative. It is given in mitral disease and cardiac dropsy ; also given in diarrhœa, dysentery, intermittent fever, colic, &c. Some believe it to be a local anæsthetic, even superior to cocaine.

Remarks.—The bark is used by the negroes as an ordeal in trials for witchcraft.

Erythrina Indica. E. Corallodendron.

Habitat.—Throughout India.

Parts used.—The leaves and bark.

Moochy wood tree. Indian coral tree (Eng.)

Vernacular.—Eng.—Moochy wood tree. India coral tree. Beng.—Palita-mandar. Burm.—Katheet, Kasi. Can.—Paravalada-mara, Harwana, Warjippe. Cing.—Erabadu. Duk.—Pangra. Hind. & Mar.—Pangra, Furrud. Sans.—Parijata, Parijataka, Mandara. Tam. — Kaliyana, Murukku. Tel. — Bad-chippa-chettu. Malay. — Kalyana-murukku.

Characters.—Fresh bark covered with smooth, grey suber and having small, corky and fissured lenticels ; outer portion of the bark granular and brittle ; odour very disagreeable ; leaves pinnately trifoliate ; leaflets entire.

Constituents.—The bark contains two resins and a bitter alkaloid erytherine.

Preparation.—Infusion of leaves (1 in 10). Dose, 2 to 8 drs. Decoction of bark (1 in 20). Dose, 2 to 4 drs.

Actions and uses.—The leaves are alterative, laxative, diuretic, galactagogue and emmenagogue ; used in syphilis, fevers, in amenorrhœa, &c. With cocoanut milk they are used as galactagogue. The bark is astringent and tonic, and given in dysentery, fevers, &c. The leaves made hot (varalians) are applied to disperse buboes. Erytherine has actions antagonistic to those of strychnine, and may be used as an antidote.

Flemingia Tuberosa.

Habitat.—The Concan.

Part used.—The tubers.

Vernacular.—Mar.—Birmova.

Characters.—Small herb in grassy places; leaves trifoliate, studded with minute golden glands ; flowers small and pea-like ; pods rounded, containing a single black seed ; roots tuberous, ovoid, oblong and tapering at the lower-end ; skin dark-brown and smooth externally, white within ; the tubers yield a sticky juice when injured ; taste sweet and astringent.

When boiled the taste of the tubers resembles that of chestnut.

Constituents.—Yellow resin 1-5 p. c., sugar and gum 25 p. c., asparagin 4-3 p. c., tannin a trace, starch 40 p. c., albuminoids 13 p.c., and ash 3·5 p.c.

Preparation.—Decoction (1 in 10). Dose, 2 to 6 drs.

Actions and uses.—Astringent. The tubers are used in dysentery and leucorrhœa.

Flemingia Grahamiana.

Habitat.—Nilgiris, Concan, Canara.

Part used.—The glands from the pods. (wars)

Vernacular.—Arab.—Wars. Hind.—Wars.

Characters.—Fruits are covered with peculiar garnet-coloured glands. Wars is obtained by drying the pods and rubbing them together over leaves. It is a granular mobile powder ; colour deep purple-red, without any odour or taste. It ignites like lycopodium. It is insoluble in water, soluble in ether, warm alcohol and caustic alkalies.

Constituents.—A trace of volatile oil, of the odour between that of carraway and lemons ; resinous colouring matter 72 p.c., the resinous matter is of a brittle consistence, soluble in ether, alcohol, benzol, chloroform, carbon sulphide, acetic acid, alkaline solution and alkaline carbonates ; also soluble in lime, magnesia. Diluted alcohol separates resinous matter into 2 resins. It also contains ash 6 p.c., albuminous matter 8 p.c., cellulose 9·5 p.c.

Preparation.—Dusting powder.

Actions and uses.—The same as those of lycopodium, used to cure scaly eruptions of the skin.

Glycyrrhiza Glabra, B. P., G. Glandulifera.

Sweet wood, Italian juice root, Spanish juice root.

Glycyrrhiza, from Glykys, sweet, and rhiza, root, from the sweet taste of the root. Glabra, from Glaber, smooth, without hair or down, leaves are smooth on both surfaces. Glandulifera—Glandula, a gland; and ferro, to bear. The pods are covered with thick glandular spines.

Habitat.– Northern Asia, Arabia, Persia, Punjab, Sindh, Southern Europe, Candia, China.

Parts used.—The peeled root and peeled subterranean stem—Glycyrrhizæ Radix, Liquorice root, B.P.

Vernacular.—Arab.—Asl-us-sus, Kobesus. Beng.—Jaishtomodhu. Burm —N'wy-K'hye, Shinbo-noegiyu. Can.—Ate-madhura. Duk.—Mithi-lakri. Eng.—Liquorice root, the juice, Spanish juice, Italian juice. Guz.—Jethi-Madh. Hind.—Jathi madha. Mar.—Jeshti-madha, Irkisus. Pers.—Bekh-Mekeh. Sans.—Yashti-madhu-kam, Madhu-yashtikam. Tam.—Ati-madhramu. Tel.—Yashti-madukam. Malay. Urith-madhuram. Cing.—Atimaduram, Velmi.

Characters.—The roots abound in saccharine and mucilaginous matter, which is slightly bitter and readily soluble in water. It is brown on the surface and yellow within; occurs in cylindrical branched pieces of various sizes, of the thickness of a finger. It is tough and friable; the taste is sweet at first, after a time it becomes somewhat mucilaginous, acrid and bitter; the odour is earthy and rather sickly; when peeled and sliced, the pieces are yellow and smooth, the fracture is coarsely fibrous. Dose, of liquorice root, 15 to 60 grs.

Constituents.—The glucoside—glycyrrhizin 6 p. c., glycyramarin, sugar, starch, resin, gum, mucilage and asparagin.

Glycyrrhizin.—The sweet principle of liquorice. To obtain it heat cold infusion of the root, add sulphuric acid, when albumen will coagulate; to dissolve the precipitate add alcohol and ether, filter and evaporate. An amorphous yellow powder, of a strong bitter taste and acid reaction, soluble in water and sparingly so in spirit and ether. In hot water it forms a jelly. It is precipitated on the addition of acid or solution of cream tartar or of neutral acetate of lead. By boiling with dilute hydrochloric acid it resolves into glycyrretin and an uncrystallizable sugar of the characters of glucose.

Glycyrrhizin combined with ammonia forms ammoniated glycyrrhizin or glycyrrhizic acid. A glucoside prepared by treating liquorice root with water and ammonia and precipitating with sulphuric acid and redissolving in dilute ammonia and allowing it to dry. Dark brown or red garnet coloured scales, taste sweet, soluble in water and alcohol, One grain flavours six ounces of water; the sweet taste of the root is due to this glucoside. Dose, $\frac{1}{2}$ to 5 grs.

Preparation.—Pulvis Glycyrrhizæ Compositus, B.P. Compound liquorice powder.

Senna 2, Liquorice root 2, Fennel 1, sublimed sulphur 1, and sugar 6. Dose, 60 to 120 grs. For constipation and hepatic disease. Extractum Glycyrrhizæ B. P. extract of Liquorice. Dose ad libitum. Extractum Glycyrrhizæ liquidum. B. P. Fluid extract of glycerrhiza. Dose, ½ to 1 fld. dr. Decoction (1 in 10). Dose, 4 to 12 fld. dr. Mistura glycyrrhizæ Composita—Compound mixture of Glycyrrhiza. Brown mixture—Liquorice extract 3, Syrup 5, acaciæ 10, Tinctura opii camphorata 12, Vinum antimoniales 6, spirit etheris nitrosi 3, water 100. Dose 1 to 4 dr.

Action and uses.—Demulcent, expectorant, and a mild laxative, also local stimulant. When chewed or sucked it increases the flow of saliva and mucus, hence acts as a throat emollient. It stimulates the mucous membrane, especially of the air passages where its action is more local than general. It is given in inflammatory affections, catarrhs, cough, hoarseness of voice, asthma, and in irritation of the larynx, bronchi and of the urinary passages. The compound powder is used as a laxative in constipation. Glycyrrhizic acid is used for flavouring decoctions, also covering the taste of nauseous drugs in a liquid form as quinine, chloride of ammonium, sulphate of magnesia, senna, senega, hyoscyamus, ipecacuanha, aloes &c. The powder is used as an excipient in pills.

Remarks.—The Indian liquorice is the root of Abrus Precatorius, Rab-us-sus ; kubas-susa (Arab.) ; the inspissated juice of Glycyrrhiza Triphylla is sold in the bazaar in the shape of black pencils. It is an ingredient in various laxative powders, confections and lozenges.

Hardwickia Pinnata.

Habitat.—Ghats of Canara, Travancore and Carnatic.

Part used.—A dark red balsam.

Vernacular. — Can. — Yenne. Mal. — Kalla, shurale. Tam. — Madeyan, Sampirani. Tinnevelly—Kolavu.

Characters.—The tree yields an oleo-resin—a black or yellowish transparent viscid fluid of the smell and taste of copaiba. A deep notch is made into the heart of the tree, and after a time the balsam begins to flow. Dose, 20 to 60 ms.

Constituents.—An essential oil 25 p. c. similar in composition to that obtained from copaiba, and 2 resins, of which one has acrid properties—does not contain any copaivic acid.

Actions and uses.—Demulcent, stimulant and expectorant ; like copaiba, used in gonorrhœa, gleet. leucorrhœa, bronchorrhœa, etc.

Hæmatoxylon Campechianum, B. P.

The Logwood tree.—

Syn.—Black wood, campeachy wood.

Hæmatoxylon from Hæma, "blood," from blood like colour of the heart wood ; Logwood—wood being imported in logs.

Habitat.—W. Indies, Jamaica, India.

Parts used.—The Heartwood—Hæmatoxyli Lignum, B. P.

Characters.—Wood in chips or coarse powder, thick, heavy and hard, externally of a purplish red colour, internally reddish brownish, marked with irregular concentric rings, odour faint and agreeable, taste astringent and sweet. Dose of the powder, 10 to 30 grs.

Constituents.—Hæmatoxylin, 12 p. c. volatile oil, tannin, fat, resin. Hæmatoxylin.—To obtain it mix powdered extract with sand and exhaust with ether, add water and crystallize. A crystalline principle, pale yellow, sweet like liquorice, soluble in alcohol and ether.

Preparations.—Decoctum Hæmatoxyli B. P. (1 in 20). Dose, ½ to 2 fld. ozs. Logwood chips 50, cinnamon bark 8, and water 1000; boil. Given in diarrhœa and hæmaturia. Extractum Hæmatoxyli liquidum. Dose, ½ to 2 drs. It contains Hæmatoxylin, hæmatein and other astringent properties of the wood unchanged.

Actions and uses.—Astringent and tonic ; under its use fæces becomes dark and urine blood red and sweet. Given in chronic diarrhœa, dysentery and hæmorrhages ; also in atonic dyspepsia.

Indigofera Tinctoria, Indigofera Sumatrana, Indigofera Indica.

Habitat.—W. India, Bengal, Madagascar.

Part used.—The plant and the expressed juice.

Vernacular.—Arab.—Nilaj. Beng.—Nil Guli. Burm.—Mai may. Shan—May. Can.—Nili. Cing.—Nila. Chin.—Lan-tian Duk.—Nil. Eng.—Dogbite shrub. Guz.—Gali, Nil. Hind.—Nil. Mah.—Nili, Guli. Malyal.—Nilam, Ameri, Tarun. Pers.—Nilaha-Ausârahenil, Sans.—Nilam Banig Bandhu. Tam.—Nilam Avari-ekli Tayum. Tel.—Nili-mandu, Aviri. Panj.—Wasma, Basma.

Shrub 2 to 3 feet high. Leaves pinnate ; leaflets in pairs, cuneate at the base, rather pointed towards the apex, of dark green colour. On squeezing a dark green juice oozes out ; flowers many, of a pink or purple rose colour ; legumes nearly cylindrical, deflexed and curved upwards ; seeds truncated at both ends. Dried juice or extract met with in hard pieces of an indigo colour. When mixed with water it forms a mixture of blue and purple. To obtain Indigo.—The plant is cut, steeped in water, and kept or allowed to ferment till the liquid becomes charged with the colouring matter. The liquid on evaporation is mixed with air with the result that oxidation takes place and the indigo is set free, which is next collected in shallow wooden boxes and moulded into small pieces one inch square. Dose, 1 to 3 grains.

Constituents.—Indican (a glucoside).

Preparations.—Decoction of the plant (1 in 10). Dose, 2 to 8 drs.

Actions and uses.—Plant stimulant, alterative and purgative ; used in enlargement of the liver and spleen, dropsy, affections of the lungs and kidneys, whooping cough and palpitations of the heart.

Indigo is given in epilepsy and erysipelas and also in amenorrhœa. The natives apply indigo to the navel with castor oil in constipation also to the pubes and hypogastrium in relieving retention of urine. A poultice of the plant is used to relieve hæmorrhoids. Indigo is a soothing application to burns and scalds, and the juice of the leaves is used as a poultice externally and given internally as a prophylactic against bites of venomous animals and hydrophobia.

Indigofera Aspalatboides. Aspalathus Indicus. Lespedeza Juncea.

Habitat.—Ceylon, Carnatic.

Parts used.—The plant.

Vernacular—Maleal.—Manili, manneli. Mar.—Shiva nimb. Sans.—Shiva nimba. Tam.—Shevenar vaymbu.

Characters.—A low shrub; branches slender, one flowered; leaflets pale green, oblong and lanceolate. Pods straight, glabrous, turgid, 6 to 8 seeded Flowers, rose coloured.

Preparation.—Decoction of the plant (1 in 20). Dose, 1 to 2 fld. ozs. Oil extracted from the root. Paste and ashes.

Actions and uses.—Cooling, demulcent and alterative. The paste of the plant is used to reduce œdematous swellings. The ashes of the burnt plant are used to remove dandruff from the hair. The decoction is used in cancerous affections and leprosy. The root is chewed to relieve toothache and aphthæ. The oil is used in erysipelas.

Indigofera Trifoliata.

Habitat.—Ceylon.

Part used.—The seeds.

Vernacular.—Guz.—Vekari.

Characters.—Seeds oblong, very smooth, shining and beautifully mottled with dull red or black points; colour varying from yellow to dark red or pink. In size they resemble mustard seeds; cotyledons of a yellow colour; taste that of Maga-ni-dala (Phaseolus mungo).

Preparations.—Confection 1 to 2 drs. and decoction (1 in 10). Dose, 4 to 12 fld. drs.

Actions and uses.—Tonic and restorative. A confection of these seeds with other mucilaginous drugs is used in rheumatism, lumbago, general debility after delivery, in seminal weakness and leucorrhœa. The decoction is used for relieving pain in the back and waist.

Indigofera Paucifolia.

Habitat.—Bengal, Madagascar.

Part used.—The plant.

Vernacular.—Tam.—Kuthekar, summattee.

Characters.—Leaves covered with a hoary pubescence; root small and twisted.

Preparation.—Decoction. (1 in 10). Dose, 1 to 2 oz.

Actions and uses.—Alterative, antiphlogistic, antisyphilitic and deobstruent. The decoction is used locally to foment the joints and internally in rheumatism.

Jonesia Asoka.

J. Pinnata. Saraca Indica. S. Arborescens.

Habitat.—Himalaya, Ceylon, East Indies.

Parts used.—The bark.

Vernacular.—Beng.—Jasundi, Asoka. Burm.—A-thau-ka-pho. Can.—Asoka, ashunkar. Cing.—Diya-rat mayl. Chin.—Wu-yu-wha. Eng.—The Asoka tree. Guz.—Asupâla. Hind.—Jasundi, Asok. Mar.—Jasundi, Asoka. Sans.—Asoka, Gundapushpa, Kankeli, Anganapriya. Tam.—Ashogam.

Ashoka—a "without," and "shoka," sorrow or pain, meaning free from pain. Gundapushpa—Gundh smell or odour, and pushpa flowers. It means odorous flowers. Angana-priya—dear to women. It is an emblem of love.

Characters.—Bark externally smooth, of a dark brown or ash colour. Internally fibrous and of a pale reddish colour. Taste, astringent.

Constituents.—Tannin and catechin.

Preparation.—Decoction (1 in 10) made in milk. Dose, 2 to 6 drs.

Actions and uses.—Astringent : the decoction with a number of aromatics is given in uterine affections. Chiefly in menorrhagia.

Remarks.—Jasundi is the name for Hibiscus Rosa sinensis, for which it should not be mistaken.

Lupinus Albus.

Habitat.—Egypt, Italy, Sicily, and Mediterranean countries.

Parts used.—The seeds.

Vernacular.—Arab, Hind.—Turmus, Bâkila-i-misri, Zurmish. Eng.—White lupine, Horse beans. Pers.—Tira misha.

Characters.—Seeds white outside and yellow internally, globular and hard, with a depression at the centre of both surfaces. They have a hole on the top, taste bitter. Dose, 10 to 15 grs.

Constituents.—Malic, oxalic and citric acids ; a golden yellow oil 5 p.c. and wax containing a little phosphorus, no starch, no inulin, but a peculiar substance related to dextrine (a white hygroscopic powder soluble in water and insoluble in ether). Galactane, a hydrocarbon, a principle similar to galactine obtained from Lucerne ; also a hydrocarbon Paragalastine—which is soluble in water; and when boiled with acid it is converted into galactose. The albuminous portion of the seeds consists of conglutin, legumin and vegetable albumen, also three alkaloids, namely, luzinine, luzanine and lupulidinol. Germinated seeds contain asparagin, phenyl amido-propionic acid, amido-valerianic acid, leucine, tyrosin, xanthine, hypoxanthine, lecithine, peptone, arginine, and choline, also vanillin.

Preparation.—Decoction (1 in 10). Dose, 2 to 8 drs.

Actions and uses.—Carminative and emmenagogue. The decoction with rue and pepper is given in fever, loss of appetite and nausea, also in leprosy. As an emmenagogue it is given in disordered menstruation; boiled in vinegar the seeds are applied to disperse swollen, scrofulous or parotid glands.

Vicia Faba.

Habitat.—Persia.

Part used.—The beans.

Vernacular.—Eng.—Field bean. Pers.—Bakila.

Constituents.—The beans contain proteids, phosphoric acid, also amylaceous and saccharine matter.

Actions and uses.—The beans are nutritive, tonic and expectorant. The root is diuretic.

Mimosa Pudica.

Habitat.—Hotter parts of India.

Parts used.—The leaves and root.

Vernacular.—Eng.—Sensitive plant. Beng.—Lajak, Lajiwant. Burm.—Hte-ka-yung. Can.—Mudugudavre. Hind.—Lajâlû, Lajuk, Lajwanti. Mar.—Lâjri. Sans. — Khaderi, Anjali-Karika. Tam. — Totavadi. Tel. —Attapatti, Pedda-Nidra-kante.

Anjali-karika—Joining hands as in prayer or worship; the leaves join together on the slightest touch.

Characters.—Flowers purple or pale pink; root fibrous; leaves pinnate, falling off on the slightest touch. Taste pungent.

Constituents.—The root contains tannin 10 p.c. and ash 5.5 p.c.

Preparations.—Infusion of leaves (1 in 20). Dose, 4 to 8 drs. Decoction of root (1 in 10). Dose, 2 to 6 drs.

Actions and uses.—Alterative given in torpor of the liver, fever, piles, and jaundice. The decoction of the root is given in urinary diseases.

Mucuna Pruriens, M. Prurita, Dolichos Pruriens.

Habitat.—India, Ceylon and Burmah.

Part used.—The seeds and hairs covering the pods.

Vernacular.—Eng.—Cowage or Cowitch. Beng.—Bichhoti, Alkusi, Kâmâch. Bomb.—Kuhili, Kavacha. Burm.—Khwæ-læ, Khu-e-le. Can.—Nasa-guni-Turâchi. Cing.—Achâryâ. Duk —Kânch-kûri. Guz.—Kávânch. Hind.—Káwâcha. Mar.—Kuhili, Kavacha. Pers. —Hub-el-Kulai, Sans.—Atmagupta, Kopikach-chhu, Vanary. Mal.—Nayi, Karona. Tam.—Puna-Kali. Tel.—Pelliadugu Kaia, Dûlagondi.

Atma Gupta—Having hidden properties, Kapikachchhu—monkey's itch. Vanari—monkey plant.

Characters.—Pods curved like the letter *f.* 3 or 4 inches long, covered with rigid brown hairs and filled with brown matter which soon penetrate the skin and irritate it if handled. Skin of the pod hard and of a dark colour ; seeds 3 to 5, dark brown or dark coloured, kidney-shaped, compressed, shining and smooth ; some mottled on the surface each having large white oblong ring, wrinkled at the margin and occupying the hilum ; testa thin and brittle ; cotyledons greyish-white, hard ; of a disagreeable smell and taste.

Constituents.—Resin, tannin and fat, and a trace of manganese.

Preparations.—Hairs of the pods or powder. Confection (1 in 2). Mucuna seeds boiled in milk, then decorticated pounded and fried in clarified butter, and made into a confection with twice the weight of sugar and aromatics. Dose, 60 to 180 grs. A compound powder, Kavacha Pushtika—contains Mucuna seeds, Tribulus Terrestris, root of white silk tree, Asparagus adscendens, Emblic myrobalans, Tinospora, starch, sugar candy in equal proportion. Dose, 10 grs. in milk for spermatorrhœa.

Actions and uses.—The seeds are nervine tonic, emmenagogue and aphrodisiac, used in leucorrhœa, menstrual derangements, and paralysis. The confection is given in paralysis and seminal debility. The hairs of the pods are vermifuge and given in round worms. They work mechanically by injuring the worms and promoting their expulsion. When applied to the skin or to the mucous membrane, the hairs produce a painful irritation and eruption, and hence are very dangerous if left in the intestines. In such cases their administration should always be followed by a purge of calomel and jalap. Dose of the hairs, 1 to 3 grs.

Mucuna Monosperma.

Habitat.—Eastern Himalaya, tropics, Western Peninsula, Ceylon.

Part used.—The seeds.

Vernacular.—Mar.—Songaivi, Mothikuhili. Tam.—Thelukodi.

Characters.—The seeds are large, flat and circular; testa rough and of a black colour. The whole convex margin is occupied by the hilum ; pods one-seeded, semioval, and armed with bristly hairs of a brown colour. Used as paste.

Actions and uses.—Expectorant and sedative, given in cough and asthma ; externally as a sedative it is applied to painful joints.

Myroxylon Pereiræ B. P. Toluifera Pereiræ.

Habitat.—Central America (Salvador.)

Part used.—A balsam exuded from the trunk after the bark has been beaten and scorched. Balsamum Peruvianum. Balsam of Peru, B. P., Black balsam, Balsamum Indicum.

Characters.—It occurs as a thick, viscid, brownish liquid of a benzoin and vanilla odour, and persistent bitter taste. It is black when in bulk, but in thin layers it is deep orange-brown or reddish brown and transparent. Insoluble in water, soluble in chloroform and alcohol and in spirit (1 in 5). Dose, 5 to 15 ms. in emulsion.

Constituents.—Cinnamein, Metacinnamein, a crystallizable solid. Resins, cinnamic acid, styracin (which is cinnamate of cinnyl), &c.

Cinnamein or benzyl cinnamate obtained by treating the balsam with potash, is a colourless aromatic oil, known as Peru balsam oil; on dry or fractional distillation the oil yields benzyl alcohol, benzylic benzoate, benzylic cinnamate, all colourless aromatic oils. With potash it saponifies and yields benzalcohol 20 p.c. and cinnamic acid 40 p.c.

Preparation.—Syrup, emulsion, solution, ointment.

Actions and uses.—In small doses antiseptic, disinfectant, vascular and nervine sedative, tonic, expectorant, diaphoretic, and diuretic. It stimulates the mucous membranes. Its action closely resembles that of styrax and benzoin. In large doses it causes nausea, vomiting, stomach pain, intestinal colic and diarrhœa.

Therapeutics.—As a disinfectant stimulant and expectorant it is used in catarrh of the mucous membranes, as in chronic bronchitis, asthma, phthisis, gonorrhœa, gleet and leucorrhœa; used externally as a stimulant in chronic skin diseases, to relieve itching in indolent ulcers, eczema, sore nipples, freshly-made wounds, also in otorrhœa and alopecia.

Remarks.—The balsam partially covers the odour of iodoform.

Myroxylon Toluifera, B. P.

Habitat.—Central America, Carthagena, Mountains of Tolu.

Part used.—The balsam, obtained by making incisions in the trunk, Balsamum Tolutanum, Balsam of Tolu, B. P.

Characters.—It occurs as a soft, tenacious solid, in thin film of a yellowish brown colour and transparent. Becoming harder and brittle on keeping; odour highly fragrant; taste acid and aromatic; soluble in alcohol and ether, insoluble in water. Dose, 5 to 15 grs.

Constituents.—Styracin, cinnamic acid, resin, and a volatile oil. Resin—amorphous, black, brittle, soluble in alcohol.

Preparation.—Syrupus tolutanus, B. P., syrup of balsam of Tolu (1 in 38). Dose, ½ to 1 dr. Tinctura tolutana, B. P. (1 in 10), Tincture of balsam of Tolu. Dose, ½ to 1 dr. An ingredient in the preparation of Tinctura benzoini composita. Dose, ½ to 1 dr.

Actions and uses.—Stimulant, and expectorant, used, like balsam of Peru, in bronchial affections, catarrh, coughs, &c. The syrup is used in cough mixtures.

Remarks.—The syrup is used to cover the taste of chloral hydrate.

Ormocarpum Sennoides.

Habitat.—Western Peninsula, Ceylon.

Part used.—Young shoots and flowering parts.

Vernacular.—Tamil.—Katmorungi, Can.—Kadunugge. Tel.—Adavimunga.

Characters.—Young shoots are covered with soft glutinous hair, and a glutinous secretion of a gold yellow colour ; leaves pinnate ; leaflets alternate, oblong, obtuse and membranous. Racemes short axillary. Flowers yellow.

Preparations.—Decoction of the root (1 in 10). Dose, 2 to 6 drs. Liniment—made by boiling the flower tops and young shoots in sweet oil.

Actions and uses.—Tonic and stimulant; the decoction is given in fevers. The liniment is used in paralysis and lumbago.

Physostigma Venenosum B. P.

Calabar bean, ordeal bean, chop nut.

Physostigma from physa an " air bubble " or " bladder " and stigma a " mark by a pointed instrument." The stigmatic appendage is hollow and inflated like a bladder. Venenosum from Venum a poison—the plant is poisonous.

Habitat.—W. Africa, India, Brazil, Calabar.

Parts used.—The ripe seeds or bean—physostigmatis semina, Calabar bean, B P.

Characters.—A woody creeper ; seeds thick, oblong and reniform ; testa hard, granular and of chocolate brown colour ; hilum broad and black with a groove along the whole length of the convex edge ; cotyledons two, firm, white, starchy and convex ; without any odour and of a bean-like taste. Dose, dry powder 1 to 4 grs. The ripe seeds contain in the integument physostigmine to which alkaloid its poisonous properties are due.

Constituents.—Calabar bean contains physostigmine or eserine ; and calabarine or eseridine ; Phytosterin, starch 48 p. c., proteids 23 p.c., mucilage, fat and ash 3 p.c.

Physostigmine or eserine.

It is obtained from the alcoholic extract of the seeds by treating it with an alkali and dissolving the alkaloid in ether. Colourless or pinkish rectangular crystals slightly soluble in water, freely soluble in alcohol, ether, chloroform and dilute acids. The solution rapidly becomes red by exposure to air and light. Dose, $\frac{1}{100}$ to $\frac{1}{50}$ of a gr. Physostigminæ Hydrobromidum. Physostimine Hydrobromide, Eserine Hydrobromate—an hygroscopic white amorphous powder, very soluble in water. Dose, $\frac{1}{60}$ to $\frac{1}{20}$ gr.

Physostigminæ Salicylas Physostigmine Salicylate. Colourless shining needle-shaped crystals without odour, of a bitter taste and neutral reaction, soluble in water (1 in 150) in alcohol (1 in 12) becoming red on exposure to air. Dose, $\frac{1}{60}$ to $\frac{1}{20}$ gr. Solution 5 p.c. is used as Injectio Physostigminæ Salicylas Hypodermica (1 in 100). Dose 1 to 6 minims. Physostigminæ Sulphas B. P. Physostigmine sulphate or Eserine sulphate, a deliquescent amorphous powder or yellow-whitish minute crystals, becoming red by exposure to air and light, of bitter taste, very soluble in water, soluble in alcohol. Dose, $\frac{1}{60}$ to $\frac{1}{20}$ of a gr. Used as *Guttæ Physostigminæ* (2 grs. to 1 ounce). *Guttæ Physostigminæ cum Cocaina*—1 gr. of sulphate of physostigmine, 5 grs. cocaine Hydrochloras to water one ounce. *Lamellæ Physostigminæ* B. P. Discs of Physostigmine, physostigmine sulphate $\frac{1}{1000}$ gr. in each. *Injectio physostigminæ sulphatis Hypodermica*—4 grs. to 1 ounce. Dose, 1 to 4 discs.

Calabarine or Eseridine—Eseridina—An alkaloid antagonistic to physostigmine and allied to strychnine in its action. Exists ready formed in Calabar bean; also obtained from the mother liquor by precipitation with subacetate of lead and ammonia. It is a white crystalline powder, sparingly soluble in water and ether, soluble in dilute acids. Dose, $\frac{1}{32}$ to $\frac{1}{16}$ of a gr.

Phytosterin.—Obtained by exhausting beans with petroleum ether. Resembles cholesterine. Has $\frac{1}{6}$ the toxic action of physostigmine, has a tetanic action on the spinal cord and produces abundant mucous discharges from the intestines

Preparations.—Of Calabar bean. Extractum physostigmatis, B.P. Extract of Calabar bean, an alcoholic extract, containing milk sugar 75 p.c. Dose, $\frac{1}{4}$ to 1 gr. given in tetanus. Tinctura physostigmatis 5 p.c. Dose, 5 to 15 ms.

Physiological action.—Physostigma is a powerful nervine sedative, myotic, paralyzant of the spinal cord, antiseptic, emetic, purgative and diaphoretic. In large doses poisonous. It produces complete paralysis with abolition of reflex sensibilities, but does not affect the brain. In medicinal doses it stimulates the secretions of the skin, the lachrymal and salivary glands, the stomach and intestines, setting up nausea, vomiting, purging, increased intestinal peristalsis, salivation and diaphoresis It is eliminated in the urine. It raises the arterial tension and increases the heart beats. Its action on the muscles of respiration is at first to cause spasm setting up dyspnœa followed by paralysis of respiration. It also causes carbonic acid narcosis, and death. The alkaloids physostigmine and calabarine have different actions. They produce contradictory results. Physostigmine paralyses the nerve centres and stimulates the muscular fibres, calabarine causes convulsions and is allied in action to strychnine. Physostigmine acts on the cord like gelsimium, but is antagonistic to strychnine and picrotoxine; Calabar acts on the cord like strychnine and picrotoxin.

Therapeutics.—The preparations of physostigma and its alkaloid physostigmine, applied locally to the eyes, contract the pupils and are antagonistic to atropine. The extract of physostigma may be given by the mouth, anus or subcutaneously in tetanus, and the dose should be repeated and increased every hour till paralysis short of arrest of breathing is produced. In chorea it may be given in small doses. In paralysis it arrests muscular wasting, and improves muscular power. In obstinate constipation it is sometimes given combined with nux vomica and belladonna. Locally it is applied to neuralgic and rheumatic painful parts. Physostigmine should be used with great care and should be at once stopped if paralysis sets in. It contracts the pupils and is antagonistic to atropine, and hence used in eye diseases to diminish reflex excitability. Physostigmine is given in large doses gr. $\frac{1}{16}$ to $\frac{1}{2}$ by the mouth, rectum or subcutaneously in tetanus, chorea and tonic convulsions. In small doses it is of benefit in locomotor ataxia, writers' cramp and progressive paralysis of the insane and paraplegia due to myelitis; often given in profuse sweating in phthisis. Hydrobromate or salicylate of eserine is preferable to the sulphate for hypodermic purposes. It is also locally applied in affections of the eye as glaucoma. in scrofulous ulcers of the cornea, in presbyopia and in iritis. Eserine drops ($\frac{1}{4}$ to 2 grs. of physostigmine sulphate to an ounce of water) cause contraction of the pupils and are antagonistic to atropine. Eserine salicylate is a spinal depressant, antitetanic and myotic, used hypodermically in tetanus, chorea, atonic convulsions. In South Africa calabar bean is used as an ordeal for witches. Taken internally, if vomiting occurs it establishes innocence of the accused.

Piscidia Erythrina. The fish catching coral tree.

Piscidia.—Piscis a fish—its effect on fish being intoxicating.

Habitat.—West Indies, chiefly growing in arid districts on the mountains of the Antilles. Most common in Jamaica.

Part used.—The root bark.

Character.—The bark is tough and fibrous, in pieces of two to four inches in length, from one to two inches wide and about one-eighth of an inch in thickness. The outer surface is dark grey or brown frequently studded with flattened protuberances of a lighter colour than the surrounding bark; central portion much lighter coloured, and when wet or freshly broken of a peculiar blue green colour; its inner surface is dark brown and very fibrous; odour narcotic, strong, disagreeable and opium like. When chewed it produces a burning sensation in the mouth and pharynx. Dose of the powder, 20 to 60 grs.

Constituents.—The active principle Piscidin, a yellowish resinoid amorphous powder.

Preparation.—Extractum Piscidiæ liquidum, fluid extract of Piscidia, not miscible with water. Dose, 20 to 120 ms. Extractum Piscidiæ, an alcoholic extract. Dose, 2 to 5 grs.

Physiological actions.—Narcotic, general sedative, anodyne and hypnotic, similar in many properties to opium, but free from its objectionable after-effects, viz., constipation, disturbance of the secretory organs, headache and other nervous symptoms; also free from the liability to the formation of a habit. It differs from opium in that it dilates the pupils; as an analgesic and anodyne it is inferior to opium, yet its hypnotic action is more decisive; as a narcotic it relaxes the muscles, produces inco-ordination of movements, lowers the sensibility, stimulates the vasomotor centre and thus increases the arterial tension and also the action of the heart. Its action on the spinal cord is to stimulate the cord with lowering of its reflexes. It increases the secretion of the skin and salivary glands.

Therapeutics.—It is given as nervine sedative in delirium tremens, sleeplessness, also in painful and neuralgic affections, whooping cough, facial neuralgia, headache, and sciatica. In uterine diseases such as dysmenorrhœa and uterine displacements it is given to relieve pain. It is a good soporific for those who are addicted to alcoholic drinks. It is also given in bronchitis, phithisis and asthma to allay irritative cough. Locally it allays toothache.

Poinciana Pulcherrima, Cæsalpinia Pulcherrima.

Habitat.—India, Ceylon.

Parts used.—The bark, leaves, and flowers.

Vernacular.—Arab.—Gula-mohara. Beng.—Gul-i-turaha. Can.—Konjige. Eng.—Small gold mohar. Hind.—Gul-i-turah, Krishna Chura. Mar.—Shankeshwar Shankeshwar. Tam.—Mail, Kannai, Komri. Guz.—Gulmohor.

Characters.—A beautiful tree; leaves doubly pinnate ; leaflets oblong oval and emarginate, surface smooth; flowers of an agreeable odour in loose spikes at the extremity of the branches, of a beautiful orange or deep red colour, or yellow with some spots of green. Bark ash coloured, smooth, and studded with elliptical corky wart-like growths. Internally pinkish; taste nauseous and very astringent.

Preparations.—Infusion of bark (1 in 10). Dose, 2 to 8 drs. and paste of leaves.

Actions and uses.—Antispasmodic, uterine sedative and laxative, given in amenorrhœa, dysmenorrhæa, colic, tympanitis, &c.

Remarks.—Allied species—Poinciana Regia or Royal Poinciana, yields a kind of gum in irregular granular warty tears ; the colour is yellowish or reddish brown. With water it forms a thick opaque mucilage. It contains a large quantity of oxalate of lime.

Pongamia Glabra.

Habitat.—Near the coast of India.

Parts used.—The leaves, root bark and leaves pod, seeds and oil (Pongamia oil).

Vernacular.—Beng.—Dahara-karanj. Burm.—Tha-wen, Pirnizu. Can.—Houge kanuga. Cing.—Mogul-karanda. Duk.—Karanj. Eng.—Karunj oil, Houge oil. Guz.—Karanj. Hind.—Kira-mâla, sukh chen, Karanj. Mar.—Karanj. Malay —Punnam, Unna. Panj.—Shook-chain. Sans.—Naktamalaka. Tam.—Pungam. Tel.—Kaggera, Krânuga, Nakta mâlâ.—Garland of the night. The pods are worn round the neck in whooping cough.

Sukh-chen—sukh, happiness, and chen, rest to the senses, meaning affording perfect satisfaction to the senses. The beautiful drooping branches, shining green leaves and rose-coloured flowers give happiness to the sense of sight.

Characters.—Leaves large and pinnate ; leaflets opposite 2 to 3 pairs, oval, pointed, smooth and shining. The taste is acrid and bitterish. Bark externally smooth, of an ash or yellowish green colour, and here and there marked with tubercles or scars. Internally green or greyish white, very tough and fibrous. Odour very disagreeable and heating. Taste bitter and pungent. Seeds larger than the kernels of the almond, of a brownish red colour, rather kidney shaped and compressed. Testa wrinkled, very thin and papery ; cotyledons oily and yellow, odour and taste resembling those of the bark.

Constituents.—The seeds contain a bitter and pale sherry coloured oil 27 p. c., known as Pongamia oil or Honge oil. The bark contains a bitter alkaloid, resin, mucilage, sugar but no tannin.

Preparation.—Infusion of leaves (1 in 10). Dose, 2 to 6 drs. Decoction of the root (1 in 20). Dose, 2 to 8 drs.

Actions and uses.—The oil is stimulant, parasiticide and non-irritant; it does not stain the skin ; used in scabies, herpes, porrigo capitis, piyriasis versicolor, psoriasis and other skin affections ; generally used combined with an equal quantity of lemon juice ; also used as an embrocation in rheumatism. The leaves are stimulant, carminative and alterative and are used in dyspepsia, diarrhœa, flatulency, also in leprosy, epilepsy and abdominal enlargements. The juice of the root is demulcent and cooling, and used in gonorrhœa and to clean foul ulcers and fistulous openings.

Psoralia Corylifolia. Trifolium Uniflorum.

Habitat.—Himalaya, Ceylon.

Part used.—The seeds.

Vernacular. — Beng.—Hakucha, Lat-a-Kastury. Guz.—Bâvachi. Duk.—Bukchi, Bâvanchiyan. Hind.—Bavanchiyan. Maleal.—Karkal. Mar.—Bavachya. Sans.—Vakuchi Somaraja Kushta-Nasini, Lala Kasturika. Tam.—Kârpokarishi. Tel.—Bapunga, Bavanchi, Kala ginja.

Characters.—Seeds, kidney-shaped, flat, oblong, rough, and of a dark brown colour; hilum situated at the lower end of its concave margin, somewhat bifid. At its upper end there is a small pointed projection, which is the remainder of the style. In some seeds the five partite calyx is found adherent ; surface highly reticulated, unctuous to the touch ; dermis oily and sticky, easily separable from the testa ; odour faintly aromatic and agreeable, resembling that of Bael fruit and elemi; taste aromatic, pea-like, pungent and bitter ; testa of a brown colour and rather horny ; cotyledon of a yellow colour and dry.

Constituents.—A colourless oil, extractive matter, 13·5 p.c. albumen, sugar ; ash 7·5 p.c. containing a trace of manganese.

Preparations.—Tincture (1 in 20). Dose, ½ to 2 drs. Extract—oleo resinous ethereal extract. Medicated oil—Oleate of Bavanchi—obtained from the seeds by soaking them for a few hours in linseed oil or karanj tel.

Actions and uses.—Seeds are alterative, nervine tonic, laxative, aphrodisiac and stimulant ; given in leprosy and chronic skin diseases. A paste of them is applied externally to leucodermal patches and scaly eruptions of the skin. The powder is given internally with small doses of arsenic in leucoderma and leprosy with good results. The medicated oil is rubbed over the patches. The oleo-resinous extract is more efficacious as an application than any other preparations. In hopeful cases, after a few days the affected patch becomes studded with red points, which gradually spread and coalesce ; sometimes pimples and small vesicles appear, which dry up and leave dark spots behind. The discoloration gradually disappears and a normal colour of the skin takes its place.

Pterocarpus Marsupium B.P., P. Indicus.

Habitat.—East Indies, Ceylon, Bengal, W. Peninsula.

Part used.—The juice obtained from incisions in the trunk and evaporated to dryness—Kino, B. P.

Pterocarpus—Pteron, a wing, and carpos, a fruit. The fruits or legumes are winged. Marsupium—a pouch, bag, or purse. The fruit is of the shape of a purse or a bag.

Vernacular.—Arab.—Dammul, Akhvayen-e-hindi. Beng.—Pita sala. Can.—Bibla Honne. Cing.—Gammalu. Duk.—Bijesara. Eng.—Indian kino, Malabar kino. Hind.—Hira-dokhi, Ranga-barota,Bejesar. Malyal.—Vennap-pasha. Mar.—Asan. Pers.—Khuneseyi, Aonshan-e-hindi. Tam.—Kândâ Miragu. Tel.—Gândâm ruyam.

Characters.—A tall tree—the juice is met with in brittle, small, dark coloured or dried-blood-like augular fragments, or pieces, or thin transparent ruby red coloured slices. Taste sweetish and astringent, and no odour ; when chewed it tinges the saliva blood red and adheres to the teeth. It is collected in little cups made with leaves, and is thus in the form of concavo-convex cakes. It is slightly soluble in water, soluble in alcohol and in boiling water (80 p. c.). In fluid state it resembles black currant jelly. Dose, 5 to 20 grs.

Constituents.—Kino-tannic acid, 75 p.c., pyrocatechin (catechol), a crystalline neutral substance kinoin, kino red·gum, pectin and ash 1-5 p.c.

Kino-tannic acid is similar to catechuic acid, found always mixed with colouring matter and pectin. It gives a greenish precipitate with persalts of iron.

Pyrocatechin—Treat kino or the aqueous solution of kino with ether. It is soluble in water, ether. Kinoin. Boil kino with dilute hydrochloric acid, and agitate the solution with ether. White crystals slightly soluble in ether, and cold water.

Preparations.—Tinctura kino, B. P. Tincture of kino (1 in 10). Dose, ½ to 1 fld. dr. Pulvis kino compositus B. P. compound powder of kino (opium 5, kino 75, cinnamon bark 20), contains opium 5 p.c. Dose, 5 to 20 grs. Infusion kino (1 to 40). Dose, ½ to 1 oz.

Actions and uses.—Astringent, tonic and hæmostatic, less powerful than tannin; used in chronic diarrhœa, dysentery, menorrhagia, pyrosis also in leucorrhœa and sore throat. Chiefly used for astringent gargles and as an ingredient in diarrhœa mixtures. Catechin acts only on the lower bowels.

Pterocarpus Santalinus, B. P.

Habitat.—Madras, Western Peninsula, Ceylon.

Parts used.—The heart-wood—Pterocarpi lignum, B. P. Red sanders wood, Red sandal wood.

Vernacular.—Arab.—Sundul, Atamar. Beng.—Rakto chonadon. Duk.—Lâl-chandan, Tambara chandana. Eng.—Red dye wood, Red sandal, Ruby or red sanders wood. Guz.—Ratanjali, Lâl chandan. Hind.—Ragata chandana. Burm.—Nasaphia. Can.—Kempu gaudhachekke. Maleæl.—Uruttah-Chandanam. Mar.—Tâmbara chandana, Ratanjali. Pers.—Sandal-surkh, Bukum. Sans.—Agaru-gandhaka-Ashtaka. Tam.—Shen-shandanam. Tel.—Rakta, Gandham.

Rakta chandan, Rakta, blood-like colour. Chandan, sandal-wood. The colour of the wood is like that of blood.

Characters.—Wood dark red with black streaks, heavy, sinking in water, taste slightly astringent, smell somewhat aromatic. The cells of the parenchyma contain large crystals of oxolate of lime. The colouring matter is soluble in alcohol, ether and alkaline solutions, and gives a red colour. Does not give any red colour to water.

Constituents.—Santalin, Santal, Pterocarpin, Homopterocarpin, Santaline or Santalic acid. To obtain it precipitate the alcoholic solution with acetate of lead, wash the precipitate, decompose it with sulphuretted hydrogen and evaporate. Red crystalline needles or resinoid colouring matter without any odour or taste. Insoluble in water and soluble in alcohol. Pterocarpine and Homopterocarpine are allied to coumarin.

Preparations.—Infusion (1 in 10). Dose, 1 oz. to 2 ozs. Tinctura Lavandulæ composita, B. P.

Actions and uses.—Refrigerant and astringent. A paste of the powder is used as a cooling application to the head, in headache and to inflamed and swollen limbs. As an astringent it is used in combination with other astringent medicines in dysentery, diarrhœa &c. Its chief use, however, is as a colouring agent in Pharmacy.

Remarks.—There are 3 kinds of sandal wood—white (shri khanda), yellow (pita chandana) and red (rakta chandana). The white and yellow varieties are one and the same wood of santalium album, only differing in colour.

Pueraria Tuberosa.

Habitat.—Western Himalaya, Western Peninsula, Orissa.

Part used.—Tubers.

Vernacular.—Hind.—Sural, Siali. Paharea.—Debrelara. Sans.—Shurava. Tel.—Dâri, Gumodi.

Characters.—Tubers pyriform or spindle shaped; size varying from a small pear to a turnip. They are composed of woody layers with a large quantity of cellular tissue. Externally brown and scurfy. Internally white and spongy. Taste acrid, bitter and mucilaginous.

Constituents.—A principle allied to Inulin, ash 18 p.c., a saccharine matter, a bitter principle, an easily oxidizable resin and a resin acid.

Actions and uses.—The root is acrid, used as a cataplasm to reduce swellings of joints.

Cytisus Scoparius, B. P.

Habitat.—Europe, W. Asia.

Part used.—The fresh and dried tops—Scoparii Cacumina. Broom tops, B. P.

Scoparius from scopæ, twigs or "broom." The tops are composed of twigs like a broom.

Characters.—Common garden shrub; leaves, small and downy. Flowers, golden yellow. Tops in thin flexible branched twigs of a dark green colour, usually free from leaves, of a peculiar odour and disagreeable bitter taste. Dose of the tops, 10 to 30 grs.

Constituents.—Sparteine; a neutral crystallizable principle, scoparin, a volatile oil, tannin, fat, wax, sugar and ash 5 to 10 p.c. Sparteine—sparteina, a volatile liquid alkaloid. To obtain it distil infusion of branches or exhaust the plant with vinegar, add liquid soda and distil. It is a colourless, viscid oily liquid, heavier than and insoluble in water, becoming brown on exposure to the air, aniline odour, taste bitter, soluble in alcohol, ether, chloroform. It contains no oxygen, possesses basic qualities, and is very poisonous. Oxysparteina. Oxysparteine,—an oxidation product of sparteine, occurs in white granular crystals, easily soluble in water, alcohol, ether, chloroform and strong alkaline solutions. Dose, ½ to 1½ gr. Oxysparteinæ hydrochloridum, oxysparteine hydrochloride—occurs in transparent crystals, freely soluble in water; may be given hypodermically. Dose, ½ to 1½ gr. Sparteinæ Sulphas, sparteine sulphate. To obtain it neutralize sparteine (alkaloid) with sulphuric acid and crystallize. Colourless or prismatic rhombic crystals or powder of saline bitter taste; it absorbs moisture on exposure to the air. It is soluble in water, 3 in 2, and in alcohol, used as a solution 5 p. c., also hypodermically or as lamels or tabloids. Dose, ¼ to 1 gr. Injectio Sparteinæ Hypodermica contains 1 gr. in 6 ms. Dose, 2 to 6 ms.

Scoparin—a glucoside. To prepare it concentrate into jelly the decoction of the plant, express and purify. It occurs in pale yellow and amorphous masses without any taste or odour.

Preparation.—Of broom tops. Infusum Scoparii, B. P. (1 in 10). Dose, 1 to 2 fld. ozs. Decoctum Scoparii (1 in 20). Dose, 2 to 4 oz. Succus Scoparii, B. P. Dose, 1 to 2 fld. drs. Extractum Scopari fluidum, fluid extract of scoparius. Dose, ½ to 1 dr. Hypodermic Tablets, ½ gr. of sparteine in each.

Physiological action.—Broom tops. In small doses, diuretic and narcotic. In large doses emetic and cathartic, paralyzing motor and respiratory centres. Sparteine sulphate, the salt, mostly used medicinally. Is similar in action to conine and digitalis. It paralyzes the end organs of motor nerves, and vagi, and the respiratory centre in the medulla. In small doses, it is a cardiac tonic, strengthening the heart beats and pulse. It increases the secretion of the skin and kidneys, giving rise to diaphoresis and diuresis. The respiration is quickened at first, but soon becomes slow and laborious, and there is a feeling of general warmth over the body. Under its use the feeling of distress and dyspnœa is relieved. Given in large doses, it causes palpitation of the heart, a sense of tightness about the chest, with muscular trembling and death by asphyxia, or from depression of the respiratory centres.

Therapeutics.—In small doses as a mild narcotic, given in asthma, palpitation, &c. Its use is contraindicated in acute renal affections. Sparteine and its salts are given in angina pectoris, weak heart, dropsy, for the relief of dyspnœa, præcordial pain, palpitation and œdema. Its action is not cumulative like that of digitalis. It is equal to that of digitalis or convallaria, but its effects are more lasting. In mitral regurgitation and in mitral stenosis with small irregular pulse, and in aortic regurgitation it quiets the heart. In ex-ophthalmic goitre and in asthma it gives marked relief. Externally applied it lowers the temperature, and hence used in erysipelas.

Sesbania Grandiflora, Agati Grandiflora.

Habitat.—W. Peninsula, India.

Part used.—The bark and flowers.

Vernacular.—Beng.—Bak. Can. — Agashi. Guz. — Agasthio. Hind.—Basna. Mar. — Agasta. — Sans.—Agasti, Vranâri, Koka Sthula pushpa. Tel.—Avisi. Tam.—Agâth.

Sthulapushpa—Large flowered. Vranari—Enemy of sores.

Characters.—Leaves pinnate, oblong, ovate, of acrid and astringent taste. Flowers papilionaceous, white or red, large and fleshy, calyx, two lipped, racemes axillary. Taste mucilaginous and bitter. Legumes pendulous, very long and contracted between the seeds. Bark fissured longitudinally—externally greyish brown. In the fissures numerous small tears of a red colour and becoming black on exposure to the air are seen. The outer portion of the bark contains the same kind of gum, but softer.

Constituents.—Tannin and gum.

Preparations.—The juice of the root 1 to 2 drs.; paste of the root locally.

Actions and uses.—The root is expectorant. The bark astringent bitter tonic. The juice of leaves and flowers is blown up the nostrils in nasal catarrh and headache with relief. The juice of the root is given with honey in catarrh. A paste of the root with the stramonium root is applied to painful swellings.

Sesbania Ægyptiaca, Æschynomene Sesban, Dolichos Saiseban.

Habitat.—India.

Parts used.—The bark and seeds.

Vernacular.—Arab.—Hab-el-fakd. Beng.—Jayante. Can.—Kariji-nange. Hind.—Jêt, Râsin. Mar.—Shevari. Pers.—Sishiban. Sans.—Jaya, Jayanti, Nâdeyi, Vaija Yanta. Tam.—Champai. Tel.—Somanti. Jaya—Victorious ; Jayanti—daughter of Indra. Nadeyi—River-born.

Characters.—Leaves abruptly pinnate, 3 times longer than broad. Leaflets 10 to 15 pairs. Legume tomentose, linear, slender, and much contracted between the seeds. Seeds oblong, kidney-shaped and smooth, taste bland, odour peculiar. It is difficult to powder. Dose of the seeds, 10 to 20 grs.

Constituents.—The seeds contain a fixed oil, an odorous body, resin, sugar, an organic acid, gum, proteids and ash 5 p.c.

Actions and uses.—The seeds and the juice of the bark are astringent and given in diarrhœa. The leaves are used as a poultice to promote suppuration. The powdered seeds are applied to relieve the pain of scorpion bites.

Tamarindus Indica B. P. T. officinalis.

Habitat.—India, cultivated throughout the tropics, East and West Indies.

Parts used.—The leaves, seeds, and the fruit freed from the brittle outer part of the pericarp and preserved with sugar—Tamarindus, Tamarinds, B. P.

Vernacular.—Arab.—Tamar-hindi, Humara Sabara. Beng.—Tentula, Tetai, Tintri Amali. Burm.—Magye. Can.—Hunase. Cing.—Mahasi, Ambala. Eng.—Tamarind, Indian dates. Guz.—Amali, Kachika. Duk., Hind.—Ambli, Imli. Mah.—Chinchoka. Malay.—Neghka. Pers.—Ambala. Sans.—Amalika, Tintidi. Tam.—Pulic, Puliyam. Tel.—Chinta pundoo.

Tamar-hindi—Indian date. Tamarind is derived from Tamar, a date, and Ind, Indian. It was supposed to be a product of an Indian palm-tree.

Characters.—A large tree, leaves pinnate, linear oblong, obtuse, and of a dark green colour, leaflets linear, very short, petioled and oblique at both ends. Fruit a pendulous legume, from 5 or 6 inches long, linear-oblong, slightly compressed, curved or nearly straight, as thick as the middle finger, and supported by a woody stalk. Outer shell, or epicarp thin and hard, brittle and of a cinnamon colour, containing within the shell the acid and juicy pulp of a dark, red or brownish dark colour. It is traversed by strong woody ramifying fibres, which, starting from the stalk, extend along the edges and sides. One of them extends along the concave edge ; and two others on either side of the convex edge ; between these are 2, 3 or 4 slender fibres all running towards the apex and throwing out filaments. Diffused in water, the pulp forms a glutinous turbid liquid, owing to the presence of pectin. Seeds 10 or 12, enclosed in a tough membranous cell, flattened, of an irregular outline, obtusely furrowed, roundish or obovate and exalbuminous. Surface glabrous, shining, and of a dark brown colour, having on both faces scars conforming to the outline of the cells. Scars of a dark colour and marked with transverse parallel ribs. Cotyledon ivory white and hard, sometimes a peculiar exudation of oxalate of lime flows from the tree in a liquid form and on drying forms white crystalline masses. Varieties. (1) These are ; West Indian, brown or red ; (2) E. Indian, black ; (3) Egyptian—flat round cakes.

The Indian variety forms a firm black sticky mass. The pulp is mixed with seeds, fibres and pieces of shell. It is usually salted. Dose of the pulp, 2 to 4 drams ; of the seeds, 10 to 30 grs.

Constituents.—The pulp contains tartaric 5 p.c., citric, 4 p. c., malic and acetic acids, bitartrate of potassium, sugar, gum and pectin, the seeds' testa contains tannin, a fixed oil, and insoluble matter.

Preparations.—Syrup. Dose, 1 to 2 drs. Confectio sennæ. Dose, 1 to 2 drs.

Actions and uses.—Pulp—antiscorbutic, refrigerant, and laxative ; used in fever to quench thirst, in sunstroke and in bilious vomiting. As an aperient, it is given in habitual constipation. The pulp and leaves made hot are applied locally to inflammatory swellings. A gargle of it is given in aphthous sores, and for the relief of sore throat. The seeds are given in dysentery. The ash obtained from the suber is used as an alkaline medicine in acidity of urine and in gonorrhœa.

Tephrosia Purpurea, T. Lancifolia, Galega Purpurea.

Habitat.—Tropical countries.

Parts used.—The plant.

Vernacular—Beng.—Ban nila. Duk.—Jangli Kulthi, Hunnai. Eng.—Purple Goat's Rue. Guz.—Surpankho, Gadâ-kâ-kân. Hind.—Sarphunká. Mar.—Unhali Sirpakhá. Malyal.—Kolinil. Sans.—Sharapunkkha, Punkhi. Tam.—Kalluk-kây velai. Tel.—Bonta Vempali. Surpunkh.

Surpunkha Sur, an arrow, and pankha—the pinion or wing—the pinion of an arrow. The pinnate leaf of the plant is like the wing of an arrow.

Characters.—Root, hard, woody and as thick as a finger, colour dirty white, smell aromatic, taste slightly bitter, stem slender, angular, furrowed and hairy; colour greyish brown, leaves pinnate, in 5 to 7 pairs, leaflets oblong, obovate, shortly petioled and hairy, especially on their under surface ; veins running parallel to one another on each side of the midrib. Each fresh leaf when torn asunder breaking off with a lower portion pointing at two ends, leaving the gap in the form of letter V. This portion resembles horse's ears when pricked, and hence called Gada ka-kan. Flowers, small and purple ; pods compressed and curved. Each pod 5 or 6 seeded, smell like that of senna, taste bitterish.

Constituents.—The extract contains chlorophyll, brown resin, a trace of wax, a crystalline principle, allied to quercitrin, gum, a trace of albumen and colouring matter, ash 6 p. c. containing a trace of manganese.

Preparations.—Decoction and infusion (1 in 10). Dose, 1 to 4 drs.

Actions and uses.—Alterative, tonic, and diuretic ; used in cough derangements of the liver, spleen and kidneys As a diuretic it is given with black pepper in gonorrhœa ; in bleeding piles it is administered with cannabis Indica leaves. An infusion of it is given in fevers. The juice of the leaves is used over swollen hands and feet and also over swelling or puffiness of the face. Decoction is given in dyspepsia and tympanitis.

Trachylobium Hornemannianum.

Habitat.—Africa.

Parts used.—The gum resin.

Vernacular.—Sandarus.

Characters.—The resin is met with in yellowish brown masses, surface wrinkled, of a chonchoidal fracture and glossy, and without odour or taste, soluble in alcohol and oil of turpentine. Dose, 20 to 40 grs.

Actions and uses.—Astringent, anthelmintic, diuretic, demulcent and emmenagogue. Wi h honey it is applied by the natives to opacities of cornea ; and with olive oil dropped into the ear, in earache ; an ointment is applied to promote the healing of wounds and to ringworm. It is also given to stop hæmoptysis. Other uses are similar to those of copaiba but milder.

Trigonella Fœnum Græcum.

Habitat.—Cashmere, Punjab, widely cultivated.

Part used.—The seeds and herb.

Vernacular.—Eng. Fenugreek. Arab.—Halbah Shimlet. Beng., Hind , Guz., Duk.—Mêthi. Burm.—Penan-ta-zi. Can.– Menthya, Mente. Cing.—Ulawa. Malyal.—Ulava. Pers.—Shembalita. Sans.—Mêthi. Tam.—Vendayam. Tel.—Mentula.

Characters.—Pods sickle shaped, 2 or 3 inches long, flattened and ending in a point ; seeds rhomboid, semi-transparent, somewhat compressed and of a greenish yellow or yellowish brown colour, hilum on the sharper edge, channel extending along the middle of the seed and dividing it into two irregular bodies, surface of the testa tubercular ; taste bitter, odour aromatic.

Constituents.—The cells of the testa contain tannin. The cotyledons contain a yellow colouring matter, but no sugar ; seeds contain a fœtid bitter, fatty oil 6 p.c., also resin and mucilage 28 p.c , albumin 22 p.c., two alkaloids—choline (a base found in animal secretions), and trigonelline. Trigonelline occurs in colourless prisms, possessing a weak saline taste. It is hygroscopic, easily soluble in water and insoluble in ether, chloroform and benzol. It is isomeric with pyridine—betain. By heating trigonelline with caustic potash pyridine distils over. The seeds on incineration leave ash 7 p.c. containing phosphoric acid 25 p.c.

Preparations.—Compound confection, known as methi modak or svalpa methi modak. Dose, 2 to 4 drs.

Actions and uses.—Demulcent, tonic and carminative ; given in dyspepsia with loss of appetite, rheumatism and to puerperal women during confinement. In leucorrhœa the pessaries of methi powder are used.

Trigonella Uncata, Melilotus Officinalis, M. Alba, M. Parviflorus, T. Corniculata.

Habitat.—Persia and India.

Parts used.—The seeds and pods.

Vernaculars.—Arab.—Aklil-ul-Malika, Giah-i-Kaisara. Bomb.—Iklil-ul Mulk, Aklula mulka. Beng.—Tairapa Sano Mâlya. Eng.—Sweet cloves.

Characters.—Pods, small crescent or sickle-shaped, greyish yellow with a beak slightly curved outwards, an inch in length, grooved on both sides, with a central partition divided into two cells, each cell containing a single row of seeds—seeds hard, rhomboidal or roundish and small, like those of fenugreek, of a yellowish colour. Deeply notched on one side and marked with numerous black spots. Odour like that of fenugreek and taste pea-like.

Constituents—Coumarin, (anhydride of coumaric acid) the odorous principle of malilot.

Coumarin is obtained from T. Unctata, also from Tanka or Tonquin beans,—the fruit of Coumaruna odorata. In the wood of asperula odorata, anthoxanthum odoratum, &c. It is first digested in strong alcohol, evaporated and purified with charcoal. Also prepared synthetically from salicylol or salicylic aldehyde. It occurs as colourless triclinic crystals of an agreeable aromatic odour and a bitter burning taste. Insoluble in cold water, soluble in boiling water.

Preparation.—Infusion. Decoction (1 in 10). Dose, 2 to 4 drs.

Actions and uses.—Alterative and stimulant. A poultice of the buds is applied to disperse swellings and to allay local pains.

Internally they are given in colic, diarrhœa, dysmenorrhœa and rheumatism ; also used in scrofula, syphilis, &c.

Coumarin is a narcotic. It stimulates the heart at first, then causes great depression; a dose of 30 to 60 grains causes great depression, vomiting and giddiness. Used to disguise the odour of iodoform.

Uncaria (Nauclea) Gambier, B. P.

Habitat.—Singapore, Eastern Archipelago.

Parts used.—An extract prepared from the leaves and young shoots. Catechu, B.P. Syn.—Catechu Pallidium.

Vernacular.—Eng.—The extract. Pale catechu. Terra Japonica. Indian—Chini Kath. Commerce,—Gambier, Druggist's Catechu in square cakes.

All the vernacular names of A. Catechu are applied to this catechu.

Characters.—Met with in cubes, reddish brown externally. Internally pale or cinnamon brown—porous and friable. Cubes composed of minute acicular crystals. Taste bitter and astringent at first and sweetish after a time. Without any odour. Almost entirely soluble in boiling water, 70 p.c. in alcohol. Dose, 5 to 15 grs.

Constituents.—Catechu. Tannic or Mimo-Tannic acid ; Catechin or Catechuic acid ; Catechuic acid by the action of alkalies splits up into japonic and rubinic acids.

Preparations.—Pulvis Catechu compositus, B. P. Catechu 4, Kino 2, Krameria root 2, Cinnamon bark 1, and nutmeg 1. Dose, 10 to 40 grs. Trochischus Catechu, B. P., 1 gr. in each. Tinctura Catechu, B. P., (1 in 5). Dose, $\frac{1}{2}$ to 1 fluid dr.

Actions and uses.—Astringent ; similar to those of Acacia Catechu. Given in diarrhœa, passive hæmorrhage, &c.

Remarks.—The plant properly belongs to Nat. O. Cinchonaceæ.

Uraria Lagopoides, U. Picta.

Habitat.—Nepal, Bengal.

Parts used.—The root bark.

Vernacular.—U. Lagopoides, Beng.—Chakuliâ. Hind.—Pithvan. Mar.—Duvala, (U. Picta) Sankarjata. Guz.—Pilavana, Dabra, Prisniparni, Rana Gânju. Sans.—Pris-niparani, Atiguha.

Prisnia parni—Spotted leaf. Atiguha—great mystery. Rânâ gânjâ. Wild cannabis.—The spikes and seeds resemble cannabis.

Characters.—Plant from 3 to 4 feet high, young parts clothed generally with minute hooked hairs. Leaves simple, oblong and ovate; upper ones or the leaflets compound linear and lanceolate ; flowers in racemes, terminal, very long and spike-like, legumes small, often pale, and of a purple or reddish colour ; seeds shining, and of a dull grey colour, thus resembling Cannabis seeds.

Preparation.—Compound decoction (1 in 10). Dose, 1 to 2 fld. oz.

Actions and uses.—Alterative, tonic and astringent; given in fevers, catarrh of the air passages and in general debility. Rânâgânjâ is used as an antidote to the poison of Phursa Snake (Echis Carinata).

Moringaceæ.—The Shengata or Bennut family.

General characters.—Trees large, leaves, bi-pinnate or tri-pinnate, Flowers white, irregular; capsules, pod-shaped, three-valved. Seeds winged, numerous, without albumen.

Habitat.—Arabia, East Indies.

Properties—Slightly aromatic and stimulant.

Moringa Pterygosperma. Guilandina Moringa. Hyperanthera Moringa.

Habitat.—India.

Parts used.—The bark, root, fruit, seeds and gum.

Vernacular.—Arab.—Habulbau. Beng.—Sohanjana. Bomb.—Sekta, Segat. Burm.—Da-tha Jwon. Can.—Nugge-gida. Cing.—Sanmurungay. Duk.—Mungey. Eng.—The Horse-radish tree. Guz—Saragavo. Sekato. Hind.—Shajanah, Sengva. Mar.—Soigut, Bododi. Malay.—Murinna. Pers.—Bân, Sajna. Sans.—Shobhana-jana, sigru Muringi, Dansha-mula-sveta, Maricha (the seeds). Tam—Murungai Tel.—Munaga, Sveta Maricha—white pepper, Doonsha, Mula. Pungent root.

Characters.—Root bark light brown, external surface reticulated; internally white, soft and thick, smell and taste pungent owing to its containing an essential oil; leaves large and bi-pinnate or tri-pinnate, leaflets, small, oblong, obtuse or rounded and smooth, green above and pale beneath; smell acrid, taste very hot and burning. Fruit a foot or several feel long, greenish or light brown when ripe, triangular and ribbed, consisting of 3 valves, each containing a soft white pulp and from 12 to 15 seeds. Seeds roundish and winged, taste of fresh kernel bitter and oily. Dried seeds, dark brown externally, white within, and resembling Amali. They yield a fixed oil. Fresh gum pink or brick red in colour. Dried specimens of a yellowish or reddish colour; met with in pieces or masses formed of agglutinated tears, pieces translucent, of variable sizes, generally vermicular in form and easily broken. Taste mucilaginous and astringent; on section the interior is white. A good substitute for horse radish. Dose, 5 to 30 grs.

Constituents.—The root yields an essential oil which is very pungent and has a very offensive odour. The husked seeds yield oil 36 p. c. The bark contains a white crystalline alkaloid, two resins, an organic acid, mucilage, and ash 8 p.c.

Preparations.—Paste. Moringa bark 4 ozs., Moringa nuts 4 ozs., tobacco 2 ozs., gunpowder 2 drs. Mix with water, make paste to rub over scorpion stings or bites. Decoction of the root (1 in 20).

Dose, 2 to 6 drs. Compound spirit (1 in 8). Moringa root, orange peel 20 ozs., nutmeg 5 drachms, spirit 160 ozs., water 4 ozs. Distil to 8 pints. Dose, 2 to 4 drs.

Actions and uses.—Antispasmodic, stimulant, expectorant, and diuretic. The root is very irritating to the skin. The decoction is a stimulant, given with asafetida and rock salt in internal deep-seated inflammation, in calculous affection, in hysteria, epilepsy, paralysis, rheumatism, dropsy, in cough and in flatulence in children, also in ascites due to enlargement of the liver. As a diuretic it is given in uric acid diathesis. The pods are taken as preventive against worms. Externally the oil from the seeds is used as a stimulant application to rheumatic joints and to gouty and other painful parts. The bark is acrid. With cumin seeds it is applied locally to gum-boils and toothache with relief. It is applied to the temples in headache, and on venereal nodes and syphilitic buboes. The decoction of the root is used as a gargle in sore throat. The bark is abortifacient, and is used to procure abortion, and is a good substitute for laminaria to dilate the os. The gum with milk or sweet oil is poured into the ear in earache. Poultice of the leaves is used in reducing glandular swellings. It always produces a blister.

Rosaceæ.

The Gulâba or Rose family. Trees, shrubs or herbs with prickles and warts on woody surfaces. Leaves simple or compound, alternate, and usually stipulate ; flowers, regular, rarely unisexual, of different lovely colours and highly odoriferous; fruit entire, a drupe, an achænium, a follicle or a pome ; seeds exalbuminous.

Habitat.—Temperate climates.

Properties.—Some are astringent with succulent and edible fruits. Others are poisonous, as they yield hydrocyanic acid.

Agrimonia Eupatorium.

Habitat.—Temperate Himalayas, Persia, Europe.

Parts used.—The herb and fruit.

Vernacular.—Arab.—Shajrat-el-Barâghit, Ghafith, or Shaukat-el-Muntineh. Eng.—Agrimony. Pers.—Gulkalli.

Gulkalli—used to cure kalli or ringworm of the scalp.

Characters.—Fruit rough and bristly, generally inverted when ripe, adhering to the clothes, stem ligneous, hairy and swarthy. Leaves indented at their edges, downy and swarthy.

Constituents.—Tannin, 4·75, yellow fragrant volatile oil, a bitter principle and a colouring matter.

Preparations.—Infusion (1 in 10). Dose, 4 to 12 fld. drs.

Actions and uses.—Aromatic, astringent, diuretic and tænicide. Agrimony tea is used in dyspepsia and taken hot to induce perspiration in fever, also as an antiscorbutic. The seeds with wine are used in dysentery.

Brayera Anthelmintica, B. P. Hagenia Abyssinica.

Habitat.—Abyssinia, mountainous districts.

Parts used.—The dried panicles of pistillate flowers. Cusso Kousso, B. P.

Vernacular.—Bom.—Kousso. Guj.—Kussu.

Characters.—The drug is gathered before the seeds are quite ripe, of a light or reddish brown colour, usually in cylindrical rolls of compressed and broken branches of long panicles of flowers, mixed with some entire flowers. The bunch is sometimes a foot or more in length. The panicle consists of a hairy stalk which is twisted and more or less branched. There are large bracts at the base of each branch. At the base of each flower there are 2 or 3 smaller ones between which is the calyx which is 5 partite and arranged in double rows. Each segment of the calyx is ovate and reticulated. The drug has a fragrant balsamic or tea-like odour, and an acrid, nauseous and disagreeable taste, difficult of retention by the stomach. Dose, $\frac{1}{4}$ to $\frac{1}{2}$ ounce.

Constituents.—A volatile oil, a bitter acrid resin 6·25, called koussin; tannin 24 p.c.; ash 15·7 p.c., a tasteless resin, chlorophyll, wax, sugar and gum.

Koussin, Kosin, Brayerin. Heat Cousso with alcohol, add calcium hydrate, boil the residue with water, filter and distil. Treat the residue with acetic acid. It is a crystalline principle, resin like floccutant precipitate, or yellow rhombic crystals; it is probably an ether of Isobutyric acid. Taste, bitter, acrid; odour leathery; insoluble in water, soluble in chloroform, ether, benzol, bisulphide of carbon, less soluble in glacial acetic acid, sparingly soluble in cold alcohol.

Volatile oil is obtained by distillation of flowers with water. The distillate also contains traces of valereanic and acetic acids.

Preparations.—Extractum Cusso fluidum. Dose, 1 to 6 drs. Compound emulsion; a 6 p. c. infusion with castor oil, yolk of egg, a few drops of ether, oil of anise and oleo-resin of male fern. Infusion (1 in 4) of flowers.

Actions and uses.—Anthelmintic; especially useful for tape worms but it rarely expels the head. It has no purgative action. In large doses it produces nausea, vomiting, colic and diarrhœa; oleo-resin of male fern is more reliable than cusso.

Cotoneaster Nummularia.

Habitat.—Persia.

Parts used.—The manna.

Vernacular.—Eng.—Blackwood tree. Guz.—Sira Khista Maiyû (Manna). Pers.—Shirkhisht, Shirkhushk, Bhaklu (Manna), Siah Chob, Kashiru.

Shirkhushk—Shir, milk, and Khushk, dried milk. Dried stems contain milk and when dry they are used for walking sticks.

Four varieties of manna are met with in India.

Turanjbin.—The product of Alhagi maurorum (Leguminosæ).

Gazanjbin.—The product of Tamarix Gallica (Tamaricaceæ).

Shakr-ul-Ashar or shakar tagar, the product of calotropis Procera, Asclepiadaceæ.

Shirkhisht.—The product of Cotoneaster Nummularia (Rosaceæ).

Characters.—The manna exudes or oozes out of the leaves, the bark of the trunk and large branches ; sometimes it bursts through large pores spontaneously. It occurs in flat viscid pieces or yellowish white granules of the size of millet seeds. Each piece from 2 to 4 inches in length, and 1 to 1½ inches in breadth, and resembling ordinary camphor, odour sugary. It easily melts in the mouth leaving a sweet cool taste. Dose, 1 to 2 drs. in children ; 1 oz. for adults.

Constituents.—Glucose 8·3 p.c., cane sugar 4·1 p.c. or an analogous sucrose and a new sugar 50 p.c. called chirkhestite which belongs to mannite group and is nearly related to sorbite.

Actions and uses.—A mild aperient, demulcent and expectorant ; given to new-born infants if the meconium has not come away freely ; also to delicate persons, females and children, in torpid liver, deranged stomach, and intestines ; also given as demulcent and expectorant in cough and sore throat.

Heuchera Americana.

Alum Root (Eng.).

Habitat.—United States.

Parts used.—The Rhizome.

Characters.—Plant viscid, pubescent ; leaves wide, crenate, flowers purple white. Root long, moderately thick, several headed, radicles thin, and many, and brownish purple. Bark thin, without any odour and astringent bitter taste. Dose, 10 to 40 grs.

Constituents.—Contains tannin 20 p.c., starch 12 p.c. Decoction (1 in 20.) Dose, 4 to 12 drs.

Physiological action.—The root is astringent, tonic and antiseptic. In small doses it is styptic to the taste and causes constriction in the throat and checks the mucous secretions and passive hæmorrhages and mucous fluxes.

Therapeutics.—Given in diarrhœa menorrhagia, and as a lotion or injection in leucorrhœa and gleet. The ointment is applied to hæmorrhoids. As a dusting powder it is applied to aphthæ, ulcers, &c.

Potentilla Canadensis, P. Sarmentosa, P. Tormentilla. P. Nepalensis.

Binta falun (Hind.); Cinque foil (Five fingers.)

Habitat.—United States, N. India, Himalaya.

Parts used.—The plant, rootlets and rhizome.

Characters.— Herbaceous plant, handsome when in flower, under surface of the leaves covered with a fine dust which, when the plant is shaken, causes sneezing ; rhizome 2 feet long and ½ foot thick, tuberculate and brownish red. Dose, 10 to 30 grs.

Constituents.—Tannin and red colouring matter.

Preparations.—Fld. Extract 10 to 30 ms. Infusion of the vine leaves and root (1 in 20). Dose, 1 to 2 ozs.

Actions and uses.—Astringent and tonic ; useful in night-sweats of phthisis and succeeds when atropine and other remedies have failed. It is also useful in diarrhœa, dysentery and acidity of the stomach. Locally as a gargle for spongy and bleeding gums.

Prunus Amygdalus, Var. Amara, B. P., P. Amygdalus, Var. Dulcis, B. P., Greek nuts.

Habitat.—Persia, Syria, Barbary, Asia ; cultivated in Europe especially Spain.

Parts used.—The almonds shell. The ripe seed. Amygdala amara, bitter almond, B. P. Amygdala dulcis, sweet almond, B. P., and oil, expressed from bitter or sweet almond, oleum amygdalæ, almond oil, B. P.

Vernacular.—Eng.—The common almond. Arab—Louza Loaz-el Murr-Louz-ul hala (Bitter almond). Beng.—Belâti badám. Can.—Badami (Ticktu badam, Bitter almond). Duk., Guz., Hind., Mar.—Badâm. Pers.—Badam. Sans.—Bada mitte. Tam.—Vadam Kottai. Tel.—Badam Vittulu.

To the common Vernacular names, the word sweet or bitter is affixed according as the Vernacular is for sweet or bitter almond.

Characters.—Fruit drupe, ovate, sarcocarp green and leathery, splitting and falling from the stone when ripe. Stone or nut is otherwise known as commercial almond. Its outer shell pale brown, porous and hard ; within the nut are one or sometimes two kernels or seeds, which when in pairs are in juxtaposition to one another. Seed about an inch in length, flattened, lanceolate, ovate, compressed and with 16 lines radiating from blunt end, rounded at one end and pointed at the other, testa or endocarp of a cinnamon brown colour and astringent as it contains tannin. The endocarp, or outer brown skin can easily be removed by keeping the seeds in hot water ; kernel is rose coloured or white, blanched and fleshy.

Amygdala Dulcis, Jordan almond, sweet almond. The seed is one inch long, oblong, compressed, pointed at one end and rounded at the other. Testa cinnamon brown, thin and rough, seed exalbuminous composed of two large plano-convex, oily cotyledons ; taste bland, without any marked odour even if triturated into emulsion with water.

Amygdala Amara, B. P. Bitter Almond,—The seed resembles sweet almond in general appearance, but is shorter and proportionately broader. The embryo has a bitter taste; when triturated with water it forms an emulsion of the characteristic odour of hydrocyanic acid.

Constituents.—Sweet almonds contain a fixed oil, oleum amygdalæ B. P. 56 p.c.; an albuminous principle or ferment emulsin, (which is soluble in water); mucilage, 3 p.c.; sugar 6 p.c; proteids (myrosin, vitellin and conglutin) 25 p.c., and ash 3 to 5 p.c., containing potassium, calcium, and magnesium, phosphates.

Bitter almonds contain a fixed oil 45 p. c.; amygdalin 1 to 3 p.c.; proteids 25 p.c.; emulsin, sugar 3 p.c.; mucilage 3 p.c., and ash 3-5 p.c. The ash contains potassium, calcium, and magnesium phosphates.

Amygdalin, a crystalline substance, a glucoside not found in sweet almonds, soluble in water and alcohol. To obtain it, boil in alcohol almond cake of bitter almond to the consistence of syrup, add yeast to set up fermentation, then filter and evaporate to syrupy consistence and add alcohol to precipitate amygdalin. Amygdalin is found in many plants belonging to Drupaceæ, Pomaceæ and amygdalaceæ orders, in kernels of peach 2·35 p.c.; cherry ·96 p.c.; plum ·82 p.c. and apple pips, ·6 p.c. in the leaves of cerasus laurocerasus, in the bark, flowers and leaves of Prunus Padus, in the seeds and bark of Sorbus Aucuparia, hawthorn, &c.

Oleum amygdalæ, B. P. Almond oil—oleum amygdalæ expressum.

The oil is expressed from sweet or bitter almonds.

Characters.—The oil is a pale yellow clear liquid, more thickly fluid than poppy seed oil, and more thinly fluid than olive oil, without any odour and of a nutty, very agreeable and mild taste; it socn becomes rancid if exposed to the air. It becomes thick and solidifies to a white butter at a very low temperature. It is soluble in ether and chloroform. It is composed chiefly of oleine and traces of palmitin, also contains traces of cholesterine, thus distinguished from sesamum, rape, poppy or olive oil. Dose, 1 to 4 fluid drachms—used as an application in skin affections.

Oleum amygdalæ amara.—The volatile or essential oil of bitter almonds. Obtained by trituration or maceration of bitter almonds with water and subsequent distillation. It is one of the products of reaction between amygdalin and emulsin acting upon one another. It contains hydrocyanic acid and volatile oil. The hydrocyanic acid is removed by distillation with caustic potash.

It is a clear-pale, cherry-coloured thin liquid, of an aromatic bitter odour and bitter burning taste, neutral reaction, soluble in water (1 in 300), but freely so in alcohol and ether. It contains hydrite of benzyl, benzaldehyde, and hydrocyanic acid. Benzaldehyde on exposure to air is converted into Benzoic acid. Dose, ½ to 1 m. Hydrocyanic acid is also found in cherry laurel, prunus Mahalib, prunus pudum and other species of prunes—in the juice of bitter cassava &c.

Emulsin or Synaptase, an albuminous principle or ferment found in both the varieties. It is extracted by water. It is coagulated by heat, and precipitated by alcohol, but not by acetic acid. In the case of bitter almonds, in the presence of water, it acts upon amygdalin forming glucose, hydrocyanic acid and benzoic aldehyde (oil of bitter almonds).

Preparations.—Of the seeds. Almond bread made from the almond cake. The sweet almond is first triturated and the fixed oil expressed, leaving almond cake. This is ground into a meal or flour and made into bread. This contains no starch and hence very useful in diabetes.

Preparations.—Of the seeds. Bitter almonds—Syrupus Amygdalæ 4 p. c. Dose, 2 to 4 drs. Sweet almonds—Pulvis Amygdalæ compositus B. P. Dose, 1 to 2 drs. Emulsum Amygdalæ contains sweet almonds 6 p. c. Mistura Amygdalæ B. P. (1 in 8) a vehicle for cough mixtures. Dose, ½ to 1 oz. Of the shells, when calcined, tooth powder.

Actions and uses.—Both the varieties differ in their physiological actions. Sweet almond is demulcent, nutritive and emollient. The oil is used like olive oil for application and internally given for pulmonary troubles and also used as a laxative. Externally the oil or the emulsion is used as an application for acne on the face, for excoriations, chapped hands and nipples, and for earache. Almond cakes made from almond meal are given as substitute for bread in diabetes.

The bitter almond oil is used for flavouring choice dishes and for scenting soap and other delicacies. It may be used as a sedative in coughs &c.

Prunus Insititia, Prunus Bokariensis.

Habitat.—Bokhara, Persia.

Parts used.—The dried plum deprived of seeds.

Vernacular.—Arab.—Alu Bokhara, Ijasa. Beng., Duk.—Alu Bokhara. Eng.—Bokhara plum. Hind.—Alu Bokhara. Pers.—Alu.

Characters.—Fruit globular, sweetish, acidulous and succulent; surface rather compressed and wrinkled, colour reddish yellow or brown, smell like that of dates. Inside the fruit is an almond-like nut, which is obliquely ovate, convex on both surfaces and marked with three prominent ridges at one of its margins. The nut when broken contains a kernel which resembles sweet almond in all its characters.

Constituents.—Malic acid, citric aid, sugar, albuminoids, pectin and ash.

Preparation.—Confection.

Actions and uses.—Demulcent and nutrient; uses similar to those of the official variety.

Prunus Armeniaca, Armeniaca Vulgaris.

Habitat.—Himalaya, Dekhan, Mysore.

Parts used.—The fruit and seed.

Vernacular.—Arab.—Binkook Tuffa armina. Bokhara.—Baboor-Kohani. Eng.—Apricot. Himalayas.—Chulu, chinaru. Hind.—Zardalu-Khubani. Pers.—Mish mish. Sutlej.—Jaldaru.

Characters.—Fruit sweetish, acidulous and succulent ; form almost globular, surface reddish yellow. Inside is a nut which contains a kernel.

Preparation.—Confection. Dose, 1 to 2 drs.

Actions and uses.—Nutrient and tonic; used in fevers to allay thirst ; the seeds form an ingredient in some of the nutritive confections.

Prunus Sp.

Habitat.—Western Asia.

Parts used.— The stones.

Vernacular.—Arab.—Jerasaya, Kerasya. Hind.—Alubalu. Pers.—Alubalu. Japan.—Sakura.

Characters.—A small tree—fruits of a light brown colour ; seeds embedded in them and resembling those of common cherry ; odour of bitter almond seeds, taste bitter and aromatic.

Constituents.—The kernels contain a volatile oil and hydrocyanic acid.

Preparation.—Confection.

Actions and uses.—Nutritive and tonic. The natives give the kernels with other tonic and aphrodisiac medicines in nervous debility and nervous exhaustion.

Prunus Domestica, Var. Juliana, B. P.

Habitat.—Persia.

Parts used.—The dried ripe fruit; Prunum—Prunes, B. P.

Vernacular.—Arab.—Barkook, Bargoog. Eng.—Common plum, Prunes. Hind.—Aru, alu, Aluchah, Shan alu.

Characters.—Ovoid or oblong, about $1\frac{1}{4}$ inch long, black and shrivelled. Pulp brownish, without any odour and of a sweet, bland, acidulous taste. The finest and sweetest variety is used as dessert. The smaller kind, which is more acid and less pleasant, is used in medicine. Dose, 2 ozs.

Constituents.—The pulp or sarcocarp contains a little malic acid, sugar 25 p. c., pectin, albumen and salts. The seeds contain a fixed oil, amygdalin and emulsin.

Preparations.—Confectio sennæ, B. P. Dose, 1 to 2 drs.

Actions and uses.—The sarcocarp is laxative, demulcent and nutrient ; taken in excess it causes griping and flatulence. It is given with purgatives as senna &c. It quenches thirst in fevers.

Prunus Laurocerasus, B. P.

Habitat.—Asia Minor.

Parts used.—The fresh leaves—Laurocerasi folia, cherry laurel leaves, B. P.

Characters.—Leaves thick, coriaceous ; petioles short and strong, oblong, obovate, 5 to 7 inches long, tapering towards each end, serrated at the apex and revolute at margins. Dark green, smooth and shining above, much paler beneath. Midrib prominent with one or two glandular depressions on each side ; odourless, but emitting smell of bitter almond seeds, when bruised.

Constituents.—On distillation with water the leaves yield Laurocerasin, identical with amygdalin ; a bitter principle, tannin, sugar and a ferment, by the action of which on laurocerasin is produced a volatile oil consisting of benzaldehyde and prussic acid.

Preparations.—Aqua Laurocerasi, B. P.—it shall be made of the strength ot $\frac{1}{10}$ p. c. of hydrocyanic acid. Dose, $\frac{1}{2}$ to 2 fld.

Actions and uses.—Sedative, anodyne, antispasmodic and narcotic ; same as those of Hydrocyanic acid.

Prunus Mahalib.

Habitat.—Central Asia and Europe.

Parts used.—The kernels and oil.

Vernacular.—Arab.—Hab-ul-mahaliba. Eng.—Perfumed cherry tree. Mar.—Gahula. Pers.—Paiwand-e-maryam.

Characters.—Shell of a dark brown or light buff colour, of an oval or ovate shape and very fragile. Seeds of a pale buff colour, testa thin and striated, kernel of a light brown colour. It has a bitter almond-like taste. The oil is rancid ; in flavour like that of hydrocyanic acid.

Preparation—Confection. Dose 1 to 2 drs.

Actions and uses.—Stomachic ; used in dyspepsia, anorexia, and general debility.

Prunus Pudum, P. Sylvetica, Cerasus Pudum.

Habitat.—Central Asia.

Parts used.—The wood bark.

Vernacular.—Guz.—Padmakasta, Padma-nulakarun. Hind.—Padmakasta. Mar.—Padma Kashtha, Chamari Jhelum.

Characters.—The wood of a light reddish brown colour, sometimes covered with a brownish thin bark which peels off in flakes. It has a faintly almond-oil like taste, and odour. Dose—Powdered bark, 15 to 25 grs.

Constituents.—Amygdalin.

Preparations.—Of the bark, decoction (1 in 10). Dose, $\frac{1}{2}$ to 2 fld. drs. Confection known as Mâhajam-e-til containing Padma Káshtá

4, Lavanga 4, Darunaj-e-abrabi 4, Behaman-e-Sapheda 3, Behaman-e-Surkha 3, Taja 2, Jâephala 2, Jâvantri 2, Jatamanansi 2, Zara Kachura 2, Jaramabáda 2, Pipali 2, Pipali mula 2, Kesara 1½, Ispanda 3, Kabâba chini 3, Elachi 1, Kulpha 3, Sugar 2, mix and make a confection. Dose 1 to 4 drs. Used in dyspepsia, congested liver, anorexia, &c.

Actions and uses.—The bark is used as a bitter tonic and sedative. It is given during convalescence from acute diseases and in palpitations of the heart.

Prunus Serotina, B.P. Wild Cherry.

Habitat.—N. America, Canada.

Parts used.—The bark—pruni virginianæ cortex. Virginian Prune Bark, B. P.

Characters.—Curved pieces or irregular fragments; young bark covered with reddish brown papery cork, thin and smooth, presenting a greenish brown inner layer, and breaking with a short granular fracture. Taste astringent, aromatic and bitter; odour in the presence of water that of bitter almonds.

Constituents.—The bark contains amygdalin, emulsin, a bitter principle, a volatile oil, hydrocyanic acid, tannin, gallic acid, resin, and starch. In the presence of water it yields hydrocyanic acid and volatile oil resembling that of bitter almonds. The root bark contains a glucoside phloridzin which is also found in the root bark of apple, pear and plum trees.

Amygdalin, a bitter uncrystalline glucoside obtained by the action of alcohol. It is not precipitated by ether.

Bitter principle—To obtain it, mix aqueous extract with alcohol, and milk of lime, evaporate, filter, boil the residue with alcohol and again evaporate. It is a brown gelatinous mass, taste bitter.

Preparations.—Syrupus pruni virginianæ, B. P. (1 in about 7). Dose, ½ to 1 fld. dr.

Prunin or Cerasin—obtained by evaporating the tincture and powdering the extract. Dose, 1 to 5 grs.

Tinctura Pruni Virginianæ, B. P. (1 in 5). Dose, ½ to 1 fluid dr.

Physiological actions.—Sedative, pectoral, tonic, and astringent. In moderate doses it is an aromatic bitter tonic, stimulates the stomach, increases appetite, aids digestion, and thus promotes constructive metabolism. The volatile oil is a stimulant of the alimentary canal. Hydrocyanic acid acts as a sedative, lessens irritation and impairs nervous excitability. Large doses depress the heart's action. Phloridzin produces glycosuria in man and animals.

Therapeutics.—Given in cough, hectic fever, scrofula, in bronchial catarrh, phthisis, and irritation of the throat. As a stomachic tonic it is given in dyspepsia, palpitation and general debility; also during convalescence from acute diseases. The volatile oil is an intestinal stimulant and acts like cascarilla, serpentaria, &c.

Pyrus Cydonia. Cydonia Vulgaris.

Habitat.—Central Asia, temperate climates.

Parts used.—The seeds.

Vernacular.—Arab.—Muzz, Hubbul, Sapharjala. Can.—Shime dalimba bija. Duk.—Bihi danah. Eng.—Quince seed. Hind.—Mogloi behedana. Pers.—Beha-danah, Tukhm-e-abi, Karabadin. Tam.—Shimai-ma-delaivirai. Tel.—Shima-dalima-Vittulu.

Characters.—10 or 15 seeds are contained in one cell of the fruit; seeds irregularly ovoid, flattened and angular or three-sided, adherent to one another by mucilage and covered by a membrane; colour of the testa, dark brown, that of the kernel, yellowish white. The seeds have the odour and taste of bitter almonds.

Constituents.—The seeds contain a mucilage named cydonin, albuminous matter, fixed oil, an oily liquid which contains ænanthic ether, and ash 3-5 p. c., containing alkalies, alkaline earths, iron, &c.

Mucilage contained in the epithelial cells is in very large quantity, and coagulates 40 times its weight of water. It has little adhesive power and is not thickened by borax. It is a compound of gum and cellulose. The fragrance is due to the presence of ænanthic ether.

Preparations.—Mucilago cydonii (1 in 50).

Actions and uses.—Cydonium or quince seeds are nutritive, astringent, demulcent, and emollient, and given with sugar in cough, dysentery, catarrhal affections of the throat and pulmonary mucous membrane; also used as a vehicle for injection in gonorrhœa and urinary disorders. Externally the mucilage is applied to burns and scalds.

Bandoline, a preparation used as a hair dressing, is identical with mucilage of cydonin.

Quillaja Saponaria, B. P.

Habitat.—Chili, Peru, N. Hindustan.

Parts used.—The inner bark—Quillaiæ cortex. Quillaia bark, B. P. Syn.—China bark or murillo bark, Panama bark, soap bark.

Quillaya means a wash, as this bark is good for washing.

Saponaria, sapo, soap. Its mucilaginous juice forms lather with water.

Characters.—Bark in flat thick pieces $\frac{1}{6}$ of an inch thick, 2 feet long and 4 inches wide, brownish white externally, smooth, white or yellowish white within. Fracture splintery, fractured surface laminated, exhibiting under a lens, glistening prismatic crystals; without any odour, of an acrid persistent taste. Wood very hard.

Constituents.—A glucoside saponin, starch, gum, calcium oxalate, and calcium sulphate crystals. Saponin—obtained by exhausting the bark with hot alcohol. A white amorphous powder without any odour and of a sweetish taste; soluble in water and dilute alcohol; it acts as a sternutatory. It consists of 2 glucosides—Quillaic acid, soluble in alcohol and precipitated by lead acetate; and Quillaia-sapotoxin, neutral insoluble in alcohol and not precipitated by acetate of lead.

Preparations.—Tinctura Quillaiæ B. P. (1 in 20). Dose, ½ to 1 fl. dr. Decoctum Quillaiæ (5 to 200). Dose, 1 to 2 dr. Fluid extract. Dose, 15 to 30 ms. Syrupus Quillaiæ. Dose, 1 to 3 drs.

Physiological Action.—Detergent, stimulant, diuretic, expectorant and irritant of the respiratory organs. The powder is sternutatory; macerated in water, the water froths like soap; it forms emulsions with oils owing to the presence of saponin. In large doses it is a local anæsthetic and antipyretic, paralyzant of the heart and respiration and a poison to the voluntary muscles. It does not produce vomiting or purging.

Therapeutics.—The decoction of the bark is given like senega in chronic bronchitis, cough, coryza and in dropsy. The powder of the bark is used as a dusting powder or snuff in rhinitis; locally an infusion is used to dispel fœtor of feet or armpits; also in alopecia as a hair tonic or detergent to remove scurf and renew the growth of hair. It is contra-indicated in irritation and inflammation of the mucous membranes. A dry extract causes the water in which it is macerated to froth, and hence used for making emulsions of fixed oil. The tincture is an ingredient in Liquor Picis carbonis, B.P. It is also used for washing purposes.

Rosa Damascena, B. P. R. Moschata. R. Sempervirens.

Habitat.—Syria, Africa, Balkan Mountains, Roumelia.

Parts used.—The flowers, flower buds, petals, stamens and a volatile oil, oleum rosæ, attar or otto of rose, B. P.

Vernacular.—Arab.—Wardel, chamak Julanja-bin (conserve). Beng.—Gulap. Can.—Gulab. Duk., Guz., Hind.—Gulab-kali, Gulkand (conserve). Mar.—Gulaphâ. Pers.—Gule-gulaba, Gule-shakar (conserve). Sans.—Sata pattri. Tam.—Gulappu, Irojappu. Tel.—Rosa-puvou. Eng.—Damask Rose.

Characters.—It is the source of the official oil of rose. Flower buds oblong of a brownish light red colour when fresh, but if old perfectly deep brown; sepals five partite, of a greenish brown colour, viscid, and ciliated. Below the sepals is an ovary resembling a thick stalk of a flower, very viscid, greenish brown; petals over-lapping one another to form a cone, of an aromatic agreeable smell and a bitterish taste.

Gulaba-ke-bija. These are not seeds but the compressed, two-lobed, oblong, reniform or roundish, small, dark coloured anthers.

Constituents.—Volatile oil, fat, resin, malic, tartaric, and tannic acids. Volatile oil—oil of rose distilled from the fresh flowers with calyx. It is colourless at first, but becomes after short time a pale yellowish, transparent liquid, with a strong, fragrant odour of roses. Taste mild and sweetish; slightly soluble in acetic acid and alcohol.

Preparations.—Aqua Rosæ Fortior. Strong or triple rose water Water saturated with the volatile oil of rose petals; obtained as a by-product in the distillation of oil of rose; used as excipient and flavouring agent. Dose, ½ to 1 dr. Unguentum Aquæ Rosæ, B. P. cold cream, ointment of rose water. Stronger rose water 7 ozs., oil of almond 9 ozs. spermaceti 1½ ozs, white wax 1½ ozs., oil of rose 8 ms., for externa application. Aqua rosæ B. P., Gulab, (Hind.) prepared by diluting Aqua Rosæ Fortior with twice its volume of distilled water. Oleum Rosæ B. P. oil of rose—attar or otto of rose—volatile oil distilled from the fresh flowers. A pale yellow crystalline semi-solid; odour strong and fragrant, taste sweet, slightly acid in reaction, sparingly soluble in alcohol. It is adulterated with a volatile oil derived from a species of Andropogon and known as oil of geranium, Idris oil, or ginger oil. It consists of an aromatic oxygenated elæopten, and an odourless solid stearopten or rose camphor. Gulkhand, a conserve of rose petals with sugar, to which cannabis Indica is sometimes added. Gulanjabin, a conserve of rose petals with honey. Medicated oil of roses, Duhn-i-ward-i-kham—sweet oil added to rose petals and exposed to the sun. Duhu-i-ward-i-matbukh—rose petals added to sweet oil and heated over the fire. The natives use the above as liniments in sprains, bruises, &c.

Actions and uses.—Mildly astringent, carminative, and refrigerant; used as basis for bitter medicines and as pill bases. Rose water is used as a cooling and astringent excipient for lotions, collyria and urethal injections and in irritability of the mucous membranes. The ointment is a soothing emollient and protective for the skin, in chapped hands, cracked nipples. Rose buds are used along with other purgative decoctions by the natives in constipation during fevers and hepatic derangements.

Rosa Gallica, B. P.

Habitat.—South of Europe, Western Asia.

Parts used.—The fresh and dried unexpanded petals, Rosæ Gallicæ petala.

Characters.—Cone-like masses, sometimes separate and more or less crumpled; petals, velvety, of a deep, purplish red colour; odour fragrant. Taste somewhat bitter. Feebly acid and astringent.

Constituents.—Red colouring matter, tannic and gallic acids, and a volatile aromatic oil (a trace), mucilage, sugar, quercitrin, salts &c.

Preparations.—Infusum Rosæ Acidum, B. P. (Red rose petals ½ ounce, diluted sulphuric acid 2 fluid drachms, boiling distilled water 1 pint). Dose ½ to 1 fld. oz. Extractum Rosæ Fluidum. Dose, 5 to 50 ms. Confectio Rosæ Gallicæ, B. P. (1 in 4). Dose, 60 grs. or more. Mel Rosæ—honey of rose, fluid extract 12, and honey 100. Dose, 1 to 2 drs. Syrupus Rosæ, B. P. (1 in 23). Dose, ½ to 1 fld. dr. Red rose is an ingredient of Pilulæ aloes et mastiches.

Actions and uses.—Tonic, mild astringent and carminative; used frequently as a colouring and flavouring agent. Flowers when full blown are laxative. The infusion containing dilute sulphuric acid is a good gargle and used in sore throat, aphthæ, ulcers of the mouth &c.

Rubus Chamæmorus.

Norwegian blackberry. Marsh raspberry. Yellow raspberry, cloudberry, dwarf mulberry.

Habitat.—Europe.

Parts employed.—The fruit and leaves.

Preparations.—Fluid Extract. Dose, ½ to 1 dr. Infusion of leaves (1 in 12). Dose, 2 to 6 drs.

Physiological action.—Leaves diuretic. They act on the kidneys without influencing the beat of the heart. Given in nephritis, cirrhosis of the liver, cardiac affections, chloro-anæmia with œdema, hysterical epilepsy, palpitations of the heart, and cancer of the stomach. The fruit is antiscorbutic, and is used in hæmoptysis.

Rubus Canadensis. Dewberry.

R. Villous, the common blackberry. R. trivialis, the bush blackberry.

Habitat.—Southern States.

Part used.—The bark of the root.

Characters.—Bark thin tough, flexible bands, colour blackish grey externally and pale brown within. Without any odour, taste astringent, bitter. Dose ½ to 2 drs.

Constituents.—Tannin, 10 p. c., gallic acid ½ p. c., villosin 0.8 p. c., ash 3 p. c. Villosin is a bitter crystalline glucoside, soluble in alcohol, ether, chloroform.

Preparation.—Extractum Rubi fluidum.—Dose, 10 to 60 minims, Syrupus Rubi aromaticus, contains rubus, cinnamon, cloves, and mace. 30 gr. each in one ounce. Dose, 1 to 8 drs. Syrupus Rubi (1 of the fluid extract to 3). Dose, 1 to 6 drs. Decoction. Dose 1 to 2 ozs.

Actions and uses.—Astringent and tonic; given in bowel complaints, such as summer and infantile diarrhœas.

Rubus Idæus, Raspberry, hindberry; Rubus strigosus, wild red raspberry; Rubus occidentalis, Thimble berry.

Habitat.—Europe, Asia.

Part used.—The fruit.

Characters.—Fruit, a receptable, conical, hollow at the base, hemispherical, red, hairy, composed of 20 to 30 drupes, small and coalesced; each drupe crowned with withered style. Juice red coloured, odour agreeable, taste sweet and pleasant.

Constituents.—Volatile oil, citric acid, malic acid, sugar 5 p. c. pectin, proteids, colouring matter &c.

Preparation.—Syrupus Rubi Idæi. Colour bright red, odour fruity, agreeable taste pleasant, acidulous. Reaction acid. Dose, 2 to 6 drs. or more. Infusion of the leaves of red raspberry (1 to 20). Dose, 6 to 12 drs.

Actions and uses.—Refrigerant, laxative and dietetic; given in fevers. Infusion of the leaves of red raspberry is used for diarrhœa.

Spiræa Tomentosa, Hard hack.

Habitat.—North America.

Part used.—The root.

Characters.—The root consists of brown bark which is bitter and astringent. The wood is hard and without any taste. Flowers fragrant. The fragrancy is due to the presence of coumarin.

Constituents.—Contains tannin, coumarin, a bitter principle and a volatile oil. Used as infusion. Decoction (1 in 2c). Dose, 4 to 6 drs. Extract. Dose, 2 to 5 grs.

Actions and uses.—Astringent and tonic; given in diarrhœa cholera infantum, also in hæmorrhages, gonorrhœa, ulcers &c.

Portulacaceæ.

The Purslane or the Kulpha family.

Succulent herbs or shrubs. Leaves exstipulate, entire. Flowers unsymmetrical. Fruits capsular, usually dehiscing transversely or by valves or by a lid. Seeds solitary or numerous. Albumen farinaceous. Root fleshy.

Habitat.—Cape of Good Hope and S. America.

Properties.—Some possess cooling and antiscorbutic properties, some bear edible roots.

Portulaca Oleracea, Portulaca Quadrifida, P. Maridiana, Illicebrum Verticulatum.

Habitat.—All warm climates.

Part used.—The seeds and herb.

Portulaca.—Porto, to carry, and lac, milk. The herb abounds in milky juice.

Vernacular.—Arab.—Baklat-al Humaka, Kurfah. Beng.—Buro Luccia. Burm.—Mya-by eet. Can.—Dooda Gorat. Cing.—Genda-kola. Duk.—Chorote. Eng.—Purslane. Guz.—Loni. Hind.—Kulpha, Linria, Moucha. Malyal.—Karichira. Mar.—Bhnigholi. Panj.—Limak, Kakeba. Pers.—Turuk, Kurfah. Sans.—Lonika, Lunia, Oopadyki. Tam.—Karil Kiraj. Tel.—Bodda-aveli-kura.

Characters.—An annual succulent creeper; fresh leaves, fleshy, entire, cuniform, succulent, oblong and flat; flowers sessile, small and yellow; capsules globose or ovate; one-celled; seeds numerous resembling those of Hura hura but smaller and of a fainter colour, black reinform and minutely tubercled. The plant has a disagreeable smell and an acid mucilaginous taste.

Constituents.—The leaves contain acid potassium oxalate, and mucilage.

Preparation.—Infusion of the leaves and seeds. Dose, 2 to 8 drs. Juice of leaves. Dose, 2 to 8 drs. Compound Tincture (1 in 10), containing bitter purslane 100, rum 150, Bordeaux wine 850, citrate of iron 5. Dose. 60 to 100 ms.

Actions and uses.—Both the varieties are bitter, diuretic and demulcent; also refrigerant and alterative; used in scanty and high coloured urine, albuminuria, cystitis, and chronic bronchitis. The compound tincture with citrate of iron is used as a bitter tonic during convalescence from acute fevers and other diseases. The bruised leaves are used as a cooling application in erysipelas, burns, scalds and other inflamed and swollen parts. The seeds are vermifuge, diuretic and demulcent, and given in hæmorrhages. The natives give the powder of the seeds in hæmoptysis.

Saxifragaceæ.

Herbs; leaves alternate, entire or lobed, stipulate or exstipulate. Flowers unsymmetrical; calyx inferior 4 or 5 partite, stamens perigynous or hypogynous. Fruit capsular, 1 to 2 celled. Seeds numerous, small, albumen, fleshy.

Habitat.—Mountainous districts of northern countries.

Properties.—Astringent.

Dichroa Febrifuga.

Habitat.—Himalaya, Java, China, Khasia mountains.

Part used.—The root bark.

Vernacular. — Bhutan. — Sing-namook. Cochin-China — Cay-thuong-son. Cham-chau. Hind.—Basak. Lepcha.—Gebokanak.

Characters.—Root bark in chips, light yellow coloured, soft and corky; externally fissured longitudinally, internally smooth and waxy; almost tasteless, odour faintly aromatic.

Constituents.—A crystalline glucoside termed Dichroin. It is allied to æsculin; another crystalline principle of the nature of wax, insoluble in water and soluble in alkaline fluids; also starch, but no tannin.

Preparation.—Decoction with liquorice (1 in 20). Dose, $\frac{1}{2}$ to 1 fluid oz.

Actions and uses.—Febrifuge and aperient; given in ague and other malarial fevers; in large doses it acts as an emetic and causes depression of the circulation.

Hydrangea Arborescens.

Wild Hydrangea, Leven bark.

Habitat.—United States.

Part used.—The root.

Characters.—A plant with white, tough root.

Constituents.—Gum, albumen, starch, resin, ferrous salts and other salts.

Preparation.—A compound powder containing Hydrangea, benzoic acid and salicylate of lithia. Dose, 20 to 60 grs. Fluid extract, 20 to 60 ms. Decoction of the root (1 in 20). Dose, 1 to 2 ozs.

Actions and uses.—Tonic, sialagogue, diuretic, stomachic and lithontriptic ; given in calculous affections and other abnormal conditions of the kidneys, chronic gleet, prostatitis and bladder irritation. It increases the flow of urine and hence is useful either in retention or suppression of urine. The powder has been regarded as a soothing alterative and antilithic in urinary calculus, diabetes, gout, cystitis, rheumatism, hæmaturia, Bright's disease, and vesical irritations generally. It promotes the removal of gravel from the bladder and relieves the pain during the passage of concretions through the ureters.

Saxifraga Ligulata.

Habitat.—Temperate Himalaya.

Parts used.—The rhizome.

Vernacular.—Beas.—Mokhan. Chenab.—Batpia. Hind.—Dakachru, Batpia. Ind. Bazaar—Pashanbhed, Pakhanbheda, Jhelum-Popal Ban, Patrak. Khasia.—Atia, Torongsingh. Nepal.—Sohanpe-soah. Panj. Shaproki. Ravi.—Saprotri. Pashanbhed means stone breaker. It dissolves stone in the bladder.

Characters.—Rhizome in small pieces 1 or 2 inches long and about ½ inch in diameter, externally brown, wrinkled and scaly, bearing scars of rootlets ; substance dense, hard and of a reddish colour. Taste astringent and odour slightly aromatic.

Constituents.—Tannic and gallic acids, starch, mineral salts, metarabin, albumen, glucose, mucilage, wax and an odorous principle. Ash 12·87 p. c., containing calcium oxalate.

Actions and uses.—Diuretic, demulcent and astringent ; given in diarrhœa and cough and in uric acid diathesis ; with honey it is applied to the gums in teething in children to allay irritation. Dose, 5 to 20 grs.

Crassulaceæ.

The house leek, stone crop or the zakhme hayata family ; plants generally succulent ; herbs or shrubs, with exstipulate, entire or pinnatifid leaves. Flowers cymose, perfectly symmetrical ; fruits dehiscent, consisting either of a whorl of follicles or a capsule ; seeds very small, albumen fleshy ; embryo in the axis of albumen.

Habitat.—Generally in dry situation, Cape of Good Hope.

Properties.—Astringent, refrigerant and acrid.

Sedum Acre.

Syn.—Wall pepper, Mossy stone crop, small house leek.

Habitat.—Europe. Runs wild in some places in North America.

Part used.—The entire plant.

Characters.—Moss-like spreading plant, growing in dry fields and on old walls. Leaves one-eighth to a quarter inch long, alternate, nearly imbricate, in about six spirally turned rows, ovate, thick, convex on the back, punctate and smooth. Flowers in scorpoid cymes, petals yellow, pistils 4 to 5, stamens 8 to 10. The plant is inodorous and has a mucilaginous and acrid taste. Dose, 10 to 15 grs.

Constituents.—Much mucilage and malates. Its active principle rutin has not been isolated.

Preparations.—Fl. extract of the whole plant. Dose, 15 to 30 grs.

Actions and uses.—The bruised plant or its juice is emetic, the emesis being copious and causing little pain, and is employed for removing the false membranes in diphtheria. It is used as an application to scrofulous, cancerous, and scorbutic ulcers, as a resolvent to enlarged lymphatic glands and a dressing to chronic diseases of the skin ; also used to remove warts and corns.

Kalanchoe Lanciniata. K. Pinnata. K. Spathulata. Bryophyllum Calycinum.

Habitat.—Deccan Peninsula, Bengal.

Parts used.—The leaves.

Vernacular.—Beng.—Hamsâgar. Bomb.—Pervur sàla, Airavana Nairavana. Burm.—Ywet-kya-pen-ponk. Can.—Kalnaru, Haradha-chchaka. Duk.—Gha-e-mari. Hind.—Ghai-mari, Parnabija, Zakhm-hyata, Ghai-oat, Aran-maran, Hemsagar. Mar.—Varnaby, Ghaimari, Ghaipat. Sans.—Aimasa-gara, Ashti-bhaksha. Panj.—Talara, Haiza-ka-patt, Parna-veja. Tam.—Malla-kulli.

Parnabija—Parna means leaf, and bija, a seed ; this is in allusion to the character of the plant, the crenulations of whose leaves in contact with the damp soil give rise to fresh buds which take roots and develop new plants.

Zakhm-e-hayata—Zakhm, a wound, and Hayat to heal, A healer of the wound. Wound heals at once and no trace of any morbid condition is left behind.

Characters.—B. Calycinum. Plant erect, tall, fleshy, and suffruticose ; leaves thick, ovate, crenated ; leaflets one large and two smaller ones ; petiole and margin of leaf purple ; flowers yellowish red ; taste acid and astringent. Dose of the juice, 30 to 40 ms. K. Lanciniata—Leaves decompound and pinnatifid ; segments, oblong, acute toothed ; flowers yellow.

Constituents.—Chlorophyll, fat, a yellow organic acid, cream of tartar, sulphate of calcium and free tartaric acid ; calcium oxalate is found in the leaves.

Actions and uses.—The leaves are styptic and applied hot to contused wounds, bruises and boils. By their application the edges of incised wounds heal generally by first intention ; when applied to unhealthy wounds and foul ulcers they allay irritation and inflammation, and facilitate cicatrization. It is used as an application to bites of venomous insects, as gnats, house leek, &c. The juice of the leaves with butter is astringent and given in diarrhoea, dysentery, cholera and phthisis.

Droseraceæ.

Sundew family. Herbs growing in marshy places, frequently glandular. Leaves alternate, exstipulate, with a circinate vernation; flowers regular, symmetrical and hypogynous; fruit, capsular, one-celled with loculicidal dehiscence; seeds numerous, albumen fleshy, embryo small.

Habitat.—Found everywhere except the arctic regions.

Properties.—Slightly acid and acrid. This family is characterized by having glands on their leaves or hairs with peculiar irritability which enables them to entrap insects. Example, Sundew or Venus's flytrap.

Drosera Peltata, D. Lunata, D. Rotundifolia.

Round Leaved Sundew.

Habitat.—Himalayas, Neilgherry. N. Europe.

Part used.—The whole plant.

Characters.—Herb of a dark olive green colour, growing in marshy places; stem erect, and glabrous; leaves scattered with glandular hairs which close when flies and insects alight upon them; long petioled, peltate with two long horns pointing upwards; style pencil-shaped. Capsule globose; seeds, oblong, numerous and small. Flowers yellow. Paper, cloth, or even wood is stained of a deep red colour by the plant if allowed to dry upon them; it has the odour of sour milk.

Constituents.—A crystalline colouring matter; a resin (having blistering property) and ash containing persalts of iron.

Preparations.—Fluid extract 5 to 20 ms. Tincture (1 in 10). Dose, 5 to 10 ms.

Actions and uses.—The expressed juice is acrid and caustic and applied to warts and corns; applied to the skin it sets up inflammation and causes a blister. Internally the fluid extract of the leaves has been used in asthma, chronic bronchitis, phthisis and whooping cough; also in gastric disorders and in flatulence. In whooping cough it lessens the violence of the paroxysms and relieves harsh and loud cough. It also prevents bleeding from the nose and vomiting.

Remarks.—It is said that animal substances if used as manure are digested by the sundews and they thrive upon such food and produce more capsules and seeds. It is used by the natives to reduce gold to powder. A paste of the plant is used to cover a sovereign which is then enclosed in an earthen pot, cemented with clay and put in fire and thoroughly burnt. Gold is then reduced to powder and used as antisyphilitic, alterative and tonic in various chronic diseases.

Liquidambaraceæ or Altingiaceæ.

Trees balsamiferous.—Leaves simple, lobed and alternate; stipules deciduous. Flowers unisexual, involucrate and amentaceous. Fruit cone-shaped; capsules two-celled enclosed in hard scales; seeds winged, peltate and albuminous. Embryo inverted. Radicle superior.

Habitat.—Natives of warm part of India, America and South of Europe.

Properties.—Remarkable for fragrant balsamic properties ; they have warm bitter barks.

In the United States it is called sweet gum, and the fragrant balsam juice which exudes from stems by incision is called liquidamber, oil of amber, or copalm balsam.

Liquidamber Altingia, Altingia Excelsa.

Habitat.—Java, Tenasserim

Parts used.—Resin, liquid storax.

Vernacular.—Arab—Meaohe-sayelah. Burm.—Nan-tayok. Eng. —Rosa malloes, liquid storax. Java.—Rasa mala. Malay.—Rasa mala.

Characters.—Bark when wounded yields a resin which is employed to mix with balsam of Peru.

Actions and uses.—The bark is bitter, aromatic and stimulant of mucous membranes, chiefly of the air passages.

Liquidamber Orientalis, B. P.

Habitat.—Forests in Asia minor.

Part used.—The Balsam obtained from the trunk, purified by solution in Ethylic alcohol, filtration and evaporation of the solvent. Styrax præparatum, prepared storax, B. P.

Vernacular.—Arab.—Meahsayelah, Lubni, Dukhan-el-daru. Bom. Burm.—Inyok. Eng.—oriental sweet gum, gum storax, Tar-wood. Guz.—Silarasa. Hind.—Silarasa Asht-loban. Ind.—Silaras, Malay.—Rosa Malay. Pers.—Asli, Lubni. Sans.—Silhaka. Tam.—Nare-arishippal. Tel.—Shila rasam. Ast loban.—Western frankincense.

Characters.—A soft or semi-liquid viscid balsam resembling honey. When in thin layers, transparent, of a greyish brown colour and heavier than water. On heating, it becomes dark brown. The smell is pleasant and balsamic. Taste pungent, burning and aromatic ; insoluble in warm water, soluble in hot alcohol, in ether, or chloroform, glacial acetic acid, bisulphide of carbon and in most of the essential oils. The bark occurs in half quills, several inches long, of a light brown colour ; externally soft and corky ; internally resinous and aromatic. Dose, 5 to 20 grs.

Constituents.—A volatile oil styrol (cinnamene); a crystalline solid styracin or Cinnamate of Cinnamic ether, two resins, one hard and the other soft ; and Cinnamic acid.

Styrol.—A hydrocarbon obtained by distilling storax with water It is a colourless thin liquid of a fragrant odour and burning taste; also synthetically obtained by heating acetylene gas, or from ethylbenzol bromide by heating it with baryta. When heated to a very high temperature it is converted into metacinnamene which is a colourless amorphous solid, insoluble in alcohol and ether. When distilled it is reconverted into styrol.

Cinnamic acid.—Closely allied to benzoic acid, obtained by heating storax with solution of sodium carbonate and precipitating by hydrochloric acid. It is colourless crystalline body, without any odour. It is excreted in the urine as hippuric acid. It is a constituent of balsam of Peru and Tolu.

Preparation.—Tinctura Benzoini composita, B. P. Dose, ½ to 1 dr. Mostly used externally.

Actions and uses.—Stimulant, expectorant, diuretic, antiseptic, disinfectant and astringent. As an expectorant it is given in pulmonary affections, chronic bronchitis, chronic catarrh of the genito-urinary organs, as cystitis, pyelitis, gonorrhœa, amenorrœa, leucorrhœa, and gleet ; in affections of the throat, and in copious perspiration. An ointment is used as a parasiticide for scabies, phthiriasis &c. It acts like Benzoin, balsams of Tolu and Peru, and copaiba. The Hindus use it for perfuming medicinal oils. Dose, 5 to 30 grs.

Liquid Amber Styraciflua.

Habitat.—North America, United States.

Part used.—The Balsam exuding spontaneously or from incisions made in the trunk.

Characters.—Thick, transparent yellowish brown liquid ; of a strong odour of liquid storax ; taste aromatic and acrid. It solidifies on exposure to the air ; soluble in alcohol, ether and chloroform. Dose, 5 to 30 grains.

Constituents.—Styracin, storesin, a hydrocarbon 3.5 p.c., almost identical with styrol and cinnamic acid 5½ p.c.

Preparation.—Emulsion, ointment, cerate.

Actions and uses.—Same as those of Liquidamber altingia ; stimulant, expectorant and diuretic.

Hamamelidaceæ.

Witch hazel family; small trees; leaves alternate; stipules deciduous; flowers perfect or unisexual; calyx superior, 4 or 5 lobed ; petals 4 or. 5 ; fruits capsular, 2 valved with a loculicidal dehiscence. Seeds pendulous and albuminous.

Habitat.—Temperate climates and tropics, Japan, China, Madagascar, Assam.

Properties.—Astringent, acrid, bitter and balsamic.

Hamamelis Virginiana, B. P.

Syn.—Winter bloom ; Witch hazel, so called from the twigs being used in the days of witchcraft as divining rods to indicate hidden springs, ores, &c.

Habitat.—United States.

Part used.—The fresh and dried leaves. Hamamelidis folia—Hamamelis leaves, witch hazel leaves, B. P., and the dried bark—Hamamelidis cortex, Hamamelis bark, witch hazel bark, B. P.

Characters.—Leaves ovate, pinnately veined with stellate hair, 3 to 6 inches long, upper surface dark green or brownish green, under surface paler ; apex obtuse, margins sinuate, petiole short; without any odour and of an astringent taste. Cortex in curved pieces $\frac{1}{16}$ inch thick, 2 to 8 inches long, sometimes covered with silvery grey or dark grey cork or warty scars ; inner surface pale reddish pink or cinnamon colour and finely striated longitudinally. Fracture laminated and coarsely fibrous. Taste astringent and bitter and without any odour. Dose, 20 to 60 grains.

Constituents.—Hamamelis Folia contains tannin, a volatile oil and a bitter principle. The bark contains tannin 8 p.c., bitter principle, resin, wax, sugar and ash 6 p.c.

Preparation.—From the bark—Tinctura Hamamelidis B.P. (1 in 10). Dose, $\frac{1}{2}$ to 1 fl. dr. Decoction (1 to 20) for external use. From the leaves—Extractum Hamamelidis Liquidum, B.P.—liquid extract of Hamamelis. Dose, 5 to 15 ms. Hamamelidin or Hamamelin, an uncertain powdered extract of a purple brown colour. Dose, $\frac{1}{2}$ to 2 grs. Suppositories of 3 grs. each of the extract with cocoa butter, useful for piles. Liquor Hamamelidis B.P. (leaves 5, water 10, alcohol 1, distil to one half) for external use. Unguentum Hamamelidis, B.P., liquid extract 1, Hydrous wool fat 9. Hazeline, an American speciality. A pleasant clear liquid, slightly sweetish, of a fragrant odour. Obtained by distillation of the twigs. Dose, $\frac{1}{2}$ to 2 fluid drs.

Physiological Action.—Anodyne, sedative, cooling, antiseptic, astringent and styptic ; used both internally and externally. All these properties are mostly due to tannin, but it appears to have some special influence over the venous circulation, somewhat like that of aconite on the arterial system. In full doses it causes throbbing in the head. As a sedative it is used locally in cutaneous inflammations. It is a good application as an injection for hæmorrhoids of a bleeding variety, for varicose veins (varicocele) erysipelas, ulcers, sprains and abrasions, also pruritus and eczema. In 1 to 3 ozs. of water it is used as an enema. Internally it is given to check passive hæmorrhages as hæmorrhage from the lungs, nose, stomach, kidneys, uterus, rectum, &c. In threatened abortion it is beneficial. It is given in excessive mucous discharges as gonorrhœa and leucorrhœa ; or as a gargle or steam inhalation used in stomatitis, aphthæ, sore throat, toothache, &c

Combretaceæ.

The Himaja or myrobalan family.

Trees or shrubs, leaves exstipulate entire without dots. Flowers perfect or unisexual, beautiful and red, white or greenish yellow. Fruits indehiscent and generally winged or obtuse angled, one seeded ; seed, exalbuminous.

Habitat.—Asia, Africa, America.

The plants are remarkable for their astringent properties.

Anogeissus Latifolia, Conocarpus Latifolius, A. Villosa, A. Parvifolia.

Habitat.—Himalaya, Ceylon.

Part used.—The gum.

Vernacular.—Can.—Dinduga. Cing.—Madhura-twacha. Eng.—Crane tree. Guz.—Dhaval. Hind.—Dhaya, Dhaura, Bakl. Sans.—Vakavriksea, Dhaval. Tam.—Vellanaga, Vakalee. Tel.—Shertinam, yella-muddi.

Vaka vrikaha, Crane tree, the fruit resembles the head of a crane (vaka); Dhava from dhva to flow: a large amount of gum flows from it like milk from the breast.

Characters.—Leaves short petioled, ovate, smooth generally, and marginate, 1 to 4 inches long, and ½ to 2 inches broad. Taste very astringent, the leaves of A. villosa are rusty and villous on both surfaces. Those of A parvifolia are small and silky. The gum from the bark resembles ghatti gund and is in vermicular or elongated tears, colourless or of a pale yellow colour, rough and of a glassy fracture, free from cracks and transparent. It darkens by keeping; with water it forms a highly viscid mucilage.

Constituents.—The leaves contain tannic acid 15·5 p. c. The ash contains carbonate of potash.

Preparations.—Decoction of the leaves (1 in 10). Dose, ½ to 1 fld. oz.

Actions and uses.—Demulcent and astringent; the gum is used as a substitute for gum arabic. The decoction is astringent, and is given in diarrhœa and gonorrhœa.

Calycopteris Floribunda.

Habitat.—W. India, Assam.

Parts used.—The leaves, root and fruit.

Vernacular.—Can.—Marsada, Bâguli. Hind.—Kokoranj. Mar.—Bâguli, Ukshi. Tel.—Bandi-Murudu.

Characters.—Leaves opposite, having on the upper surface thinly scattered long hairs; under surface rusty, tomentose. Taste astringent and bitter. Fruit ovoid, 5 ribbed and villous.

Constituents.—Tannin 6·86 p. c.

Preparation.—Juice of leaves; infusion (1 in 20). Dose, 2 to 8 drs. Paste of the root.

Actions and uses.—Stimulant and astringent. The juice of leaves or infusion is used in colic and dyspepsia. The root paste, mixed with that of croton oblongifolium is used for bites of Phoorsa snake (Echis carinata). The fruit is used along with other carminatives in jaundice. The fruit is rubbed with the root of Grewia Pilosa and the paste mixed with honey is applied to ulcers.

Quisqualis Indica. Q. Villosa.

Habitat.—Malaya and India.

Parts used.—The seeds.

Vernacular.—Duk.—Rangûn-ki-bel. Eng.—Rangoon Creeper, Chinese honeysuckle. Hind.— Rangûn-ki-bêl. Malay.—Sun-sung, aroos. Mar.—Vilayati Chumeli. Tam.—Irangûn-Malli. Tel.—Rangunu-malle-chettu.

Characters.—Dry seeds black, yellowish and oily internally. Fruits oval or oblong, pointed at either end and sharply pentagonal. They dehisce from the apex. Pericarp woody, thin, fragile and of a mahogany colour and enclosing a seed.

Constituents.—Fruits consist of shells 41 parts, and kernels 59 parts in 100 parts; they contain a fixed oil 15 p.c. of a yellow colour, a sugary substance, similar to levulose, and an organic acid similar to cathartic acid. The seeds afford an alkaline ash.

Actions and uses.—The bruised seeds are anthelmintic and given in expelling lumbrici. Dose, 4 or 5 seeds.

Terminalia Arjuna, Pentaptera Arjuna, P. Glabra, P. Angustifolia.

Habitat.— Deccan, Ceylon, Bengal, Punjab, N.-W. Provinces.

Parts used.—The bark.

Vernacular.—Beng.—Arjun. Bom.—Arjun Ladara. Burm.—Tonk-kyan. Can.—Toru Billimatti. Duk.—Arjuna. Hind.—Arjan, Kahu, Jamla. Malyal.—Vella-maruta. Mar.—Kowa, Shârdul. Pinjal, Arjun. Panj.—Jumla, Kukhsoba. Sans.—Arjuna, Kakubha. Tam.—Veellai-Maruda-maram. Tel.—Tella-maddi-chettu.

Characters.—Bark, in quills, brown, soft, scabrous and corky, easily separable from the wood, and breaking with a short fracture, taste astringent and odour aromatic.

Constituents.—The ash of the bark contains 34 p.c. of almost pure calcium carbonate. The bark also contains tannin.

Preparation.—Decoction (1 in 10). Dose, $\frac{1}{2}$ to 1 fld. oz.

Actions and uses.—Astringent, and tonic; given in heart disease. Locally used as a wash for wounds, ulcers, contusions, and specially used in promoting union of fractures and dispersion of ecchymosis; internally largely used by the natives in hæmorrhagic and other fluxes and as a lithontriptic.

Terminalia Bellerica.

Habitat.—India, Ceylon, Coimbatore, Peshawar.

Parts used.—The dried pulp of the fruit without stones.

Vernacular.—Arab.—Balilaj. Beng.—Bohorâ, Baherâ. Bom.—Behedân. Burm.—Phankha-si-tit-sein. Bankha. Can.—Tari-kâyi. Cing.—Bulu. Duk.—Bâlarâ, Balda. Eng.—Beleric myrobalan,

Bastard myrobalans, Bedda-nuts. Guz.—Behdân. Hind.—Bharla, Bahera, Balra. Mar.—Behadâ, Karsba-phal, Bhulvaso. Malyal.—Tani. Pers.—Balileh. Sans.—Vibhitaka, Anilaghnaka, Bahira. Tam.—Tanrik-kây. Tel.—Tandra-kayi, Bahadraha.

Anilaghnaka means Windkilling.

Characters.—Two varieties, one with nearly globular fruit, the other ovate and much larger. The dried fruit, larger in size than a jaephala and obtusely angled ; external surface brown, velvety or silky, slightly wrinkled, having a small stalk at the bottom and a depression on the top ; interior containing a dried pulp, yellow and brittle, and easily removable from the stone ; stone hard, woody, oval in shape, of a pale yellow colour and containing an almond-like seed, very much wrinkled ; seed when fresh oily and having the taste like that of filberts, and intoxicating when eaten in quantities. Bark when wounded giving out insipid gum in tears and vermiform pieces ; colour dark brown, surface smooth, free from cracks, very little soluble in water, and forming a tough mass. It contains crystals of oxalate of lime.

Constituents.—Gallo-tannic acid, colouring matter, resins and a greenish yellow oil.

Preparations.—Powder of the pericarp. Dose, 10 to 40 grs. and decoction of fruit (1 in 10). Dose, ½ to 1 fld. oz. Linctus or lozenges.

Actions and uses.—Astringent, tonic and laxative ; with salt and long pepper it is given as an expectorant in the form of electuaries in cough, hoarseness of voice, sore throat and dyspepsia. The dried pulp roasted is kept in the mouth as lozenges in sore throat. The fruit is given in diarrhœa, dropsy, piles, leprosy, &c., also in enlargement of the spleen.

Terminalia Chebula, T. Reticulata, Myrobalan.

Habitat.—Tablelands of India, Ceylon, Punjab.

Parts used.—The dried fruits—myrobalans and galls.

There are four varieties of chebulic myrobalans used medicinally in India, but they are the same fruit at different stages of maturity. Very large fruits fetch a fancy price.

Vernacular.—Quite mature or ripe fruits.—Arab.—Halital-i-Cabuli. Beng.—Hara, Haritaki. Can.—Alale-kayi. Cing.—Aralu. Duk.—Hardâ, Harlâ. Guz.—Sardari harade, Mohoti Harade. Pile harade. Kabuli Harade. Hind.—Harpile, Harja umbedhur, Harda. Lepcha—Silimking. Malyal.—Kulukka. Mar.— Hàrapa. Pahari-Hana. Pers.—Halilohei, Zarda. Sans.—Haritaka, Abhaya, pranada pathiya, sudha, Bishak priya vigia, Amruta chetaki. Tam.—Kadukkay. Tel.—Karakkaya.

Fruit when arrived at or near maturity and yellow. Arab.—Habileh-i-Asfar, Halileh-i-chino. Bomb., Hind.—Haradan, Rangari hirade. Pers.—Rohini, Halileh-e-asfar.

Young fruit when dried becoming black and brown and of the size of a raisin.—Arab.—Halileh-i-Zangi, Halibche siyah, Halilaji asvad. Bomb.—Bôla harade. Can.—Alsle-pinda. Duk.—Balhalre, Zangi-hârle. Eng.—Black myrobalans. Guz —Himaja, himaji harade. Hind.—Bâlhâr, Langi-hâr, kâlihâr. Pers.—Halilahe sibajâh. Sans.—Bala-haritaka, Himavali Patanâ Abhayiâ. Sind.—Imachi. Tam.—Kadak-kay. Tel.—Pinda Karak-kâya.

Fruit very young about the size of a grain of barley. Arab.—Halileh-i-Jawi. Guz.—Java harade. Mar.—Javasa, fruit about the size of a cinnamon seed. Arab.—Halileh-i-zira.

Gall-like excrescenses. Incorrectly considered as flowers. Beng.—Haritaki-phul. Can.—Alale-havon. Duk.—Halre-kè-phûl. Guz.—Harle-phûl, pilo harle phûl. Malyal.—Katukka-pû. Mar.—Hirada-phule. Sans.—Haritaki pushpam. Tam.—Kadu-kai-pu. Tel.—Karak-kayu-puvvulu Aldicai.

Pranada life giver. Sudha, Nectar. Bhishakpriya, Physician's favourite. Shakra—Shrista, created by Indra. Pathya, a corruption of paraiya or Paharija or paharej—abstinence from unwholesome or luxurious living. This drug can be given with benefit to persons who may be suffering from the ill effects of reckless eating and drinking.

Characters.—Halileh-i-kabuli, sarwar-i-Hindi, survari harade—a very large sized fruit of an ovoid form, smooth, dense, readily sinking into water and heavy ; about 2 inches long, and tapering, especially at the lower end ; 5 or 6 sided, furrowed longitudinally and highly wrinkled ; epidermis yellowish brown. When cut into, it shows a yellowish or darkish brown pulp and stone; pulp astringent and somewhat sticky to the taste. The best quality of harade contains a large, rough, bony one-celled endocarp and largest quantity of pulp. The epidermis when chewed is smarting to the tongue, the stone is insipid, the pulp is bitter and somewhat sour. Dose, 2 to 10 grs. Haradan, Rangari hirade. These are smaller in size, wrinkled and less furrowed than survari harade. In length each is about an inch or more. The epidermis is yellow. When cut into, it presents a yellow dried pulp and a stone. Bâla harade. These are unripe fruits, smaller in size than the above two varieties, and ovoid ; colour deep brown or black, wrinkled, tapering, epidermis dark or brown. On section, in the interior is found a pulp which is dark and homogeneous. There is no stone. It has a shining fracture and an astringent taste. Dose, 30 to 60 grs. Java harade. It is the most diminutive of all. The word Java means barley, and it is so called as in size it resembles Java ; other characters are similar to those of himaja. Galls. These are produced by the tender leaves being punctured by an insect, and its eggs deposited therein which by extravasation of the sap became enlarged into hollow glands of various shapes and sizes. Dose, 1 to 3 grs.

Constituents—Myrobalans contain astringent principles—tannic acid (45 p. c.) and gallic acid, mucilage, a brownish yellow colouring matter. Chebulic myrobalans also contain an organic acid named chebulinic acid, which, when heated in water, splits up into tannic and gallic acids.

Chebulinic acid.—To the extract of chebulic myrobalans, add sodium chloride solution. Dissolve the matter that separates in water, shake the solution with acetic ether. Evaporate the ether, dissolve the residue in water—chebulinic acid crystallizes out in rhombic prisms. It is an acid without any odour. Taste sweet, freely soluble in alcohol and hot water, sparingly so in ether and in cold water. The myrobalans also contain an oleo resin of a green colour, soluble in alcohol, petroleum spirit, and oil of turpentine. It is called myrobalanin.

Preparation.—Survari harade—a confection, paste and electuary of the fruit deprived of stone. Infusion or decoction (1 in 10). Dose, 4 drachms to 1 ounce.

Himaja powder fried in ghee or in castor oil. Dose, ½ to 2 drs. Java harade, the same as those of himaja ; a compound powder—Amrita haritaki and a decoction pathyadi kuâtha.

Actions and uses.—Purgative, astringent and alterative. The ripe fruits are generally purgative and the unripe ones astringent and aperient. Survari harde freed from the stone (the pulp and the cortex being only used) is used as a laxative generally combined with aromatics as fennel seeds and carraway and given in chronic bronchitis, asthma and in gastric intestinal disorders. Combined with embelic and beleric myrobalans, it forms the well known Indian preparation called Triphala, meaning the three fruits, which is used as an alterative, tonic and stomachic.

Rangari hirade—alterative, stomachic, laxative and astringent ; given in fevers, piles and intestinal disorders ; chiefly used by tanners.

Bâla harade, a mild and safe aperient, and astringent. Like rhubarb, it causes one free motion, and then regulates the bowels. Fried in ghee over a fire it is largely used in chronic diarrhœa, choleraic diarrhœa and dysentery ; also in flatulence, vomiting, hiccough and colicky pains. Java harade.—Its actions and uses are similar to those of himaja. Galls on the leaves are powerfully astringent and given in dysentery and diarrhœa in children.

Many imitations of survari harade are sold by Jogis and Mâravaries who sell them at very high or fanciful prices ; spurious preparations often weighing as much as 6 to 12 ozs., are prepared by over-lapping diminutive survari harade (taken as a nucleus) with several slices of other survari harade, the whole being cleverly glued together and made to resemble a natural big-sized fruit. The high price fetched for survari harade is said to be due to its rarity and also to the fanciful medicinal properties attributed to it. It is said that Rajas and others who have a repugnance to take medicine internally, are made to keep survari harade in their hands for a few minutes, when it acts as a purgative. In order that the public may give ready credence to such fanciful virtues, the Jogis who prepare fictitious harade generally paint them with some highly irritant cathartics under the belief that when held in the hand the irritants become absorbed and produce purgative effects.

Terminalia Catappa, T. Myrobalans.

Habitat.—All over India.

Parts used.—The fruit or nut, bark and oil.

Vernacular.—Eng.—Indian almond tree, leaf-nut. Beng.—Benglâ-bâdâm. Cing.—Kotamba. Can.—Nat-badami. Guz.—Nât-ni-bâdâm. Hind. and Duk.—Jangli-bâdâm. Mar.—Nât-bâdâm. Malyal.—Kâtta-kurn. Catappa. Pers.—Badame-hinde. Sans.—Jugudi-phallaani Desha-bâdâmitte. Tam.—Nattu Vadam-kottai. Tel.—Nattu-Badam-Vettichi.

Characters.—Fruit, a drupe, oval, smooth, compressed or flattened, of a dull purple colour when ripe. Nut rough, hard and thick ; kernel cylindrical, edible and resembling almonds, and hence called country almonds or 'leaf nut' amongst the Europeans.

Constituents.—The seeds contains 50 p. c. of the oil resembling almond oil, in flavour and mildness. It is of a pale yellowish colour and without any odour, and composed of stearine and oleine. The bark yields a black pigment used by the natives to colour their teeth.

Preparations.—Decoction of the bark (1 in 10). Dose, ½ 1½ fld. oz.

Actions and uses.—The bark is astringent and given in atonic dyspepsia, diarrhœa, gonorrhœa and leucorrhœa. The fruit has the same properties as those of almond.

Terminalia Paniculata, Pentaptera Paniculata.

Habitat.—Malabar, Nilgherries and Coorg.

Parts used.—The flowers and bark.

Vernacular.—Can.—Honal Huluwa. Mar.—Kinjal, Kindal. Tam.—Maruthu, Matti, Maida. Tel.—Nei-muri.

Preparation.—Powder.

Actions and uses.—Stimulant. The flowers are used by the natives with the root of cissampelos pareira in cholera. The juice of the flowers or bark with that of guâvâ bark is used as an antidote in opium poisoning. The same juice melted with butter and rock-salt is applied externally in parotitis.

Terminalia Tomentosa, Terminalia Glabra, T. Alata, T. Crenulata.

Habitat.—India.

Parts used.—The bark.

Vernacular.—Beng.—Ashân, Piasal. Can.—Mutti karai. Cing.—Koombuk. Duk.—Jangli-karanj. Hindi.—Asan. Mal.—Tambavu, karu-maruta. Mar.—Ain. Tam.—Kurrupu-maruta, Kara-marada. Tel.—Nalla-maddi-chettu.

Characters.—The bark is thin, yellowish brown.

Constituents.—The ash of the bark contains much potash and tannin.

Preparations.—Decoction (1 in 10). Dose, 1 to 2 ozs.

Actions and uses.—Astringent ; used in diarrhœa, dyspepsia, and leucorrhœa, like the bark of T. catappa.

Myrtaceæ.

The Jâmbu or Myrtle family. Trees or shrubs, with opposite, alternate, entire, exstipulate and usually dotted leaves. Flowers white or scarlet, generally brown. Fruits dry or succulent, dehiscent or indehiscent, seeds numerous, exalbuminous.

Habitat.—Temperate climates and tropics.

Properties.—The trees are remarkable for pungent and aromatic properties due to their containing volatile oils. Many of these oils are used as stimulants, antispasmodics, diaphoretics, aromatics and carminatives. Some species are astringent and others secrete a saccharine matter; some bear edible fruits, some are used as spices, and others are used in preparing perfumery. Some are used as timber.

Careya Arborea.

Habitat.—Throughout India.

Parts used.—The dried calices of flowers and the bark.

Vernacular.—Beng.—(The dried calices) Bakumbha. Burm.—Bambhooai, banubwai, ban. Bomb.—Bakumbha. Cing.—Kahaatta. Eng.—Wild guava. Guz.—Vakumbha.—Kumbha. Hind.—Kamba, kumbhee. Malyal.—Peloa. Mar.—Vâkumbha, kumbha. Sans.—Kumbhi. Tam.—Ave-mavo, Ayama, putatanni. Tel.—Kumbhi, Dudippi. Can.—Kumbhia, gouju. Mal.—Peru. Guz.—Vakumbha. Beng.—Bakumbha.

Kumbhi means a jar, a pitcher, or a water pot ; this is in allusion to the hollow on the top of the fruit resembling in appearance a water pot.

Characters.—The calices about an inch or 1½ inches long, of a brownish dark colour, and of the shape of cloves ; epidermis deeply furrowed and much wrinkled. It has a very small stalk at the bottom. On the top of the fruit there are diverging four scaly calyx-lobes. In the middle of these there is a cup-shaped depression, from the centre of which a long, slender, and wire-like curved style projects. On transver se section the ovary presents cavities in the interior of which abortive seeds are attached, taste faintly aromatic, aciduous, and astringent; odour aromatic. Bark rough, red and fibrous within. On moistening it much mucilage is given out. An astringent gum exudes from the fruit and stems.

Constituents.—The thick red bark contains tannin, 8 p.c. The liber contains calcium oxalate in large simple crystals.

Preparations.—Decoction (1 in 10). Dose, 4 to 12 drs.

Actions and uses.—The bark and calices of the flowers are astringent, demulcent, and aromatic. The decoction is used in indigestion, and also as a demulcent in coughs and colds. The bark is used in preparing emollient embrocations.

Remarks.—Vakumbha is erroneously called by the druggists vavani phula.

Eugenia Caryophyllata, B. P., Caryophyllus Aromaticus, Myrtus Caryophyllus.

Habitat.—Malacca, East and West Indian Islands, Sumatra, Penang, India, Ceylon, Travancore.

Parts used.—The fruit ; the dried flower-buds—Caryophyllum, cloves B. P., and oil—oleum Caryophylli, B. P.

Caryophyllus from caryon, a nut, and phyllon, a leaf, in allusion to the nut-like appearance of flower buds which are like leaves. Clove, from clavus, a nail. The dried flowers resemble nails.

Vernacular.—Arab.—Karanaphal. Beng.—Lovanga, long. Bom.—(the fruit) nara lavanga. Burm.—La-nyen-pwen. Can.—Lavanga. Chin.—Tkeng-hia, Ting-hisug. Cing.—Karambu krabugaha, Warrala. Duk.—Ranjambool lavanga. Eng.—Cloves. Guz.—Lavanga. Hind.—Laung, (the fruit) nara lavanga, (the clove stalks) vikunia. Malay.—Karampu bunga chanke. Mal.—Bunga lavanga, Ran-jambul. Pers.—Mykek. Sans.—Lavanga. Can.—Lavanga. Tel.—Davanga-pu. Tam.—Kirambu Karuvap-pu. Ind.—(bazar, the fruit), naelnaug.

The dried unripe fruits are known as mother cloves.

Karanphul is derived from karan, an ear, and phul, a flower. It means a flower ornament for the ear, gold or silver ornaments used for the ear resemble cloves in shape and size, hence the ornament is often call lavong or karanphul.

Early writers call Lavang by the name of karanphul. This is due to the practice of keeping lavang in the hole in the lobe of the ear to prevent it from closing.

Narlavang—Nar, a male, and lavang, a clove—mother-clove, because of the erroneous notion among the native that the seed-bearing organ is always the male.

Characters.—A handsome evergreen. The dried unexpanded flowers (cloves) consist of calices, ovary and flower buds $\frac{5}{8}$ of an inch long, of a rich or darkish brown colour, and very oily. In form resembling vakumbhá; calyx tube tapering below, terminated by four thick rigid teeth which diverge at the top of the ovary. Within them are four imbricated petals forming small globular balls, enclosing numerous stamens and a single style. Below the teeth of the calyx is a club-like stalk which is the unripe ovary, surface much wrinkled, smell strong, fragrant and spicy, taste aromatic and very agreeably pungent. All parts of the clove abound in oil cells ; when scratched the oil exudes. Dose, 5 to 20 grs.

Mother cloves are ovate, oblong, about an inch long, containing two dark brown oblong, starchy, cotyledons, in size resembling pipli, they abound in starch but contain less essential oil; it has the odour of cloves.

Constituents.—A heavy volatile oil 18 p. c., Caryophyllin—a camphor, resin 6 p. c. Caryophyllic acid or eugenic acid; eugenin, a crystalline body, tannin, woody fibre, gum, &c.

Oleum Caryophilli. B. P. The oil distilled from cloves with water or steam. A colourless or pale yellow oily liquid when fresh, becoming thicker and reddish brown by keeping. Odour strong, pungent and aromatic, taste, pungent and spicy—soluble in alcohol and glacial acetic acid. It consists of a light and a heavy portion. The light portion contains sesquiterpene caryophyllene. The heavy portion contains eugenol, a phenol-like compound and caryophilline. Dose, $\frac{1}{2}$ to 3 ms.

Caryophyllin—obtained by treating ethereal extract of cloves with water, the precipitate is next filtered and treated with ammonia. It occurs in silky stellate needles.

The oil of cloves of the Indian bazaars is prepared by steeping cloves in sweet oil and keeping them for some days.

Preparation.—Of the clove buds—Infusum caryophilli, B. P. (1 in 40). Dose, $\frac{1}{2}$ to 1 oz. Infusum auruntii composita. Dose, $\frac{1}{2}$ to 1 oz.

Physiological action.—Antiseptic, local anæsthetic, general stomachic, carminative, aromatic, antiemetic and antispasmodic; externally rubefacient, anæsthetic and antiseptic; internally, it increases the circulation and raises blood-heat, promotes digestion and nutrition, and relieves gastric and intestinal pain and spasm. It stimulates the skin, salivary glands, kidneys, liver and bronchial mucous membrane. It is excreted in the breath, perspiration, bile, milk and urine.

Therapeutics.—Given as a flavouring agent to correct griping caused by purgatives, to relieve flatulence and to increase the flow of saliva. In combination with other spices and rock salt it is given to relieve colic, indigestion, vomiting and thirst. Externally it is used as an application in rheumatic pains, sciatica, lumbago, to the head in headache, and to the tooth in toothache; roasted in the flame of a candle and kept in the mouth it improves the breath, relieves sore throat and strengthens the gums. The powdered clove is a chief ingredient of a native preparation—lavangâ-di-churana, which is given in cough, asthma, &c. A paste of them applied to the forehead and to the nose is a popular remedy among the natives in headache, coryza &c.

Eucalyptus Globulus, B. P., and other Species.

Gum wood, Australian fever tree, Australian blue gum tree, iron bark, woolly butt.

Habitat.—Australia, Italy, Algeria, Europe, United States, California.

Parts used.—The dried leaves, Eucalypti folia; and oil, oleum eucalypti, B. P.

Characters.—Leaves smooth, entire, ensiform, 6 to 12 inches in length and 1 inch in breadth; glaucous when fresh; yellowish green and coriaceous when dry. Held up to the light they ara found to be studded with oil glands; odour strongly balsamic and camphoraceous, taste astringent, pungent, bitter and aromatic. Dose, 5 grs. in powder.

Constituents.—The leaves contain a volatile oil 6 p. c., tannin, cerylic alcohol, a crystallizable fatty acid, and a resin composed of three resinous bodies. No alkaloidal principle.

Volatile oil—oleum eucalypti, B. P. The oil is distilled from the fresh leaves of E. globulus, E. gracilis, E. incrassata, E. amygdalina (wanting in eucalyptol), E. dumosa, E. oleosa, E. cneorifolia, E. uncinata and E. odorata. It is a colourless or pale yellow liquid, of an aromatic camphoraceous odour and pungent spicy taste, leaving an after-sensation of coldness in the mouth. Sp. gr. 0·900 to 0·920.

It is not caustic and does not cause much coughing when inhaled; nor does it irritate the skin or the mucous membrane when applied. It is destructive to low organisms. It is insoluble in water and freely soluble in alcohol, oils, fats, paraffins, glacial acetic acid and carbon bisulphide. Dose, ½ to 3 ms. in capsules or emulsion.

The oil dissolves camphor, pine resins, elemi, sandarac, dammar, asphalt, copal, benzol, dragon's blood, amber, shellac, caoutchouc, wax, &c.

The volatile oil consists of different bodies which distil over at varying temperatures, viz. cymene, eucalyptene, terpene and eucalyptol; also small amount of valeric, butyric and capronic aldehydes.

Eucalyptol.—A neutral body obtained from the volatile oil, principally obtained from eucalyptus cneorifolia, E. dumosa and E. oleosa; other plants also yield it, viz.—santonica, rosemary, curcuma, mentha, cajuput salvia, laurus, and canella. It is identical with cineol or cajuputol. By the action of phosphoric acid it is converted into eucalyptene a substance allied to cymene and eucalyptolene. It is a colourless liquid of aromatic, camphoraceous odour, and pungent, cooling taste; soluble in alcohol, carbon bisulphide, and glacial acetic acid. Dose, 3 to 10 ms.

Eucalyptene or eucalyptia. A purified oil distilled from the leaves for internal use. Eucalyptene hydrochloride—eucalypteol. In white crystalline scales of a bitter taste; soluble in alcohol, ether and chloroform, nearly insoluble in glycerin and water, decomposed by alcohol and alkalies. Dose, 2 to 6 grs., used as an enema—eucalypteol 30 grs., olive oil 2 ounces, and yolk of egg, one; mix; also given in diarrhœa, typhoid fever, and in cough in phthisis.

Eucalyptus honey, an Australian product, produced by a small bee Apis Nigra Mellifica, which feeds on the flowers of eucalyptus tree. It is used as a bactericide in phthisis, and in diseases of the kidneys and bladder, and in scrofulous affections, as a substitute for cod liver oil.

Preparations.—Inhalation, eucalyptus oil 5, acid carbolic 10, liquor ammoniæ 12, alcohol 25, used in diphtheria, bronchitis, ozæna, &c.

Unguentum iodoformi et eucalypti: iodoform 1, eucalyptus oil 9, paraffin 20, vaseline 20. Unguentum eucalypti, B. P. (1 in 10): hard paraffin 4, soft paraffin 5, oil of eucalyptus 1, used as an antiseptic dressing. Tinctura eucalypti foliorum (1 in 5). Dose, 15 to 120 ms. Infusum eucalypti (1 in 10). Dose, 2 to 6 fl. drs. Emulsio eucalypti, contains eucalyptus oil, powdered gum Arabic, equal parts and water 40, used as an urethral injection or as a lotion in gonorrhœa and may be taken internally. Dose, 1 to 4 drs. Extractum eucalypti fluidum, fluid extract of eucalyptus. Dose, 10 to 60 ms. Vapour eucalypti 40 ms. to 1 oz. with carbonate of magnesia. Dose, 1 drachm in 1 pint of water.

Eucalyptus gauze contains eucalyptus oil, 6 p. c. It is also known as carbasus eucalypti. The cotton gauze impregnated with oil of eucalyptus 1, dammar resin 3, paraffin wax 3. Cremor eucalypti compositus, an emulsion containing 50 p. c. of cod liver oil and 5 minims of eucalyptus for each drachm—valuable for phthisis. Dose, 1 to 2 drs. Euc-alembroth gauze, contains sal alembroth, castor oil, and eucalyptus oil. Eucalyptus sawdust (1 in 9) used to deodorize the air of rooms. Eucalyptus wool, 5 p. c. of oil.

Physiological action.—The dried leaves are febrifuge, stimulant, expectorant, diaphoretic and antiseptic. The anti-malarial properties of the trees are chiefly due to the volatile oil, and partially to the great avidity they have for water when growing. Eucalyptus increases the flow of saliva, gastric and intestinal juices and hence when taken into the stomach it increases the appetite and digestion. It increases the heart beats and lowers the arterial tension. It is eliminated by the skin, kidneys, bronchi and may be found in the perspiration, urine, breath, milk, &c. In large doses it is an irritant of the alimentary canal, producing eructation, indigestion, nausea, vomiting and purging. It lowers the body heat, causes great weakness of the muscles, and often leads to congestion of the brain and kidneys. In toxic doses it is a narcotic poison. It paralyzes the respiratory centre in the medulla.

Therapeutics.—It stimulates the mucous membrane and hence given in chronic bronchitis, chronic catarrh of the genito-urinary organs, in broncho-pulmonary catarrh, and during convalescence from acute diseases. In influenza the oil is very useful. As antimalarial the leaves or the oil are given to reduce the size of the spleen by absorbing the noxious germs; by draining the soil of its water and by its antiseptic emanations, the tree purifies the malaria stricken atmosphere in its vicinity. It is given as a stomachic in chronic dyspepsia and in worms. In ague and other malarial fevers, an infusion of the leaves is largely used in place of quinine. It is also tried in septic fevers, remittent fevers, and in later stages of typhoid. The leaves with belladonna or stramonium leaves, or the oil are smoked to relieve asthma and whooping cough. The oil is a powerful antiseptic and has an ozonising influence on the atmosphere while it oxidises. It is inhaled or used as a spray in influenza. Given both internally and applied externally it does not irritate the skin or the mucous membranes. The oil mixed with olive oil is used as a rubefacient in rheumatism. The leaves, coarsely powdered, are smoked in cardiac asthma, ozæna, bronchitis, phthisis, and diphtheria. Externally the oil is used as a substitute for carbolic acid, as a spray, as an inhalation or as an antiseptic solution, or as a stimulant disinfectant in stomatitis, pharyngitis, tonsillitis, &c.; as a wash to ulcers and wounds and as an injection in gonorrhœa, leucorrhœa, &c. It prevents putrefaction and hence used as a vehicle for alkaloids to prevent the development of penicillium. It is used as a spray deodorizer to remove fœtid odours. It is added to cod liver oil to remove its fishy flavour. It prevents moths entering woollen clothes. Eucalyptol is given in bronchitis, phthisis, typhoid fever and diarrhœa. The E. amygdalin and E. globulus oils differ. The oil obtained from E. globulus contains eucalyptol but no phellandrene. That obtained from E. amygdalinæ contains phellandrene as its principal constituent and no eucalyptol.

Eucalyptus Rostrata, B. P., and other species.

Habitat.—Australia, Malay Peninsula, Nilgherry Hills.

Parts used.—The bark. The gummy exudation from the bark. Eucalypti gummi B. P., eucalyptus gum, red gum.

A ruby coloured exudation, in grains or small pieces of various sizes and of a deep red or garnet colour and shining; thin fragments, which are tough and difficult to powder are transparent and of a ruby red colour. Taste highly astringent. If chewed the gum adheres to the teeth and tinges the saliva red. It is soluble in cold water 80 to 90 p. c., entirely so in alcohol. Used as pills. Dose, 2 to 5 grs.

Preparations.—Tinctura eucalypti gummi (1 in 4). Dose, 20 to 40 ms. 1 of tincture to 7 of water forms a very astringent gargle.

Trochisci eucalypti compositi, Eucalyptus gum 1 gr., chlorate of potash 2 grs., and cubeb powder, ¼ gr. in each. Trochiscus eucalypti gummi, B. P. One grain in each. Dose, 1 to 2.

Extractum eucalypti gummi liquidum. Dose, 20 to 60 ms.

Syrupus eucalypti gummi (5 of the liquid extract to 3 of sugar). Dose, ½ to 1 dr.

Decoctum eucalypti gummi (1 in 40). Dose, 2 to 4 drs. used as a gargle. Internally given for diarrhœa. Insufflatio eucalypti gummi, eucalyptus gum, in powder and starch equal parts, a powerful astringent applied through an insufflator to the relaxed larynx.

Actions and uses.—A powerful astringent both internally and externally; given in diarrhœa and dysentery. The extract, if injected into the nostrils at once, stays bleeding from the nose. It is injected into the vagina or the rectum in cases of excessive mucous and sanguineous discharges. If applied on lint it arrests hæmorrhage from wounds. Suppositories are used for relaxed condition of the rectum and vagina. Red gum lozenges or the diluted extract of it are used in relaxed sore throat. It checks the diarrhœa due to mercury, when given in syphilis.

Remarks.—This gum should not be confounded with common Australian gum or Botany Bay kino gum, which is the product of eucalyptus resinifera. The latter is resinous, and is hardly soluble in water.

E. Robusta. The leaves yield an essential oil. It is like cajuputi oil and very fragrant.

Eugenia Jambolana, E. Fruticosa, Syzygium Caryophyllifolium, Syzygium Jambolanum.

Habitat.—India, Coimbatore, Bengal, Camaon, East Indies.

Parts used.—The fruit, leaves and dried seeds (jambolanæ semina) and bark.

Vernacular.—Beng. — Kâlâ Jam. Bomb.—Jambul. Can.—Nerala. Cing.—Madang. Duk.—Sittala-chini. Eng.—Java-plum, Jamun, Jambul. Guz.—Pâras, Jambul. Hind.—Jamuna. Mar.—Jâmbu. Sans.—Jambu, Megha-varna, Rajaphala, Nilaphala, Jambva (spirituous liquor). Tam.—Nawal. Tel.—Naregar.

Meghavarna means Cloud coloured. Nilaphala means black fruit. Meghaba—Cloud-like: Rajaphala means royal fruit.

Characters.—The fresh bark is grey, or of a pale brown colour ; surface fissured and scabrous ; internally red and fibrous or pale white, soft, brittle, and full of starch-like granules ; wood tough and fibrous, juice rather sticky. Taste acidulous and astringent. Leaves—oblong, acuminate, smooth, shining, and glabrous, or of a green or darkish green colour, of an aromatic odour and taste ; fruit of a purple colour, subacid, sweetish and astringent. When eaten unripe it imparts a dark colour to the lips, teeth and tongue. When very large and of the size of a pigeon's egg it is called paras jambudo. Epidermis smooth, shining, and very thin, and can be easily removed by scratching ; pulp, of a dark reddish colour. A vinegar is prepared from it. The seed when fresh of a pinkish colour which becomes brown on drying ; testa thin and brittle, enclosing thick, hard, and wrinkled cotyledons ; taste of the seed is aromatic. Dose of the powdered fruit stone, 5 to 30 grains, in cachets, powder or pills.

Constituents.—The seed contains jambulin, a glucoside; also a trace of essential oil, chlorophyll, fat, resin, gallic acid, albumen &c. The bark contains tannin 10 p.c. and a kino-like gum.

Preparations.—Extractum Jambul liquidum. (Take fresh seeds, discard the pericarps and exhaust in alcohol, without heat.) Dose, ½ to 1 dr. Syrup from the ripe fruit. Dose, 2 to 4 drs. Jambul and gluten biscuits, 30 grs. in each. Dose, 4 to 6 biscuits. Decoction of the bark (1 in 10). Dose, 2 to 4 drs. Pancha Rasa. The five astringent juices. Obtained by macerating in water the bark of Kâlâ Jam, Rakto Sumul, Lâl barjala, Jujube and Jayanti.

Actions and uses.—The juice of the ripe fruit or syrup is stomachic, astringent, and diuretic and given in scanty urine. The decoction of bark is astringent, and used in diarrhœa of children, in chronic dysentery, as a gargle mixed with Dhumâso for the relief of spongy gums, and sore, cracked or irritable tongue. A paste of leaves is used to promote healthy discharges from indolent sores or from unhealthy ulcers. The extract of powdered seeds and dried fruits is used in diabetes. It checks diastatic conversion of starch into sugar in cases depending on increased production of glucose.

Myrtus Chekan, Eugenia Chekan.

Syn.—Cheken, Chequen, Aroyan.

Habitat.—Chili.

Parts used.—The leaves and shoots.

Constituents.—A volatile oil resembling that of eucalyptus, a volatile alkaloid, checkanine, and tannin.

Preparations.—Extractum Chekan Liquidum. Dose, ½ to 3 fl. dr. Infusum Chekan (1 in 10). Dose ½ to 2 oz.

Actions and uses.—Aromatic, antiseptic, expectorant, diuretic and tonic; given in chronic bronchitis and catarrh of the bladder. As an inhalation, it is given in diphtheria, laryngismus stridulus, and as an injection in leucorrhœa and gonorrhœa; also employed in phthisis and pulmonary hæmorrhages. Dose of the leaves, 1 to 2 drs.

Melaleuca Leucadendron, B. P., M. Cajuputi, M. Minor.

Mela-leuca from melan, black, and leukos, white. The trunk of this tree is black and the branches white. Leucadendron from leukos, white, and dendron, a tree.

Habitat.—Molucca Islands, Indian Archipelago, and the Philippines.

Parts used.—A volatile oil distilled from the leaves—oleum cajuputi, B. P

Vernacular.—Burm.—Thit-tha-hputshi (the tree). Eng.—Cajuput oil. Guz.—Kajuputi-tela. Hind., Beng., Mar.—Kayakuti-tel Malay.—Kayu-puteh (the tree). Tam.—Kayapudai-tailam (the oil).

Characters.—Oleum cajuputi—a light thin liquid of a bluish green colour. Rectified oil is yellow. It is transparent and mobile, of an agreeable but penetrating, warm camphoraceous odour, and a bitter, cooling and aromatic camphoraceous taste and of a neutral reaction; its green tint is often due to the presence of copper; freely soluble in alcohol.

Constituents.—The oil contains bihydrate of cajuputine or cajuputol about ⅔, and several terpenes; also acetic, butyric and valerianic ethers of turpineol. Soluble in alcohol (1 in 1). Dose of the oil, ½ m. to 3 ms. The green colour has been attributed to chlorophyll or to copper which is present in it.

Preparations.—Spiritus cajuputi B. P. (1 in 10). Dose 5 to 20 ms. Emulsion, pills and linimentum.

Actions and uses.—The oil is like other volatile oils, a powerful stimulant sudorific, carminative, diuretic, and antiseptic ; externally parasiticide and anthelmintic, rubefacient and counter-irritant to the skin. Taken internally it produces a sense of warmth in the stomach and increases the pulse beat. Used externally over rheumatic and painful joints, in paralysis, muscular rheumatism, chilblains and neuralgias, or given internally, in spasmodic affections of the stomach and bowels, as colic, flatulency, and in dysmenorrhœa, dropsy, syphilis and cholera. As a stimulant and diaphoretic it is given in low states of the system and in hysteria, nervous vomiting, hiccough and dyspnœa. In elephantiasis and other skin affections it is given with benefit. With olive oil it is dropped into the ear in deafness and earache. It forms an ingredient of croton oil liniment.

Myrcia Acris.

Myrcia—surname of Venus—the plant is beautiful. Acris, from acer, sharp, pungent—odour of the leaves is pungent.

Syn.—Wild clove or wild cinnamon, Jamaica bay berry.

Habitat.—West Indian islands, Jamaica, Trinidad, Venezuela.

Parts used.—A volatile oil distilled from leaves, oil of Myrcia, oil of Bay.

Characters.—Leaves entire, long, ovate obtuse, coriaceous, strongly veined, pellucid, punctate and shining. Odour aromatic when bruised.

Constituents.—Volatile oil and tannin. The volatile oil—Myrciæ Oleum, oil of Myrcia, obtained by distillation from the leaves with water or steam. A yellowish liquid ; odour clove-like, taste pungent and spicy; slightly acid in reaction, becoming turbid with alcohol, glacial acetic acid and carbon bisulphide. It contains eugenol, myrcene, chavicol, methyl eugenol, methyl chavicol, a turpene (phillandrene) and citral.

Preparations.—Spiritus Myrciæ, spirit of myrcia. Bay rum contains oil of myrcia 16, oil of orange peel 1, oil of pimenta 1, alcohol 1,220, water to 2,000.

Actions and uses.—Astringent, tonic and stimulant ; used externally to the forehead in nervous headache, faintness and on cracks and fissures, also as hair washes. It is principally used as perfume.

Myrtus Communis.

Habitat.—Europe, cultivated in India.

Parts used.—The berries, leaves, bark and oil (myrtol).

Vernacular.—Arab.—The berries, Hab-el-aas, Asbiri, murad, Isbar Ismar, Isfaren. Bomb.—Velayati Mhendi. Eng.—Myrtle. Guz.—Matli, Makli. Hind.—Sata sova, Baragasha, the leaves, Vilayatimehndi. Pers.—Barg-i-murad (leaves).

Characters—Berries black, pear-shaped, and slightly sweet ; seeds yellowish white, hard, kidney-shaped, and 6, 8 or 12 in number ; taste bland; leaves small, lanceolate, and dotted, margins revolute, very agreeably aromatic when bruised. Dose, 10 to 60 grs.

Constituents.—The ripe berries contain a volatile oil, myrti oleum—oil of myrtle, resin, tannin, citric acid, malic acid, sugar, &c. The oil is distilled from the leaves. It consists of a mixture of pinene, another hydrocarbon and cineol—the active principle, identical with eucalyptol. Dose, 1 to 3 ms. in capsules.

Preparations.—Infusion (1 in 10). Dose, 4 to 12 drs. Powder of leaves and berries.

Physiological action.—The plant is stimulant and astringent. The volatile oil is antiseptic, parasiticide and rubefacient ; applied to a raw surface it sets up irritation and inflammation but it does not affect the unbroken skin. Internally it is a stimulant of the alimentary canal, produces warmth in the mouth and increases the flow of saliva and gastric juice. In full doses it is a nervine sedative, and in very large doses an irritant. It is an antiseptic and stimulant to the mucous membrane of the excretory organs, as the lungs and kidneys, and is eliminated in the expectoration and urine.

Therapeutics.—In small doses it aids digestion and is given internally like copaiba, to check profuse expectoration in chronic fœtid bronchitis, bronchorrhœa, gangrene of the lungs, whooping cough, asthma and in chronic inflammation of the bladder and urethra; also in passive hæmorrhages. An infusion of the berries is used as rectal injection against round and thread worms, as an injection in leucorrhœa and prolapsus of the uterus and vagina. The powder of the leaves is used as an application in eczema, intertrigo and for wounds and ulcers. As an antiseptic it is used as a wash for fœtid ulcers and as an injection for deep sinuses. Locally it is used in favus, pityriasis, herpes and parasitic skin diseases, also in otorrhœa, ozæna and other foul discharges from fœtid ulcers.

Pimenta Officinalis, B. P., Eugenia Pimenta.

All-spice, Pimento, Jamaica pepper.

All-spice—as it was supposed that it combined at one time the odour of all the important spices, such as cinnamon, clove, and nutmeg.

Habitat.—S. America, W. Indies, Jamaica.

Parts used.—The dried full-grown unripe fruit.

Characters.—Fruit thick, brownish, nearly globular, $\frac{1}{5}$ to $\frac{1}{3}$ of an inch in diameter crowned with a short calyx and short style. Two-celled, one-seeded. Seed brown and reniform ; odour clove-like, taste pungent and aromatic. Dose, 5 to 15 grs.

Constituents.—The berries contain a volatile oil 3-4 p.c., probably identical with oil of cloves, also a fixed oil, 6-8 p. c., resin, gum, sugar, fat, tannin, ash, 4 p. c.

Oleum Pimentæ, B. P., oil of all-spice—oil of pimenta. This oil is distilled from Pimento with water or steam. It is a yellow or yellowish red liquid when fresh, gradually becoming darker; odour aromatic and taste pungent. Reaction faintly acid, heavier than water. Dose, ½ to 3 ms.

Preparations.—The oil is a constituent of Bay Rum; Aqua Pimentæ, B. P. from the fruit (1 in 40). Dose, 1 to 2 fl. ozs. It is also prepared from the oil (1 in 500).

Actions and uses.—All-spice is a stomachic, carminative, aromatic and stimulant; also used as a condiment. It increases the vascularity of the gastric mucous membrane, and stimulates the salivary secretion; hence it improves digestion and increases saliva. The oil is used in dyspepsia, flatulence, intestinal colic and as a corrective to griping medicines. It is also used as a flavouring agent to cover the taste of nauseous drugs.

Psidium Pyriferum and P. Pomiferum. P. Guava.

Habitat.—America, naturalized in India.

Parts used.—The bark, fruit and leaves.

Venacular.—P. Pyriferum—the white guava. P. Pomiferum—the red guava.

The fruit.—Arab.—Amarude. Beng.—Goáchhi-phál, peyara. Burm.—Malaka. Can.—Shibe hannu. Cing.—Suda-pera. Duk.—Jáma. Eng.—Guava. Guz.—Piyara, peru, Jamaruda. Hind.—Amrud, saphri âma, safrijam. Mar.—Tupa-pela, peru. Malyal.—Pela-Jambu. Pers.—Amrude. Sans.—Amaruta bahu bija phallama. Tam.—Koia-maram, goyyâ-pazham. Tel.—Jama-chettu.

Characters.—Bark smooth, brown, and externally marked with superficial scars showing the separation of squamous plates of the dead bark. On removing the epidermis, the bark is green. Internally marked with striæ of a light brown colour; taste astringent and somewhat acid. Fruit edible; when unripe, it is of a green colour and highly astringent. Pulp, hard and containing numerous seeds; rind very thin. Ripe fruit has a faintly yellow colour, pulp soft and delicious to the taste, of a strong aromatic flavour. Leaves aromatic, egg-shaped or oblong, short stalked and covered with soft down.

Constituents.—The bark contains tannin 27·4 p.c. Resin and crystals of calcium oxate.

Preparations.—Decoction (1 in 10). Dose, 2 to 8 fluid drachms.

Actions and uses.—Astringent; the unripe fruit is indigestible, and often causes bilious vomiting and feverishness. The ripe fruit is edible but produces costiveness. The bark of white guava is astringent, and the decoction is used along with other astringents, for chronic diarrhœa of children. It is also used as a wash in prolapsus. The leaves are astringent and stomachic, and are used to arrest vomiting in diarrhœa. The bark and leaves of the red variety are used to allay vomiting and diarrhœa of cholera.

Barringtoniaceæ.

The Samudara-phala family—trees or large shrubs, very much allied to myrtaceæ. Leaves alternate and serrated, flowers scarlet, finely long or racemose, fruits drupaceous.

Habitat.—Tropical regions in all parts of the world.

Properties.—Rather intoxicating and dangerous. Some have faintly aromatic, bitter, aperient and acrid bark.

Barringtonia Acutangula, Eugenea Racemosa. Stravadium Rubrum.

Habitat.—Throughout India.

Parts used.—The seeds.

Vernacular.—Beng.—Hijjul. Bomb.—Samudar-phala, Tiwvur. Burm.—Kyaitha. Cing. –Ella-Midella-gass. Hind., Guz.—Samudar-phala. Hind.—Hijjula. Malay.—Sjeria, Samstravad. Mar.—Pivar Sath-phal, Dhatri-phal. Sans.—Hijja or Hijjala. Tam.—Kadapum. Tel.—Kanapa, Kanagi.

Characters.—Seeds hard and resembling nutmeg or haradan in shape and size, dark brown compressed and marked with longitudinal striæ. Internally hard, horny and brittle. Put into water it becomes soft. It consists principally of a homogeneous, pale white substance (starch); odour very agreeable or faintly aromatic, taste sweet at first but soon becoming acrid and nauseating. Dose, 2 to 6 grs.

Constituents.—A body allied to saponin, which is the active principle, starch, proteid, cellulose, fat, caoutchouc and alkaline salts.

Actions and uses.—Emetic and carminative; used with the juice of fresh ginger in catarrhs of the nose and respiratory passages, and to relieve flatus from the bowels. Externally rubbed with water it is applied to the chest to relieve pain and to the abdomen to relieve colic and flatulence.

Barringtonia Racemosa.

Habitat.—Ceylon.

Part used.—The root.

Vernacular.—Cing.—Deya-midella. Malayl.—Samudrapu. Tam.—Samudra-pallam.

Characters—The root is slightly bitter but not unpleasant.

Preparations.—Infusion of the root (1 in 10). Dose, 2 to 6 drs.; and snuff.

Actions and uses.—A cooling refrigerent and aperient; given in fevers. The powdered seed is used as a local sedative snuff in cold and catarrhs of the nose; also as a dusting powder, in sore throat and cutaneous eruptions.

Melastomaceæ.

Mela from melan, black, and stoma, mouth; from property of the species, dyeing the mouth black. Trees, shrubs or herbs; leaves opposite, ribbed and dotless; calyx 4, 5 or 6 lobed, adherent to the ovary and imbricated, petals twisted in œstivation; ovaries adherent, many celled. Fruit either dry or distinct from the calyx and dehiscent or succulent, or united and indihescent; seeds numerous, small and exalbuminous. Flowers beautiful.

Habitat.—Tropical regions and all parts of the world.

Properties.—Slightly astringent; many produce edible fruits, and some are used for dyeing black and other colours.

Memecylon Edule. M. Tinctorium.

Habitat.—Eastern and Western parts of India, Ceylon.

Parts used.—The plant.

Vernacular.—Can.—Surpa. Cingh.—Dodi-gaha, Serookaya. Eng.—Iron wood tree. Mal.—Kashawa, Kana-yavu. Mar.—Anjan, yalki, kurpa, Lokhando. Sans.—Anjani. Tam.—Kayampoo-voo. Tel.—Alli-cheddu.

Characters.—The plant has bright green foliage with purplish blue flowers. Berries globose, deep purple and crowned with four toothed limbs of the calyx; leaves entire, firm and leathery; taste acrid, bitter and astringent.

Constituents.—The leaves contain chlorophyll, resins, malic acid 6·48 p.c., glucose 6·25 p.c., gum, colouring matter, starch, crude fibre' and inorganic matter containing silica.

Preparations.—Infusion of the leaves (1 in 20). Decoction of the root (1 in 10). Dose, ½ to 1 fld. oz.

Actions and uses.—Demulcent and astringent. The infusion of the leaves is used as collyrium for the eyes in conjunctivitis. The decoction is used in menorrhagia. Pounded bark with aromatics like ajwan, pepper and zedoary, is used as fomentation or lep to contusions, bruises, &c. The leaves are also used in gonorrhœa.

Lythraceæ.

The Loosestrife, Mendi or Henna family.

Herbs, shrubs or trees; leaves opposite, rarely alternate, and exstipulate; flowers regular or irregular and of a white, red or yellowish colour; fruit capsular, dehiscent and membranous; seeds numerous with or without wings, and exalbuminous.

Habitat.—Temperate climate.

Properties.—Generally astringent and used in dyeing.

A. Baccifera. Ammannia Vesicatoria,

Habitat.—Tropical India.

Parts used.—The herb and leaves.

Vernacular.—Beng.—Ban marach. Bomb.—Agiya. Duk.—Agin buti. Hind.—Dad mari. Mar.—Agaya, Guren, Bhar-jambul. Mal.

—Kallarvanchi. Sans.—Agnigurbha. Tam.—Kallurivi, nirumel-nir-appu. Tel.—Agni-vendapaku. Agni gurbha. Agni, fire, and gurbha, a womb The plant is pregnant with fire.

Characters.—Herb erect, and much branched; stems four-sided; leaves sessile, opposite, and lanceolate, about 1 inch long and 1 inch broad ; calyx four cleft to the middle ; lobe acute. Flowers minute, sessile and red. Smell muriatic, agreeable and aromatic.

Constituents.—Resin, glucoside, and perhaps an active principle, allied to plumbagin.

Preparations.—Ethereal tincture of the leaves (1 in 2). Decoction of the dried plant (1 in 20). Dose, 4 to 6 drs.

Actions and uses.—Leaves irritant, acrid and vesicant. The leaf or the tincture when applied to the skin raises a vesicle within half an hour or an hour, and is applied to the joints in rheumatism and to the neck in fevers with cerebral symptoms. In action it is similar to cantharides and may be used as a substitute for it. In obstinate spleen diseases the juice of the leaves is administered internally. Its decoction with ginger and cyperus root is given in intermittent fevers. The ash is applied with oil in herpetic eruptions.

Lawsonia Alba, L. Spinosa, L. Inermes.

Habitat.—Western India, cultivated throughout India.

Parts used.—Dried leaves, flowers and seeds.

Vernacular.—Arab.—Hinna. Beng.—Mehedi. Chin.—Hai-nah Shudu. Bur.—Dan. Can.—Garante. Cing.—Maritondi. Eng.—Eygptian privet, Henna. Hind. and Guz.—Henna, Mendi. Mar.—Mendi. Mal.—Pontaletshi, Mail-linshi. Pers.—Hina. Sans.—Kura vaka, Mendika Sakachara, Raktagarbha. Southern India—Iswan. Tam.—Marudam. Tel.—Goranta, Iveni.

Iswan, a corruption of Isband, the seeds of peganum harmala. Raktagurbha, from rakta, red, and garbha, a womb, meaning the plant pregnant with red colouring matter.

Characters.—Leaves opposite, smooth, lanceolate, oblong and pointed at both ends; about one inch long and ½ inch broad; flowers terminal, globular, panicles of a greenish white colour and very fragrant; fruit rounded, four grooved, apex, depressed and 4 celled; seeds irregular angular and marked with prominent ridges with intervening depressions, of a reddish brown colour and somewhat rugous; taste bitter. The plant contains a colouring matter of a deep orange red colour which stains the skin and does not disappear until the epidermis is removed.

Constituents.—Henno-tannic acid—a kind of tannin, resin and a colouring matter.

Preparations.—Paste or powder of dried leaves. Decoction of leaves and of bark (1 in 10). Dose, ½ to 1 fld. oz.

Actions and uses.—The bark is alterative, sedative and astringent; given in jaundice, enlargement of the spleen, and calculus affection: as an alterative in leprosy and skin diseases; also in spermatorrhœa, leucorrhœa, &c. Externally the fresh leaves are applied with vinegar and catechu to burning of the soles of the feet. A powder of the leaves is used as suppository in prolapse of the rectum and vagina. A paste of the leaves with oil and resin is applied to the head in headache ; they also increase the growth of the hair. Decoction of the bark is applied to burns and scalds. Infusion of flowers is used as an application to bruises.

Punica Granatum, B.P.

Habitat.—Subtropical countries, throughout India, Persia, China, Japan, E. and W. Indies, Arabia, and Socotra.

Parts used.--The flowers, rind of the fruit, and juice; and the dried bark of the stem and root.—Granati cortex—pomegranate bark, B.P. Punica from puniceus, scarlet, the colour of its flowers. Granatum, having many grains or seeds. The fruit is many seeded. Pomegranate—Pomum, a fruit ; and granatus, grained.

Vernacular.—Arab—Ruman, Kilkul, Rana, the flowers, Julnâr, Gulnar. Beng.—Dalim. Bur.—Tha-lai. Can.—Dalimbe. The flowers Hastu-dalimbe. Cing.—Delumghedi. Duk.—Anar. Eng. —Pomegranate, Carthaginian apple. Guz.—Dadam. Hind.—Anar. The flowers, Gulnar. Mal.—Dalima. Maleal.—Madala, Rumonpais. Mar.—Dalimba. Pers.—Rumon, Anar. Sans.—Dadima Shukadana, Kuchaphala. Tam.—Madalam, mogilam. The flowers Rimadalai. Tel.—Danimuca. The flowers—Pevadanimma.

Shukadana means Parrot's food ; Kuchaphala means Breast fruit.

Characters.—A small tree; flowers of a reddish colour and very showy. Fruit globular, resembling orange or tomato, somewhat flattened and obscurely six-sided, short necked at the top and crowned with from 5 to 9 toothed thick and tubular calyx, fruit divided into 5 or 6 compartments, each containing numerous grains. Each grain consisting of a thin transparent vesicle which contains a sweet, red, juicy pulp, surrounding a small angular seed. The juice is acid, sweet and sour ; dried seeds, sticky, lumpy, and black. Rind or the skin of the fruit in thick fragments, hard and brownish, yellow, or reddish in colour. External surface or the epidermis shining and tubercled. under surface of a yellow colour, rugous, concave, and marked with depressions conforming to the marks of seeds. It can easily be powdered. The taste is astringent. The root is heavy, knotted and of a yellow colour. Bark in thin quills, in strips or fragments. Externally greyish yellow, warty and longitudinally ridged. Inner surface smooth and yellow; taste, slightly bitter and astringent, without any odour. When chewed it colours the saliva yellow.

Constituents.—The bark contains tannin and punico-tannic acid 22 p.c., mannit, sugar, gum, pectin, ash 15 p.c., an active liquid alkaloid Pelletierine and isopelletierine, and two inactive alkaloids.

Pelletierina—Pelletierine—to obtain it mix the root bark with milk of lime, add water, and percolate with chloroform. It has strong basic properties, and occurs as colourless, minute crystals, soluble in water, alcohol, ether, chloroform, &c., Dose, 3 to 6 grs as an anthelmintic.

Pelletierinæ sulphas.—In minute white acicular crystals which on keeping become brown and moist or viscid and syrupy; soluble in water and alcohol. Dose, 5 to 8 grains to be followed by a purge. As subcutaneous injection. Dose, 5 grs

Pelletierinæ Tannas, Pelletierine Tannate—a greyish white amorphous powder, soluble in alcohol (1 in 800), water (1 in 900). Dose, 5 to 8 grains as an anthelmintic. Pelletierinæ hydrobromidum—a brownish viscid liquid. Dose, 5 to 8 grains ; used in cases of paralysis of the muscles of the eye.

Preparations.—Decoctum granati corticis B.P. (1 in 5). Dose, ½ to 2 fl. ozs. Juice of grains. Dose, 1 to 4 drachms. Extractum granati liquidum made from the root bark. Dose, ½ to 1½ drachms. Rind. Dose, 20 to 30 grains.

Physiological Actions.—Granatum and its alkaloids are astringent, anthelmintic and tænifuge. The flowers and rind of the fruit are astringent and stomachic. The decoction in full doses causes diuresis. It produces nausea and vomiting, often purging, flatulence and cramps in the legs with giddiness, dimness of sight and numbness of the limbs. The juice of the fruit is cooling and refrigerant.

Therapeutics.—The juice is given in dyspepsia and fevers; flowers and rind of the fruit mixed with aromatics and astringents, such as cloves, cinnamon, coriander, pepper, &c., are given in chronic diarrhœa of children and in chronic dysentery unaccompanied with tenesmus. The juice of the flowers with durva root juice (cynodon dactylon) is used to stop bleeding from the nose. The decoction of root bark is vermifuge and is used for expelling tape worms. The alkaloid Pelletierine is used in leucorrhæa, and passive hæmorrhages and as a gargle in relaxed sore throat. Pelletierine sulphate is used as a vermifuge against tape worms and is also used subcutaneously in 5 grains doses for paralysis, vertigo, menier's disease, tetanus and hydrophobia.

Remarks.—The native use dalimba juice in the preparation of Loha bhashma to facilitate its powdering.

Woodfordia Floribunda, Lythrum fruticosum, Grislea Tomentosa.

Habitat.—Throughout India.

Parts used.—The flowers.

Vernacular.—Beng.—Dhai, Dhonga. Bomb.—Daite, Dhanen. Can.—Dhatake. Eng—Downy Grislea. Hind.—Dhaiti, Chotadhaon, Dhava, Devti, Gul-bakar, Gul-dhaur. Mar.—Dhaite, Dhaoshi, Phulsatti. Sans.—Dhataki, Dhayatia-pushpika, Tamra-pushpi, Guchcha pushpi, Parvati, Aganijvala. Tel.—Dhataki Kusumaum. Gaji, Godari Serinji.

Tamra pushpi means red flowers. Guchchha pushpi, from Guchcha, a cluster of hair, having clusters of blossoms or of numerous small flowers arranged like Guchcha—clusters of hairs on the temple. Parvati from parvata, a hill. It means hill born, in allusion to the plant being common in mountainous tracts. Agni Jvala—agni, a fire, and jvala, a flame, the colour of flowers being like that of a fire flame.

Characters—Flowers brownish red, long and covered with calices; calices red, containing mature capsules, slightly channelled on both sides, membranous, and containing many seeds—seeds very minute, numerous, of a brown colour, shining and angular. Taste, highly astringent, smell somewhat aromatic. Dose, 10 to 20 grs.

Constituents.—Tannin 20 p. c.

Preparations.—Confection—Dhauriphula, bela, lodhra, valo, gâjâpipali, honey, each 2 drs. mix. Dose, 1 to 2 drs.

Actions and uses.—Stimulant and astringent; given in dysentery beaten up with honey; also in checking hæmorrhages, and chronic discharges, such as menorrhagia and leucorrhœa. The powder of flowers is sprinkled over vesicular eruptions and foul ulcers to diminish the discharges and promote granulations.

Umbelliferæ or Apiaceæ.

The ajamoda or Parsley family.

Umbelliferæ—umbella, a little shade or umbel, or from umbra, a shade, and fero, to bear. The flower stalks are in umbels or heads.

General Characters—Herbs, shrubs or rarely arborescent plants, with hollow or solid furrowed stems; leaves alternate, divided, generally sheathing at the base and compound, exstipulate; Flowers small umbels of yellow, white, pink or blue colour with or without an involucre. Fruits diachænium or cremocarp, consisting of two carpels (mericarp) adhering by their face to a common axis (carpophore) from which they ultimately separate. Each mericarp is indehiscent, one seeded and on its dorsal surface marked with five primary longitudinal ridges or nerves and four alternate secondary ridges, separated by interstices or channels in which are longitudinal, oily receptacles or canals called vittæ. containing a gummy, resinous, aromatic juice; seed solitary, pendulous and firmly adherent to the pericarp—embryo minute, albumen, horny.

Habitat.—Temperate climate.

Properties.—Many are edible, such as celery, parsnip, carrot, parsley, fennel, &c.; some are aromatic, carminative, tonic and stimulant; they abound in resins and contain an essential aromatic volatile oil, as anethinum, daucus, coriander &c., others are poisonous owing to their containing an acrid narcotic juice as conium; the rest are antispasmodic and contain a fœtid gum resin. The fœtid gum resin is composed of a volatile oil, gum and resin. These include galbanum, ammoniacum, oppoponax, segapenum, and assafetida, and are used as stimulant in nervous disorders.

Archangelica Officinalis, and A. Atropurpurea, Garden Angelica, European Angelica.

Habitat.—Northern parts of Europe, Asia and America.

Parts used.—Root, herb and seeds.

Characters.—Leaves double pinnate, flowers greenish-white stem, purplish, smooth, hollow-pointed. Root long and fleshy, thick, annulate, fusiform, juicy, resinous and pungently aromatic. Dose, 10 to 30 grs.

Constituents.—Volatile oil, resin, valerianic acid.

Preparations.—Infusion (1 in 10). Dose, ½ to 1 oz.—Tincture (1 in 10). Dose, ½ to 1 drs. Juice (succus). Dose, ½ to 1 dr. Fluid extract of root 30 to 60 ms. Fluid extract of seed, 5 to 30 ms.

Actions and uses.—The root is pungent, aromatic, stomachic tonic, stimulant, carminative, diaphoretic and diuretic, giving tone to the stomach and increasing appetite ; combined with tonis, it is given in typhoid condition, bronchitis, intermittents, flatulent colic and pain in the stomach. The fruit has similar properties, and syrup or candied angelica is taken as dessert as a very agreeable stomachic in rheumatism, gout, painful and swollen parts.

Remarks.—Large quantities of Angelica are used in the preparation of London gin, and the liqueur known as bitters.

Anthriscus Cerefolium.

Habitat.—Europe, cultivated elsewhere.

Parts used.—The fruit.

Vernacular.—Eng.—Chervil. Ind. Bazar—Atrilal. There are two kinds: True atrilal, Khalal-i-Khalil, and Egyptian kind, Rijl-el-Ghurab, Rijlel-tair, Harjes Shayatin. Atrilal means devil's bane.

Characters.—Fruit lanceolate, laterally compressed, almost cylindrical, black, terminating in a short 5 angled beak. The seeds in the Egyptian variety are dark coloured, resembling in size the celery seeds, and in shape the cumin seeds, and are very bitter ; in the true atrilal the seed is light coloured, the fruit is aromatic, and free from bitterness.

Preparations.—Infusion (1 in 20). Dose, 2 to 6 drs.

Actions and uses.—Diuretic, stomachic, and deobstruent; used as a stimulant to reinvigorate the body when exhausted by venereal excesses or by old age. In white leprosy the seeds are rubbed down over the patches, and also administered internally with pyrethrum and honey. The patient is then made to sit in the hot sun with the parts exposed and uncovered when the patches show blisters, and the new skin appears in its natural colour.

Remarks.—The fruit of vernonia anthelmintica is often sold for atrilal. The leaves are used for flavouring soup, salads, &c. The genuine article is difficult to obtain.

Apium Graveolens.

Habitat.—S. Europe.

Parts used.—The fruit.

Vernacular.—Arab.—Buzz-ul-Karaphs. Beng.—Chanoo Rhadodni. Can.—Ajmoda, Voma. Duk.—Ajmudah, Ajvân. Eng.—Celery. Guz. —Bori Ajmud. Hind.—Ajamo, Ajmud, Bhut-jata. Mar.—Ajamoda-Nova. Pers.—Tukhin-e-Karaphas. Sans.—Ajamoda. Tam.—Asham-tagam. Tel.—Ashu-Madaga-vomam.

Characters.—Fruit long, small and ovate or globular. Surface hairy, slightly tubercled, wrinkled, and marked with prominent ridges. Colour greenish yellow or brown ; 2 mericarps, 5 ribs and 12 oil tubes. Taste aromatic, somewhat pungent and slightly mint-like at first, then bitterish ; odour coriander-like, faintly terebinthaceous. Seeds like those of parsley. Dose, 5 to 30 grs.

Constituents.—The seeds contain apiin—a glucoside, a jelly-like substance which when boiled with dilute sulphuric acid splits up into, apigenin, and glucose. Apiin is slightly soluble in cold water, easily soluble in hot water, more easily in hot alcohol and insoluble in ether. Also volatile oil, apiol or apiolum, &c.

Preparations.—Infusion (1 in 10). Dose, ½ to 2 fluid ozs.

Actions and uses.—The fruit is carminative, aromatic, stimulant, tonic and emmenagogue. Its infusion is given in bronchitis and intermittent fevers ; as an adjunct to purgatives, it is given in constipation ; as a deobstruent and resolvent, with linseed or barley meal it is used as a poultice on swollen glands.

Carum Carui, B. P.

Carum Nigrum, C. Gracile.

Habitat.—Europe, Cashmere, Western Thibet, Persia, S. and W. Asia.

Parts used.—The dried fruit. Carui fructus, B. P., Caraway seeds, caraway fruits.

Vernacular.—Arab.—Curwiya, Kamune rumi. Beng.—Shia-jira. Bomb.—Kurwa-jira. Can.—Shime jirige. Cashmere.—Guinyun. Cin.—Rata-Dam. Duk.—Karoyat. Eng.—Black cumin, Indian carraway. Guz.—Kâlun-jira. Hind.—Siyah zirah. Panj.—Umbhu. Maleal.—Shima-jirakam. Mar.—Sa-jiri, Kalijiri, Pers.—Zirâhe rumi. Panj.—Umbo. Sans.—Sushava, Krishna jiraka. Tam.—Delappu. Tel. —Sinajila-kara. European caraways. Hind., Mar., Guz.—Vilayite-jira. Tam.—Kekku-Virai, Shiwai-Shonabu. Tel.—Kekku-Vittulu Shuna-Sapu. Can.—Shune-sapu. Beng.—Bilati-jira.

Characters.—Fruit brown, 2-seeded, ovoid ; cremocarp, slightly arched, laterally compressed ; mericarp, too commonly called caraway seeds, separate curved and narrowed at both ends with five yellowish foliform ridges and oil tubes, having an agreeable aromatic odour and a sweet spicy taste. Dose, 5 to 30 grs.

Constituents.—A volatile oil 6 p. c.; fixed oil, wax, resin, sugar, mucilage, tannin and ash 5 p. c.

Oleum Carui, B. P.—Oil of caraway, the volatile oil, is the active principle to which its medicinal properties are due, and obtained by distillation of the seeds. It is a limpid, thin liquid, colourless or of a pale yellow colour, odour aromatic, taste spicy and pungent, soluble in alcohol (1 in 1). It becomes brown by keeping. Dose, ½ to 3 ms. It contains carvene, 35 to 50 p. c., isomeric with turpentine, an unoxidized product chemically identical with citrene, hesperidene and dextrogyrate limonine; carvol, isomeric with thymol, an oxidized product closely related to menthol, myristicol and cumin alcohol; and is identical with carvicrol. Carvicrol—to obtain it distil a mixture of carraway oil with potash or soda, when carvene is separated. To the residue add sulphuric acid. It is a viscid yellowish oil, odour and taste like that of creasote.

Preparations.—Aqua carui, B. P., from the oil (1 in 500). From the fruit (1 in 20). Dose, 1 to 2 ozs. Spiritus Juniperi compositus, $\frac{1}{20}$ p. c. Dose, ½ to 1 oz. Tinctura Cardamomi composita, B.P. Dose, ½ to 1 dr. Infusum carui (1 in 40). Dose, 1 to 2 ozs.

Actions and uses.—Diuretic, stomachic, stimulant and carminative; given to expel wind, allay hiccough and pain of flatulent colic in infants. As a carminative and stomachic it is added as an adjunct to purgative mixtures to prevent griping and nausea. Locally the oil acts as an anæsthetic, and its poultice is applied over painful piles; other actions are similar to those of dill and anise. Carvacrol is useful in toothache and is inserted into the cavity of the teeth.

Remarks.—The name Krishna Jiraka is also applied to the seeds of Nigella Sativa. Karwajirah is also the name for Kali jiri (vernonia anthelmintica). Both are similar in colour, being darkish brown or black. Karvâ jirah differs, however, from Kali jiri, in the former being larger and rounder than carum nigrum. Shajira, carum nigrum, differs from vilayati jirun (carraway) in that the former has more slender and darker coloured fruits than carraway.

Coriandrum Sativum, B. P.

Coriander, from koris, a bug. The leaves have the odour of a bug, Sativum, from sativus, sown or cultivated. It is a cultivated plant.

Habitat.—Cultivated in India, Europe, China, Southern Asia.

Parts used.—The fruit—Coriandri Fructus, B. P., coriander fruit.

Vernacular.—Arab.—Kezirah. Beng.—Dhanyaâ. Burm.—Nannan. Chin.—Sheh-lo Can.—Kottumbari. Cing.—Kattumbaru, Dhanalu. Duk.—Dhanyân. Eng.—Coriander seeds. Guz.—Dhânâ Kothamiri, the plant. Hind.—Dhanyâ. Mah.—Dhane. Malyal.—Meti, Kottampâlare. Pers.—Kitnu, Kushuiz. Sans.—Kushthumbari, Dhânyâ-Kam. Tam.—Katta-malli. Tel.—Danyalu, Kotimiri.

Characters.—Fruit, of a pale, yellow colour, plump, and oval or ovoid in form, resembling inflated balloons, in size resembing gahula seeds ; surface marked with 10 ridges ; between every two ridges are tubercles, with undulated or longitudinal lines. Apex crowned with two prominences, base presenting a hole from which the stalk is removed ; mericarp adherent at the base by two joining ridges. Each mericarp has two oil tubes, odour like that of limbu, and the taste aromatic and oily.

Constituents.—The fruits yield a volatile oil 1 p. c.; fixed oil 13 p.c.; fatty matter 13 p. c. ; mucilage, tannin, malic acid, and ash 5 p. c.
Oleum Coriandri B. P.—Oil of coriander, distilled from the fruit with water or steam. The essential oil is isomeric with borneol, and is a yellowish liquid, odour characteristic and aromatic, taste spicy and warm ; soluble in alcohol, and glacial acetic acid. It consists of linalool or coriandrol. Dose, ½ to 3 ms.

Preparations.—Of the fruit. Infusum coriandri (1 in 40). Dose, 1 to 2 ozs. Of the oil.—Confectio sennæ, B.P. Dose, 1 to 2 drs.; syrupus sennæ, B.P. Dose, ½ to 2 drs. Compound Powder—Dhanâ-ni-dâl.—The fruits are fried lightly and pounded (husks being removed). To this is added jiruh, kálá miri, lavanga, and nimakha. The whole is stirred together, lime juice being subsequently added, and the mass dried in the sun.

Dhânâ Asva—A cooling drink, containing coriander, fennel fruits, poppy seeds, kanchan flowers, rose buds, cardamoms, cubebs, almonds, and black pepper, sweetened with sugar. Dose, 1 to 2 drs., given in colic, dyspepsia &c.

Actions and uses.—Aromatic, stimulant, carminative and stomachic ; used in sore throat, dyspepsia and common catarrh, but chiefly as a flavouring agent and as a corrective to griping medicines as jalap, rhubarb and senna. With barley meal, the leaves (kotha miri. Hind.) form a useful application for indolent swellings. Dhána disguises the odour and taste of senna and of other purgatives. The oil is a carminative and aromatic, and is used in flatulent colic ; also in rheumatism, neuralgia, &c. The fresh herb is called kothamiri and is used to flavour vegetables and curry.

Conium Maculatum, B. P, Spotted Hemlock.

Habitat.—Waste places and along streams, Europe, N. Asia.

Parts used.—The dried full grown unripe fruits, conii fructus, B. P., and fresh leaves and young branches, conii folia, B. P.

Vernacular.—Arab.—Banj-e-rumi, shokran. Bomb.—Kirdâman. Eng.—Athenian state poison, common or spotted hemlock, poison-hemlock, cow bane, beaver poison. Hind.—Kurdumana. Ind. Bazaar.—Khorasain-Ajwan. Pers.—The root, Bikhi-i-Tafti, the fruit, Duras-i-Tafahati, the seeds, Tukum-i-Tokhra, Karvaya-i-dashti, Yezd-Duras.

Characters.—A full grown fruit, gathered while green. Fruit, a cremocarp of a dark, grey colour, laterally compressed, small and elongated with vertical ridges on its outer surface. The ridges are of a pale or grey colour, 2 mericarps with 5 crenate ribs, but no oil tube. In form it resembles anisum, but is rather larger. When crushed the odour is offensive and acrid ; on section the interior is resinous, yellowish black, and oily. Taste, slightly bitterish, somewhat acrid and oily. Green, unripe fruits are the most active part of the plant. Fresh leaves decompound, smooth, arising from stems which are smooth and with dark purple spots. Leaves deep green, shining, tripinnate with leaflets pinatifid. Petioles furrowed and sheathing at the base, those of the lower leaves hollow, odour strong and disagreeable. Dose of the leaves, 1 to 5 grs.

Constituents.—The leaves contain a volatile oil to which the smell is due. The leaves and fruit contain 3 alkaloids known as coniine ($\frac{1}{5}$ to $\frac{1}{2}$ p. c.,) liquid and volatile; methylconiine, and conhydrine, both solid and volatilizable, and pseudo conhydrine ; a volatile oil, fixed oil, conic acid or malic acid, and ash 6 p.c. Conine or coniine, cicutine conicine. Dextro-a-prophl piperidine—is obtained synthetically from alpha picoline, also obtained by distilling the fruit with an alkali or adding ammonia to the extract, passing sulphuretted hydrogen over the mass, thus converting ammonia into sulphate, then exhausting it with alcohol and ether, leaving ammonia sulphate undissolved, finally distilling with alkali when conine is liberated. It is a colourless, inflammable, yellow, oily fluid of a penetrating odour, compared to that of urine of mice, and acrid taste. Like ammonia it forms dense fumes with volatile acids. It is soluble in ether, alcohol, chloroform, benzol, benzine and fixed oils. Freely soluble in carbon bisulphide, slightly so in water (1 in 100). It is quickly decomposed by heat. By long keeping it becomes inert. Dose, $\frac{1}{80}$ to $\frac{1}{10}$ gr. or $\frac{1}{10}$ to 2 ms.; too irritant for hypodermic use. Coninæ Hydrobromidum—colourless and odourless crystals, resembling magnesium sulphate in appearance. Insoluble in ether, and freely soluble in water. Dose, $\frac{1}{12}$ to 1 gr. Pilula coninæ Hydrobromidi, $\frac{1}{3}$ gr. in each pill. Injectio coninæ hydrobromidi hypodermica, 1 gr, in 20 ms. Dose, 1 to 3 ms. Conium Hydrochlorate. Dose, $\frac{1}{12}$ to $\frac{1}{4}$ gr. Paraconiine is artificially prepared by the reaction between butyric aldehyde and alcoholic solution of ammonia. It is isomeric with coniine, but not identical with it.

Preparations.—Of the fruit. Tinctura conii, B.P. (1 in 5). Dose, $\frac{1}{2}$ to 1 fld. dr. Of the leaves and young branches, succus conii, B. P., contains one volume of alcohol for every three of the juice. Dose, $\frac{1}{2}$ to 2 fld. drs. Extractum conii, 1 gr., is equal to 1 gr. of the drug. Dose, 2 to 5 gr. Extractum conii fluidum. Dose, 2 to 5 ms. Vapor coninæ—succus conii, $\frac{1}{2}$ oz., solution of potash 1 dr., water 1 oz. Dose, 20 ms, for inhalation to be put on a sponge and vapour of hot water passed over it. Unguentum conii, B. P., prepared from the juice, 88 parts evaporated to 11 parts, to this add hydrous wool fat 33 parts ; used in pruritus ani, piles, &c.

Physiological actions.—Sedative antispasmodic, anodyne, soporific and antaphrodisiac. Like curare it paralyses the end organs of motor nerves, without affecting sensation or consciousness. If given for some time it afterwards paralyses the motor centres in the brain and spinal cord. The muscular irritability remains intact. It is a direct sedative to the respiratory centres, and death is due to paralysis of the respiratory muscles.

Methyl coniine is a stimulant of the spinal cord and produces convulsions as seen in cases of coniine poisoning. The sensibility is impaired, and there is a feeling of numbness in the limbs and paralysis of reflex action. In full doses conium gives rise to gastric irritation, increased vomiting, followed by numbness in the legs, sense of fatigue, staggering gait, dilated pupils, impaired speech, and laboured breathing. In poisonous doses it acts as a direct sedative to the muscles of respiration, leading to paralysis of the voluntary muscles; there is paraplegia, loss of speech and sight. Death may be due to asphyxia. The cerebral functions are not affected by it, and the mind remains clear to the last. It has no action on the heart.

Therapeutics.—Coniine is indicated in diseases characterized by excessive motor activity as in neurosis, tremors, chorea, paralysis agitans, hysteria and muscular twitching; also to relieve spasmodic cough in bronchitis, pertusis, asthma and phthisis; sometimes it is given with morphinæ in convulsive affections, such as tetanus, hydrophobia, epilepsy, acute mania and delirium tremens. Locally it is a resolvent and discutient. In enlargement of the breasts with profuse lacteal secretion, its application produces atrophy and the secretion of milk becomes scanty and even suspended. As an anodyne application it is useful in tender glandular enlargements, and scrofulous and painful growths; also in cancer, and rheumatic joints. The ointment is used for painful affections of the rectum and anus such as piles, pruritis ani, &c.; conine vapour is a palliative in the tickling cough of phthisis, or of acute bronchitis. In pneumonia and pleurisy, an hypodermic injection of coniine by inducing paresis of the respiratory muscles, reduces the temperature and thus gives relief.

Remarks.—Kirda māna is often mistaken for kira mani ová, the flower heads of a composite plant, which is not poisonous.

Cuminum Cyminum.

Habitat.—Africa, cultivated in India.

Parts used.—The fruit.

Vernacular.—Arab.—Kamûn, Kemun. Beng.—Jirâ, Zirâ. Burm.—Zee-yâ-, Dze-ya. Can.—Jirga. Cing.—Duru. Duk.—Shâhjira. Eng.—Cumin seed. Guz.—Sapheda jirun. Hind.—Safed jirâ. Malay.—Jintan, Mar.—Jirê, Jirû. Pers.—Jira-i-safed. Sans.—Jirana, jira, kunchicka, jirakaha, Ajaji, Ajmoda. Tam.—Shiragam. Tel.—Jila kara, jirana.

Ajaji, from, Aj, a goat, meaning that which overcomes goats. Ajmoda—goat's delight. Jerûn is derived from jri, to digest, in allusion to the digestive properties of the seeds.

Characters.—Fruit of a light brown colour, elongated, cylindrical, and ovoid in shape, smaller in size than variali, surface rugous, hairy and marked with longitudinal ridges ; at the apex, the fruit is surrounded by two small acute projections which are the remains of the styles attached to each mericarp. On bruising, the odour is disagreeable. Dose ½ to 2 drs.

Constituents.—The seeds yield 7·7 p.c. fat oil, 13·5 p.c. resin, 8 p.c., mucilage and gum, 15·5, protein compounds, malates and an essential oil on which the peculiar aromatic odour and taste depends. This essential oil contains cuminol or cuminaldehyde 56 p.c. a mixture of hydrocarbons, cymene or cymol, terpene, &c.

Actions and uses.—Carminative, aromatic, stomachic and stimulant ; used in hoarseness of voice, dyspepsia, flatulence aud diarrhœa.

Daucus Carota, Daucus Vulgaris.

Habitat.—Cashmere, W. Himalaya, N. Asia.

Parts used.—The root and fruit.

Vernacular.—Arab.—Ista flim Jazr, jazr-ul bostani. Beng.—Gajara Can.—Gajjari. Chin.—Hu-lo-peh. Duk.—Gajara, jugur. Eng.—Common or wild carrot. Guz.—Gâjar. Hind.—Gajra, jugur, gajur. Mar.—Gâzara. Pers.—Zir duk. Punj.—Marmuj, Bal-kach. Sans.—Grinjana, Garjara, Garjarama, Shikha-mulama. Tam.—Gâjjar. Tel. —Gajjara-gadda, Shekka-mulamu.

Characters.—Fruit pale, dull brown, oval, and compressed from the back, longer than suvà bij ; mericarps adherent. At the apex of the fruit are two prominences, the remains of styles ; surface rugous, marked with ridges, three on the convex back, two on the plane of the commissure, ridges distinctly winged. Wings fringed with white teeth or bristles. When crushed, the fruit emit an acrid or balsamic odour, taste balsamic, acrid, bitter, and oily. On expression they yield an essential oil. Root fusiform 6 to 12 inches long, and of a reddish yellow colour ; parenchyma fleshy and edible. It has a sugary and mucilaginous taste, and a feebly aromatic smell.

Constituents.—The root contains carotin, hydrocarotin, oil, sugar, pectin, nitrogen compound and volatile oil. The fruit contains volatile oil and a fixed oil.

Preparations.—Infusion (1 in 10). Dose, ½ to 1 fl. oz. Fluid extract. Dose, 5 to 30 ms.

Actions and uses.—Fruit stimulant, laxative, emollient, antiseptic diuretic and emmenagogue. As a diuretic it is given in nephritic affections, dropsy, strangury and amenorrhœa. This property is due to its containing the volatile oil which acts locally upon the nervous structures of the kidney during the excretion ; as an antiseptic, a poultice of the root is used to correct fœtid discharges from eczema, unhealthy sores, carcinoma, &c., the root is saccharine and edible. The seeds are said to cause abortion.

Dorema Ammoniacum, B. P., D. Glabrum, Ferula Orientalis, F. Tingitana and probably other species.

Habitat.—Persia, Afghanistan (on silicious soil, deserts and barren regions).

Parts used.—The gum resin exuded from flowering and fruiting stem ; Ammoniacum, B. P.

Vernacular.—Afghan —Kandal. Arab.—Fashuk, Ushá shaka· Bomb.—Ushaka. Eng.—Ammoniac. Guz.—Ushaka, Astrak, Gunda. layaka. Hind.—Samagh Hamama. Pers.—Ushna ooshak. Tam.—Kandal. Afghan—Gama Nayakan. Tel.—Gama Nayakam.

Characters.—Gum resin in roundish tears, agglutinated masses, or cakes ; tears of a pale cinnamon or brown colour, breaking into an opaque shining or yellow conchoidal white fracture, and having a faint odour and a bitter nauseous taste. The cakes resemble in appearance and smell hinga cakes, giving with water a milky emulsion ; an inferior variety is obtained from the base of the stem, often mixed with vegetable fragments and earthy matter. It softens by handling. The root called Boi is fibrous, of a loose, spongy texture, and of a faint aromatic odour, often mistaken for sumbal. Dose, 5 to 15 grs.

Constituents.—Gum, 18 to 26 p. c. ; resin, 70 p. c. ; volatile oil, 1·4 p. c.; moisture, 5 p. c.; Ash, 3 p. c. The volatile oil differs from that of asafetida in that it does not contain sulphur or phosphorus. The resin does not yield umbelliferon. It consists of an acid and two resins, one soluble and the other insoluble in ether, the latter is soluble in volatile and fixed oil.

Preparations.—Emplastrum ammoniaci cum hydrargyro, B. P. ammoniac plaster with mercury, ammoniac 12 oz., mercury 3 oz., olive oil 56 grs., sublimed sulphur 8 grs. Mistura ammoniaci, B. P. (1 in 33) with syrup of Tolu. Dose, ½ to 1 fld. oz.

Actions and uses.—The root, Boi, is used as a fumigation. The gum is a stimulating expectorant and laxative ; also rubefacient and resolvent. A plaster of it promotes nitrition in the part to which it may be applied. As an irritant it produces papular eruptions. Internally its action is like that of asafetida but less powerful ; given in chronic pulmonary catarrh of the aged with profuse secretion, and attended with difficult expectoration and without fever ; generally combined with ammonium chloride. It gives tone to the feeble pulmonary circular muscular fibres and hence in asthma it is very useful. It removes the exciting cause of the nervous paroxysm. Its use should not be long continued as it leads to a dry and irritable state of the bronchi. In hysterical asthma it is used when combined with asafetida. It is sometimes given in chronic catarrh of the urinary passages. Externally as a resolvent, it is used as a plaster in asthma, in indolent tumours and glandular swellings, in enlargement of the liver and spleen and as an irritant in chronic muscular rheumatism, in chronic bronchial catarrh and chronic pleurisy.

Ferula Alliacea.

Habitat.—Balkh, Persia.

Parts used.—The gum resin from the root.

Vernacular.—Arab.—Hiltit, Tyih. Eng.—Indian Asafetida. Guz. —Hing. Vagarni. Ispahan,—Angusht,—Gandah,—Pers.—Angozah Kema. Sind.—Hinga, Vaghaunni. Sans.—Bhût nasan, Sula-nasan, Nasana Hinguhu.

Bhutnasan, from Bhut, demon, and nâsana, nasvun, to fly away or run away or to destroy. It dispels demons. Sula nasana from sula, pain in the stomach, to destroy, or drive away pain from the stomach.

Characters.—It is semifluid at first, of an opaque white colour, but gradually becomes dull yellow or darker; met with in irregular masses of opaque tears moist or dry and imbedded in a yellowish or brownish grey sticky mass. It has a strong fœtid garlic-like alliaceous persistent odour and an acrid bitter taste. With water it forms a white milky emulsion. The odour is due to the volatile oil it contains. It dissolves entirely in rectified spirit. Dose, 3 to 5 grs.

Ferula Fœtida, B. P., Narthex Asafetida, Ferrula Narthex, Ferula Scorodosma.

Habitat.—Persia, Afghanistan, Panjab.

Parts used.—The gum-resin obtained by incision from the root. Asafetida, B. P.

Vernacular.—Arab. Hiltit Sujadân, Shamagh-ul-Mahrus, Juwifeh. Beng.—Hing. Burm.—Singu or Shinkhu. Can.—Ingu. Cing.—Pirunka yam. Duk.—Hing. Eng.—Devil's dung, asafetida. Guz.—Hingra, Vagârnihing. Hind.—Hingu, Hingiseh Anguza. Maleal.—Parungayam. Pers.—Angoyah, angustagooda anjadana. Sans.—Romatham, Bhuta nasana, sula nasana, hinguhu. Tel.—Juguva, Hingu-patri.

Characters.—A perennial herb ; the gum resin is met with in moist, flaky, pieces or tears of a dull yellow colour, becoming darker on keeping, tough when fresh, internally yellowish and translucent, or milky white and opaque, odour, strong, persistent and alliaceous, taste bitter and acrid, soluble in alcohol 65 p. c. ; with water it forms a milk-white emulsion. Dose, 5 to 15 grs.

Constituents.—A sulphuretted volatile oil, 3 to 9 p. c., consisting chiefly of allyl sulphide, resin 50 to 70 p.c., soluble in ether ; gum, 30 p. c., saline matters and ash ; 3 to 4 p.c., also ferulaic, malic, acetic, formic and valerianic acids.

Volatile oil.—The odour and stimulant property of asafetida are due to this oil which may be obtained by distilling asafetida with water or alcohol. It contains several sulphides of ferulyl, two terpenes which yield sesquiterpene and a blue coloured oil.

The resin on dry distillation yields umbelliferon, which is not found in the Indian variety. When fused with potash, it yields resorcin and pyrocatechuic acid.

Preparations.—Pill of asafetida—containing Hing 1, Camphor 1, Opium 1, and black pepper 1, made into one pill. Hinga ashtaka churana, a compound powder, Hinga 4, Shajira 5, Pipali 4, Ajavana 4, Bodi Ajamoda 5, Sonachola 4, Miri 3, and Suntha 3, mix and make a powder, to this, sometimes Afima 2 is added. Dose, 10 to 20 grains—used as a carminative and digestive in dyspepsia, vomiting, colic, flatulence, &c. Hinga-Vadi-Varati Suppositories—Hinga 5, Madha 6, Sindhava 4—mix and make a suppository in kokumtel, used in constipation, piles, &c.

Enema asafetidæ, 30 grains in 4 ounces. Pilula Aloes et Asafetidæ, B.P. (1 in 4). Dose, 4 to 8 grs. Pilula Galbani composita, B.P. (2 in 7). Dose, 4 to 8 grs. Spiritus ammoniæ Fetidus, B. P. (1 in 13). Dose, 20 to 40 ms. Tinctura Asafetidæ, tincture of asafetida, B. P. (1 in 5). Dose, ½ to 1 fld. dr. Emulsum asafetidæ, milk of asafetida, 4 p.c. Dose, 4 to 12. Mistura magnesiæ et asafetidæ, Dewee's carminative—magnesium carbonate 5, tincture of asafetida 7, tincture of opium 1, sugar 10, water 100. Dose, ½ to 4 drs.

Physiological Actions.—Among the natives, Hing is usually fried before being used as medicine, as they believe that raw hing causes vomiting. It is a most powerful fœtid gum resin, a valuable stimulant acting on the organs of circulation and secretion; also a nervine and pulmonary stimulant, and a powerful antispasmodic. It is also carminative, tonic, laxative, diuretic and emmenagogue, also anthelmintic and aphrodisiac. In small doses and if long continued, it produces a sense of warmth without any rise of temperature. It impairs digestion, gives rise to alliacious eructations, acrid irritation in the throat, flatulence, diarrhœa and burning in the urine. In large doses it stimulates the secretion and excretion and increases the sexual appetite. The volatile oil is rapidly excreted and may be found in the urine, milk and sweat. It also increases the menstrual flow.

Therapeutics.—It is given in nervous and neurotic diseases, as hysteria, and hypochondriasis; as an expectorant, in habitual cough, chronic catarrh, bronchitis and asthma; as a carminative in dyspepsia, colic and other gastric affections, and to expel worms. It is said to ward off malaria if taken with food in malarious districts. It relieves gaseous distension of the bowels. An enema of hinga is the best form in which it is exhibited in convulsions. It is a useful remedy in habitual constipation. With myrrh and ammoniac it is given in tympanitis of typhoid fever. An enema of hinga with castor oil and turpentine is very beneficial in intestinal colic and worms. In habitual abortion it is a very reliable remedy.

Varieties.—Khandari asafetida—this is superior to hingra, but inferior to the Indian hing. Stony asafetida is a mixture of hingra with sand, clay, &c. It is the most inferior of all the varieties.

Ferula Galbaniflua, B. P., and probably other species.

Habitat.—Persia, Smyrna, India, coasts of the Mediterranean.

Part used.—The gum resin Galbanum, B. P.

Vernacular.—Arab.—Barahada Kinneh. Bomb.—Javashira. Duk.—Barija-gonda. Eng.—Galbanum. Hind.—Birejâ, Ganda-biroza. Pers.—Biriz, Jhav-shira, Berazadd, Gaoshira, Barazahd-i-gaoshir. Javashira, a corruption of the Persian Gaoshira. Jao or gao means a cow, and shira, milk ; in allusion to the milky nature of the juice.

Characters.—Yellowish brown externally, and milk-white within, often mixed with stems fruits and flowers. Found in minute tears or agglutinated hard masses or granules of the size of a pea. The odour resembles that of ushaka or celery, taste balsamic and rather acrid. With water it gives milky emulsions. Dose, 5 to 15 grains.

Constituents.—Volatile oil, 6 to 9 p. c., isomeric with turpentine, resin 60 to 66 p.c. ; gum 15 to 20 p. c. ; it yields on dry distillation, a blue oil and umbelliferon, a tasteless substance in satiny crystals. The oil contains no sulphur.

Preparations.—Pilula galbani composita—compound pill of asafetida (2 in 7), asafetida 2. Galbanum 2, myrrh 2, syrup of glucose 1. Dose 4 to 8 grs. Emulsion, Tincture (1 in 10). Dose, $\frac{1}{2}$ to 1 dr., and Plaster.

Actions and uses.—Stimulant, expectorant, and antispasmodic ; similar to those of ammoniac, but is less powerful than asafetida. Locally it is used as a stimulant application to indolent glands, boils and tumours, combined with other gum resins ; an ointment is used for acne Internally it is given in hysteria, chlorosis, asthma, rheumatism, chronic bronchitis and catarrh of the mucous membranes generally. It has a stimulant action upon the uterus and is given in vaginal and uterine catarrh, and in amenorrhœa and chronic rheumatism.

Ferula Persica, F. Sagapenum.

Habitat.—Persia.

Part used.—The gum resin.

Vernacular.—Arab.—Sakabinaja, Sugabinaja. Bomb.—Easus. Eng.—Sagapenum. Hind.—Kundel. Pers.—Suga fium, Iskabinah.

Characters.—Gum resin in masses forming brown cakes, principally in tears of a greenish hue, closely resembling javashira ; odour like that of garlic, taste acrid, and terebinthaceous.

Constituents.—Volatile oil, resin and gum. Same as those of galbanum, but it also contains sulphur.

Preparations.—Plaster ; Segapenum pills—containing Aloes 1, Segapenum 1, Bdellium 1, and Agaric 1, given in flatulence and dyspepsia. Dose, 4 to 8 grs.

Actions and uses.—Stimulant, emmenagogue and anthelmintic ; given in flatulent dyspepsia, and in chronic bronchitis, with profuse secretion ; externally it is used as a stimulating plaster.

Ferula Sumbul, B. P.

Sumbul from arabic sumbul which means a spike. The appearance of the flowering stem is like that of a spike.

Habitat.—Northern Asia.

Parts used.—The dried transverse slices of the root, Sumbul Radix, B. P.

Vernacular.—Arab.—Sumbul. Eng.—musk root.

Characters.—A large plant ; root large, thick, fusiform, light and spongy, but longitudinally wrinkled, bark thin, brown and fibrous, interior whitish with yellow dots and irregular fibres—odour strong and musk-like, taste bitter and aromatic. Dose, 5 to 30 grs.

Constituents.—A volatile oil, of a bluish colour, balsamic resin 9 p.c, obtained by distillation and containing umbelliferon, sumbulic or angelic acid, valerianic acid, methyl crotonic acid, a bitter extractive ; sugar and starch.

Preparations.—Infusum Sumbul or Decoctum Sumbul (1 in 20). Dose, 2 to 6 drs. Tinctura Sumbul, B. P. (1 in 10). Dose, ½ to 1 dr. fl. Extract. Dose, 3 to 5 grs.

Actions and uses.—Stimulant, nervine tonic and antispasmodic like musk and valerian ; given in hysteria, nervous disorders, chlorosis, also in leucorrhœa, gleet, hypochondriasis, delirium tremens, and epilepsy. In chlorosis it is often combined with iron, arsenic, &c. Also given as a substitute for musk in cholera, typhoid and other adynamic conditions, asthma, &c.

Fœniculum Capillaceum, B. P., F. Vulgare, Fœniculum Panmohuri.

Habitat.—W. Asia, cultivated in India and Europe.

Parts used.—The dried ripe fruit, Fœniculi fructus, B. P. Fennel fruit ; and root.

Vernacular.—Arab.—Razeeanej and distilled water Arak-i-badiana. Bomb.—Sonpha. Cing.—Devaduru, Rataenduru. Beng.—Panmohuri, Moorie, Goowamooree. Can.—Somp. Eng.—Sweet or wild fennel. Guz.—Variari. Hind—Bari, Sonpha, Panmohuri, Mayuri. Mar.—Bari Sonpha. Pers.—Badian, Karafah. Tam.—Perun. Sheragom. Tel.—Shohi Kire. Pedda-gilla kara. Sans.—Mudorika.

Characters.—Fruit, cremocarp of a bright yellow colour changing to dark brown by keeping, from ⅕ to ⅖ of an inch long, and $\frac{1}{10}$ inch in diameter, oblong, more or less curved, having a long slender thread-like stalk at the bottom, apex slightly pointed, surface smooth, deeply channelled, and marked with ten prominent ridges, separable into two prominent mericarps. It exhibits on transverse section 4 oil tubes on the back, and 2 or 4 on the flat surface ; odour agreeable and aromatic, taste sweet and aromatic. Indian sweet fennel is smaller and straighter than the European article. Dose, 5 to 30 grs.

Constituents.—A volatile oil 2 to 6 p.c., united with a terpene, and almost identical with oil of aniseed; fixed oil 12 p. c., mucilage, sugar and ash 7 p. c.

Oleum Fœniculi.—Volatile oil of fennel. To obtain it distil the fruit or entire plant with water or steam. A pale yellow liquid, almost identical with anise oil, odour and taste peculiar and characteristic, neutral in reaction, soluble in alcohol (1 in 1) and glacial acetic acid (1 in 1). Dose, 2 to 4 ms. The oil contains pinene, phellandrene (isomeric with oil of turpentine), dipentene, fenchone and anethol, or anise camphor. Anethol consists of a liquid portion eleopten and a solid stearopten.

Preparations.—Aqua Fœniculi, B. P. (1 in 10), of the fruit, or 1 in 500 of the oil. Dose, 1 to 2 fld. ozs.—pulvis glycyrrhizæ compositus, B. P. Dose, 60 to 120 grs.

Actions and uses.—A mild stimulant, carminative, aromatic, stomachic, emmenagogue and galactagogue; employed like other carminative and aromatic medicines. It acts as a diuretic and diaphoretic in children and infants, promoting the secretion of urine and perspiration. It is also given for the relief of nausea, flatulency and colic. As an emmenagogue its hot infusion is given in amenorrhœa. As a galactagogue it is used in re-establishing lacteal secretion when wanting or suppressed. As a corrective, the oil is useful in flatulence and in arresting griping of purgatives. It is a common ingredient in confections. The root is used in native practice in the form of infusion for similar purposes, and as an enema to expel flatus in infants.

Remarks.—Fennel is often confounded with anise.

Hydrocotyle Asiatica.

Habitat.—India, Ceylon, Southern Africa.

Parts used.—The leaves and root.

Vernacular.—Arab,—Brahami Artâniyâ-a-hindi. Beng.—Thol-kuri. Bomb.—Brahami. Burm.—Minkhuâ-bin. Can.—Unde-lagâ. Cing.—Hingotu-kola. Duk.—Vallari-kâ-patta. Eng.—Asiatic or Indian Pennywort, Indian Hydrocotyle. Guz.—Khara brahami. Hind.—Brahami, Khula Khudi. Maleal.—Kodagam. Mar.—Karivana. Sans.—Brahami, Mandukaparni. Tam.—Vallarâi-kire. Tel.—Manduka-brummi, Bokkudu, Babassaielaka.

Characters.—Creeping herb, sending out large runners which produce leaves, roots and fruits at the joints; leaves with long stalks, reniform, crenate, glabrous or hairy on the under surface, and cordate at the base. Stem slender and longitudinally furrowed. Fruits, clustered at the joints, small, laterally compressed and furrowed or ribbed longitudinally; when bruised, the odour is aromatic, taste pungent, nauseous and bitter.

Constituents.—An oleaginous substance vellarine, having the odour and bitter persistent taste of the fresh plant, resin, and some fatty aromatic body, gum, sugar, albuminous matter, salts, mostly alkaline sulphates, and tannin.

Preparations.—Powder. Dose, 5 to 10 grains. Cataplasma, fluid extract. Dose, 2 to 5 ms.

Actions and uses.—Alterative, tonic, diuretic and local stimulant. It has a special influence on the urino-genital tract. It sets up urinary and ovarian irritation and itching over the whole body. The root is given with milk and liquorice, in fever and dysentery. As a stimulant and alterative the powder is given in chronic skin diseases, such as eczema, lupus, psoriasis, secondary syphilitic sores or skin eruptions ; also in anæsthetic leprosy, elephantiasis and scrofula. As a snuff, it is used in ozæna. The poultice or cataplasm is applied in syphilitic and other forms of ulcerations. The powder is dusted over ulcers.

Peucedanum Grande and Pastinaca Grande.

Habitat.—Hills of Western India.

Parts used.—The fruit.

Vernacular.—Bomb.—Baphalli. Eng.—Wild carrot. Hind.—Dukkû ; Daku. Pers.—Duku.

Characters.—Fruit resembling gajara, large, broadly elliptical, compressed, convex in the middle, with a dilated border and marked with ridges, and reddish yellow all over. The seed is of a pale yellow or brown colour adhering to the margin ; odour lemon like, and taste pungent bitterish.

Constituents.—An essential oil, of a light yellow colour.

Preparations.—Infusion (1 in 10). Dose, ½ to 1 fld. oz.

Actions and uses.—Similar to those of fennel, and used as carminative, diuretic and stimulant in flatulency, gastric and intestinal disorders &c.

Peucedanum Graveolens, B. P.

Anethum sova. A. graveolens—Pastinaca graveolens.

Habitat.—S. Europe, Asia, cultivated in India.

Parts used.—The dried ripe fruit, anethi fructus, dill fruit, B. P.

Vernacular.—Arab.—Shabbit. Beng.—Sovalakinda, shova sulpha. Burm.—Tsa-mont Sanun, Tsa-Morihpyn. Can.—Sabba-sagi. Cing. —Hinen dura, sata, kuppi. Duk.—Soyi. Eng.—Common dill fruit. Hind.—Sawa, soyah, suichuka. Guz.—Soova. Mar.— Suva, shepu. Malayal.—Jemuju adas-manis, anisi. Pers.—Valane khurda, shada. Sans.—Sita, siva, misreya, shatapushpa. Tam.—Sadakuppi. Tel.—Soyikura, vittulu. Unani—anitun.

Characters.—Fruit broadly oval, oblong, rather flat and smaller than variâli, composed of two mericarps which are usually separate and freed from pedicel ; each broadly oval $\frac{1}{10}$ of an inch long and $\frac{1}{8}$ inch broad, with smooth surfaces and containing oil tubes, and having a slender, long stalk at the base. At the apex are two small projections, the remains of the styles. Surface rugous darkish, or greyish yellow, or brown, with two thick ridges, united together from the apex to the base, forming a thick margin on both sides, three thin intervening ridges occupying their surfaces. On bruising, the odour is like that of peppermint, taste warm somewhat pungent, and spicy like that of caraway. Dose of the seed, 5 to 30 grs.

Constituents.—Volatile oil 3 or 4 p.c., and fixed oil. The volatile oil is composed of anethene, carvol and another hydrocarbon.

Oleum anethi, B. P. The volatile oil to which its medicinal properties are due is obtained by distillation of the seeds. It is a limpid, thin, yellowish or colourless liquid, odour aromatic, taste spicy, soluble in alcohol. Dose, ½ to 3 ms.

Preparations.—Aqua anethi, B. P., from the fruit (1 in 10); of the oil (1 in 500). Dose, 1 to 2 fld. ozs.

Actions and uses.—Carminative, stomachic, aromatic, stimulant, and galactagogue. Women use it as a cordial drink after confinement to stop a tendency to vomiting and hiccough, and in indigestion and flatulent colic; it is also given in amenorrhœa. With methi the seeds are fried in butter and used to check diarrhœa.

Remarks.—The natives use this drug very freely as a carminative in various prescriptions.

Petroselinum Sativum.

Syn.—Apium Petroselinum, Carum Petroselinum.

Habitat.—Southern Europe.

Parts used.—The root, fruit or leaves, and Apiol—an oleo-resin obtained from the fruit.

Vernacular.—Beng.—Bilati Pitursilli. Eng.—Common Parsley, Hind.—Pitar Saleri.

Characters.—A biennial plant, leaves radical 3 pinnate, flowers yellow, fruit long, ovate, greenish brown, mericarp with 5 ribs and 6 oil tubes; root conical, yellowish, 6 inches long and ½ inch thick.

Constituents.—The root contains a volatile oil, a gelatinous substance apiin and starch. The fruit also contains Apiol (an oleo-resin) which is the true active principle.

It is a greenish brown oily liquid of a peculiar odour and a disagreeable pungent parsley-like taste, readily soluble in alcohol, ether, chloroform and glacial acetic acid. Insoluble in water. Dose, 2 to 6 ms.

The name apiol is also given to a kind of camphor. It occurs in white needles, odour feeble and parsley-like, insoluble in water, freely soluble in alcohol or ether. Dose, 15 grs. as an antiperiodic, 10 grs. as an emmenagogue against dysmenorrhœa.

Preparations.—Extractum Apii Radicis Liquidum. Dose, 15 to 60 ms. Extractum Apii Fructus Liquidum. Dose, 15 to 60 ms. Infusum Apii of the root (1 in 20). Dose, 1 to 2 fld. ozs

Physiological action.—Parsley is aperient, diuretic, diaphoretic, expectorant and carminative ; also emmenagogue and febrifuge ; used in dropsy, gravel, strangury, gonorrhœa, uric acid diathesis and in ague. Apiol in small doses is carminative, diaphoretic, diuretic, also expectorant and vascular stimulant. In large doses it is emmenagogue and febrifuge. Its action is similar to that of quinine. Like quinine it produces headache, giddiness, ringing in the ears, &c. In over doses it is decidedly narcotic.

Therapeutics.—Apiol is given in intermittent fevers, and in malarial neuralgias, but chiefly given in amenorrhœa if due to anæmia, in dysmenorrhœa when the discharge is fœtid, and in accidental suppression of menses ; as an abortifacient, it is quite useless. Locally parsley leaves applied to the breasts suppress secretion of milk.

Pimpinella Anisum, B P.

Anisum officinalis.

Habitat.—Persia, Egypt, S. E. Europe.

Parts used.—The fruit, Anisi fructus, B. P., and oil, Oleum Anisi, B. P.

Vernacular.—Arab.—Anisum, Shamâr. Beng.—Mahoori, Mitha jira. Bom.—Ervados. Burm.—Tsa moun-tsa-bah, team-sompu. Can.—Sompu. Cing.—Sinhala-asamodayan. Duk.—Sonf. Eng.—Common Anise. Guz.—Ervadosa. Hind.—Sonf. Malay.—Jira-manis, Adis-manis, Perinchirakam. Mar.—Somp. Portuguese Herba-doce. Pers.—Raziyan-i-rumi, Vâlâne Buray. Sans.—Awak-pushpi Karavasata-puspha. Tam.—Shombu. Tel.—Kuppi-chattu Pella Jillakara. Ervadosa is a corruption of Herba-doce. The native names are involved in great confusion, many of them being wrongly applied to several other fruits and seeds.

Characters.—Fruit $\frac{1}{6}$th of an inch long, a cremocarp, ovoid, rough, compressed at sides, of a greyish brown colour and hairy, mericarp usually remains united or attached to the pedicel ; primary ridges, pale, slender and entire containing 15 to 20 oil tubes ; on crushing the seeds they give out an agreeable aromatic odour, and a sweet spicy taste. The volatile oil resembles oil of fennel. It becomes dark by keeping. Dose of the fruit, 10 to 20 grs.

Constituents—Volatile oil, 1 to 3 p. c., fixed oil 3 to 4 p. c., sugar, mucilage, and ash 7 p. c.

Oleum Anisi, B.P., Oil of anise—a volatile oil obtained by distilling the fruit with water or steam, used medicinally. It is a colourless. yellowish, thin liquid, of a sweet, mild, aromatic taste, soluble in alcohol (1 to 1). Solidifies into white crystals if kept for some time. It contains a terpene—phellandrene 10 to 20 p. c., a stearopten—anethol or anise camphor 80-90 p. c. Dose, $\frac{1}{2}$ to 3 ms. Anethol by oxidation is converted into anisic acid which resembles salicylic acid.

Preparations.—Spiritus Anisi, B. P. (1 in 10). Dose, 5 to 20 ms. Tinctura Camphoræ composita, B. P. Dose, $\frac{1}{2}$ to 1 dr. Aqua anisi,

B. P., anise water, from the fruit (1 in 10), and of the oil (1 in 500). Dose, one to two fluid ounces.

Preparations.—Of the fruit, infusum anisi (1 in 40). Dose, 2 to 8 drs.

Actions and uses.—The volatile oil which is the active medicinal agent, is aromatic, slightly stimulant of the heart and digestive organs. It liquefies the bronchial secretion, hence it is used as expectorant; it is also carminative and stomachic, and is used as a corrective to allay griping of purgative medicines. It is given in flatulence, intestinal colic and in bowel complaints. It has a special influence on the bronchial tubes, and is given in infantile bronchial catarrh, after the acute stage has passed away. In large doses it is slightly narcotic. Locally the oil is applied to the head to relieve headache and to the abdomen to expel flatus, to the joints in rheumatism, and round the ear in earache.

Prangos Pabularia.

Habitat.—North of India, Thibet and Cashmere.

Parts used.—The fruit and root.

Vernacular.— Arab.— Phatara-e-Saleyuna. Afghan.—Badian-e-Kohi. Bomb.— Phatarasaliuna, Fiturasaliyun. Hind.— Komal. Eng.—Silphium Parsley. Ind. Bazaar.—Fiturasaliyun. Mar.—Phatura Salyuna. Sans.—Komal, Avipriya. Thibet.—Prangos.

Characters.—Root conical, thick and yellow, becoming darkish brown when long kept. Fruit, a pair of mericarps, oblong, rather compressed and larger than varialee; surface rugous, marked with 5 convoluted ridges, on the top of each mericarp are two curved prominences, the remains of the styles; mericarps with 5 ribs and 6 oil tubes separate from below where the stalk is jointed. Odour resembling that of caraway. When kept for a long time the smell resembles cats' urine, taste pungent and resembles that of an inferior variety of Hinga.

Constituents.—The dried fruit contains an essential oil, a trace of fixed oil, resins, traces of an alkaloid, quercitrin in large amount, and an ethereal salt of valeric acid.

Preparations.—Of the fruit. Infusion (1 in 20). Dose, 1 to 2 fld. ozs. Decoction of the root (1 in 20). Dose, 1 to 2 fld. ozs.

Actions and uses.—The root is diuretic, and the fruit is carminative and stimulant; given in urinary diseases, gravel, strangury and dyspepsia, also in dropsy and gonorrhœa.

Remarks.—The fruit phatare saliyun, is sold as a substitute for petroselinon or rock parsley of the Greeks, and Karafs-el-jibali of the Arabs.

Ptychotis Ajowan Levisticum, Ajowan, Carum Ajowan, Carum Copticum, B.P., Ajwain Omum.

Habitat.—India, Southern Asia, Africa.

Parts used.—The fruit.

Vernacular.—Arab.—Kâmun-el-mulûki, Amus. Beng.—Ajwain, Juvân, Baro-joan. Bomb.—Ova. Burm.—Samhume. Can.—Omu, Voma. Cing.—Assumoda. Duk.—Ajvan. Eng.—Lovage, Bishop's weed, King's cumin. Guz.—Ajamo. Hind.—Ajvayan, Ajamoda. Mar.—Ova, Ajma vovasieda. Malay.—Homama Azamoda Kam. Pers.—Zhinyan, Nânkhâh. Sans.—Yavani Ajmodam, yavanika. Tam.—Omam. Tel.—Vaman Chettu.

Characters.—Mericarps adherent by a bright yellow stalk or separated, colour pale brown, resembling that of anisum, in size smaller than anise. Adherent mericarps, broadly ovate, pointed, stalked and conical, streaked with yellow stripes ; separate mericarps, compressed or arched on one side, and convex on the other. Surface highly tubercled, marked with five or ten prominent ridges, the intervening spaces being dark brown ; on bruising the odour is strong, resembling that of Thymol or origanum. Taste peculiarly heating, pungent and also aromatic. Dose of the fruits, 10 to 40 grs.

Constituents.—An aromatic volatile oil and a crystalline substance which collects on the surface of the distilled water. This stearopten, known under the Hindustanee name of Ajawankaphul, flowers of ajowan or ajwon camphor, is identical with English thymol contained in Thymus vulgaris. Dose, (stearopten) ½ to 2 grs.

Preparations.—Oleum Ptychotis—oil of ajwan—oil of omum. Dose, 1 to 3 ms. in emulsion. Medicated oil for application in rheumatism, bruises, lumbago, &c. Extractum Ptychotis liquidum, not miscible with water. Dose, 10 to 30 ms. Araka—Aqua Ptychotis, ajwan or omum water. Dose, 1 to 2 ozs.

Actions and uses.—Diffusible stimulant, stomachic, carminative, antispasmodic and antiseptic. The fruit combines the powerful stimulant qualities of mustard or capsicum, the bitter property of chiretta and the antispasmodic virtues of asafetida, and is of great service in cholera. As an antiseptic, it removes offensive smell from foul ulcers. As a stomachic, it increases the flow of saliva, augments the gastric secretion, and hence is given in diarrhœa, dyspepsia, acid eructations, heartburn, &c. As an antispasmodic it is given in flatulency, colicky pains, hysteria, stoppage of urine and tympanitis. In bronchitis, with profuse expectoration, it lessens the sputum. A poultice of crushed fruits is applied to painful rheumatic joints, and fomentation of hot seeds to the chest in bronchitis, asthma, and to the cold hands and feet in cholera, fainting and syncope. Ajama-na-phula, is antiseptic and germicide. With camphor and other antispasmodics it is given in cholera, diarrhœa, intestinal colic, spasm of stomach, asthma and dysmenorrhœa. The oil is applied as a stimulant embrocation for the relief of pains in the limbs or rheumatism, and also given internally for colic, tympanitis, &c. Aqua ptychotis is used to disguise the taste of nauseous drugs.

Trachydium Lehmani.

Habitat.—Persia, Kashmir, Egypt.

Parts used.—The root.

Vernacular.—Arab.—Shirza. Eng.—Egyptian Misree. Ind. Baz.—Secacul misree. Pers.—Sakakul, Kirsygeyah. Shiraz.—Badran.

Characters.—Root resembling small carrots in shape and size. Externally, longitudinally furrowed, highly wrinkled and of a light brown colour; surface marked with scars of fallen rootlets. On section it is resinous, or sugary looking, and of a dark amber colour. The taste is sweetish and starchy.

Constituents.—The root contains saccharine matter, starch, &c.

Preparations.—Confection. Dose, 1 to 2 drs.

Actions and uses.—Tonic and aphrodisiac. It resembles in its actions sapheda musali and is given in seminal debility and leucorrhœa.

Thapsia Garganica

Habitat.—Northern Africa, Southern Europe, Arabia.

Parts employed.—The root and resin.

Preparations.—Fluid ext. 10 to 30 minims. Plaster from its resin.

Actions and uses.—Counter-irritant. It relieves the localized pains of rheumatism, gout, bruises and bronchitis. Like croton oil, its action is limited to the spot of its application. Internally it acts as tonic in small doses, but in large doses it is an irritant cathartic.

Trianthema Monogyna, T. Obcordata, T. Pentandra.

Habitat.—Throughout India.

Part used.—The root.

Vernacular.—Beng.—Sâbuni, Lal and Lovet sabuni, Gado-Cunya. Guz.—Satudo. Hind.—Nâsur Janghi, Bish Khapra. Mar.—Vish Khâpra. Sans.—Punarnava. Tam.—Sharvalay-Kiray. Tel.—Ambati-maddu, Bodo-pail-kura, Ghalijeroo.

Characters.—Plant, diffused, glabrous and fleshy; root of a dirty brown or brownish white colour, 3 to 4 inches long and as thick as a crow's quill; smell aromatic; taste astringent, bitter, pungent, and acrid; leaves succulent, thick, smooth, obovate or obcordate, margin red. The flowers of a light pink colour. Dose, 30 to 120 grs.

Constituents.—A glucoside, similar in properties to saponin.

Preparations.—Infusion (1 in 20). Dose, 1 to 2 ozs.

Actions and uses.—Cathartic and irritant; given in constipation, jaundice, strangury and dropsy; it is also used in torpid liver, asthma and amenorrhœa. Among the natives the plant is boiled and eaten as a vegetable.

Onagraceæ.

Evening primrose, or Singoda family.

Herbs or shrubs, with simple exstipulate, alternate, dotless leaves; fruit capsular, succulent and dehiscent or indehiscent; seeds numerous without albumen.

Habitat.—India, temperate parts of North America and Europe.

Properties.—The plants of this order are harmless. They possess mucilaginous properties. The fruits are acid and edible. The roots are also edible; some are astringent.

Œnothera Biennis.

Habitat.—Europe, North America, &c.

Part used.—The flowering tops.

Characters.—A shrub with simple, alternate or opposite, exstipulate leaves without dots; flowers axillary, almost sessile; calyx, superior 2—4 lobed, in æstivation valvate; petals, large, showy, regular and twisted in æstivation. Dose, 10 to 30 grs.

Preparations.—Decoction as a wash. Fluid extract, 20 to 60 ms. ointment.

Actions and uses.—Sedative and antispasmodic; indicated in pulmonary and gastric affections, depending on a morbid sensitiveness in the laryngeal, pulmonary or gastric branches of the pneumogastric nerve. It is beneficial in whooping cough, and spasmodic asthma—externally, a decoction is used as a wash in infantile eruptions and as an application to ulcers; the roots are edible.

Jussiæa Suffruticosa, J. Villosa, Epilobrium Fruticosum, J. Exaltata.

Habitat.—India, Ceylon.

Part used.—The plant.

Vernacular.—Beng.—Lâl-ban-Lavanga. Ceylon—Hæmorago. Can. —Kava cula. Cing.—Hœmarago. Hind.—Ban Laung, Kanchana. Maleal.—Carambu. Mar.—Pâna Lavanga. Sans.—Bhàllavi-anga, Tel.—Nirbatsala. Tam.—Nirkirambu, Niruaghendra-paku.

Pâna Lavanga means water-clove—indicating, the habitat of the plant.

Characters.—Herb erect pubescent or villous, leaves broad, lanceolate, sometimes linear, acuminate, shortly petioled; flowers sessile, capsule, linear, 1 or 2 inches, cylindrical, more or less villous, 8 ribbed fruit large, yellow, resembling a clove.

Preparations.—Decoction (1 in 20). Dose, $\frac{1}{2}$ to 1 fl. dr.

Actions and uses.—Astringent, carminative, diuretic and vermifuge; given in flatulence; powder steeped in butter milk, is given in diarrhœa and dysentery. As an astringent it is given in hæmoptysis, and in leucorrhœa.

Haloragaceæ, Mare's Tail, or Water Chestnut family.

Herbs or shurbs, generally aquatic ; upper leaves and petioles tomentose, lower leaves opposite ; calyx minute, villous ; seeds solitary and pendulous ; albumen fleshy or exalbuminous, nearly allied to onagraceæ, merely an imperfect form of onagraceæ. Edible seeds ; found in all parts of the world.

Trapa Bispinosa, T. Natans, T. Bicornis, Tribulus Aquaticus.

Habitat.—Peninsulas of India, Bengal, Cashmere, Peshawar Nepal.

Parts used.—The fruit, or nut, or seeds.

Vernacular.—Eng.—Water chestnut, 2 spined water caltrop, Jesuit nut. Chin.—Ling. Beng.--Pâni phala. Bomb.—Singora. Guz.—Singoda. Duk.—Pani-phal. Hind.—Singhârah, Pâni phal. Maleal.—Karim polam. Mar.—Singàdá. Panj.—Gaunri. Sans.—Seringata, Tel.—Parike-gadda. Tam.—Pauri-mattai.

Characters.—Fruit or nut is dark green, externally marked with horns. very conical in shape and barbed backwards as projecting spines, Seeds large, amygdaloid with unequal cotyledons ; nuts abounding in starchy fecula of a white colour, and of a sweetish taste ; seeds edible ; those of Trapa Natans are known as Jesuit's nuts at Venice.

The dried fruit deprived of husk is dull brown externally and white within. In shape, it is compressed, and like an obtuse angled triangle. On section it is hard and brittle. Dose, 1 to 2 drs.

Constituents.—Contains manganese and starch.

Preparations.—Confection. Dose, 2 to 4 drs.

Actions and uses.—Nutritive, tonic, and cooling ; given in diarrhœa and dyspepsia, and with milk, in nervous and general debility, seminal weakness and leucorrhœa. Fresh fruits are edible—dried ones are baked, and then eaten. Powder of the dry fruits is used to prepare bread.

Samydaceæ, Samyda Family.

Trees or shrubs ; leaves alternate, simple, evergreen stipulate, and marked with round or linear transparent dots. Flowers perfect. Fruit capsular and leathery, one-celled. Seeds numerous and arillate, albumen fleshy or oily.

Habitat.—Tropical—principally America.

Properties.—Bitter and astringent.

Casearia Esculenta.

Habitat.—Southern India and Ceylon.

Parts used.—The bark of the root.

Vernacular.—Goa.—Sataganda. Hind.—Chilla, Chilara, Bairé. Mar.—Mora-âgeru, Bithori, Pingri, Mormassi. Tam.—Kaddla Shingi. Tel.—Gundu gungura.

Morâ-ageru—morâ, a pile, and ageru, the rectum. This medicine is used for the treatment of piles. Sâtagunda—sâta, which means seven, and gonda, a ring, the transverse section of the root bark shows seven concentric rings. Moramassi, mora pile and mashi, flesh, or a soft tumour. It is a cure for piles or soft tumour.

Characters.—A small shrub; root crooked, forming angular bends; bark very hard, of a dull red colour, and covered with thin papery suber of a yellow colour; taste astringent.

Constituents.—The bark contains tannin, similar to Ratanhio-tannic acid, and a principle allied to cathartic acid.

Preparations.—Decoction (1 in 20). Dose, 1 to 2 fld. ozs. Extract. Dose, 10 to 20 grs., and syrup (1 of extract in 6). Dose, 1 to 2 drs.

Actions and uses.—Laxative and alterative; used for hepatic enlargement, and for piles, both internally and externally. Its action on the liver is very marked. It is also given in diabetes.

Papayaceæ.

The Papaw family. Trees or shrubs, with acrid milky juice; leaves on long petioles, lobed, and alternate; flowers, unisexual or hermaphrodite. Fruit succulent and dehiscent; seeds many and albuminous.

Habitat.—India, South America.

Properties.—The plants of this order contain an acrid, milky juice Some plants are deadly poisonous; the unripe fruit and juice of some are anthelmintic. Ripe fruits are edible.

Carica Papaya, C. Vulgaris.

Habitat.—Native of America, cultivated throughout India.

Parts used.—The milky juice, seeds, and pulp.

Vernacular—The fruit. Arab.—Anabahe-hindi. Beng.—Popo-yiâh. Bom., Hind.—Arand-Kharbuza, papaya. Burm.—Tienbaw, then, thin-baw. Chin.—Muhkwa. Can.—Parangi. Cing.—Papal. Duk.—Popaiyah, Popâl. Eng.—Papaw. Guz.—Papâyi. Mar.—Popayâ. Malay.—Papâya-papa, Bate. Maleal.—Papeta, umbbalay. Pers.—Anobahe-hindi. Sind.—Katha Chibhadu. Tam.—Peppah-maram. Tel.—Madhurnakam, Bapaia pandu.

Characters.—Ripe fruit, succulent, oblong, furrowed, yellowish green, and containing numerous slimy, round, coloured albuminous grey seeds. The seeds smell like Asâlio; the unripe fruit, wood and leaves contains a large quantity of thick, milky juice, of a gelatinous consistence—and which contains a digestive ferment, which is the active principle called Papain.

Constituents.—The juice contains an albuminoid, digestive, or milk-curdling ferment—Papain or Papayotin. The fresh fruit contains a caoutchouc-like substance; a soft, yellow resin, fat, albuminoids, sugar, pectin, citric, tartaric and malic acids, dextrine, &c. The dried fruit contains a large amount of ash, 8·4 p. c., which contains soda, potash and phosphoric acid. The seeds contain an oil, Papaya oil, or caricin, an oil-like substance of a disagreeable taste and smell, soluble in ether and alcohol; and several acids; similar to palmitic acid, carica fat acid, and a crystalline acid called papayic acid. These are insoluble in cold water, but soluble in hot water and alcohol, also a resin acid, having an irritant and bitter taste, insoluble in water and ether, and soluble in alcohol and alkalies; and a soft resin. The leaves contain an alkaloid called carpaine, which with hydrochloric acid forms carpaine hydrochloride, soluble in water; used hypodermically as an injection. Dose, $\frac{1}{30}$ to $\frac{1}{15}$ of a grain. As a cardiac tonic, it may replace digitalis. Papayotin—a concentrated, active principle, obtained from the juice by precipitation with alcohol. A whitish, amorphous, hygroscopic powder, soluble in 75 p.c., of absolute alcohol, water and glycerine. Dose, 2 to 10 grs. It is capable of digesting 200 times its weight of fresh pressed blood fibrin. Its action is quicker than that of pepsin at a higher temperature, and does not require an addition of free acid. Seven grains of papayotin can digest one pint of milk. It acts as a solvent in alkaline solutions, and like pepsin it curdles milk. Dose, 1 to 8 grains.

Preparations.—Of the unripe fruit—succus, or papaw juice. Dose 1 to 4 drs. Papaw Spray (2 drs. in 4 ozs.) contains in addition three grains of Hydro-naphthol, and 15 minims of dilute hydrochloric acids. Pigment.—Contains papain, 12 gr.; borax, 5 gr.; water, 2 drs. Lozenges.—$\frac{1}{4}$ to $\frac{1}{2}$ gr. of papain with $\frac{1}{18}$ of cocaine in each. Elixir Papain. Dose, 1 dr.

Physiological Actions.—The action of the milky juice of the unripe fruit upon raw meat is well known among Indian cooks. It is an enzyme, similar to pepsin, acting as a solvent in alkaline, acid or nentral solutions. It is a powerful digestive of meat albumen, forming true peptones. As a solvent of fibrin and other nitrogenous substances, the juice makes the meat tender, and is used as an anthelmintic, and for dyspepsia. Externally it is applied for ringworm and psoriasis, sometimes it is given as an emmenagogue. It is not precipitated like pepsin on boiling, but is precipitated by mineral acids, iodine, mercuric chloride.

Therapeutics.—Acid glycerole of papain is largely used in dyspepsia as it dissolves mucus in the stomach which prevents the absorption of food in cases of indigestion, colic, flatulence, gastric ulcers, and as an aid to the nutrition of patients suffering from phthisis. As a solvent of albuminous bodies, papaine solution is used to dissolve fibrinous membrane, or to remove exudation in diphtheria, croup, swelled mammary and axillary glands &c. A 5 p. c. solution with $2\frac{1}{2}$ p. c. of bicarbonate of sodium, is used as drops into the ear in chronic otorrhœa. A pigment, well rubbed is used to remove corns, warts, or any hardness of the skin and in chronic eczema. Its solution in glycerine is applied to ulcers and fissures of the tongue. The lozenges are recommended for syphilitic ulcers of the tongue and throat. The milky juice and the seeds with honey are anthelmintic, and are given to expel lumbrici ; also useful in dyspepsia, in hepatic and splenic enlargements. The seeds are used as emmenagogue ; made into pessaries they are used in India to procure abortion—locally with glycerine a paste of seeds, or the juice is used as a cure for ringworm and psoriasis.

Turneraceæ.

The Turnera family. Herb, or shrubs. Leaves alternate, exstipulate and hairy. Flowers axillary ; calyx inferior, 5-lobed, petals 5, equal, twisted and perigynous. Stamens 5, alternate with the petals, filaments distinct. Ovary, one-celled, superior. Fruit capsular one-celled, 3-valved, dehiscing in a loculicidal manner. Seeds slightly curved, embryo, in the midst of fleshy albumen.

Habitat.—South America and West Indies.

Properties.—Astringent, tonic, expectorant and aromatic.

Turnera Aphrodisiaca. T. Microphylla.

Habitat.—California and Mexico.

Parts used.—The leaves and tops.

Characters.—Damiana is a small mint-like plant, bearing yellowish white fragrant flowers, and growing near the western coast of Mexico. The leaves are small, serrated, about one-fourth to one-third of an inch long, light green in colour, with a faint aromatic odour, and slightly bitter taste.

Constituents.—A volatile oil and a resin.

Preparations.—Extractum Damianæ Liquidum. Dose, $\frac{1}{2}$ to 2 drs. Extractum Damianæ. Dose, 2 to 10 grs. Aphrodisiac pill :—Damiana Extract 2 grs., Nux Vomica Extract $\frac{1}{8}$ gr., Phosphorus $\frac{1}{100}$ gr., Coca Extract $\frac{1}{2}$ gr., Reduced iron 1 gr.—for one pill.

Actions and uses.—Tonic, aphrodisiac, nervine, laxative, cholagogue and diuretic. It has specific action in seminal emissions, loss of seminal power, prostatitis, prostatorrhœa, and enlargement of the prostate gland. It has been largely employed as an aphrodisiac as it has a special tonic and stimulant effect over the genito-urinary organs. It is useful in exhaustion from excesses. As a general nervine tonic it is given in cerebral exhaustion, general atony of the nervous system, sick headache, hemiplegia and paraplegia.

Cucurbitaceæ.

The gourd, dodhi, or kâkady family. Herbs, generally succulent, prostrate or climbing with tendrils. Leaves alternate, more or less lobed, and scabrous. Flowers unisexual, monœcious or diœcious, and of a yellow or white colour. Fruit a pepo, or a succulent berry. Seeds numerous, more or less flattened and exalbuminous ; testa, horny or leathery.

Habitat.—Common in the tropics.

The pulp surrounding the seeds is edible. It sometimes possesses acrid, bitter, and purgative properties. Some species are poisonous. The seeds are generally harmless. By cultivation, the fruits lose their acridity, and become edible.

Benincasa Cerifera, Cucurbita Cerifera.

Cucurbita Hispida, C. alba (white pumpkin), C. Pepo (common pumpkin).

Habitat.—Tropical Asia, India.

Parts used.—The seeds and juice of the fruit.

The word red or white or black is affixed to the vernacular name for Pepo.

Vernacular.—Arab.—Majda bab (C. Pepo). Bomb.—Pandri chiki Kohala. Beng.—Komra, chal-kumra. Burm.—Shwapha young. Chin.—Tung Kwa. Can.—Kumbala-kaya. Duk.—Kaddu, Pethah. Eng.—Chinese pumpkin, Pepo, White tallow gourd. Guz.—Bhopala Dangara, Bhurûn-Kohalun. Hind.—Kâshi-phal, Hulwâ, Mitha Kaddoo. Mar.—Koholum. Sind.—Prata-Kalu. Maleal.—Kumbulum, Kuvaly Punj.—Pitha. Pers.—Kodu. Sans.—Kush manda. Tam.—Pushinikkaya kumbuli. Tel.—Budide-gum madi.

Characters.—Fruit large, yellowish, red or white, longitudinal or cylindrical, externally smooth, covered with obtuse ribs; pulp, yellowish red or white, marrow-like, and juicy; seeds pale yellow or white, flat, thick, broad, ovate and acuminate, taste sweet, refreshing, cooling or bland and oily. No odour. Dose of the seeds, 1 to 2 ozs. Given as an emulsion with sugar. Dose of the resin, 10 to 15 grs.

Constituents.—Fixed oil, 44 p. c.; starch 32 p. c. an alkaloid cucurbitine, an acrid resin, proteids, myosin, vitellin, sugar, ash, 4 p.c.

Preparations.—Emulsion and Confection. Pushtik conserve. Take Bhurun Kohalu, cut in small pieces, dry them in shade and powder, fry the powder in butter and add almonds, quince seed, cloves, cardamoms, nutmegs, asparagus sarmentosus, satawari seeds, seeds of mucuna pruriens; musk, curculigo archioidis, akalkaro, assan, Tejbal, Behman, (safed and surkh), Tamal patra, agar, nag kesor equal parts; add sugar to make a confection. For spermatorrhœa, with cumin seeds; and as a galactagogue with coriander and fenugreek seeds. Dose, ½ to 1 dr.

Actions and uses.—Fruit is nutritive, tonic and diuretic. The seeds deprived of the outer covering are vermifuge, and are given in tape-worms and lumbrici; as a diuretic it as given in gonorrhœa and urinary diseases. The oil has been used for the same purposes.

The confection is alterative, tonic, diuretic and restorative, and given in impotence, phthisis, dyspepsia, anorexia, and to check internal hæmorrhages such as hæmoptysis, &c. Given to children in marasmus and for the relief of cough and asthma. The fresh juice with sugar and saffron is given in insanity, epilepsy, nervous diseases, and in diabetes.

Bryonia Alba, B. Dioica.

B. Alba—White bryony. Vitis alba—Wild hops—Tetter berry, wood vine. B. Dioica—Red bryony, devil's turnips.

Habitat.—S. Europe in thickets and hedges, East Indies.

Parts used.—The root.

Characters.—Perennial plant. Root spindle-shaped, long, 2 inches in diameter. Bark—thin, yellowish grey, or brown. The interior is made up of numerous small wood bundles in radiating lines. The centre is white, fleshy, and lactescent; taste bitter and acrid; odour nauseous. Dose, powdered root, 10 to 60 grs.

Constituents.—It contains an active principle, Bryonin—a glucoside, starch, sugar, gum, fatty matter, malates and other salts.

Bryonin—To obtain it exhaust the root with alcohol, add tannin, and evaporate the precipitate. It is soluble in alcohol, and in water, insoluble in ether. Boiled with diluted sulphuric acid we get glucose, bryoretin and hydrobryoretin. Dose, $\frac{1}{8}$ to $\frac{1}{4}$ gr.

Preparations.—Tinctura Bryoniæ, from fresh-bruised roots (1 in 10). Dose, 1 to 10 ms. or more. Infusum Bryoniæ (1 in 20). Dose, 4 to 12 drs.

Physiological action.—Emmenagogue, hydragogue, cathartic, vesicant, emetic and styptic. It is a cardiac depressant, lowering the heart's beats. As an irritant, the fresh plant sets up cutaneous inflammation with fever, and also produces vesication. It is a violent irritant of the mucous membranes. In small doses it irritates the stomach, intestines, and the bronchi, causing gastritis, and dry hacking cough, with pain and soreness in front of the chest, and behind the sternum. As an irritant of the serous membranes it sets up pleuritis with fibronous effusion. It leads to congestion of the brain, liver, kidneys and bladder, producing frontal headache, vertigo and sometimes epistaxis; also pain and tenderness in the liver, bilious vomiting and even jaundice, and pain and tenderness in the bladder with profuse secretion of urine. As a hæmostatic its infusion (1 in 10) causes progressive contraction of the capillaries. In large doses it is a drastic purgative, and acts like jalap. It is also emmenagogue and emetic.

Therapeutics.—In small doses Bryonia is given in the advanced stage of serous inflammations after the fever has subsided, as in pleurisy, pleuropneumonia and pericarditis. It promotes absorption of the effused products. It is given in hysteria, epilepsy, enlarged spleen, and swelled glands. An infusion of Bryony is styptic, and is used to arrest metrorrhagia. In rheumatic fever, it relieves the pain and stiffness. It should be given after the swelling has been reduced. It relieves the pain, soreness and dry hacking cough in persons suffering from cold in the chest. In bilious fevers, in bilious headaches, in gastralgia with pyrosis, in congestion of the liver, and in croup its use is very beneficial. Bryonin is given in dropsies; it acts as a diuretic and as a drastic purgative.

Bryonia Epigæa, Corallocarpus Epigæa.

Habitat.—Punjab, Sind, Guzerat, Deccan.

Parts used.—The root.

Vernacular.—Arab., Pers.—Lûf—or Lûfa. Bomb.—Kavale-chedole. Can.—Akashu garuda-gadde. Duk.—Akâsa gaddah, Gâraja phala. Guz.—Karvi-nai. Hind.—Akàsa gaddah, chhilihinda. Mar.—Siva Linga. Sans.—Chhili-hinda, Pàtàla-garuda, Mahamula. Tam.—Gollan-kovaiks-kizh-angu. Tel.—Akàsa-garuda-gaddalu, Nâgadouda. Maha mula, the great root. Akâs, the sky; Gadda, the tuberous root. Linga Shiva—the linga of Siva, in allusion to the shape of the fruit.

Characters.—Root turnip shaped, very large and heavy, met with in pieces, or slices resembling kalamba. Each piece from 1 to 4 inches in length, and from 1 to 1½ inches in thickness, in colour resembling that of Bhui koholâ, outer surface brownish, and marked with four circular rings; on section it yields a viscid juice, which hardens into gum; taste very bitter, mucilaginous and subacid; odour somewhat acrid. Dose, of the powder, 10 to 30 grs.

Constituents.—A bitter glucoside—Bryonin, starch, resin and mineral matters.

Preparations.—Tincture (1 in 10). Dose, 10 to 30 ms.

Actions and uses.—Alterative and laxative; given in rheumatism, syphilis and other venereal complaints; also in the later stages of dysentery. It has a reputation in India as a remedy in snake bites, and is given internally and applied to the bitten part. It is also used as an anthelmintic. Locally a liniment of the root, combined with onions, cumin and castor oil, is used as an embrocation for chronic rheumatism and painful joints. It is also used as a substitute for Bryony.

Bryonia umbellata, Gowala-kakri (Hind). Mohakri (Hind). On the Sutlej the root is given for spermatorrhœa.

Bryonia Laciniosa.

Habitat.—India, Ceylon, Pegu.

Parts used.—The plant.

Vernacular.—Beng.—Mala. Can.—Lingatondi. Dutch.—Slitten. Hind.—Bajgureya, Ghurga-Nâru. Mal.—Nehoe maka. Mar.—Kavadori. Sans.—Baja. Tel.—Linga-douda. Portuguese—Nohla. Gharu-Naru, string of ankle bells, used by dancing girls, these bells have vertical slits, resembling the vertical lines on the fruit.

Characters.—Climbing shrub, common in hedges; leaves palmately, 5-lobed, and deeply divided; under surface studded with white, jointed, calcareous hairs. Flowers small, and pale yellow. Fruit round, smooth and marked with white vertical stripes. The whole plant is very bitter.

Constituents.—A bitter principle similar to bryonin, fat and colouring matter.

Preparations.—Infusion (1 in 10). Dose, ½ to 1 fld. ozs.

Actions and uses.—Laxative ; given in vomiting and in fevers, accompanied with flatulence and constipation.

Cephalandra Indica.

Habitat.—Throughout India.

Parts used.—The leaves, root and fruit.

Vernacular.—Beng.—Tela kucha. Can.—Tonde konde. Guz.—Gholi. Hind.—Kanduri. Mar.—Tondali, Rân-tondla. Sans.—Vimbaja, Vinba, Tundkeri, Vimboshta, Tundika. Tam.—Kavai. Vimboshta, means red, or cherry lipped.

Characters.—Plant, a creeper cultivated for its edible fruits. Fruits oblong, 2 inches long, green or yellowish green, with white stripes intervening ; leaves 5-lobed, somewhat thick, green, or darkish green ; flowers white ; root spindle-shaped, yellowish grey on the outside, interior white and fleshy ; odour nauseous, taste bitter, acid and astringent.

Constituents.—The dried powder contains resin and an alkaloid, starch, sugar, gum, fatty matter, an organic acid, and ash 16 p.c., which contains no manganese.

Preparations.—Tincture (1 in 10). Dose, ½ to 1 dr. Decoction (1 in 10). Dose, ½ to 1 fld. oz. ; and juice of the root, 60 to 180 grs.

Actions and uses.—Alterative ; given in diabetes, enlarged glands, and in skin deseases such as pityriasis.

Citrullus Colocynthis, B. P., Cucumis Colocynthis.

Citrullus, from Citrus, orange or citron, in allusion to orange red colour of the fruit when cut.

Habitat.—India, Japan, Asia, Africa, Spain, and Asiatic Turkey.

Parts used.—The fruit, deprived of its rind, the root and the dried pulp of the fruit, freed from seeds, colocynthidis pulpa, B. P.

Vernacular.—Arab.—Hanzal, Aulqam. Duk.,Beng.—Indrayan, Mâkkâ. Baluchistan.—Khar Khusta. Bomb.-Guz.—Indrayana. Burm.—Kayâ-si. Can.—Hava, mekke-kayi. Cing.—Yekka-madu. Eng.—Bitter apple, bitter cucumber, Indian or wild gourd ; colocynth apple. Hind.—Indarayan, Hanzil, Maqal. Mar.—Indrâyana, Karuvrandâwan, Indrâvana. Pers.—Kabiste talkh, Kharbuzahe-rubah. Sans,—Indravaruni, Vishâla. Maleal.,Tam.—Peykomatti. Tel.—Eti-puchcha, Patsa kaia, Papara budama.

Characters.—Fruit of the size of a small orange, thick and globular, greenish, mottled, containing whitish, light and spongy pulp, embedded in which are numerous small, ovate, oblong, compressed, smooth, brown seeds which should be rejected before the pulp is used. When dry, the external surface of the fruit is smooth, yellowish brown and tubercled. The rind is brittle, and breaks into three wedge-shaped pieces. The inner surface of the rind is covered with a soft spongy, white substance ; taste intensely bitter; root woody, brownish white and tapering ; wood fibrous, and containing a bitter starchy substance ; top of the root is semi-globular, tubercled and giving off several diverging slender stems. All parts of the plant are inodorous, but very bitter, the pulp more so than the seeds. Dose, of the pulp: 2 to 10 grs.

Constituents.—The pulp contains colocynthin, also colocynthein (a resin), colocynthitin, pectin, gum, no starch, ash 11 p.c. The seeds contain a fixed oil 17 p.c., albuminoids 6 p.c., and ash 3 p.c.

Colocythin.—A crystallizable glucoside, is the chief cathartic bitter principle. To obtain it, exhaust with water an alcoholic extract, precipitate with acetate and subacetate of lead, filter. Treat the yellow filtrate with sulphuretted hydrogen and precipitate with tannin—dissolve tannate of colocynthin in alcohol, add lead subacetate to precipitate tannin. Digest with animal charcoal and evaporate. A yellow mass, readily soluble in water. Boiled with diluted acids, it splits up into sugar and resinous colocynthein. Dose, 1 to 6 grains. Hypodermically, $\frac{1}{8}$ to $\frac{1}{4}$ gr.

Colocynthitin.—A tasteless crystalline powder, soluble in ether, insoluble in water. It has a purgative action.

Preparations.—Extractum Colocynthidis. Dose, $\frac{1}{2}$ to 2 grs. Extractum Colocynthidis compositum, compound extract of colocynth B. P.—Colocynth pulp 6 ozs. Extract of Barbados aloes 12 ozs., Scammony resin 4 ozs., curd soap 4 ozs., Cardamom seeds 1 oz., alcohol one gallon. Dose, 2 to 8 grs. Pilula Colocynthidis composita, B. P.—Colocynth pulp 1 ounce, Barbados aloes 2 ozs., Scammony resin 2 ozs., potassium sulphate $\frac{1}{4}$ oz., oil of cloves 2 drs., Distilled water q. s. Dose, 4 to 8 grs. Pilula Colocynthidis et Hyoscyami B.P.,—Compound pill of colocynth 2, and extract of hyoscyamus 1. Dose, 4 to 8 grs. *A compound purgative pill*—contains pârâkajali 1, Colocynth pulp 4, Sulphur 4, Cardamoms 4, Long pepper 4, Chebulic myrobalans 4, Pellitory root 4. Mix, make a mass. Dose, 3 to 5 grs.

Physiological action.—Drastic hydragogue, cathartic and diuretic, in large doses emetic and irritant ; in moderate doses it increases peristalsis and the intestinal glandular secretions, producing rapid watery evacuations with griping pains. As a purgative its action is very powerful and it acts even if applied to the abdomen. In large doses it is a gastro-intestinal irritant and leads to gastro-enteritis, irritation of pelvic organs and even death from prostration. It is an indirect diuretic.

Therapeutics.—It is given in constipation with other purgatives in febrile affections, in amenorrhœa, jaundice, ascites or dropsy, and in elephantiasis. It is also a vermifuge. It is a valuable evacuant, producing rapid derivation in coma, apoplexy and recent paralysis due to congestion of the brain. Its irritant action on the bowels extends to the urethra and bladder and leads to strangury. A snuff of the powdered root is irritating to the eyes and nostrils. In India the root is given in rheumatism and enlargements of the abdominal viscera in children; a paste of the fruit or root with that of nux vomica is applied to boils and pimples to hasten maturation. In minute doses, it is very beneficial in colic, sciatica, ovarian and other neuralgias; and also to relieve pain of glaucoma.

Citrullus Vulgaris, C. Cucurbita, Cucurbita Citrullus, Cucumis Citrullus.

Habitat.—Cultivated throughout the East Indies.

Parts used.—The seeds (deprived of testa) and pulp of the fruit.

Vernacular.—Arab.— Belikh-Zichi. Beng.—Tarmuj, Titoolaoo. Bomb. and Mar.—Kalingada. Burm.—Pha-rai. Cing.—Pilcha ghadi, Komordu. Eng.—Water melon. Guz.—Kârigu. Hind.—Samoka. Jamauka, Tarbuz. India—Dilpasand. Malay.—Mandeki Patak, somangka. Pers.—Hinduaneh Tarbuz. Sans.—Chaya-pula, Kuttoo wombi. Tam.— Pitchakai. Tel.—Darbuje.

Dilpasand—Dil, heart, and Pasand, to have a liking for. Water melon is taken with great fondness.

Characters.—Fruit sweet. The bitter fruit is C. Amara. Seeds flat, and of a reddish or blackish colour, ovate or oblong, and marked with two small channels running from both sides of the apex downwards about the middle of the seeds. Surface smooth, testa brittle, cotyledons white and oily, and of an almond-like taste. Dose, $\frac{1}{2}$ to 1 dr.

Constituents.—The seeds yield a fixed oil and proteids.

Preparations.—Cold infusion (10 in 10) Dose, 2 to 4 drs.

Actions and uses.—The seeds are nutritive, cooling, diuretic and demulcent, and used in strangury and affections of urinary organs and form an ingredient of tonic confections, given in general debility. The pulp, like vegetable marrow, is cooling and diuretic, and is given in gonorrhœa, hepatic congestion and intestinal catarrh.

There are 5 cucurbitaceous seeds, used as cooling, diuretic and nutritive. These are Citrullus Vulgaris, Tarbuz; cucumis, sativus, cucumber, kâkadi; cucumis citrullus, melon or khurbuz; Lagenaria vulgaris clavata, bottle gourd, or Dudhi; and Benincasa cerifera Koholun.

Cucumis Melo.

Habitat.—Throughout India.

Parts used.—The seeds.

Vernacular.—Arab.—Betika. Bomb.—Kharabuza. Burm.—Tha-khwamwœ. Chin.—Then kwa, Hiang-kwa. Cing.—Rata-komadu. Eng.—Musk melon. Hind.—Kharabuza. Malay.—Labo-frangi. Maleal.—Baka-kaia. Panj.—Gilas, Girasa. Pers.—Kharbuzeh. Tam., Tel.—Mulam.

Characters.—Seeds greyish brown, oblong, or rather ovate, smaller in size than Kâkari bija, acute at the apex with a small circular ridge. At the base testa is tough, cotyledons white ; taste sweet and resembling that of almonds.

Constituents.—Fixed oil, starch, resin and sugar.

Preparations.—Cold infusion (1 in 10). Dose, 2 to 6 drs.

Actions and uses.—Nutrient, demulcent and cooling ; like the other four cucurbitaceous seeds they are used by native Hakims in gonorrhœa and as a cooling diuretic in fevers and general debility.

Cucumis Sativus, C. Utilissimus.

Habitat.—India.

Parts used.—The seeds.

Vernacular.—Arab.—Kusud. Beng.—Kankur Karkti. Burm.—Thkhwassi. Can.—Mullu Kusud. Cing.– Pipingya-Rata Kikari. Duk. —Kankari. Eng.—Cucumber. Guz.—Kakri. Hind.—Kira, Susa. Mar. —Kâkadi. Malyal.—Mullen-velleri. Mal.—Antimun, Timmun. Pers.—Khiyâr. Panj.—Khira. Sans.—Mutrulla Sookasa. Tel.—Dosakaia. Tam.—Mullu Veleri. Velleri Kai. Tel.—Dosa Kala.

Characters.—The seeds are brownish white, linear, oblong, and pointed at both ends, slightly notched at the apex ; testa rough, cotyledons oily and sweet.

Constituents.—Fixed oil, starch, resin and sugar.

Preparations.—Cold infusion (1 in 10). Dose, 2 to 4 drs.

Actions and uses.—Nutritive and demulcent. The seeds resemble in action and uses the five cucurbitaceous seeds.

Cucumis Trigonus, C. Pseudo Colocynthis, C. Pubescens.

Habitat.—India.

Parts used.—The fruit.

Vernaculars.—Arab.—Kiza-ut-taul. Beng.—Kankur, Karkti. Burm.—Tha-khwa. Can.—Hal-mekki. Eng.—Bitter gourd, Squirting cucumber. Hind., Mar.—Pee Ransha, Bislambhi, Katvel, Karit Takmakis. Pers.—Khyar-i-badrang. Sans.—Vishâlâ. Tam.—Bislambi. Tel.—Kodinella.

Characters.—Cucumis Trigonus, the wild form. Fruit smooth, velvety, of the size and shape of a small egg and marked with green or yellow streaks ; ripe fruit sweet. Dose, 2 to 15 grs.

Preparations.—Decoction (1 in 10). Dose, ½ to 1 oz.

Constituents.—Both contain resin similar to that found in colocynth and a bitter crystalline principle.

Actions and uses.—Purgative and diuretic. The fruit pounded and boiled with milk is used in medicine ; other properties are similar to those of colocynth but milder and less irritating.

Ecballium Elaterium, B. P.

Habitat.—S. Europe, N. Asia.

Part used.—A sediment from the juice of the fruit, known as Elaterium B. P.

Vernacular.—Arab.—Khiyar-i-Khar, Katha-el-himar. Eng.—Squirting or wild cucumber, balsam apple. Ind. Bazaars—Kâtr. Indrayani. Ind.—Kitrana. Pers.—Khiyar-i-Khar, Katha-el-himar Katha-el-himar, ass's cucumber ; Khiyar-i-khar, khiarzeh, little cucumber.

Characters.—Fruit an elliptical pepo, pale green, covered with fleshy prickles, 3-celled and containing mucilaginous, watery, bitter juice seeds many, and light brown. Ripe fruit falls from its attachment to the ground when the contents are violently expelled, hence called squirting cucumber. Elaterium.—A substance deposited by the juice ; of the fruit, is in light, friable, flat cakes $\frac{1}{10}$th of an inch thick, pale green or yellowish green, and of a granular fracture. The odour is faint, and tea-like ; taste bitter and acrid ; it should yield from 20 to 25 p. c. of elaterin. Dose, $\frac{1}{10}$ to $\frac{1}{2}$ gr.

Constituents.—A neutral, active, principle. Elaterin B. P. 25 to 33 p. c. ; chlorophyll 10 p. c. ; prophetin, ecballin, hydro-elaterin, and elaterid ; Elaterinum, elaterin B. P.—Elaterin, Momordicin—to obtain it exhaust elaterium with chloroform, add ether, when the crystals of elaterin are deposited ; met with in small hexagonal prisms or scales, without odour and of bitter acrid taste and neutral reaction ; almost entirely insoluble in water, sparingly soluble in hot alcohol (1 in 337), readily so in alkaline solution and in chloroform. Dose, $\frac{1}{40}$ to $\frac{1}{10}$ of a gr.

Preparations.—Pulvis Elaterini compositus, B. P. (1 of elaterin with 39 of milk-sugar. Dose, 1 to 4 grs. Tinctura Elaterii composita. Dose, 10 to 30 ms.

Physiological action.—Elaterium is a most powerful hydragogue cathartic, but is very depressant, and should be used with caution. It has some reputation in malarial fevers. It wards off paroxysms. In large doses it causes prostration, gastro-intestinal irritation with nausea, vomiting, and also acts as an irritant poison.

Therapeutic uses.—Given to produce free watery motions in ascites, anasarca, especially depending upon renal and cardiac disorders, uræmia and congestion of the lungs and brain.

Lagenaria Vulgaris.

Habitat.—Cultivated throughout India.

Parts used.—The seeds and the pulp.

Vernacular.—The bitter variety. Beng.—Kadu, lan. Bomb.—Karava bhopalá. Eng.—White pumpkin, the bitter-bottle gourd. Guz.—Karavi tumbadi. Hind.—Tamra Kaddu, Jangali Kadu, Belas-chora-tumbi. Mal.—Gara-dudi, Labo ambon. Maleal.—Bella Shora.

Mar.—Kadu bhopalá. Sans.—Tikta tumbi. Tam.—Shoriaikai. Tel.—Shora kaia. *The sweet variety.*—Arab.—Charrah. Bomb.—Dudhi. Eng.—Calabash—white pumpkin. Hind.—Mitha Kadu, Dudhi. Mah.—Dudhi. Sans.—Tumbi, Alabu.

Characters.—There are two varieties, sweet and bitter. The bitter fruit varies much in shape and size, and is generally bottle-shaped ; rind, hard and lignous ; fresh pulp, white, spongy and very bitter ; dry pulp, a soft powdery substance; seeds grey, about $\frac{1}{2}$ to $\frac{3}{4}$ of an inch long, and about 3 lines broad at the base ; kernels white and oily on expression ; oil bland and of an olive colour, soon getting rancid. The sweet variety. Fruit bottle-shaped or oblong, rind soft, pulp white spongy, and sweet.

Preparations.—Infusion of seeds (1 in 10). Dose, $\frac{1}{2}$ to 1 fld. oz. The dried pulp of the bitter variety. Dose, 4 to 10 grs.

Actions and uses.—The pulp of karavi tumbadi is emetic and purgative. The oil is used as a cooling and emollient application for the head. The pulp of sweet dudhi is an ingredient in various confections. The seeds are nutritive and diuretic and constitute one of the five cucurbitaceous seeds.

Luffa Amara, L. Fœtida, L. Acutangula.

Habitat.—Throughout India.

Parts used.—The fruit, seeds and root.

Vernacular.—Beng.—Jhingo (L. fœtida) Ghoshá lata Tito-dhundhul. Bomb.—Rana turai. Burm.—Tha-bwat-nha-wai. Can.—Hâre-balli. Duk.—Karvi-turai. Guz.—Kadavi-Hind.—Karvi turai Kurella, Chaul turai (L. fœtida) Maleall Pechingab (L. fœtida). Mar. —Kadavi ghisodi, Kadudorkâ, Kadu-siro-a. Sans.—Kosha taki, Dalika Ghoshaka. Tel.—Adavi-bira, Sendu-bira-kai.

Kosha—the cocoon of a silkworm ; the seeds are enclosed in a fibrous network.

Characters.—Fruit smooth, ovoid and marked with ten prominent ridges, about 4 or 5 inches long with white and spongy pulp ; odour resembling that of kakadi seeds, dark brown in shape and size and resembling Tarabuza bija ; epidermis or testa, highly tubercled and wrinkled.

Preparations.—Infusion of the ripe fruit (1 in 80). Dose, 1 to 2 ozs.

Actions and uses.—Every part of the plant is bitter, tonic and diuretic, and combined with nitro-hydrochloric acid, is given in dropsy and in enlargement of the liver and spleen due to malarial poison. The juice of the leaves is applied to sores and to the bites of venomous animals. The root combined with that of Hibiscus Rosa sinensis root and that of hemidismus indicus, cumin seeds, sugar and milk is given in gonorrhœa. The pulp is emetic and cathartic. The infusion of ripe seeds is used as a purgative and emetic. The dried fruit powdered is used as a snuff in jaundice.

Luffa Echinata, L. Pentandra, L. Patola.

Habitat.—Guzerat, Sind, Bengal.

Parts used.—The fruit and seeds.

Vernacular.—Bomb-Guz.—Deodal Kukadavela, Bindâl, Vaplâ. Burm.—Tha-bwat. Beng.—Dhundhul ghoosal by (L. Pentandra). Can.—Deodal. Dukh.—Gusali turai (L. Pentandra). Hind.—Deodail, Ghia Turai (L. Pentandra) parol. Pers.—Khyar. Tel.—Neli bira. Mar.—Kukadavela, Deodangri. Sans.—Vâpo vrata kosha, Devadale, Garâ-jimuta, Jâlani.

Vâpo—weaving, cocoon-like network in which the seeds are imbedded or interwoven.

Characters.—The fruit, oval, of the size of a large nutmeg, covered with several long, broad based, stiff bristles; colour brownish yellow, three-celled, each being separated from the other by tough, fibrous walls, cell triangular; cell wall consisting of tough fibres, within it, is a soft spongy pulp containing seeds which fall off when the cell dries up; seeds ovate and oblong, compressed of a pale, yellowish colour and marked with tubercles.

Constituents.—The dried fruit, deprived of seeds, contains a principle allied to colocynthitin and a gelatinous principle named luffein. The seeds contain a bland fluid oil.

Preparation.—Infusion and decoction (1 in 20). Dose, ½ to 1 oz.

Actions and uses.—Emetic and purgative; also abortifacient; given in bilious fevers, colic and jaundice; also for snake bites and in cholera. In putrid fever, the infusion is applied to the whole body, and in jaundice to the hepatic region.

Momordica Charantia, M. Muricata, M. Balsamina.

Habitat.—Throughout India.

Parts used.—The fruit, seeds, and leaves.

Vernacular.—Arab.—Karavalla, Kessâul-barri. Beng.—Uchchhell. Duk., Bomb.—Karela. Burm.—Kyet-hen-kha. Chin.—Kukwa Lai-pu-tan. Can.—Kâyi gida. Cing.—Karawila. Eng.—Balsam apple. Guz.—Karelân. Hind.—Karelâ. Maleal.—Pandi-pavel, Kaippa-valli. Mar.—Pavakkâ-cheti Mar. Karli. Pers.—Simahang. Sans.—Sushavi, Karaval-lkandira. Tam.—Poda langkai, Pavakkap Chedi. Tel.—Kâkara.

Characters.—Leaves palmately five-lobed, sinuate, toothed and villous on the under surface. When young, peduncles are slender. Fruit oblong, 10 to 14 inches long, and 2 to 4 inches in diameter; edges curiously notched or ridged, tubercled and of the size of kakadi, taste extremely bitter. In young fruits the pulp over the seeds is whitish, becoming red after a time.

Constituents.—A bitter glucoside, soluble in water, insoluble in ether, a yellow acid, resin, ash 6 p.c.

Preparations.—Juice of leaves. Dose, ½ to 2 drs. Compound ointment, contains powdered fruit, Taja, long pepper and oil of hydnocarpus wightiana.

Action and uses.—Stimulant and alterative; the ointment is applied in psoriasis, scabies and other skin diseases. The fruit pulp and juice of leaves and also seeds are anthelmintic and given in lumbrici. The fruit is also tonic and alterative and given in rheumatism, gout and diseases of the liver and spleen. The whole plant powdered is used for dusting over leprous and other intractable ulcers.

Momordica Cochin Chinensis, Muricia Cochin Chinensis.

Habitat.—Deccan Peninsula, Canara, Bengal.

Parts used.—The seeds.

Vernacular.—Beng.—Gol-kakra. Hind.—Kakrol. Sans.—Karkataka.

Karkataka.—The shell of a crab. The seeds resemble the shell.

Characters.—Flowers cream coloured; fruit large, red and thorny. Pulp yellow, insipid; seeds ½ inch in diameter and ¼ of an inch thick, ovate compressed and black; margins, corrugated; shell fragile, kernel oily. Dose, 5 to 30 grs.

Constituents.—The seeds deprived of the husk contain a greenish oil 43·7 p. c., and a bitter glucoside. The oil possesses very powerful siccative properties.

Preparations.—Confection. Dose, 1 to 2 drs.

Actions and uses.—Demulcent, stimulant and aperient; given in cough and to women immediately after parturition. As an aperient, the seeds are given in hepatic diseases, lumbago, &c., externally applied in procidentia uteri, prolapsus ani, fractures, &c.

Remarks.—It is an ingredient of a hot stuff, known in Bengal as Jhal, and given to women after delivery.

Momordica Dioica.

Habitat.—Throughout India.

Parts used.—The fruit and tuberous root.

Vernacular.—Bomb.—Karatoli. Burm.—Sa-byet. Can.—Madahagala. Cing.—Tumba-karawilla. Mah., Guz.—Kantolan. Hind.—Dhâr-karela. Mar.—Karantali. Mal.—Erima-avel. Sans.—Vâhassa Tam.—Paloo paghel. Tel.—Potu kakara.

Characters.—Fruit ovate, muricated, and somewhat tapering at the base. When ripe, it bursts irregularly showing red or yellow arillus of the seeds; seeds black, shining and almost spherical; tubers of the fresh female plant yellowish, smooth, of the size of a turnip, or even large, and irregular in shape; dry and sliced pieces, resembling those of kolamba. When reduced to powder it becomes yellow; the taste of the fruit as well as of the tuber astringent and bitter. Dose, ½ to 1 dr.

Constituents.—An alkaloid, a fragrant extractive matter, and ash 3·4 p.c. The ash contains a trace of manganese.

Preparations.—Electuary of tuberous root. Dose, 1 to 2 drs.

Actions and uses.—Stimulant and astringent; locally the powdered root with cocoanut, pepper, and red sandal wood is applied to the head in headache and to the skin to render it soft and supple and to lessen sweat; the electuary is given in bleeding piles.

Momordica Umbellata, Zehneria Umbellata.

Habitat.—Throughout India.

Parts used.—The leaves, fruit and root.

Vernacular.—Beng.—Kudari. Goa.—Popinho do Patare. Hind.—Tarali. Mar.—Gometta. Malabar.—Gomth Karwi-valli. Sans.—Gumthi. Tel.—Tid-däuda.

Characters.—Common on hedges; leaves short, petioled, cordate, or sagittate, palmately, lobed, lobes 3 to 5, longer than petiole, 5 partite, sinuate and toothed; root or tubers brown externally and white within, of a faint nauseous odour. Berries oval oblong, of the size of pigeons' eggs, smooth and red when ripe.

Preparations.—Confection of powdered root. Dose, 1 to 2 drs. Powder. Dose, 3 to 10 grs.

Actions and use.—Stimulant and demulcent. The juice of the leaves is used as a soothing application to the skin, inflamed by the application of bhilamo. The root is stimulant and invigorating. In confections it is generally combined with onions, cumin, sugar and butter. It is also given in gonorrhœa and dysuria.

Mukia Scabrella.

Habitat.—Throughout India.

Parts used.—The plant in fruit.

Vernacular.—Hind.—Agamaki. Mal.—Mucca-piri. Mar.—Chirati. Sans.—Ahilaykum, Ghantali. Tam.—Mosum-daki, Mosumuski. Tel.—Puten-budinga, Nûdhosa.

Ahilaykum, a corruption of ahilakhâna, meaning marked like snake. The fruit being marked with vertical white stripes. Ghantali—Ghant, a bell. It means a row or string of bells as worn by dancing girls having vertical slits like vertical stripes on the fruit.

Characters.—Fruit marked with vertical white stripes. Plant scabrous; leaves cordate; berries globular, of the size of a pea, when ripe of a scarlet colour and sprinkled with few bristly hairs. Plant and fruit are bitter.

Preparations.—Infusion (1 in 20). Dose, 1 to 2 ozs.

Actions and uses.—Aperient and stomachic, given in dyspepsia, especially to children.

Trichosanthes Cucumerina, T. Dioica, T. Cordata.

Habitat.—Northern India, Guzerat to Assam, Bengal, Ceylon.

Parts used.—The plant in fruit.

Vernacular.—Beng.—Patel. Bomb.—Kadu padavala. Burm—Tha-b'hot-kha, Tópelen-moye. Chin.—Ko-lau, Kwa-lau. Can.—Bettada-padaval. Cingh.—Dumma-ala. Eng.—Bitter Gourd. Guz.—Jangali parula, parwar. Maleal.—Podavalam. Hind.—Jangli Chichôndâ, Chuchinga. Mal.—Kaippam-patolam. Mar.—Karuparval. Punj.—Gwal-kakri. Sans.—Patolaka. Tam.—Pudal, Kattup-pepudal. Tel.—Patola, Adavi Pottâ.

Characters.—Plant fœtid, leaves harsh, broad, sinuate, or cordate; five lobed and serrated; upper surface downy, tendrils bifid; flowers white and fringed; fruit oblong, acute, or pointed at both ends, 3 to 6 inches long, glaucous, of a greenish white colour and marked with irregular, longitudinal stripes; stem rather quadrangular, twining and striated, sometimes woolly and scabrous. Fruit, 2 to 3 inches long, oblong, acute and red; seeds, minute, compressed and corrugate on the margin.

Preparations.—A compound decoction (1 in 20)—contains Patola 5, Ratanjali 4, Kadu 5, Galo 4, Jethi madha 5, Vinevela 5, Pashana bheda 5, and Water 100. Make decoction. Dose, 1 to 2 ounces, or Patola, cyperus, chiretta, neem bark, catechu, oldenlandia, root bark of adhatoda equal parts, water 1 oz. Dose, 1 to 2 ozs. Extract—Dose, 3 to 5 grs.

Actions and uses.—The unripe fruit is laxative, hydragogue, alterative and antiperiodic; the tender shoots and capsules are bitter, stomachic and laxative. The seeds are stomachic and anthelmintic and given in disorders of the stomach. As an alterative, the decoction is given in syphilis, rheumatism, fever and general weakness. The extract is a powerful and safe cathartic, and recommended as a substitute for elaterium. The natives use it in leprosy, and as a febrifuge and general tonic. In chronic fevers it is given in combination with aromatics and bitters.

Trichosanthes Palmata.

Habitat.—India.

Parts used.—The fruit and stem.

Vernacular.—Arab.—Anbaghôl. Beng.—Makal. Bomb.—Kaundal. Can.—Avagude-hannu. Cing.—Titta-hondala. Duk.—Gudá-pandû. Hind.—Kaundala. Lal Indrayan. Mal.—Kekapelam. Mar.—Kaundal. Pers.—Hanzal-e-surkh. Sans.—Mahákâla. Tam.—Shavari pauham. Tel.—Avvagûda-pandu.

Kondala means a circle, pendant or an ear-ring, and the plant is so named in allusion to the shape of the fruit, which is like Lulaka or kundal and used by Dukhnee Hindus as a pendant for their God Ganesh or Ganpaty.

Characters.—Fresh fruit round, oval or pyriform and resembling a small apple or orange; pulp like cow-dung and of a dull orange colour; fruit dry, shell thin, brittle, and very bitter; seeds and pulp lie loose, so that the contents when shaken produce a rattling sound; seeds blackish, flat, irregular and generally triangular; kernel sweet and oily.

Constituents.—The rind and pulp contain an amorphous, bitter principle, trichosanthin, resembling colocynthin. It is soluble in water, alcohol and slightly so in ether. The green pulp in the interior of the fruit contains a colouring matter.

Preparations.—Medicated oil contains fruit mixed with warm cocoanut oil. Decoction or infusion of root (1 in 20). Dose ½ to 1 fld. oz.

Actions and uses.—Tonic and stimulant. The oil is dropped into the ear in otorrhœa, into the nose in ozœna and for other fœtid discharges. The natives sometimes smoke the rind of the pounded fruit in asthma and use as a fumigatory in ozœna and other discharges from the nose: a paste of the root with colocynth root is applied to carbuncles. In gonorrhœa it is given with triphla and turmeric. The root is reputed to be a tonic similar to calumba.

Zanonia Indica.

Habitat.—Assam, Bengal, Ceylon, Malabar Coast.

Parts used.—The leaves.

Vernacular.—Eng.—Bandolier fruit. Hind, Mar.—Chripota Mal.—Penar-valli. Sans.—Chirpota, Dirgh patra, Kuntali, Tiktaka, Pindavalli.

Characters.—Leaves 6 inches long, 3 inches broad, and acute; petiole 1 inch; fruit three-celled, each cell containing two seeds—seeds compressed and minute.

Actions and uses.—Anodyne; leaves beaten with milk and butter are used as an application to quiet nervous irritation of boils, sciatica, and to the chest in cough and asthma.

Datiscaceæ. Datisca or Akalbar family.

Herbs or trees; leaves alternate, ex-stipulate; flowers declinous; fruit dry, opening at the apex; seeds numerous, minute, without albumen.

Habitat.—Widely distributed over the globe.

Properties.—Some are bitter and purgative, and others are used for their fibres.

Datisca Cannabina.

Habitat.—Himalaya, Nepal, Sind.

Parts used.—The herb and root.

Vernacular.—Hind.—Akalbâr. Punj.—Bayr-bunja, Bhang-jala.

Characters.—Stems stout and branching ; leaves pinnate, flowers simple, pedicles with linear bracts ; anthers oblong, filaments short ; capsule one-celled, open at the apex ; seeds numerous and striated. Dose, 5 to 15 grs.

Constituents.—A glucoside datiscin ; a resin and a bitter principle. To obtain datiscin, exhaust the herb with alcohol, and evaporate. Add water to the residue, to precipitate the resin, decant the fluid and evaporate. Occurs as colourless, silky needles or scales ; taste bitter, of neutral reaction ; soluble in cold water, sparingly soluble in warm water and ether.

Preparations.—Infusion (1 in 10). Dose, ½ to 1 oz.

Actions and uses.—Bitter, stomachic, alterative, expectorant and laxative ; given in scrofula, intermittent fever with vomiting and in catarrh of the throat and bronchi. As a local sedative the bruised leaves are applied to the head in headache.

Cactaceæ—The Indian Fig family.

Succulent plants, usually spiny and leafless ; stems globular, columnar, flattened or 3 or more angled ; flowers sometimes showy, sessile. Fruits succulent ; seeds numerous, parietal or embedded in the pulp without albumen.

Habitat.—The Tropics.

Fruits of some species are acid, and agreeable, and others are used as food for cattle.

Anhalonium A. Williamsii.

Habitat.—West Indies.

Parts used.—The flowers and stems.

Characters.—Stems stout and branching, flowers simple, with short filaments, anthers oblong.

Constituents.—An alkaloid pellotine, yielding salts with acids. Pellotine Hydrochloride. Dose, ⅓ to 1 gr. ; and Mezcaline, another alkaloid.

Action and uses.—Pellotine is hypnotic and analgesic, and used as hypodermic injection to procure sleep and to relieve pain of locomotor ataxia, neuritis, &c.

Cactus Indicus, Opuntia Dillenii.

Habitat.—India, South of Europe, America, Punjab.

Parts used.—The fruit, flowers and stems.

Vernacular.—Hind., Duk.—Chappal send. Beng.—Nâgphunee. Can.—Kattali-papas. Cing.—Kodu-gaha. Eng.—Prickly pear. Maleal.—Naga Mulla. Mar.—Vilayati Nevarung. Panj.—Kabuli-tsui, Kangi-chii. Portuguese.—Palmatoria d'inferno. Sans.—Vidara-Vuhra-sâreka. Tam.—Nâga-kali. Tel.—Nagadali. Palmatoria d'inferno means punishment on the palm of the hand, the flat branches resembling flat pieces of wood used at school to beat children upon the palm of their hand.

Characters.—A plant on which cactus insects thrive and multiply abundantly.

Constituents.—Soluble malate of manganese, a fluid fatty acid, a trace of citric acid and wax, resinous matter, sugar &c.

Preparations—Syrup (1 in 10). Dose, 1 to 4 fld. drs.

Actions and uses.—Antispasmodic, expectorant and alterative; given in whooping cough, asthma and bronchial catarrh; also in hepatic congestion.

Ficoidæ.

Ice plant, Fig-marigold, or the Satodo family.

Plants generally succulent. Herbs or shrubs with opposite or alternate and stipulate leaves. Flowers small. Fruits, capsular or indehiscent, many-celled. Seeds, few or numerous with a curved or spiral embryo. Albumen mealy.

Habitat.—The Tropics.

Properties.—Some plants are edible, others yield an abundance of Khâr when burnt, roots of some are cathartic.

Gisekia Pharnaceoides.

Habitat.—The Punjab, Sind, Ceylon.

Parts used.—The plant.

Vernacular.—Cing.—Et-eilla-pala. Beng. Hind. Duk.—Bâluki. Mar.—Valuchi. Sans.—Bâlu, Voôlukâ, Elavâluka. Tam.—Manalikire. Tel.—Esuka dantikura.

Valuka, Bâluka means sand or sandy, in allusion to the number of large raphides contained in the leaves and which give them the appearance of being full of sand.

Characters.—Leaves opposite, fleshy, oblong or elliptical, narrowed at the base; carpels 5; seeds blackish, smooth, minutely glandular and punctate; embryo curved. Dose of the plant, 1 oz.

Constituents.—The seeds contain tannin-like principles, provisionally named Alpha Gisekia, and Beta Gisekia, both having probably anthelmintic properties.

Preparation.—Draught made by grinding the plant in a mortar with water.

Actions and uses.—Aperient and anthelmintic, given in tænia.

Mollugo Stricta, M. Spergula.

Habitat.—India.

Parts used.—The plant.

Vernacular.—Beng.—Ghimshak. Burm.—Gyen-ga. Can.—Parpaehtaka. Duk.—Hazandanah. Hind.—Jim, Jani. Mar.—Jharasi. Maleal.—Kaipa Jira. Sans.—Grishma-Sundaraka, Phanija. Tam.—Parpadagum. Tel.—Parpataka.

Characters.—Stem glabrous, branching and leafy ; leaves whorled opposite, lanceolate, elliptical, acute, much narrowed at the base ; cymes compound ; capsules globose ; seeds many, covered with tubercles and short bristles, dark chestnut coloured ; embryo curled. The dried herb during the process of combustion deflagrates owing to the presence of alkaline nitrates.

Constituents.—A bitter principle, a bitter resin, gum, ash 68 p.c. containing alkaline nitrates

Preparation.—Tinctura (1 in 10). Dose, ½ to 1 dr.

Actions and uses.—Stomachic, uterine stimulant, and aperient ; given to promote menses and lochia ; the juice made warm is dropped into the ear in earache ; also applied to itch and other skin diseases with relief.

Araliaceæ, the Ivy Family.

Trees, shrubs or herbs ; leaves alternate without stipules. Flowers perfect, rarely unisexual. Inflorescence in umbels or capitate. Fruit 3 or more celled, dry and succulent. Seeds pendulous, albumen fleshy,

Habitat.—Found universally.

Properties.—Stimulant, aromatic, diaphoretic and tonic. They are not poisonous.

Aralia Guilfoylia.

Habitat.—India.

Parts used.—The leaves.

Vernacular.—Tâpmari. Tâp, fever, and mari to kill. The drug is supposed to be a fever killer.

Characters.—Leaves alternate, exstipulate, when crushed they have a strong odour of ivy or fenugreek. Root fusiform with a rounded head externally, closely annulate and wrinkled ; on section brownish yellow, or white, and breaking with a mealy fracture ; odour faintly sweet ; taste slightly aromatic.

Constituents.—The leaves contain an alkaloid, two odorous principles, one of which is of the odour of fenugreek, resin and sugar, and ash 15·2 p. c. containing alkaline salts.

Preparations.—Syrup of the leaves (1 in 10). Dose, ½ to 2 fluid drs. Decoction or infusion (1 in 20). Dose, 2 to 6 drs.

Actions and uses.—Stimulant, stomachic tonic and febrifuge. The syrup is given in cough, seminal debility, and to reduce heat of skin in fevers. Also given in dyspepsia and vomiting.

Panax Pseudo Ginseng, P. Quinquifolium.

Habitat.—Nepaul.

Parts used.—The root.

Characters.—The stalks glabrous, straight, single, and terminating in 3 leaves, each composed of 6 uneven leaflets, and toothed at the edges. Flowers in an umbel ; berries kidney-shaped, compressed ; seeds, semi-circular. The root is of the thickness of a finger like that of parsley. Externally brownish yellow and white within, 2 or 3 inches long, wrinkled and often divided into two branches, rarely into 3 or 4, presenting a slight resemblance to a human form, hence the Chinese name. The parenchyma is horny and compact, with some resinous points. Odour sweet, somewhat aromatic, Taste saccharine like that of liquorice, subsequently becoming bitter.

Constituents.—Starch, gum, albumen, resin, and a sweet principle—Panaquelon.

Preparations.—Tincture (1 in 10). Dose, ½ to 1 dr. Infusion, 1 in 20. Dose, ½ to 1 oz.

Actions and uses.—It is regarded as a powerful restorative, stimulant and aphrodisiac, given in cough, seminal debility and fevers.

Cornaceæ—The Dogwood order.

Shrubs, trees, or rarely herbs. Leaves simple, opposite, rarely alternate, exstipulate. Flowers perfect, arranged in heads, corymbose or umbellate ; calyx superior, 4-lobed ; stamens 4 ; ovary inferior, 2 celled ; ovule, pendulous, solitary ; style and stigma simple. Fruit a drupe crowned with the remains of the calyx. Seed solitary, pendulous. Embryo, fleshy, albuminous ; cotyledons large and leafy.

Native of temperate parts of Europe, Asia and America.

Properties.—Tonic, febrifuge and astringent.

Cornus Florida.

Flowering Cornet, Boxwood, Dogwood.—C. Sericea, Swamp Dogwood.—C. Circinata, Round-leaved Dogwood.

Habitat.—Sutlej Valley, Punjab, N. America.

Parts used.—The inner bark of the root.

Vernacular.—Hind.—Kandar, Kaksh. Panj.—Kasir, Kagshi Haleo, Harin, Hadu, Mang.

Characters.—Bark deprived of the corky layer, in curved pieces of various sizes, about one-eighth of an inch thick, of a pale reddish colour, striated, transverse and with a short longitudinal fracture ; taste astringent and bitter. Dose, in powder, 15 to 60 grains.

Constituents.—Cornin, or cornic acid, tannin, 3 p. c. and resin, Cornin, a bitter, crystallisable active principle, soluble in water and alcohol. Heat destroys the active principle and hence the decoction is useless.

Preparations.—Solid extract. Dose, 2 to 8 grs. Fluid extract, 10 to 60 ms.

Actions and uses.—Bitter tonic, antiperiodic ; given in fevers as a substitute for calumba or Peruvian bark. As a stomachic bitter given in debility, neuralgia, dyspepsia and during convalescence from many acute diseases. As an astringent, used in leucorrhœa, chronic diarrhœa and dysentery. The twigs are dentifrice and used to rub the teeth.

Alangiaceæ.—The Alangium or the Ankola Family.

Trees or shrubs, leaves alternate, entire and exstipulate, without dots ; calyx, superior, 5-10 ; petals, 5-10 linear reflexed ; stamens twice or four times the number of petals, and toothed ; ovary inferior, 1-2-celled ; ovules solitary pendulous ; fruit drupaceous and 1-celled ; seeds solitary ; albumen fleshy ; cotyledons, large, flat and leafy.

Habitat.—Native of East Indies and United States.

Properties.—Some species are purgative and aromatic. Fruit succulent and edible. The fruit of Nyssa Capitata is succulent and used as a substitute for lime fruit and hence it is called ogechee lime.

Alangium Lamarckii. A. Hexapetalum. A. Tomentosum.

Habitat.—Throughout India, Khassya Hills, Ceylon and Gujerat.

Parts used.—The roots, bark, seeds and leaves.

Vernacular.—Beng.—Bâgh-ankrâ, Dhalâ-kura. Burm.—To-sh-on-bin. Can.—Anisaruli-mara, Ecpaata. Cing.—Ecpaatta. Guz.—Duk.—Dhera, Akola. Eng.—Sage leaved alangium. Hind.—Akola, Akarkanta. Mar.—Ankulo. Malyal.—Kara angolam. Sans.—Ankolamu, Ankotha, Gupta Sneha, Niko-chaka, Ankota. Tam.—Allangi. Tel.—Uduga.

Characters.—Wood heavy, close grained, of an oily appearance. Bark of a yellow or whitish brown colour, corky, and covered with circular warts ; taste nauseous and bitter, odour nauseous ; leaves alternate, narrow, oblong or ovate, lanceolate, of a green or darkish green colour, 3-nerved, persistent at the base. Fruit, a berry ; seeds, oblong, albumen ruminate ; cotyledons leafy and crumpled. Dose, 3 to 10 grs.; as an emetic 30 to 60 grs.

Constituents.—Non-crystallizable, bitter alkaloid, alangine.

Preparations.—Decoction of the root bark (1 in 10). Dose, $\frac{1}{2}$ to 1 fld. oz. Medicated oil and paste of the root.

Actions and uses.—The leaves are used as a poultice to relieve rheumatic pains, and the medicated oil is applied to indolent ulcers. The decoction is given internally in pyrexia, as an alterative in chronic skin diseases, syphilis and leprosy ; the powdered root bark is a safe emetic and a good substitute for ipecacuanha.

Caprifoliaceæ.

The Honey-suckle family. Caper, a goat, and folium a leaf. The plant has a climbing or capering habit (tendency) like a goat. Shrubs or rarely herbs, leaves opposite and exstipulate. Flowers corymbose, showy, sweet scented. Calyx 4-5 superior ; ovary, usually 3-celled, inferior. Fruit indehiscent, succulent or dry, berry or a drupe ; seeds solitary, or numerous ; albumen fleshy.

Habitate.—Native of temperate climate.

Properties.—Some species are emetic, purgative ; others astringent, diuretic, sudorific or acrid, and a few again are poisonous.

Sambucus Nigra, B. P., S. Canadensis.

Habitat.—Europe and Western Asia. N. America.

Parts used.—The flowers, elder flowers, Sambuci flores, B.P., berries and bark.

Characters.—Flowers small ; calyx, 5-toothed, superior ; corolla flat rotate, of a cream white colour, also 5-lobed with five stamens inserted in the tube ; anthers yellow ; odour peculiar, sweet, faint and agreeable ; taste bitter and aromatic. Fruit indehiscent ; seeds solitary. Dose, 30 grs.

Constituents.—Flowers contain volatile oil, ½ p.c. Resin, fat, mucilage, valerianic acid, wax, sugar and tannin. The volatile oil is a yellowish, limpid liquid of butyraceous consistence, of a strong odour and warm bitter taste. The bark contains valerianic (viburnic) acid, potassium and calcium malates, &c.

Preparations.—Aqua Sumbuci, B.P. (flowers 1 in water 5 to distil down to one-fifth). Dose, 1 to 2 fld. ozs.

Decoction of bark (1 in 5). Dose, 2 to 4 fld. ozs. Poultices, ointment of flowers. Wine (Elder. wine).

Actions and uses.—Stimulant, carminative, diaphoretic diuretic and laxative ; used locally in rheumatism to relieve local pains, in burns and scalds, for blisters, hæmorrhoids, abscesses, &c. The bark is a hydragogue cathartic, emetic and given in dropsy, rheumatism, syphilis, &c. The berries are diaphoretic and laxative. The juice of the berries is given in rheumatism and syphilis.

Viburnum Fætidum.

Habitat.—Western India, Burmah.

Parts used.—The leaves and the plant.

Vernacular.—Bomb.—Narvela. Can.—Naruval. Sans.—Shirparna, Jaya.

Characters.—Leaves usually ovate, lanceolate and serrated, colour darkish green. Flowers greenish white. Berries small, ovoid and of a red colour. All parts of the plant emit a peculiarly fœtid odour.

Constituents.—A fœtid volatile oil and an alkaloid, gum resin and ash, 12 p.c. The oil is the odorous principle, in white, greasy flakes. The fœtor can be removed by distillation. The alkaloid is a whitish powder of a peculiar sharp taste, soluble in alcohol and chloroform, slightly so in ether and water.

Preparations.—The juice of the leaves. Dose, 4 to 8 fld. drs. Decoction of the plant (1 in 18). Dose 4 to 8 drs.

Actions and uses.—Uterine astringent and sedative, given in menorrhagia, post partum hæmorrhage and in threatened abortion; also in dysmenorrhœa and after pains.

Hindu women during confinement hang a branch of the plant over their door, to prevent demons from causing illness.

Viburuum Opulus—Cramp Bark.

High cranberry, guelder rose, squaw bush, whitten tree. Cramp bark, socalled as the bark relieves cramps.

Viburuum Prunifolium.

Sweet viburuum, stag bush, blackhaw.

Habitat.—United States.

Parts used.—The bark of the stem and root.

Characters.—The bark in flat thin curved bands, with transverse brownish warts and longitudinal black lines or thin ridges. Internally brownish red, and of a tough fracture—without any odour and bitter astringent taste. Dose, 20 to 60 drs.

Constituents.—Viburnin, viburnic acid, identical with valerianic acid, sugar, tannin, oxalic, citric and malic acids, earthy chlorides, sulphates, phosphates and ash, 8 to 9 p.c. Viburnin.—Bitter principle is a greenish yellow or whitish powder, resinous, soluble in alcohol, sparingly so in water.

Preparations.—Fluid extract. Dose, 15 to 60 ms. Extract. Dose, ½ to 10 grs. Decoction Viburni and Infusum Viburni (1 in 10). Dose, ½ to 1 fld. oz.

Celerina is a speciality said to contain Viburnum, celery, cocoa and kola. Used as a nervine tonic, given to promote corpulence. Malto Viburnin, a combination of viburnum and extract of malt. Dose, 1 to 4 drs.

Actions and uses.—Bitter, nervine tonic, antispasmodic and astringent. As a powerful uterine sedative it is used to check uterine hæmorrhages, and to prevent threatened abortion. In spasmodic dysmenorrhœa, in uterine or ovarian irritations, in subinvolution and even in vomiting of pregnancy it is given with cannabis, morphine and other nervine sedatives or aromatics, with benefit. As a sedative it is given in neurotic condition, as hysteria and in asthma. In large doses it excites nausea and vomiting.

Rubiaceæ—The Majitha or Madder Family.

Herbs, shrubs or trees; leaves opposite, entire, whorled, having inter petioler stipules. Flowers white, blue, pink, red or yellow. Fruit berry, capsular, drupaceous, dry or succulent, inferior, edible, 2 to 10 celled; seed one or more in each cell; albumen horny or fleshy.

Habitat.—Native of temperate climate and tropics.

Properties.—Many species are tonic, febrifuge, astringent, emetic and purgative; also diuretic and emmenagogue; some are dyeing and tanning agents, others are intoxicating and in rare cases even poisonous.

Adina Cordifolia.

Habitat.—Throughout the hilly parts of India.

Parts used.—The bark.

Vernacular.—Beng.—Keli-Kadam. Can.—Hedde, Yet-tega. Hind.—Haldu. Mar.—Hedu. Sans.—Dhâra-Kadûmba. Tam.—Manja-Kaambe. Tel.—Dudagu.

Characters.—Bark in thick curved pieces, dirty white externally. Inner surface reddish-brown and fibrous. Taste bitter and astringent.

Constituents.—Cincho-tannic acid, a red oxidized product, a bitter principle, starch, and calcium oxalate.

Preparations.—Decoction (1 in 10). Dose, 1 to 2 fld. ozs.

Actions and uses.—Bitter tonic and febrifuge. Like cinchona it is used in fevers, dyspepsia, anorexia.

Anthocephalus Cadamba—Wild Cinchona.

Habitat.—Himalaya, Ceylon, Darjeeling, Terai.

Parts used.—The fruit and bark.

Vernacular.—Beng., Hind.—Kadamb. Can.—Cadavâla mara. Sans.—Kadamba, Halipriya, Sisupâla. Tam.—Vella Kadamba. Tel.—Kadambe.

Sisupâla, protecting children. Hali-priya, dear to agriculturists.

Characters.—Flowers, night scented; flower heads large, globular and lemon coloured; fruit about the size of an orange, edible; bark in thick flat pieces, externally grey and studded with small corky lenticels, inner surface red and fibrous; taste bitter and astringent. Dose of the bark 10 to 20 grs.

Preparations.—Decoction of the bark (1 in 10). Dose, 1 to 2 fld. ozs.

Actions and uses.—Tonic. The juice is given to children with cumin and sugar in gastric irritability. The fruit is cooling, refrigerant and febrifuge, and given in fever with great thirst.

Canthium Parviflorum, C. Umbellatum, C. Didymum, C. Cymosum.

Habitat.—W. Peninsula, Ceylon.

Parts used.—The shrub.

Vernacular.—Cing.—Poruwa. Hind.—Ursool. Malyal.—Kanden, Khara. Mar.—Varsangi, Ursool. Tam.—Karai cheddi, Nella Balsu. Tel.—Ballusoo Rura, Naum papal.

Characters.—A small thorny shrub. Leaves opposite, ovate and attached to young shoots ; flowers small and yellow ; fruit with 2 seeds, obovate,compressed, a drupe,colour reddish-brown, of the size of a horse bean ; nut 2-celled. The leaves and seeds smell like coriander. The fruit has a sweet taste.

Preparation.—Decoction of leaves and root (1 in 20). Dose, ½ to 1 fld. oz.

Actions and uses.—Astringent, given in dysentery, diarrhœa, and leucorrhœa. The root is anthelmintic ; and given to expel worms.

Coffea Arabica, B. P.

Habitat.—Tropical Africa, Abyssinia, S. E. Asia, South Arabia, E. and W. Indies, Assam, Nepaul, Khassya hills.

Parts used.—The seeds.

Vernacular.—Arab.—Bûn, Kahwa. Bom.—Boon. Eng.—Coffee caffea Hind.—Coffee, Kawa. Ind. Bazaar.—Kahvah. Maleal.—Kawa. Tam.—Capie cottay.

Seeds large, solitary, rounded on the back, and flat on the ventral surface, where there is a deep narrow fissure, oval, longitudinally grooved upon the flat side, albumen is horny, the colour yellowish or greenish. Raw coffee has a faint odour and a sweetish astringent bitter taste. When roasted part of the caffeic acid is converted into methylamin, the sugar is changed into caramel, and several volatile substances are formed known as Caffeone to which the aroma is due. Dose, 30 to 60 grs.

Constituents.—Seeds contain an alkaloid, caffeine, 1 to 3 p.c. ; proteid 6 to 13 p.c. ; sugar, legumin, glucose, dextrine 15 p.c. ; caffeo-tannic acid 1 to 2 p.c. ; volatile oil and ash, 3 to 5 p.c. Caffeine B. P. is identical with Theine guaranine, Methyl-Theobomine, or Trimethylxanthine. To obtain caffeine, add acetate of lead to the infusion, filter, add sulphuretted hydrogen to decompose excess of acetate of lead and neutralize with ammonia.

Caffeine is found in various substances besides coffee. These are dried leaves of camelia thea, pulp or seeds of paullinia sorbilis (guarana), the leaves and twigs of Ilex paraguayensis, kola nuts, the seeds of sterculia acuminata, and cocoa.

Caffeine is in colourless, silky acicular crystals without odour and bitter taste, neutral reaction ; soluble in cold water (1 in 80) easily soluble in boiling water, alcohol or chloroform, sparingly soluble in ether ; given in solution or pill. Dose, 1 to 5 grs.

Preparations of Caffeine.—Caffeinœ citras, B. P., a white powder, without any odour and of faintly bitter taste and acid reaction, soluble in water (1 in 32) and also in a mixture of chloroform alcohol (2 to 1). Dose, 2 to 10 grs. Caffeinæ citras effervescens, B. P. 4 p.c. Dose, 60 to 120 grs.

Caffeine Hydrobromide and C̈. Hydrochloride—Occur in glass-like crystals, becoming greenish or reddish on exposure to air ; soluble in water (1 in 50). Decompose by keeping. Dose, ½ to 5 grs.

Bromo Caffeine.—A proprietary preparation often confounded with caffeine hydrobromate.

Caffeine Chloral.—A compound ot caffeine and chloral. Occurs in small white granules or colourless shining scales of the acrid taste of chloral, soluble in water. Dose, 3 to 8 grs. A nice analgesic and laxative used hypodermically in sciatica and rheumatism.

Iodo Caffeine or Sodium Caffeine Iodide. Contains 65 p.c. of caffeine. A white powder without any odour or taste, sparingly soluble in water. Dose, 2 to 10 grs. A good diuretic given in dropsy and pleurisy with effusion. Does not affect or disorder respiration or digestion.

Caffeine sodio benzoate, caffeine sodio cinnamate and caffeine sodio Salicylate—Prepared by dissolving caffeine in solution of sodium benzoate or sodium cinnamate, or sodium salicylate respectively, these act like digitalis but more rapidly. Dose, 1 to 4 grs.

Chloro Caffeine—One atom of chlorine introduced into the caffeine molecule ; diuretic and cerebral stimulant, given in nervous affections.

Caffeine Sulphas—A crystalline powder slightly soluble in water. Dose, ½ to 5 grs. Caffeine Valerianas. Dose, ½ to 3 grs. Hypodermic tablets given in hysterical vomiting.

Physiological action.—Cerebro spinal, gastric and renal stimulant laxative, highly antiseptic, efficient diuretic and antilithic. Roasted coffee if moderately taken as a food or beverage acts as a stimulant, it assists assimilation and digestion, promotes intestinal paristalsis, lessens tissue waste and decreases the excretion of urea. It allays the sense of prolonged bodily and mental fatigue and keeps off sleep for some time without exhaustion. It increases the reflex action and mental activity. Given in excess it disorders digestion and leads to headache, vertigo and palpitation of the heart, great restlessness, convulsions and paralysis. Coffee is more stimulating, but less sustaining than cocoa.

Therapeutic uses.—Coffee is given in prolonged bodily fatigue, and in mental and cardiac depression ; as an analgesic it is given with guarana in neuralgic and nervous headache, in insomnia of chronic alcoholism, to stop vomiting, to check diarrhœa and to allay spasms in asthma ; also given in cases of narcotic poisoning. In heart disease caffein is given with paraldehyde, with benefit.

Cinchona Succirubra B. P.

Habitat.—Slopes of Chimborazo, S. America, S. India, Sikkim and Ceylon.

Part used.—The dried branch of the stem and branches. Cinchonæ Rubræ cortex, Red Cinchona Bark, B.P.

Cinchona was first introduced into Europe from Peru, America, by the Jesuit missionaries, hence known as Jesuit's bark, Peruvian bark ; also called Countess's powder from a countess of Cinchon, the wife of a viceroy of the colony of Peru, having been cured of fever by this bark.

Succi Rubra, succus, juice, and ruber, red. The sap is colourless at first, on exposure it becomes white and finally red.

Characters.—Occurs in quills or in curved pieces coated with periderm. It varies in length from 2 inches to a foot or more, in thickness from 2 lines to ¼ of an inch, coluor reddish-brown or brownish; epidermis rough with longitudinal ridges and warty. Inner surface brick red or deep reddish brown and striated, of a fibrous fracture, without odour, and of a bitter astringent taste. Dose, 10 to 60 grs. Contains largest percentage of total alkaloids. It should yield from 5 to 6 p.c. of total alkaloids, of which half should be quinine and cinchonidine. Other varieties are also in use, which are given below.

C. Officinalis.—The pale crown loxa bark, var. condaminea, Bonplandia and Crispa. The original Peruvian bark occurs in quills. It contains ½ to 1½ p.c. of the alkaloid, and a little quantity of quinine.

C. Peruviana, C. Nutida, C. Micrantha—grey or Huanuco bark. It contains from 1½ p.c. to 2 p.c. of the alkaloids, chiefly cinchonine and quinidine.

C. Calisaya, C. Ledgeriana. Calisaya bark, quinine bark. Native of Sikkim, exclusively of the Himalayas, Southern India, Bolivia, Peru and Java. The most valuable of all the cultivated varieties of cinchona bark. It occurs in quills and contains 5 p.c. of alkaloids and from 2½ to 4 p.c. of quinine.

C. Lancifolia, and C. Cordifolia, Columbian or Carthagena bark,—A soft bark, occurs in quills or broken pieces with whitish epidermis. It contains mostly cinchonidine and a small quantity of quinidine.

C. Pitayensis—Pitayo bark; occurs in short, curly pieces of a brownish colour, rich in alkaloids, especially quinine and quinidine.

Remjia Pedunculata. Cuprea bark or copper coloured bark. It is not a true cinchona bark. It contains cupreine, cinchonamine, an alkaloid hydro-quinine, 3 p.c., quinine 2 p.c., but no cinchonidine.

Remijia Purdieana. Remija bark contains quinine, quinidine, cinchonine, but no cinchonidine, also an alkaloid cupreine which in combination with quinine is known as homo quinine or ultra quinine.

Constituents.—Alkaloids quinine, quinidine, cinchonine and cinchonidine; quinamine, a crystallizable alkaloid; aricine, also kinic and kinovic acids, kinotannic, and kinovotannic acids, a red colouring principle; starch, volatile oil, gum, sugar, wax, ash 2 to 3 p.c.

Cinchonina—cinchonine—an amorphous feeble alkaloid, isomeric with cinchonidine, having half the activity of quinine. It occurs in white shining prisms or needles, taste bitter, not fluorescent. Insoluble in water. Dose, 1 to 10 grs.

Preparations of cinchonine.—Pulvis cinchoninæ compositus (1 in 5). Cinchona with bicarbonate of sodium and sugar of milk. Dose, 3 to 10 grs Cinchoninæ Hydrochloridum, soluble in water and spirit. Dose, 2 to 10 grs. Cinchoninæ Sulphas, Cinchonine sulphate. Hard, colourless, prismatic crystals, of vitreous lustre, soluble in water (1 in 66). Absolute alcohol (1 in 10), and in dilute acids, sparingly soluble in ether and solution of ammonia. Dose, 2 to 10 grs. Cinchonine iodomercurate, yellow powder, used externally as an antiseptic.

Cinchonidinæ Sulphas. Sulphate cinchonidine. Colourless, acicular, silky. crystals. Taste bitter, soluble in water (1 in 100), sparingly soluble in chloroform and ether and in rectified spirit (1 in 60). Dose, 1 to 10 grs. used like quinine. Cinchonidine Salicylate—tonic and antiperiodic; given in neuralgia, rheumatism, intermittent fever, &c. Dose. 5 grs. in pills or cachets.

Quinidina—Quinidine—White prisms, without any odour, taste nauseous and bitter, almost insoluble in water, soluble in dilute acids, partially soluble in ether and in benzol. Dose, 1 to 20 grs.

Quinidinæ Sulphas—Quinidine Sulphate. Conquinine or conchinin sulphate. An alkaloid obtained from cinchona pitayensis or cinchona caprea. In white acicular crystals like those of quinine sulphate. Soluble in water (1 in 100), in absolute alcohol (1 in 32) freely in dilute acids. Dose, 1 to 20 grs.

Quinquinina—Quinetum—Cinchona febrifuge, contains 50 to 70 p.c. of cinchonidine extracted from red cinchona bark by acidulated water, precipitated by soda and dried. A greyish, white amorphous powder, slightly soluble in water, easily dissolved in dilute acid, and in alcohol (1 in 10). Dose, 1 to 5 grs. Quineti Sulphas—Quinetum sulphate. Closely resembles quinine sulphate. In crystals, soluble in water Dose, 1 to 5 grs.

Quinina—Quinine—obtained from the bark of various species of cinchona and Remijia. It occurs as a white amorphous or minutely crystalline powder, very sparingly soluble in water (1 in 1670), freely soluble in alcohol (1 in 6), in ether, chloroform, benzene, aqueous ammonia and dilute acids. Heated with glycerine it is converted into an isomeric base quinicine. Dose, 1 to 10 grs.

Preparations of Quinine.—Quininæ Arsenas—quinine arsenate, small white crystals, sparingly soluble in water—contains quinine 67 p.c. and arsenic acid 29 p.c. Dose, $\frac{1}{8}$ to $\frac{1}{2}$ gr. Quininæ Bisulphas—Quininæ sulphas acida—neutral quinine or soluble sulphate of quinine. In large, colourless crystals, or small needles, efflorescing and becoming opaque on exposure to the air, without any odour. Has a strong acid reaction, soluble in water (1 in 10). Dose, 1 to 5 grs. As an hypodermic injection 1 gr. in 12 ms. Dose, 4 to 15 ms. Quininæ Carbolas—In crystals—containing quinine 77 p.c., and carbolic acid 23 p.c. Given in diarrhœa. Dose, 2 grs. Quininæ Carbonas—in fine needles, soluble in water. Dose, 1 to 3 grs. Quininæ Chloras—Quinine Chlorate, in acicular crystals, sparingly soluble in water, explodes when heated. Dose, 1 to 5 grs. Quininæ Citras—Quinine Citrate, in acicular crystals of very little taste, sparingly soluble in water (1 in 900), used in pill or powder. Dose, 1 to 5 grains. Quininæ Fluoridum, sparingly soluble in cold water, more freely in hot water. Dose, $\frac{1}{24}$ to $\frac{1}{2}$ gr. In combination with fluoride of ammonium it is used in enlarged spleen due to malaria. Quininæ Hydrobromidum—Quinine Hydrobromide—In colourless lustrous needles, without any odour, of bitter taste and alkaline reaction, soluble in water (1 in 54), produces less cinchonism than quinine. Dose, 1 to 6 grs. Syrupus Ferri et Quininæ Hydrobromatum— Syrupus Ferri Bromidi cum Quinina. Dose, ½ to 1 dr. Syrupus Ferri Quininæ et Strychninæ Hydrobromatum, each dr. contains 1 gr. of quinine hydrobromide. Dose, ½ to 1 dr. Quininæ Hydrobromidum acidum.—Yellowish crystals, freely soluble in water (1 in 6), richer in alkaloids than the quininæ sulphate. Dose, ½ to 2 grs. in tablets ½ gr. each. As hypodermic injection 1 gr. in 6 ms.

Quininæ Hydrochloridum B. P.—Quinine Hydrochlorate, Quinine Muriate—In filiform, silky, white crystals, contains 83 p.c. of quinine against 75 in the quinine sulphate, soluble in water (1 in 35), in cold alcohol (1 in 3), very soluble in boiling water and in boiling alcohol. Dose, 1 to 10 grs. used as solution 1 in 800 as a germicide ; hypodermic injection containing quinine hydrochloride 3, antipyrin 2 and water 10. Dose, 2 to 5 ms. Quinine Hydrochloridum Aceticum—A white crystalline powder, soluble in less than its own weight of water. Dose, 1 to 10 grs. Vinum Quininæ, B. P.—1 gr. quinine hydrochloride to 1 oz. of wine Dose, ½ to 1 oz. Tinctura Quininæ B. P.—1 gr. in 50 of tincture of fresh orange. Dose, ½ to 1 dr. Quininæ Glycero Phosphas—A white powder, soluble in alcohol, slightly soluble in hot water. Containing 68 p.c. of quinine. Dose, 2 to 8 grs.

Quininæ Hydrochloridum Acidum, B. P.—Acid quinine hydrochloride, quinine dihydrochloride. White yellowish crystals soluble in water (1 in 1). Dose, 1 to 10 grs.; used hypodermically ½ to 2 grs. Quininæ Hydrochloro Sulphas—In small needles or reduced to powder ; soluble in water (1 in 1). Contains 74 p.c. of alkaloid. Dose, 1 to 10 grs Injectio Quininæ Hydrochloro Sulphatis Hypodermica, 1 gr. in 4 ms. More suited than the sulphate or the hydrochloride. Dose, 2 to 12 ms. Quininæ Hydrochloro Carbamidum—Urea Quinine—a new compound of quinine and urea, in small prisms, non-irritant. Soluble in water (1 in 1). The solution (50 p.c.) is used as hypodermic injection. Dose, 5 to 15 grs. Quininæ Iodas—Quinine Iodate. White silver needles, soluble in water (1 to 250). Dose, 1 to 5 grs. Quininæ Hydriodum—Quinine Hydr Iodide—Quininæ Iodidum—Quinine Iodide. A neutral salt in pale yellow crystals, sparingly soluble in water. Dose 1 to 5 grs. Quininæ Hydridum Acidum—Quininæ Iodidum Acidum—Acid Quinine Iodide.—An acid salt in large yellow crystals freely soluble in water. Dose, 1 to 4 grs. Syrupus Ferri et Quininæ Iodidi—A saturated solution of quinine 2 grs. in an ounce of syrup of ferrous iodide. Dose, 1 dr. Quininæ Lactas—Quinine Lactate.—A white amorphous powder soluble in water (1 in 10). Dose, 1 to 5 grs. Easy of digestion—used as solution 1 p.c. for hypodermic injection. Quininæ Oleatum (1 to 3). Locally used as inunction in fevers. Quininæ Phosphos—Quinine Phosphate. In acicular crystals. Dose, 1 to 6 grs. Quininæ Salicylas—Quinine Salicylate.—An anhydrous salt, crystallizes in white silky needles, of a bitter taste, sparingly soluble in water (1 in 1225), Ether (1 in 120), Chloroform and rectified spirit (1 in 24), contains 70 p.c. of quinine. Dose 2 to 6 grs. given in pills or in cachets or suspended in water. Quininæ Sulphas B.P. Disulphate Quinine—Quinine Sulphate, In light filiform, silky, white crystals ; taste intensely bitter, soluble in water (1 in 800), alcohol (1 in 65), glycerine (1 in 40), entirely soluble in ammonia and acidulated water—given in solution, pills, powder, or cachets. Dose, as a tonic, 2 to 5 grs., as an antiperiodic 5, to 20 grs. Febricide Pills—containing quinine sulphate, antefebrin, each 2 grs and cocaine hydrochlorate ⅙ grs. Dose, 1 to 2 pills in malaria.

Tinctura Quininæ Ammoniata B.P.—Quinine Sulphate 2, solution of ammonia 10, and alcohol 90, soluble in aerated water—not miscible with plain water. Dose, ½ to 1 dr.

Collunarium Quininæ—Quinine nasal douche—Quinine Sulphate in water (1 in 875).

Mistura Chlori cum Quininæ. Mix potassium chlorate 30 grs. and hydrochloric acid 60 ms., add water 11 ounces. Then add Quinine Sulphate 24 grs. and syrup of orange 1 oz. Dose, 1 oz.

Warburg's Fever Tincture—Tinctura Pyrexialis—contains quinine sulphate (1 in 50), Socotrine Aloes (1 in 40), opium (1 in 4000), rhubarb root (1 in 125), camphor (1 in 500), and saffron and other aromatics. Dose, 1 to 4 drs.

Quininæ Sulphas Acidus—Acid quinine sulphate, neutral or soluble quinine sulphate. In large rectangular prisms or crystalline masses, soluble in cold water (1 in 12). Dose, 1 to 10 grs. Hypodermic injection, 1 gr. in 12 ms. Dose, 4 to 15 ms.

Quininæ Sulpho-carbolas—An amorphous white powder, sparingly soluble in water sometimes known as carbolate of quinine. To obtain it make a combination of quinine sulphate with phenol. In the case of true carbolate of quinine the combination is of quinine alkaloid and phenol. It combines the action of quinine with that of sulphocarbolate—given in diarrhœa and fever. Dose, 1 to 6 grs.

Quininæ Tannas.—A white amorphous powder, sparingly soluble in water, quite tasteless. Dose, 1 to 4 grs.

Quininæ Valerianas.—White pearly lustrous crystals, sparingly soluble in water (1 in 100); boiling water (1 in 40); alcohol (1 in 5) and slightly soluble in ether—odour of valerian. Dose, 1 to 4 grs.

Preparations.—Of the bark. Infusum Cinchonæ Acidum, B.P., red cinchona bark 1 ounce, aromatic sulphuric acid 2 fld drs. ; distilled water 20 fld. ounces. Dose, ½ to 1 fld. oz. Extractum cinchonæ liquidum, B. P. (5 grs. of the total alkaloids in 110 ms.). Dose, 5 to 15 ms. Tinctura Cinchonæ, B. P. (1 in 5) containing 1 p.c. of alkaloids. Dose, ½ to 1 fld. dr. Tinctura Cinchonæ Compositæ, B. P., contains tincture of red cinchona bark 10 ; dried bitter orange peel 1 ; sepentary root ½ ; with cochineal and saffron for 1 pint. Dose, ½ to 1 dr. Decoctum Cinchonæ (1 in 16). Dose, 1 to 2 fld. ozs. Elixir Cinchonæ. Dose, ½ to 1 dr.

Physiological action.—Cinchona is a general tonic, bitter stomachic, astringent, febrifuge and antiperiodic. In small doses it increases appetite, assists digestion, increases the flow of saliva and the gastric juice. It augments the force of heart's action. If continued for a long time, it acts as a gastric irritant, impairs digestion, produces gastric, catarrh and even constipation. In large doses it causes flatulence, eructation, rise of body heat with chill, and fever. Quinine is a bitter tonic, antiseptic, most powerful antiperiodic and antipyretic; also analgesic. In small doses it stimulates the heart and increases the arterial tension. In large doses, it has direct action on the cardiac ganglia, and thus slows the pulse beat, and lowers the arterial tension. It is a protoplasmic poison. It prevents the development of the plasmodium and hence the most important agent in malaria. It is rapidly diffused. In the blood it increases the number of white corpuscles, but prevents or arrests their movements, it lessens oxidation, and in fever it lessens the body heat. It lessens the size of the spleen when enlarged from fever. As an antiseptic it is an active destroyer of low organisms (1 in 500), it destroys fungi, checks fermentation and putrefactive decomposition; it sometimes produces sexual excitement. In the urine it lessens the excretion of uric acid but not of urea. It often acts as an uterine stimulant if long continued and in large doses. It causes quinism or cinchonism, a set of symptoms characterised by fulness and constriction in the head, buzzing in the ears, vertigo, reeling gait, deafness, amblyopia, &c. In excessive doses, it leads to dilated pupils, delirium and even convulsions..

Therapeutics.—Quinine is given in 10 grain doses to bring down fever. It is also given in whooping cough, hay fever, enlargement of liver and spleen, hemicrania, and other localized neurotic pains. In small doses it is given as a tonic in dyspepsia, gastric catarrh, adynamia and convalescence from fevers and in weak and flabby subjects. In remittent fever, large doses of 15 or 25 grs. of quinine may be given once or twice a day. In chronic cases, large doses of chinchonine are safer than quinine. Quinine is also used as antipyretic in typhoid fever, variola, septic fevers pneumonia, acute rheumatism, in acute tonsillitis, acute nasal catarrh, pyæmia and in surgical operations. The indiscriminate use of quinine, if taken regularly and in large doses, for a long time weakens the heart and produces restlessness and cachexia. In obstinate cases of ague with persistent vomiting, in malarial fevers, in irritability of the rectum or where the patient is insensible or cannot swallow and in all cases where it cannot be given by the mouth, hypodermic injection of quinine may be used, generally combined with guaiacol, with benefit. It should be injected deeply into the gluleal or scapular muscles or in the arm. Locally as an antiseptic injection, it is used in cystitis and abscess cavities, as a wash for wounds and ulcers, and as a gargle in sore throat. It is an ingredient in dentifrice. The ill-effects could best be avoided by giving it with diluted hydrobromic acid. Warburg's Tincture is given in remittent and continued fevers, even during the pyrexial period. In severe attacks of influenza, in chronic bronchitis of old age, in asthma, and in phthisis, ½ fld. oz. may be given after any convenient purgative, to be repeated in 3 hours. No food or drink to be given from the first dose to an hour after the second; for ordinary cases 2 fld. drs. may be given for a dose.

Diplospora Sphærocarpa—Wild Coffee.

Habitat.—Western Ghats.

Parts used.—The seeds.

Characters.—Seeds round, flattened and glossy, of a light brown colour. Albumen horny. The roasted powder resembles coffee in aroma.

Constituents.—An alkaloid, an astringent acid, an aromatic body, fat, sugar and mineral matter.

Preparations.—Decoction (1 in 10). Dose 2 to 6 drs.

Actions and uses.—Nervine tonic and stimulant like coffee ; given in low states of the system, in acute fevers, in hemicrania and neuralgias.

Galium Aparine.

Syn.—The plant Cleavers, goose grass (Eng.)

Habitat.—Europe and United States.

Parts used.—The herb and inspissated juice.

Preparations.—Succus Galii—dose 1 to 2 drs. Extractum Galii—dose, 5 to 20 grs.

Actions and uses.—Acid, astringent, alterative and diuretic ; given in dropsy, jaundice, suppression of urine, gravel complaints and skin diseases ; also in scrofula, epilepsy, and obesity. A poultice of the herb is used in obstinate psoriasis. The inspissated juice is locally applied in lepra, eczema, and acne, and to promote healthy granulations in wounds and cancerous ulcers ; also used as a styptic for bleeding wounds.

Gardenia Gummifera. G. Resinifera. G. Arborea and G. Lucida. G. Campanulata, G. Florida.

Habitat.—Western Peninsula, Ceylon, Burma, Chittagong, India.

Parts used.—The resinous exudation from the fruits.

Vernacular.—Arab.—Kala-loxada, Kimk-kham. Burm.—Tsay-tham-by-ah. Can.—Tella-manga, Chinaka-ringuva. Cing., Duk., Guz., Hind., Mar.—Dika-mâle. Sans.—Hingu-nadika, Pindahva. Tam.—Kumbi. Tel.—Chiribikki, Tella-manga.

Characters.—The exudation occurs in masses or irregular flat cakes, opaque, of a dull olive green colour, often mixed with soft bark leaf buds and pieces of stem, &c. The smell is very fœtid like that of cat's urine. Dose, 1 to 2 grs.

Preparations.— Emulsion with water (1 in 50). Dose, 1 to 2 drs., and paste.

Constituents.—Gardenin—a crystalline resin of a gold yellow colour, another resin soft and of a greenish colour.

Actions and uses.—Antiperiodic, cathartic, anthelmintic, alterative, and antispasmodic ; given in intermittent fevers, dyspepsia, flatulence, and chronic skin diseases. A paste of it is applied for cleaning foul ulcers and for the relief of itching in piles. It keeps away flies or maggots from sloughing sores. As an antispasmodic the root of G. Florida is given alone or combined with bharangi in hysteria. As a cathartic and anthelmintic it is given to expel worms.

Hymenodictyon Excelsum. Cinchona Ecelsa.

Habitat.—W. Himalaya, Chittagong, Deccan, C. India, Tenasserim.

Parts used.—The bark.

Vernacular.—Duk., Hind.—Bhaulan, Kàlâbachnak. Mar.—Kálâkadva, Bhoursal. Panj.—Barthoa, Thab. Tam.—Sagapu-maram. Tel.—Burija, Bandâru.

Characters.—Inner coat of the bark resembles cinchona and is bitter and astringent ; outer coat spongy, light and tasteless ; wood fine close-grained, colour pale, mahogany-like. Dose, 5 to 20 grs.

Constituents.—A bitter neutral principle, and an alkaloid hymenodictyonine, allied to quinoidine, berberine paricine, and a glucoside.

Preparation.—Infusion (1 in 10). Dose, ½ to 1 fld. oz.

Actions and uses.—A bitter tonic and febrifuge ; used during convalescence from acute diseases and fevers.

Ixora Parviflora, I. Alba.

Habitat.—South of India.

Parts used.—The bark and flowers.

Vernacular.—Beng.—Rangan. Can.—Gorabi. Eng.—Torch tree. Hind.—Kotha-gandhul, Runghun. Mar.—Kura-Kurat, Raikura, Makadi. Sans.—Ishwara. Tam.—Shulundu. Tel.—Karivipola.

Ixora or Ishwora means a Hindu god. The plant is sacred to Iswar (Shiva). It is used as a torch in the forest.

Characters.—Flowers sweet scented ; root pale brown. The wood burns very readily and clearly, and hence post-runners make torches of it.

Constituents.—Fatty matter, tannin, red coloring matter, and ash containing a trace of ferric oxide.

Preparations.—Decoction of the bark (1 in 20). Dose, ½ to 1 fld. oz.

Actions and uses—Tonic. The flowers pounded in milk are given in whooping cough ; the bark is a bitter tonic like cinchona and given in anæmia and general debility.

Ixora Coccinea, I. Grandiflora

Habitat.—W. India.

Parts used.—The root.

Vernacular.—Hind-Beng.—Rajana. Burm.—Pan-sa-yeik. Eng.—Flame of the forest, jungle or country geranium. Mar.—Bakura, Pentgul. Maleal.—Shetti. Tam.—Vitchie. Tel.—Theti.

Characters.—Root branched. Bark thick, smooth, and brown, marked with warty prominences; on cutting it a yellow juice exudes, odour disagreeable, due to the presence of volatile fatty acids. Dose, 5 to 20 grs.

Constituents.—Tannin, saccharine matter, a little fat and coloring matter.

Preparations.—Decoction (1 in 20). Dose, ½ to 1 fld. oz.

Actions and uses.—Astringent, stomachic, and tonic; given in fevers and gonorrhœa. In dysentery it is generally combined with Nâg-kesar and cumin. As a stomachic tonic it is given in flatulence and atony of the stomach.

Pavetta Indica, Ixora Pavetta, P. Alba.

Habitat.—Ceylon.

Parts used.—The root.

Vernacular.—Beng.—Kukura, Chura. Can.—Pappadi. Cing.—Pavetta, Mar., Hind.—Kakra. Maleal.—Malia-Mothi. Sans.—Pappana, Pâpata. Tam.—Pavetti-maram. Tel.—Tella-papata.

Characters.—An ornamental shrub. Root crooked ¼ to 1 inch in diameter. Taste bitter. Bark gray, light brown, epidermis, papery. Taste sweetish and aromatic. Dose, powdered root ½ to 1 dr.

Constituents.—A green resin starch, no tannin, an organic acid and a bitter glucoside resembling salicin.

Preparations.—Decoction (1 in 10). Dose, ½ to 1 fld. oz.

Actions and uses.—Bitter tonic and aperient; given in torpor of the liver and with ginger in dropsy.

Morinda Citrifolia, M. Tin

Habitat.—Throughout India, Malwa, Malabar.

Parts used.—The leaves and fruit.

Vernacular.—Beng.—Atchhu. Bur.—Yoi-yoe, Nayhgyle. Can.—Maddi. Cing.—Ahugaha. Eng.—Indian Mulberry. Hind.—Al, atchi, ak. Maleal.—Kada pilva. Mar.—Baratundi, A'sa Nagakuda. Tam.—Manja-pavattay. Tel.—Moolugu, maddi. Sans.—Achchhuka, Uchyuta Bárátondi is derived from Bâra, twelve, and Tond a month. The fruit is marked with as many as twelve scars which represent so many months.

Characters.—Leaves oval, oblong, shining, smooth, alternate and of a yellowish green or dark green colour; taste bitter. Ripe fruit shining, fleshy, oblong, and marked with scars; emitting a fœtid odour. By keeping the seeds and pulp become black or brown and sticky, resembling seeds and pulp of dried pomegranate.

Constituents.—The root bark contains morindin, a dyeing principle.

Preparations.—Decoction of leaves (1 in 20). Dose, 1 to 2 fld. oz.

Actions and uses.—Astringent, tonic and febrifuge; generally given mixed with aromatics. Decoction is given in diarrhœa, dysentery and fevers ; the ripe fruit is an emmenagogue, and given in disordered menstruation. The juice of the leaves is used as an application for the relief of pain in gout and healing of wounds and ulcers.

Mussænda Frondosa. M. Flavescens.

Habitat.—Nepal, Ceylon and Himalayas.

Parts used.—The root, leaves and fruit.

Vernacular.—Bomb.—Sarwad, Bhooteasse, Sanchount. Hind.—Bebina, Sribar. Maleal.—Belila. Mar.—Srivardoli, Bhut-kes. Nepaul.—Asari. Tam.—Vella allay. Sans.—Shrivati, Nagavalli.

Characters.—Leaves white. Flowers deep yellow or golden coloured. Taste bitter. Root slender, long and fibrous. Dose, 20 to 60 grs.

Constituents.—Bitter principle—a glucoside, resin, sugar, mucilage and colouring matter ; the bitter principle is soluble in water and rectified spirit.

Preparations.—Juice of root or leaves. Syrup of flowers, dose, 1 to 2 drs.

Actions and uses.—Alterative, and demulcent. The root is given with milk in jaundice. The juice of fruit and leaves is used as collyrium for the eyes. Syrup of flowers is a gentle expectorant and given in coughs, asthma, flatulence, and ague. Externally the paste of the root is used as a cooling application in skin eruptions.

Oldenlandia Umbellata, Hedyotis Umbellata, H. Hispida H. Indica.

Habitat.—Peninsula of India, Coromandel coast.

Parts used.—The root and leaves.

Vernacular.—Cing.—Choya, Sayan-mul. Eng.—Chayroot, Indian madder. Tam.—Emburel chedditel, Cheri velu.

Characters.—Leaves opposite, verticillate, linear, pale on the under surface ; margins recurved, covered with bristles ; flowers white and in racemes, root slender, long with few lateral fibres of an orange colour.

Constituents.—The bark contains a colouring matter.

Preparations.—Decoction (1 in 20). Dose $\frac{1}{2}$ to 1 fld. oz.

Actions and uses.—The leaves are expectorant, and given in cough, asthma and consumption. The root is alterative and used in cutaneous diseases and applied over poisonous bites of venomous animals.

Oldenlandia Corymbosa, O. Biflora, O. Herbacea.

Habitat.—Throughout India.

Parts used.—The herb.

Vernacular.—Guz., Mar., Beng.—Khet pâpra, Pitpapara. Can.—Kalla Sabatra-sige. Eng.—Two-flowered Indian madder. Hind.—Daman-pâpra, Bakra, Parputi, Pitpâpara. Sans.—Kshetra parpâta. Tam.—Parpa dagam. Tel.—Verinella vemu.

Characters.—Annual slender herb, leaves linear, with margins recurved, nerveless ; peduncle solitary ; flower 1 to 4 ; capsule, broad, hemispherical. Dose, 1 to 2 drs.

Constituents.—An alkaloid, and a large proportion of alkaline salts.

Preparations.—A compound decoction called Pancha Bhadra, meaning five bitters, containing, parpata, mustaka, gulancha, chiretta, and ginger equal parts, given in remittent fever. Dose, 1 to 2 fld. ozs.

Actions and uses.—Tonic and antiperiodic, given in fevers with gastric irritation and nervous depression.

Ophiorrhiza Mungos.

Habitat.—Mountains of Assam, Java, Sumatra, W. Peninsula and Ceylon.

Parts used.—The root and plant.

Vernacular.—Can.—Nanjâre, Rashme. Cing.—Mendi. Guz.—Mungusvel, Nakuli. Hind., Mar.—Râsna. Java.—Kajomar. Sans.—Nagasuganda. Tam.—Keri purandan. Tel.—Nakuli Sarpashe-chettu.

Characters.—Root about 6 to 9 inches in length, and as thick as the finger, contorted and brown externally ; bark closely adherent and corky ; taste bitter, like that of gentian. Leaves opposite, lanceolate, acuminate and glabrous.

Constituents.—Starch, amorphous alkaloid, resin and fat &c.

Preparations.—Decoction (1 in 10). Dose, ½ to 1 fld. oz.

Actions and uses.—Bitter tonic like gentian, and used as a tonic in dyspepsia and diarrhœa. Among the Cingalese it has a high reputation as a remedy against bites of snakes and mad dogs.

Policuria Densiflora, or probably from a Species of Nectandra.

Habitat.—Bolivia, South America.

Parts used.—The bark—coto-bark, also para coto-bark from another plant.

Characters.—Flat curved pieces, ½ inch thick ; cork fissured, cinnamon coloured ; odour nutmeg like, pungent and agreeable ; taste pungent and bitter, when chewed it increases the flow of saliva. Dose, 1 to 8 grs.

Constituents.—An acrid bitter principle—cotoin, Piperonylic acid, volatile oil and resin, but no tannin. Paracotoin is found in parocoto bark along with hydrocotoin; it occurs in small laminar crystals, weaker and paler than cotoin ; soluble in ether, boiling alcohol, boiling water and chloroform ; slightly soluble in water. Dose, ½ to 3 grs.

Cotoin occurs as pale yellow, amorphous powder or minute curved crystalline prisms, non-volatile, of a bitter taste and irritating to the nostrils; slightly soluble in water, freely soluble in alcohol, ether, chloroform and alkalies. Dose, ½ to 2 grs.; it checks salivation and night sweats.

Preparations.—Extractum Coto liquidum—liquid extract; not miscible with water. Dose, 2 to 6 ms. Tinctura Coto (1 in 10). Dose, 10 to 20 ms.

Actions.—A powerful astringent; given in chronic intestinal catarrh, dysentery and diarrhœa of rickets, typhoid fever, and phthisis; also in diarrhœa due to teething in children—cotoin is given in the night sweats of phthisis and in phthisical diarrhœa; it is also used hypodermically in cholera, 15 ms. of a 1 in 4 solution in acetic ether as an injection.

Pæderia Fœtida, Psychotria Volubilis, Apocynum Fœtidum, Convolvulus Fœtidus.

Habitat.—Himalaya, Bengal, West Peninsula of India.

Parts used.—The whole plant.

Vernacular.—Beng.—Gandha-bhadhuli. Guz.—Gandhana. Hind.—Gandhali. Mar.—Hiranvel. Sans.—Prasarani, Gundha bhadalya. Tel.—Savirela chettu.

Characters.—The plant has a very offensive odour of bisulphide of carbon, when bruised.

Constituents.—A volatile oil of an offensive odour, 2 alkaloids, namely, Alpha Pæderine and Beta Pæderine.

Preparations.—A liquid extract and a compound syrup or electuary containing liquid extract of gandhali 1 part, ginger and pepper 2 parts, plumbago root ½ part, and sugar 5 parts. Dose, 1 to 2 fld. drs. Liniment, contains liquid extract of gandhali 1 part, oil 8 parts and camphor ½ part.

Actions and uses.—The whole plant is alterative, antispasmodic, and emetic. The root is an emetic. The compound syrup is given in colic, rheumatism, gout and spasmodic diseases. The liminent is used externally in rheumatism and over painful joints.

Pilocarpus Jaborandi, B. P., P. Pinnatifolius, P. Selloanus.

Habitat.—Brazil, in forests, and on hill slopes.

Parts used.—The dried leaflets, Jaborandi Folia, B.P.

Characters.—Leaflets, long, short stalked, oval, marked with numerous pellucid dots, punctate, entire, emarginate, oblong, lanceolate, of a dull, green colour, coriaceous and tomentose; odour aromatic, taste pungent and bitter; when chewed it increases the flow of saliva. Dose, powdered leaves 5 to 40 grs.

Constituents.—Contain 4 alkaloids, viz—1 pilocarpine, 2 pilocarpidine, 3 jaborine antagonistic in action to pilocarpine and 4 jaboridine ; volatile oil, malic acid, and salts.

Pilocarpina—Pilocarpine—a syrupy liquid alkaloid. To obtain it add to the alcoholic extract of Jaborandi at first hydrochloric acid and then any alkali, shake the whole with chloroform and finally with acidulated water. Jaborine—also present in leaves, does not form crystallizable salts ; it is colourless and more liquid, without any odour, Pilocarpidine is supposed to be dihydroxylnicotine. Pilocarpine and pilocarpidine have been synthetically prepared from pyridine. Pilocarpidine on oxidation yields jaboridine.

Volatile oil is obtained by distillation. It contains chiefly turpene and a trace of paraffin-like substance.

Pilocarpinæ Nitras B. P. Pilocarpine Nitrate.—A white crystalline powder, soluble in water (1 in 9), slightly soluble in cold and freely so in hot alcohol. Dose, $\frac{1}{20}$ to $\frac{1}{2}$ gr. by the mouth.

Injectio Pilocarpinæ Nitratis Hypodermica—used hypodermically (1 gr. in 20 ms.) Dose, 2 to 6 ms. Hypodermic lamels or tablets contain $\frac{1}{4}$ gr. each. Guttæ Pilocarpinæ. 2 grs to 1 oz. Ophthalmic discs $\frac{1}{500}$ gr. in each. Lotio Pilocarpinæ—Pilocarpine nitrate 2 grs., quinine hydrochloride 8 grs., glycerine 2 drs., rose water 6 drs., used in alopecia. Pilula Pilocarpinæ Nitratis—Pilocarpine nitrate $\frac{1}{20}$ gr. with milk-sugar and glycerin of tragacanth—to make one pill. Pilocarpinæ Hydrochloridum, Pilocarpine Hydrochloride—White crystals, deliquescent, bitter, without any odour, freely soluble in alcohol and water, insoluble in ether and chloroform. Dose, $\frac{1}{20}$ to $\frac{1}{3}$ gr., used hypodermically, $\frac{1}{18}$ to $\frac{1}{2}$ gr. by the mouth. Pilocarpinæ Phenas—Pilocarpine carbolate, aseptoline. A colourless oily liquid, soluble in alcohol and water, used as hypodermic injection in phthisis (1 in 5,000). Pilocarpinæ salicylas—Pilocarpine salicylate—colourless crystals of a bitter taste, soluble in water. Dose, $\frac{1}{20}$ to $\frac{1}{2}$ gr.

Preparations.—Of Jaborandi Folia—Extractum Jaborandi liquidum B. P. Liquor Jaborandi—Fluid extract of pilocarpine, not miscible with water. Dose, 5 to 15 ms. Extractum Jaborandi (solid). Dose, 2 to 10 grs. Tinctura Jaborandi, B. P. (1 in 5). Dose, $\frac{1}{2}$ to 1 drachm. To check night sweat. Infusion (1 in 20). Dose, 1 to 2 ozs.

Physiological action.—Powerful sudorific and sialagogue, cardiac depressant, myotic, emetic, galactagogue, and abortifacient ; taken internally it paralyses the vaso motor system and is a stimulant of the peripheral nerve ends, supplying glands and involuntary muscles. It increases the general secretions, promotes sweating, causes flushed face, increased salivation, catarrh of the nose, bronchi and of the lachrymal duct. It is rapidly eliminated by the skin and salivary glands. In large doses it causes drowsiness, contracted pupils, and impaired or want of co-ordination of reflexes, laboured respiration, contraction of the bladder, uterus and spleen.

Therapeutics.—The leaves are given in uræmic convulsions, and renal dropsy; it should not be given if the heart is weak. In albuminuria, anasarca, pulmonary œdema, diabetes insipidus, it relieves the kidneys. It stimulates the skin, and hence used in fever. As a hairwash it promotes the growth of hair in alopecia. As a galactagogue it increases the flow of milk. In ptyalism it acts specifically in minute doses on the salivary glands. In erysipelas and in diphtheria it is of great benefit in detaching the false membrane and to prevent its reformation. Its use should be supported by food and stimulants. As an absorbent it is given with iodides and mercurials, in pleuritis, meningitis, retinitis, amblyopia due to alcoholism or tobacco, iritis and in glaucoma.

Pilocarpine in small doses $\frac{1}{30}$ to $\frac{1}{24}$ gr., checks night sweats ; but in large doses it is a most powerful sialagogue and diaphoretic, and used in kidney diseases, dropsy, diabetes insipidus, intermittent fever, severe hiccough and syphilis. In hiccough $\frac{1}{4}$ gr. can be hypodermically used ; also in deafness due to affection of the labyrinth and to arrest paroxysm of spasmodic asthma.

Psychotria Ipecacuanha, B.P.

Cephaëlis Ipecacuanha, Carthagena Ipecacuanha. Two varieties—long styled and short styled.

Habitat.—Brazil, India.

Parts used.—The dried root—Ipecacuanhæ Radix, B.P., Ipecacuanha root.

Characters.—In Carthagena Ipecacuanha, the root is thicker and the annulations less marked. Ipecacuanha root occurs in tortuous pieces, 6 inches long, and $\frac{1}{4}$ inch thick, colour dark brick red or dark brown, and closely annulated, breaking with a short fracture, cortex greyish : odour slight, but disagreeable, taste bitter. Dose, as an expectorant, $\frac{1}{4}$ to 2 grs., as an emetic, 15 to 30 grs.

Constituents.—An active principle—an alkaloid, emetine, 1·3 p.c. cephaeline ·6 p.c., Ipecacuanhic acid allied to catechin, saccharose, starch, fatty or oily matter, cholin, resin, pectin &c.

Emetina—Emetine—Emetia—the commercial article is a mixture of alkaloids—pure emetine, cephaeline (both emetic) and another alkaloid. Pure emetine occurs in white amorphous powder, taste slightly bitter, sparingly soluble in water, soluble in alcohol, ether, benzin, chloroform and dilute acids, scarcely so in caustic alkalies. Dose, $\frac{1}{120}$ to $\frac{1}{40}$ gr. as an emetic ; $\frac{1}{8}$ to $\frac{1}{4}$ gr. of Ipecacuanha yields 2 p.c. of crude emetine, Vinum Emetinæ (1 gr. of hydrochloride of emetine in 8 ozs. of sherry). Dose, 5 to 40 ms. Emetine has direct nauseant and emetic properties—used in pulmonary diseases, and biliousness. It rapidly darkens on exposure to light and air, and forms crystalline salts, as the hydrochloride and hydrobromide. The salts of cephaeline are uncrystallizable. It occurs in crystals, white at first, becoming dark yellow by exposure, sparingly soluble in ether, soluble in caustic alkalies which distinguishes it from emetine.

Cephalic or Ipecacuanhic acid—An amorphous, bitter glucoside, allied to caffeotannic acid. Occurs as brown powder, soluble in alcohol.

Preparations.—Of the root—Pulvis Ipecacuanhæ Compositus, B.P. —Dover's powder—Ipecacuanha 1, opium 1, and potassium sulphate 8, dose, 5 to 15 grs. Extractum Ipecacuanhæ liquidum B.P.—Ipecacuanha percolated with alcohol, then mixed with calcium hydroxide and again percolated ; strength from 2 to 2·5 p.c. of the alkaloid. Dose as an expectorant, ½ to 2 ms. ; as an emetic, 15 to 20 ms. Trochiscus Ipecacuanhæ, B P., ¼ gr. in each with fruit bases. Trochiscus morphinæ et Ipecacuanhæ, B.P., $\frac{1}{12}$ gr. of Ipecacuanha and $\frac{1}{30}$ gr. of morphine hydrochloride in each with tolu basis. Pilula Ipecacuanhæ cum scilla, B.P. (opium 5 p.c.). Contains Dover's powder 3, squill 1, ammoniacum 1, syrup of glucose q.s. Dose, 4 to 8 grs. Syrup Ipecacuanhæ aceticus, Vinegar of Ipecac. 1 pint, sugar 2¼ lbs. Dose, ¼ to 2 drs. Acetum Ipecacuanhæ B.P. (1 in 20). Dose, 10 to 30 ms. Vinum Ipecacuanhæ, B.P. (1 in 20). Extract of Ipecacuanha 1, to sherry 19. Dose, as an expectorant, 10 to 30 ms. ; as an emetic, 4 to 6 fld. drs. Pulvis Ipecacuanhæ sine Emetina, Ipecacuanha from which emetine has been extracted. Dose, 10 to 30 grs. Emetin, an extractive substance, soluble in water, has properties like the root ; must not be confounded with the alkaloid emetine. Dose, as an expectorant, $\frac{1}{16}$ to $\frac{1}{10}$ gr.; as an emetic, ½ to 1 gr.

Actions and uses.—Emetic, nauseant, diaphoretic, expectorant, sternutatory, laxative, cholagogue, hæmostatic, and vascular depressant; as an emetic it is not so depressant as tartar emetic, but more depressant than sulphate of zinc, mustard, or common salt ; it often acts as cathartic. In moderate doses it depresses the circulation and hence allied to aconite and tartar emetic. In small doses, it is a diaphoretic and expectorant. As an emetic it is largely used, especially in sthenic cases to unload the stomach in the beginning of fever, and in indigestions and in croup and diphtheria ; in bronchitis, especially of children, it promotes expulsion of mucus from the bronchi. As a cardiac sedative it is largely used in fevers to reduce the pulse rate, and to produce gentle diaphoresis. In catarrh of the bronchi and lungs, pneumonia and phthisis, its stimulating effects on the mucous membrane are well marked. Its principal value consists in its being almost a specific in dysentery. Large doses of Ipecacuanha, as much as 20 to 30 grs., or Ipecacuanha sine emetina, are given. In order to prevent its being vomited, no liquid is allowed before or after the dose, and the dose is preceded by a morphia draught or morphia hypodermically injected. Oftentimes in such cases mustard plaster is applied to the pit of the stomach, a few minutes before Ipecacuanha is given. The dose may often be repeated 3 or 4 times.

Remarks.—The Goanese Ipecacuanha, the root of Naregamia alata, Nat. O. Meliaceæ, bears similar properties to Ipecacuanha.

Randia Dumetorum, R. Longispina Canthium, Coronatum, Gardenia Dumetorum. G. Spinosa. Posoqueria Dumetorum, Ceriscus Malabaricus.

Habitat.—Throughout India, Gujerat, Dehra Doon, Ceylon, Coimbatore.

Parts used.—The fruit.

Vernacular.—Arab.—Jouzel kowsul, Jouz-ul-kai. Beng., Bomb. —Gelaphala, Pieralu, Menphal. Can.—Mangâre. Cing.—Wali, kukuru man. Duk.—Medaphala. Eng.—The emetic nut. Guz.—Mindhal. Hind.—Mainphal, Mayina, Pinda, Mindhla. Mar.—Gehela, Piralu. Punj.—Mindhal. Sans.—Madana. Tam.—Madu-karray, maruk arang. Tel.—Mangha, manda.

Characters.—Fruit small, like Jâephala, globular or ovate, of a deep grey or reddish brown colour. At its base is a small disc-like stalk or rim of the calyx. Surface minutely and roughly wrinkled, and obtusely ribbed ; ribs varying from five to seven cells or cavities, two with thick woody walls, and covered with a yellowish grey, rather soft, and unctuous pulp. Within the cells are the seeds, small, hard, numerous, translucent, shining, and oblong, or rather kidney-shaped. Pulp is nauseous in taste, and the smell is similar to that of valerian. Dose of the pulp, 15 to 20 grs.

Constituents.—An active principle, saponin, valerianic acid, wax, resin and colouring matter.

Preparations.—Infusion of seeds (1 in 10). Dose, ½ to 1 fld. oz ethereal tincture (1 in 5). Dose, 15 to 60 ms.

Actions and uses.—A good substitute for Ipecacuanha. The dry pulp is emetic, the thick shell and hard seeds are not emetic at all. The Native Hakims give the pulp in combination with aromatics in dysentery, fever (ague), headache, &c. It contains valerianic acid, hence the tincture is used as a nervine calmative and antispasmodic, in whooping cough and mania. The shell and seeds are cathartic and anthelmintic, and used to remove biliousness and worms in children. The fruit is used to procure abortion and as a fish poison like coculus. A paste of it is locally applied as a discutient to disperse swellings and abscesses.

Remarks.—The Arabic name Jouzul-akai is also applied to nux vomica.

Randia Uliginosa, Posoqueria Uliginosa, Gardenia Uliginosa.

Habitat.—Ceylon, India, in moist places.

Parts used.—The unripe fruit.

Vernacular.—Beng.—Chuvadi alu. Can.—Kare-pindalu. Guz.—Pinglu. Mar.—Pendhâri.—Hind.—Pedalu. Sans.—Pindhaluka· Tam.—Vagata. Tel.—Guahu—Pedda-mranga ; Devota-malle ; Nalla-ika.

Characters.—Flowers large, white, and fragrant, in 2 or 3, on the top of branchlets. Berry of the size of an egg, ash coloured, or olive grey, 2-celled. Seeds flattish, adherent to the pulp fibres. Dose of the powdered fruit, 10 to 30 grs.

Actions and uses.—Astringent, roasted in hot ashes they are used in diarrhœa and dysentery.

Rubia Cordifolia, R. Munjishtha, Heart-leaved Madder, R. Tinctoria, R. Secunda.

Habitat.—Hilly districts, S. Europe, Asia, Assam, Nepal, Sind, Siberia, and China.

Parts used.—The roots.

Vernacular.—Arab.—Runas, Sabba-ghni. Beng.—Aruna, Manjith. Chin.—Si-tsau-ken. Can.—Manjushta. Guz.—Majith. Mar., Hind., Duk. —Manjita. Eng.—Indian madder. Malyal.—Pooat. Pers.—Runâs. Sans.— Kala Mashika. Tam.—Manjithi, Shevelli. Tel.—Manjishta, Mandastic, Tamravalli.

Characters.—The stem is square, rough, and covered with short prickles, root creeping, short, with numerous cylindrical rootlets of the size of quills, suber, brownish, and thin. Bark red brown, odour somewhat aromatic, taste sweetish at first, then corky and acrid. Dose of the root, 10 to 60 grs.

Constituents.—Resinous and extractive matter; gum, sugar, colours ing matter, and salts of lime. The medicinal properties are due to resinous and extractive matters. The colouring matter consists of purpurin, manjistin, garancin, alizarin (orange red) and xanthine (yellow).

Preparations.—Infusion (1 in 10). Dose, ½ to 1 fld. oz.

Actions and uses.—Alterative, diuretic, emmenagogue, and astringent. In pharmacy it is used to colour liniments and ointment. The root is given in paralysis, dropsy, jaundice, amenorrhœa, and scanty lochia; externally as an astringent it is locally applied to inflamed parts, swellings, ulcers, fractures, &c. With honey it is applied to various discolorations of the skin, as bruises, contusions, pityriasis versicolor, leucoderma and freckles.

Spermacoce Hispida, S. Scabra.

Habitat.—Throughout India.

Parts used.—The plant.

Vernacular.—Beng.—Madana-Banta-kadu. Eng.—Shaggy buttonweed. Malyal.—Thartavel. Mar.—Ghanti-chi-bâji, Dhoti, gondi. Sans.—Madan ghanta. Tam.—Nutti choorie. Tel.—Madana.

Characters.—Herb scabrous, procumbent; root fibrous; leaves obovate, oblong, or elliptical with cartilaginous edges, and coriaceous; flowers small, blue or white, and in a whorl; capsules, pubescent; seeds oblong granulate and opaque.

Preparations.—Decoction of the root (1 in 10). Dose, 1 to 2 fld. ozs. Confections of seeds. Dose, ½ to 1 drs.

Actions and uses.—Alterative and tonic. The seeds are cooling, demulcent and given in diarrhœa and dysentery. The root is alterative and used like sarsaparilla.

Vangueria Spinosa, Meynia Spinosa.

Habitat.—India.

Parts used.—The fruit.

Vernacular.—Bombay—Alu. Beng.—Mayna. Can.—Maggare-gida. Hind.—Pundrika, Pinditak, Bangariki-lakri. Mar.—Chircholi. Madandriksh. Sans.—Pinda, Pindiluka. Tam.—Pedda-munga. Tel.—Vadanike, Chega-gadda.

Characters.—Cymes of greenish flowers. Fruit a drupe, subglobose fleshy, and of the size of a cherry. Colour yellow when ripe. Odour terebinthinate.

Preparations.—Decoction (1 in 20). Dose, 2 to 6 drs.

Actions and uses.—The fruit is refrigerant and cholagogue and used in biliary complaint with hepatic congestion.

Valerianaceæ.

The jatamansi family. From valeo to be strong. In allusion to the well marked medicinal properties and powerful smell.

Herbs, leaves exstipulate, opposite ; flowers, cymose, hermaphrodite or rarely unisexual. Fruit dry and indehiscent, frequently pappose. Seed pendulous, solitary, and ex-albuminous.

Habitat.—Native of temperate climates.

Properties.—Remarkable for the presence of a strong scented volatile oil. They are stimulant, tonic and antispasmodic.

Nardostachys jatamansi, Valeriana jatamansi, Nardus Indicus, Valeriana Celtica (Nardus spica Celtica).

Habitat.—Alpine Himalaya, Asia.

Parts used.—The rhizome and oil.

Vernacular.—Arab.—Am-ul-tibe, sumbul-ul-aspire-hinde. Can.—Jata manashi. Cing.—Jara mansi. Mar., Beng., Duk.—Jhata manasi, billi lotan. Eng.—Musk root, Indian spikenard. Hind.—Jata masi, Kalichada, sumbul, Bala chari. Malyal.—Jeta manchi. Pers.—Sumbul-i-hindi, Bekh-i-sumbul, Sans.—Jata manasi Bhutakesi, Pisita, Tapasvini. Tam.—Jata mashi. Tel.—Jeta mamshi.

Billi lotan (Duk) (a name also applied to Acalypha Indica) means cat's struggle, cat is supposed to be fond of this plant. Bhûtakesi. Bhut, a demon, and kesi, hair—devil's hair—from the devilish strong smell of the rootlets which are like hair.

Characters.—Rhizome in short pieces about the thickness of goose quills, of a dark grey colour and surmounted by a bundle of reddish brown fibres ; odour heavy and peculiar like that of pâtchouli, taste bitter and aromatic. Dose, 15 to 45 grs.

Constituents.—A volatile oil, oleum jatamansi, resin, sugar, starch bitter extractive matter, and gum.

Preparations.—The oil. Dose, 2 to 6 ms. Tincture (1 in 8). Dose, ½ to 2 fld. drs. Medicated oil.

Actions and uses.—Same as those of valerian. In nervous disorders it is combined with asafetida; in chlorosis with iron and strychnine; taken habitually in small doses, it improves the appetite and digestion without confining the bowels. As an emmenagogue it is very useful in amenorrhœa and dysmenorrhœa; also used in cerebral anæmia, vertigo, or fainting, &c.

Valeriana Officinalis, B. P.

Habitat.—Europe, N. Asia, Sind, Burmah, Ceylon, New England, Vermont.

Parts used.—The dried erect rhizome and roots.

Vernacular.—Arab.—Sumbul-ul-asfar. Duk.—Vilayeti jhata manasi. Eng.—True valerian. Hind.—Sugandha bâlâ chhara. Pers. --Sumbul-ul-tib. Sans.—Bâlâ Hrivera.

Characters.—A large herbaceous plant, with small white rose-coloured flowers, rhizome short, erect, dark or yellowish brown externally and whitish or yellowish internally. Roots numerous, slender and brittle; colour same as that of the rhizome, odour aromatic and musk-like; taste camphoraceous or somewhat pungent. Dose, 5 to 30 grs.

Constituents.—A volatile oil 2 p.c., valerianic acid, formic, acetic and malic acids, chatinine, tannin, starch, sugar, resin, gum and extractive.

Oleum Valerianæ—A volatile oil obtained by distilling the root with water. A pale green liquid, of a pungent, valerian-like odour, and of an aromatic taste and acid reaction, soluble in alcohol. On exposure, it becomes viscid and yellow. By oxidation is developed valerene, valerol or baldrian camphor and valerianic acid. Dose, 2 to 5 ms.

Valerianic acid.—An oxidation product. The volatile oil on exposure to the air becomes oxidized and converted into valerianic acid. It is also obtained as a product of oxidation of amylic alcohol with sulphuric acid. It is an oily liquid, of a characteristic and sweet taste; used in preparing various valerianates, as valerianates of iron, zinc, ammonium and quinine. It also occurs in many other plants, and in cod liver oil.

Preparations.—Of valerianic acid—Validol—a combination of valerianic acid and menthol, a clear viscid liquid. Dose, 10 to 15 ms.

Preparations.—Of valerian—Extractum valerianæ fluidum. Dose, 10 to 30 ms. Infusion. Dose, 1 to 2 ounces. Tinctura Valerianæ (1 in 8). Dose, ½ to 2 drs. Tinctura valerianæ ammoniata, B. P. (1 in 5). Dose, ½ to 1 fld. dr. Zinci valerianas. Dose, 1 to 3 grs.

Actions and uses.—General stimulant, anodyne, hypnotic, antispasmodic, vermifuge and diaphoretic. It often stimulates sexual powers. As a sedative to reflex excitability, its action is opposed to that of brucine, thebaine, and strychnine. In full doses it stimulates the heart, raises the temperature, and produces exhilaration of spirits

If long continued it leads to melancholia. In very large doses it is a powerful irritant of the brain and of the gastro-intestinal tract, leading to nausea, vomiting, diarrhœa, frequent passage of urine containing lithates. The oil paralyses the brain and the spinal cord, lowers the blood pressure and slows the pulse. Valerian is used in epilepsy, hysteria, hemicrania, nervous cough and hiccough. As a tonic it is given in fevers and low states of the system ; also given in whooping cough, diabetes, dysmenorrhœa, convulsions, worms and flatulence in children. In the coma of typhus fever the oil is very efficient. As an antispasmodic it is inferior to asafetida.

Validol is used in asthma, hysteria, and as a preventive against sea-sickness. As a stimulant, antispasmodic, anodyne it surpasses valerian in energy and rapidity of action, and besides it has anæsthetic properties. As an hypnotic it produces sleep like morphia, and chloral hydrate 5 minims are sufficient to produce tranquil sleep without any depressing action on the heart. It has been found very serviciable in biliary colic.

Valeriana Wallichii, V. Hardwickii, V. Brunoniana.

Habitat.—Temperate Himalaya.

Parts used.—The rhizome.

Vernacular.—Arab.—Sumbul-jibali, Asaruma. Beng.—Taggera ganthoda. Bhutan.—Pâmpe. Can.—Naudibattal. Hind.—Bâlâ Taggar, Chhar ganthona, mushkwali. Ind.—Asarun. Panj.—Mushk-i-wali, vala. Bala. Pers.—Rishaiwâla. Sans.—Pindi-tagara, Nandyâ varta, Nandini, Varhini. Nahushakhya.

Characters.—A fragrant herb, rhizomes short, knotty and about 1 to 1½ inches long, diameter varying from that of a quill to that of a little finger, colour dark brown, surface highly wrinkled, and here and there marked with transverse ridges and prominent tubercles, or scars of fallen leaf-sheaths; lower end blunt, very hard and tough; upper end broad with traces of long stripe-like leaves ; odour, aromatic and pungent, resembling that of officinal valerian, but much more powerful; taste camphoraceous.

Constituents.—The root contains volatile oil, tannin, glucose resin, albuminoids, starch, &c.

Preparations.—Infusion (1 in 20). Dose, ½ to 1 fl. oz.

Actions and uses.—Stimulant, nervine tonic, antispasmodic and sedative ; used in hysteria; headache, epilepsy, chorea ; also in suppression of urine. As a stimulant it is given in advanced stages of fever, &c.

Compositæ or Asteraceæ. The Thistle or the Sevati family.

Shrubs or herbs, rarely trees, forming almost the tenth part of the described vegetable kingdom ; leaves opposite, alternate, and exstipulate, simple or lobed ; flowers variegated, hermaphrodite, unisexual or neuter, and arranged in capitula ; fruits achene, dry and indehiscent, one-celled ; seeds solitary, erect, and ex-albuminous.

Habitat.—Universally distributed, abundant in hot climates.

Properties.—Many are bitter and tonic; some purgative and anthelmintic; others stimulant and narcotic; some contain volatile oil and are diaphoretic, aromatic and carminative.

Achillea Millefolium, A. Moschata, A. Santolina.

Habitat.—W. Himalaya, N. America.

Parts used.—The flowering tops and leaves.

Vernaculars.—Bomb.—Roja mari. Eng.—Nose-bleed, yarrow. Egypt.—Barbara. Indian Bazars.—Biranjâsif. Panj.—Bui-Madaran, Momadra, Capendiga. Pers.—Bui-e-Madarân.

Characters.—Perennial herb, stems hairy and furrowed; leaves alter nate, soft, hairy, linear, dentate, lanceolate; globular beneath; and nine to twelve inches long, segments toothed, and of a dark green colour. Flowers white and corymbose. Fruit achene, odour feeble, aromatic, like that of chamomile. Taste bitterish, saline and aromatic.

Constituents.—Yarrow yields on distillation, a dark green coloured, butyraceous volatile oil, a bitter extractive—achillein, also resin, tannin, gum, and various salts as malates, nitrates, phosphates and chlorides of potassium and calcium, and ash, 15 to 18 p.c.

Achillea Moschata contains a volatile oil known as Jvaol, of a refreshing odour and mint-like taste; it also contains ivain, achilleine, achilletine and moschatine.

Preparations.—Infusion (1 in 10). Dose, 1 to 2 fld. ozs. Volatile oil. Dose, 10 to 20. Decoction (1 in 20). Dose, 1 to 2 fld. ozs.

Actions and uses.—Medicated vapour bath containing yarrow, lavender flowers, wheat bran, and milk is used in nasal catarrh and fever. It has a specific action on the pelvic organs and used in amenorrhœa, menorrhagia, and leucorrhœa. As a bitter tonic it is given during convalescence from fevers, and in atonic dyspepsia to promote appetite. Its chief use is in relaxation of the sphinctor ani with discharge of mucus or blood during defecation. The infusion is applied to relaxed throat and sore nipples with benefit.

Anthemis Nobilis, B.P., Matricaria Chamomilla.

Habitat.—Europe, N. India, Persia, W. Asia, and Australia.

Parts used.—The dried expanded flower heads, Anthemidis flores, chamomile flowers, B. P., and oil, oleum anthemidis, B. P.

Vernacular.—Arab—Tuffah ul-arz, Shajrat-el-kafûr, Babûnâj (flower). Chin.—Kau-kiuh-hwa. Can.—Shime-Shyâ-Mantige Eng.—True Chamomile. German Chamomile (matricaria). Guz., Mar., Hind.—Babunâ. Malyal.—Shima-Jeventi. Pers.—Bâbûnah. Tam.—Châman duppu. Tel.—Sima—chamanti push pamu.

Shajrat-el-kafur. Shajrat, plant, and Kafur, camphor. The "camphor plant," the odour of its flowers being like that of camphor.

Characters.—An annual plant. The drug contains pieces of stem mixed up with flower heads. The stalk is long, slender and furrowed; flowers hemispherical, small, white, or nearly white in colour, broad and flattish; involucre with 2 or 3 rows of oblong bracts and obtuse scales, having a membranous margin, and a conical and solid receptacle, hollow in matricaria. Florets, ligulate and white, of strong aromatic odour and bitter taste. Dose, flowers 10 to 30 grs.

Constituents.—A volatile oil 1 p.c., anthemene, anthemic acid, a bitter extractive principle, tannin, resin, malates, tannates.

Chamomile oil, oleum anthemidis, B. P. The volatile oil is a dark blue, thin, transparent, thickish liquid, by keeping becoming green and brown, of a strong odour and warm, aromatic taste. Contains anthemol. Dose, ½ to 3 ms. Anthemol—to obtain it exhaust chamomile flowers with hot acetic acid, concentrate, and precipitate the products with alcohol and evaporate—occurs as tasteless crystals, insoluble in alcohol, ether, chloroform, soluble in acetic acid. The true chamomile oil contains various ethers, as the angelates and valerianates of butyl. Dose, 2 ms. on sugar.

Preparations.—Infusium anthemidis (1 in 10). Dose, 1 to 4 fld. ozs. Extractum anthemidis, B.P. Dose, 2 to 8 grs. Tinctura anthemidis (1 in 2). Dose, 3 to 10 ms.

Physiological action.—Stomachic tonic, carminative, emmenagogue and antiperiodic. As a stimulant of the gastric mucous membrane, it increases the appetite and aids digestion.

Therapeutics.—It is given in flatulent colic, dyspepsia, chlorosis, amenorrhœa and during convalescence from acute febrile and other diseases. The warm infusion causes vomiting, hence it is given in colic, biliary derangements, periodic headache and to confirmed drunkards and heavy gluttons. The cold infusion is a stomachic tonic and given in indigestion, flatulence, and summer diarrhœa. As an antiperiodic it is given in malarious fevers. Fomentation of chamomile flowers is a very soothing application to relieve local colicky pains. The oil is a stimulant and antispasmodic and is given internally to relieve reflex cough, pulmonary catarrh, diarrhœa of children, spasmodic asthma, and whooping cough; also in dysmenorrhœa and in hysteria. With other stimulating liniments it is applied over sprains and rheumatic affections.

Anacyclus Pyrethrum, B. P.

Pyrethrum from pyros, fire. The roots having fiery spicy taste.

Habitat.—N. Africa, Algeria, and Europe.

Parts used.—The dried root, Pyrethri Radix, B.P. Pyrethrum root or Pellitory.

Vernacular.—Arab.—Akara-Karhâ, ud-el Karih-Jibbali. Hind. Guz., Mar., Duk., Beng.—Akalkara. Bom.—Mitho Akalararo. Burm. —Kûkaijâ or Kûkayâ. Can.—Akkalâkare. Eng.—Spanish pellitory,

Indian fever root, Spanish Chammonile. Malyal.—Akke Karuka. Pers.—Akar-Karah. Sans.—Akara-Karabha. Tam.—Akkira-Karam. Tel.—Akala-Karra.

Characters.—The root resembles the narrow end of sambarasinga. It is long, compact, tapering at both extremities. The crown of the root is covered with a tuft of hairs; also shrivelled and marked with a few scars of fallen rootlets; surface smooth and marked with longitudinal, or irregular furrows; colour light brown; on section homogeneous and pithy in the centre where the colour is whitish. The taste is rather sweet at first and then becomes hot, acrid or pungent, acridity depending on a fixed acrid oleo resin, deposited in vesicles in the bark. It produces a glowing heat in the mouth, followed by a tingling and pricking sensation on the tongue and lips. Dose, 30 to 60 grs. as a masticatory.

Constituents.—Pyrethrin—an acrid brown resin, Pyrethrine 5 p.c. —an alkaloid, 2 fixed oils, inulin 50 p.c., gum, salts, a trace of tannin.

Preparations.—Decoctum Pyrethri (1 in 10). Dose, 2 to 4 fld. drs. Tinctura Pyrethri B. P. (1 in 5). Dose, ½ to 1 dr. Confectio Pyrethri, "Akara Kara-bhadi churana"—contains akalkaro, kesara, jaephal, lavang, rakta chandan, each 2 drs., afim, 1 dr., dhaturâna'bij 1 dr., mix, add sâkar 6 drs. Dose, 6 grs. As an aphrodisiac.

Physiological action.—Stimulant, rubefacient, irritant and sialagogue; locally rubefacient. When chewed it at first irritates or stimulates the nerves and vessels of the mouth, salivary and buccal glands and then deadens and blunts their sensibility. In small doses it is stimulant and cordial. As a masticatory sialagogue it produces pricking sensation in the tongue, with heat, pungency and copious flow of saliva, constriction in the fauces and increased buccal mucus. In large doses it is an irritant of the mucous membrane of the intestines, causing bloody stools, tetanoid spasms and profound stupor. The pulse becomes accelerated.

Therapeutics.—The infusion is given with lesser galangal and ginger in low states of the system with drowsiness and lethargy. The tincture is given in neuralgic headache, toothache due to caries, in paralysis of the tongue and in neuralgia of the face; as a local anæsthetic gargle or lotion or a mouth wash it is used in sore throat, relaxed uvula, aphonia, &c. As a sternutatory, the powder is inhaled in chronic catarrh of the frontal sinuses. The confection is given in impotence and in chronic seminal weakness. As a sialagogue it is an efficient remedy in chronic iodine poisoning where it secures a prompt and rapid elimination.

Pyrethrum Roseum—P. Carneum. Persian Pellitory—Persian sweet powder. The plant resembles chamomile and is found in Western Asia and Persia. The powder of flower heads is used for killing insects, 4 grs. is sufficient to kill one fly.

Arctium Lappa, L. Major, L. Minor, L. Tomentosa, Lappa officinalis.

Grass Burdock, Lappa clotbur.

Habitat.—Europe, N. Asia, and United States, Temperate Zone.

Parts used.—The fruit, root and seeds.

Characters.—It is a biennial weed common on road-sides and waste places. The root is about twelve inches or more long and about one inch thick, nearly simple, fusiform, fleshy, longitudinally wrinkled and crowned with a tuft of whitish soft, hairy leaf stalks, of a grey brown colour, bark rather thick ; inner part and soft wood radically striated, parenchyma studded with cavities, and lined with snow-white remains of fibrous tissues ; odour feeble, and unpleasant, taste mucilaginous, sweetish and somewhat bitter ; seeds angular, obovate, slightly curved, flattened and brown grey mottled with black. Dose of the root, 20 to 60 grs.

Constituents.—The root contains inunlin, a trace of volatile oil, bitter extractive, sugar, resin, fat 9 p.c. tannin, glucoside and ash 4 p.c. The seeds contain oil, resins and lappin.

Preparations.—Of the root. Extractum Lappæ Fluidum. Dose, ½ to 1 fld. dr. Decoctum Lappa (1 in 20). Dose, 1 to 2 fld. ozs. of the seed. Tinctura Lappa (10 p.c.) Dose, ½ to 2 fld. drs. before meals.

Actions and uses.—Alterative, aperient, diuretic and diaphoretic; used in scrofula, constitutional syphilis, skin diseases as psoriasis, scurvy and in copious urinary deposits ; also pulmonary catarrh, gout and rheumatism ; externally the decoction is useful for baldness, hæmorrhoids and chronic sores.

Arnica Montana, B. P.

Mountain arnica, mountain tobacco, leopard's bane, accident plant. Accident plant from its use in cases of sprains, contusions, concussions due to accidents.

Habitat.—Indigenous to European Mountains, Germany, Siberia, Switzerland, Alps, Missouri, Columbia.

Parts used.—Flower heads—Arnicæ Flores ; and the dried Rhizome and roots, Arnicæ Rhizoma, B. P.

Characters.—Perennial plant, flowers large, orange yellow and broad, involucre in two rows, receptacle, flat and hairy, odour aromatic. Taste pungent and bitter. Rhizome with several rootlets thick, brown, curved and wrinkled, rough from the scars of leaflets ; dark brown, externally and whitish internally ; bark thick containing a circle of resin-cells, and a large spongy pith. Rootlets thin, not numerous ; odour aromatic, taste acrid and bitter, distinguished from valerian by its smell ; from serpentaria from the latter having many contorted rootlets ; from Veratrum, from thick rootlets. Dose—Flowers, 5 to 20 grs. Rhizome, 2 to 20 grs.

Constituents.—The flowers contain Arnicin—a glucoside, trimethylamine, an ammoniacal alkaloid and the active principle, volatile oil, resins, and salts. The rhizome contains in addition capronic and caprylic acids. Inulin 10 p.c., tannin, an essential oil, and mucilage. Arnicin. To obtain it—pass the tincture through animal charcoal and evaporate. Add ether to the residue which dissolves, arnicin and fat; shake with alcohol to dissolve arnicin. It occurs as yellow amorphous mass; of an acrid taste, soluble in alcohol, ether and alkalies, very sparingly so in water.

Preparations.—Tinctura arnicæ florum (1 in 5). Dose, 5 to 30 ms. Infusum arnicæ florum (1 in 5). Dose, ½ to 1 fld. oz. Best for local use as it does not excite dermatites. It is free from the volatile oil and from arnicin. Tinctura Arnicæ Radicis B. P. (1 in 20). Dose, ½ to 1 fld. drs. Extractum Arnicæ. Dose, 1 to 3 grs. Emplastrum Arnicæ Radicis, 33 p.c. of the root to 67 p.c. of lead plaster.

Physiological action.—Gastric and intestinal irritant, cardiac stimulant, antipyretic, and sternutatory; also diuretic and emmenagogue. In small doses taken internally it stimulates the heart beat and raises the arterial tension. In large doses it at first stimulates but soon depresses the circulation, respiration and the nerve centres; it gives rise to headache, convulsions and even unconsciousness, paralysis of motion, with dilatation of the pupils. It often leads to collapse and death.

Therapeutics.—As an antipyretic it is used in typhus and typhoid fevers, also given in concussion of the brain, in chronic catarrh, and in internal hæmorrhages as epistaxis, hæmoptysis, &c., as a diuretic it is given in gout, rheumatism and dropsy. As an emmenagogue it is given in amenorrhœa and chlorisis; also for internal bruises, in chronic diarrhœa, dysentery and in paralysis of the bladder. Locally its infusion is applied to sprains, contusions, echymosis, &c. The solution is used to promote union of cut surfaces.

Artemisia Absinthium, A. Vulgaris, A. Indica, A. Grata.

Habitat.—Waste places on chalky soils, Nepal, China, Japan. Indigenous in Europe, Asia and mountainous districts of India, cultivated in the United States.

Parts used.—The dried herb, leaves and flowering tops.

Vernacular.—Arab.—Afsantin-e-hindi, Kashus-Rumi. Duk., Guz., Beng.—Mastaru, Nagdoni. Can.—Uruvalu, Urigattige; Mâchi patri. Cing.—Walko-gundo. Eng.—Wormwood, Mugwort (A. Vulgaris). Hind.—Machiparna Gund-mar mastaru, Duna murwa. Mal.—Tiru-nitri-pachcha. Mar.—Surpana. Pers.—Barunjá-sif-i-kohi, Artemas-saya. Sans.—Indhana. Tam.—Machi pattiri. Tel.—Tartiha, Moshe-patre.

Characters.—Bundles of the dried herbs of a brownish white or ash colour, of a silky touch, leaves trifid, or simple, pinnatifid, and tomentose on the under surface; flower heads small yellow in racemes, hoary and ashy on their under surface, pannicled, and ovate; smell agreeable and aromatic, due to the volatile oil it contains, taste bitter. Dose of the herb, 15 to 30 grs.

Constituents.—Volatile oil, a bitter extractive matter—absinthin ; tannin, resin, succinic acid, matates and nitrates of potassium &c., and ash 7 p.c. The volatile oil is obtained by distillation. It is a dark green liquid of a strong camphoraceous odour and aromatic taste. It contains Thujone or absinthol, terpenes 2 p.c., and a deep blue oil. Absinthin—to obtain it precipitate the infusion with tannin. It is an intensely bitter white or yellowish brown amorphous glucoside, soluble in alcohol, chloroform, slightly so in ether, insoluble in water. The odour is camphoraceous.

Preparations.—Extract. Dose, 1 to 4 grs. Oil. Dose, ½ to 3 ms. ; Tincture (1 in 8). Dose, ½ to 2 fld. drs. Infusion (1 in 10). Dose, ½ to 1 fld. oz. Vinum Aromaticum absintheum (1 p.c.) or absinthe, a French liquor—It is an alcoholic solution of the oil containing marjoram, angelica, anise, etc.

Actions and uses.—The oil is a narcotic poison if long used. It stimulates the heart and the brain, gives use to tremors, stupor, epileptic-form convulsions, stertor, involuntary passage of urine and fæces, &c. It irritates the stomach and gives rise to morning nausea and vomiting. As a local sedative the herb steeped in hot vinegar is used as fomentation to the head in cephalalgia, to the joints in gout or rheumatism, and over painful sprains and bruises. Absinthium is a bitter, stomachic tonic; it increases appetite and promotes digestion ; given in dyspepsia ; as a febrifuge, it is inferior to clerodendron inerme. It is also given in hysteria, in spasmodic affections as epilepsy, in nervous irritability and in nervous depression ; also in mental exhaustion. As an enema its infusion is used as an anthelmintic.

Remarks.—A. Sieversiana differs from Artemisia Indica in its odour, which is more aromatic and camphoraceous, and its flowers more ashy and tomentose.

Artemisia Maritima var. Stechmanniana, B.P., A. Santonica, A. Pauciflora.

Habitat.—N. Turkestân, Khurdistan, Plains of Kirghiz, Asia Minor.

Parts used.—The dried unexpanded flowering heads and young branches (Santonica).

Vernacular.—Arab.—Shih, sariphûna, afsant-el-bahara. Eng.—Levant worm seed. Mar., Guz.—Kira-mani-ova, Kir-mani-ajmo. Hind.—Kirmalâ. Pers.—Darmanah. Sans.—Juvániya, Gadadhara.

Characters.—A small perennial plant, flowers oblong, ovoid, obtuse, smooth, glossy, greyish green, on exposure becoming light brown, yellow or brown, consisting of closely imbricated involucre 12 or 18 glandular scales with broad midrib, very small, elliptical, numerous florets buds, flowering axils and pieces of very slender stems covered with a white down ; smell agreeable and aromatic, taste bitterish and mint-like. Dose, 15 to 60 grs.

Constituents.—Volatile oil 2 p.c. (of a peculiar smell and taste) ; a crystalline substance santoninum, or santonin 2 p.c. ; resin, sugar, fat, and salts of lime.

Santoninum, santonin, B.P., a neutral principle ; to obtain it digest flower heads in alcohol and slaked lime, evaporate, then add acetic acid when santonine will be separated. Met with in white shining crystals or prisms, odourless, of bitter after-taste, neutral reaction, becoming yellow on exposure to the air and light. Scarcely soluble in cold water, sparingly so in boiling water (1 in 250), soluble in chloroform (1 in 4), in cold alcohol (1 in 40), ether (1 in 140) and in boiling alcohol (1 in 3) freely so in solution of caustic alkalies. Dose, 2 to 5 grs.

Preparations.—Infusion (1 in 20) of flowering heads. Dose, 1 to 2 fld. ozs. Trochiscus santonin, B.P. (1 gr. in each).

Physiological actions.—Taken internally it passes into the blood as sodium santoninate, and affects the sight, objects appearing blue, green, red, and lastly yellow. It renders the urine, if acid, of a green yellow colour,and if alkaline, reddish purple. It also produces eneuresis. If long continued it may lead to blindness. In large and poisonous doses it acts upon the brain, heart and respiration, disturbs consciousness, produces intoxication, tremors, cold surface, cold sweats, feeble pulse, slow respiration, vomiting, convulsions and death by asphyxia.

Therapeutics.—The infusion is given in flatulence, amenorrhœa and dyspepsia ; locally a poultice of the flower buds is used to relieve pain from the bites of scorpions and other venomous reptiles. Santonine—the active principle does not kill worms, but its presence being distasteful to them, it causes them to fly away from their resting place and lodge in the large intestines from which they are dislodged by a purgative such as calomel or castor oil the next morning. It may be used as suppository against round worms, but it has no effect against tape worms ; often given for nocturnal incontinence of urine with benefit. It should not be given to children during fever, nor in constipation.

Artemisia Sieversiana.

The fresh herb is used in Persia, and is cultivated in Bandora, near Bombay. The Portuguese know it by the name of Azarona. Stem erect, suffruticose. Leaves ashy, tomentose beneath, lower ones pinnatifid, upper trifid. Heads of flowers racemose, pannicled. Dose, 15 to 60 grs. It contains absenthate of potash, a bitter substance, and a green volatile oil ; used as an infusion (1 in 20). Dose, 2 to 6 drs. The herb is a tonic, stimulant, febrifuge, and anthelmintic—locally it is an antiseptic and discutient. It is given in jaundice, dropsy, gout and hysteria.

Artemisia Frigida.

Mountain sage, found in Western United States. Used as the powdered herb, dose, 1 to 2 drs. ; and fluid extract, dose, 1 to 2 drs.

Actions and uses.—A new substitute for quinine. It produces no head symptoms, such as ringing in the ears, deafness and temporary delirium. Given in rheumatism, sciatica, neuralgia and general malaise. In rheumatism, scarlet fever, diphtheria, &c., it is given hot until perspiration and urination are established.

Artemisia Sternutatoria, A. Ptarmica, Centipeda orbucularis.

Habitat.—Plains of India, Ceylon.

Parts used.—The plant.

Vernacular.—Arab.—Afkar. Beng.—Naka chhikani. Eng.—Sneeze-wort. Guz. — Chhikani. Hind.— Naka chhikani. Ind.—Hachitte. Mah.—Naka chinkani.

Characters.—The drug consists of broken pieces of stems or stalks of a light ash or brown colour, furrowed and woody ; of pieces of numerous wedge-shaped leaves which are sessile, dentate and villous, and of flower heads which are hermaphrodite, small, roundish, of a yellow colour, and surrounded by oval bracts. The odour is pungent, taste acrid, and bitterish.

Preparations.— Compound powder, known as Nak-chhikni, containing Nāk chhikni 2, Arithâ-Chhala 2, Navsagar, Tambâkhu, saphed miri, kadavi turai, and kali chuno, each one part—mix and make a powder.

Actions and uses.—Its powder is used as a sternutatory in headache, cold in the head, giddiness, hemicrania &c.

Blumea Balsamifera, B. Densiflora, Conyza Balsamifera, Conyza Odorata, Baccharis Salma.

Habitat.—Tropical Himalaya, Burma, Eastern Peninsula, Fiji Islands, Ceylon, and Moluccas.

Parts used.—The plant.

Vernacular.—Beng.—Kuksungh. Burm.—Pungmatheing. Chin.—Ngai. Cochin China.—Kaidaibi. Hind.—Kukronda. Java.—Sumbun. Malay.—Bonga chappa. Sans.—Kukundara Kukkura-dru. Kukkuradru—meaning dog's bush.

Characters.—Shrubby plant, branches erect, covered with coloured bark ; leaves alternate, short petioled, lanceolate, serrate and pinnatifid, downy beneath ; flowers, small and yellow, odour like that of wormwood and camphor, taste pungent. Dose, of the powdered leaves, 1 to 2 drs.

Constituents.—A volatile oil having the odour of wormwood, and a camphor, called Ngai camphor, similar to Borneo camphor.

Preparations.—Infusion of the plant (1 in 10). Dose, ½ to 1 fld. oz. A compound decoction (1 in 10) containing Blumea Balsamifera, Vitex Negundo, Careya arborea, citrus acida, of each one part. Dose 1 to 2 ozs.

Actions and uses.—Diaphoretic, expectorant, anthelmintic and astringent. A compound decoction is given in fevers and catarrhal affections; also in dysentery, diarrhœa, chronic uterine, and other discharges, leucorrhœa, menorrhagia, &c. It is used in thread worms and tinea tarsi. As a deobstruent and resolvent it is used in Bengal in disease of the nose known as *ahwah.* The oil is highly esteemed as a remedy for renal dropsy. In coryza the powder of the leaves is used as snuff, and also given internally as a stomachic and antispasmodic in colic, hysteria, &c. The camphor is used for the same purposes as officinal camphor.

Blumea Eriantha, B. Lacera, Laggera Aurita, B. Aurita.

Habitat.—Western and Southern India, Ceylon.

Parts used.—The plant.

Vernacular.—Arab.—Kamâ phitûs. Burm.—Mai-ya-gân. Duk. —Devari Muli, Jangli kasni. Guz.—Chancharmari, Kalar. Hind.— Kakrôndâ. Mar.—Nimurdo, Bhamburdi. Tam.—Kâttu Mullangi, Nárak-Karan-doi. Tel.—Kâru-pôgaku, Adavi Mullangi,

Chanchermari—Chânchar, a flea, and mari, to kill. in allusion to its property of killing fleas. Bhâmbhurdâ and Chancharmâri are names indiscriminately applied to all Blumeas. Divarimuli, from Divar or Divâl, a wall, and muli, the root, in allusion to the root or the plant being generally found near the walls of ruinous buildings or in graveyards. Adavi Mullangi—Adavi, small, and Mullan, a radish —a small radish, in allusion to the resemblance of its leaves and root to a small radish. Jungli muli—Jungli, wild, and muli, radish.

Characters.—The plant is remarkable for the clusters of globose and woolly buds near the crown of the root. Flowers yellow, odour that of carraways.

Constituents.—Resin, volatile oil, tannin, malic acid, and a crystalline principle allied to quercitrin, and ash 8·3 p.c., of brown colour, and containing a trace of manganese and iron.

Preparations.—Infusion (1 in. 10). Dose, ½ to 1 fld. oz. The herb is used to drive away fleas.

Actions and uses.—The juice is carminative, diaphoretic, diuretic and emmenagogue; given in catarrhal affections, fevers, amenorrhœa, leucorrhœa, &c. The herb with the leaves of Vitex Nugunds and Careya Arborea is used for fomentations.

Calendula Officinalis.

Syn.—Garden Marigold, Marybud Calendula.

Habitat.—S. Europe, cultivated everywhere.

Parts used.—The florets and fresh leaves.

Characters.—The florets are wide, linear, strap-shaped, 3-toothed, of an orange yellow colour, and of a slight heavy odour and a bitter saline taste. Dose, 15 to 60 grs.

Constituents.—A volatile oil, bitter amorphous principle calendulin, sugar, gum. Calendulin is a gummy principle allied to Bassorin. It is yellow and tasteless, soluble in alcohol and swells into a jelly with water.

Preparations.—Tincture (1 in 5). Dose, ½ to 1 fld. dr. Fluid extract. Dose, 5 to 30 ms. Decoction (1 in 10). Dose, 1 to 2 ozs. Ointment, 1 to 9. Insufflation contains Tincture 1 min. and boric acid 4 grs.

Actions and uses.—Stimulant, tonic aud febrifuge; given in scrofula, low fevers, amenorrhœa and jaundice; externally the lotion is used in otitis. As an embrocation the tincture is used in sprains and bruises. The ointment is used for incised wounds, burns and ulcers. It promotes cicatrization with but little suppuration.

Carthamus Tictorius; C. Oxycantha; Crocus Indicus.

Habitat.—Throughout India.

Parts used.—The plant, seeds and flowers.

Vernacular.—Eng.—Safflower, Parrot seed. Arab.—Zurtum, Usfar, Bazr-el-ahris. Beng.—Kajireh. Burm.—Hsoo. Can.—Kusumbe. Guz.—Kasumbo. Hind.—Kasumba Kar. Mar.—Kardi. Pers.—Khasaka dânâh, Kâzirah. Sans.—Kamalottara. Tam.—Sendur Kum. Tel.—Agni sikha.

Characters.—Annual herb; leaves branched, lanceolate, and spinose; flowers, orange red, corolla tubular. Flower heads of a saffron colour and surrounded by numerous leafy bracts; seeds white, angular, smooth, and shining like little conch shells, broad at the base and pointed towards the apex, apex marked with concentric rings. Near the base is a small brownish scar; cotyledons, greyish and oily; odour slight, taste bitter.

Constituents.—The flowers contain a red colouring principle carthamin, a yellow colouring matter, cellulose, extractive matters, albumen, silica, manganese, iron, &c., the seeds contain a fixed oil.

Preparation.—Infusion, and decoction (1 in 20). Dose, ½ to 2 ozs. Medicated oil—the plant boiled in sesamum oil.

Actions and uses.—The seeds are purgative. The medicated oil is locally applied to rheumatic and painful joints, paralytic limbs and intractable ulcers. The hot infusion of dried flowers is given as a diaphoretic in jaundice, nasal catarrh and muscular rheumatism. A cold infusion is used as a laxative and tonic in measles and scarlatina to favour efflorescence of eruptions.

Remarks.—The leaves have the property to curdle milk like rennet, hence it can be used in making cheese. It is also extensively used for dyeing red tape.

Centaurea Behen.

Habitat.—Persia, Syria, Armenia and Cabul.

Parts used.—The root.

Vernacular.—Arab.—Bahaman Abiad. Bomb., Hind.—Saphed bahamen. Eng.—White Rhapontic, White Behen. Pers.—Bahaman-i-suphed. Bâhman or Brâhman means supreme intelligence. Baman is also the name of the eleventh Persian month and of the second day of each month.

Characters.—The roots are of a light brown colour, and 1 or 2 inches in length. They are rather twisted, shrivelled and having two or three branches at their lower portion. The upper end of the root is blunt where it is marked with blackish rings, which are the remnants of sheath-leaves. In some the remains of leaf buds are seen resembling in shape a bunch of grapes ; on section, it is white, homogeneous, and starchy. The odour is rather aromatic ; taste mucilaginous and sweetish.

Constituents.—Fat, sugar, gum, and ash.

Preparations.—Decoction (1 in 20). Dose, ½ to 1 fld. oz. Confection (1 in 5). Dose, ½ to 2 drs.

Actions and uses.—As a diuretic, it is given in calculous affections and jaundice. As a mild aperient, it is used like rhubarb. It is a good substitute for sapheda musali, and used in seminal debility, &c.

Centaurea Benedicta, Carduus Benedictus, Cnicus Benedictus.

An annual plant cultivated in Europe. It contains cnicin, an amorphous bitter principle. It is used as tincture (1 in 10). Dose, ½ to 1 dr. Cnicus is bitter tonic, antiperiodic, and irritant of the alimentary tract, causing burning sensation and constriction in the throat, nausea, vomiting, colicky pain and diarrhœa. The seeds are used as a bitter tonic, like calumba, gentian, taraxacum, &c.

Chrysanthemum Coronarium, C. Roxburghii.

Habitat.—Mediterranean regions and India.

Parts used.—The flower heads.

Vernacular.—Beng., Hind., Guz.—Sevati, Guldâudi. Can.—Shyâvantige-huvu. Duk.—Guledâudi. Eng.—Christmas flower. Mah.—Shevanti. Maly.—Jêvanti-pûva. Sans.—Shevantikâ. Tam.—Shâmantippû. Tel.—Chêmanti.

Characters.—Dried flowering heads of a pale brown colour ; corollas in some detached, in others overlapping the whole flower heads. Within the corollas are silky bracts, large or small, and of a white or yellow colour. When fresh, the odour is very sweet and agreeable, taste bitterish and rather mucilaginous. When chewed for a long time, a tingling sensation is produced on the tongue like that produced by pyrethrum.

Preparations.—Infusion (1 in 10). Dose, ½ to 1½ fld. oz.

Actions and uses.—As a diuretic, it is given in uric acid diathesis ; combined with kálá miri it is used as a demulcent for gonorrhœa ; other uses similar to those of chamomile flowers for which it is a substitute.

Cichorium Intybus, Wild Succory or Chicory (Eng.). Cichrorium Endivia.

Habitat.—Persia and Europe, cultivated in India.

Parts used.—The seeds and root.

Vernacular—Kasani. Arab.—Shikoriah. Hind., Bomb., Beng.—Hinduba, kâsni. Chin.—Ku-tsai, ku-ku. Eng.—Endive, chicory. Mar.—Kâchani. Pers.—Kâsni, Ambuboia. Tel.—Kâsini-viltulu. Tam.—Kâshini-virai.

Hinduba is a corruption of Intuba, or Intybus.

Characters.—Seeds small, colour light or dark brown, angular, furrowed, and rather cuneate or narrow at the base, apex crowned with numerous torn calyces or teeth. Sides of the seeds rather curved, taste slightly bitter ; root of a brown colour with radiating lactiferous vessels ; bark thinner than that of taraxacum, light, soft, pithy and corky ; taste bitterish.

Constituents.—The seeds contain a bland oil. Burnt chicory contains sugar, free extractive, cellulose, ash, nitrogenous matter, fat, &c. The roots contain nitrate and sulphate of potash, mucilage, some bitter extractive principle, and inulin, 36 p.c. The flowers contain a colourless crystalline glucoside insoluble in ether, soluble in hot water and alcohol. In alkalies it dissolves and becomes yellow.

Preparations.—Decoction of seeds (1 in 20). Dose, 1 to 2 fld. ozs. Fluid extract of the root. Dose, 1 to 2 fld. drs., and powder.

Actions and uses.—The seeds are carminative and cooling, used in bilious complaints. Like taraxacum, chicory increases the secretion of bile and promotes digestion ; it also promotes the secretion of the bowels and kidneys. The decoction of the seeds is largely used in torpor of the liver, enlargement of the spleen and general dropsy. The root is bitter, tonic and demulcent, and given with other vegetable bitters in dyspepsia and fever. The dried root, roasted and powdered, is used as a substitute for coffee and for adulterating it.

Cynara Scolymus, Cynara hortensis.

Habitat.—Southern Europe, India, Dekhan.

Parts used.—Succulent receptacles, fleshy leaflets of the calyx, and leaves.

Vernacular.—Arab.—Kirshuf, Kharsjuf. Eng.—Artichoke. Hind., Pers.—Kanjir.

Characters.—The plant is perennial and so named from all its parts being sharp like dog's teeth. It has large flowers of a violet blue colour. The leaves are very bitter.

Preparations.—Tincture (1 in 10). Dose, ½ to 1 fld. dr. The juice, extract and infusion of leaves.

Actions and uses.—The juice is tonic, diuretic and astringent ; used in dropsy and ascites. The leaves contain tannin, and are used in place of galls.

Doronicum Pardalianches, Doronicum Scorpioides.

Scorpioides—The rhizome has the form of a scorpion.

Habitat.—Europe, Syria.

Part used.—The rhizome.

Vernacular.—Arab.—Darunaj-i-Akrabi. Eng.—Leopard's bane. Hind.—Darunaj-i-Akrabi, Akrabi.

Characters.—Rhizome brittle, horny and knotted. In scorpioid form, flat and jointed, greyish externally, dirty white within, upper surface scaly, under surface marked with scars of rootlets, smell aromatic, resembling that of shapeda musali, taste insipid at first, then mucilaginous and somewhat acrid or faintly bitter, and lastly giving a warm pricking sensation to the tongue.

Constituents.—A large quantity of glucose and fat.

Preparations.—Decoction (1 in 20). Dose, 1 to 2 fld. ozs.

Actions ana uses.—Stomachic and tonic ; used in dyspepsia, flatulence, nervous depression and impaired digestion. Given with milk its powder is used in seminal debility.

Echinacea Angustifolia, Nigger-head.

Habitat.—Western States, Kansas.

Part used.—The root.

In Kansas it is known as nigger head from the shape and sombre colour of its fruit.

Characters.—An herb ; root thick, of the size of a little finger, deep brown or black, wrinkled longitudinally. Woody portion consisting of medullary rays and a greenish pulpy substance, taste pungent ; stems numerous, 2 or 3 feet long, stout and bristling with hairs. Leaves 3 veined, lanceolate or linear, very slender at the base, with short petioles ; involucre consists of 2 rows of bracts. Flower disc concave at first, after a time becomes ovoid, and the receptacle assumes a conical form. The receptacle is surrounded by bracts which are boat-shaped and concave, becoming narrowed into a stiff spine-like projection. The fruit is acutely four-angled, one seeded, dry, indehiscent ; pericarp firm, tough and corklike in texture.

Constituents.—The root contains an acid organic resin, nearly colourless, and of a persistent and acrid taste.

Preparations.—Ecthol—prepared by mixing the active principle of echinacea angustifolia and thuja occidentalis in equal proportions. A faint yellowish liquid. Dose, 10 to 40 ms.

Actions and uses.—Ecthol is antispasmodic, antisuppurative and antidote to blood poisoning ; given in malarial fever, cholera, erysipelas. In pyæmia it is given internally and applied externally also. Locally applied in carbuncles, boils and bed sores. It is used as a remedy for bites of snakes, stings of insects, and for pimples. In suppurative disorders of the mucous membranes it is used as a wash or gargle. Under its use suppuration is sometimes avoided.

Echinops Echinatus.

Habitat.—Himalaya, Mysore, Rajwara.

Parts used.—The plant.

Vernacular.—Guz.—Utkatâro, utakanto. Hind.—Oontakatârâ. Sans.—Unthkantaka, Utati.

Oontakantaka is derived from oont or oonth, a camel, and kântik, kântâ, a thistle. It means camel's thistle because camels consume it readily.

Characters.—Plant thistle-like, one to two feet high, erect and much branched ; leaves pinnatifid, tomentose, cottony and spinous ; upper surface viscid, hoary, and tomentose, and cottony beneath; flowers spiny and toothed ; flower heads terminal, solitary, and globose ; root tapering and of a whitish brown colour.

Preparations.—Decoction (1 in 10). Dose, ½ to 2 fld. ozs. Expressed juice of leaves. Dose, 30 to 60 ms.

Actions and uses.—As an alterative it is given in dyspepsia, scrofula. syphilis and fever; a chief ingredient in various alterative and tonic decoctions. As a tonic it is used in seminal weakness.

Remarks.—Often mistaken for Bhuiringni, it having similar spiny leaves. In utakatára the leaves are tomentose and cottony.

Eclipta Alba, E. Prostata, E. Erecta.

Habitat.—Common weed, in irrigated fields and gardens throughout India.

Parts used.—The herb.

Vernacular.—Arab.—Kadun-el-bint. Beng.—Kesuryia. Can.—Garagada-sappu, Kâdige-garaga. Duk., Guz., Mar.—Bhangra, Markava. Hind.—Bhârângraj, Bharngraj. Malyal.—Karishánganni, Cajenneam. Sans.—Kesaraja, Brinjraj, Markava. Tam.—Kareshalanganni, Kaikeshi. Tel.—Gunta-Kalagara.

Characters.—Herb small, prostrate, or erect; colour darkish brown. The whole plant is pleasant and aromatic to the taste, covered all over with white stiff hairs ; leaves opposite, entire, lanceolate or rather waved. Flower heads axillary, or terminal in pairs, pedicelled or stalked and of a white colour. Seeds rugous of a dark brown colour, wedge shaped, or compressed and marked by a ridge in the middle of both surfaces ; taste acrid, odour disagreeable ; root white, fibrous and much branched.

Constituents.—A large amount of resin and an alkaloidal principle, ecliptine.

Preparations.—Expressed juice. Dose, 1 to 2 fluid drs. Decoction (1 in 10). Dose, ½ to 2 fld. ozs. Oil. Dose, ½ to 3 ms. A kind of khir or porridge made up of bangra juice 1 part, juice of leucas zeylanica $\frac{1}{4}$, ginger 2, vitex trifolia (juice) 1, sesbania grandiflora 3, boil in cocoanut juice and add rice and treacle. Dose, 2 to 4 fluid ozs. Given in tetanus.

Actions and uses.—Cholagogue similar in action to taraxacum. The expressed juice of leaves is tonic and alterative, and given with ajowan seeds in catarrh, cough, and enlargement of the liver and spleen. A paste of the plant is locally applied to chronic glandular swellings and to elephantiasis and in skin diseases. The expressed juice is dropped into the ears in earache. Mixed with castor oil, it is given to expel worms; also used to dye hairs black.

Remarks.—In tattooing, the natives after puncturing the skin, rub the juice of white *Bhângrâ* over the part which thus becomes indelibly blue. *Bhângrâ* is of 3 kinds: yellow, white, and black. The yellow or *Pivalâ Bhângrâ* is Wedelia Calendulacea. This herb has yellow flowers on long peduncles. White *Bhângrâ* (Eclipta prostrata) has white flowers and darkish green leaves. Black *Bhângrâ* has dark coloured stems. It is a variety of white *Bhângrâ*. It is the same plant which when in flower is called white *Bhângrâ*, and when in fruit, *Kâlâ Bhângrâ*. In the latter the white corollas having withered away, they are followed by the development of a dark green or black achenes or fruits which are mistaken for flowers by the natives.

Elephantopus Scaber.

Habitat.—Throughout India in shady places.

Parts used.—The root and leaves.

Vernacular.—Beng.—Shamdulum. Can.—Hakkarike. Eng.—Prickly leaved Elephants' foot. Hind.—Gobhi. Mar.—Go-jibha. Maleal.—Ana-shovadi. Sans.—Go-jihva. Tam.—Anashavadi. Tel.—Husti-Kasaka.

Go-jibha—ox tongue; Gojibha—Go, a cow, and jihba, a tongue.

Characters.—Root fibrous; leaves radical, and spreading flat upon the ground, wrinkled, crenulate, and very hairy. The plant is mucilaginous and astringent.

Preparations.—Decoction of the root and leaves (1 in 10). Dose, $\frac{1}{2}$ to 2 fluid ozs.

Actions and uses.—Alterative, astringent, and mucilaginous. The decoction with cumin and butter milk is used in dysuria; also in diarrhœa and dysentery.

Erigeron Canadense, E. Viscosum—Canada Fleabane (Eng.) Squaw Weed.

Habitat.—W. Himalaya, Punjab, Rohilkhand, Europe, and N. America.

Parts used.—Volatile oil distilled from fresh flowering herb (oil of Fleabane.

Erigeron.—From eri, early, and geron, hoary, aged, or an old man, in allusion to the early aged appearance of the plant before spring. Fleabane, in allusion to a supposed property of the plant to destroy fleas. Large bundles of this plant soaked in milk are suspended in the rooms to allure flies to their destruction. Squaw weed, from the weed having a special action upon the uterus.

Characters.—A flowering plant ; stem erect, striate, slender with scattered hairs ; branches numerous, ascending ; leaves radical, obovate, dentate. Flowers yellow in disks. Achenes flat, glabrous, odour mint-like ; taste astringent, bitter.

Constituents.—A volatile oil, bitter extractive principle and tannin. Oleum Erigerontis is obtained by distillation. The oil is a pale yellow liquid becoming darker and thicker by age, of a peculiar aroma and persistent odour, taste not very pungent, terebinthinate, and aromatic ; of neutral reaction, readily soluble in alcohol. Dose, 5 to 10 ms.

Actions and uses.—The drug owes its virtues to the volatile oil. It acts like turpentine, but is less irritating and less efficient. It has a special action as a hæmostatic on the uterus and intestines, and is of special value in uterine hæmorrhages, menorrhagia, intestinal hæmorrhage of passive form, and in typhoid fever. It relieves irritability of the bladder, and is given in cystitis, calculus, &c. It is also given in bronchial catarrh, in hæmoptysis without fever, and in diarrhœa, dysentery and dropsy.

Eupatorium Ayapana, E. Triplinerve, E. Aromaticus.

Habitat.—America, cultivated in India, damp and swampy places, meadows and banks.

Parts used.—The dried leaves, flowering tops and twigs.

Vernacular.—Hind.—Ayapâna. Guz.—Allepa. Tam.—Ayappanni.

Characters.—Shrub of a pleasant aromatic odour; branches reddish, and straight, with scattered hairs ; leaves triple nerved, opposite, smooth and lanceolate. Flowers yellow, taste bitter.

Constituents.—A volatile oil and a neutral crystalline principle Ayapanin. In long needles, soluble in ether and alcohol, but insoluble in water.

Preparations.—Infusion (1 in 10). Dose, ½ to 1 fld. oz. Fluid extract. Dose, 10 to 30 ms.

Actions and uses.—Bitter tonic, expectorant, antiperiodic and diaphoretic ; in full doses, aperient ; given in derangement of the stomach and bowels, dyspepsia and cough. It is also given in ague. It is very efficacious in cough. The leaves when fresh are applied to foul ulcers, and to bites of venomous animals. Its action resembles that of chamomile.

Eupatorium Cannabinum, Rusticorum Panacea, Hemp Agrimony.

Habitat.—Temperate Himalaya and Europe.

Parts used.—The root and leaves.

Characters.—Young shoots have a mealy appearance owing to the presence of white balsamic exudation. Leaves opposite, in pairs, fleshy, lanceolate and smooth ; midrib thick ; flowers purple ; odour aromatic ; taste bitter.

Constituents.—The flowers and leaves contain a bitter alkaloid.

Preparations.—Infusion (1 in 10). Dose, ½ to 1 fld. oz.

Actions and uses.—Diaphoretic, diuretic and emetic, used in fever, jaundice, scurvy, and locally for foul ulcers.

Eupatorium Perfoliatum.

Syn.—Bone-set, wood bone-set, ague weed, fever wort, vegetable antimony, sweating plant, Indian sage, thorough wort.

Eupatorium from Eu, well, easy, and pater, father, born of a noble father. Or from Mithridates Eupator, King of Pontus, who used it medicinally.

Bone-set.—It relieves the pain in bones and limbs in influenza and bone fever (Dengue).

Habitat.—America.

Parts used.—The leaves and flowering tops.

Characters.—Stems hairy, erect, much branched at summit ; leaves opposite and united at base. lanceolate, wide tapering, crenately serrate, rugosely veined, rough above, downy, resinous and dotted below. Flower heads corymbed and numerous ; florets, tubular, white with bristly pappus in a single row. The plant has a bitter astringent taste and weak, and aromatic odour. Dose, 30 to 60 grs.

Constituents.—A neutral bitter principle. Eupatorin (glucoside) a volatile oil, tannin, wax, gum, resin, sugar, ash 7.5 p.c. Eupatorin—a crystalline glucoside, soluble in water, alcohol, chloroform and ether.

Preparations.—Extractum Eupatorii Fluidum. Dose, 10 to 60 ms. Infusion (1 in 10). Dose, 1 to 2 fld. ozs.

Actions and uses.—Bitter, tonic and an efficient diaphoretic. In large doses purgative, emetic, and antiperiodic, similar to chamomile ; given during the shivering stage of fevers, acute catarrh, or general cold ; also in muscular rheumatism, bronchitis, influenza, and sore throat. As a bitter tonic it is given in dyspepsia and general debility.

Eupatorium Purpureum—Queen of the Meadow, Gravel root,

Habitat.—United States.

Parts used.—The root.

Characters.—Perennial herb, with green or purplish band at the joints. Leaves petiolate, in whorl, long, white and downy beneath; flowers purple, corymbs, wood dry. Dose, 1 to 3 drs.

Preparations.—Fluid extract, 30 to 60 ms.; solid extract, 3 to 10 grs. Eupurpurin (abstract) 1 to 4 grs.

Actions and uses.—Lithontriptic. It has a decided power over the uric acid diathesis. Given in rheumatism, gout, and acidity of the urine.

Glossocardia Linearifolia, G. Bosvallea.

Habitat.—Central India, Deccan.

Parts used.—The plant.

Vernacular.—Deccan.—Pitta-Pâpádâ. Mar., Hind.—Phatara-suvâ.

Phatara suva. Phatar a stone, or rock, and suva, anethum. It means rock anethum; Pitta papada, a name also given to Fumria as well as to some acanthaceous plants.

Characters.—Small annual plant; stems many; leaves alternate, linear at the base, and much divided; flower heads solitary and yellow, each with a short naked peduncle, taste bitter and odour fennel-like.

Constituents.—The root contains an essential oil. The leaves, stems and flowers contain a bitter alkaloid.

Preparations.—Confection (1 in 20), 1 to 4 drs.

Actions and uses.—It is used as an emmenagogue to promote the flow of menses.

Grangea Maderaspatana, G. Adansonia, Artemsia Maderaspatan.

Habitat.—Throughout India, Bengal.

Parts used.—The plant.

Vernacular.— Beng.— Namuti. Eng.— Madras wormwood. Mar.—Mâshi patri. Maleal.—Nelampata. Tam.—Mâshiputri. Tel.—Mustaru.

Characters.—Stems procumbent, diffuse and villous, growing flat on the ground; leaves solitary, sub-globose, pinnate, sinuous and obtusely lobed with terminal peduncles. Flower-heads solitary, yellow and sub-globose; odour like that of wormwood.

Preparations.—Infusion (1 in 10). Dose, ½ to 1 fld. oz.

Actions and uses.—Stomachic and uterine stimulant, combined with ginger, pepper and sugar used in obstructed menses, and in dyspepsia and hysteria. Externally it is used as fomentations to inflamed and painful parts; as an antiseptic application the powdered leaves are applied to wounds and ulcers.

Grindelia Robusta, G. Sqarrosa, Gum plant.

Habitat.—California, Mexico, N. America.

Parts used.—The leaves and flowering tops.

Characters.—Herbaceous, perennial plant. Leaves about 2 inches or less long, oblong, or lanceolate, sessile or clasping, obtuse and sharply serrated, pale green, smooth, finely dotted and brittle. Flowering tops many involucre, hemispherical, about half an inch broad, composed of numerous imbricated scales ; the involucres and often the leaves are coated with glutinous oleo-resin ; florets, yellow, ligulate ; odour balsamic, taste pungently aromatic, and bitter. Dose, 10 to 40 grs.

Constituents.—Resin, bitter principle, a fixed and a volatile oil, an alkaline principle grindeline, fat, wax, sugar, robustic acid, gum, tannin and ash 7 p.c.

Preparations.—Extractum Grindeliæ fluidum. Fluid extract of grindelia. It is alcoholic and contains much resin. Dose, 10 to 30 ms. Tinctura Grindeliæ (1 in 10). Dose, $\frac{1}{2}$ to 1 fld. dr. Infusum Grindeliæ (1 in 20). Dose, 1 to 2 fld. oz. Extractum Grindeliæ. Dose, 2 to 3 grs. Mistura Grindeliæ,—liquid extract of Grindelia 30 ms., liquid extract of liquorice 1 dr., mucilage mixture 1 oz.

Physiological Actions.—Grindelia is acrid bitter, when chewed. It increases the flow of saliva. It is antispasmodic, and a motor depressant, a powerful diuretic and mild expectorant. In large doses it is an irritant, producing scalding and high coloured urine. In small doses, it relieves prostration and quiets the nervous system. It is regarded as a palliative and specific for asthma, it gives instantaneous relief, especially when the asthmatic paroxysms recur at night. In whooping cough it modifies the intensity, and lessens the frequency of the paroxysms. In dyspnœa accompanying inveterate chronic bronchial catarrh, and in chronic bronchitis of the aged and in emphysema, given in combination with bromide of ammonium, it allays irritability. It is also used with considerable relief in dyspnœa of the heart and pulmonary diseases, and in coughs due to cardiac hypertrophy.

Therapeutics.—As a sedative it is used in chronic cystitis, in painful conditions of the sexual organs, as priapism and in vaginitis and also in cancer of the stomach. The addition of calomel in minute doses increases the expectorant effects of grindelia ; it is generally given with iodide of potassium or with bromide of ammonium. Grindelia has been regarded as a specific in the bites of venomous serpents and in the stings of insects. As a sedative lotion (1 to 9) it is used for burns and scalds when these are superficial ; if applied in the form of wet cloths, it soothes the agonizing pain in skin diseases with itching and burning sensations in vaginitis, uterine catarrh and herpes zoster. Chronic ulcerations, even when deep and fœtid and exquisitely tender, are often speedily cured by the topical use of this drug.

Guizotia oleifera, Ramtilla oleifera, G. Abyssinica.

Habitat.—Africa, cultivated in India.

Parts used.—The seeds and oil.

Vernacular.—Beng., Hind., Bomb., Guz.—Râmatil, kâlâtil. Can.—Hutchu-ellu. Eng.—Niger seed. Tam.—Oochellu. Tel.—Ulisi, valesalu.

Characters.—Seeds greyish black, somewhat angular, compressed laterally and tapering at the base; surface smooth, taste oily and nutty. The expressed oil from the seeds is sweet in taste and of a pale yellowish colour.

Constituents.—The seeds contain oil 43.2 p.c., albuminous substances 19.3 p.c., sugar, gum, 13 p.c., cellulose 14 and ash 3 p.c. The oil is light yellow or brown, solidifies at a low temperature. It contains 94 p.c. of fatty acids.

Actions and uses.—Emollient. The oil is rubbed over the painful parts in rheumatism as a substitute for linseed oil.

Inula Helenium. I. Quadrifida or Pulicaria Crispa.

Habitat.—C. Asia, S. Europe, N. America.

Part used.—The root.

Vernacular.—Arab.—Ussul-ur-rasun. Eng.—Elacampane, Syrian costus or Syrian ginger. Hind.—Phatmer or Phatmel. Pers.—ganjabil-i-shami, pil-gush. Rasan, kust-i-shami.

Pil-gush means elephant's ear. Phatmel :—phata, rent, and mel, union.

Characters.—Root 6 to 12 inches long, one inch thick, very fleshy, divided below into several branches; sliced longitudinally and transversely; bark overlapping, transverse slices concave and somewhat striated, wrinkled and brownish externally and white internally, odour slightly fœtid, peculiar and aromatic, taste bitter. Dose, 20 to 60 grs.

Constituents.—A volatile oil, an acrid resin, bitter principle, wax, helenin and inuline. Volatile oil contains Alantol or inulol and alant camphor or inula camphor. Alantol is an aromatic liquid of peppermint-like odour and taste. Inula camphor is in white crystals of camphor-like odour, very slightly soluble in water, soluble in alcohol. Inulin—a peculiar body allied to starch. It has no concentric formation and does not gelatinize. It occurs as a fine white powder and is only coloured yellow by iodine, tasteless and without odour. It is contained from 19 to 45 p.c.; also found in arnica, taraxacum, &c. Dose, 1 to 3 grs. Helenin—Alanto Lactone or Elecampane camphor, an active principle, a crystalline camphor or a stearoptene is obtained from the root, in light white acicular crystals or needles, like quinine sulphate in appearance, of a faint odour and aromatic taste—insoluble in water and soluble in alcohol. Dose, ½ to 2 grs.

Preparations.—Decoction and Infusion (1 in 10). Dose, ½ to 1 fld. oz. Ointment (1 in 8).

Physiological Action.—The root is diuretic, tonic, expectorant and emmenagogue. In large doses it is irritant and produces nausea and vomiting.

Therapeutics.—Given in cough, asthma, vesical catarrh, amenorrhœa and dropsy; also in dyspepsia, acidity of the stomach and rheumatism; an ointment is used in skin eruptions and in bites of animals. It is also used to flavour absinthe. The active principle helenin or helenina is an antiseptic and (1 in 1000) arrests putrefaction and prevents the growth of bacilli, and used as a wash in ozæna. Internally it is given in diarrhœa, malarial fevers, and tuberculosis, in tubercular infantile and catarrhal diarrhœa; also in bronchitis and spasmodic asthma to arrest profuse secretions; its chief value is in phthisis. A solution dissolved in oil is used as a paint in diphtheria. It keeps off mosquitoes and other insects. Inulin is aromatic, tonic, stimulant and expectorant; used in dyspepsia and pulmonary affections. Alantol is similar in actions to Helenin, mixed with alantic acid it is more efficacious in tuberculosis than helenin.

Lactuca Sativa, L. Scariola, L. Capitata, L. Virosa.

Habitat.—E. and S. Europe, cultivated throughout India and Persia.

Parts used.—The seeds and concrete milky juice (lactucarium.)

Vernacular.—Arab.—Bazrul-khasa. Guz., Duk.—Kahu. Eng.—Acrid garden lettuce, strong scented lettuce, prickly lettuce. Hind.—Kâhu-khaskabija. Pers.—Tukhme-kâhu. Tam.—Shallatulvirai. Tel.—Kâvu vittulu.

Characters.—A biennial plant; seeds very small, whitish brown, ribbed longitudinally, and little curved vertically, elliptical, lanceolate and compressed; apex pointed; smell slightly aromatic, taste bitterish. Lettuce opium or lactucarium—a concrete milky viscid juice of a brown colour; to obtain it wound the stems of wild lettuce and evaporate the juice. It occurs in circular plano-convex cakes, or irregular, angular pieces of a dull greyish brown colour. When cut into, it has a waxy yellowish white lustre, odour narcotic and opium like, taste bitter. It is partly soluble in alcohol and in ether; with water it forms a turbid mixture.

Constituents.—Lactucarium is a mixture of lactocin, and three bitter principles—lactucin, lactopicrin, and lactucic acid. It also contains lactucerin, an inert waxy substance about 50 p.c. and a trace of hyoscyamine; also a non-volatile acid and a volatile acid smelling like valerianic acid; albumen 7 p.c.; mannite 2 p.c.; and ash 3 to 6 p.c., which contains potash, soda, manganic oxide, ferric oxide, and lime.

Lactucin occurs as a yellowish fusible bitter waxy body, in white crystals or scales, soluble in 80 parts of cold water, moderately soluble in alcohol and acetic acid and less soluble in ether—used as a sedative and hypnotic. Dose, 1 to 5 grs. The leaves contain albuminous matter, starch, sugar, gum, cellulose, chlorophyll, fat and ash, rich in nitrates.

Preparations.—Tinctura Lactucarii (50 p.c.). Dose, 10 to 30 ms. Syrupus Lactucarii, contains 10 p.c. of the tincture. Dose, 1 to 4 drs. Extractum Lactucarii. Dose, 5 to 15 grs. The Ku-chin-kan—a Chinese preparation. It is obtained by cutting off tips of the full grown lettuce, collecting the milky juice which exudes and inspissating it by a moderate heat.

Actions and uses.—Anodyne sedative, hypnotic, diuretic, and expectorant; in action similar to opium, but it leaves no bad after-effects. It is given in palpitation of the heart and in nervousness. The seeds are cooling, demulcent and refrigerant, used in fevers, acute inflammation, and in coughs. The leaves are slightly hypnotic and sedative, and are used in wakefulness due to mental over-work. Ku-chin-kan is said to produce sleep without producing any narcotism, to prove sedative without any previous stimulation, and to afford an excellent substitute for opium where opium is inadmissible. Dose of the seeds, 2 grains to an infant.

Remarks—Kâhu is also the name of Arajuna sádrá—Terminalia Arjuna, with which it should not be mistaken.

Mikania Guaco.

Habitat.—South America and West Indies.

Parts used.—The leaves.

Preparations.—Powdered leaves. Dose, 30 to 60 grs. Fluid extract, 30 to 60 ms.

Actions and uses.—Stimulant, alterative, bitter tonic and febrifuge; also used as a preventive and cure for the bites of serpents and insects; given in chronic rheumatism, both internally and externally, and in intermittent fever and atonic dyspepsia. It is recommended as a local application in gouty paroxysms.

Saussurea Lappa, Aucklandia Costus, Aplotaxis Auriculata; Arabian Costus.

Habitat.—Cashmere.

Parts used.—The root.

Vernacular.—Arab.—Kust. Beng.—Koshta, Kust Patchaka. Can.—Koshta. Guz.—Upalet. Mar., Hind.—Kutha, Kushta Patchuk, Uplete. Malyal.—Sepudday. Sans.—Kushta-Pushkaramula. Tam.—Koshtam. Tel.—Goshtamu, Kashm Koot.—Pers. Koosht-i-shirin.

Characters.—Root very light, in crooked twisted pieces, brown externally and marked with longitudinal ridges, texture very firm. Internally lightish brown, and here and there sprinkled with resinous shining granules; odour somewhat aromatic, resembling that of Jatamasi. Taste bitterish at first, but soon becoming hot, pungent and biting on account of the resin it contains. Dose, 5 to 25 grs.

Constituents.—An odourous principle, composed of two liquid resins, an alkaloid, a solid resin, salt of valeric acid, an astringent principle, and ash which contains manganese.

Preparations.—Infusion:—containing cardamoms 1, kusht 3, water 32. Dose, 1 to 2 ozs. Medicated oil known as Dhupel Tela, lotion and paste. Dhupela tela contains *Upaleta* 1, *Kapura kàchari* 2, *Agara* 1,

Chandana 1, *Golába kali* 1, *Válo* 1, *Pátcha pándri* 1, *Nàkhalá* 1, *Gahulá* 1, *Motha* 1, *Lobana kodiun* 5, *Sisama-na-chhodan* 1. Mix and reduce to a coarse powder and then intimately mix with *Koparela tela* 40. Add to this *Vàlo*, and the whole wrap up in a piece of cloth and put in an earthen pot, invert this vessel over another earthen vessel and the two cemented together with clay, the whole is put into a fire made of fire wood for several hours, when the contents are intimately mixed together.

Actions and use.—As a stimulant it is given in spasmodic diseases, as cough, asthma, cholera, and deranged digestion. As an alterative it is used in chronic skin diseases and rheumatism. Locally a paste of it made in rose water is applied to swollen hands and feet and to swelled abdomen in obesity, and as a cooling lotion to sprains, contusion, and to the head in headache. It is also smoked like opium. Externally it is used as an astringent ointment on ulcers. Dhupel tela is used for itch, baldness, &c. Ladies use it as a hair oil to relieve headache, to remove pediculi and scurf from the head or hair.

Remarks.—It is used as an incense and a perfume, and to protect clothes or bales of cotton, or Cashmere shawls from the ravages of insects as moths. Other drugs similar in action to upaleta and used to protect clothes are kapura, miri, patchòli, kapura kachari, &c.

Siegesbeckia Orientalis.

Habitat.—Persia, throughout India and tropical climates.

Parts used.—The herb.

Vernacular.—Chin.—He-ki-en, Kau-kau. Tam.—Katampam Katampu.

Characters.—Herb erect, and much branched; leaves opposite, triangular or ovate, toothed and scabrous; flowers yellow; fruit achenes, without pappus.

Constituents.—A bitter principle, named darutyne, similar in properties to salicin, a derivative of salicylic acid. Darutyne—to obtain it treat strong decoction of leaves with acetate of lead to precipitate the colouring matter, remove the lead by diluted sulphuric acid and evaporate. Treat the extract with alcohol and water and finally crystallize. Occurs as crystals, soluble in alcohol and ether, but insoluble in cold water, dilute acids, alkalies and chloroform.

Preparations.—Fluid extract. Dose, 10 to 30 ms. Tincture (1 in 8). Dose, 10 to 30 ms. Syrup. Dose, 1 to 2 drs.

Actions and uses.—As an alterative combined with potassium iodide, it is given in scrofula, syphilis, gout, rheumatism and skin diseases. Locally the juice or tincture is used in tinea, thrush, gangrenous sores and other skin diseases; also for healing gangrenous and sloughing sores; it forms a coating like varnish on wounds and ulcers. As a stomachic tonic its properties are similar to chamomile.

Sphæranthus Indicus.

Habitat.—India.

Parts used.—The herb.

Vernacular.—Arab.—Dookkon, Kamâzariyûs. Beng.—Chagul-medi. Can.—Mundi Kasa. Duk.—Moondi. Guz.—Gorukh-mundi. Hind.—Khamadrus, Zakhim-i-hyat, Gurak moondi Moondibuti Malyal.—Adak-majyen, Atakka-mani. Pers.—Kamâdariyus. Sans.—Munditika, Bhikshu, Parivraji. Tam.—Kottak Karandai. Tel.—Boda Saram.

Characters.—A small plant. Leaves thick, sessile, obovate, covered with long white hairs. Roots fibrous ; stem slightly furrowed, oblong or perfectly rounded. Flower heads solitary, mostly terminal, and sub-globular ; flowers many, minute, in close contact with one another ; bracts hairy and ciliated ; seeds very minute and of a grey colour ; odour of the whole plant peculiarly aromatic, taste rather acrid and bitter. Dose, 10 to 30 grs.

Constituents.—The herb yields a deep cherry-coloured essential oil. The stems, leaves and flowers contain a bitter alkaloid—sphæranthine.

Preparations.—Distilled water, a paste.

Actions and uses.—As an alterative it is given in syphilis, rheumatism and boils ; as a demulcent in urethritis, frequent micturition, &c., externally a paste is applied to piles and swollen glands.

Spilanthes Oleracea, S. Acmella, S. Calva and S. Paniculata.

Habitat.—Throughout India.

Parts used.—The flower heads.

Vernacular.—Can.—Vana Mugali. Eng.—Para cress. Hind.—Pokarmul. Mar.—Acharabondi, Pipulka.

Acharhondi—achar, a breast, and Bondi, Botdi, a nipple. The flower buds resemble a well developed nipple to a breast.

Characters.—A pot herb ; stem small, smooth, succulent and highly coloured. Flower heads with long stalks, solitary, of a brown colour and conical in form. In size they resemble unâb ; smell aromatic, taste acid, pungent and warm, resembling that of the true pellitory root. Dose, 10 to 30 grs.

Constituents.—A resin similar to pyrethrin, fixed oil, yellow colouring matter, astringent organic acid, glucose, extractive matter and mineral matter.

Preparations.—Tincture (1 in 10). Dose, 10 to 30 ms.

Actions and uses.—Powerful stimulant, and sialogogue. Flower heads are chewed to relieve toothache, which they do by producing irritation of the gums and salivation ; also chewed in headache, paralysis of the tongue, cough, &c. The natives regard it as a local specific in inflammation of the periosteum of the jaw, and the application has a speedy effect in relieving pain and swelling. It is also used as a fish poison.

Tanacetum Umbelliferum, Pyrethrum Umbellferum.

Habitat.—Eastern Persia.

Parts used.—The root.

Vernacular.—Hind., Bomb.—Mitha Akalakara. Eng.—Sweet Pellitory. Pers.—Bozidan.

Characters.—The root is devoid of the acridity of the true pellitory root, which in appearance it closely resembles. It is larger and of a lighter colour than the true pellitory. It is rough and furrowed externally, and hard and whitish within ; on section it is starchy and fibrous. The taste is sweet. Dose, 15 to 60 grs.

Constituents.—Very little Pyrethrin, inuline, a trace, and sugar.

Preparations.—Decoction (1 in 10). Dose, ½ to 1 fld. oz.

Actions and uses.—As an alterative given in rheumatism, gout, and enlargement of the liver and spleen.

Tanacetum Vulgare, var. Crispum—Common Tansy.

Habitat.—Europe, Asia, N. America.

Parts used.—The leaves and tops.

Characters.—An herbaceous perennial plant. Leaves long, bipinnatifid and serrated, of a dark green colour, surface smooth and glandular. Flowers yellow. Dose, 10 to 60 grs.

Constituents.—A volatile oil, a bitter principle, called tanacetin, fat, resin, tannin, mucilage, sugar, tartrates, citrates and malates. Volatile oil—obtained by distillation of the leaves and flower tops by water or steam. It contains a terpene, ketone, tanacetone, alcohol and tanacetyle 20 p.c. It is a greenish yellow liquid, having camphoraceous odour, pungent taste, soluble in alcohol.

Preparations. — Fluid extract. Dose, 10 to 60 ms. Infusion (1 in 10). Dose, 1 to 2 fld. ozs. Oleum Tanaceti, oil of tansy. Dose, 1 to 5 ms.

Actions and uses.—Stimulant, tonic, and emmenagogue. In large doses an irritant narcotic poison ; it causes clonic spasms, disturbed respiration and cessation of the heart's action. Generally given in hysteria, for worms in children, intestinal colic and amenorrhœa. Locally the oil is rubefacient and used in rheumatism, bruises. In large doses as a narcotic it is given in wakefulness.

Taraxacum Officinale, B. P., T. Densleonis, Leontodon Taraxacum.

Habitat.—Europe, Himalaya, Nilgiris, N.-W. Provinces. N. America.

Parts used.—The fresh and the dried roots. Taraxaci Radix B. P.

Taraxacum.—Dandelion from dens, tooth ; and leo, lion. The leaves are of the shape of lion's teeth.

Vernacular.—Eng.—Swine Snout, Puff ball, Dandelion, Lion's tooth, White wild endive. Hind.—Dudhal, Baran, Kanphûl. Pers.—Tarkhash Kûn.

Characters.—Leaves direct from the root crown, 6 to 8 inches long and 2 to 3 inches broad, edges toothed, teeth bent backward 5 or 6 on a side, sessile, glabrous, colour bright green ; root nearly cylindrical, very long and thick, crowned with several short thick heads, longitudinally wrinkled, colour dark-brown ; fracture short, fractured surface exhibiting concentric rings. All parts of the plant exude from any break or wound, a bitter milky juice. When dry the root is wrinkled and shrivelled longitudinally ; axis, porous and yellow ; bark thick and white, with it are many milk vessels in concentric circles ; without any odour, taste bitter, closely resembling the Intybus root.

Constituents.—The milky juice contains a bitter amorphous principle—Taraxacin, a crystalline principle, taraxacerin, also potassium or calcium salts, resinoid and glutinous bodies. The root contains inulin 25 p.c. ; pectin, sugar, levulin, ash 5 to 7 p. c.

Preparations.—Of the fresh root : Extractum Taraxaci, B. P. Dose, 5 to 15 ms. Succus Taraxaci, B. P. Dose, 1 to 2 drs. Decoctum Taraxaci, (1 in 20). Dose, 1 to 2 ozs. Extractum Taraxaci Liquidum, liquid extract of taraxacum, B. P. Dose, ½ to 1 dr.

Actions and uses.—Diuretic, bitter tonic, and aperient ; hepatic stimulant in large doses ; given in cases of chronic hepatic and splenic congestion, hepatic inflammation, especially among residents in the tropics ; also in dyspepsia, constipation and dropsy. Used as an excipient for pills.

Tricholepis Glaberrima.

Habitat.—Central India, Marwar, the Concan and the Deccan.

Parts used.—The plant.

Vernacular.—Bomb.—Bráhámá dàndi. Mah.—Brahmo dandi. Sans.—Ajâdandi.

Characters.—Drug of a pale brown colour consisting of pieces of stems and flower heads ; stems slender, round, furrowed, slightly hairy, soft, and containing a white pith ; flower heads, conical and surrounded by numerous bristly bracts. Within these or in the middle of the flower heads are numerous down-like serrated pappus, white in colour and surmounted on seeds which are erect, wrinkled, furrowed and of a darkish brown colour ; taste bitterish. The flowers smell like chamomile.

Preparations.—Infusion (1 in 10). Dose, 4 drs. to 2 ozs.

Actions and uses.—Aromatic bitter, nervine tonic, and aphrodisiac ; recommended in seminal debility, impotence, hysteria, &c.

Tricholepis Procumbens—Volutarella Divaricata.

Habitat.—India.

Parts used.—The herb.

Vernacular.—Arab.—Shanukat-el-baida. Hind., Bomb.—Bádá-varda. Mah.—Sukayi. Pers.—Asphar-i-bari, kangar-i-supheda. Badaward.

Characters.—Plant thorny, slender, whitish, smooth, and triangular; stems tough, thick as the thumb; flower heads white, surrounded by three needle-like spines and covered with a white down resembling that of Brahama dándi; bracts not ciliated and broad, apex terminating in a long white needle shaped and channelled bristle; slightly mucilaginous and of bitter taste.

Constituents.—A green volatile oil, an acid resin, fatty matter, an alkaloid, and gum.

Peparations.—Decoction (1 in 20). Dose, ½ to 2 fld. ozs.

Actions and uses.—Stomachic, and tonic, given in dyspepsia, flatulence, nervous depression, and impaired digestion. It is also given with milk in seminal debility.

Tussilago Farfara.

Habitat.—W. Himalaya, Persia, Europe, Panjab.

Parts used.—The herb.

Vernacular.—Arab.—Fanjiun. Eng.—Colts' foot. Hind.—Watpân Afangiun. Ind. Bazaar.—Fanjiun.

Characters.—Plant mucilaginous and bitterish; a creeper with many fibres; flowers bright yellow; leaves erect, furrowed, and heart shaped, and sharply toothed, very smooth and glaucous, green above white, and densely cottony beneath.

Constituents.—The leaves contain caoutchouc, gallic and tannic acids, resin, glucoside, wax, gum and saponin.

Preparations.—Infusion (1 in 10). Dose, ½ to 1 fld. oz.

Actions and uses.—Astringent aud demulcent, given in cough. The cotton-like down of the leaf is used as a stypic dressing to wounds.

Vernonia Anthelmintica, Serratula Anthelmintica, Conyza Anthelmintica, Ascaridia Indica.

Habitat.—Throughout India.

Parts used.—The fruit.

Vernacular.—Arab.—Atarital. Beng.—Sômarâj, Bukachi, Kalijiri. Can. — Kâdu-Jirage. Cing.—Sauni-nâya. Guz., Duk.—Kadvi-Ziri. Eng.—Purple fleabane. Hind.—Bakachi. Mar.—Kâralye, Ráná-chá-jirê. Malyal.—Kattai Jirakam. Pers.—Itrital. Sans.—Vakuchi Atavi Jirâkâh, Kanana-jiraka Avalguja, Somarajin. Tam.—Kattu shiragam. Tel.—Adivi-jilakara. Kadvi Jire—Bitter jrûn.

Characters.—Fruit black or dark brown, about 3 or 4 lines in length, and 1 or 2 lines in breadth, cuneate at the base, and seated on a glabrous, sessile ring, becoming broader as it approaches the apex. Apex crowned with brownish white coloured scales the remains of the toothed calyx ; surface covered with whitish scattered hairs and marked with 10 or 12 longitudinal ribs. Seed one, small, oily of a brown or dark colour and conforming with the fruit ; taste bitter and nauseous ; odour faintly aromatic. Dose, 20 to 60 grs.

Constituents.—The seed contains resins, an alkaloid known as vernonine, an oil and ash 7 p.c., free from manganese.

Preparations.—Compound powder—Tikta Jirâkadi Churana—contains vernonia seeds 2, chiretta 4, Picrorhiza root 3, dika mâlee 1, rock salt 2, ginger 5. Dose, ½ to 1 dr. Infusion (1 in 10). Dose, ½ to 1 fld. oz.

Actions and uses.—Anthelmintic, stomachic, antiperiodic and alterative ; given in leucoderma, lepra, psoriasis and other skin diseases. As an anthelmintic, the powdered seeds are given for the removal of ascarides. As a stomachic, in loss of appetite, dyspepsia, &c.; as an antiperiodic the compound powder is given in fevers. Native women use a paste of the seeds for destroying pediculi.

Vernonia Cinerea, Conyza Cineria, C. Purpurea.

Habitat.—Throughout India and Bengal.

Parts used.—The leaves, seeds, and flower heads.

Vernacular.—Beng.—Kukseem, chota koksun. Guz.—Sâdeori. Hindi.—Sahadevi. Kak-jangi. Mar.—Sâhadevi, Sadâdi. Malyal.—Puvanku runal. Sans.—Sahadevi. Tam.—Sira-shenga-lanir, Nedsitu. Tel.—Gheritte-kamina.

Characters.—Leaves oblong, oval, roundish, or ovate, slightly toothed and of a darkish green colour ; flower heads of a pale blue colour. Dose, 10 to 30 grs.

Preparations.—Infusion of the whole plant (1 in 10). Dose, ½ to 1 fld. oz.

Actions and uses.—The seeds are alterative, and used in leprosy and chronic skin diseases. A poultice of the leaves is used as an application to guinea worms. As a diaphoretic the whole plant is given in fevers to bring on perspiration. The seeds are used to destroy vermin in the hair.

Xanthium Strumarium.

Habitat.—Hotter parts of India, Ceylon, Europe.

Parts used.—The herb.

Vernacular.—Arab.—Hasak, Hamazel, Amir. Beng.—Banokra. Can.—Kadvala mara. Chin.—Ts'angurh, Si-rh. Eng.—Broad-leaved Burweed. Hind.—Lane-tonru, Shankhahuli. Pers.—Ispahan-Harada

Khâr-i-khasak. Mar.- Shankishivar, Gokhru Kallan. Panj. and Sind. —Goghru Kallan. Sans.—Sankhini, Shankhapushpi. Tam.—Marlumatta. Tel.—Veritel-nep. Gokhru Kollan means Great Gogharu.

Characters.—The herb contains a yellow colouring matter ; stem, erect, scabrous, mottled with dark coloured spots ; leaves alternate, kidney shaped, or cordate, notched and scabrous ; flowers terminal ; fruit prickly. Dose, 3 to 15 grs.

Constituents.—The fruit contains fat 38·6 p.c., ash 5·2 p.c., albuminoids 36·6 p.c., sugar, resin, organic acids, and a glucoside named xanthostrumarin related to datiscin. Xanthostrumarin is yellow, amorphous mass, soluble in water, alcohol, ether, benzol and chloroform.

Preparations.—Decoction (1 in 20). Dose, ½ to 1 fld. oz.

Actions and uses.—Diaphoretic, diuretic and sialogogue ; given in urinary and renal complaints and long standing cases of malarial fevers ; other actions resemble those of Jaborandi.

Lobeliaceæ—The Dhavala or Lobelia family.

Herbs or shrubs abounding in acrid milky juice ; leaves alternate and exstipulate ; calyx, superior ; corolla, monopetalous, valvate; stamens 5 ; ovary, inferior 1-3 celled ; style 1 ; stigma surrounded by a fringe of hairs ; tube adherent to many seeded pod ; fruit capsular, 2-valved, dehiscing at summit ; seeds numerous, and albuminous.

Habitat.—Natives of temperate climates and tropics.

Properties.—Some species contain the milky juice, which is very acrid ; some are narcotico-acrid, others emetic, purgative and vesicant.

Lobelia Inflata, B.P.

Loobelia B.P.—Bladder podded lobelia, wild or Indian tobacco, emetic herb or weed, asthma weed, vomit wort, gag-root, Inflata from inflatus, inflated or swollen. The pod is egg-shaped and inflated.

Habitat.—N. America.

Parts used.—The dried flowering herb collected after the portion of the capsules has become inflated.

Characters.—An annual weed growing on the roadsides ; stems angular, and channelled ; leaves long, upper ones sessile, lower ones petiolate, ovate, dentate and hairy, of a pale green colour ; flowers small, in long racemes, of a pale blue colour ; calyx superior, 5 toothed, ; corolla, bilabiate ; capsules inflated, two-celled, seeds minute, oblong, brown and reticulated ; odour heavy, unpleasant, slightly irritating, and acrid ; taste nauseous, mild acrid and tobacco-like. Dose, as an expectorant, 1 to 5 grs. As an emetic, 15 to 20 grs.

Constituents.—Lobeline, a narcotic principle ; Lobelacrin, an acrid principle ; Inflatin ; also Lobelic acid, resin, wax, gum, fixed oil, lignin, salts of calcium, potassium and iron, Lobeline—Lobelinium : to obtain it triturate acetic or alcoholic tincture,or the extract with magnesia, agitate, add ether, filter and evaporate. It is a yellow, aromatic liquid, soluble in water. Dose, $\frac{1}{50}$ to $\frac{1}{20}$ gr. Lobelacrin : to obtain it, to the tincture add charcoal ash, with water and exhaust the residue with boiling alcohol. Lobelic acid—precipitate the decoction with sulphate of copper and decompose with sulphuretted hydrogen

Preparations.—Tinctura Lobeliæ Ætherea, B. P. (1 in 5). Dose, 5 to 15ms. Extractum Lobeliæ Fluidum. Dose, 1 to 10 ms. Decoction or Infusion (1 in 20). Dose, ½ to 1 oz. Acetum 10 p.c. Dose, 5 to 40 ms. Oil of the seed 2 to 5 drops.

Actions and uses.—In small doses, diaphoretic, expectorant, antispasmodic and sialogogue. In large dose emetic and purgative ; like tobacco, the leaves, when chewed, excite nausea, vomiting, giddiness headache, general relaxation, increased flow of saliva, and of gastric mucus, of urine and of perspiration; as an antispasmodic it is given in paroxysmal asthma, dry cough with tickling in the throat ; also in whooping cough, angina, influenza, chronic bronchial catarrh and pneumonia. An enema is given in twisting, or intussusception of the bowels and in strangulated hernia, in impaction of the fœces. Drop doses of the tincture every hour gives relief in habitual constipation or 10 drop doses at bed-time act favourably. As an emetic it is too depressing for children.

Lobelia Nicotianæfolia.

Habitat.—Ceylon, Travancore, Bombay.

Parts used.—The plant.

Vernacular.—Can.—Kadahoge Sappu. Eng.—Indian wild tobacco. Mah —Bokenul, Deonul, Dhaval. Tam.—Kottu popillay. Tel.—Adavi pogaku.

Characters.—An annual plant, studded with granules of resinous exudation. Leaves large, resembling those of tobacco, finely serrated, and covered with simple hairs ; dried stalks hollow in the centre; flowers white, in spikes, and supported on a tubular stem ; fruit globular ; capsules about the size of a pea, two-celled ; seeds many, very small, oval, flattened and marked with delicate lines ; colour light brown ; taste hot and acrid. Dose, as an emetic 10 to 20 grs. As an expectorant 1 to 5 grs.

Constituents.—Two alkaloids, Lobeline and Inflatine.

Preparations.—Infusion (1 in 20). Dose, ½ to 1 fld. oz. Tincture (1 in 10). Dose, 10 to 30 ms.

Actions and uses.—Seeds are extremely acrid ; infusion of leaves is expectorant, diaphoretic and antispasmodic ; in large doses emetic and purgative, producing much depression, cold sweats &c. ; used in spasmodic asthma, laryngial and bronchial catarrh, whooping cough, and in dyspnœa.

Ericaceæ—Heath family.

Trees or shrubs ; leaves ever green, opposite or whorled and exstipulate ; calyx inferior ; corolla regular, hypogynous ; ovary 3 to 10 celled, surrounded by a disk or scales ; fruit a capsule, baccate or berry, generally edible ; seeds numerous, small ; albumen, fleshy.

Habitat.—Found universally.

Properties.—Many species are astringent, tonic, and diuretic ; some narcotic, others poisonous ; fruits of many are edible.

Arctostaphylos, Uva Ursi, B. P.

Bear berry ; wild cranberry ; bear's grape.

Arctostaphylos-arctos a bear ; and staphyla, a bunch of grapes. The fruit is rough like a bear, and the berries occur in clusters like grapes. Uva ursi—uva, a grape ; ursus or ursi, bear ; the berries are rough or bearish.

Habitat.—Europe, Asia, mountains, dry and rocky soil, N. America.

Parts used.—The dried leaves—Uvæ ursi folia, B. P. Bearberry leaves.

Characters.—Low, evergreen shrub. Dried leaves, yellowish, green, obovate, long, broad and short-stalked ; coriaceous and obtuse ; margin revolute ; upper surface shining, glabrous with depressed veins ; lower surface reticulate ; odour faint, hay-like ; taste very astringent and bitter. Dose, 10 to 30 grs.

Constituents.—Arbutin, Ericolin, bitter and amorphous ursone, also tannin 6 to 7 p.c., gallic acid, volatile oil a trace, and ash 3 p.c.

Arbutin is a bitter neutral crystalline glucoside ; to obtain it precipitate the decoction with lead acetate, add sulphuretted hydrogen, filter, evaporate and crystallize. It occurs in needles, insoluble in ether, soluble in warm water ; freely soluble in hot water and alcohol. Dose, 3 to 5 grs. Ursone—a resinous crystalline principle ; to obtain it exhaust the decoction by ether and evaporate. Fine needles of a neutral reaction, without any taste ; insoluble in water, sparingly so in ether and alcohol.

Preparations.—Infusum Uvæ Ursi, B. P. (1 in 20). Dose, ½ to 1 fld. oz. Extract of leaves. Dose, 2 to 10 grs.

Actions and uses.—In small doses diuretic, sialogogue and antilithic. In large doses it produces vomiting and purging. It has a specific action on the urinary organs. Arbutin splits up in the system into glucose and hydro-quinone. Uva Ursi is given in cystitis, urethritis, urinary gravel, nephritis, incontinence of urine and dysuria ; also in obstinate gonorrhœa, gleet and leucorrhœa. Arbutin is given in cardiac dropsy and in urethritis with success.

Chimaphila Umbellata, Pipsissewa Chimaphila.

Prince's pine, rheumatism weed, king's cure, bitter winter green. noble pine, pine tulip. Chimaphila means winter loving. The leaves remain green all the winter as though loving that season.

Habitat.—N. America, certain parts of Europe, Asia.

Parts used.—The leaves.

Characters.—An evergreen plant. Leaves long, sharply serrated above ; wedge shaped, nearly entire towards the base ; coreacious, smooth, and of a dark green colour, of no odour, and of a bitter astringent taste. Dose, 10 to 60 grs.

Constituents.—Chimaphilin, a neutral yellow and crystalline principle. Arbutin, a crystalline but colourless substance ; ericolin ; urson, tannin 4 p.c. ; resin, sugar, gum and ash 5 p.c.

Preparations.—Liquid extract. Dose, ½ to 2 drs. Decoction (1 to 17). Dose, 1 to 3 ozs.

Actions and uses.—Similar to those of buchu, uva ursi, pareira, scoparius. As an agreeable gastric tonic, it increases the appetite and aids digestion. As a stimulant of the kidneys, it is given in dropsy, lithic acid gravel ; also in hæmaturia and chronic cystitis attended with albuminuria. It lessens uric acid secretions and hence useful in gout and rheumatism. It has a peculiar influence upon the lymphatics. If used for a long time it causes atrophy of the testes and mammæ. Fresh leaves bruised and applied are rubefacient.

Gaultheria Fragrantissima, G. Procumbens, Andromeda Leschnaultii. G. Leschnaultii.

Habitat.—Hills of India, Nilgheries, Burmah, Ceylon, Himalaya.

Parts used.—The volatile oil distilled from the leaves—oleum gaultheriæ.

Vernacular.—Bomb., Hind.—Jav, Gandapuro. Eng.—Winter green.

Characters.—An aromatic evergreen shrub ; branches glabrous ; leaves 3 cornered, ovate, thick and coriaceous ; contain an essential oil of a yellowish or reddish colour ; flowers in white racemes, axillary; berries of a blue colour.

Constituents.—Volatile oil, arbutin, ericolin, ursone, resin, tannin 6 p.c. ; ash 5 p.c.

Volatile oil, Oleum Gaultheriæ—oil of winter green, is a liquid of a peculiar brick-red colour, owing to the presence of iron ; of an aromatic odour, sweet, warm taste and acid reaction ; readily soluble in alcohol. The oil furnishes carbolic acid identical with that obtained from coal tar. It contains methyl salicylate 90 p.c., gaultherilene—a hydrocarbon, 10 p.c. Dose, 3 to 10 ms.

Salicylic acid.—To obtain it add to Gaultheria oil, diluted caustic alkali, saponify by heat and dissolve. Decompose the solution with mineral acid, separate the methylic alcohol, evaporate and crystallize.

Spiritus Gaultheriæ, Spirit of Gaultheria (1 in 20) of the oil. Dose, ½ to 1 dr. used for flavouring.

Actions and uses.—Like other aromatic essential oils it is antiseptic, carminative, stimulant, diuretic ; in large doses it is a gastric irritant. The oil is used as a flavouring agent in dentifrice preparations. As a caustic, it is locally applied to warts, corns, &c. Like salicylic acid it is given in gout, rheumatic fever, migraine, sciatica, diabetes, cystitis and diphtheria. Locally an ointment is used in eczema and other cutaneous eruptions.

Primulaceæ—The Primrose Family.

Herbs ; leaves, simple and exstipulate ; flowers regular, perfect ; calyx 4-5-cleft and persistent ; ovary superior ; fruit capsular, dehiscent, transverse or valvular ; seeds numerous ; albumen fleshy.

Habitat.—Native of cold and temperate regions, rare in the tropics.

Properties.—The flowers of the cowslip are sedative and diaphoretic, the roots of some are purgative and emmenagogue.

Anagallis Arvensis, A. Cærulea.

Habitat.—India, Europe, W. Asia, Nepal, Kamaon, Khassya.

Parts used.—The herb.

Vernacular.—Arab.—Marijaneh. Eng.—Scarlet Pimpernel. Hind.—Jonk mari, Jam ghani. Kashmir—Kálá-Changra. Pers.—Geah Surkh gul. Jonk mari—Jonk, a leech, and mari, to kill. The herb is given to kill leeches.

Characters.—Herb, male with red flowers and female with blue flowers ; root small ; stem more or less procumbent ; leaves sessile, many ribbed, dotted with purple at the back ; fruit pale, of the size of a pea ; taste bitter and acrid.

Constituents.—A substance identical with saponin to which its poisonous properties are due ; and a strong smelling, volatile oil of a pungent and acrid taste.

Preparations.—Infusion (1 in 10). Dose, 2 to 4 drs. ; a medicated oil.

Actions and uses.—As an alterative given in melancholia, epilepsy, hydrophobia and gout ; as a local sedative it is applied to relieve the pain in the liver and kidneys ; also used in bites of rabid animals.

Cyclamen Persicum.

Habitat.—Persia, Levant.

Parts used.—The tubers.

Vernacular.—Pers.—Azarbu, Chabok-Punjeh-Marium, Ushnan. Eng.—Sow bread. Hind.—Hathajoree. Ind Bazaar—Bakhûr-i-Miryam.

Characters.—Root roundish and tuberous ; leaves roundish, ovate, margins sometimes angular ; capsule 5 valved, coiling up spirally with the seed vessel in the centre.

Constituents.—Cyclamin—an active principle similar to saponin. Taste bitter and acrid. Forms a soapy mixture with water. Boiled with acid it is converted into glucose and a resinous substance named cyclamireten.

Preparations.—Ointment (1 to 40).

Actions and uses.—Locally used as a resolvent of tumours. As an irritant applied to the abdomen to cause vomiting and purging and to the pubes to induce diuresis.

Dionysia Diapensiæfolia.

Habitat.—Persia.

Parts used.—The plant and the seeds.

Vernacular.—Ind.-Bazaars, Hamâma. Pers.—Mahilû.

Characters.—A small shrub like a bunch of intertwining woody stems. Flowers small, like wall flowers ; leaves like those of moss ; seeds 2 lines in length, elliptical, concave on one side and keeled on the other, of a brown colour. Dose, 15 to 30 grs.

Constituents.—A light brown resin ; a crystalline body ; and free fatty acid. The resin on exposure to the air becomes covered with a glaucous film. It is soluble in sulphuric acid and in alkaline solution, The taste is pungent or acrid. It increases the secretion of saliva.

Preparations.—Poultices ; Infusion (1 in 10). Dose, ½ to 1 fld. oz.

Actions and uses.—Local sedative applied to boils and scorpion bites. Internally the infusion is given as an alterative in gouts torpor of the liver and in enlarged spleen.

Plumbaginaceæ—Lead wort or thrift, or Chitraka family.

Herbs or under shrubs ; leaves entire, exstipulate, and generally covered with white or brownish powdery bloom. Flowers regular, rose white or blue coloured ; calyx tubular, 5 partite ; corolla membranous ; fruits utricular, or dehiscing by valves at the apex ; seeds solitary, embryo straight, albumen mealy.

Habitat.—Found in seashore salt marshes and in temperate regions.

Properties.—Most species are acrid and astringent. In some species the roots, applied to the skin when fresh, cause blister.

Plumbago Zeylanica and P. Rosea.

Habitat.—Sikkim, throughout India.

Parts used.—The root.

Vernacular.—Arab.—Shitaraj. Mar., Bom., Guz., Duk., Beng.—Chitra-mul Burm.—Ken-ky-ok-Phyoo. Can.—Chitra mula. Cing.—Sudu nitual. Eng.—White lead wort. Hind.—Chitro, chitraka,

Malyal.—Tumba-Kodivali. Pers.—Shitarah. Sans.—Chitraka, Druna, Tam.—Codiveli, chitra mulum. Tel.—Agni mata, Yarra Chiitra Moolin.

P. Rosea bears the same vernacular names as above with the addition of adjective red, insteadof white.

Characters.—The fresh root exudes a yellow juice. The dried root is in pieces from 2 to 4 inches long, cylindrical, and as thick as the little finger ; bark thick, brittle, smooth of darkish brown colour and marked with small scars of fallen rootlets ; surface marked with irregular fissures ; wood hard, tough, and of a brownish colour ; odour acrid and disagreeable. Red chitraka—the roots are very short and the flowers of a red colour, and hence the name.

Constituents.—Plumbagin, an acrid principle. To obtain it boil the ethereal extract of the root with water, allow it to cool, and crystallize. In delicate needles or prisms, taste saccharine at first, then acrid and biting, melts readily and volatilizes, leaving no residue ; of neutral reaction. Insoluble in cold, mor esoluble in boiling water, freely soluble in alcohol and ether, with strong nitric acid it changes into yellow, with alkalies to cherry red.

Preparations.—Paste, made with vinegar ; Tincture (1 in 10). Dose, 10 to 30 ms. Compound powder :—contains chitrak root emblic myrobolans, himaj, long pepper, piplimula, rhubarb, rock salt, each equal part. Dose, 20 to 140 grs. Shaddharanayoga, a compound powder. It contains chitrak, inderjav, cessampelos pareira, kudu kutaki, ativisi, and Himaj equal parts. Dose, 1 dr. given in flatulence.

Actions and uses.—Alterative and gastric stimulant ; given in chronic diarrhœa, dyspepsia and general anasarca. Locally as a vesicant the root causes more pain than the ordinary blisters and the vesication does not heal readily. A paste of the root is used as a stimulant application to rheumatic joints, leprosy paralytic limbs and to abscesses to promote suppuration. The compound powder is alterative and given in flatulence, rheumatism. The root is acrid and if introduced into the os uteri causes abortion. Lal chitraka is a more powerful vesicant than chitro or safed chitraka, and is used in the preparation of caustic application. Taken internally it is said to expel the fætus whether dead or alive. In large doses it is a narcotico-irritant poison

Apocynaceæ.—Dog bane family.

Trees or shrubs, usually with acrid milky juice ; leaves entire, exstipulate, commonly opposite, sometimes whorled or scattered, generally smooth and with parallel veins ; flowers of rose white or yellow colour ; calyx 5 partite ; corolla 5 lobed ; ovary 2 celled ; style 2, stigma 1 resembling in shape an hour glass or dumb bell ; ovules, numerous. Fruit, 1 or 2 follicles, a capsule, drupe or berry ; seeds albuminous.

Habitat.—Found in tropical regions, Asia, Arabia, Ceylon, Peninsula of India, Malacca, Bengal, Java.

Properties.—They abound in milky juice with which some acrid principle is frequently combined, hence many of them are intensely poisonous. The fruits of a few species are edible, of others are drastic purgative. The bark and seeds in some are tonic, febrifuge and astringent. India-rubber is obtained from the juice of many species.

Allamanda Cathartica, A. Aubletii, A. Grandiflora, A. Verticellata, A. Angustifolia.

Habitat.—America, cultivated in India, growing wild on the Western coast and in Goa.

Parts used.—The leaves and bark.

Vernacular.—Burm.—Pha yung Chan. Mar. and Bomb.—Jheri Sontaka. Can.—Arasina. Malyal.—Arali.

Characters.—Climbing shrub; leaves elliptical, lanceolate, and on short petioles, arranged in fours round each stem; flowers large and funnel or chimney-shaped.

Constituents.—An alkaloid and a glucosidal acid, similar in action to cathartic acid.

Preparations.—Infusion of the leaves (1 in 20). Dose, ½ to 1 fld. oz. Extract of the bark. Dose, 1 to 2 grs.

Actions and uses.—Hydragogue cathartic, in large doses, emetic. Used in lead or painter's colic, biliousness, and constipation.

Alstonia Constricta, Australian or Queen's land fever bark.

Habitat.—East Indies, Australia.

Parts used.—The bark.

Bark in flat pieces about quarter foot in length, one to two inches broad and about ¼ of an inch in thickness, highly fragile, very light and of a soft spongy texture; colour deep brown externally, yellowish brown internally, with deep longitudinal fissures on its outer surface; smell rather disagreeable; taste acrid and bitter. Dose, 3 to 5 grs.

Constituents.—Alkaloid—Alstonine or chlorogenine.

Preparations.—Tincture (1 in 10). Dose, ½ to 2 fld. dr. Fluid extract. Dose, 2 to 5 ms.

Actions and uses.—Astringent bitter tonic and antiperiodic; it possesses the combined properties of quinine and nux vomica, and is an excellent substitute for cinchona bark; especially indicated in remittent fevers which do not yield to the salts of quinine. It is also useful in chronic diarrhœa and as an anthelmintic in worms. It is however inferior to dita bark.

Alstonia Scholaris, A. Oleandrifolia, Echites Scholaris.

Scholaris—school board; in allusion to the planks prepared from the bark of this species and covered with sand being used as a school board. In old days children used to trace letters upon these planks.

Habitat.—Drier forests of India, Travancore, Assam, Coromandel, Bengal, South Konkan, Western Africa, Moluccas, Phillipine Islands.

Parts used.—The leaves and bark, "Dita bark."

Vernacular.—Burm.—Lik-htuk. Can.—Jan thalla. Cing.—Rook-tanna-gass. Eng.—Dita bark. Beng., Hind.—Datyûni, Chhatiân. Malyal.—Pâla, mukan-pâla. Bomb., Mar.—Satavin, Hori kowan. Sans.—Sapta-chhada, sapta parna, vishala tváka, vrihat, tvaka, guchha pushpa. Tam.—Ezhilaip pâlai. Tel.—Edâkulapâla, Pâla-garuda.

Satvin from Sat, seven, and vin, leaves. Satvin is a corruption of the *Sapta párná*, septa, seven, and parna, leaves, in allusion to the plant having verticels, each bearing from 5 or 7 leaves. *Vishála tvak* or vrihat tvak. Vishála or vrihat means "broad or large"; and tvak, dark, the satavina bark being large or broad, and of a dark colour.

Characters.—Leaves, 5 to 7 in a whorl, obovate, oblong, obtuse. Dita—bark, in flat pieces or irregular fragments of from 2 to 4 inches long, one to two inches broad, and about ¼ of an inch in thickness, very light, and of a spongy texture; external surface darkish brown, and deeply longitudinally fissured; internal surface, pale or yellowish brown, spongy and resinous looking; smell disagreeably acrid; taste bitter like gentian. The milky juice furnishes gutta percha.

Constituents.—An alkaloid ditamine; two bases echitamine and echitenene; also echicaoutchin, an amorphous yellow mass; echicerin, in acicular crystals; echitin, in crystallized scales; echitein, in rhombic prisms; and echiretin, an amorphous substance.

Ditamine.—To obtain it exhaust the powdered bark with petroleum ether, and add boiling alcohol. An amorphous, or crystalline powder, having alkaline reaction and bitter taste, similar to quinine. Dose, 5 to 15 grs.

Preparations.—Tincture (1 in 10.) Dose, 1 to 2 fld. drs. Infusion (1 in 20). Dose, 1 to 2 fld. ozs. Liquid extract. Dose, 3 to 8 ms. A compound decoction (1 in 10). It contains alstonia scholaris (bark). Tynospora cordifolia (stem); Azadirachta Indica (bark) and Betula Bhojpatra (bark) equal parts. Dose, 4 to 12 drs. in dyspepsia.

Actions and uses.—As an alterative, the bark is given in gout, rheumatism, skin diseases, &c. As an astringent in chronic diarrhœa, and in advanced stage of dysentery. As a bitter tonic, in convalescence from exhausting diseases and fevers. The compound decoction is given in dyspesia and in cachexia due to enlarged spleen. The alkaloid is regarded as febrifuge equal to quinine in efficacy, and is given in all forms of malarial fevers. It is also a decided galactagogue.

Apocynum Cannabinum. A Androsæmifolium.

Canadian hemp, Indian Physic.

Habitat.—Canada, United States.

Parts used.—The root.

Characters.—An indigenous perennial plant. Root cylindrical, somewhat branched, thick, brown or brownish grey, longitudinally wrinkled and transversely fissured; the bark is thick, abounding in milky juice ; without any odour and of a bitter agreeable aromatic taste. Dose, as a diuretic 1 to 5 grs., as an emetic 10 to 30 grs.

Constituents.—Apocynin : Apocynein ; gallic acid, tannin, resin, bitter extractive, wax, caoutchouc, starch and ash, 1 p.c. Apocynin —a peculiar active principle, not a glucoside, but a resin amorphous mass, insoluble in water, soluble in alcohol and ether. Dose, $\frac{1}{4}$ to $\frac{1}{2}$ gr. Apocynein—A glucoside of a yellowish colour, soluble in alcohol and water, acts like Digitalin.

Preparations.—Liquid extract, 5 to 20 ms. Tincture (1 in 10). Dose, 20 to 60 ms. Decoction (1 in 40). Dose, $\frac{1}{4}$ to $\frac{1}{2}$ fld. oz.

Actions and uses.—The root is a powerful emetic and hydragogue cathartic ; in small doses antiperiodic, diuretic and diaphoretic, similar in action to strophanthus, adonidin and digitalis ; given in dropsy, ascites and anasarca of Bright's disease. Apocynin is a nauseating expectorant and soporific ; it induces drowsiness and diminishes the frequency of the pulse. As a hydragogue carthartic and diuretic, it is given in uræmia. Under its use albumen and casts are decreased. It is given as a resolvent in pleuritic effusions, in hydrothorax and as an anthelmintic for destroying worms.

Aspidosperma Quebracho-Blanco, White Quebracho.

Habitat.—South America, chiefly in Chili and the Argentine Republic.

Parts used.—The bark.

Characters.—A large evergreen tree. The wood is white ; bark in flat, or curved pieces, $\frac{1}{2}$ to 1 inch thick, yellowish grey, deeply fissured externally reddish, yellow and striated within, fracture, granular ; without any odour and with bitter aromatic taste. Dose, 15 to 60 grs.

Constituents.—It contains 6 different alkaloids, *aspidospermine*, aspidospermatine, aspidosamine, quebrachine, quebrachamine, hydroquebrachine : a peculiar sugar called quebrachit ; and tannin, 3—4 p.c.

Aspidospermine and quebrachine represent the activity of the drug.

Aspidospermine—a crystalline body only soluble in oils and fats as cod liver oil, from 6 to 8 p.c. With acids it forms salts as sulphate or muriate which are freely soluble in water.

Preparations.—Tincture (1 in 5). Dose, $\frac{1}{2}$ to 1 fld. dr. Liquid extract, not miscible with water. Dose, 10 to 60 ms. Solid extract ; Dose, 2 to 8 grs. Vinum quebracho. (6 p.c.) Dose, 1 dr. to 1 oz.

Actions and uses.—In small doses, a bitter tonic, antispasmodic and antiperiodic, assists the oxygenation of blood, stimulates the respiratory centres and promotes digestion. It is known as digitalis of the lungs. It is given in dyspnæa due to phthisis, bronchitis, emphysema uræmic and spasmodic asthma and spasmodic cough. It should be avoided in dyspnæa, due to heart disease or in old persons. It enables one to endure fatigue, to climb elevations ; it decreases the sensation of need of air during faitguing exercise ; it is also given in typhoid and other fevers. The solution is used as a protective to wounds. Aspidospermine sulphas has been used hypodermically in cardiac neurosis and in asthma. Dose, $\frac{1}{64}$ to $\frac{1}{32}$ gr.

Carissa Corundas, Capparis Corundas, Echites Spinosa.

Habitat.—Throughout India, dry, sandy or rocky grounds. Kangra and Katah jungles.

Parts used.—The fruit, bark, and leaves.

Vernacular.—Beng.—Karamoha. Cing.—Maha-karomba. Eng.—Bengal currants. Malyal.—Keelay. Hind., Guz., Mar.—Karwando, Karonda Timukhia. Sans.—Karamardaka, Krishna pal. Tam.—Perin-kalak-phallam. Tel.—Pedda kalivi pandu.

Characters.—A large, thorny bush. Fruits oval, resembling large olives; unripe fruits milky and of a greenish colour, surface shining and smooth, taste astringent and acid; ripe fruits, purple, dark purple, or black, and contain a delicious sweet pulp ; leaves subsessile, coriaceous, base rounded or retuse, top rarely mucronate ; root bark with large stony cells forming a network round the wood.

Constituents.—The root contains a fixed oil, a volatile oil, a dark yellowish resin and an alkaloid.

Preparations.—Syrup of fruits. Dose, 1 to 2 fld. drs. Juice of fruits. Dose, 30 to 90 ms. Decoction of leaves (1 in 5).—Dose, 1 to 2 fld. ozs.

Actions and uses.—The fruits are stomachic, antiscorbutic, and digestive. The unripe fruits are astringent, used for preserves and pickles, and as an antiscorbutic. The ripe fruit is cooling, digestive and refrigerant. The juice of ripe fruits mixed with sákara and elachi is a cooling drink, during hot weather and in biliousness. The decoction of the leaves as a refrigerant is used in fevers. A paste of the root is applied with lime juice and camphor in itch.

Carissa Schimferi Acocanthera Ouabaio.

Habitat.—Somali Coast.

Parts used.—The root and wood.

Constituents.—A glucoside ouabain; in white, transparent, rectangular crystals, bitter to the taste, sparingly soluble in cold water, much more readily soluble in hot water, insoluble in ether and chloroform, soluble in stong alcohol, homologous to digitalin and strophanthine, being more powerful cardiac tonic but less cumulative. Dose, $\frac{1}{1000}$ to $\frac{1}{250}$ of a gr.

Preparations.—Watery extract of the root. Dose, $\frac{1}{25}$ to $\frac{1}{16}$ gr.

Actions and uses.—Ouabain, a direct heart sedative, paralysing the cardiac muscle. Hypodermically it is used as a powerful emetic. As a local anæsthetic it is even superior to cocaine. In medicinal doses it increases the secretion of urine, stimulates the intestinal peristalsis and promotes defecation. It chiefly acts on the respiratory centres, hence given in whooping cough to cut short the attack, to reduce the violence and to hasten convalescence. In diabetes it lessens the quantity of sugar in the urine. It promotes the action of the skin and produces perspiration. Generally given with potassium bromide or chloral hydrate. The juice is used as an arrow poison by the Somalis in East Africa.

Cerbera Odollam, C. Manghas, C. Quaternifolia.

Habitat.—Salt swamps in Malabar and creeks on the sea coast of India, Ceylon, Laccadives.

Parts used.—The seeds.

Vernacular.—Can.—Honde. Eng.—Odallam tree. Beng.—Dabûr, Dhakur. Burm.—Kullua. Hind.—Pili Kirbir. Mal.—Odallam. Mar.—Sukanu. Pers.—Kaner zard. Tam.—Kat arali.

Characters.—Carpels ripe, ovoid, fibrous and woody within ; seed one, broad, white and compressed ; cotyledons two and oily. The seeds yields 55 p.c. of a bland fixed oil of a pale yellow colour. Dose, of the kernel, 1 to 4 grs.

Constituents.—A poisonous glucoside identical with thevetine.

Actions and uses.—The bark, leaves and milky juice are emetic and purgative. Like thevetia neriifolia, the kernel is emetic and purgative, in large doses irritant and used for criminal purposes to procure abortion. The natives use the fruit combined with dhatura seeds in hydrophobia.

Holarrhena Antidysenterica, H. Pubescens, Echites Antidysenterica, Chensmorpha Antidysenterica.

Habitat.—Throughout the drier forests of India.

Parts used.—The bark and seeds.

Vernacular.—Arab.—Lisan ul asfir-al-mur. Zabân-i-gungishk-i-talk. Beng.—Kurchi. Can.—Kodasiga. Bomb., Guz ,Duk.—Pandhra-koora, Karva indarjaw, Kudabija, Dholakuda. Eng.—Conessi or Téllicherry bark. Goa.—Khao, Kurro. Hind.—Kueya, Kaureya. Portuguese.—Codagapala, corte de pela. Malyal.—Kotakap-päla. Mar. —Pandhra Kuda. Panj.—Kuro. Pers.—Zabane kunjashke. Sans.—Kutaja—Kalinga, Vatsaka Giri-walika, Sakra sakhin and sakra sána, Bhadrayava Vatsa, Kavya-sakravija. Tam.—Veppa larishi. Tel.—Amkudu.

Vatsaka—cow tree, Sakra sakhin—Indra's tree, Sakrâ sana —Indra's food. Sakrâ vija—Indra's seed. Indrajav or Indrayana, the name of a small hand instrument used by the Hindu god Indra. The instrument resembles in shape a barley seed or Java. Zabân-i-gangish-i-talkha — Jabân a tongue, gangish a sparrow, and talkha, which means bitter. In allusion to the bitter taste of the seeds resembling in shape the sparrow's tongue.

Characters.—Stem bark, brittle, thick, often twisted or quilled, colour dirty white or snuff like. Surface rugous, soft internally; taste slightly bitter at first which soon becomes intensely increased, and resembles that of Ránajái. Root bark, reddish brown, less thick than that from the stem, and studded with prominent small warty growths; taste very bitter; seeds whitish, resembling oats, or of cinnamon brown colour, narrow, elongated, about ½ to ¾ of an inch long, compressed and chanelled on one side, with tuft of hairs on the end most remote from the root stock ; convex on one side, concave and marked by a pale line on the other, easily broken between fingers; taste bitter; odour unpleasant, resembling that of Wrightia Tinctoria.

Constituents.—A non-oxygenated alkaloid. Wrightine.

Wrightine—To obtain it treat powdered seeds with carbon disulphide ; remove the fat oil, then dry, and exhaust with alcohol ; add hydrochloric acid and mix with ammonia, when a copious flocculent precipitate is thrown down. It is an amorphous powder insoluble in ether and in carbon disulphide, soluble in water and alcohol ; also in dilute acids.

Preparations.—Decoction (1 in 10), Dose. ½ to 2 fld. drs. Tincture (1 in 8). Dose, ½ to 2 fld.. drs. Vine Kutej arishta. Dose, ½ to 1 dr. Compound Powder, Pathâ dya Churana :—Contains Indrajav 5, Lodhra 4, venivel 4, bela 5, lâl chitrak 2, trikatu 4, jâmbul chhál 3, dâlimb chhâl 5, dhâuriphul 4, kutaki 5, ativish 5. Jirûn 5, Nâgar moth 5, dâru halad 4, Kariâtu 5, kuda chhâl equal in weight to all the above ingredients Dose, 1 to 2 drs. Confection "Kutajaleha":—To decoction of kudâchhal 20, add jaggary 5, Rasavanti 2, mocharus 2, trikatu 2, triphlâ 2, chitrak 1, venivel 2, bela phal 3, Indrajav 5, vekhând 2, bhilâmo 1, ativish 5, vàvading 4, vâlo 4, madh 12 parts. Dose, ½ to 1 to be given in milk or chhás.

Actions and uses.—The bark and seeds are antiperiodic, similar to cinchona alkaloids, but do not produce nausea, vomiting or headache. They are given in fever, chronic diarrhœa, dysentery, worms, internal hæmorrhages; also in chronic chest diseases, as asthma, in renal colic, and to allay the vomiting in cholera. They are used after delivery to give tone to the genital soft parts (vagina). It is seldom given alone, generally in combination with a number of aromatics and astringents. Pathadya churana is given in dysentery and itnestinal worms. The confection in piles, chronic dysentery and the vine in dysentery and diarrhœa.

Ichno Carpus Frutescens, Apocynum Frutescens, Echiles Frutescens.

Habitat.—W. Himalaya, Bengal, the Deccan and Concan.

Parts used.—The root.

Vernacular.—Beng., Hind., Bomb.—Syamlata. Can.—Kareumbu. Duk.—Krishna Sariva. Malyal.—Palvulli. Tel.—Nallatiga, Moonlagajja namu.

Syamlata—black creeper.

Characters.—The plant a creeper, roots similar in appearance to those of hemidesmus indicus ; bark dark-brown, closely adhering to the wood, harder than that of H. Indicus and having a central pith; taste almost absent.

Constituents.—Acid, allied to cincho tannic acid—a red colouring matter: resin, a small quantity of coumarine and a caoutchouc like substance.

Preparations.—Decoction (1 in 10). Dose, 1 to 4 drs.

Actions and uses.—Alterative, tonic, diuretic and diaphoretic, similar to Indian sarsaparilla, given in syphilis, scrofula, skin diseases. convalescence from fevers and other dyspeptic affections, and in uric acid diathesis.

Nerium Odorum, N. Oleander (Rose-berry Spurge.)

Nerium from Neros, humid, the habit of the species.

Habitat.—Central India, Baluchistan, Afghanistan W. Himalaya, Levant, moist places.

Parts used.—The root and root bark.

Vernacular.— Arab.— Sumul-himar. Beng.—Karabi. Can.—Kanagila. Chin.—Kiah Chuh-au. Duk.—Ganer. Eng.—Sweet scented oleander, solander laurel. Mar., Bomb., Guz., Hind.—Kaner, Khasuba, Khar Zahra. Malyal.—Aralu. Pers.—Khar Zahrah. Sans.—Sveta Pushpa, Rakta Pushpa Prati Lasa, Ashva Maraka, Karavira. Tam.—Arali. Tel.—Kasturi Patte.

Sveta Pushpa, white flowered ; Rakta Puṣhpa, red flowered ; Prati Lasa, laughing. Ashva Maraka—Ashva a horse and Maraka, a killer. The root if given to a horse will kill the animal. Sumul-Himar or Khar-zaharah means asses' bane.

Characters.—Root crooked ; bark of a pale white colour, externally thick and corky and marked with very small longitudinal fissures ; internally very white; wood pale yellow and porous; odour acrid, taste bitter. Dose, 1 to 3 grs.

Constituents.—The tuber contains two bitter non-crystallizable principles. Neriodorin and Neriodorein (both powerful heart poisons) ; a glucoside. Rosaginine; an essential oil; and a crystalline body, neriene identical with digitaleine ; tannic acid—wax. The leaves contain an alkaloid oleandrine ; a glucoside pseudocurarine ; also Neriene and Neriantine.

Preparations.—Medicated oil 116. To prepare it boil oleander root karaveradya-taila in tila oil 8 and add chitraka root and vavadinga seeds each ½. Decoction or infusion (1 in 10). Dose, ½ dr. to 2 drs. Paste.

Actions and uses.—Oleanderin, if hypodermically injected, causes the heart's beats to fall from 75 or 80 to 10 or 12, if continued for some time the heart ceases to beat and with it the respiration. Both the root and the root bark are powerful diuretic and cardiac tonic, like strophanthine and digitalin—an infusion is given in cardiac systole as well as in dropsy. The root is often used to procure abortion and for the purposes of self-destruction. Villagers use the powder of the dried leaves as a remedy for colic, and as an errhine. The wood is employed as rat's-bane, the oil is used as a local application in skin diseases such as itch, herpes, eczema, impetigo, &c. The paste is applied to chancres and ulcers on the genitals and on ringworm.

Plumeria Acuminta, P. Acutifolia, P. Alba.

Habitat.—Throughout India.

Parts used.—The bark, flowers, leaves and juice.

Vernacular.—Beng.—Gabar Champa. Duk.—Gulachin. Eng.—Jasmine tree, Pagoda tree. Bomb., Hind., Guz., Mar.—Dholo Champo Khair Champa. Pers.—Aachin. Sans.—Kshira Champa. Tel.—Vadaganneru.

Characters.—Plant with milky juice and several blunt truncated branches, the leaves long, lanceolate, acuminate, smooth and with parallel veins; flowers, delicate and of an orange colour; root with blunt-ended branches. Dose of the juice, 5 to 10 ms.

Constituents.—The juice contains calcium salt; a kind of caoutchouc, resins, and plumeric acid.

Preparations.—Decoction of the bark (1 in 80). Dose, ½ to 1 fld. oz.

Actions and uses.—The leaves are used as a poultice to reduce indolent swellings. The juice, like gamboge, is counter-irritant, and in combination with sandal-wood oil and camphor it is applied to relieve rheumatic pains, to dispel swellings, and to cure itch. The root bark is a violent cathartic. As a demulcent it is largely used in gonorrhœa and gleet. The flowers are used as antiperiodic. Its branches are used like those of chitraka to procure abortion.

Ranwolfia Serpentina, Ophioxylon Serpentinum.

Habitat.—Throughout India, Ceylon.

Parts used.—The root.

Vernacular.—Beng.—Chandra. Bomb.—Harkai. Can.—Sutrunabhi. Cing.—Avulpori Jovana. Hind.—Chhota Chand. Malyal.—Chivan Avelpori. Sans. Sarpagandha, Chandraka. Tam.—Chivan Melapodi. Tel.—Patalagandhi.

Characters.—Root in pieces, each from 3 to 5 lines in diameter crooked, and somewhat tapering; bark soft, corky, of a light brown colour, and marked with longitudinal fissures, cut portion presenting the appearance of a honeycomb; wood brittle; odour acrid, taste very bitter.

Constituents.—Alkaloid ophioxylin, an orange coloured crystalline principle, resin, starch and wax. The ash contains iron and manganese.

Preparations.—Decoction (1 in 10). Dose, 1 to 2 ozs.

Actions and uses.—The root is a bitter tonic and is an antidote to snake bites and scorpion stings. It is given in colic, dysmenorrhœa, dysentery, diarrhœa and cholera. In cholera it is given combined with aristolochia indica. It promotes the expulsion of the fœtus.

Strophanthus Kombe, B. P.

S. Hispidus, known in Africa as onage or orage. Strophanthus—strop—turning, to turn, to twist; and anthos a flower. The corolla is twisted and tailed lobed. Hispidus—Hairy, bristly; seeds covered with long, coarse hairs.

Habitat.—Tropical and sub-tropical regions, Africa, Java, Sumatra, Asia, Zambesi, Guinea, Senegambia.

Part used.—The mature ripe seed, freed of its long awn. Strophanthi semina, B. P.

Characters.—A climbing plant, pods scimitar shaped ; seeds $\frac{3}{4}$ inch long, $\frac{1}{6}$ inch broad; each seed has a compressed comose appendage attached to the apex resembling that of Taraxacum but longer. It is oval, flattened, obtusely edged, of a greenish fawn colour, covered with silky hairs and with longitudinal ridge on one side ; kernel white, oily ; cotyledons straight ; odour characteristic; taste bitter. All parts of the fruit are poisonous.

Constituents.—Strophanthin, Inein, combic acid, oil, &c., but no alkaloid. Strophanthin strophanthinum—a neutral active principle, a glucoside. The seeds contain it 8 to 10 p.c. To obtain it add acidulated hydrochloric acid and alcohol to powdered seeds, and evaporate and treat the extract with water. White shining colourless or yellowish crystalline powder. Taste bitter, slightly acid ; freely soluble in water and alcohol. Insoluble in ether, chloroform and benzin. With hot diluted sulphuric acid it splits up into strophanthidin and glucose. Dose, $\frac{1}{200}$ to $\frac{1}{30}$ of a grain used hypodermically. Strophanthin Tannas—an amorphous yellowish white powder, soluble in alcohol, contains 58 p.c. of strophanthin, used in a toxic preparation known as the kombe arrow poison.

Preparations.—Extractum strophanthi, B. P. Percolate the seeds with ether and the residue with alcohol, mix with milk sugar 2 to 1 and concentrate. Tinctura strophanthi, B. P. (1 in 40). Treat the seeds with ether to remove the oil, add spirit (1 in 10). Dose, $\frac{1}{2}$ to 1 dr. Decoction (1 in 150). Dose, $\frac{1}{2}$ to 1 dr. Tabellæ. Mix the tincture with chocolate. Each contains 2 ms. of the tincture. Dose, 1 to 3.

Actions and uses.—Strophanthus is like digitalis—a powerful diuretic and cardiac stimulant. In small doses it increases the force and lessens the rate of the heart's action, it is not cumulative, does not cause any gastric or intestinal irritation. It has a powerful effect over rigors; it cuts them short and prevents their recurrence. In large doses it paralyses the heart in systole, and leaves the cardiac muscle in a state of powerful contraction, thus relieving cardiac dyspnœa. In chronic Bright's disease with dropsy, in uræmia, in valvular diseases of the heart with anasarca, in palpitation, in pulmonary œdema, in exophthalmos with tumultuous heart, in asthma &c., it well replaces digitalis. Is is useful in endocarditis, atheroma of the arteries, hysteria, chlorosis and in rigors following operations on the urethra. In tetanus 2 minims of the tincture is found useful.

Remarks.—In America arrow poison is prepared from S. Hispidus. The extract is used to coat hunting arrows. It kills the game but the flesh is not injured by the poison.

Taberna Montana Caronaria, Nerium Divaricatum and T. Heyneana.

Habitat.—Cultivated in India, Australia, Tropical Asia.

Parts used.—The milky juice and root.

Vernacular.—Can.—Nandi-battal. Eng.—Ceylon Jasmine. Hind., Guz.—Tagar. Malyal.—Karata pala. Sans.—Nandi Vriksha. Tam.—Ghandi Taggarapu. Tel.—Nandi Vardhana Chettu.

Characters.—Shrub 6 to 8 feet, much dichotomously branched; bark pale ; leaves glossy, cariacious ; flowers, pure white, often double and sweet-scented or fragrant; all parts of the plant abound in a bitter cream-like sap or milky juice which is free from acridity.

Constituents.—The root contains resin, extractive matter, and an alkaloid. The milky juice contains caoutchouc and resin.

Actions and uses.—Local anodyne, the root when chewed relieves toothache. The juice is very cooling, and is used as an application with lime juice in opacity of the cornea, in ophthalmia and wounds. The flowers are also used in inflammation of the eyes.

Thevetia Neriifolia, Cerbera Thevetia.

Habitat.—West Indies, India, Calcutta.

Parts used.—The bark and oil of seeds.

Vernacular.—Beng.—Kolkaphul. Burm.—Molamiyai-pan. Eng.—Exile or yellow oleander. Guz., Hind., Duk., Mah.—Pivala Kaner. Malyal.—Pachcha-Arali. Tam.—Pach-ch-ai-alari. Tel.—Pach-cha-gan neru.

Pivala Kaner—Pivla, yellow, and kaner, the plant ; the colour of its flowers which is yellow and saffron like. The colour of the foliage resembles that of oleander.

Characters.—All parts of the plant abound in a milky venomous juice, of an acrid smell. Flowers large, saffron coloured, bell-shaped. Foliage like that of the oleander. Fruits fleshy and contain a hard stone ; kernels of the seeds are extremely bitter when chewed, and produce numbness on the tongue. The oil expressed from the kernel is of a yellow colour, taste agreeable, and mild like that of almond oil. Bark in quills, of the thickness of cinnamon, externally of an ash colour, soft, corky and brittle. Internally white, also soft and full of milky juice, taste bitter. Odour disagreeable. Two grains of this bark is equal to 10 grains of cinchona bark.

Constituents.—The seeds contain 41 p.c. of a bland oil. Thevetin; theveresin the active principles, and pseudo Indican. The bark contains thevetin. The oil is limpid, almost colourless. Taste mild and agreeable like that of fresh almond. Exposed to cold it becomes pasty, and even entirely solid at a very low temperature. It consists of triolein 63 p.c., tripalmatin 23 p.c., and tristearin 27 p.c. Thevetine, a glucoside, is obtained from the cake after expression of the oil.

Preparations.—Tincture (1 in 5). Dose, 5 to 15 ms. as an antiperiodic ; 20 to 60 ms. as a cathartic and emetic.

Actions and uses.—The bark is bitter, antiperiodic ; it is given with benefit in remittent and intermittent fevers. In large doses, it acts as an emetic and purgative, and in poisonous doses as an acrid poison. The oil is emetic and purgative. Like olive oil, it is used externally.

Wrightia Tinctoria, Nerium Tinctorium, W. Rothii.

Habitat.—Central India, W. Peninsula, Burma, Coromandel, Coimbatore, Godavery.

Parts used.—The seeds, bark and leaves.

Vernacular.—Arab.—Lasânul-aasâ-fer. Beng.—Inderjou. Bomb.—Kâlâ kura, Bhurkury. Cing.—Vepâl-arsi. Eng.—Sweet Indrajao. Hind., Mar., Guz.—Mithâ Indrajav, Kâlâ kudu, Gode Indrajava. Malyal.—Kota kappâla. Pers.—Tukhme-ahare-shirin, Zabâne kunjashke shirin. Sans.—Hya-maraka. Tam.—Vetpâla-Verai. Tel.—Ankudu Kodisha.

Characters.—Leaves pale green, soft, elliptical, lanceolate, ovate or oblong, acuminate or glabrous ; panicles terminal ; flowers white, follicles in pairs, jasmine-like, and fragrant. Tube of corolla twice as long as the calyx ; bark over the stem free from red colouring matter and smooth ; root bark, dark brown or black, and here and there marked with warty growths. It is not distinctly sweet, but is free from bitterness and tinge the saliva red ; seeds greyish brown, more pointed at the ends than those of karava indrajava, and marked with irregularly longitudinal fissures, some having a tendency to become channelled ; interior is homogeneous, and of a darkish red or brick-red colour.

Preparations.—Decoction of leaves and bark (1 in 10). Dose, ½ to 2 fld. ozs.

Actions and uses.—Stomachic tonic and febrifuge in combination with other vegetable bitters, given in bowel complaints and during convalescence from fever, and other acute diseases. The seeds are tonic and are given in seminal weakness. Leaves when chewed relieve toothache. The bark is confounded with that of Holarrhena, antidysenterica.

Asclepiadaceæ—The Upalasari, Asclepias, or milk-weed family.

Asclepiadaceæ—Æsculapius, Asclepias, tutelary god of medicine. Shrubs or herbs, generally milky, succulent, and frequently of a twining habit; leaves opposite, entire and exstipulate; flowers regular, pink, greenish yellow, white or purple; calyx and corolla 5 partite; stamens 5, alternate with the lobes of the corolla; fruit with two follicles, running when ripe at an acute angle, and thus resembling the two horns of a calf; seeds woody and frequently comose with thin albumin. Other characters and properties are allied very nearly to those of Apocynaceæ. It is a native of Tropics, Southern India, Arabia, Ceylon, Assam, China, Japan.

The roots of this whole order contain chiefly a bitter acrid juice which renders them stimulant, emetic, acrid, purgative, and diaphoretic; some species are used as antidotes to poisoning by snake bites. The roots of some are aromatic and alterative. The root bark of Mudar is a good substitute for ipecacuanha; and that of upalasari for sarsaparilla. The milky juice of several species yield caoutchouc, while others afford indigo.

Asclepias Curassavica.

Blood-flower; wild or bastard Ipecacuanha; Indian root or yellow milk weed; silk weed or wild cotton. Blood-flower because the herb or the leaves have the property of checking capillary hæmorrhages when applied on a fresh wound. Bastard Ipecacuanha, the root is employed in some of the West Indian islands as an emetic like ipecacuanha.

Habitat.—Central America and West Indies, introduced into India and has run wild over all the Peninsula.

Parts used.—The root and juice.

Vernacular.—Bomb.—Kurki, Kakatundi.

Characters.—Herb with oleander-like leaves; flowers red, saffron or orange coloured; seeds and hairs glossy, hence called vegetable silk; root stock short, abruptly divided into yellowish brown rootlets; bark thin, and when fresh exuding a milky juice; taste bitter and some what acrid. Dose, 15 to 60 grs.

Constituents.—An active principle, Asclepiadin, a glucoside, closely resembling emetin.

Preparations.—Fluid extract. Dose, 20 to 60 ms. Decoction (1 in 20). Dose, ½ to 1 fld. oz. Syrup of the juice—Dose, 2 to 6 fld drs.

Actions and uses.—In large doses it gives rise to vomiting, diarrhœa; in small doses powdered dried root is an emetic like ipecacuanha. Syrup of the expressed juice of the leaves given on an empty stomach acts as a very prompt tæniacide (anthelmintic). Decoction is used with benefit as an injection in vaginal leucorrhœa.

Asclepias Curnuti, A. Syriaca, Common milk-weed, silk-weed.

Habitat.—United States.

Parts used.—The rhizome.

Characters.—Root wrinkled, knotty, brownish ; bark, thick with lactiferous vessels ; wood with wedges, yellow ; taste bitter and nauseous. Dose, 15 to 40 grs.

Constituents.—Asclepion, a tasteless crystalline bitter principle ; caoutchouc 6 p.c., milk juice, resin, tannin and starch.

Preparation.—Tincture (1 in 10). Dose, 5 to 40 ms. ; and dusting powder.

Actions and uses.—Alterative, expectorant and emetic, given in asthma, cough, fever, &c. The powder is used locally to promote cicatrization of wounds, ulcers, &c.

Asclepias Incarnata, flesh-coloured asclepias, swamp silk-weed.

Habitat.—United States.

Parts used.—The root.

Characters.—Root knotty, oblong, brownish ; bark thin with central pith, emitting milky juice when wounded; taste sweet and bitter. Dose, powdered root, 10 to 40 grs.

Constituents.—Volatile oil, two acrid resins, and asclepiadin.

Preparations.—Fluid extract. Dose, 15 to 40 ms. Tincture (1 in 10). Dose 5 to 40 ms. Infusion and Decoction (1 in 10). Dose, 2 to 6 drs.

Actions and uses.—As an alterative, given in scrofula, rheumatism as an emetic in asthma, etc., as an anthelmintic to kill worms.

Asclepias Tuberosa.

Pleurisy root or butterfly weed, silk weed, colic root, orange swallow wort, white root, wind root.

Habitat.—United States.

Parts used.—The root.

Characters.—Root large, fusiform, from 1 to 6 inches long, and about three-quarters of an inch or more in thickness, head knotty and slightly but distinctly annulate, and longitudinally wrinkled, externally orange brown, internally whitish, tough, and having uneven fracture. Bark thin, in two distinct layers, the inner one whitish with large white medullary rays, inodorous and of a bitterish somewhat acrid taste. Dose of the powdered root, 20 to 60 grs.

Constituents.—Wood contains two resins, a crystalline glucoside Asclepedin, gum, salts, a volatile odorous fatty matter, starch, tannin, gallic acid, albumin, pectin. Asclepedin is freely soluble in alcohol and ether, sparingly so in water.

Preparation.—Tincture (1 in 10). Dose, 5 to 30 ms. Infusion or Decoction (1 in 20). Dose, ½ to 1 fld. dr. Liquid extract. Dose, 20 to 60 ms. Infusion (1 in 15). Dose, 1 to 2 drs.

Actions and uses.—Diaphoretic, expectorant, emetic, cathartic, and heart sedative. It is used as a specific in pleurisy. It should be given in frequent doses till it produces free perspiration and expectoration. Asclepidin is very useful in pneumonia, asthma, hepatic derangements, diarrhœa, dysentery, rheumatism, amenorrhœa. It promotes the eruption in exanthematous fevers. Generally given with gelsimin, veratrin, hyoscyamin, podophyllin, sanguinarin, &c. Its power is increased by administering it in warm water.

Catotropis Gigantea, C. Procera, Asclepias Gigantea (White variety).

Habitat.—Throughout India, Malay Islands, Persia, Africa, S. China.

Parts used.—The dried root bark (catotropis cortex), milky juice, leaves and flowers.

Vernacular.—Arab.—Ushar. Beng.—Shwet-akund. Burm.—Mayo-bin. Can.—Yakke-gida. Cing.—Varâgahâ. Eng.—Gigantic swallow wort. Bomb., Mar., Guz., Hind.—Akadâ Mundâr Akund, Rui. Malyal.—Erika. Panj.—Pachkand. Pers.—Khark, Drakhte-zahrnak, Shakar-di-Tighal. Sans.—Arka, Rudra Aditya, Surya pâtra, Mondara shri-ai, Taur-kam. Tam.—Erukku, Arka Vella yercam. Tel.—Tella Jelledu.

Drakhte Zahrnak—poison tree. Alarka, or white, and arka, or red, the colour of their flowers.

Characters.—Most acrid of all the asclepeas; every part of the plant abounds in an acrid milky juice. Shrub 6 to 10 feet, of an ash colour and of a peculiarly fœtid odour. Root tapering and thick; bark small, flat or arched and in pieces, brownish or pale white externally, yellowish grey internally. It is corky, soft and fissured longitudinally; taste mucilaginous, bitter, acrid; odour peculiar. Wood porous, yellowish and light; leaves thick, oblong, ovate, wedge-shaped, rather acuminate; stem-clasping at the base, upper surface smooth, under surface pale and clothed with woolly down; flowers star-shaped, of a pink or dark purple colour, rather large and showy; leaflets, keel-formed, circinately recurved at the base. Dose, as an emetic ½ to 1 dr., as a diaphoretic and alterative, 5 to 10 grs.

Constituents.—Mudarine, caoutchouc, yellow bitter acrid resin. Mudarine an active principle, soluble in alcohol and ether, insoluble in cold water, and olive oil, possesses the singular property of congealing by heat and becoming again fluid on exposure to cold.

Preparations.—Powder. Dose, as an alterative 3 grs., as an emetic 30 to 60 grs. Infusion (1 in 10). Dose, ½ to 1 fld. oz. Aquæ (1 in 50). Dose, 1 to 2 ozs. Bougies. Medicated oil (arka taila). Boil together the juice 16, sweet oil 8, and turmeric. Used in eczema.

Actions and uses.—As an alterative the root with calomel and antimonial powder is given internally, and the bark made into paste applied to the legs and scrotum, in elephantiasis, to leprous ulcers, leucoderma and other skin diseases. The root bark, powdered, soaked in the milky juice, dried, and made into cigars, is smoked as an inhalation in coughs and asthma. Dried bark is an emetic. a very good substitute for ipecacuanha, and with opium it is used like Dover's powder in dysentery. The leaves are deobstruent, with rock salt are roasted in a close vessel and the ashes given with whey by the natives in enlargement of the liver and spleen, in intestinal worms, ascites, anasarca, and in dysentery. As rubefacient the leaves are smeared with oil, and used as varalians, to relieve colicky pain and tympanitis. As a poultice, they give relief to inflammatory swellings. The flowers are tonic, stomachic and digestive, and used in cough, asthma, &c. The juice is drastic purgative and caustic, in combination with the juice of Euphorbia neriifolia applied to caried teeth to relieve pain and dropped into the ear in earache. Also applied to the cervix to procure abortion. Given in rheumatism, malarial and low hectic fevers ; and largely used in syphilis, hence known as vegetable mercury. The juice mixed with powdered wood of Berberis asiatica and the juice of Euphorbia Neriifolia made into tents, and introduced into the rectum to relieve tenesmus. In scorpion and insect bites, it relieves the pain and burning. As a depilatory it is used by tanners, and also by women for removing hair from the pubes and other parts. It is a useful local application for the relief of painful joints and swellings, and for ringworm of the scalp. In combination with the juice of Nateio Thuhar and with the wood of Berberis Asiatica it is used as a caustic for closing sinuses and fistula in ano.

Ceropegia Acuminata et Bulbosa, C. Tuberosa.

Habitat.—W. India, Punjab, Upper Gangetic plain, Malabar Hill.

Parts used.—The bulbous root.

Vernacular.—Mah.—Pátála tumbadi. Mar.—Khappar kadu. Punj.—Galôt. Tam.—Bach-chalimanda. Tel.—Manchi Manda.

Characters.—A creeper. Roots bulbous, as large as a small apple ; tubers fleshy, when fresh taste like turnip, of a dark colour and smooth externally, apex slightly depressed with a constriction at the other end. On section white, pith-like and starchy. When chewed they are mucilaginous like salep, and somewhat bitter. Dose, 1 to 2 grs.

Constituents.—A bitter alkaloid ceropegin, fat, sugar, gum, albuminoids, starch. The ash contains manganese.

Actions and uses.—All parts of the plant are edible. The tubers are nutritive tonic, given in leucorrhœa, seminal debility, bowel complaint of children &c. It forms an ingredient of aphrodisiac and tonic confections.

Cosmostigma Racemosum.

Habitat.—W. India, Ceylon, Chittagong.

Parts used.—The root.

Vernacular.—Can.—Ghârahuvvu. Goa.—Gharphul. Mal.—Vattu valli. Mar.—Shendvel, Shendari, Mârvel.

Characters.—Climber running over high trees. Leaves large, coriaceous, smooth, sometimes rounded with a group of dusty brown prominent glands at the junction of the petiole with the leaf; root light brown, externally and scabrous, of a starchy and friable fracture. Without any taste, but a faint odour like ipecacuanha. Dose, of the root bark, 5 to 10 grs.

Constituents.—Crystalline fatty acids, soluble in cold rectified spirit and aqueous alkalies; an acid resin which is glucocidal related to jalapin, gum, sugar, and carbo-hydrates, etc., having the properties of dextrin; on incineration the roots leave inorganic matter.

Preparations.—Decoction (1 in 10). Dose, 4 to 6 drs.

Actions and uses.—The root bark is an efficient cholagogue and given in dyspepsia with fever and clay-coloured stools. It restores the natural colour to stools even in cases where euonymin or mineral acids, &c., have failed.

Dœmia Extensa, Asclepias Echinata, Cynanchum Extensum, C. Cordifolium, C. Bicolor.

Habitat.—Throughout India.

Parts used.—The root and leaves.

Vernacular.—Beng.—Chhâgul. Can.—Kutinga-Juttuve, Talavarnaballi. Duk.—Utran, Jutuk. Guz.—Nâgala-dudheli. Mar.,-Hind.—Utrañ, Ságaváni. Malyal. — Velip-parutti. Sans. — Phala-Kantak. Tam.—Uttâmani, Velipparutti, Tel.—Jittu-paku.

Utran, or Uttara, means ejecting or vomiting, or antagonist.

Characters.—Twining plant; flowers dull white and drooping; follicles with curved beak and covered with soft bristles; leaves roundish, cordate, acuminate, and pubescent, auricled at the base; odour mousy and peculiar; taste faintly bitter and nauseous, when ignited evolve alkaline fumes like that of tobacco or adhatoda. The root is long, slender, and of a dirty white colour; root bark wrinkled and longitudinally fissured, marked with scars of fallen rootlets; wood whitish, porous, and arranged in wedges. Dose, 5 to 10 grs.

Constituents.—Alkaloid Dœmine—soluble in ether, alcohol and water; ash, 15·5 p.c.

Preparations. Decoction (1 in 10). Dose, ½ to 1 fld. oz. The juice of the leaves. Dose, ½ to 1 dr.

Actions and uses.—Emetic and expectorant, given to children in pulmonary bronchial catarrh and in asthma. The juice of the leaves is used as an anthelmintic. Locally the juice mixed with lime (chunam) is applied to rheumatic swellings, boils and abscesses with relief. In large doses it acts as a purgative.

Like Dœmea Extensa, the leaves of hoya viridiflora are employed by the natives as an application to boils and abscesses and as an emetic and expectorant.

Dregea Volubilis var. Lacuna.

Habitat.—Bengal, Assam, Peninsula.

Parts used.—The root, herb and fruit.

Vernacular.—Beng.—Tita kanja. Hind.—Nak chikni. Mar.—Hirandadi, ambri. Tam.—Kodi-palai. Tel.—Dudhi palla.

Characters.—Large climber with green flowers in drooping umbels; bark smooth and ash coloured ; leaves coriaceous, at the base rounded or cordate; follicles obtuse, and covered with brown mealy substance which consists of moniliform hairs. Dose of the root, 10 to 40 grs.

Constituents.—The fruit contains a glucoside Dregein, in light coloured transparent scales, of peculiar bitterish sweet taste, neutral or slightly acid reaction, soluble in water.

Preparations.—Decoction (1 in 10). Dose, ½ to 2 ozs.

Actions and uses.—Emetic, diaphoretic, expectorant, diuretic and sternutatory. The root and tender stalks are intensely bitter and nauseant. As a diuretic they are given in dropsy. The leaves are employed as poultices to boils and abscesses. The root is applied to snake bites.

Gonolobus Condurango.

Habitat.—Equador, Peru and Central America.

Parts used.—The bark.

Characters.—Bark in quills, or curved pieces ; periderm, ash grey colour, wrinkled, warty and with greenish black lichens attached ; liber pale, brown and striated ; odour slight, taste bitter and acrid. Dose, 15 to 60 grs.

Constituents.—A glucoside, condurangin, resin, alkaloid, starch, tannin, gum, &c.

Preparations.—Liquid extract. Dose, 3 to 60 ms. Vine (1 in 10). Dose, 1 to 4 fld. drs. Infusion (1 in 20). Dose, ½ to 2 fld. ozs. Tincture (1 to 8). Dose, 1 to 4 fld. drs.

Actions and uses.—Alterative, tonic and diuretic ; emetic in large doses, given in chronic syphilis, rheumatism, almost as a specific in cancer of the stomach, it mitigates cancer pain, improves the appetite and increases strength considerably. Condurangin is a nerve poison.

Gymnema Lactiferum.

Cow plant, Ceylon cow tree. Beng.—Kiri Hanguna.

Cow tree derives its name from producing a juice similar to milk in colour and consistence. The leaves are administered to nurses to increase the secretion of milk.

Gymnema Gymnos, naked; and nema a thread—in allusion to the peculiar structure of the stamens. Lactiferum—Carrier of milk. The shrub is milky.

Gymnema Sylvestre, Asclepias Geminata, Periplaca Sylvestris.

Habitat.—Deccan Peninsular, Bengal, Nepaul, Assam, East Africa, East Indies.

Parts used.—The root and leaves and the acid principle.

Vernacular.—Ben.—Merasingi. Hind. and Bomb.—Meshasingi. Can.—Sennagerse. Cin.—Binnûg. Duk.—Parpatrah. Mar.—Kavli Wakandi. Sans.—Mesharingi. Tam.—Shiru-kurunja. Tel.—Poda patra.

Meshashringi :—Mesha, a sheep (ram), and shringi horns, in allusion to the follicles resembling the horns of a sheep.

Characters.—Milky shrub of a twining habit; leaves from 4 to 5 inches long, ovate, lanceolate, and of a dark green colour, shining above and pale beneath; flowers small, yellow, with globular apex of white stigma; root about the size of the little finger and resembling Hemidesmus root; wood tough; bark spongy and of a reddish brown colour; taste acrid and saltish.

Constituents.—The sun dried leaves contain resin; a bitter neutral principle; albuminous and colouring matters; pararabin, glucose, carbohydrates, tartaric acid, gymnemic acid 6 p.c. and ash. The bark contains starch and a large amount of calcium salts and other crystalline concretions.

Gymnemic acid:—Triturate the leaves in water, add sulphuric acid and precipitate the extract. In appearance it resembles chrysophanic acid. It forms insoluble salts with alkaloids, a fact which accounts for its property of masking the taste of quinine and of sweets.

Preparations.—Decoction (1 in 10). Dose, ½ to 1 fld. oz.

Actions and uses.—Astringent, stomachic tonic, and refrigerant, given in fever, cough. The root powder mixed with castor oil is applied externally like Ipecacuanha to snake and insect bites. The leaves are applied like varalians to enlarged liver or spleen; the leaves when chewed benumb for a time the taste for sweets and bitters such as sugar and quinine.

Hemidesmus Indicus, B. P., Periploca Indica, Smilax Aspera, Asclepias Pseudosara var. Latifolia.

Habitat.—N. W. and S. India, Bengal and Bombay.

Parts used.—The roots. Hemidesmi Radix, B. P.

Vernacular.—Arab.—Anslabatunnâr. Cing.—Irimusu. Can.—Duda-sali, Sugade Karibanta. Beng.—Anantamool. Duk.—Sugandhi-pâlâ, Natkâ-aushbah. Eng.—Indian scented and country Sarsaparilla. Hind.—Anantamula, Magrale—Jangali Chambeli, Kural. Hindi—Salsa. Malyal.—Narsoninti, Nannari-Kizhanna. Guz., Mar.—Gopa-Kanga Uperasâra, Dudhsali. Goa.—Upercao. Pers.—Aushbahe-hindi, Yâsa mine-barri, Mugraboo. Sans.—Anantamula, Gopi mulama, sugandhi-utapala, sariva. Naga Jihva (snake tongue) Shadipa. Tam.—Nannâri. Tel.—Gadi-Sughandi.

Characters.—Plant twining ; root cylindrical and tortuous ; stem glabrous, long and rigid ; root-bark fissured, longitudinally and cracked or broken transversely ; wood hard and of a yellow colour ; bark wood reddish, brown or dark brown coloured ; odour aromatic and camphoraceous like that of sassafras, tonka bean, or mellilot. Taste sweet but somewhat acrid.

Constituents.—Coumarin. The aroma and taste of the drug are due to this constituent ; a volatile oil, a crystallizable principle hemidesmine ; and a crystalline stearopten called smilasperic acid.

Preparations.—Infusion (1 in 10). Dose, 1 to 2 fld. ozs. Syrupus Hemidesmi, B. P. (1 in 10½). Dose, ½ to 1 fld. dr.

Actions and uses.—Valuable alterative, diaphoretic, diuretic, tonic; the powder fried in butter is given to children in thrush. With honey it is given in rheumatic pains and boils. As a diuretic, its infusion with cows milk is given in scanty and high coloured urine, strangury and gravel. As a diaphoretic and tonic, it is given in fevers with loss of appetite and disinclination for food. As an alterative it is given in chronic rheumatism, skin diseases, scrofula, syphilis, cachexia, constitutional debility &c. Infusion with onion and cocoanut oil is given in piles. It is a good substitute for sarsaparilla. Often mistaken for Ichnocarpus Frutescens (apocynaceæ). Both are called in Sanscrit Sariva. Barleria preonitis.—Karanta (Hind), is frequently sold by druggist. for upalasari.

Pentatropis Microphylla, Asclepias Tenuiflora, Asclepias Microphylla, P. Spiralis.

Habitat.—Tropical plant.

Parts used.—The root.

Vernacular.— Guz.—Shingroti. Ind. —Amber vel. Malyal. —Perpada gum. Punj.—Pushpi. Tam.—Ambar-vel. Tel.— Pulapala.

Characters—A creeper. Leaves thick, smooth and fleshy, from 1 to 2 inches long and from 1 to 1¼ inches broad, cordate, ovate, and with a very small sharp point at the apex ; stem very slender ; root thick as the little finger, of a pale brown colour externally, and white within ; smell of the root camphoraceous, and taste acrid.

Preparation.—Decoction of root (1 in 10). Dose, 1 to 2 fld. ozs.

Actions and uses.—Alterative, a constant ingredient in native alterative decoctions, used in gonorrhœa, syphilis, rheumatism and general debility.

Tylophora Asthmatica, Asclepias, asthmatica, cynanchum, Ipecacuanha, C. Vonutorium. Tylophora Pubescens.

Habitat.—Bengal, Madras, Ceylon, Southern India.

Parts used.—The dried leaves and the root.

Vernacular.—Beng., Hind.—Jangali-pikwâna, antamul. Cing.—Bin-Nuga. Duk.—Pitkâri. Malyal.—Valli-Pàla. Sans.—Gandhana kuli, Anterpachak. Tam.—Codegan, Nanga Murich cham, Nay-palai. Tel.—Kukka-pala. Bomb., Mar.—Pittkari, Kharaki, kharaki rasna. Can.—Adumuttoda

Khadaki Rasna, Khadaki or khadak, a rock, and rasana, a brownish coloured fictitious root, in size resembling the little finger ; the root grows in the crevices of rocks. Antamul, anta or anterdun means entrails, and mula the root ; the root is the remedy to clear or to free or empty, the intestines from dysenteric motions. Anter patchak—anter, intestines, and pachak, to digest. The root is intended to digest or assimilate what may be in the intestines.

Characters.—The leaves 2 to 3 inches long, opposite, entire, ovate, roundish, acuminate, cordate at the base, glabrous above and downy below; dried leaves yellow, brittle, thick and harsh; odour disagreeable when bruised and taste nauseous. Root twining, fleshy, whitish; each being 6 to 7 inches long, of a pale white or brown colour, slender, brittle and wiry : thickest root about two to three lines in width ; root bark wrinkled, longitudinally fissured, and here and there marked with scars of fallen rootlets ; wood light and porous with a somewhat aromatic and acrid smell ; taste slightly bitter. In general appearance, it resembles valerian root.

Constituents.—An alkaloid tylophorine and an emetic principle.

Preparation.—Decoction of leaves (1 in 10). Dose, ½ to 1 oz. Infusion of root bark (1 in 10). Dose, ½ to 1 fld. oz.

Actions and uses.—Emetic, diaphoretic, expectorant, stimulant and alterative. A good substitute for ipecacuanha, given in dysentery, catarrh and fever. As an alterative in syphilitic rheumatism and as a bitter aromatic and stimulant to increase lochia in parturient women. Locally it is soothing and applied to relieve gouty pain. As an emetic the powdered leaves 25 to 40 grains is combined with ½ or 1 grain of tartar emetic, and as an expectorant powdered leaves, 3 to 5 grains is generally combined with opium. The root bark may be given in similar doses and for similar purposes.

Loganiaceæ, Spigelia Strychnos, Niramali or Kuchala family.

Shrubs, herbs, or trees ; leaves opposite, entire, and stipulate, stipules sometimes in the form of raised line or ridge ; ovary 2, to 3 or 4 celled ; style simple below and as many divisions above as there are cells in the ovary. Fruit capsule, or a drupe ; seeds generally peltate, sometimes winged, fleshy, or cartilaginous and albuminous. Natives of tropical regions.

Properties.—Almost all the plants are poisonous. They act on the nervous system and produce frightful convulsions. Some are used in torpid or paralytic conditions of the muscular system ; others are tonic and anthelmintic, but their use requires much caution. They require generally to be given in very small doses.

Gelsemium Nitidum, B. P., Gelsemium Sempervirens, Yellow Jasmine, Wild Jasmine.

Habitat.—Southern States of N. America.

Parts used.—The dried rhizome and roots—Gelsemii Radix, B. P.

Characters.—A climbing plant ; flowers showy, yellow, and forming festoons from one tree to another ; rhizome, cylindrical, long and thick, fracture splintery. Root thin, of a yellowish brown colour and tough ; bark thin and silky, closely adherent to the pale yellow porous wood ; odour aromatic, taste bitter. Dose, 2 to 20 grs.

Constituents.—Two alkaloids, Gelsemine and gelseminine ; also Gelseminic or gelsemic acid ; a volatile oil, resin and starch. Gelsimina Gelsimine—an active principle. To obtain it add acetic acid to the tincture; the resin is precipitated; concentrate the filtrate, and add ether or chloroform, when gelsemic acid will be precipitated ; next add potassium carbonate to precipitate Gelsemine, which is extracted by adding chloroform, ether or benzene. It is an amorphous alkaline very bitter mass, or a pale yellow amorphous solid of intensely bitter taste ; possessing strong basic properties, neutralizing the strongest acids and forming soluble salts. It is sparingly soluble in water. Dose, $\frac{1}{60}$ to $\frac{1}{20}$ of a gr. Gelsiminæ Hydrochloridum. It is freely soluble in water. Dose, $\frac{1}{60}$ to $\frac{1}{20}$ of a gr. Liquor Gelsiminæ Hydrochloride, 1 gr. in 1 dr.

Preparations.—Alcoholic extract. Dose, $\frac{1}{2}$ to 2 grs. Tinctura Gelseminii, B. P. (1 in 10). Dose, 5 to 15 ms. Fluid extract (not miscible with water). Dose, 1 to 10 ms.

Actions and uses.—Similar to those of conium, digitalis, aconite veratrium and antimony. As a motor depressant it acts on the spinal cord. In medicinal doses it lowers the temperature, impairs sensibility, leads to diaphoresis, gives rise to languor, feeble muscular action, slowing of the pulse, drooping of the lids and dilated pupils. In large doses it paralyses motion and sensation, produces complete anæsthesia vertigo, staggering gait, extreme prostration, loss of speech, cold sweats and death by asphyxia or by paralysis of respiration. As a nerve sedative it acts primarily on the nerve centres, affecting both motion and sensation, but not on the nerve ends as is the case with conium. Gelsimine is singularly efficient in antagonizing the mental condition, in removing the state of abnormal fear of any approaching ordeal or any ordinary trial of life. It entirely relieves a woman of her fear of impending confinement or a student from his fear for examinations. Gelsimine Hydrochlorate dilates the pupils like atropine, over which it has the advantage of quicker action and of a more rapid passing off of the dilatation. It is contraindicated whenever there is a weak heart. As an antispasmodic, it is given in intercostal neuralgia; in neuralgia of the fifth nerve, sciatica, rheumatism, muscular spasms, in toothache, spasmodic asthma, dysmenorrhœa, sick headache, chorea, hysteria, sunstroke, pruritis, eczema, epilepsy, tetanus, also in insomnia, delirium tremens, and irritable bladder. As an antiperiodic and also on account of its property of lowering the pulse, it is used in remittent and typhomalarial fevers. It should not be given in a weak heart.

Spigelia Marilandica.

Spigelia anthelmia or Demarara pink root; Carolina pink; Worm grass.

Habitat.—United States, Maryland, Guiana.

Parts used.—The rhizome and roots.

Characters.—A perennial worm grass. Flowers large, showy, scarlet or crimson externally, and yellow within. Rhizome is horizontal, long, thick, of a purplish brown colour; upper surface cup-shaped, and marked with scars; lower surface having many thin brittle rootlets; odour aromatic. Taste, sweetish bitter. Dose, 1 to 2 drs.

Constituents.—A bitter principle Spigiline, a volatile oil, resin, tannin, lignin, wax, salts and gum. Spigeline, an alkaloid. To obtain it distil the tincture with milk of lime and add hydrochloric acid, evaporate to dryness. It is soluble in water, alcohol, insoluble in ether.

Preparations.—Liquid extract. Dose, 10 ms. to 1 fld. dr. Compound infusion of spigelia—worm tea—contains senna, 10; fennel, 10; manna, 30; spigelia, 15; water, 500. Dose, 1 to 2 ozs.

Actions and uses.—Anthelmintic or vermifuge. In large doses, irritant cathartic; in poisonous doses, narcotic. In small doses it is given with cathartics, as senna, calomel, &c., to expel round worms. In large doses it is an uncertain cathartic and may produce vertigo, dilated pupils, spasms and convulsions. It is usually given with an active purgative in mitral, or aortic disease, in palpitation of the heart and dyspnœa.

Strychnos Calubrina, S. Rheedii, Lignum Colubrinum.

Habitat.—Malabar Coast, drier parts of Ceylon, W. Deccan, Peninsula, Cochin.

Parts used.—The wood and root.

Vernacular.—Hind., Beng.—Koochilalata. Eng.—Snake wood, serpents' wood. Guz.—Goagari-lakri. Malyal.—Modira Kaniram. Mar—Deva kadu. Tel.—Naga-musadi, Tansoopaum. Rumphius Arbor ligni colubrini. Tansoopaum—tân-soor, dancing, and paum, a serpent. In allusion to the serpent cobra de capello, which is known for dancing. It erects its head and moves it from side to side at the sound of music.

Characters.—Wood of a light brown colour, knotty and crooked, sometimes covered with a scabrous soft bark which is porous and hard; smell acrid; taste very bitter.

Constituents.—Alkaloids—Strychnine and Brucine.

Preparations.—Tincture (1 in 10). Dose, 2 to 10 ms.

Actions and uses.—As a febrifuge it is given in obstinate intermittent fever and quartan agues. As a tonic, it is given in dyspepsia and malarial cachexia. Largely used by the natives as a remedy in the bites of Nag (snake) both internally and externally. In skin affections it alleviates pain and removes swellings.

Strychnos Castelnæana and other species. Best known as Curare, Urari, Woorara, or Wourala.

Habitat.—Brazil, Guiana.

Parts used.—A resinoid extract from the bark ; also obtained from paullinia curare and other plants of the strychnos family.

Constituents.—Curarina or curarine, resin and fat—Curarina, an alkaloid, an active principle, a yellowish brown powder, or in crystals; soluble in water and alcohol. It contains no oxyzen. Dose, $\frac{1}{400}$ to $\frac{1}{40}$ gr. Resin :—a blackish brown extract, bitter and friable ; soluble in water (3 in 4). Dose, of curare hypodermically $\frac{1}{20}$ to $\frac{1}{6}$ gr. ; of curarine $\frac{1}{200}$ to $\frac{1}{100}$ gr. hypodermically, and $\frac{1}{100}$ to $\frac{1}{40}$ gr. by the mouth.

Actions and uses.—Sedative and antispasmodic and a powerful motor depressant. Like coniine and gelsimine, it paralyses the end organs of the motor nerves and through them the voluntary muscles. The brain, cord, and sensory nerves are subsequently affected. The heart is stimulated at first, then depressed; eyelids droop, the eyeballs protrude, the vision is disordered, and curara diabetes sets in. The absorption is very slow, hence it is eliminated by the kidneys without any change. Hypodermically injected it is promptly absorbed. Hence tried with some success in tetanus, hydrophobia, chorea, epilepsy and other convulsive and spasmodic nervous affections, as much as 4 grains of curare having been injected subcutaneously in 24 hours.

Strychnos Gautheriana, Strychnos Malaccenses.

Habitat.—Tropical districts of Laos, Anan, and Tonquin mountains.

Parts used.—The bark.

Vernacular.—Eng.—Tropical Bindweed. Chin.—Hoang-nan or Hwang-nao. A creeping vine.

Constituents.—Allied to nux vomica and ignatia. It contains alkaloids strychnine and brucine, the latter predominating in very large quantity. In nux vomica and in ignatia, strychnine predominates.

Preparations.—Powdered bark. Dose, 1 to 5 grs. Tincture (1 to 5 p.f. s.p.) Dose, 5 to 30 ms., freely diluted with water, and best given before meals.

Actions and uses.—Like nux vomica it is a general tonic, active tetanizer. It stimulates the nervous system, without causing any depression, strengthens the muscular and glandular apparatuses and the heart. Given in chronic alcoholism, to remove the tremor and prostration which follow a debauch. In anæmia it may be given with iron ; as an alterative it is given in leprosy, syphilitic and scrofulous sores and tumified glands, in bites from dogs, venomous serpents and other reptiles, in seborrhœa of the scalp; also in alopecia, its use benefiting the growth of the hair. In hyperoidrosis it checks morbid excess of perspiration. Good results have been obtained in pustular eczema, acne, sycosis, furuncles, and carbuncles. In malarial fever it is given instead of quinine.

Strychnos Ignatii—Ignatia Amara.

Habitat.—The Philippine Islands.

Parts used.—The seed, St. Ignatius' bean.

Vernacular.—Arab.—Papita. Bomb.—Papetan. Eng.—St. Ignatius' bean. Hind.—Papeeta. Tam.—Kayappan Kottai.

Characters.—A small tree; fruit of the shape and size of a pear; pericarp brittle; seeds 24, embedded in bitter pulp; each seed about an inch in length, in form ovoid, or triangular, or bluntly angular, and covered with silvery hairs; epidermis brown, or of a dull grey colour; albumen, horny; intensely bitter and of an earthy smell.

Constituents.—Strychnine, 1 p.c.; Brucine, 1 p c. and Proteids.

Preparations.—Powder ½ to 3 grs. Tincture of Ignatia (1 in 10). Dose, 2 to 20 ms.

Actions and uses.—Similar to nux vomica, but more active, as it contains larger quantity of strychnine. It is, however, not used in European medicine, though in native practice it is still used in cholera. In plague and other infectious diseases, in intercostal neuralgia, convulsions in children, hysteria, hyperæsthesia, insomnia, aphonia, and in hypochondriasis it is used with good results.

Strychnos Nux Vomica, B.P.

Nux Vomica. Nux, a rent; and Vomere, to vomit. Excessive dose may vomit or require vomiting to save life, small doses allay it.

Habitat.—Throughout Tropical India, E. I. Cochin China Island, Tanjore, Malabar, Ceylon, Java.

Parts used.—The stem bark, the dried ripe seeds called nux vomica, B.P.

Vernacular.—Arab.—Falus Mahi, Khane-kul-kalb. Beng.—Kuchila. Burm.—Khaboung. Can.—Hemmushti-caniram. Cing—Kudaka-dornatta. Eng.—Dog, Quaker or Bachelor's button, vomit nut, dog poison, rats' bane, deal root, poison nut, false angustura bark, snake wood tree. Duk.—Coochla. Hind.—Kuchila, Karerua. Malyal.—Kannirak. Mar.—Kâjrâ-Jher-katchura. Pers.—Fuloose mahi. Sans.—Visha mushti, Kulaka Kura chilla, Vishatin duka, Kupilu, kunch. Tam.—Yettik Kottai. Tel.—Musædi, Mushte-vettulu.

Kulaka—a kind of ebony. Kuruchilla, crab seeds, bear resemblance in shape to a crab. Kunch—to make crooked.

Characters.—All parts of the tree are bitter and poisonous. Fruit of the shape, size and colour of an orange; round, smooth, polished, pulpy and indehiscent; on section large quantities of bitter sticky, gummy fluid escape. Within the pulp are from 1 to 5 seeds—seeds are flattened, disc-like or roundish, of the size of a quarter to half a rupee piece, about an inch in diameter, and about 3 or 4 lines in thickness, slightly concave on the dorsal, and convex on the ventral surface, with a depression in the centre. Outside the edge is bevelled with a small protuberance from which a raphe projects to the hilum. Structure hard and horn-like. Colour light grey, or greenish; surface shining, covered with satiny hairs. Internally translucent, tough and horny with a large cavity; cotyledons, small and leafy, homogeneous and of a pale white colour. Even with direct heat, the seeds are very difficult to powder; without any odour; taste persistent, and very bitter; wood in slices about an inch in length, and covered with a light brown bark which is rough and warty in some parts, taste exceedingly bitter.

Constituents.—Seeds contain Strychnine; $\frac{1}{2}$ p.c.; Brucine, $\frac{1}{4}$ to 1 p.c.; Igasurine or impure brucine in combination with igasuric or strychnic acid. Loganin, a glucoside; proteids 11 p.c.; yellow colouring matter, a concrete oil or fat; gum, starch, sugar 6 p.c.; wax, earthy phosphates and ash 2 p.c. The wood bark and leaves contain brucine, but no strychnine.

Strychnine B.P.—Strychnina—strychnia:—an alkaloid, to obtain it boil powdered seeds with hydrochloric or sulphuric acid, to liberate, igasuric, acid, mucilage, colouring matter, &c. To the chlorides and sulphates of the alkaloids thus formed, add milk of lime which will precipitate strychnine and brucine. To separate strychnine boil the residue with alcohol, purify with animal charcoal and reprecipitate with ammonia. Colourless, 4 sided, rhombic prisms without any odour and of an intensely bitter taste even in 1 in 700,000 solution of alkaline reaction, soluble in water (1 in 6,700), soluble in cold alcohol (1 in 150), in boiling alcohol, more freely in chloroform (1 in 6), slightly soluble in cold absolute alcohol (1 in 400), and in boiling absolute alcohol (1 in 40), nearly insoluble in ether. Dose, $\frac{1}{60}$ to $\frac{1}{15}$ gr.; fatal dose, $\frac{1}{2}$ gr.

Strychninæ Hydrochloridum, B. P.—Strychnine Hydrochlorate. Small colourless prisms, readily efflorescing in the air, soluble in water (1 in 35), in alcohol (1 in 60), used as liquor strychninæ hydrochloratis (1 p.c. solution). Dose, 5 to 10 ms.

Strychninæ acetas:—colourless crystals—soluble in water (1 in 80). Dose, $\frac{1}{60}$ to $\frac{1}{12}$ of a gr.

Strychninæ arsenas, Strychnine arsenite:—crystals—soluble in cold water (1 in 35). Dose, $\frac{1}{60}$ to $\frac{1}{15}$ of a gr. Solution $\frac{1}{2}$ p.c. in liquid vaseline is injected hypodermically in phthisis. Dose, 4 to 15 ms. Strychnine Hydrobromidum, soluble in water (1 in 60). Dose $\frac{1}{90}$ to $\frac{1}{12}$ of a gr. Strychninæ Nitras, Strychnine Nitrate:—crystals or colourless needles of silky lustre and bitter taste, soluble in water (1 in 70), alcohol (1 in 70), glycerine (1 in 26). Insoluble in ether, contains 84 p.c. of strychnine, used as solution 2 p.c. Dose, $\frac{1}{60}$ to $\frac{1}{15}$ gr. Being less irritant than the sulphate it is preferred for hypodermic injection; solution 1 p.c., given in incontinence of urine. Dose, 1 to 4 ms. Strychninæ Phosphas, soluble in water (1 in 31). Dose, $\frac{1}{60}$ to $\frac{1}{15}$ gr. Strychninæ sulphas, Strychnine sulphate.—Large prismatic crystals, efflorescent, without any odour, intense bitter taste, neutral reaction, slightly soluble in water (1 in 50), in alcohol (1 in 100), insoluble in ether; contains 75 p.c. of strychnine. Dose, $\frac{1}{60}$ to $\frac{1}{20}$ gr. Strychninæ sulphas acida—soluble in water (1 in 36), used as solution (1 in 40). Dose, $\frac{1}{60}$ to $\frac{1}{15}$ gr. of the solution for hypodermic injection 1 to 3 ms.

Brucina—Brucine—with alkaloid strychnine, it is found in the seed of strychnos nux vomica and alone in the bark of strychnos Ligustrina. It occurs in prisms, pearly flakes or masses, less bitter and weaker than strychnine, slightly soluble in water (1 in 850), freely soluble in alcohol (2 in 3), chloroform, ammonia, creasote and essential oils, insoluble in ether and fatty oils; seldom used. Dose, $\frac{1}{12}$ to $\frac{1}{2}$ gr. Liquor Brucinæ 1 p.c. Dose, 10 ms.

Ignasurin or Ignasuria occurs in the liquors from which strychnine and brucine have been precipitated by lime, in white crystals; Loganine a bitter glucoside in white prisms, soluble in water, alcohol.

Preparations.—Of the seeds (nux vomica) : Powder. Dose, 1 to 4 grs. Extractum nucis vomicæ, B.P., contains 5 p.c. of strychnine and 15 p.c. of total alkaloids. Dose, $\frac{1}{8}$ to $\frac{1}{4}$ gr. Extractum nucis vomicæ fluidum, B.P., contains $1\frac{1}{2}$ p.c. of total alkaloids. Dose, 1 to 5 ms. Tinctura nucis vomicæ, B.P. 0·3 p.c. of total alkaloids or $\frac{1}{4}$ gr. of strychnine in 110 ms. Dose, 5 to 15 ms.

Strychnine. Hypodermic tablets, $\frac{1}{60}$ to $\frac{1}{30}$ gr. each. Syrupus Ferri Phosphates cum Quinina et Strychninæ, B.P., Syrup of phosphate of iron with quinine and strychnine, "Easton's syrup," Compound syrup of hypophosphites hydrobromatis. Phosphorus pills.

Actions and uses.—The seeds are nervine stomachic, tonic and aphrodisiac. Externally the paste is antiseptic; the solution is highly irritant to the tissues. If injected subcutaneously it is poisonous. The action of nux vomica is that of strychnine. In small doses it stimulates the stomach and intestines, increases the gastric, the pancreatic, the intestinal and the biliary secretions. Strychnine promotes digestion, sharpens appetite, increases peristalsis and acts as a purgative. It stimulates the uterus and the genito-urinary organs, promotes menstruation and increases virile powers. It increases the flow of urine and is often found in the urine, saliva and sweats. It is a cumulative poison. it contracts the renal arteries and thus hinders its own excretion by the kidneys. In large doses it produces tetanic spasms with relaxation between the paroxysms. During the paroxysm it causes contraction of the arterioles and thereby raises the blood pressure. The pupils are dilated, there are jerking movements of the limbs, the respiration becomes spasmodic, the lower jaw becomes stiff, and there is risus sardonicus, or an unmeaning smile depicted on the face.

In poisonous doses there is in addition a sense of suffocation, great dyspnœa and rigidity of the limbs (which are stuck out), the hands are clenched, the feet arched, and the belly tense. There is oposthotenos, and the breathing becomes arrested. In the height of the paroxysm the face becomes cyanosed and the eye-balls protrude. The pulse is frequent, there is increased blood heat, but the intellect remains clear to the last. There is a feeling of a sense of approaching death. In the interval of the paroxysms there is great prostration with profuse sweating. Any slight cause, as a breath of wind, some noise, or even bright light, brings on the recurrence of the paroxysm. Death may be due to exhaustion or asphyxia, due to prolonged rigidity of the respiratory muscles.

As a general stimulant it is given in acute or chronic fevers, anæmia, chlorosis, wasting and other exhausting diseases ; also in hysteria, chorea, epilepsy, infra-orbital neuralgia or in neuralgia of the viscera, &c. In local paralytic affections it should be given only after the acute stage has passed away. In prolapsus ani, in incontinence of urine, due to atony of the bladder, and sometimes in impotence and spermatorrhœa it may be given with benefit. It is administered internally or injected subcutaneously in impending cardiac failure from any cause. With an imperceptible pulse, clammy breath and cold extremities, liquor strychninæ has been given with advantage. It is a nice bitter tonic, in atonic dyspepsia. Given as an adjunct to purgatives in constipation, it increases their peristaltic effects. In vomiting of pregnancy and of phthisis it is the best agent. In torpid liver with foul breath, coated and furred tongue, pale coloured and offensive stools, if given with blue pill it is very useful. In sick headache or in headache occurring in women at the climateric period it is a very valuable agent. As a neurotic it influences the pneumogastric nerve and is useful in cough of phthisis, in bronchitis, pneumonia, emphysema ; also in bronchial asthma, in cardiac or pulmonary dyspnœa, cardiac palpitation with irregular heart and in hypochondriasis ; strychnine is of great service in acute and chronic alcoholism, under its use the morning vomiting, dyspepsia of drunkards and delirium tremens disappear. It removes the craving for stimulants.

Strychnine is an antagonist to poisoning by chloral, morphine, physostigmine and by cobra (serpent) venom. Brucine is a powerful local anæsthetic. A 10 p.c. solution is useful for chronic pruritus, and 5 p.c. solution for inflammation about the external ear. The natives use nux vomica seeds as a vermifuge. Its efficacy is much increased by giving it with Dariâi narel. Paste of the wood with Dariâi narel is used as a domestic remedy for application to the head in headache, to the body in intermittent fevers, and to the bites of venomous snakes.

Strychnos Potatorum.

Habitat.—Deccan, Peninsula, India, Ceylon.

Parts used.—The seeds.

Vernacular.—Beng.—Induga. Burm.—Kamouye-kyie. Can.—Chillibij. Cing.—Inginiatta. Duk.—Chil-binj. Eng.—Clearing nut. Maleal.—Tetram-kotta. Hind., Mar.—Katak, chilbij, nirmali. Sans.—Ambu prasada. Tam.—Tetran-koltai. Tel.—Indugu, kata kamu.

Niramali is derived from Nira, not, and Mal or Mel, dirt or mud. The seeds are used for purifying muddy water. This property is due to their containing albumen and caseine. Ambu prasâda, from amb, water, and prasada, clearness. An ignorant man is compared to muddy water. He is refined by the society of the learned as dirty water is cleared by the presence of the nut.

Characters.—Fruit shining and black; seeds orbicular, button shaped and smaller in size than those of kuchala. Each having at its border a projecting ridge. Integument yellowish and covered with hairs. Albumen copious and horny, but not so hard as that of nux vomica. No taste. Dose of the powder as an emetic, ½ dr.; as a demulcent, 10 to 15 grs. Contains no strychnine but brucin is present.

Preparations.—Infusion (1 in 10). Dose, ½ to 1 fld. oz.

Actions and uses.—Alterative, tonic, stomachic and demulcent, rubbed down with honey and camphor it is applied to the eye to prevent lachrymation, and to remove opacities; also applied to the abdomen to relieve colic. Its infusion is recommended in irritation of the urinary organs, as gonorrhœa, diabetes and as an emetic in cough.

Gentianaceæ.

The kariatu or Gentian family. Herbs, rarely shrubs; leaves usually smooth, generally exstipulate, glabrous, opposite, simple, entire, sessile and strongly ribbed; flowers regular, showy, of a yellow rose, blue or white colour, axillary or terminal; fruits capsular or berry, 1 to 2 celled, 2 valved; seeds many and small; embryo, minute; albumen, fleshy. Found universally, the properties of this order are bitter, tonic, febrifuge, and stomachic. Bitter principles pervade in them universally.

Canscora Decussata, Pladera Decussata.

Habitat.—Throughout India.

Parts used.—The plant and the fresh juice.

Vernacular.—Beng.—Dankuni. Mar., Hind.—Saukahuli, Dânipola, Dânkuni. Malyal.—Causjun-cora. Sans.—Sankha-pushpi, kambu maleni, Dandot pala.

Characters.—Stem erect, 4 sided, angles very sharp and smooth, branches opposite, cross armed; leaves opposite, sessile, sharp pointed, smooth, entire; flowers white terminal and peduncled; capsule 1 celled, many seeded.

Preparations.—The juice, ½ to 1 fld. oz. Infusion (1 in 80). Dose, 1 to 2 ozs.

Actions and uses.—Laxative, alterative and nervine tonic. Fresh juice is given in insanity, general debility, scrofula, dyspepsia, &c.

Enicostema Littorale, Exacum Hyssopifolium, Cicendia Hyssopifolia, Stevoglia Orientalis, Hippion Orientale.

Habitat.—Throughout Southern India.

Parts used.—The plant.

Vernacular.—Beng.—Kirota. Bomb.—Chhota kirayata. Guz.—Mamijwa. Tam.—Vellurugu. Tel.—Chevu kurti.

Characters.—A small plant growing in damp places, about a foot or more in height, leafy from the base ; leaves opposite, lanceolate or oblong ; flowers small white and sessile. A substitute for andrographis paniculata, known in Mangalore as country creat.

Constituents.—A bitter principle of a glucosidal nature.

Preparations.—Infusion (1 in 20). Dose, ½ to 1 fld. oz.

Actions and uses.—Bitter, laxative and stomachic; a good substitute for kadavi-nai—used like other vegetable bitters, in dyspepsia, gastric, vomiting, &c.

Exacum bicolor—grows in the Deccan and Mangalore, possesses same bitter, stomachic properties as exacum littorale.

Exacum tetragonum, Sebœa carinata—purple chiretta (Eng.), koochuri (Beng.), Ooda chiretta (Hind.), found in the Concan and above the Ghauts ; possess same properties as above.

Erythrœa Roxburghii, E. Centauria, Chironia Centauroides.

Habitat.—Mysore, Deccan and Bengal.

Parts used.—The plant. Veru Lantak, Kauturiyun.

A delicate plant 4 to 10 inches high ; root small and fibrous ; stem quadrangular and winged ; leaves ovate, oblong and obtuse, those on the stem linear acuminate. Flowers pink, star-like ; capsules oblong, mucronate. A most powerful bitter ; an excellent substitute when chiretta is not obtainable.

Gentiana Dahurica, G. Olinieri.

Habitat.—Persia.

Parts used.—The flowering tops.

Vernacular.—Hind.—Gul-i-Ghafis. Pers.—Ghapitha ; Gul kalli.

Characters.—The quadrangular flower stalks, terminating in five flowers ; corolla, funnel-shaped, erect, five partite ; calyx, five partite ; stamens, five ; style, single ; stigmas two. Fruit one-celled, containing numerous seeds.

Constituents.—A bitter crystalline principle, gum; wax and colouring matter.

Preparations.—Infusion (1 in 40), Dose, ½ to 1 fld. oz.

Actions and uses.—Bitter tonic, diaphoretic and alterative, used in dyspepsia, fever and general debility.

Gentiana Kuroo.

Habitat.—N.-W. Himalaya, Cashmere.

Parts used.—The root stock.

Vernacular—Eng.—Himalaya Gentian. Hind.—Karu, Nilkant.

Characters.—Root creeping, terminating in knotty crowns from which spring numerous vertical rhizomes, each bluntly quadrangular, as thick as a goose quill, and marked with projections, the remains of rootlets. On section, there is a central woody portion surrounded by a thick cortex ; colour yellow, odour and taste similar to that of gentian root.

Constituents.—A bitter principle ; a yellow transparent resin, resembling mastic, which softens in the mouth ; it is without any odour or taste.

Preparations.—Infusion (1 in 80). Dose, ½ to 1 fld. oz.

Actions and uses.—Bitter stomachic, tonic, and appetizer ; Like European gentian it forms an efficient substitute for chiretta.

Gentiana Lutea, B. P., G. Catesbœi—an American species—(Blue Gentian).

Lutea, Lutens, golden yellow. The golden yellow flowers.

Habitat.—Central and Southern Europe mountains.

Parts used.—The dried rhizome and root. Gentiana radix, B. P.

Vernacular.— Arab.— Jintiyânià. Duk.— Juntyana. Eng.—Blue Gentian, Common, pale or yellow gentian, bitter root. Hind.—Pakhânbhêd. Pers.—Gintiyana, Koushâd.

Characters.—Large perennial herb, with a thick hollow and yellowish green stem : leaves entire, 5—7 nerved, long ovate, glabrous and yellowish green. Flowers numerous, in cymes ; rhizome in cylindrical pieces, entire or longitudinally split, yellowish brown, wrinkled longitudinally, and covered over by leaf scars; tough when moist, and brittle when dry ; surface reddish yellow, odour peculiar faint, taste sweet at first and bitter afterwards.

Constituents.—Gentopicrin ; Gentianic or Gentesic acid (an inert amorphous body) ; gentianose (uncrystallizable sugar) 14 p.c., pectin, gum, sugar, a trace of volatile oil 6 p c., ash 8 p.c. No tannin.

Gentopicrin or gentianin, a bitter glucoside—to obtain it add charcoal to the concentrated alcoholic extract, boil with alcohol, treat with oxide of lead to remove colouring matter, precipitate the lead with sulphuretted hydrogen, agitate with ether and crystallize. It is soluble in water and dilute alcohol. With dilute acid it splits up into glucose and gentiogenin. Gentianic acid—to obtain it wash the alcoholic extract with cold water to remove bitter principle, then wash with ether to remove fat, and crystallize ; yellow tasteless amorphous body, sparingly soluble in alcohol and ether.

Preparations.—Of the root. Infusum Gentianæ compositum, B. P. Gentian root, ¼ oz., Dried bitter orange peel, ¼ oz., Fresh lemon peel, ½ oz., Distilled water, 1 pint. Dose, ½ to 1 oz. Extractum Gentianæ, B. P. —Dose, 2 to 8 grs. Tinctura Gentianæ composita, B. P., Gentian root, 2 oz., Dried bitter orange peel, ¾ oz., Cardamom seeds, ¼ oz. Alcohol 45 p.c. 1 pint. Dose, ½ to 1 dr.

Actions and uses.—Like calumba, it is a simple bitter without astringency or aroma. As a valuable stomachic tonic, it is given in dyspepsia, gout, hysteria, jaundice &c. It increases the appetite and strengthens digestion, but does not constipate. As a febrifuge it is used in low malarial fevers. It is a good vehicle for administering chalybeates, mineral acids, neutral salts, and also cod liver oil. The discoloration of iron salts by gentian is due to gentesic acid, and not to any tannin, as it contains none.

Remarks.—The term Pakhanbhed is also applied to a mineral clay.

Swertia Decussata, Ophelia Elegans, O. Multiflora.

Habitat.—N. Circars, West Deccan, Peninsula, Mahableshwar.

Parts used.—The plant-stems and root.

Vernacular.—Duk.—Salaras or Silajit. Tel.—Shilajatu. Hind.—Kadu.

Characters.—Plant 6 to 20 inches long; leaves sessile, narrow, lanceolate or ovate, tapering to a point, opposite and five nerved; stem quadrangular, clasping, smooth and rather thick. From their axils several small white or pale blue, sessile flowers are given off. The whole plant is very bitter and is an excellent substitute for gentian.

Preparations.—Infusion (1 in 80). Dose, ½ to 2 ozs.

Actions and uses.—Like chiretta, a bitter stomachic tonic, febrifuge, and laxative; as an antiperiodic with neem bark and black pepper, it is given in fevers. Hakims use it with aromatics as an aperient in internal piles before operation. The term salaras (Dukani) is also applied to storax, and silajit to mineral clay, Armenian bole, or to bitumen.

Swertia Chirata, B.P., Ophelia Chirata, Agathotes Chirata.

Habitat.—India, Temperate Himalaya, Nepaul, Kumaon.

Parts used.—The entire dried plant, Chirata, B.P.

Vernacular.—Arab—Kasab-ud-daura. Beng., Hind., Mar., Guz., Bomb.—Chirata; Kalapnath, kalamegh. Burm.—Tou-kha-kyi. Can.—Nila bevu. Cing.—Bin-cohamba, atadi. Duk.—Kreat. Eng.—Chirayit, Bitter stick. Malyal.—Nila Veppa. Pers.—Dowa-i-pechish. Sans.—Kirata-tikta; Anârya tikta; Bhu-nimba, Kuch-chi. Tam.—Shirat. Tel.—Nila Vembu.

Kirata tikta is derived from kiratta, kiratas, an out-caste race of mountaineers in India, and tikta, bitter. The plant is very bitter and common over the mountains. Anarya tikta, the bitter plant of the Non-Aryans.

Characters.—Several plants closely allied in medicinal properties to gentian are known by the name of kiriat. The drug is generally sold in bundles. It consists of the whole plant except the coarser woody stems. Root is woody and knotty irregularly, giving off several small rootlets; bark pale brown; wood, pale yellow; stem, single, varying in thickness from 2 to 5 lines, orange brown or dark purple, about 2 or 3 feet long, cylindrical in the lower and quadrangular in the middle and upper part, jointed and pithy; branches decussated, angular at the extremities. Surface smooth; flowering portion yellow (sometimes present in the drug); flowers in cymes of a dark-brown colour. No odour. Taste intensely bitter. The intensity being most marked in the flowers and root. Dose, 15 to 30 grs.

Constituents.—Ophelic acid, an amorphous bitter principle; chiratin, a yellow bitter glucoside; resin, gum, carbonates and phosphates of potash, lime and magnesia; ash 4—6 p.c.; no tannin. Ophelic acid, a syrupy liquid, bitter. soluble in water, alcohol, and ether. Not precipitated by tannin. Chiratin—Hydroscopic, crystalline, yellow powder; soluble in alcohol, ether, warm water, precipitated by tannin. By hydrochloric acid it is decomposed into chiretogenin oophelic acid.

Preparations.—Liquor chiratæ concentratus B.P. (1 in 2). Dose, ½ to 1 dr. Extractum chiratæ fluidum. Dose, 10 to 30 ms. Infusum chiratæ, B.P. (1 in 20). Dose, ½ to 1 oz. Tinctura chiratæ, B.P. (1 in 10). Dose, ½ to 1 dr. Drogue amere—a tincture—contains mastich, frankincense, resin, myrrh, aloes and chirata root, equal parts, steeped in brandy for a month and strained; used in apthæ. Chirattine tablets or Saccharo chirettine; it is prepared without heat. It is soluble in water, and can be given with alkaline carbonates, tannin, and iron. Three grains is equal to 1 grain of quinine—used as a tonic and febrifuge. Compound powder.—Sudarashana churana—Sudarashana is the name of the principal implement of war used by the Hindu god Vishnu. The shape of the weapon is like that of a carriage wheel (chakra) and is mythologically supposed to be the only powerful instrument to cut off or to remove devil's heads. Churana a powder. Sudarashana churana is a powder, which is supposed to be so efficacious as to suppress, dispose of or to cure any or every bad or virulent fever. It contains Kariátun 5, Triphala 6, Trikatu 5, Kâsni 4, Chud 3, Aftimun 3, Kulfah 3, Kâhu bij 2, Sáthra 2, Lavang 5, Harade 4, Dáruhalad 3, Kuchala 3, Pipali mula 4, Moravel 4, Gulvel 3, Dhamaso 4, Kutaki 6, Motha 4, Limado 3, Kutha 3, Jethi madha 5, Kudá chhála 4, Ajamoda 4, Indrajava (bitter) 6, Bharingani mula 3, Vekhanda 5, Padma kashatá 3, Valo 4, Ativisha 6. Dose, 20 to 60 grs. Used in chronic fevers.

Actions and uses.—Like cinchona and other bitter tonics, it is bitter stomachic, laxative, anthelmintic and febrifuge. It excites the appetite strengthens digestion, but does not constipate; it diminishes flatulence and hyperacidity; removes biliousness; given in atonic dyspepsia, liver troubles, acidity of the stomach and flatulence, gout in intermittent and other fevers. In combination with acids, alkalies and aromatics, it is given in bilious affections, and in burning heat of the body. A compound powder sadurashana-churana is a popular native remedy for chronic fevers; as a laxative and alterative it is given in scrofula and general malaise.

Convolvulaceæ—The Nishotara, Bindweed or Convolvulus family.

Convolvulaceæ—Convolvere, roll together, entwine—stems having a twining habit. Twining, trailing or milky herbs, or shrubs; roots generally containing milky acrid juice; leaves exstipulate, alternate, simple, or lobed, sometimes parasitic; flowers generally large, bell-shaped, and of a beautiful pink purple, blue, red, yellow, or white colour. Fruit often globular, capsule, 2 to 4 celled; seeds generally hairy; cotyledons, foliaceous and crumpy. Albumen small and mucilaginous—found in the plains and valleys of tropics and temperate climates. This order is remarkable for the presence of an acrid, milky, purgative juice, which is contained in the roots of many of its species. Seeds of some are purgative. This property is due to a resin and a glucoside in their juice. In some roots the resin is entirely absent, or in very small quantity. In them starch and sugar predominate, and thus render them edible. They are allied to solanaceæ and scrofuleriaceæ.

Argyreia Speciosa, Ipomœa Speciosa, Convolvulus Speciosus, C. Nervosus, Lettsomia Nervosa.

Habitat.—Throughout India.

Parts used.—The leaves and root.

Vernacular.—Beng.—Bechotârok. Guz., Mar., Hind., Bomb.—Samudra shokha. Can.—Chandrapoda. Duk.—Samander-kâ-pattâ. Eng.—Elephant creeper. Malyal.—Samudra-yogam. Sans.—Vriddha-dâraka. Tam.—Shamuddirap-pachchai. Tel.—Chandra-poda.

Characters.—Leaves large, heart-shaped, and ovate; under surface covered by a thick layer of silky hairs; upper surface dark green and smooth; roots long, woody and tough; bark dark brown; stems marked with furrows; root in the middle portion porous, and resinous at the margin.

Constituents.—Tannin, amber coloured acid resin which is soluble in ether, benzole and partly soluble in alkalies.

Preparations.—Decoction (1 in 20). Dose, $\frac{1}{2}$ to 1 fld oz.

Actions and uses.—Alterative tonic, given in rheumatism, and syphilis. The under surface of the leaf is irritant, and is used to hasten maturation and suppuration, it sometimes acts as a vesicant—the upper surface is cooling and supposed to possess healing properties.

Convolvulus Scammonia, B.P.

Habitat.—Western Asia, Syria, Levant, Kaira in Gujerat.

Parts used.—The root scammoniæ radix, B.P. A resinous, gummy exudation from the root, scammonium; and a resin, scammoniæ resina, B.P.

Vernacular.—Arab.—Sakamunia, mahamooda, sogmoonia.—Eng.—Virgin scammony, Aleppo scammony. Guz., Bomb., Hind.—Saka muniya. Pers.—Mahmudah. Tam.—Mâmûdâ. Tel.—Shakumuniyâ.

Characters.—Roots contorted or cylindrical and tapering, brown without and white within, surface longitudinally furrowed.

Constituents.—Resin 75 to 90 p.c., gum 3-8 p.c., sugar, starch. The root contains an active principle, Jalapin—identical with con volvulin of Jalap.

Scammonium, B.P., Scammony—a gum resin obtained by incising the fresh root—occurs in flattened cakes, or irregular pieces of a brown, dark grey, or nearly black colour, and often covered with a greyish black powder, brittle and glossy ; when broken, the surface is resinous, porous and dark brown. Ash grey when reduced to powder, triturated with water yields greenish emulsion ; odour characteristic, and taste acrid ; soluble in ether (3 in 4). Dose, 5 to 10 grs.

Scammoniæ B.P. Resina,—Scammony resin, a resin obtained from the gum resin scammonium by means of rectified spirit ; brown, translucent pieces, brittle, resinous in fracture and of a sweet fragrant odour, almost entirely soluble in alcohol, ether and benzene ; it is identical with orizabin of ipomœa orizabin. Dose, 3 to 8 grs.

Preparations.—Pilula scammonii composita, B.P. Scammony resin 1 oz., jalap resin 1 oz, curd soap 1 oz., tincture of ginger 3 fld. oz., mix and evaporate. Dose, 4 to 8 grs. Pulvis scammonii compositus, B P. Scammony resin 4 ozs.. jalap powder 3 ozs., ginger 1 oz. Dose, 10 to 20 grs. Extractum colocynthidis compositum (1 in $6\frac{3}{4}$). Dose, 2 to 8 grs. Pilula colocynthidis composita, B.P. (2 in $5\frac{1}{2}$). Dose, 4 to 8 grs. Pilula colocynthidis et Hyoscyami B.P. Dose, 4 to 8 grs.

Actions and uses.—An active hydragogue or cholagogue cathartic. and anthelmintic ; when baked scammony loses its aperient properties and acts as a powerful diuretic. It is more active than jalap; it acts very promptly, causes much griping, colic and watery stools ; it stimulates the liver and the intestinal glands ; it combines with soda in the bile with which it forms a solution. As an anthelmintic it is given against tape worms. The taste being insipid it can be given to children in constipation and as a vermifuge in lumbrici ; it is seldom given alone, but is generally associated with potassium sulphate, jalap, colocynth, calomel, aromatics and demulcents. It is given as a derivative in dropsy, cerebral affections, torpid liver and in intestinal catarrh with shiny intestinal mucus. Its use should be avoided if there is any irritability of the stomach or bowels.

Artificial scammony is made from the juice of calotropis gigantea, mixed with flour of a kind of pulse called in Persian karasanah. Baked Scammony :—The powdered drug is enclosed in a bag, the bag is then placed inside an apple or quince, hollowed out for the purpose. The apple is covered over with dough like a dumpling and baked in an oven.

Cressa Cretica.

Habitat.—Throughout India.

Parts used.—The plant.

Vernacular.—Hind., Beng.—Rudravanti. Guz.—Una. Mar.—Khardi, chavel. Sans.—Rudantika, Amrit srava. Sindi.—Una.

Amrit Srava. Amrit, Amrut, sweet ; Srava, moist. Believed to cause moisture which is sweet, because ants are found near it.

Characters.—Plant very small, shrubby and diffuse ; leaves ovate, sessile, very small, and acute ; of an ash colour ; flowers numerous, small, subsessile, and of a white or pink colour.

Preparations.—Decoction (1 in 20). Dose, ½ to 1 fld. oz.

Actions and uses.—Alterative, tonic and expectorant, given in bilious affections, cough and in general debility.

Evolvulus Alsinoides, E. Hirsustus.

Habitat.—Throughout India, Ceylon.

Parts used.—The herb.

Vernacular.—Can.—Vishnu Krandi. Hind.—Sankha-pushpi. Mar. Shankavalli. Sans.—Vishnu Gaudhi. Tam.—Vishnu Karandi.

Characters.—Herb procumbent, covered with hairs; leaves ovate, oblong, baccous plant; flowers small, ½ inch long, beautiful, of a deep blue.

Constituents.—A yellow neutral fat, an alkaloid, an organic acid and saline substance.

Preparations.—Infusion (1 in 40). Dose, ½ to 1 fld. oz.

Actions and uses.—Tonic, alterative and febrifuge, used in fever, nervous debility and loss of memory, sometimes used in syphilis, scrofula, &c.

Ipomæa Digitata, Batatas Paniculata.

Ipomæa—a worm, a bind weed. From its twisting habits.

Habitat.—Tropical India.

Parts used.—The tuberous root.

Vernacular.—Beng.—Bhui Kumrâ. Can.—Buja.—Gumbala. Hind.—Bidâri Kand. Malyal.—Palmodekka. Guz., Mar.—Bhui-Kohala, Pattâna. Sans.—Kshira-Vidâri, Bhumi Kushamanda, Payas vini. Tam.—Nelli Kumbalu Tel.—Matta-paltiga.

Characters.—Fresh root milky, a simple or forked tuber and rather wrinkled. Dry roots, warty, scabrous, of a greyish white or dark brown colour externally; and white within; cut surface presenting concentric, rings formed of lacticiferous vessels from which a viscid milky fluid exudes; taste astringent and somewhat acrid, not unlike that of raw potatoes. The whole tuber consisting of starchy parenchyma about 10 or 12 lbs. in weight.

Constituents.—A resin, sugar, and starch.

Preparations.—Powder, decoction (1 in 10). Dose, ½ to 1 fld. oz. Confection.—Vidari, wheat flour and barley, and milk, butter and honey.

Actions and uses.—Tonic, alterative, largely used in several restorative aphrodisiac and demulcent preparations. It checks excessive menstrual discharges. As a lactagogue, given with wine, it promotes the secretion of milk in women after delivery. The confection is recommended for emaciated children suffering from debility, diarrhœa and want of digestion.

Remarks.—In Singapore the foreigners who pose as lion-hunters deceive rich and credulous people by passing off pieces of Bhui Kohala for lioness milk. The price paid for these tubers is the same as that paid for an equivalent weight of opium.

Ipomœa Hederacea. Pharbitis Nil.

Habitat.—Throughout India.

Parts used.—The seeds.

Vernacular.— Arab.— Habbun-nil. Beng.—Nila Kalomi. Duk.— Zirki-kê-binj. Hind., Guz.—Kâladana. Mar.—Nilâpushi. Pers.— Tukhm-i-nil. Tam.—Jiriki-virai, Kodi Kakkatan virai. Tel.—Kolli vittulu.

Characters.—Fruit globular; made up of four distinct seeds arranged in a spherical form. Each seed of the form of a quarter segment of a sphere. Its two sides flat and compressed, so as to adapt themselves to the flat surfaces of the adjacent seed. Their junction is marked by a scar which is near the hilum and by a thin edge resembling the border of a wedge. The convex surface is marked by a flat or broad groove; kernel yellowish brown and oily; taste oily and somewhat acrid; odour earthy. Dose, 5 to 8 grs.

Constituents.—A thick oil, 14·4 p.c.; mucilage, albuminous matter in tannin and Pharbitis, an active resinous principle, identical with convolvulin, a light yellowish friable mass, of a nauseous acrid taste, and an unpleasant odour, soluble in alcohol and insoluble in ether, benzol, chloroform, and sulphide of carbon.

Preparations.—Compound powder contains kaladana, sindhalona equal parts, and suntha or kalanjan $\frac{1}{8}$ part. Dose, 30 to 50 grs. Tincture (1 in 8). Dose, 2 drs., and the resin 4 to 8 grs.

Actions and uses.—Drastic purgative and anthelmentic used in constipation.

The name, kaladana is often applied to the seeds of clitorea ternata, a good substitute for jalap; Garanibija or Gokaranibija being similar in colour and properties; Kalonji seeds, which are dark brown and similar in shape; in ipomæa muricata, the seeds are reddish brown, glabrous, spiny, smooth and larger than those of kaladaná, but not grooved like kaladânâ on their convex surface. Ipomæa muricata is a native of Persia (a garden weed in many parts of Concan) and is known as Bârik Bhauri or the lesser Bhauri or Tukm-i-nil.

Ipomœa Pescapræ, I. Biloba, Convolvulus Pescapræ, Ipomœa Brasiliensis.

Habitat.—Coast of India, Ceylon.

Parts used.—The root and leaves.

Vernacular.—Beng. — Chhagulkhuri. Can. — Adambu-balli. Eng.—Goat's foot creeper. Guz.—Ravara patri. Hind.—Dopâlteluta. Mar.—Maryad vela. Sans.—Marajâd vela, Vriddha-dâraka. Tam.— Adapu-kadi, Tel.—Bala bandi tige.

Characters.—Stems creeping; root twisted upon the broken ends and containing a black concrete juice; leaves thick, smooth, long petioled and deeply bifid at the apex; flowers large and rose-coloured. Dose of the dried juice, 5 to 15 grs.

Constituents.—A resin and an alkaloid.

Preparations.—Decoction (1 in 20). Dose, 1 to 2 fld. ozs.

Actions and uses.—Alterative, tonic, and purgative ; used in rheumatism, gout, gonorrhœa, &c. The juice is purgative and given in dropsy. The leaves boiled in water are locally applied as varalians to painful joints in rheumatism and to the abdomen in colic. The paste of the leaves is applied to boils and carbuncles.

Ipomæa Purga, B.P., Exogonium Purga, Ipomæa Jalapa Veracruz.

Habitat.—E. Mexico, shady woods in Mussoorie and in the Nilgiris.

Parts used.—The dried tubercles. Jalapa, Jalap, B.P.

Jalapæ from Xalapa, a city in Mexico, from which it is imported.

Characters.—Perennial herb ; stems numerous, twisted, slender, furrowed, smooth and twining round other objects. Root pyriform, oblong, thick ; dried roots or tubercles, ovoid, fusiform or oblong, of the size of a nut or orange, also wrinkled, dark brown, hard and compact ; internally yellowish grey or dingy brown with numerous concentric circles composed of small resin cells. The fracture is resinous, not fibrous ; odour sweetish and smoky ; taste sweetish but acrid. Dose, 5 to 20 grs.

Constituents.—Resin 17 to 20 p.c. starch, gum, sugar and colouring matter. Resin composed of convolvulin 90 p.c. and jalapin 10 p.c. The latter is the principal constituent of spurious Jalap (Ipomœa orizabensis), identical with scammonin.

Jalapin or orizabin consists of mixed decolorized, soft resins. It is a whitish amorphous powder, brittle, breaking with a resinous fracture, easily pulverizable, of a sweetish fragrant odour and of an acrid taste ; soluble in alcohol or potassa insoluble in turpentine, acids, and warm water, soluble in ether (1 in 30). Dose, 1 to 5 grs.

Jalapæ resina B. P.—Macerate the root with alcohol and percolate, throw the residue into water, precipitate the resin and dry. A yellowish brown mass or powder of a peculiar odour and acrid taste—soluble in alcohol. Dose, 2 to 5 grs.

Convolvulin or Jalapurgin, a glucoside, hard, insoluble in ether, soluble in alkalies—more active than jalapin.

Preparations.—Pulvis Jalapæ compositus, B.P. Jalap 5 ozs., acid potassium tartrate 9 ozs., ginger 1 oz. Dose, 20 to 60 grs. Extractum Jalapæ, B.P. (Hydro alcoholic). Dose, 2 to 8 grs. Resina Jalapæ. Dose, 2 to 5 grs. Jalap is an ingredient in the preparation of pilulæ cathartica composita and of pil-catharticæ vegetabilis. Tinctura Jalapæ, B.P. (1 in 5). Standardized to contain $1\frac{1}{2}$ gr. of resin in 110 ms. or 1·5 p.c. of resin. Dose, $\frac{1}{2}$ to 1 fld. dr. Sapo Jalapinus—jalap resin 4, soft soap 4, alcohol 3, dissolve and evaporate. Dose, 2 to 6 grs. Abstractum Jalapæ. Dose, 1 to 5 grs.

Actions and uses.—Jalap is an active hydragogue cathartic, vermifuge and diuretic. It is more drastic than senna, and less irritating than gamboge, podophyllin, or scammony and produces copious watery stools with nausea, griping and great tenesmus. It increases the intestinal and biliary secretions, but it does not cause congestion of hæmorrhoidal vessels. In over doses it is a dangerous hypercathartic. Convolvulin is an irritant poison, producing gastro-enteritis. It does not irritate the skin, conjunctivæ or the nasal mucous membrane. It is not eliminated by the urine or fœces. It is given in dropsy and in inflammatory affections; also in fevers with constipation and in head troubles. As a vermifuge it is given with calomel and santonin against lumbrici. In ascites and anasarca it is much employed.

Ipomœa Quamadit.

Vernacular.—Sita-che-kes (Mar.) Sita's locks. Kamalata (Sans.) or Cupid's flowers—a small twining plant found in Nilgiri. Leaves filiform, punctate. Flowers small, bright crimson or white; pounded leaves are used as refrigerant and cooling application to bleeding piles and as a lep to carbuncles.

Ipomœa Reniformis.

Habitat.—Nilgiris.

Parts used.—The plant.

Vernacular.—Bomb.—Undirkani, mushkani. Sans.—Mûshakarani. Tam.—Perretay-keeray.

Undirkani, from ûndar, a rat, and kani, like an ear. The leaves of this plant resemble in form rat's ears.

Characters.—A creeper with many roots from the joints; stem creeping; petioles hairy, slender, wiry, and furrowed longitudinally; leaves kidney-shaped, dentate towards their margins and obtuse; flowers small, taste mucilaginous.

Preparations.—Decoction (1 in 20). Dose, ½ to 1 fld. oz.

Actions and uses.—Purgative and alterative, given in rheumatism, neuralgia, headache, &c.; the juice is given in rat-bites. It is also used for ulcers in the ear. In large doses it acts as a purgative. This plant is often mistaken for Bhrahami—Hydrocotyle Asiatica. The leaves of both are of the same shape and generally used for the same purposes.

Ipomœa Sp.

Varadharo (Guz.) the root is in pieces of from 4 to 5, or 6 inches long; the root bark longitudinally furrowed, and slightly twisted; colour brownish. On section the wood is porous and whitish, and between it and the bark a resinous matter exudes; the smell is disagreeable, taste somewhat acrid. Used as decoction (1 in 10). Dose, ½ to 1 fld. oz. It is an alterative and tonic and given in chronic nervous diseases and rheumatic affections, scrofula, syphilis, &c. Sanscrit writers attribute high medicinal virtues to this drug. In Bombay, the root of samudra sokha is substituted for varadharo. In Bengal, the root of argeria spiciosa is sold as vardharo.

Ipomœa Turpethum—Convolvulus Turpethum.

Habitat.—Throughout India, Ceylon.

Parts used.—The bark of the root and stem.

Vernacular.—Arab.—Hud-ul-zangi. Beng.—Dood-kalmee. Teori. Can.—Dike-puti-gadi. Cing.—Trista-vàlu-mûl. Duk.—Tikrâ. Eng.—Turpeth root. Guz.—Nishotara, Turbad. Hind.—Pitôhri, Nâk-patar, Nishot-Tarwai. Malyal.—Chivâka-véra. Mar.—Nishottar, Shetvara, Phutkari. Sans.—Trivrit, Triputa, Kutaruna Kaloparni, Kalameshi (black variety). Tam.—Shivadai-vér. Tel.—Tegada-vêru.

Nasotara, from Nasa, a nerve, and tara or trana, three, in allusion to the stem of the plant being three nerved, or three winged. Triputa—tri, three, and puta, angle. The stem is three angled. Trivrit, tri, three, and Vrit, folds which are spiral or circular, the stem being provided with three spiral folds or wings. Turbad is a corruption of the Sanscrit word Trivrit.

Characters.—The root and stem about 2 to 4 inches or more in length, and ½ to 2 inches in diameter, twisted like a price of rattan cane, or columnar; bark, dark brown, or pale, rough, longitudinally fissured, and here and there deeply furrowed. Transverse section shows a porous surface of a dirty white colour, and here and there loaded with a pale yellowish white resin; smell slightly agreeable, taste nauseous, or feebly acrid. The acridity is only perceptible after it has been kept for some time in the mouth. Dose, 20 to 40 grs.

Constituents.—Turbeth resin consists of a soft resin soluble in ether, and of a substance insoluble in ether, benzine, sulphide of carbon, and essential oils. This substance is called Turpeth or Turpethine; a volatile oil, and yellow colouring matter. Turpethin, a resin, a grey substance, analogous to jalapine and convolvuline. It is named as having some resemblance in colour to turpeth mineral. Alkaline bases convert it into turpethic acid and mineral acid into glucose and turpetholic acid. The root contains it to the extent of 4 p.c.

Preparations.—A compound powder. Nishut 3, Pancha-lavana 2, Java-khára 2, Himaja 3, Hinga 1, Ajavân 3, vavading seeds 2, Tejabal 3, Kapilo 2, Palas-bij 2. Dose, 40 to 60 grs. Used in habitual costiveness, flatulence, tape worms, colic and sluggish liver. Confection—Contains Nishotar 4 ozs., Scammony 1 oz., Surijan 3 ozs., Saffron 2 ozs., Costus ½ ozs., Sugar 12 ozs., Cinnamon 1 oz., Honey 60 ozs. Dose, ½ to 2 drs. Used as a purgative, for children in sluggish liver, deranged digestion, flatulence, &c.

Actions and uses.—Turbeth is cathartic—given either alone, or in combination with other purgatives. With Harade, it is particularly beneficial in rheumatic and paralytic affections, melancholia, gout, dropsy and leprosy; it is more powerful and drastic than jalap.

Boraginaceæ—The Borage or Gaozabana order.

Herbs, shrubs or trees, with more or less rounded stems ; leaves alternate, entire, or toothed, usually thick and rough, and generally covered on both sides with white glands; flowers regular, and of a red, blue or whitish colour—fruits 2 to 4 seeded, Native of N. temperate regions. The plants are mucilaginous.

Cordia Myxa, C. Domestica, C. Obliqua, C. Latifolia.

Habitat.—Throughout India, Egypt, Cochin China, Australia, Punjab, Ceylon.

Parts used.—The fruit and bark.

Vernacular.—Arab.—Dibka, Mokhitah. Beng.—Bahubara. Burm.—Tana-si-thanat. Can.—Doduchallu. Cing.—Lolu. Duk.—Gôndni. Eng.—Sebestan plum. Guz.—Sapistan, Gondni, Burgund. Bomb.-Hind.—Bhokur Lasora. Malyal.—Viri kottâ. Mar.—Shelvant. Pers.—Slesha mataka. Sans.—Selu, Bahu Vara. Tam.—Naru Villi. Tam.—Nakkeru chettu.

Sebesten or sapistan is an abbreviation of sagpistan, derived from sag, a dog, and pisatan, dugs. The fruit resembles bitches' dugs in shape. Dibk and Mukhitah means mucilaginous, in allusion to the glutinous character of the pulp.

Characters.—Dry fruit a drupe, irregular, oblong, colour darkish brown, surface rugous, and highly wrinkled. In size, resembling jaephal; rind tough and sticky, pulp not easily separable from the seed; odour like that of cassia pulp, or decayed date, taste mucilaginous rather aciduous and disagreeable.

Constituents.—The pulp of the fruit contains sugar, gum, extractive matter, ash ; the bark contains a principle allied to cathartin.

Preparations.—Decoction of the fruit or bark (1 in 10). Dose, 1 to 2 oz.

Actions and uses.—Demulcent and mucilaginous, used in coughs, chest affections and in irritation of the urinary passages, and as a laxative in bilious affections. The bark is a mild astringent and tonic, and used in general debility and convalescence. The decoction also is used as a gargle in sore mouth.

Heliotropium Indicum, H. Cordifolium, Tiaridium Indicum.

Habitat.—Throughout India.

Parts used.—The herb.

Vernacular.—Hind., Beng.—Hathisura. Eng.—Indian turn-sole. Guz.—Hâthi-sundhâna. Mar.—Burûndi. Malayal. — Tetkatukka. Sans.—Hoste sunda, shri-hastine. Tam.—Tel-kodukki. Tel.—Nagadonti.

Hathi sundhana is derived from hathi, an elephant, and sundha, a trunk, in allusion to the spikes of the flowers being curved like the trunk of an elephant.

Characters.—Herb erect, or rather procumbent, generally hairy all over ; leaves cordate, ovate, oblong ; surface, much wrinkled and rugous, taste bitter ; colour green, or darkish green ; flowering spikes, scorpioid and longer than the leaves, densely flowered at one side ; flowers very small and tubular; tubes 4-sided and hairy, colour pink or pale blue ; fruit mitre-shaped, odour fœtid, like that of stramonium ; taste bitter.

Constituents.—Tannin, an organic acid and an alkaloid.

Preparations.—The juice.

Actions and uses.—Local anodyne. The juice boiled with castor oil is used to allay the pain of the sting of a scorpion and to cure the bite of a mad dog. The leaves are applied to painful gum boils and pimples on the face with benefit.

Coccinia glauca, Onosma Bracteatum.

Habitat.—Persia.

Vernacular.—Hind., Bomb., Beng., Tam.—Gaozaban. Arab.—Lisan-uth thour.

Parts used.—The herb known in Persia as gaozabana ; and flowers.

Gaozaban—Gao, a cow and Zabana, tongue, in allusion to the leaves being covered with tubercles and tapering points which resemble the enlarged papillæ on the tongue of a cow.

Various plants are sold in the Indian bazaar under the name of Gaozaban. These are onosma bracteata, cacalia kleinia ; Anisomeles Malabarlica, and Trichodesma Indicum.

Characters.—The drug consists of broken pieces of the stems and leaves; the colour is greyish brown ; stem in pieces, pale brown, channelled or compressed, longitudinally furrowed, fissured, and marked with broad based white hairs. Hairs generally get broken off, leaving white scale-like tubercles ; leaves thick, procumbent, brittle, rough and greyish green, or black like bullock's tongue, covered on both sides with similar white calcareous glands, from which calcareous hairs $\frac{1}{8}$ inch long arise ;* surface much wrinkled ; odour disagreeable, sometimes resembling that of tea; taste mucilaginous; flowers of a brownish pink or blue colour, wide mouthed, about 1 to $1\frac{1}{2}$ inches long, hairy and tubular, taste sweetish and mucilaginous, odour tea-like; calyx 5 partite and set with calcareous hairs. Stamens 5. If long kept the flowers turn reddish.

Constituents.—A nitrogenous substance, forming a jelly on cooling from a boiling solution ; the ash contains silica, alumina, traces of iron, lime, &c.

Preparations.—Decoction (1 in 20). Dose, 2 to 4 ozs.

Actions and uses.—Alterative, tonic, diuretic and demulcent, given in chronic fevers, rheumatism, syphilis, leprosy, hypochondriasis, diseases of the kidneys, gonorrhœa, and dysuria. It might be substituted for sarsaparilla.

Trichodesma Indicum, T. Zeylanicum, Borago Indica, B. Zeylanica.

Habitat.—Throughout India, Ceylon.

Parts used.—The herb.

Vernacular.—Mar., Hind.—Jhingi, Chhota Kulpha. Punj.—Rat mundu. Sans.—Jhingi, dubala, ambu sirishika. Sind.—Pabarpam. Tam.—Nilakai. Tel.—Guva gutli.

Jhingi Jhinga, means shrimps or prawns, with rough tubercles or bristles. The covering of the herb is bristly and covered with hairs and tubercles.

Characters.—Leaves opposite, sessile, cordate, lanceolate; stem clasping, tuberculate on the upper surface. Flowers pale blue ; calyx villous, cordate ; corolla tube-like.

Preparations and actions.—Similar to those of gaozaban.

Hydrophyllaceæ—Water-leaf family.

Hydrophyllaceæ, so called from each leaf having a cavity for holding water.

Herbs, bushes, or small trees being hairy and juicy; leaves hairy, toothed, lobed and alternate. Flowers either solitary stalked, axillary, and regular, or scorpoidal, and arranged in circinate racemes or spikes; calyx persistent; corolla regular, ovary simple, 1—2 celled; styles and stigmas 2 ; ovules 2 or many. Fruit capsular, 2 valved, 1 to 2 celled ; seeds netted, albumen hard and abundant. Grows in a temperate climate and is used as stimulant and astringent.

Eriodictyon Glutinosum.

Yerba Santa, holy herb, sacred herb, bear's-weed, consumptive or tar weed, mountain balm.

Habitat.—California and Mexico.

Parts used.—The leaves.

Eriodictyon—means wool and a net, the leaves are woolly and net veined. Glutinosum from glutiosus, meaning gluey or viscous, the leaves and stems are resinous and sticky.

Characters.—A perennial evergreen shrub 3—5 feet high ; bark smooth, green and herbaceous along the stem and branches; leaves lanceolate, pointed at the apex, elliptical, petiolate, finely or serrately dentate, 1—3 inches in length, alternate with 1 to 3 or more, growing from axil ; upper surface green, smooth, perfectly varnished with the resinous principle as to present a most gorgeous spectacle ; under aspect minutely reticulated, presents a silvery appearance which is due to its pubescency; flowers pinkish, purple, blue, densely clustered, in raceme ; odour aromatic, taste balsamic and sweetish, like that of tolu.

Constituents.—An acrid gum resin 30 to 40 p.c. eriodictyonic acid, a bitter principle, gum, tannin, a fixed and an aromatic volatile oil, ericolin, a peculiar saccharine and crystalline principle.

Preparations.—Fluid Extract. Dose, 1560 ms. Syrup (1 in 10). Dose, ½ dr. Velatine—a combination of glycyrrhizin and yerbasanta.

Actions and uses.—Demulcent, diuretic, bitter tonic, sedative and expectorant. It does not cause nausea. It covers the taste of quinine. The resin is sedative and balsamic, and exerts decidedly soothing and stimulating effect upon the bronchial tubes; given with grindelia for cough and cold; also given in chronic bronchitis, pneumonia, phthisis, aphonia, hay asthma, pertussis, chronic gastric catarrh, hæmorrhoids and in catarrh of the genito-urinary tract &c.

It has the power of completely covering the bitter taste of quinine and its salts. The taste is also obviated by giving it in the pill form with glycerin, or liquorice, chocolate and velatine.

Cuscutaceæ—The Amaravela, Kasusa or Dodder family.

Allied to or a sub-division of convolvulaceæ. The plants are distinguished by their parasitic habit, by the absence of leaves; stems generally yellow, wiry and succulent; flowers have scales alternating with the corolline lobes; seeds small, resembling those of convolvulus plants. Natives of temperate climates; having purgative properties.

Cuscuta Reflexa.

Habitat.—Persia.

Part used.—The fruit.

Vernacular.—Arab.—Tukhm-i-kasusa; kushooth. Eng.—Dodders. Hind., Guz.—Amaravela, Akasaveli. Pers.—Tukhm-i-kasusa.

Kushooth—Having neither root, fruits, leaves, nor any fragrance. Akásavela, Akása, sky, and Vela, a twiner. The plant is parasitic and grows on other plants, viz. the Amaranthus, Euphorbia, Erythema, Acacia, &c. It has no root under the ground, but only grows as a dodder, and hence the natives call it sky-twiner or Akásavela.

Amaravela, Amara, immortal, and Vela, a twiner. It is an immortal twiner. It grows during the rains and every year the growth is afresh on the same plant, hence it is called Amaravela.

Characters.—The drug is generally mixed with spines, pieces of stems, small oblong leaves, broken up flowers, seeds &c., of the plant on which it has grown. It is of a brownish yellow colour, of an aromatic odour, and a bitterish taste, the stems are slender, wiry, and longitudinally furrowed; flowers pedicelled and cupped. Each cup has several teeth. Within the cup there is a corolla—the seeds are four, small, light brown, convex on one side and concave on the other, and enclosed in a round capsule; they resemble kála danah. In size, they resemble mustard or radish seeds, taste bitter.

Constituents.—Quercetrin, a bitter glucosidal resin, a trace of alkaloidal principle, astringent matter, wax and oil. The resin is insoluble in ether, soluble in amylic alcohol and in water.

Preparations.—Decoction (1 in 20). Dose, ½ to 2 ozs.

Actions and uses.—Alterative, purgative, and anthelmintic, used in constipation, liver diseases, and bilious affections. Varáliáns of the dodder are used in piles.

Remarks.—Akásavela is also the name of Cassytha filiformis of the natural order Lauraceæ. Both are parasitic plants of a yellow colour.

Cuscuta Sp.

Habitat.—Europe and Western and Central Asia.

Parts used.—The stem.

Vernacular.—Arab.—Aftimun. Eng.—Lesser Dodder. Hind.—Aphatimuna.

Characters.—A parasitic plant growing on thyme or a shrub growing upon bushes and thorns. Flowers small, whitish ; seeds round, and reddish yellow ; stems in pieces, of a light brown colour. Each piece is wiry, compressed and striated. The plant has a somewhat aromatic odour, and an astringent bitter taste.

Constituents.—Preparation and properties are the same as those of cuscuta reflexa.

Myrsinaceæ—The Myrsine or Vavading family.

Trees or shrubs—leaves coriaceous, smooth, exstipulate. Flowers small, unisexual or perfect ; calyx and corolla, 4 to 5 partite, anthers longitudinal and dehiscent—ovary, superior, one-celled. Fruit fleshy, pungent; albumen abundant and horny. Natives of India. The fruits and seeds of some are anthelmintic, aromatic and astringent.

Embelia Ribes, E. Glandulifera, Embelia Ribesioides.

Habitat—Throughout India, Bombay.

Parts used.—The berries.

Vernacular.—Pers., Arab.—Biranj-i-kabuli. Duk., Beng.—Babarang. Can.—Vâyubliaga. Eng.—Embelia fruit. Bomb., Guz., Hind.—Vayvarang. Mar.—Vâvadinga. Malyal.—Visha-al. Sans.—Vidanga, Vrisha nâsana, Chitra tandula. Tam.—Vâju Vilangam. Tel.—Vayu Velangam.

Vrisha nusana—destroyer of the enemy (worms) ; chitra-tandula having variegated seeds.

Characters.—The berries angular, globular and in large bunches ; fresh ones, of a reddish dark colour, and of the size of a peppercorn or chini kabab, and contain a whitish and fleshy pulp. At the base is a fine toothed calyx, with a small adherent stalk. Where the calyx is absent a hole is apparent. At the apex is a short beak from which five prominent ridges run downwards and outwards, and converge towards the base. Between the ridges are several longitudinal ribs or nerves. The pericarp is brittle ; the seeds are embedded in the pulp. The seeds are hard, oily, of a pale brown colour, and covered with a thin membranous reddish testa ; taste is aromatic. Dose, of the powdered seeds, 1 to 4 drs.

Constituents.—Embelic acid, a volatile and fixed oil, colouring matter, tannin, a resinoid body and an alkaloid called christembine. Embelic acid—small orange red crystals, insoluble in water and soluble in alcohol, used for tape-worms.

Preparations.—Ammonii embelas, ammonium embelate or ammonium salt of embelic acid—found in needle-shaped crystals of a red colour, tasteless. Dose, 3 to 6 grs. Liquid extract. Dose, 1 to 4 drs. Decoction (1 in 10). Dose, ½ to 1 fld. oz. Fruit preserved in syrup. Confection of preserved fruit, freed from nuts. Dose, 1 dr. Compound pill—sajivani gotika—Sajivan, to restore, and gotika, pills, Medicine to restore digestion—contains vai-vairung, suntha, pipali, bâlaharade, âmalâ, bahedânâ, vehkanda, galo, bhilâmo, each 5 parts, bachanâg 1½ part. Triturate and add madha. Dose, 5 grs. To be given in the juice of adraka.

Actions and uses.—The pulp is purgative, the fresh juice cooling diuretic and laxative. The fruit is carminative, anthelmintic, alterative and stimulant ; mixed with ervados and pipli, the pulp is given to children in habitual constipation and in acute capillary bronchitis; as a carminative the fruit is given in dyspepsia and flatulence ; as an alterative in skin diseases and rheumatism. When taken for a long time it is found to turn the urine acid and red. As an vermicide, embelic acid or the ammonii embellas is used in tape-worms—the worms are killed, and to remove the dead mass, castor oil is given the next morning. A paste of it is used locally in ringworm and other skin diseases. The compound pill is given in dyspepsia and to check diarrhœa.

Sapotaceæ,—The Sapota or Sapodilla or Mohawa family.

Trees or shrubs often with a milky juice; leaves simple, entire, alternate, coriaceous and exstipulate ; flowers hermaphrodite, white, pale yellow or pinkish; calyx 5, persistent; ovary, 4 to 12 celled. Fruit fleshy, containing large seeds with a shining bony testa ; embryo large, albuminous; the bark is bitter, astringent and febrifugal; the milky juice of some yield caoutchouc or India rubber. Native of tropical parts of Asia, Africa, America—many species yield edible fruits. The seeds of several contain a fatty oil.

Achras Sapota.

Habitat.—West Indies, India, China.

Parts used.—The bark, fruit and seeds.

Vernacular.—Bomb.—Keweet. Burm.—Thwool-ta-bat. Cing.—Ratami. Eng.—Sapodilla plum, Bully tree (the wood). Mar.—Chiku. Tam.—Simielupei. Tel.—Simaippa—Chettu.

Characters.—Bark red, outer coat grey and tuberous, of a strong bitter and astringent taste. Fruit delicious, ovoid, rusty brown and rough externally, yellowish white, soft and pulpy within; seeds black, elongated, shining and ovoid. Taste every bitter. Dose of the seeds, 1 to 5 grs.

Constituents.—The bark contains 2 resins, tannin, and an alkaloid sapotine, soluble in alcohol, ether and chloroform, and precipitated from its salts by ammonia.

Preparations.—Decoction of the bark (1 in 10). Dose, ½ to 1 fld. oz.

Actions and uses.—The bark is tonic and febrifuge, and used as a substitute for cinchona bark. The seeds are aperient and powerfully diuretic. The fruit is refrigerant and given in fevers. Achras or sapota mulleri, a native of Guiana yields a kind of gutta percha known as Balatas.

Bassia Latifolia (Mohwa tree), B. Longifolia (Wild sapota or Ellopa tree), B. Butyracea (Butter tree).

Habitat.—Central India, Malabar Coast, Kumaon, Bengal, Ceylon, Terai, Oudh, Gwalior, Nagpore, Gujerat, Almora and Nepaul.

Parts used.—The flowers and oil of the seeds.

Vernacular.—B. Longifolia: Burm.—Kan-zan. Can.—Ippagida. Cin.—Migass-telmi. Eng.—Mohwah, Guz.—Mahovudûn (B. Latifolia). Hind.—Mohwa. Bomb.—Mohra. Beng.—Mauh Sans.—Madhuka, Mar.—Maha pushpa. Pers.—Drakhte-gul-chakan. (B. Butyracea) Hind., Duk., Beng.—Falwa, Falawara. Malyal.—Poounam; Madhu sravas, Madhu-madhavi. Madhu-vasavd, Madhu druma, Guda pushpi. Tam.—Ennai, karrai maram. Tel.—Ippa Chettu.

Madhu druma, from madh, honey, and druma, a tree. Parts of this tree are sugary. Madhu-sravas, means sugar flower; Madhuka sara, means concrete oil of the seeds or the milky juice of the bark. Madhuva sava, spirituous liquor prepared from the flowers. Madhu Madhavi, fermented juice of the sugary flowers. Guda pushpi. Guda, gode means treacle, and pushpi, flowers. The flowers have a sweet taste. Darakht-i-gulchakan—in allusion to its deciduous flowers.

Characters.—Small white flowers, generally deciduous; the ripe flowers are fleshy and smell like that of jaradalu and have a sickly acid and sweet taste. The dry ones resemble dried raisins in appearance and colour; fleshy, sticky, and compressed or hollow, with an aperture at both ends; upper end much larger and many toothed. Within the hollow are several light brownish or pink coloured hairy anthers, which soon wither, and are found in large quantities under the tree every morning. The taste is like that of figs. Fruit large, containing two white kernels or cotyledons, which yield above 50 p.c. of greenish yellow fatty oils which becomes buttery in cold weather. The oil is known as mawah oil or yellah oil. That obtained from B. Butyracea is called Fulwa Butter.

Constituents.—Flowers contain cane sugar, cellulose, albuminous substances, and ash. The seeds contain oil, fat, tannin, extractive matter, bitter principle, probably saponin, albumen, gum, starch and ash. The ash contains silicic acid, phosphoric acid, sulphuric acid, lime and iron, potash and traces of soda. The juice contains caoutchouc from which gutta percha can be manufactured, tannin, starch, calcium oxalate, gum, resins, formic and acetic acids and ash. The oil is yellowish, but becomes colourless after exposure to the light. It has a faint agreeable odour. Sparingly soluble in alcohol, readily so in ether. By saponification it yields oleic acid, glycerin, and two fatty acids; the oil is used in the preparation of country soap.

Preparations.—Concrete oil from the seeds; spirituous liquor from flowers; milky juice of the bark; decoction of the bark (1 in 20). Dose, ½ to 1 fld. oz. Infusion of flowers (1 in 20). Dose, 1 to 2 fld. ozs.

Actions and uses.—The fresh juice is alterative and given in scrofula, and rheumatic affections. The fermented juice of the sugary flowers is stimulant and appetizing and may be substituted for rum. The fruit serves as food to man and is cooling and refrigerant. The flowers are nutritive, tonic and demulcent; and also intoxicating, and form a vehicle in many cooling and demulcent mixtures. By distillation they yield an alcoholic spirit. They are largely used in India, in diarrhœa and dysentery, and as food. An infusion of the flowers is given with sugar, for the relief of thirst, burning of the body, and giddiness. They are also used in coughs. The concrete oil is used as an application to the head in headache, to wounds, and as a lubricant in rheumatism and contraction of the limbs, in cutaneous affections, and also as an ointment base like kokam butter. The fatty oils are used in the manufacture of coarse soap and in India for lamps and for culinary purposes.

Palaquium Oblongifolium, Isonandra Gutta.

Habitat.—Malay Peninsula and Sumatra.

Parts used.—A concrete exudation, Gutta Percha.

Vernacular.—Eng.—Gutta percha or Taban tree.

Characters.—Obtained by incision in or felling trees, removing the bark, the juice being collected in cocoanut shells, in which it coagulates. The inspissated juice is in tough pieces, very flexible, of a yellow or grey colour, plastic, heavier than water, without any odour or taste—insoluble in alcohol or water, soluble in chloroform, oil of turpentine, carbon bisulphide, benzin and benzol.

Constituents.—Gutta 80 p.c.—a hydrocarbon, a fine white powder; two resins (fluavil, a yellow resin, and alban, a white resin); volatile oil, salt, fat and colouring matter.

Preparation.—Liquor gutta perchæ contains gutta percha 9, carbonate of lead 10, and chloroform 91. As a protective to the skin it soon evaporates, leaving thin adhesive pellicles. Gutta percha splints. Traumaticin, a solution of gutta percha in chloroform (1 in 10).

Actions and uses.—Gutta percha solution is used as a protective application to wounds and eruptions ; also used for the preparation of plints, pessaries, &c. Traumaticin is used as a coating in skin diseases and slight wounds. The application does not contract the skin. It is an excellent basis for chrysarobin application in psoriasis, and as an adhesive film in wounds, abrasions, sore nipple, &c.

Mimusops Elengi.

Habitat.—Deccan Peninsula, Nagpore, Khandalla.

Parts used.—The bark, flowers, fruit.

Vernacular.—Beng.—Bakul, Woula. Burm.—Kya-ya. Can.—Mugalimara. Cing.—Moone-mal-gass. Duk.—Taindu. Eng.—Bakula tree. Bomb., Guz., Hind.—Maulsari, Bakuloli, Bolsaree. Mar.—Voula, ovali. Central Provinces—Taindu. Mal.—Elengee. Portuguese.—Pomme de Adami. Sans.—Vakula, Kesara, Sinha Kesara, Tam.—Moga-dam. Tel.—Pogada Manu.

Sinha Kesara, from Sinha, Sihen, a lion and Kesara, the mane—the lion's mane. Burmese ladies use small delicate scented blossoms, made in strings in chaplets like lion's name for the head.

Characters.—Bark like quills, darkish brown, tough, fibrous, rather scabrous and marked with short irregular fissures. Internally reddish brown, brittle and breaking transversely ; smell rather disagreeable ; taste slightly bitter and astringent ; flowers small, pale, brown or white, powerfully aromatic, sweetish smelling ; an oil is distilled from them. Berry oval and smooth, unripe fruit astringent and full of milky juice. The ripe fruit contains no milk, but a yellow pulp, which is sweet and astringent ; the leaves produce an extraordinary noise when burnt.

Constituents.—Tannin, some caoutchouc, wax, colouring matter starch and ash.

Preparations.—A fragrant water from flowers. Decoction of the bark (1 in 10). Dose, 4 to 12 drs.

Actions and uses.—The bark is astringent and given in catarrh of the bladder and urethra ; also used as a gargle in salivation, sore mouth, loose teeth, and in spongy gums. The unripe fruit when chewed is said to strengthen loose teeth. A snuff made of the powdered flowers produces copious discharge from the nose and relieves headache and fever.

Mimusops Hexandra.

Habitat.—Deccan Peninsula, Ceylon, N. India.

Parts used.—The bark and seeds.

Vernacular.—Beng.—Khira. Bomb.—Ahmedâbâdi mevo (truit). Hind.—Rana Kakodio, Kshiri. Mar. and Guz.—Ranjana. Sans.—Rájadani, Kheri. Tam.—Pall. Tel.—Palla.

Khsheri or Kheri—means milky or deliciously juicy; Râja-dâni, Râjah, king, and Adani, an edible substance, or fruit—an edible fruit highly prized by the rajas.

Characters.—Pretty trees ; leaves broad and wedge shaped ; bark in several layers, most external layer smooth and of an ash colour; next to it green, and within it the innermost red layer which contains milky juice. Wood very tough, seeds darkish brown, smooth and shining; testa brittle and breaking with a crackling noise; kernel reddish brown and oily; taste of the bark, bitterish and pungent ; that of the seeds oily and acrid. The oil is obtained by expressing the seeds.

Constituents.—The bark contains tannin, resin, wax, a colouring matter, starch and mineral matters. The seeds contain a fixed oil. The fruits contain sugar, caoutchouc, pectin, coloring matter and tannin.

Preparations.—Decoction of the bark (1 in 10). Dose, ½ to 1 fl. oz

Actions and uses.—The bark is astringent and used for the same purposes as mohvara and bakuli. A paste of the seeds is used to procure abortion. The oil from the seeds is demulcent and emollient. The ripe fruit is deliciously sweet and restorative.

Ebenaceæ—The Ebony family.

Large trees or shrubs, without milky juice. Leaves leathery, alternate, entire, thick, coriaceous, and exstipulate. Flowers polygamous, calyx 3-7 partite, inferior, persistent. Fruits fleshy and edible in some ; seeds large and albuminous. Wood hard and black as ebony and iron woods.

Habitat.—Native of Tropical India.

Properties.—Some have astringent bark, many have edible fruits, others are remarkable for the hardness of their wood, known as ivory and iron wood.

Diospyros Embryopteris, D. Virginiana, D. Glutinosa, D. Ebenum (Abnus), Embryopteris Glutinosa—Indian Persimmon.

Habitat.—Throughout India, United States.

Parts used.—The unripe fruit and dried seeds.

Vernacular.—Arab.—Abnes-e-hindi. Beng.—Gâb. Burm.—Yendaik. Cing.—Tumbiri. Hind., Guz.—Temru, Gâb. Duk., Mar.—Timburni. Malyal.—Vanan chikka maram. Sans.—Tumbiri Tinduka Kinkini Kankr. Tam.—Tumbilikkay. Tel.—Tumiki, Tinduki.

Characters.—Fruit, plum like, 1 inch thick, sub-globose, glandular, rusty, and yellow ; when ripe 4-lobed ; calyx at the base, covered, 6-celled, with rust coloured clubbed hair ; seeds reniform and arranged round the central core, pulp glutinous. Dose, 15 to 60 grs.

Constituents.—Tannin, pectin and glucose.

Preparations.—Tincture (1 in 10). Dose, 10 to 30 ms. Extract Dose, 1 to 5 grs. Infusion (1 to 10). Dose, ½ to 1 oz.

Actions and uses.—Astringent ; given internally in gonorrhœa, leucorrhœa, uterine hæmorrhage, sore throat, diarrhœa, and dysentery. A lotion (2 drs. to 1 pint of water) is a valuable injection in leucorrhœa. Abnus is astringent and lithontriptic.

Styracaceæ—The Lobana or Storax family.

Trees or shrubs. Leaves simple, alternate and exstipulate ; flowers axillary, calyx 4 or 5 partite, almost entire, and persistent. Fruit drupaceous, more or less fleshy, seed one in each cell, albumen abundant and fleshy.

Habitat.—Found in tropics and temperate climate.

Properties.—This order is remarkable for yielding stimulant balsams and resins. The bark of some plants is astringent.

Styrax Benzoin, B. P.

Habitat.—Sumatra, Java, Siam, Borneo and Islands of Eastern Archipelago.

Part used.—Balsamic resin flowing from the incision of the bark, Benzoinum B. P. Benzoin,

Vernacular.—Arab.—Hasi-luban-el-Javi, Bakkur, Kunnuk. Guz., Beng.—Lôbân, Sambarani. Burm.—Lobân. Mar.-Can.-Cing.—Sambroan. Hind.-Duk.—Luban, ood. Eng.—Gum Benjamin, storax, Benzoin laurel. Malay.—Konim Jan. Malyal.—Konimjan. Pers.—Dur-i-haskhak. Sans.—Dêva-Dhupaha. Tam.—Dupani. Tel.—Tam brani.

There are two varieties—Siam Benzoin which is highly fragrant, and occurs in masses of a dark brown colour mottled with white ; and Sumatra Benzoin, in tears of a greyish colour but inferior. The superior variety is called Karis lobân from the fact of its containing tears which are similar in size and somewhat in shape and colour to kawri, a small shell.

Characters.—Benzoin, a Balsamic resinous exudation indurated in the air, obtained by longitudinal or somewhat oblique, incisions in the bark of the stem, is met with in separate flattened agglutinated tears or drops, yellowish or reddish brown externally and milky white within, or in masses pitch dark or amber brown, exudation adulterated with wood bark and other impurities, very brittle, with a slightly waxy and transparent glossy fracture, readily softening in the mouth like mastick, odour balsamic, vanilla like, and fragrant, taste slightly balsamic ; soluble in 5 parts of warm alcohol or fixed alkaline solution ; on heating it evolves fumes of benzoic acid. Dose, 5 to 30 grs.

Constituents.—Three resins, Benzoic acid, cinnamic acid, vanillin and volatile oil.

Acidum Benzoicum, B.P.—Benzoic acid, Benzoyl Hydrate. Flowers of Benzoin—an organic acid obtained from Benzoin by sublimation; also artificially prepared from tuluol, hippuric, or phthalic acid or from other organic compounds. It occurs in yellowish or white lustrous scales or friable needles ; when pure it has no odour generally ; when obtained from benzoin it has the odour of benzoins, and a warm acid taste, soluble in cold water (1 in 400), in boiling water (1 in 17), absolute alcohol (1 in 1), alcohol (1 in 3), ether (1 in 2·5), chloroform (1 in

7), soluble in fats and fixed and volatile oils and in alkaline solutions. With alkaline solution forming benzoates,such as benzate of ammonium, lithium and sodium. Dose, 5 to 15 grs. in wafers. Resins—these are extracted from benzoin by sublimation or by adding boiling solution of caustic potash. Vanillin—treat benzoin with caustic lime, precipitate benzonic acid with hydrochloric acid, shake the liquid with ether.

Preparations.—Of the gum resin—Tinctura Benzoini composita B. P.—contains Benzoin 2 oz., prepared storax 1½ oz., balsam of tolu ½ oz., socotrine aloes 160 grs. alcohol to produce 1 pint. Dose, ½ to 1 fld. dr. Adeps Benzoatus B. P. (3 gr. in 100.) Trochiscus acidi Benzoici, B. P. ½ gr. in each with fruit basis. Tinctura camphoræ composita, B.P. Dose, ½ to 1 dr. Tinctura opii ammoniata. Dose, ½ to 1 dr.

Actions and uses.—Benzoin like balsams is an antiseptic, disinfectant, stimulant and expectorant. It stimulates the skin, kidneys, salivary glands and the bronchial mucous membrane. It renders the urine acid and increases its quantity. It is excreted by the kidneys as hippuric acid in combination with glycocoll. If inhaled, it irritates the nose and fauces, and causes sneezing and cough; taken into the stomach it causes epigastric pain. It is used extensively as an incense. Its tincture 1 dr. to 1 oz. is added to a pint of hot water, and the fumes inhaled in laryngeal affections and in sore throat and bronchitis. Lobana is often used as a stimulant expectorant in phthisis, asthma, pulmonary catarrh, chronic laryngitis, chronic diarrhœa, and dysentery. It should never be used in acute inflammatory diseases or in cases of gastric irritability. A healing and protective paste of lobana made in Movarano daru or the compound tincture is applied to foul and indolent ulcers, over cut surfaces, sore nipples, chaps of hand and feet, and over contused wounds. Benzoic acid as antiseptic and is given in genito-urinary diseases, to neutralize morbid alkaline fœtid urine, in chronic cystitis, phosphatic gravel, in copious uric acid deposit, in gonorrhœa and Bright's disease; also in albuminuria and incontinence of urine. A solution (1 in 20) relieves urticaria and may be used as an antiseptic application on freckles and other skin diseases.

Symplocos Racemosa, S. Theofolia.

Habitat.—Burma and N. India.

Parts used.—The bark, lotur bark.

Vernacular.—Can.—Jalariya med. Beng., Hind., Guz., Mar.—Lodhra, Hoora. Sans.—Lodhra, Tilaka, Shrimata, Savura Lodhra. Tam.—Erra lodduga. Tel.—Lodduga.

Characters.—Bark in pieces or in quills; colour light or brick brown, external surface rugous, very soft, friable and easily pulverizable; on section, marginal portion reddish and very soft, that about the middle yellowish and fibrous looking; fibres very soft, taste sweetish, balsamic, and astringent; odour agreeable and aromatic. Dose, 5 to 15 grs.

Constituents. — Three alkaloids. Loturine, colloturine and loturidine; and ash, which contains carbonate of soda.

Preparations.—Decoction (1 in 10). Dose, ½ to 1 fld. oz.

Actions and uses.—Astringent and tonic; with bael and nux vomica, given in diarrhœa, dysentery, menorrhagia and other chronic discharges. The decoction is used as a gargle in relaxed uvula and bleeding gums; as a plaster it is used to promote maturation of boils. It is one of the constituents of *lep*.

Oleaceæ—The Olive family.

Trees or shrubs; leaves alternate, simple, entire, exstipulate; flowers small, axillary, perfect, rarely unisexual; calyx persistent, monosepalous, generally enlarging so as to cover the fruit, inferior and 4-cleft—corolla regular, 4-cleft, or in four distinct petals; ovary free. often embedded in the disk, superior, 2-celled, with two suspended ovules in each cell. Fruit drupaceous, fleshy, or dry, often one-seeded; seed with integument, solitary and pendulous; albumen fleshy, embryo straight.

Habitat.—Native of tropical and temperate regions.

Properties.—The barks of some are tonic and febrifuge; some yield manna. The common olive yields the well-known olive oil.

Chionanthus Virginica.

Fringe tree, old man's bread.

Habitat.—United States.

Parts used.—The bark of the root.

Preparations.—Fluid extract. Dose, 15 to 60 ms. Solid extract. Dose, 3 to 12 grs. Tincture (1 to 8 of proof spirit) ½ to 2 fld. drs.

Actions and uses.—Alterative, and cholagogue; a stimulant of the lymphatic system and slightly diaphoretic and diuretic. It is highly spoken of as a remedy in cases of jaundice, in bilious and remittent fevers and as a tonic, after convalescence from debilitating diseases. Locally it is used as a poultice over ulcers and inflammatory swellings.

Fraxinus Ornus, Ornus florifera, F. Rotundifolius, Flowering Ash.

Habitat.—Mediterranean, Sicily, Asia Minor, South of Europe.

Parts used.—The concrete saccharine exudation.

Vernacular.—Eng.—Manna Flowering ash. Guz.—Mâûn, Malyal.—Manna. Pers.—Shirkhisht. Tam.—Ménâ. Tel.—Menâ.

Characters.—The juice or sap oozes out of the leaves, bark of the trunk and large branches. It also bursts through large pores spontaneously. It occurs in flat friable pieces, concretes on exposure to the sun; each piece varies in size, occasionally 8 inches long and 2 inches broad, usually smaller; externally yellowish white, or white, porous and crystalline; within, brownish white and glutinous; taste sweet, bitter and slightly acrid; odour honey-like. In appearance it resembles country kapura. Dose, 4 to 12 drs.

Constituents.— Mannit 60—90 p.c., mucilage which does not undergo vinous fermentation, glucose 15 p.c.; fraxin, and an acrid resin. Mannit or manna sugar—boil the exudation with alcohol and crystallize.

Preparations.—An ingredient in infusum sennæ compositum.

Actions and uses.—A mild laxative, demulcent, expectorant and cholagogue. In large doses it causes flatulence and colic. Combined with senna, rhubarb and magnesia, it is given to disguise the taste and to promote the purgative action ; as a demulcent it is given in piles, irritation of the genito-urinary tracts, and cough, and as a mild laxative to delicate persons and children, and to new-born infants, if the meconium do not come away freely.

Olea Europæa, B.P.

Habitat.—S. Europe, California, Algeria, Australia, Asia.

Parts used.—A fixed oil expressed from the ripe fruit, oleum olivæ, olive oil, B. P.

Characters.—The ripe fruit is a drupe, long, ovoid and pointed, and of a deep purple colour. Sarcocarp, firm, fleshy and full of oil. The stone is thick, and one-seeded, the oil is expressed from the fruit. Olive oil—a pale yellow, or greenish yellow oily liquid, of a faint nutty odour and an nutty oleaginous bland taste, and of a neutral reaction ; sparingly soluble in chloroform and alcohol, readily so in ether ; becomes acrid by keeping. Dose, 4 to 8 drs.

Constituents.—A fluid oil as olein, 72 p.c. and palmitin 28·p.c. (a solid oil or stearopten). Both are compounds of the base glyceryl with oleic and palmitic acid respectively. It also contains arachin, stearin, and cholesterin; olive oil is often adulterated with sesamum, oil ground nut oil and cotton-seed oil.

Preparations.—Sapo durus, B.P., hard soap, sodium oleate, white castile soap, made by mixing olive oil and sodium hydroxide until saponified, a solid mass, colour whitish, odour faint and peculiar, taste disagreeable, alkaline reaction, soluble in water, alcohol, &c.

Sapo mollis, B.P., soft soap, made of olive oil with potassium hydroxide. Ceratum cetacei contains 55 p.c. of olive oil. Emplastrum Ferri 5 p.c., Emplastrum Picis Burgundicæ 5 p.c., Emplastrum Plumbi 60 p.c., Unguentum Diachylon 50 p.c., Emplastrum Saponis, B.P., soap plaster, contains hard soap 6 ounces, lead plaster 2¼ ounces and resin 1 ounce. Pilula Saponis composita, B. P., compound pill of soap contains 20 p.c. opium Dose, 2 to 4 grs. Linimentum Saponis B.P. soap liniment—tinctura Saponis Camphora—liquid opodeldoc—camphorated tincture of soap, contains soft soap 2 ounces, camphor 1 ounce, oil of rosemary 3 fluid drachms, alcohol 16 fluid ounces, distilled water 4 fluid ounces. Linimentum Potassii Iodidi cum Sapone B.P., contains curd soap 2 ounces, potassium iodide 1½ oz., glycerin 1 fld. oz., oil of lemon 1 fld. dr. distilled water 10 fld. ozs.

Actions and uses.—Laxative ; rubbed into the skin it is absorbed by the lymphatics, and hence directly nutritious ; locally demulcent and emollient ; a nice protector of the mucous membrane against any acrid or poisonous substances. It renders the skin soft and supple. In the intestines, it is partly emulsified, and partly saponified ; its glycerin is set free, its fatty acids combine with the free alkalies to form soap. The emulsion enters the blood through the lacteals and is finally oxidized into carbonic acid and water, the excess of it is excreted by the urine. It thus increases the fat of the body and lessens the waste of nitrogenous tissues and supplies heat. As a laxative it is given in enema, or internally during constipation and as a specific in biliary and renal colic, gall stones, and acrid poisons. Locally applied it protects the wounds and sores from the action of the air, and hence applied to burns, acute inflammatory affections of the skin, to bites, stings, bruises, sprains and wounds ; as a diluent and a lubricating agent it facilitates friction over stiff joints. It is of benefit in removing desquamation of the skin in scarlet fever. In corrosive poisoning it is a good protective of the gastric mucous membrane and prevents absorption.

Jasminaceæ —The Jasmine, or Chambeli order.

Shrubs, often twining. Leaves opposite, flowers very fragrant, calyx persistent, 5 to 8 divisions; corolla regular, 5 to 8 partite; fruits capsules, or berries ; seeds with little or no albumen.

Habitat.—Native of warm regions.

Properties.—The leaves of some species are astringent, bitter and tonic. The flowers are fragrant and abound in a volatile oil; those of J. Sambac are reputed have the power of arresting the secretion of milk.

Jasminum Grandiflorum—Spanish Jasmine.

Habitat.—Cultivated all throughout India.

Parts used.—The leaves and flowers.

Vernacular.—Bur.—Myat-lœ. Beng., Bomb., Hind.—Chambeli, Jati. Sans.—Jati.

Characters.—A twining shrub ; leaves opposite and pinnatifid ; leaflets, pointed and entire ; flowers large, white and very fragrant. From the flowers a perfumed oil is prepared. The drug has a bitter and astringent taste.

Constituents.—Resin, salicylic acid, an alkaloid—named Jasminine and an astringent principle.

Preparations.—The juice of the leaves.—Dose, 3 to 12 ms. and oil.

Actions and uses.—Astringent. The juice of the leaves, or the oil is dropped into the ear in otorrhœa. The leaves are chewed, or locally applied to aphthous sores or ulcers in the mouth. As uterine sedative a poultice of the leaves and flowers is applied over the genitals, pubis and loins, in painful menstruation, and in loss of venereal desire. The fresh juice of the leaves is applied to soft corns with relief.

Jasminum Sambac, J. Undulatum, Nyctanthes Sambac, Mogorium Sambac.

Habitat.—Cultivated everywhere.

Parts used.—The flowers.

Vernacular.—Arab.—Varde-abyaz. Burm.—Sabay malee. Can.—Mallige huvvu. Cing.—Pich-chi-mal. Bomb., Beng., Hind., Guz., Duk., Mar.—But Mogrâ, Hazarea mugra. Malyal.—Tejerijam mulla. Pers.—Zambak. Sans.—Vara shiki, nava malika. Tam.—Mallegaippu. Tel.—Boondoo.

Characters.—Flowers white and large, of a delicious fragrance; corolla double; calyx, greenish yellow with many slender teeth.

Actions and uses.—Lactifuge. Flowers, bruised and applied to the breasts, arrest the secretion of milk in the puerperal state, and prevents formation of mammary abscesses. The oil is cooling and used for hairs.

Nyctanthes Arbortristis.

Habitat.—Central India, Mussoorie, cultivated throughout India.

Parts used.—The fruit and leaves.

Vernacular.—Beng.—Singahar. Burm.—Hseik-ba-lu. Can.—Harsinghar. Cing.—Sepala. Duk.—Keysur. Eng.—Night Jasmine, weeping or sorrowful Nyctanthes. Guz.—Parbuttee. Hind.—Harasinghara, Kersu Dundee. Mal.—Munja-pumerum. Mar.—Paharbutte. Panj.—Pakûra. Sans.—Sephalica, Parijatak, Rajani hano, Atyûha. Tel., Tam—Pagala-mully.

Characters.—Flowers, numerous, of a dull whitish yellow or red colour; calyx companulated, 5-notched and downy; corolla tubular, cylindrical and orange red, very fragrant and opening at sunset and withering before morning; leaves opposite, short, petioled, oblong, scabrous, pointed and coarsely serrated; fruit when dry flat, oblong and divided into two cells, each containing a seed; seeds dark-brown, bitter and very astringent. The leaves when chewed, stain the saliva yellow.

Constituents.—Resin, colouring matter, an alkaloid. (Nyctanthine) and an oily principle, similar to the oil of peppermint.

Preparations.—Decoction of seeds (1 in 10). Dose, $\frac{1}{2}$ to 1 fl. oz. Infusion of leaves (1 in 10). Dose, $\frac{1}{2}$ to 1 fld. oz.

Actions and uses.—As anteperiodic, the fresh leaves bruised are given with sugar or fresh ginger, in obstinate intermittent fevers. The powdered seeds are used locally to remove scurf from the head. The decoction or the infusion is used as an alterative in obstinate cases of sciatica and rheumatism.

Salvadoraceæ—The Khakhana family.

Shrubs or small trees; leaves opposite, entire, and leathery. Flowers small, pannicled, greenish, yellow, or white; fruit, fleshy, of white, black or red colour, one-celled; seeds solitary, erect and exalbuminous.

Habitat.—Native of India, Syria and N. Africa.

Properties.—Some species are acrid and stimulant.

Azima Tetracantha, Monetea Barberioides.

Habitat.—The Deccan and Ceylon.

Parts used.—The leaves, root and the juice obtained from the root bark.

Vernacular.—Beng.—Trikanta-juti. Hind.—Kanta-gur-kamai. Mar.—Sukkapât. Tam.—Sungham-cheddi. Tel.—Tella upi.

Characters.—Herb thorny; branches innumerable, forming an impenetrable bush. Thorns, axillary, fourfold spreading and very sharp. Leaves opposite, reflexed, oval or acute. Flowers axillary, fruit a berry, globular, of the size of a pea, white and succulent, seeds two; root dark brown and juicy.

Preparations.—Decoction (1 in 10). Dose, 1 to 2 fld. ozs. Compound decoction—Sukka pât 10 ozs. Tribulus Terrestris, the root of trianthema, monogyna, cephalandra indica, each one oz. Beleric and chebulic myrobolans each ½ oz., water 6 pints. Dose, 4 to 12 drs.

Actions and uses.—A powerful diuretic; given in rheumatism, dropsy, dyspepsia, and chronic diarrhœa, and as stimulant tonic after confinement.

Salvadora Persica, S. Indica, S. Wightiana and S. Oleoides.

Habitat.—W. India, Ajmere, dry parts of India, Arabia, Persian Gulf.

Parts used.—The bark, leaves, oil, and fruit.

Vernacular.—Arab.—Khardak. Beng., Guz., Bomb.—Khakhana, Pilu. Hind.—Mithijar, Kaurijal. Mar.—Kaugani. Pers.—Darakhte miswâka. Sans.—Pilu, karambha-priya. Sind.—Kebbar. Tam.—Karkol. Tel.—Chuma-varu gogu.

Drâkhte miswak, Tooth brush tree—pieces of the stem are used as tooth brush.

Characters.—Stem dark brown, cracked and covered with numerous whitish brown scars; root bark smooth, of a light brown colour and studded with scabrous, corky warts; odour pungent and heating; taste acrid and warm; leaves petioled and shining on both surfaces, oval or oblong and fleshy. In length 1 to 2 inches; in breadth about one inch; smell acrid like that of cress; fruit small, red or pink-coloured, globular and juicy; taste sweet; seeds erect, resembling grape (currants), when chewed acrid and pungent; taste like garden cress, and having aromatic smell.

Constituents.—The seeds contain an oil, a greenish yellow fat of the consistence of butter and of an acrid pungent smell and taste. The root bark contains resin, colouring matter and an alkaloid called salvadorine; also trimethylamine, and ash containing a large amount of chlorine. The fruit contains a large amount of sugar, fat, a colouring matter and an alkaloid.

Preparations.—Decoction of the leaves and root bark (1 in 10). Dose, 4 to 12 drs.

Actions and uses.—The shrub is given to buffaloes as fodder to render their milk rich and thick. The fruit is edible, digestive, carminative and diuretic, and is used in enlarged spleen, lithiasis and rheumatism; a decoction of the leaves is used in asthma, cough, &c., and poultice of the leaves is applied to painful tumours, rheumatic joints, piles, &c. The bark is used as a tooth brush to strengthen the gums. A decoction of the bark is given as a tonic and stimulant in low fevers, and in amenorrhœa. The freshly pounded bark of the root acts as a rubefacient and vesicant due to the presence of trimelhylamine. The oil—Khakhantel is used as a stimulant application to painful rheumatic affections, and as an inunction to the body after child-birth.

Solanaceæ—The Bhuiringni, Potato or night-shade family.

Solanum from sol, the sun, plants dislike the sun and best grow in the shade, hence night-shade, or from solor to comfort, from some of the plants having a soothing and narcotic effect.

Herbs or shrubs, leaves alternate, often geminate; inflorescence, axillary or extra axillary; flowers isomerous, ovary, usually two-celled; style simple; stigma, two-lobed. Fruit capsular or baccate, 2-celled; seeds numerous and albuminous; embryo, straight or curved in an annular or spiral form.

Habitat.—Universal in the Tropics.

Properties.—The plants possess harmless as well as poisonous and narcotic properties, but less powerful than those of the atropaceæ, some are pungent and stimulant, owing to the presence of an acrid resin; others contain a bitter tonic principle; a few bear edible fruits and tubers. The roots of some are febrifuge, astringent and alterative.

Capsicum Nipalensis.

Most acrid and pungent. Found universally. The fruit is chiefly used medicinally.

Vernacular.—Arab.—Filfil ahmer. Beng.—Lanka morich. Duk—Lalmorich. Burm.—Ngayonkthi. Can.—Menashina-kâya. Cing.—Rata mirich. Eng.—Red pepper chillies. Guz., Hind.—Lal mirch. Malyal.—Chabe sabrong. Mar.—Tambari mirchi, mirsingha. Pers.—Fiffel-i-Surkh. Sans.—Brahu maricha. Tam.—Golakonda. Tel.—Mirapa-kaya.

C. Frutescens.—Cultivated throughout India, America.

Vernacular.—Beng.—Lâl lâmba mircha. Eng.—Nepal chilli, Golconda chilli, goat pepper, bird pepper. Hind.—Lanka mirch.

C. Minimum B. P.—Cultivated in India, Birds-eye pepper. Hind.—Gach-mirch, Kafri-mirch. Tam.—Oosi mulaghai. Tel.—Sudi mirapa-kai.

C. Annuum.—Cultivated in South America, Mexico, India. Eng.—Common capsicum, common pepper, pod pepper. Malyal.—Kappal melaka. Tam.—Mallagu. Tel.—Mirapa Raia.

C. Fastigatum.—Imported from Zanzibar and Tropical Africa Cing.—Kaffru marich, Negro-pepper. Eng.—Nepaul, Guinea pepper, red pepper. Cayenne, Negro or African pepper. Tam.—Usari mallaghai.

Characters.—C. Minimum. The shell of the fruit is fleshy and coloured and contains a pungent principle. Fruits oblong, pendulous, or erect, and conical, and seated on a slightly curved stalk; ½ to ¾ inch long and ¼ inch in diameter, colour orange red. When fresh the colour is generally green which changes to red on ripening. The surface is smooth and glabrous, skin thin, about 2 or 3 lines in thickness, tears very readily and shrivels on drying. The fruit, 2-celled, containing numerous seeds, flattened, somewhat roundish, or reniform, and of a yellowish white colour with a central placenta; smell peculiar and acrid, taste highly pungent and burning. The powder of the seeds of capsicum fastigiatum is dark, orange red and called cayenne pepper.

C. Annuum.—Fruit 2-4 inches long, and 1—1½ inch thick, small, conical, oblong, sometimes curved or sub-globular, yellow or orange coloured, becoming brown, when dry, shining externally, with spongy pulp within; seeds 2-celled, white, flat and reniform. Dose, ½ to 1 gr.

Constituents.—Capsicin a volatile alkaloid; capsaicin—a crystalline substance; a volatile oil, fixed oil, fatty acid, resin, red colouring matter, and ash, 4—5 p.c.

Capsaicin mostly found in the pericarp and placenta. To obtain it, to the petroleum extract add diluted alkaline solution, pass carbonic acid and crystallize; occurs as colourless, prismatic crystals, insoluble in water, soluble in alcohol, ether, benzene, and fixed oils. The red colouring matter is sparingly soluble in alcohol and readily so in chloroform.

Volatile oil—obtained by distillation gives to the fruit its odour.

Capsicin—It is a volatile alkaloid—occurs as a thick red oily liquid, insoluble in water, soluble in alcohol, ether and oil of turpentine, having the odour of conine and is devoid of pungency.

Preparations.—Of the fruit. Fluid extract (alcoholic). Dose, 1 to 5 ms. Infusion (1 in 40). Dose, 2 to 4 dr. Tinctura Capsici, B.P. (1 in 20). Dose, 5 to 15 ms. Tinctura Capsici Fortior, (1 in 3). Dose, 1 to 3 ms., chiefly used externally. Linimentum Capsici (1 in 10). For chest affections, rheumatism, &c. Tinctura Capsici Etherea—made with pure ether instead of spirit of wine, used externally as a rubefacient and a liniment (1 in 4) with ammonia, turpentine and linseed oil. Collodium capsici, 15 grs. to 1 oz. Unguentum capsici B.P. (1 in about 5). Snuff. consisting of cayenne pepper, borax and carbonate of ammonium. Emplastrum capsici, $\frac{1}{4}$ of a gr. of oleo resin on each square inch of muslin.

Actions and uses.—A powerful local irritant; applied for a long time to the skin, it produces visication. In medicinal doses it stimulates the alimentary canal, gives rise to a burning sensation in the mouth, increases the flow of saliva and gives sensation of warmth in the stomach, promotes the gastric juice, aids appetite and digestion, and increases the peristalsis of the intestines. It stimulates the heart, skin and kidneys; as an aphrodisiac, it stimulates the nervous and genital system. Like ergot, it acts as a styptic upon the unstriped muscular fibres of the blood vessels. As an aphrodisiac tonic, it is given in functional impotence, spermatorrhœa, in chronic cystitis and catarrh of the prostate. In parenchymatous nephritis it checks the waste of albumen. As a stomachic tonic with nux vomica, it is used in atonic dyspepsia, chronic diarrhœa, colic, tympanitis, ague, and extreme prostration; in dipsomania it allays the craving usual in ch ronic alcoholism. It is given in delirium tremens in large doses with good results, also in opium habit. In sea-sickness, in malarial and other low fevers, gout, in habitual constipation, hæmorrhoids, in cholera it acts as a stimulant. It also checks uterine hæmorrhages such as menorrhagia, or those due to endometritis; also in tuberculous dysentery, internal bleeding from piles, &c. As a local stimulant, a gargle of the tincture (1 in 50) is used in tonsillitis, pharyngitis, malignant sore throat, diphtheria, &c. Externally, as a counter-irritant capsicum is too irritating. The snuff is used for hay fever. Externally the chillies diluted with soap liniment or til tel, is painted on the skin or applied to painful areas, as in sciatica, lumbago, rheumatic joints and chest affections. The etherial tincture is applied locally to the joints in gout, chronic rheumatism and to the chest in bronchitis and bronchial catarrh.

Datura Stramonium B.P.—Thorn apple.

Habitat.—Europe, South Russia, Himalaya, Afghanistan, and Persia, United States.

Parts used.—The dried leaves. Stramonii Folia, B.P. The dried ripe seeds. Stramonii Semina, B.P.

Datura Alba.—White flowered, Datura. The capsules are small, sub-globular, seeds triangular, rough and yellowish brown. In India, the seeds are used for criminal purposes.

Datura Fastuosa.—Purple flowered, black variety, native throughout India.

Dhatura Tatula.—Purple stem, purple flowers, and anthers, and dark green leaves.

Dhatura Metel.—Native of Western Himalaya, Deccan Peninsula. The root, leaves and seeds are used in medicine.

Vernacular.—The adjective white, Safed, is affixed for D. Alba, and black, Kala, for D. Fastuosa. Arab.—Jous-ul-mathel. Beng.—Dhutûra. Burm.—Padayin Khatta. Can.—Vummattee. Cing.—Anhenta-sudu attana. Eng.—Downy thorn apple. Hind.-Guz.—Kanak bij-Dhatura. Malyal.—Rotiku bung. Mar.—Kanto Dhatura, Pisotu Dhatora. Pers.—Kovz-masale. Sans.—Hênukâ, kanaka, unmeta, sveta. Tam.—Vumattai. Tel.—Ummetta.

Pisotu or Pisna means to pound, hurt or injure; the seeds, like those of rice, or wheat grains, are pounded or hurt between two stones. The effect of Dhatura is to pound his enemy.

Characters.—Annual plant; fruit prickly, about the size of a walnut, nearly globular, ovate, or obtusely quadrangular, covered with sharp tubercles or short unequal rigid spines ; capsule, 4-celled dehiscing half-way down and splitting in an irregular manner into numerous fragments ; pulp white and soft ; seeds ear-shaped, or reniform, of a light yellowish brown, or black colour, and hard pitted or compressed on both surfaces, with a groove on its wall and edges ; embryo curved and embedded in a whitish oily albumen. The seeds have no marked odour, but a slightly bitter taste Near the hilum the pulp is adherent, but it can easily be removed by scratching ; leaves dark green above, lighter underneath, smooth, very brittle, ovate, acuminate, unequal at the base and very coarsely dentate ; taste bitter and nauseous. The root is light brown, tapering and giving off root fibrils ; stem green and succulent. The flowers are large and white, the whole plant has a very disagreeable noxious fœted or rank odour ; taste nauseous and bitter. Dose, of the leaves, 2 to 5 grs.; of the seeds. 1 to 3 grs.

Constituents.—The leaves contain an alkaloid—daturine, mucilage, albumen and ash, 17 p.c. which contains potassium nitrate 25 p.c, The seeds contain daturine, resin, mucilage, proteids, malic acid, scopolamine, and ash, 3 p.c. Daturina—Daturin, an alkaloid identical with atropine, combined with malic or daturic acid and consisting of hyoscyamine and atropine. It is a tropate of tropin and occurs in light feathery crystals. Dose, $\frac{1}{120}$ to $\frac{1}{40}$ gr. in solution generally given with dilute sulphuric acid.

Daturinæ Sulphas.—Daturine sulphate in minute white granular crystals, readily soluble in water. Dose, $\frac{1}{120}$ to $\frac{1}{60}$ gr.

Guttæ Daturinæ.—2 grs. to 1 ounce. Ophthalmic discs $\frac{1}{2000}$ gr. in each combined with gelatine.

Preparations.—Of the leaves, Tinctura stramonii B.P., (1 in 5). Dose, 5 to 15 ms. Extractum Stramonii, B.P. Dose, $\frac{1}{4}$ to 1 gr Medicated oil—obtained by boiling the seeds with petroleum. is of a greenish yellow colour and a slight odour of valerianic acid ; on exposure to the air it becomes thickened. Compound, powder. Pulvis stramonii compositus—contains stramonium, lobelia, potassium nitrate, anise, &c., similar to Himrod's cure. For asthma it is burnt on a plate and fumes inhaled. Compound pill : Svalpajvaran kusa, contains Dhatura bija ; Para kajali, ; Trickatu ; Bachanaga ; mix, rub the whole together with lime juice, and make a pill mass. Dose, 2 to 4 grs.

Actions and uses.—Narcotic and anodyne; other and properties are similar to those of belladona, but stronger. It affects the sympathetic nervous system, but not the motor or the sensory nerves. In full doses, the heart's action becomes irregular, and there is furious delirium. Like atropine, hyoscyamine, and duboisine it acts as a mydriatic. As an antispasmodic, it is given in hepatic colic, laryngeal cough, chorea, stammering, &c. In dysmenorrhœa, neuralgia, ticdouloureux and sciatica it is very useful. In nymphomania and in puerperal mania with a tendency to suicide it is given with benefit. Pulvis stramonii compositus is burned on a plate and the fumes inhaled. Cigarettes ofdhatura tatula are used in nervous attacks of asthma. Externally a pasteof the seeds is used in urticaria and other skin diseases, due to the presence of lice, or other animal parasites. It is also applied to decayed teeth and to relieve toothache. Dhatura seeds are frequently used in India for criminal purposes. Toddy, a country drink for natives of India, is made more intoxicating by placing some of the seeds upon red-hot charcoal and inverting an earthern vessel (Ghârian) over them. The vessel full of dhatura smoke, is next filled with toddy which imbibes some of the qualities of dhatura. The natives apply a medicated oil to the head in headache, to enlarged testicles and boils, and to the skin in skin diseases as pediculi, lice, and psoriasis. Dhatura juice with the root of boerhavia diffusa (satodi) and opium is used as an application for the relief of rheumatic pains, and swelling over the hands and feet. In hæmorrhoids, fissures, and other painful diseases of the rectum, leading to tenesmus, its application as a local anodyne ointment gives relief. Sval pajvaran kusa is used in fever and cough.

Duboisia Myoporoides.

Habitat.—N. S. Wales and Queensland.

Parts used.—The leaves.

Characters.—Leaves entire, 3 or 4 inches long, broad, petiolate with prominent midrib ; taste bitter. Dose, 1 to 3 grains.

Constituents.—Duboisine—a volatile poisonous alkaloid, identical with Hyoscyamine and isomeric with atropine.

Duboisinæ sulphas, Duboisine sulphate, Amorphous Hygroscopic powder, very soluble in water. Dose, $\frac{1}{120}$ to $\frac{1}{80}$ gr.

Preparations.—Fluid Extract. Dose, 1 to 5 ms. solid extract. Dose, $\frac{1}{4}$ to $\frac{1}{2}$ gr. Tincture (1 in 10). Dose, 5 to 20 ms. Guttæ, 1 gr. to 1 oz. of water ; Ophthalmic discs, $\frac{1}{5000}$ gr. combined with gelatin.

Actions and uses.—A mild mydriatic ; its action is rapid and of short duration. It does not produce conjunctival inflammation. It is more calmative and hypnotic and less cerebral excitant than belladonna. It is superior to atropine in relieving the excitement of the insane. It is given to check morphine habit, paralysis agitans, puerperal mania, hysteria, headache, delirium of typhoid fever, night sweats of phthisis, and in vesical tenesmus. It is a very good antagonistic to morphine or muscarine.

Fabiana Imbricata.

Syn.—Pichi, Pichu.

Habitat.—Chili, South America.

Parts employed.—The stems and leafy branchlets.

Characters.—A shrub ; leaves thick, broad, ovate, barely pointed, a line long, and closely imbricated upon minute branchlets, densely crowded ; their bases and margins and all the tender parts to some extent, the wood and the bark are covered with ash grey, minute gland-like protuberances which exhibit under the lens a peculiar resinous lustre ; the resin is quite dry and brittle, and forms a greyish powder.

Constituents.—An active principle, a fluorescent glucoside, volatile oil and a crystalline neutral oleo-resin.

Preparations.—Fluid extract from the leaves not miscible with water, but miscible by the addition of an alkali. Dose, 10 to 60 ms.

Actions and use.—Pichy is diuretic and sedative. Its virtues reside in the oleo-resin. In urinary calculi it disintegrates the calculi by dissolving the mucin that keeps the particles together. It thus facilitates their expulsion in the shape of a harmless pulp. It is especially efficacious in hæmaturia, gonorrhœa, cystitis, vesical catarrh (acute or chronic). In uric acid diathesis, it should be given with a potassium salt to dissolve the urates. It should not be given in organic disease of the kidney and in albuminuria. As a diuretic and cholagogue it has some action on the liver ; also used in rheumatism, lumbago and sciatica in the course of which urates are precipitated from the urine in large quantities.

Hyoscyamus Niger, B.P.

Habitat.—Beluchistan, West Punjab, Sind, Khorasan, W. Himalaya, Europe, Northern United States.

Parts used.—The leaves with flowering tops or the fresh leaves, and flowers with the branches—Hyoscyami Folia, B.P. Henbane leaves and seeds.

Vernacular.—Arab.—Bazrul-banj. Can.—Khurasânin Vadakki. Cing.—Dungazha. Eng.—Common Henbane, Hagbean, poison tobacco, fœtid night shade. Duk., Guz , Hind.—Khurasani-ajvayan kôhi-bang. Mal.—Puka-yila. Mar.—Khorasani-vova. Pers.—Sickran, Banga. Sans.—Parasica, Khorasani Yamani, Syrians Azmâblus. Tam.—Pugai Ilai, huyamani. Tel.—Pogaku Dhumra pattram u.

Characters.—A biennial plant, leaves ovate, sessile, long and broad, lower ones largest, sinuately toothed, triangular, of a greenish grey colour with prominent midrib on the under surface, glandular, hairy, or woolly ; odour heavy, and narcotic ; taste bitter, and somewhat acrid; flowering tops numerous, nearly sessile, erect, arranged on simple terminal spikes of a straw colour ; fruit globular, capsule, 2-celled and many seeded ; seeds black, small, reniform, laterally compressed, of a dirty brown or grey colour ; in shape and appearance resembling those of kâkanaj ; albumen, oily ; surface beautifully pitted ; taste acrid ; odour resembling that of dammar. Dose, 1 to 10 grs.

Constituents.—The leaves contain Hyoscyamine, Hyoscine scopolamine, hyoscipicrin, choline, fatty oil, mucilage, albumen, and potassium nitrate 2 p.c. The seeds contain hyoscyamine, a fixed or fatty oil 25 p.c., an empyreumatic oil (obtained by destructive distillation) and ash 4-5 p.c.

Hyoscyamine—an alkaloid isomeric with or readily convertible into atropine, and identical with daturine and duboisine. It is the chief constituent of the leaves, juice and seeds of hyoscyamus, and is also found in datura stramonium, Duboisia myoporoides, in Atropa Belladona, Scopola Carniolica and in S. Japonica. To obtain it, treat the seeds with ether to remove the oil, then add hydrochloric or sulphuric acid, exhaust with alcohol and benzene. To decolorize saturate with ammonia, shake out the alkaloid with chloroform, and evaporate. An oily liquid or deliquescent, minute white silky needles or prisms, colour yellow, becoming brown by exposure to air ; more soluble in hot water, ether and dilute alcohol than atropine. It is converted into atropine by heating it to a high temperature. By boiling it with dilute hydrochloric acid, or baryta water, it splits up like atropine into tropine and tropic acid. Dose, $\frac{1}{120}$ to $\frac{1}{40}$ gr. In acute mania, $\frac{1}{8}$ to $\frac{1}{4}$ gr.

Amorphous Hyoscyamine, an uncrystallized dark brown extract-like substance of a strong and disagreeable odour; it contains Hyoscine, to which its activity is chiefly due. Dose, $\frac{1}{6}$ to $\frac{1}{8}$ gr.

Hyoscyaminæ Sulphas, B. P.—Hyoscyamine sulphate.—A deliquescent granular crystalline powder without any odour and of a bitter acrid taste; freely soluble in water (2 in 1), alcohol (1 in 2-5), slightly so in ether and chloroform. Dose, $\frac{1}{200}$ to $\frac{1}{100}$ gr. ; used as Injectio Hyoscyaminæ Hypodermica (1 in 120). Dose, 1 to 2 ms. Pills and Granules. Dose, $\frac{1}{100}$ gr., used for sea-sickness. Hypodermic Lamels, $\frac{1}{50}$ gr. combined with gelatin. Ophthalmic doses, $\frac{1}{5000}$ gr.

Hyoscyaminæ Hydrobromidum, Hyoscyamine Hydrobromide—it is similar to Hyoscyaminæ sulphas. A deliquescent yellowish white amorphous mass or crystals ; odour like that of tobacco, taste acrid, nauseous and bitter ; sparingly soluble in water (3 in 1), and alcohol (1 in 2). Dose, $\frac{1}{200}$ to $\frac{1}{100}$ gr.

Hyoscina—Hyoscine. An alkaloid isomeric with atropine—a syrupy brown or colourless semi-liquid substance found in hyoscyamus niger, different species of scopola, and other solanaceous plants. It is believed by some to be the chief constituent of amorphous Hyoscyamine. Boiled with water it splits up into tropic acid and pseudotropine. Hyoscinæ Hydrobromidum, B.P., or scopalamine Hydrobromide. It is in colourless, transparent, rhombic crystals without any odour, and of an acrid bitter taste, soluble in cold water (1 in 1), in alcohol (1 in 13), slightly so in ether and chloroform. Dose, $\frac{1}{200}$ to $\frac{1}{100}$ gr. Injectio Hyoscinæ Hypodermica, 1 gr. in 200 ms. Dose, 1 to 2 ms. Hypodermic tablets $\frac{1}{200}$ gr. each, combined with gelatin, Hyoscine Hydrochloride and Hyoscine Hydro-iodide are in large crystals. Dose, $\frac{1}{200}$ to $\frac{1}{100}$ gr. Pilula Hyoscianæ Hydrobromidum, $\frac{1}{200}$ to $\frac{1}{100}$gr.

Hyoscipicrin is a bitter glucoside, precipitated by tannin ; with Hydrochloric acid, it is converted into fermentable sugar and a yellowish acrid bitter resin.

Preparations.—Of Hyoscyamus, Extractum Hyoscyami Viride, B. P. Dose, 2 to 8 grs. Succus Hyoscyami. B.P. Dose, ½ to 1 fld. dr. Tinctura Hyoscyami, B.P. (1 in 10). Dose, ½ to 1 fld. drs. Abstractum Hyoscyami. Dose, 3 to 5 grs. Infusion (1 in 20). Dose, 2 to 4 drs.

Actions and uses.—The leaves are anodyne, hypnotic, mydria tic and antispasmodic, like duboisia, belladonna and stramonium ; but most calmative and least irritant of the group. The delirium is never furious and is generally accompanied by insomnia. As a vasomotor and cardiac stimulant it is superior to stramonium. As a laxative its action is chiefly confined to the intestines. It is a marked sedative of the urinary passages. Hyoscyamus being a non-irritant and hypnotic, it could be used hypodermically like belladonna. As a narcotic, it is given to children or in cases where opium is contra-indicated. Hyoscyamus is given in acute mania, insanity, delirium tremens, dry tickling night cough, asthma, chorea, &c. Like atropine, hyoscyamine is injected hypodermically in epilepsy, obstinate insomnia, hallucinations, in tremors of paralysis agitans, or in mercurial tremors, to relieve pain and disordered co-ordination as in locomotor ataxia. In constipation, Hyoscyamus is given with other purgatives to prevent griping and to render them less drastic. In irritation of the bladder from any cause it is a safe remedy and is given with carminatives and aromatics in colic and dyspepsia. Hyoscine is used in the morphine habit to control restlessness and insomnia, resulting from the withdrawal of morphine and in paralysis agitans. It is chiefly used in violent and abusive restlessness in mania. Locally the seeds mixed with barley and hot brandy are applied to inflammatory swellings. As a local anodyne mixed with tobacco, belladonna, stramonium and nightshade, it relieves swollen testicles, inflamed breasts and enlarged and painful gouty joints. Pessaries made of Hyoscyamus with poppy seeds are used in painful uterine complaints.

Nicotiana Tabacum, N. Havanensis.

Habitat.—Throughout India, Tropical America, Cuba, Virginia, &c.

Parts used.—The dried leaves and stalks, and herb.

Vernacular.—Arab.—Taubâk Bujjir bhang. Mar., Bom., Guz, Duk., Hind., Beng.—Tâmáku. Burm.—Se. Tsha Can.—Hage sappu. Cing.—Dimgazha. Eng.—Virginia Tobacco. Malyal.—Puka-yila.

Pers.—Tanbâbkû. Sans.—Dhuma pataram, Támara kûta. Tam.—Pugai-Ilai. Tel.—Dhumrâ.

Characters.—Annual plant; herb pubescent and glutinous; stems erect, tapering, branched above; leaves very large, oblong, lanceolate, acuminate, narrowing at the base and sessile; leaves when fresh darkish green, viscous to the touch, and of a fœtid odour, and containing a very poisonous oily fluid, irregularly angled, brittle, light, and of a brown colour; taste heating and acrid; dry leaves and stalks of a yellowish light or dark brown colour.

Constituents.—Nicotine—a liquid alkaloid, Nicotianin a volatilisable camphoraceous principle, resin, albumen, gum, extractive matter and ash, containing a large amount of salts as sulphates, nitrates, chlorides, phosphates, malates and citrates of potassium, ammonium, calcium &c.

Nicotina, Nicotine or Nicotia is the poisonous principle. Its quantity varies greatly in different specimens. To obtain it add potassa to concentrated acidulated infusion of the leaves, shake with ether to dissolve thealkaloid, add oxalic acid to form nicotine oxalate; this is precipitated by ether. It is a colourless volatile oily liquid; taste acrid, odour strong and disagreeable; exposed to the air it rapidly becomes brown. It forms soluble salts with acids; soluble in water, also in alcohol and ether. Dose, $\frac{1}{10}$ to $\frac{1}{6}$ gr., given in tetanus and strychnine poisoning.

The quantity of nicotine in different specimens varies. It is 6 to 8 in 100 in French tobacco; and is 2 p.c. in Havana tobacco; Turkish tobacco contains little or none. According to some, tobacco smoke contains no nicotine, but in its stead it contains a series of empyreumatic decomposition products as pyridine, picoline, collidine, parvoline, &c. In the smoke of tobacco used for pipe, pyridine is found in the largest quantity; whereas in cigars, where there is free access of air, collidine predominates. Tobacco smoke also contains about 9 p.c. of carbon dioxide; and such substances as hydrocyanic acid, creosote, hydrogen sulphide gas and acetic, carbolic and valerianic acids.

Ncotinæ tartras. In fine white crystals, freely soluble in water. A suitable form for administration in tetanus or strychnine poisoning.

Preparations.—Enema, 20 grs. infused in 8 ozs. oil—a most virulent poison obtained by distilling leaves with water or collected from Hooka pipe. It is a black tarry substance of an empyreumatic odour. Poultices of leaves, used for orchitis. Gurako—a mixture containing coarse sugar or molasses with apple, sumbul, the root of Jatamansi and tobacco. Tapkhir (or snuff), a very fine powder of the leaves.

Actions and uses.—The juice of the leaves is sedative and antispasmodic. Dry leaves are irritant, nauseating, emetic, and sometimes purgative. In small doses, tobacco stimulates the secreting glands as the saliva, the intestinal secretions and the urine. It lessens the sense of excessive exertion and fatigue. It keeps the bowels free. In some persons it usually causes vomiting. In large doses and if taken for a long time it produces tremors, clonic spasms, contracted pupils, depression of the heart, cold skin and profuse sweats. In toxic doses, it leads to coma and death by paralysis of the heart and respiration.

Smoking or chewing tobacco leaves to excess, causes irritation of the fauces, pharynx and stomach, leading to dyspepsia, to great nervous depression, impaired sexual appetite, and even to angina. It interferes with nutrition, digestion and assimilation, and hence smoking is very injurious in the young. In a few cases, it leads to cardiac hypertrophy, cardiac dilatation, and even cardiac valvular lesion.

Nicotine is a violent gastric irritant. It often leads to vomiting and collapse. Its action is very rapid, and fatal results follow in a few minutes. Given in minim doses internally, or 2 minims by the rectum, it relieves spasms in tetanus, and in strychnine poisoning. $\frac{1}{24}$ gr. hypodermically injected is also very effective. Tobacco may be given as a diuretic in renal dropsy and as an antispasmodic in emphysema, asthma, whooping cough, obstinate hiccough, nymphomania, chordee, and to relieve colic. It may also be used as inhalation, in nasal polypi, nasal catarrh, headache, chronic giddiness, and fainting. The leaves are made hot and applied to the abdomen in colic and gripes, and to the spine in tetanus. The upper surface of the leaf painted with silarasa is used as an application to the painful swelling of the testes in orchitis. Fresh leaves when bruised are locally applied as a palliative in urticaria, gouty and rheumatic painful joints, and to the abdomen in lead colic. The natives use a coarse powder or thin slices of the leaves to smoke in hukka, or to chew it in the mouth. Moderate tobacco smoking is considered to be calmative and cardiac, sedative, disinfectant, and good for fumigating rooms. A very fine powder of the leaves known as tapkhir (snuff) is often used as a tooth powder.

Physalis Alkekengi.

Habitat.—Europe, United States, Persia.

Parts used.—The berries and juice.

Characters.—Berries or fruits, baccate, 2 or more celled, spherical, smooth, and marked with stripes of greenish yellow colour; seeds reniform, many, and albuminous; taste bitterish, and somewhat acidulous.

Constituents.—The berries contain sugar and citric acid. The leaves contain a bitter principle called physalin.

Preparations.—Extract—Dose, 5 to 15 grs. Tincture (1 in 4). Dose, ½ to 1 dr.

Actions and uses.—Hepatic stimulant, alterative and diuretic; the juice and seeds are given in strangury due to cantharides, in dropsy, rheumatism, and gout and in skin diseases.

Physalis Minima.

Habitat.—Throughout India.

Parts used.—The fruit.

Vernacular.—Beng.—Bantepariga. Can.—Bandula. Hind.—Tulati-pati. Mar.—Thânmori, chirboti. Sans.—Tankâri. Tel.—Kupante.

Characters.—Plant pubescent, or glabrous; fruit globular,

about the size of a pea, or about $\frac{1}{2}$ inch in diameter ; seeds numerous, reticulated.

Preparations.—Medicinal oil—it contains Tankari, Pokharmul, Hing, Hirdân, long pepper, black salt, sindhava, rock salt, Java khara, ginger, and butter or ghee.

Actions and uses.—Alterative, diuretic, and aperient ; used in dropsy, urinary diseases and gout. The medicated oil is used as an application in the enlargement of the spleen.

Scopola Carniolica, S. Atropoides, S. Japonica.

Habitat.—Bavaria, Hungary, Central Europe, Nepaul, Sikkim, Central Himalaya.

Parts used.—The rhizome and leaves.

Characters.—Plant downy; leaves resembling those of Datura, of a pale green colour, with tobacco-like odour. Flowers solitary, drooping, of a greenish purple or lurid yellow colour ; fruit globose ; seeds numerous and reniform.

Constituents.—Hyoscyamine 5 p.c., a trace of Hyoscine ; vegetable cholesterin and a fluorescent alkaloidal substance, scopolamine or scopoleine. Scopalamine is found in the rhizome of scopala ; also found in belladonna root, in stramonium seeds and in duboisia. It is allied to atropine and hyoscyamine.

Preparations.—Liquid extract standardized to contain 0·25 p.c. of the alkaloid. Dose, 1 to 5 ms. Liniment (4 of liquid extract in 25). Extract contains 2 p.c. of this alkaloid. Dose, $\frac{1}{8}$ to $\frac{1}{2}$ gr. Onintment contains alcoholic extract 1 in 10. Emplastrum—liquid extract 1 in 5 of lead plaster.

Actions and uses.—Sedative, diuretic and mydriatic ; used for the same purposes as belladonna. It does not produce dryness of the mouth and throat. Scopolamine is preferred to atropine in the treatment of keratitis, corneal ulcers and iritis. The liniment is used in reducing pain and swelling in rheumatism.

Solanum Dulcamara.

Habitat.—Europe, Asia, N. America.

Parts used.—The young branches.

Vernacular.—Eng.—Violet bloom, scarlet berry. Fever twig, nightshade vine. Hind.—Ruba barik. Indian Bazaar.—Inabes-thâlib,

Characters.—Twigs or branches of the size of a goose quill, thick, striate, angular and warty ; on section hollow ; bark thin, pale brown or greenish, marked with alternate leaf scars ; odour slight, taste bitter at first, then sweet ; Dose, 1 to 2 drs.

Constituents.—Dulcamarin—a glucoside, picroglycion—a peculiar principle, solanin—an alkaloid, resin, gum, starch, wax and calcium lactale. Dulcamarin—to obtain it, digest the infusion with animal charcoal, exhaust with boiling alcohol, evaporate, dissolve the residue in water, precipitate with subacetate of lead, digest the precipitate with alcohol and decompose it with sulphuretted hydrogen. A yellowish powder, soluble in alcohol, or water ; taste bitter, then sweet. By acids, it splits up into sugar and dulcamaretin. Solanin also axists in S. Tuberosum, S. Nigrum, S. Lycopersecum, etc. It occurs in minute crystals, or prisms ; taste bitter, reaction alkaline ; soluble in boiling alcohol (1 in 125), insoluble in water. It exists in very small quantity. Dose, 1 to 2 grs.

Preparations.—Fluid extract. Dose, ½ to 1 dr. Decoction (1 in 10). Dose, 1 to 2 ozs. Infusion (1 in 10). Dose, 1 to 2 ozs.

Actions and uses.—In small doses alterative, anaphrodisiac, and deobstruent ; in toxic doses narcotic. Under its use the respiration is lowered, the circulation becomes languid and there is a dusky colour of the fingers and lips. As an irritant of the mucous membranes, it produces nausea, vomiting, vertigo, erythematous eruptions, convulsions in children, gastro-enteritis, a feeling of heat in the throat and chest, and extreme prostration. As an alterative it is given in herpes, pityriasis, psoriasis, acne and eczema ; also in diarrhœa, jaundice, gout, rheumatism, chronic bronchitis, and in whooping cough. As a diaphoretic, it is used in catarrh of the nose, bladder or of the lungs. As an anaphrodisiac it is given in mania with excessive venereal desire.

Solanum Indicum.

Habitat.—Throughout India.

Parts used.—The fruit and root.

Vernacular.—Beng.—Byâkura. Cing.—Tibbatu. Can.—Gulla. Duk.—Kôlse-kâ-jhâr. Eng.—Indian night-shade. Mar., Guz.—Ubhi ringni, mothi ringni. Hind.—Barhanta. Malyal.—Cheru Chunta. Sans.—Bhantaki, Vrihati, Mahati. Tam.—Pappara mulli. Tel.—Tella-mulaka,

Characters.—Root, of a lightish yellow colour ; stem with numerous branches; young parts downy and armed with very acute, somewhat curved spines ; leaves solitary, or in pairs, petioled, and ovate, on both sides downy, sinuately lobed and armed with a few straight spines on both surfaces; berries round, smooth, of the size of a mokai, of a yellow colour when fresh ; taste pungent, almost acrid ; tasteless when dry.

Constituents.—Wax, fatty acids, and an alkaloid, solanin.

Preparations.—Decoction (1 in 10). Dose, ½ to 1 fld. oz. A compound decoction (1 in 10), containing the root of Solanum Indicum, Solanum Xanthocarpum, sida cordifolia, justicia adhatoda and raisins equal parts. Dose, ½ to 1 fld. oz.

Actions and uses.—Diaphoretic, stimulant, diuretic and expectorant; used in fevers, coughs and dysuria. Solanum Indicum is an ingredient in Dasa mula-di-kvath.

Solanum Jacquini, S. diffusum, S. Xanthocarpum.

Habitat.—Throughout India, Coromandel, Travancore.

Parts used.—The plant.

Vernacular.—Arab.—Hadak-i-barri. Beng.—Kântâ kari—Jangli began. Burm.—Khayân Kazo. Can.—Nelagulla. Cing.—Katu valbatu.—Eng.—Wild egg plant, bitter sweet, woody night-shade. Ind.—Cundun ghatrievayr. Hind.—Laghu Khatai. Guz., Duk., Mar.—Bhuiringni, Kante ringni, Dorali. Pers.—Badingân-i-barri. Sans.—Nidig-dhika, Kântâ kini, Tam.—Kandan Kattiri. Tel.—Vakudu.

Characters.—Root biennial, long, and of a light brown colour; stem prostrate or diffuse, branched and covered with long broad-based, tapering spines; leaves frequently oblong, sinuately pinnatifid, lanceolate, smooth, and armed on both surfaces with long strong spines; flowers in racemes, prickly, pedicelled, large, and of a beautiful light yellow or bright blue côlour; berries spherical, very smooth, drooping and marked with variegated stripes, generally greenish yellow; taste acrid and pungent; fruit small with spines; seeds reniform, compressed and of a light brown colour.

Constituents.—The fruit contains fatty acids, wax and an alkaloid. The dried leaves contain an alkaloid and an organic acid.

Preparations.—Decoction (1 in 40). Dose, ½ to 1 fld. oz. Medicated oil. To prepare it, boil pounded seeds or juice of leaves in sweet oil —Kanta kary aveleha or electuary. To prepare it, take Tinospora cordifolia, piper chaba, plumbago zeylanica, chavak, cyperus rotundus, rhus kakrasinghi, black pepper, ginger, alhagi maurorum, clerodendron siphonanthes, vanda Roxburghii and zedoary, sugar; mix, and make a fine powder. To this add kanta kari, boiled in water and made into an extract. Next add ghee and water, and boil the whole over a fire till reduced to the consistence of an extract; when ready add honey and vanslochan, long pepper, to make an electuary. Dose, 4 to 6 drs.

Actions and uses.—Aperient, carminative, expectorant, and diuretic. The confection is given in asthma, cough, catarrhal affections of the lungs, fever, flatulence and pain in the chest; as a diuretic, the decoction is given in dysuria, cystic calculi and dropsy; also given in costiveness. It is seldom given alone and is generally combined with other expectorant, demulcent and aromatic medicines. A paste of the seeds is locally applied to promote the suppuration of boils, buboes and other indolent chronic abscesses. The oil is applied to the chest to relieve the pain of bronchitis, and to the skin in chronic skin diseases. Fumigation of the fruits is largely used by the natives as sialogogue, and applied for the relief of pain in caried teeth. Bhuiringani is one of the ingredients of Laghu panch mula of Dasa mula-di-kvatha.

Solanum Nigrum.

Habitat.—Throughout India and Ceylon.

Parts used.—The herb.

Vernacular.—Arab.—Inabes-thaliba. Beng.—Kakamachi Kovidaraha. Burm.—Simani-gahâ. Can.—Kanchi-Ganikê. Cing.—Semanigaha. Duk.—Udi-Kamanê. Guz.—Makoy, Kâlopilludo. Hind.—

Makô, Gurkamai, udâ-maki. Malyal.—Manatta Kali. Mar.—Kamuni Ghati, Kâlâ kanguna. Pers.—Rubah turbak ; angûrê rûbah, Sagangura. Sans.—Kôvidâraha, Krishna-kô Vidâraha, Dhvanksha machi, Jaghana Khal or Kinkini-Kakamachi, Kakamâta. Tam.—Karuppu. Tel.—Kâmanchi chettu.

Characters.—Small shrub ; stems erect, branches many, irregular, spreading, glabrous or pubescent ; wood on section greenish yellow, with one or two concentric rings, angles of the branches somewhat swollen ; leaves ovate, oblong, attenuated at both ends, entire or slightly toothed, and of a dark green colour. Flowers dirty white, small, and generally attached to the swollen parts of the branches ; berries small, globular, and of a greenish yellow, brown or black colour; seeds numerous, compressed and reniform ; smell acrid, taste biting and pungent.

Constituents.—The berries contain solanin, which is a compound of sugar and solanidine—an aikaloid having the property of dilating the pupils.

Preparations.—Expressed juice. Dose, 1 to 4 oz. Fluid extract. Dose, $\frac{1}{2}$ to 1 fld. dr. Decoction (1 in 10). Dose, $\frac{1}{2}$ to 1 fld. oz. Infusion (1 in 10). Dose, $\frac{1}{2}$ to 1 fld. oz. Syrup. Dose, 1 to 2 fld. drs.

Actions and uses.—The herb is alterative, sedative, diaphoretic, diuretic, hydragogue and expectorant ; locally anodyne. Solanine is a powerful, protoplasmic poison, acting upon amœboid organisms and ciliated epithelial cells. Its solution 1 p.c., prevents the growth of bacteria. It coagulates albumen. If kept for some time in contact with blood, it dissolves the red corpuscles. As an alterative the herb is given in skin diseases such as psoriasis, eczema and in syphilis ; as a diuretic in gout, rheumatism, dropsy, gonorrhœa, renal and vesical catarrh, coughs, splenic and hepatic enlargements, &c. The syrup is used as a cooling drink and as a diaphoretic in fevers. The leaves made hot are applied to painful and swollen testicles and on swelled legs and hands.

Solanum Tuberosum.

Habitat.—Temperate climates.

Parts used.—The tubers, stem and leaves.

Vernacular.—Cing.—Ruta-innala. Hind.—Puttata, alu. Malyal.—Ubi kantang. Pers.—Seb-zamini. Tam.—Kelangu. Tel.—Ooralay gadda.

Constituents.—Solanina starch, which can be removed by process of boiling.

Preparations.—Decoction of the stem and leaves (1 in 20). Dose, 2 to 8 drs.

Actions and uses.—Alterative ; given in skin diseases. Solalina starch is nutrient and used like arrowoot.

Withania Somnifera, Physalis Fluxuosa.

Habitat.—Dry sub-tropical India, Coromandel, Concans, West Coast, Travancore.

Parts used.—The root and leaves.

Vernacular.—Bomb., Beng.—Asvagandha. Can.—Herimaddina. Goa.—Fatar Fodá. Duk., Hind., Guz.—Asagandha, Asana. Malyal. —Pevetti. Mar.—Tula, Kanchuki Dorgunj. Sans.—Ashvagandha, Varàha Karni Vrisha, Turagi gandha. Tam.—Amkoolang. Tel.—Penerr.

Turagi gandha, smelling like a horse or mare. Varaha-karni, Boar-eared. Ashvagandha is derived from Ashva, a horse, and gandha, smell. It is said that the root smells like the skin of a horse.

Characters.—Plant 2 to 4 feet high; branches very slender; leaves alternate, petioled, obtuse, ovate, oblong, and sometimes oblique at the base; young parts and nerves of the leaves covered with whitish starry tomentum; root, hard, tapering and branched, below whitish brown, woody, and thick as the little finger; root bark round, thick, smooth, giving off irregularly branched fibrils; wood hard, of a white colour and not easily broken; on section it presents an outer thin ring within which is a homogeneous, starchy, crystalline, white substance; taste intensely bitter, odour resembling that of bhuikohola.

Constituents.—An alkaloid Somniferin having hypnotic property, resin, fat and colouring matter.

Preparations.—Decoction (1 in 10). Dose, ½ to 1 fld. oz. Medicated oil. "Narayen tel" contains Ashagandh, Chikaná-pát-mul, Bela, Venivel Bhui-ringani, Ubhá gokharu, Limado, Tetu mul, Puneranavá, Arani, each 2 parts. Make a decoction. To this add Til tel 40 parts, and a paste of Dudh 10 parts, Kátho Elachi, Jatámánasi, Vekhand, Moravel, Rakta-chandan, Sindhav, Asan, Rásaná, Variáli, Devadár, Sálavan, Pitavan, Tagar, each 2 parts. Boil the whole for one hour.

Actions and uses.—Tonic, alterative and sedative; a paste of the root taken with milk and clarified butter helps the nutrition of weakly children. As an alterative, a confection is given in consumption, debility from old age and rheumatism. Native women combine it with various restoratives in nervous debility and leucorrhœa; as a sedative and hypnotic, the leaves moistened with castor oil are applied to carbuncles. Narâyan tel is dropped into the nose in deafness, and is used as an inunction over the body in hemiplegia, tetanus, rheumatism and lumbago and as an enema in dysentery, and anal fistula. It is given internally in 15 to 60 ms. doses in consumption, emaciation of children, debility from old age, leprosy, nervous diseases and rheumatism.

Withania Coagulans.

Habitat.—Persia, Punjab, Scinde, Baluchistan.

Parts used.—The fruit.

Vernacular.—Afghan.—Spin bajja. Arab.—Kâk-najê-hindi. Beng.—Ashva ganda. Eng.—Vegetable rennet. Duk.—Nâl-ke-as-gand. Bomb., Hind.—Kâknaj, panir-phota, panir-bandâ, Akri. Panj.—Khamjari. Pers.—Arusaka-pas-i-paradah. Sans.—Râjâputrika. Sinde.—Panirjafota. Tam.—Amuk-kura-verai. Tel.—Penneru jodda vittulu.

Panira Banda. Panira, means cheese, and Banda to bind, or coagulate ; this fruit coagulates milk into cheese ; one ounce of the decoction of the fruit will, like rennet, coagulate a gallon of warm milk in about half an hour.

Characters.—Shrub stellately tomatose, resembling harmal (Paganum Hamâlâ); fruit rather larger in size than, but similar in shape to Makoya, brownish yellow or reddish brown, and much shrivelled; epidermis, rugous and rather shining; seeds many, flattened, reniform, pitted, light reddish brown, compressed, sticky, and resembling Bhuiringani bija ; odour fruity, taste aciduous and acrid. The berries contain a ferment similar in action to animal rennet in its coagulating power.

Preparations.—Infusion (1 in 10). Dose, $\frac{1}{2}$ to 1 fld. oz. ; and confection (1 in 5). Dose, 1 to 2 fld. drs.

Actions and uses.—The ripe fruit is emetic. The dried fruit is diuretic, alterative, carminative and stomachic, and is given in chronic congestion of the liver, in skin diseases, jaundice rheumatism, urinary diseases, dyspepsia and flatulent colic. In large doses it is narcotic.

Scrophulariaceæ—The Fig-wort family.

Herbs or rarely shrubs ; leaves opposite, entire, or toothed, some times parasitical on roots. Flowers irregular, beautiful, and of a blue yellow, or pink colour; calyx 5-lobed, corolla, irregular, 2-lipped; stamens 4, didynamous; ovary, sessile, 2-celled; fruits capsular, baccate, 2-celled; seeds numerous, albumen fleshy.

Habitat.—Found everywhere.

Properties,—The plants are bitter, astringent, emetic, purgative and diuretic; some are narcotic poisons.

Digitalis Purpurea, B. P.

Habitat.—South and Central Europe.

Parts used.—The dried leaves, Digitalis Folia, B. P.

Fairy gloves, folks or ladies' glove, dog's finger, dead men's bells. Digitalis, from digitus, a finger—coralla is finger shaped or thimble shaped. Purpurea—Purpureus, purple coloured, its flowers are purple. Foxglove—corruption of folk's glove. Folk synonym of fairies.

Characters.—Biennial plant. The drug consists of dry leaves from the wild indigenous plant when $\frac{2}{3}$ of flowers are expanded. The dried leaves are dull green, long, ovate, contracted at the base into a winged petiole, downy, wrinkled above, and reticulate beneath ; odour slight and tea-like ; taste, bitter and nauseous ; flowers purple, in spikes ; seeds are known to contain the active principle in larger proportion than the leaves but are never used. Leaves if imperfectly dried are subject to decomposition, so also the tincture of the leaves if mixed with water, or syrup, the active principle being destroyed. Dose, of the leaves, $\frac{1}{2}$ to 2 grs.

Constituents.—5 principles, Digitalinum or Digitalin (at one time thought to be the active principle), Digitonin, Digitin, Digitalein, and Digitoxin; Digitalosmin (a stearoptin) ; Digitoleic acid, extractive, mucilage, gum, pictin, &c. Digitalin—a granular glucoside, soluble in alcohol, almost insoluble in water, sparingly soluble in ether, or chloroform. Dose, $\frac{1}{60}$ to $\frac{1}{30}$ gr. Digitoxin, a crystalline glucoside. Light crystals, insoluble in water, soluble in alcohol, sparingly so in chloroform, most toxic and cumulative in action Dose, $\frac{1}{250}$ to $\frac{1}{60}$ gr. Digitalein—an amorphous powder, soluble in water, alcohol and insoluble in ether or chloroform. Non-cumulative and non-irritant, hence used hypodermically. Dose, $\frac{1}{60}$ to $\frac{1}{20}$ gr. Digitonin—a crystalline glucoside, soluble in water, insoluble in cold alcohol, ether, or chloroform—similar in action to saponin—a good diuretic. Digitin—a crystalline body, insoluble in ether and chloroform, sparingly soluble in water, readily soluble in alcohol ; generally inert.

Preparations.—Extractum Digitalis. Dose, $\frac{1}{6}$ to $\frac{1}{2}$ grs. Extractum Digitalis fluidium ; macerate the leaves, percolate in alcohol and water and evaporate. It contains mostly Digitalin and Digitalein with trace of Digitoxin. Dose, $\frac{1}{2}$ to 3 ms. Infusum Digitalis, B.P. 60 grs. to 1 pint. Dose, 2 to 4 fld. drs. It contains mostly Digitonin, little Digitalein, but no Digitalin or Digitoxin, hence used best as a diuretic. Tinctura Digitalis, B.P. (1 in 8). Dose, 5 to 15 ms. It contains Digitalin, Digitoxin and Digitalein; used best as a cardiac stimulant. Abstractum Digitalis. Dose, $\frac{1}{4}$ to 2 grs.

Actions and uses.—Digitalin contracts the blood vessels generally; Digitoxin, Digitalein and Digitonin dilate the renal arteries, thereby increasing the arterial tension and blood pressure in the glomeruli. In medicinal doses Digitalis is a diuretic, hæmostatic, cardiac and vascular stimulant ; in large doses an irritant, causing sneezing, nausea, vomiting, and dark green bilious stools ; it gives rise to headache, giddiness and irregular pulse. Under its use the heart contracts more powerfully but slowly. It is largely used in cardiac affections, functional or organic, as in cardiac hypertrophy with dilatation, in mitral regurgitation, accompanied with venous congestion, in irregular, intermittent, and feeble pulse and in œdema of the lungs. Digitalis prolongs the cardiac diastole ; it thus gives time for the dilated auricle to empty itself through the incompetent orifice, strengthens the contraction of the left ventricle and brings about better approximation of the mitral valve flaps. There is, therefore, less regurgitation and less venous congestion and more blood is forced into the arterial system. In mitral constriction, in tricuspid regurgitation and constriction, in dilatation of the right side of the heart with rapid and feeble pulse, cough, dyspnœa, pulsating jugulars, dusky face, scanty, high coloured urine and dropsy, it is given with great benefit. It should not be given in aortic disease as it prolongs the diastole, gives more time for the blood to regurgitate and thus increase the danger of fatal syncope. It is equally dangerous in atheroma, fatty degeneration of the heart, and chronic Bright's desease. If given for a long time it causes extreme contraction of the renal vessels, stops the renal circulation and secretion of urine, and thus instead of the elimination of digitalis by excretion, it is accumulated in the blood and acts as a cumulative poison. The excretion of urea is increased at first, but is subsequently diminished; respiration, which may be slow at first, soon becomes rapid and feeble. There is paralysis, cyanosis, coma, and convulsions followed by death. Digitalis being an uncertain diuretic, it is safe to give it with sodium nitrite, which dilates the renal vessels. As an antipyretic in fevers, in the first stage of pneumonia and in other acute inflammatory affections, as rheumatism, in acute bronchitis, pleurisy and in specific fevers, its use is of great benefit. As a hæmostatic, large doses of digitalis are given with ergot and strychnine in menorrhagia, hæmoptysis, &c. In dyspnœa and orthopnœa, due to loss of tone in the vascular system, digitalis has proved very beneficial and gives quiet sleep. As an anaphrodisiac combined with potassium bromide, it is given in spermatorrhœa with feeble erections, frequent emissions, and cold hands and feet.

Franciscea Uniflora.

Habitat.—Brazil.

Parts used.—The root—Manaca, also called mercurio vegetal or vegetable mercury.

Characters.—Shrub; leaves, alternate, oblong, acuminate; petiole, short; stem, tough and woody; internally yellowish; bark thin and dark.

Constituents.—An active principle, Franciscеine.

Preparations.—Fluid extract. Dose, 10 to 60 ms.

Actions and uses.—Alterative, antisyphilitic, emmenagogue, cholagogue and diuretic. The root stimulates the lymphatic system, and thus eliminates morbid matters from the blood by the skin and kidneys. In acute and chronic rheumatism, in rheumatic arthritis it eliminates the urates and prevents their being deposited in the joints. It also stimulates the lymphatics and acts as an absorbent to remove exudation products. It stimulates the liver and lessens jaundice associated with constipation. As a tonic and alterative like nux vomica, it is used in scrofula, in Bright's disease, with scanty urine and in syphilis, even after such remedies as iodides, stillingea and berberis have failed. On this account, it has been termed mercurio-vegetal.

Herpestis Monniera, Bramia Indica, Gratiola Monniera.

Habitat.—Throughout India, in marshy ground near streams and borders of tanks.

Parts used.—The herb.

Vernacular.—Beng.—Shwete chamini. Cing.—Sunn-véla. Bomb., Hind.—Bâma, Nir-brami, Jala-brahmi. Malyal.—Beami. Mar.—Nir-brami, Bâmbâ. Sans.—Jalla-brahmi, Jali-nim. Tam.—Neerpirimi. Tel.—Sambrâni-âku.

Characters.—Plant annual and creeping. Stems several, round jointed, smooth and succulent; leaves linear, or obovate, also entire, wedge shaped, or oblong, smooth, succulent; opposite, sessile and dotted with minute spots; peduncles, axillary, solitary; flowers blue; capsules, ovate, 2-celled, 2-valved; seeds numerous; taste saline.

Constituents.—A trace of oily matter—which is soluble in alcohol and of an acid reaction; tannin, an alkaloid, soluble in ether and chloroform; an organic acid, 2 resins, both soluble in alkaline solutions and one readily soluble in ether.

Preparations.—Infusion (1 in 20). Dose, ½ to 1 fld. oz.

Actions and uses.—Diuretic, aperient and tonic; given in stoppage of urine with costiveness; also in nervous debility, seminal weakness, epilepsy, &c. With petroleum, the juice is rubbed on rheumatic painful parts. The plant is applied hot to the chest in bronchitis and cough in children.

Limnophila Gratioloides and L. Gratissima.

Habitat.—India, swampy places.

Parts used.—The plant.

Vernacular.—Beng.—Karpur. Hind.—Kuttra. Mal.—Mânga nâri. Mar.—Ambuli. Sans.—Ambuja, Amragandhaka.

Ambuja, water-born. Amra-gandhaka, having odour of mangoes.

Characters.—The plant has a grateful odour and aromatic taste. Leaves whorled, pinnatifid, ¼ to ¾ inch long, opposite, entire at the top of the stem and numerous and multifid at its base. Stems simple, hairy.

Preparations.—Medicated oil of the plant with cocoanut oil—used as liniment.

Actions and uses.—Local stimulant and antiseptic; the juice is rubbed over the body in infectious diseases, as fevers, measles, small-pox, &c. The liniment is used as an application to the legs or scrotum in elephantiasis.

Picrorrhiza Kurroa, Veronica Lindleyana.

Habitat.—Shady woods of mountains in Europe and Nepaul.

Parts used.—The rhizome.

Vernacular.—Arab.—Asava, Khar-baka. Beng.—Kutki Tita. Cing.—Kalû-rana. Guz., Bomb., Duk.—Kâli-kutaki, karu. Eng.—White

Christmas rose. Hind.—Kutki, Pathanbed. Mar.—Bâlakadu. Pers.—Karatika. Panj.—Karrooa. Sans.—Katu-rôhani, Kutaki-Dhauvan tari grasta Krishna bhedi, Ashaka-rohini chakranga. Tam., Tel.—Katuka rôgani.

White Christmas rose is so called from the flowers appearing in winter during Christmas time. Bal kadu—from Bal, a child, and Kaddu, bitter ; it means a child's bitter, being used as a laxative for children.

Characters.—Two varieties—*kadu* occurs in short broken pieces, from 1 to 3 inches long, resembling goose quills, externally smooth, and of a brownish white colour ; slightly shrivelled, knotty, and marked here and there with scars of fallen rootlets ; very fragile, light and soft, and can be compressed between the fingers ; cut surface black and presenting the appearance as if made up of layers or scales. It has a white broken ring between the centre and the external surface. In *Kâli kutaki* the pieces are knotty, and resemble in size those of kadu, but somewhat thicker ; colour, brownish dark ; externally each piece is covered over with 3 or 4 scales, which are the marks of leaflets ; on section, the cut surface resembles kadu ; in colour, appearance, &c., both have a smell somewhat like that of Majitha, or tobacco, and a very bitter taste. Dose of the root, as a tonic, 10 to 20 grs. ; as aperient 2 drs., as an antiperiodic, 20 to 40 grs.

Constituents.—A bitter principle Picrorhizin, Picrorhizetin, cathartic acid, glucose, wax, &c. Picrorhizin is a glucoside and obtained by exhausting the powdered drug with ether. It is soluble in water and alcohol, and insoluble in ether.

Preparations.—Decoction (1 in 20). Dose, 1 to 2 fld. ozs. Tincture (1 in 10). Dose, ½ to 1 dr.

Actions and uses.—Alterative, bitter, stomachic and cholagogue; given in dyspepsia, chronic dysentery, asthma, hepatic derangements, jaundice, &c. Its action on the liver is similar to, but milder than that of colocynth. It is a valuable antiperiodic in low continued fevers ; it is given to children in worms.

Remarks.—The root is confounded with black Hellebore.

Schweinfurthia Sphærocarpa.

Habitat.—Sind, Beluchistan, Afghanistan.

Parts used.—The herb, with broken-up fruits.

Indian Bazars—Sannipât, Sannipât nud. Hind.—Nepal nimb, Eng.—Nepal bitter.

Characters.—Fruit globular, capsule papery, mucronate ; seeds 5 angled, mumerous, wedge-shaped, with longitudinal ridges ; testa tubercular ; calyx 5 partite, upper segment large, extending over the fruit like a hood. Leaves ovate, leathery, with short blunt hairs ; margin lighter in colour than the rest of the leaf ; whole plant bitter with a tea-like taste.

Constituents—An alkaloid ; fatty saccharine matter, mineral matter &c.

Preparations.—Infusion (1 in 30). Dose, 2 to 4 fld. drs.

Actions and uses.—Powerful stimulant and diaphoretic ; given in typhoid condition during fevers and other acute diseases—largely used by the natives.

Verbascum Thapsus, V. Indicum.

Habitat.—Europe, Siberia, Caucasus, Himalaya.

Parts used.—The root, leaves and flowers.

Vernacular.—Arab.—Mahizahraj Labidah-el-baida. Adaned-dubb Eng.—Great mullein weed, cow's lung wort. Hind.—Phùlla Ban Tambâku. Pers.—Busir.

Characters.—Leaves large, woolly, oblong, upper ones acuminate and sessile, those on the stems more or less crenate and covered with soft whitish stellate hairs ; taste, bitter, mucilaginous ; odour disagreeable ; flowers in a spike, bright yellow, 5 lobed, smooth above and tomentose beneath; seeds cone-shaped, finely pitted, very tough and horny, of an acrid taste and without odour. Dose, 15 to 20 grs.

Constituents.—The flowers contain a volatile oil, a fatty acid, free malic acid, malate and phosphate of lime, acetate of potash ; also phosphoric acid, sugar, gum, chlorophyll and a yellow resinous colouring matter. The leaves contain a crystalline wax, volatile oil, resin, tannin, a bitter principle, sugar, mucilage and ash, 12·6 p.c.

Preparations.—Tincture (1 in 8). Dose, ½ to 1 fld. dr. Infusion (1 in 5) of milk. Dose, 4 to 6 ozs.

Actions and uses.—Expectorant, nutritive, emollient, demulcent and anodyne; given in phthisis and in wasting diseases. Under its use the expectoration becomes easy, cough is lessened, and like cod-liver oil it improves the weight and general condition. It is also given in diarrhœa, in gout and rheumatism, generally in combination with aperients. Dried leaves are smoked in nasal catarrh ; the seeds are antispasmodic and used in asthma and infantile convulsions ; in Northern India, the roots are used as febrifuge.

Veronica Virginica.

Habitat.—N. America, Canada.

Parts used.—The rhizome and rootlets—Leptandra.

Syn.—Culver's physic, Culver's root, black root, purple Leptandra.

Characters.—Perennial plant ; rhizome horizontal, thick and flattened, of a blackish brown colour, marked with cup-shaped scars on the upper surface ; the bark is thin, wood yellowish, pith purplish brown. Roots thin, wrinkled and fragile, without any odour and a bitter acrid taste. Dose, powdered rhizome 20 to 60 grs.

Constituents.—Leptandrin, an active principle—a glucoside, resin, 6 p.c., saponin, tannin, mannit, gum, citric acid, and a volatile alkaloid. Leptandrin—Precipitate the infusion of the root with acetate of lead, add sodium carbonate to remove the precipitate, add alcohol, then wash with water, add alcohol, filter and evaporate. Needle-shaped crystals, bitter, soluble in ether, alcohol, water.

Preparations.—Fluid extract. Dose, 20 to 60 ms. Solid extract. Dose, 1 to 3 grs. Tincture (1 in 8). Dose, ½ to 1 dr.

Actions and uses.—Like other resin-bearing purgatives, it is emetic, cathartic and efficient cholagogue, alterative and tonic. It excites the liver and promotes the flow of bile without any irritation of the bowel. It is given in duodenal indigestion, chronic constipation with deficiency of bile and intestinal secretions; in action, it resembles podophyllin.

Bignoniaceæ, the Bignonia, Trumpet flowers or Tetu family.

Trees, or twining, or climbing shrubs; leaves exstipulate, usually opposite, simple, conjugate, compound, very large as in Tetu. Flowers irregular and often beautifully yellow, brown, red, pink, or purple; capsules compressed, seeds many and winged.

Habitat.—Native of tropical countries.

Properties.—These plants are very little used in medicine; the barks of some are anthelmintic and astringent.

Crescentia Cujete, Calabash tree (Eng.).

Habitat.—Native of S. America, cultivated in India.

Parts used.—The fruit.

Characters.—Fruit large, gourd-like, and green; shell, woody; pulp, slightly acid, and white and containing flattened cordiform seeds.

Constituents.—The pulp contains crescentic acid; also tartaric, citric and tannic acids, 2 resins, a bitter aromatic extractive, and colouring matters, resembling indigo.

Preparations.—Syrup (1 in 10). Dose, 1 to 2 drs.

Actions and uses.—Demulcent and expectorant; given in dysentery and cough. In the form of poultice the pulp is applied to the chest.

Oroxylum Indicum, Calosanthes Indica.

Habitat.—Throughout India.

Parts used.—The root bark.

Vernacular.—Beng.—Nasona. Guz., Bomb.—Tetu. Hind.—Arlu, Sona, Phalphal. Mar.—Kharasinga, Bahman-tetu. Malyal.—Peiani. Panj.—Talpalanga. Sans.—Syonaka, Prathu Simbih, sukâ nasa, Arall, Bhalluka-priya. Tam.—Vanga-adanthay. Tel.—Dundillam.

Prathu Simbih, having broad pods; sukâ nasa, having nose like a parrot's beak. Bhalluka priya, dear to bears.

Characters.—The tree is remarkable for terminal spikes of large lurid fleshy flowers, and large, transversely compressed, somewhat curved pods. The root bark is of a light yellow colour, of an offensive smell and an acrid taste ; bark of the stem, rough and marked with large scars of fallen leaves, thickly studded with wart-like protuberances ; internal surface, very yellow. Dose, 5 to 15 grs.

Constituents.—Oroxylin, an acrid principle, pectin, extractive matter, fat, wax, &c.

Preparations.—Infusion (1 in 10). Dose, ½ to 1 fld. oz. Decoction (1 in 10). Dose 4 to 8 drs. Medicated oil—boil Teel oil in the decoction of Tetu bark over a fire till the watery portion is evaporated.

Actions and uses.—As an anodyne the oil is dropped into the ear in otorrhœa. The powder and infusion of the bark combined with opium are sudorific, better than Dover's powders. As an anodyne, a bath prepared with the bark is frequently employed in acute rheumatism. It is also used in dropsy. The root bark is an ingredient of the Dasa mulâ dekvâtha.

Stercospermum Suaveolens, S. Chelonioides. Heterophragma Suaveolens. H. Chelonioides.

Habitat.—India, throughout the moist parts.

Parts used.—The root bark and flowers.

Vernacular.—Can.—Hudai. Guz.—Pandan. Beng., Hind.—Parul, Kashta-pâtali. Mar.—Kâlgori, Padri. Sans.—The tree, Pâtálá Patali, Kama duti, Madhu duti, Patala. South India.—The flowers Madan—Kamapu. Tam.—Padri. Tel.—Kalgoru Padari.

Kama duti, Cupid's messenger; Madhu duti, messenger of spring Patala, light, red or rose coloured.

Characters.—Flowers large, of dark dull crimson colour, highly fragrant, corolla light purple above, brownish purple below, hairy at its convexity ; bark ash-coloured, and somewhat scabrous.

Constituents.—The flowers contain albuminous, saccharine and mucilaginous matters and wax.

Preparations.—Infusion of the bark (1 in 10). Dose, ½ to 1 fld. oz.

Actions and uses.—Refrigerant and diuretic ; used in dyspepsia, fever, cough, dropsy &c. The flowers with honey stop troublesome hiccough.

Remarks.—The bark is one of the ingredients of Dasa mula dekvath.

Stercospermum Xylocarpum, Bignonia Xylocarpum.

Habitat.—Deccan Peninsula.

Parts used.—The tar.

Vernacular.—Can.—Ghansing. Mar.—Kharsing.

Characters.—Wood hard, internally presenting a yellow, resinous surface. The tar obtained from the wood is a thick fluid of the colour and consistence of ordinary Stockholm or pine tar. Dose, 3 to 10 grs.

Actions and uses.—Stimulant, expectorant and parasiticide. The tar is useful in the treatment of skin eruptions. Other properties are similar to those of pine tar, for which it may be used as a fair substitute.

Pedaliaceæ—the Pedalium or Tila family.

General Characters.—Glandular and often glutinous herbs; leaves entire, dentate or lobed, and exstipulate. Flowers axillary, large, tubular, irregular, and of a pink, white or other variegated and beautiful colours; ovary on a glandular or fleshy disk, 1-celled, sometimes 4-celled. Fruits bony, or capsular; seeds wingless, without albumen, cotyledons large.

Habitat—Natives of tropical countries.

Properties.—The plants are remarkable for their oily seeds; leaves are demulcent and mucilaginous; the capsules of some species are diuretic and demulcent.

Martynia Diandra.

Habitat.—Concan, India.

Parts used.—The nuts.

Vernacular.—Eng.—Tiger's claw, devil's claw. Guz.—Vichhida. Mar.—Vinchhu, Vecchhu. Vinchhu, scorpion, so named because of the resemblance of the fruit to a scorpion.

Characters.—The fruit is a green, fleshy capsule, and contains a hard, black, woody, wrinkled nut with two hooks which are sharp and curved, thus resembling a beetle.

Actions and uses.—A paste is used as a local sedative; the nut, rubbed down with water and applied, is said to have a curative effect upon the bites of venomous reptiles such as scorpions, &c.

Pedalium Murex.

Habitat.—Deccan Peninsula, Madras Peninsula, Ceylon, Coromandel, Cape Comorin.

Parts used.—The fruit and leaves.

Vernacular.—Arab.—Khussuke Kabir. Cing.—Cet-neringi. Can.—Annegalugida. Bomb., Hind., Guz.—Kadava gokharu, ghati gokharu, Bara gokhru. Malyal.—Kattu nerumil. Mar.—Ubha gokhru, karonta. Sans.—Ghilja-sudu-moostra. Tam.—Kaka-mulu. Tel.—Yea nuga palleros.

Characters.—Plant low, spreading and succulent; leaves smooth, truncate, oval, dentate and obtusely pointed. Fruit a drupe, pendulous, and four-angled, or winged with a sharp spine at the base of each angular ridge; fresh fruit, green and succulent, dry fruit, corky. Nut 2-celled, 2 seeded; seeds arillate, 4 in number, elongated and narrow. Under surface of the leaves and of immature capsules present a frosted appearance, due to the presence of numerous small, brilliant crystalline glands. Agitated with water they produce white viscid mucilage, like white of eggs. The glandular bodies are the source of mucilage. The plant has a peculiar, disagreeable, musk-like odour.

Constituents.—An alkaloid, fat, resin, gum and ash 5 p.c.

Preparations.—Infusion (1 in 10). Dose, 1 to 4 fld. ozs. Decoction, (1 in 10). Dose, 1 to 2 fld. ozs.

Actions and uses.—The infusion is a favourite and excellent demulcent and diuretic in dysuria and gonorrhœa, and for gonorrheal rheumatism. It is also used as a diuretic, and lithontriptic. The fresh leaves and young shoots, dipped in boiling milk and kept for a few minutes give the milk a bitter and mucilaginous taste and are used in gonorrhœa. The decoction is given in seminal debility, nocturnal emission, impotence and incontinence of urine, and as a diuretic in dropsy. Chota Gokhru is the fruit of Tribulus terrestris.

Sesamum Indicum, S. Orientale, S. Trifoliatum, S. Luteum.

Habitat.—Throughout India, cultivated in the South of United States.

Parts used.—The seeds, and the fixed oil expressed from the seeds.

Vernacular.—Arab.—Sunsin Burm.—Huan, Huonma goshya. Bomb.—Goda-tela. Can.—Valley-ennê. Cing.—Teel-tel. Eng.—Gingili oil, Teel oil, Benne oil, Sesame oil. Beng., Guz., Hind. —Mitha tel, Teel-katal, Berik-tel, Krishna, tel. Mal.—Eloo, Chirettâ. Malyal.—Nallena. Mar.—Chak-ka tel. Pers.—Râghanê-Kunjad. Sans.—Teela-telam, Telaka telam. Tam.—Nal-yennai. Tel.—Manchi-noovay.

Characters.—Sesamum or Benne plant. Tila seeds as met with are black, white and red. The red seeds are minute and flat; taste oily and sweet. The black and white only are used in medicine. They yield the largest quantity of the oil. The black seed or kala tila must not be confounded with "Ramtila." Dose, 30 to 90 grs.

Constituents—Fixed oil, 50 to 60 p.c.; proteid, 22 p.c., mucilage 4 p.c., and ash, 4·8 p.c.

Oleum Sesami—Obtained by expression of seeds, or extracted by carbon bisulphide. A clear bland fixed oil, similar to olive oil. It is a yellowish, non-drying oil without any odour and of a bland, nut-like taste, neutral reaction; and less liable to become rancid or thick. It contains olein 76 p.c.; myristin, palmitin, stearin, resinoid compounds, higher alcohol, sesamin, and an uncrystallizable thick oil. Dose, 2 to 6 drs.

Preparations.—Confection of seeds. Dose, ½ to 1 dr.

Actions and uses.—The seeds are used as food. A laxative they are used in removing constipation and in piles. As demulcent they are given in dysentery, and as diuretic in urinary diseases. The oil is used as hair oil in place of olive oil, for which it is a very good substitute. It is useful in preparing plasters, ointments and other medicated fragrant or scented oils.

Acanthaceæ—The Acanthus or Adusâ family.

General Characters—Herbs or shrubs; leaves opposite, simple, rarely lobed, exstipulate. Flowers irregular, bracteated, white, purple, red or yellow; calyx 4 to 5 partite; sepals 4 or 5, much imbricated; inflorescence, terminal; corolla, 2-lipped, stamens, 2 or 4, didynamous, axillary or in spikes; ovary in a disk, 2-celled; fruit capsular, and 1 or 2-celled; seed one, or more, suspended by hard, cup-shaped, or hooked projections; no albumen; cotyledons, large and fleshy, radicle, inferior.

Habitat.—Natives of tropical countries.

Properties.—Some are tonic and mucilaginous; others bitter and stomachic; the leaves of Barleria are highly astringent; those of the Rhinocanthus are used in ringworm.

Acanthus Ilicifolius, Dilivoria Ilicifolia.

Habitat.—Malabar, Ceylon (sea coasts, marsh and salt lakes).

Parts used.—The plant and root.

Vernacular.—Hind., Beng.—Hârkûch Kanta. Goa.—Moranna. Mal.—Paina Schulli. Mar.—Marandi. Sans.—Harikasa. Eng.—Holly-leaved Acanthus.

Characters.—Stems erect and numerous; bark smooth, very sharp, four-fold and covered with prickles; leaves opposite, short petioled, oblong, waved, spinous and dentate; spikes terminal, sometimes axillary. Flowers solitary, opposite and large; capsule, 2-celled; seeds 2 in each cell, obliquely cordate and compressed.

Constituents.—A bitter alkaloid, an organic acid, fatty matter, chlorophyll, and soft resins.

Preparations.—Decoction (1 in 20). Dose, $\frac{1}{2}$ to 1 fld. oz.

Actions and uses.—The tender shoots and leaves are used locally for snake bite. The root is expectorant and used in cough and asthma. As a stimulant, the decoction is given with cumin seeds in dyspepsia with acid eructations.

Acocanthera Ouabaio—Arrow poison.

Habitat.—Native of Somali coast.

Part used.—Ouabain, a glucoside; also obtained from the seeds of Strophanthus Glabrus and Carossa Schimperi.

Characters. In white and odourless crystals, of a bitter taste, slightly soluble in cold water, more so in hot water, insoluble in alcohol, chloroform and ether. Dose, $\frac{1}{1000}$ gr.

Actions and uses.—Used by the Africans as an active poison, paralyzing the heart muscle. Hypodermically injected it acts as a powerful emetic. It also acts as a local anæsthetic for the eye, and is superior to cocaine. As a stimulant to the kidneys and intestines it acts as a diuretic and promotes defœcation. It does not affect the body temperature. In small doses it stimulates the heart like Digitalis. In pertussis it may be used with benefit.

Adhatoda Vasica, Justicia Adhatoda.

Habitat.—India, Punjab, Assam, Bengal, Nepaul, Ceylon.

Parts used.—The leaves, root and flowers.

Vernacular.—Burm.—Mesan-bin. Beng.—Bâkas. Cing.—Adatoda Pâvatta. Can.—Adasôge-sappu. Bomb., Mar., Duk.—Adalsâ, Arusâ. Eng.—Malabar nut. Guz., Hind.—Arusa, Bânsa, Asganda. Malyal.—Atalôta kam. Panj.—Bhekkar. Sans.—Vasaka, Sinha mukhi, Sinha parni, Utarosha Vaidyamâtru, Vrikshaha. Tam.—Adâtodai. Tel.—Addasaram. Sinha-makki, lion mouthed. Senha-parni, lion-leaved.

Characters.—Shrub bushy; leaves opposite, short, petioled, broad, lanceolate, long, tapering or pointed, smooth on both surfaces, and of a yellowish, green or dark green colour. Flowers whitish, spotted, sulphur coloured; taste bitter and aromatic; odour strong and peculiar.

Constituents.—An odorous principle, fat, resin, a bitter alkaloid vasicine, an organic acid, adhatodic acid, sugar, gum, colouring matter, salts.

Preparations.—Infusion (1 in 10). Dose, ½ to 2 fld. ozs. Aqueous extract. Dose, 4 to 10 grs. Juice of the leaves. Dose, 2 to 4 drs. Tincture (1 in 10). Dose, ½ to 1 fld. dr.

Actions and uses.—Expectorant, antispasmodic, and alterative; the flowers and roots with ginger and sitab are given in ague, rheumatism, consumption, asthma, chronic bronchitis and other chest affections; the root is a fair substitute for senega. The leaves are often smoked in asthma.

Andrographis Paniculata, Justicia Paniculata.

Habitat.—East Indies, China, shady places throughout India.

Parts used.—The herb, dried stalks and root.

Vernacular.—Arab.—Vizra-ufar, Vasab-buvâ. Hind., Beng.—Kalo megha; Cherota, Mahatela. Can.—Nela bevinagida. Cing.—Hamba Kalpa. Duk.—Kalafnâth. Eng.—Kreat. Guz.—Kiryâta. Mar.—Olen Kirayata. Malyal.—Nila Veppa, Kiryattu. Pers.—Nain chânvandi. Sans.—Bhunimbaha. Tam.—Nella Vemboo. Tel.—Kari-vemu.

Characters.—Plant annual, stem, with the root attached, occurs in pieces of about a foot in length, quadrangular, pointed, smooth, of a light brown colour; taste persistent, and bitter; leaves opposite, smooth and on short petioles; calyx 5-cleft; corolla, bilabiate, lanceolate; upper surface dark green and shining; under surface pale; flowers, remote, alternate on long petioles, downy, panicled and rose coloured, streaked with purple; capsules, erect, cylindrical; seeds 3 to 4 in each root, fusiform, simple and woody; taste intensely bitter. It yields its properties readily to water and spirit.

Constituents.—A bitter principle, and a considerable quantity of sodium chloride.

Preparations.—Succus—concentrated expressed juice of fresh leaves and stalks (1 part represents 4 of the drug). Dose, 10 to 60 ms. Compound infusion (1 in 20). Contains olen kariat, 4 drs. ; orange peel, 1 dr. ; coriander, 1 dr. ; boiling water, 10 fld. ozs. Dose, 1 to 2 fld. ozs. Compound Tincture (3 in 20), contains olen kariyat, 6 ozs. ; myrrh and aloes, each 1 oz. ; brandy 40 fld. ozs. Dose, 1 to 4 fld. drs. Pilulæ Alui compositus known as Halviva (Beng.). It contains cumin, aniseed, cloves and greater cardamoms equal parts ; mix in the juice of kalmeg. Dose, 2 to 5 grs. in milk.

Actions and uses.—Bitter tonic and stomachic, like quassia and chiretta. The expressed juice of the fresh leaves or the compound infusion is given with cardamom, cloves and cinnamon to infants, in general debility, in convalescence after fever, and for the relief of griping pain with irregularity of the bowels and loss of appetite, and in advanced stage of dysentery. It is used as a substitute for quinine.

Asteracantha Longifolia, Barleria Longifolia, Ruelia Longifolia, Hygrophila Spinosa.

Habitat.—Throughout India, Ceylon, Western coast, watery places and ditches, paddy fields of Bombay.

Parts used.—The plant, root and seeds.

Vernacular.—Beng.—Kuliakhara. Burm.—Supadân. Can.—Bahel shulli. Cing.—Katu-Ikkiri. Guz.—Ekharo (seeds), Talamkhânâ. Hind.—Goksura, Phulmakhânâ, Ik-chura. Duk., Bomb., Mar.—Talimkhana, Kolista, Kolsunda. Malyal.—Vayal schulli. Sans.—Koklilâksha, Ikashugandha, Ikshura-Gokantaka. Tam.—Nir muli. Tel.—Vayroo Gobbi.

Characters.—Plant annual, erect, 3 to 4 feet high ; roots biennial. tapering, with numerous rootlets ; stem erect, bluntly quadrangular, branches opposite, jointed, flattened, hairy and often coloured ; leaves sessile, opposite, long, rather wavy and inserted in pairs at the joints of the stems ; flowers awl-shaped and spreading, calyx 4-cleft, corolla, funnel-shaped, 5-cleft, flowers on whorls, axillary, numerous, sessile, and of a bright, blue or rose colour ; seeds small and compressed, pointed at the apex and broad at the base where they are oblique; colour, brownish red. When placed in the mouth they immediately become coated with a large quantity of extremely tenacious mucilage which adheres to the tongue and palate. Dose of the seeds, 10 to 20 grs.

Constituents.—The seeds contain mucilage, albuminoids, traces of an alkaloid and a yellow fixed oil. The root and stem exhausted with alcohol deposit red shaped crystals.

Preparations.—Decoction of the root (1 in 20). Dose, ½ to 1 oz. Infusion (1 in 10). Dose, ½ to 1 fld. oz. ; acetum of the leaves (1 in 8) of vinegar. Dose, 1 to 4 fld. drs. The natives use ashes of the burnt dried plant. Dose, ½ to 1 dr.

Actions and uses.—The root is demulcent and diuretic, and given in dropsy, gonorrhœa, hepatic obstruction, rheumatism, and in urinary affections. The seeds are used as aphrodisiac ; a paste of the seeds is applied to rheumatic joints.

Barleria Prionitis.

Habitat.—Tropical India.

Parts used.—The plant.

Vernacular—Hind., Beng.—Kanta-Jâti, Jhinte. Can.—Goratige. Malyal.—Kaletta vitla. Guz., Mar.—Kanta-shelio, karántá, pivala-karânta, vajradanti, kulsunda. Sans.—Kurantaka, Mahasaha, Pitaj linta; Awlana. Tam.—Vara mulli. Tel.—Pachcha.

Characters.—Root brownish, smooth and rather knotty ; stem short and erect with numerous, opposite, round and smooth branches ; leaves of a yellowish green or dark green colour, decussate, opposite, short petioled, oblong, rather waved, glabrous, and smooth. From the axils of the leaves spring up 2 or 3 sharp spines ; flowers axillary, generally solitary, sessile, large and yellow.

Constituents.—Neutral and acid resins, soluble in petroleum and ether.

Preparations.—Juice of leaves. Dose, 2 to 4 fld. drs. Decoction of the root (1 in 10). Dose, ½ to 1 fld. oz. Medicated oil.

Actions and uses.—The plant is slightly bitter and astringent. and given in catarrhal affections of children accompanied with fever ; also in anasarca. Locally the juice of the leaves is applied to the feet to prevent the cracking of the soles and with common salt to strengthen the gums when spongy. The paste of the root is applied to boils and glandular swellings to cause their dispersion. The medicated oil is used as an application to unhealthy wounds.

Blepharis Edulis—Acanthodium Hirtum.

Habitat.—Egypt, Persia, Sind and Punjab.

Parts used.—The seeds.

Vernacular.—Arab.—Kariza. Hind., Bomb.—Utingana. Pers.—Anjurah.

Characters.—Capsules hard, glabrous, shining, and in colour mahogany-like ; in broken pieces, mixed with few entire fruits and seeds ; compressed, smooth, shining, longer than those of sesamum, obtusely pointed at the apex and broad at the base, where they are oblique. The surface is covered with bristles or long coarse hairs ; colour pale brown ; cotyledons black and homogeneous ; seeds mucilaginous. This is due to the desintegration of the bristles, when soaked in water.

Constituents.—A bitter crystalline principle, soluble in water, amylic and ethylic alcohol, but insoluble in ether ; mucilage, albumen and ash.

Preparations.—Decoction (1 in 10). Dose, ½ to 1 fld. oz.

Actions and uses.—Demulcent, diuretic, nervine tonic and expectorant ; given in seminal debility, coughs, gonorrhœa, high coloured urine, &c. The seeds are an ingredient in numerous aphrodisiac confections.

Acanthus Roseus.

Habitat.—W. India.

Parts used.—The root.

Characters.—Root tuberous, spindle shaped, thick as a quill, bark dark brown. Dose, 20 to 60 grs.

Preparations.—Decoction (1 in 20), 1 to 2 fld. ozs.

Actions and uses.—Astringent and nervine tonic ; the root boiled in milk is largely used in leucorrhœa and general debility.

Justicia Procumbens, Rostellularia Procumbens.

Habitat.—S. India, Deccan, Ceylon.

Parts used.—The herb.

Vernacular.—Mar.—Ghati pitpapra. Tam.—Nerei poottie.

Characters.—A small plant of a bitter, disagreeable taste ; stem procumbent, diffuse ; leaves rounded, glabrous and somewhat hairy ; spikes compressed, slender ; flowers small, pale, purple ; root slender, woody ; taste bitter.

Constituents.—A bitter alkaloid.

Preparations.—Infusion (1 in 20). Dose, 4 to 6 drs.

Actions and uses.—Alterative and expectorant ; given in asthma, cough, rheumatism, &c. The herb is used as substitute for fumaria.

Rhinacanthus Communis, Justicia Nasuta.

Habitat.—Deccan, Ceylon, cultivated throughout Western India.

Parts used.—The leaves, root and seeds.

Vernacular.—Can.—Nâga-mallige. Chin.—Tong-pong-chong. Cing.—Anitta. Duk.—Kabûtar. Hind.—Pâlak-jôhi. Guz., Mar.—Gajakarni. Malyal.—Pushpa-kedol. Sans.—Uthika-parni. Tam., Tel.—Nâga mulli.

Nâga-mulli.—Naga, a snake, and mulli, a root ; the root is used by the natives against the bites of poisonous snakes.

Characters.—Shrub thin ; stem erect, green and shrubby ; bark smooth and ash coloured ; young shoots jointed ; leaves opposite, short petioled, broad, lanceolate, obtusely pointed, smooth above and a little downy below ; panicles corymbose, axillary and terminal ; pedicels short and downy ; flowers white ; leaves when chewed having a pungent taste, somewhat resembling that of cinnamon ; odour disagreeable.

Constituents.—Rhinacanthin, apparently related to crysophanic acid. It is a dull cherry red resinous substance obtained by exhausting powdered root fibres with dilute alcohol.

Preparations.—Expressed juice.

Actions and uses.—Parasiticide and stimulant; a paste of the leaves, seeds and fresh root is applied with pepper and lime juice or sulphur for several successive days in parasitic diseases, as ring-worm, dhobie's itch, Malabar itch, eczema and other skin diseases. Leaves and roots are regarded as antidotes to snake poisons.

Verbenaceæ—The Vervain, or Niragundi family.

Trees, shrubs or herbs; leaves generally opposite, rarely alternate, exstipulate; calyx persistent, tubular ; ovary, 2 or 4-celled ; flowers, red white or blue, generally irregular ; fruits dry or drupaceous ; carpels 2 to 4 when ripe, separating into as many one-seeded achænia ; seed erect, with little or no albumen, radicle inferior.

Habitat.—Native of temperate and trop ical regions,

Properties.—The plants are slightly bitter, aromatic, febrifuge and alterative ; some have edible fleshy fruits ; some are fragrant and have beautiful flowers ; the leaves of a few are used as substitutes for China tea.

Callicarpa lanata, C. Cana, C. Tomentosa, C. Americana.

Habitat.—Deccan, Ceylon.

Parts used.—The root, bark and leaves.

Vernacular.—Beng.—Masandari, Muttura. Hind.—Bastra. Malyal. —Tondi, Teregam. Mar.—Pondi Karavati, Iswar. Tam.—Kat komul.

Characters.—Young branches, cinnamon like, shaggy and woolly ; leaves ovate, lanceolate and tomentose beneath ; on the removal of tomentum, numerous oil glands are visible ; taste bitterish, odour faintly aromatic. It affords considerable mucilage when boiled.

Preparation.—Decoction of the root and bark (1 in 20). Dose, 1 to 2 fld. oz.

Actions and uses.—Refrigerant, hepatic stimulant, demulcent and emollient. The decoction of the root is used to lessen fever and high temperature, and to remove hepatic obstruction ; also given in skin diseases. It is also used as a wash for aphthæ in the mouth.

Clerodendron Inerme, Valkameria Inermis.

Habitat.—Ceylon, India, near the sea-coast.

Parts used.—The leaves and juice.

Vernacular.—Eng.—Garden Quinine. Ceylon—Wolbu-ronda. Beng.—Banjuen. Bomb.—Dariai jai, vanjai. Can.—Naituk-kille. Hind., Duk.—Sangan-kuppi, chhoti-arni, Isamdhari. Mar.—Vanajai, khari narvel. Java.—Gamber laut. Malyal.—Nirnotajil. Sans.—Kundali. Tam.—Pina Shengam kooppi. Tel.—Tak-kalapu, Eru-Pichha.

It is called garden quinine, on account of its intense bitter taste.

Characters.—Shrub slender, zig-zag, with white fragrant irregular flowers, bearing beautiful long purple stamens, growing near the sea-shore and common in large gardens; leaves opposite, rarely ternate, small, one or two inches long, smooth, shining, oval, and often fleshy; margins reflex, with numerous dark green dots studding both the surfaces; odour agreeable and apple-like, taste intensely bitter.

Constituents.—A bitter principle similar to that found in Chiretta, a fragrant stearopten to which its apple-like odour is due, resin, gum and a brown colouring matter and ash containing a large amount of sodium chloride.

Preparations.—Infusion and decoction (1 in 10). Dose, ½ to 1 fld. oz. Tincture (1 in 8). Dose, ½ to 1 fld. dr.

Actions and uses.—Tonic, febrifuge and alterative; given in intermittent and remittent fevers; also as an alterative in scrofulous and venereal diseases. A poultice of the leaves is used to resolve buboes; a bath of the leaves is recommended in itch.

Clerodendron Phlomoides, Valkameria Multiflora.

Habitat.—Tropical countries.

Parts used.—The root.

Vernacular.—Bomb., Guz., Hind.—Arani. Mar.—Tâkali. Sans. —Aguimantha, Gani kârikâ. Tam.—Telutala. Tel.—Tekkar, Tilaka.

Characters.—The root is thick and of a lightish brown colour. It is slightly aromatic. The taste is astringent and somewhat bitter.

Preparations.—Decoction (1 in 10.) Dose, 4 to 12 fld. drs.

Actions and uses.—Alterative, bitter tonic and demulcent; given to children during convalescence; as a demulcent it is useful in gonorrhœa.

Remarks.—It is one of the five roots, Vrihata Panchmuli of Dasa mula dikvath.

Clerodendron Serratum, C. Macrophyllum, Valkameria Serrata, C. Siphonanthus.

Habitat.—Salsette, Nepaul.

Parts used.—The root.

Vernacular.—Duk., Mar., Hind.—Gant Baharangi. Malyal.—Jarutika. Sans.—Bhargi. Tam.—Chirudekku. Tel.—Brah-mari.

Characters.—Root light colored, often contorted about an inch in thickness; bark thin, of a brown colour, within which the wood is tough and marked with medullary rays and concentric rings. Taste faintly bitter, no peculiar odour. Dose of the powdered root, 10 to 20 grs.

Constituents.—Starch, a peculiar bitter principle, acrid resin and fatty matter.

Preparations.—Decoction (1 in 20). Dose, 1 to 2 fld. ozs.

Actions and uses.—Stimulant, tonic, and alterative; given in dyspepsia, catarrhal affection of the lungs, scrofula and rheumatism. It is often confounded with Premna Herbacia—Knotted Bharangi.

Clerodendron Infortunatum, C. Viscosum, Valkameria Infortunata.

Habitat.—Throughout India, Belgaum, Bengal.

Parts used.—The leaves.

Vernacular.—Hind., Beng.—Bhant, Ghantu. Burm.—Bughyee. Can.—Kare. Malyal.—Peragu. Bomb., Mar.—Bhandira, Kari. Nepaul. —Chitu. Sans.—Bhandira. Tel.—Manduka bramhi. Bokada, Sorasvati aku, gurrapu.

Characters.—Shrub 3 to 4 feet high, dark green and spreading by underground suckers; leaves 8 to 10 inches long, and 6 to 8 inches broad at their base, round or ovate, and with long petioles, edges dentate, covered on both surfaces with white and jointed hairs; branches quadrangular, panicle large, terminal and naked; odour very disagreeable, taste bitter; flowers white, tinged with pink. It is a cheap substitute for chiretta.

Constituents.—Resinous matter, bitter principle, and tannin.

Preparations.—Infusion (1 in 10.) Dose, 1 to 2 ozs.

Actions and uses.—Bitter, tonic, antiperiodic and vermifuge; also a good laxative; a decoction is sometimes given as a rectal enema for worms; also given as a bitter tonic during convalescence from acute diseases. As an antiperiodic it is given in malarial fever.

Gmelina Arborea.

Habitat.—N. W. Himalaya, Deccan Peninsula, Coromandel, Neilgherries, Ceylon.

Parts used.—The root, bark and fruit.

Vernacular.—Burm.—Yemaneh. Can.—Shivan. Cing.—Atdemmata. Beng., Guz., Mar., Hind.—Shevana, Kambhari, Gumhar, Joogani, Chookur. Malyal.—Cumbulu. Sans.—Shriparani, Kasa mari, Gamabhari. Tam.—Tagvomooda. Tel.—Pedda Gumudu.

Characters.—Bark, covered with powdery tomentum, thick, rather brittle and mucilaginous, colour lightish brown, taste astringent; fruit a drupe, ovoid, 2-seeded, sweetish bitter, cooling and mucilaginous.

Constituents.—The root contains a yellow viscid oil, resin, an alkaloid, a trace of benzoic acid, and ash free from manganese; the fruit contains butyric and tartaric acids, an alkaloid, saccharine matter, resin, and a trace of tannin.

Preparations.—Decoction of the bark (1 in 20). Dose, 1 to 2 fld. ozs. A compound decoction of the fruit contains shivan, parûshaka, liquorice root, red sandal wood and ushera, equal parts and water 16 parts, the whole quantity reduced to one half. Dose, 1 to 2 fld. ozs.

Actions and uses.—Demulcent, stomachic, tonic, refrigerant, and laxative. The root bark is given in fevers, indigestion and anasarca. With liquorice, it is given to increase the secretion of milk in women. The juice of the leaves is demulcent and given in gonorrhœa; other properties are similar to those of arani. The fruits are bitter and cooling, and given in fever and burning heat of the body. The bark is used to regulate fermentation of toddy. The wood is used for making artificial limbs, stethoscopes, etc. The root is also one of the ingredients of the Vrahata pancha mula of Dasa mula di kvatha.

Gmelina Asiatica, G. Parviflora.

Habitat.—Travancore, Coromandel.

Parts used.—The root, leaves and young shoots.

Vernacular.—Can.—Kumatha. Cing.—Gatta-demata. Hind.—Shiri-gumudu. Malyal.—Nilak-kumagh. Sans.—Biddarie. Tam.—Nilak-kimnizh. Tel.—Challa-gumudu.

Characters.—Leaves opposite, petioled, ovate and tomentous; underneath a sharp short lobe on each side; spines horizontal, opposite, axillary; flowers large, on peduncles from the end of tender twigs; fruit a berry or drupe.

Preparations.—Infusion (1 in 10). Dose, 1 to 2 fld. ozs.

Actions and uses.—The root is demulcent and mucilaginous, and given in dysuria and gonorrhœa.

Lippia Nodiflora.

Habitat.—Throughout India, Ceylon.

Parts used.—The herb.

Vernacular.—Guz., Bomb.—Ratalyo, Ratavalio. Beng., Hind.—Bukkan, Bhui-okra. Mar.—Vakkan, Ratolia. Sans.—Vâshira, Yasuka. Tam.—Podutalai. Tel.—Boke-naku.

Characters.—Small herb; stem creeping and somewhat coloured; leaves opposite, small, cuneate at the base, and dentate towards the apex, somewhat hairy; flowers axillary, very small, whitish or rose coloured, and arranged on cylindrical spikes, from 1 or 2 inches long. When the flowers have withered away the spikes with fruits look like long *Pipali*. The plant is slightly bitter.

Preparations.—Decoction and infusion (1 in 10). Dose, $\frac{1}{2}$ to 1 fld. ozs.

Actions and uses.—Demulcent and antiperiodic; given to children in indigestion, dysuria and malarial fevers. It is commonly given in combination with *Jirun* or *Suvá* in gonorrhœa with scalding in the urine; also used in intermittent fevers. A poultice of it is used in swollen cervical glands. Chronic indolent ulcers heal readily under its use. A paste of it is applied to promote suppuration in boils.

Premna Herbacea.

Habitat.—Himalayas, Deccan.

Parts used.—The root and leaves.

Vernacular.—Beng.—Bhooi-jam. Can.—Nayit-yaga. Cing.—Siribekku. Mar., Hind., Guz.—Bharangi. Malyal.—Tajeru-teka. Noar. Circars.—Gunta Bharinjie. Sans.—Bhoomi Jambuka, Bhooi-jam, Hangika, Bririgaja, Nardhaka. Tam.—Shiru-tek. Tel.—Gunta Baringa, Gunta Bharingi.

Characters.—Root in pieces, from ½ to 1 inch in thickness, with numerous woody knots of a whitish brown colour; root bark scabrous and brittle; taste peculiarly bitter and pungent; wood hard, tough, arranged in concentric rings, and of a whitish colour, leaves cuneate, ovate and dentate at their margins; when fresh of a darkish colour.

Constituents.—The root contains an orange brown, acid resin, soluble in ether, alcohol, and alkaline solutions, traces of an alkaloid, also a quantity of starch, but no tannin.

Preparations.—Decoction (1 in 20). Dose, 1 to 2 fld. ozs.

Actions and uses.—The root is stimulant, alterative, and bitter tonic, and used in catarrhal affections of the lungs, asthma, cough, fever and scrofulous diseases. The leaves are alterative and used in fever, cough, rheumatism, &c. As a poultice, the leaves are used in promoting the suppuration of boils.

Premna Integrifolia.

Habitat.—Coast of India, Ceylon.

Parts used.—The root and leaves.

Vernacular.—Beng.—Bhut-bhiravi. Guz., Bomb.—Airana-mula, Arani. Can.—Takkile. Hind.—Ganiari, Agetha, Arani. Malyal.—Appel. Mar.—Takali, Chamaree. Sans.—Arani, Agani, Mantha, Hari-mantha, Vahni-mantha, Gani-karika. Tam.—Munnay. Tel.—Ghebu-nelli.

Characters.—Root thick, of a lightish brown colour; bark smooth, and light brown; leaves opposite, petioled, serrated at the margins and smooth.

Constituents.—A resin, a bitter alkaloid, and tannin.

Preparations.—Infusion of leaves, and decoction of the root (1 in 10). Dose, 1 to 2 fld. ozs.

Actions and uses.—Stomachic, alterative and tonic. The infusion of the leaves is used in eruptive fevers, colic and flatulence; the decoction of the root is given in gonorrhœa during convalescence from fevers; also in rheumatism and neuralgia.

Premna Taitensis.

Habitat.—Fiji Islands.

Parts used.—The root bark and leaves.

Constituents.—The leaves contain starch, potassium chloride and a volatile alkaloid—tongine. The bark contains sugar, pectin, volatile oil, &c.

Preparations.—A compound fluid extract known as Tonga—a proprietary nostrum—prepared from this root as well as from the roots of Raphidaphhora vitensis and Epipremium mirabile. Dose, ½ to 2 fld. drs.

Actions and uses.—Antineuralgic and analgesic; given in hemicrania, tic-douloureux, occipital and trifacial neuralgias, painful affections of the eyes, &c It is superior to quinine, gelsemium and croton chloral. But recently it has been superseded by the new analgesic remedies, such as antipyrine, phenacetin, exalgene &c.

Tectona Grandis.

Habitat.—Concans, W. Deccan Peninsula, Central India, Burmah, banks of Taptee and Godavery.

Parts used.—The fruit, wood and tar.

Vernacular.—Arab.—Sâj. Beng.—Segun. Burm.—Ky-won. Can.—Jaddi, Tegu. Cing.—Tekka. Eng.—Teak tree, Indian oak. Guz., Mar., Duk., Hind.—Sâgûn, Sagwan, Sàkhû. Malyal.—Têkka-maram, Jati. Pers.—Sâl. Sans.—Saka. Tam.—Teku-manna. Tel.—Tekkoo chetu.

Characters.—Wood hard; colour light, or yellowish; odour somewhat aromatic; wood tar, black and opaque; bark scaly, scabrous, of an ash or light brown colour; flowers small and white, panicles large and terminate; fruits drupaceous and covered with enlarged membranous calices; seeds very oily, of the size and shape of sesamum seeds.

Constituents.—The wood contains in its cavities, white crystalline deposits of calcium phosphate, silica and ammonium and magnesium phosphate. It also contain a resin; the seed contains a bland fatty oil.

Preparations.—Paste of wood.

Actions and uses.—Local refrigerant and sedative. The wood brayed in water is used as a local application for the relief of headache, toothache, and to subdue the inflammation and irritation of the skin set up by the use of marking nuts and cashewnuts; it is also used for dispersing inflammatory swellings. The oil of the nuts is used to promote the growth of hair and also to cure itchiness of the skin. The bruised seeds with palasa papada are used as varaliâns over the pubes, in partial suppression or retention of urine.

Vitex Agnus Castus.

Habitat.—India, Syria and Persia.

Parts used.—The berries.

Vernacular.—Pers.—Panjangusht. Arab.—Athlak. Mar.—Ranuka bija, Sambhalu, Ka-lija.

Characters.—The drug consists of very grey small and extremely hard fruits, resembling fresh figs, obovate or globular, lower half covered with a tomentose calyx; apex of the calyx dentate, base presenting a small stalk; berry wrinkled, smooth, of a brownish colour, consisting of small 4-celled cavities, each containing one yellowish brown small seed; taste of the seed oily and pungent.

Constituents.—Bitter principle, called castine, a volatile acrid substance, a free acid and fat oil.

Preparations.—Decoction (1 in 10). Dose, ½ to 1 fld. oz.

Actions and uses.—Stimulant, diuretic and alterative; given in enlargement of the liver and spleen and in dropsy. They are given with pipali in hiccough.

Vitex Negundo, V. Paniculata.

Habitat.—Ceylon, throughout India.

Parts used.—The root, fruit and leaves.

Vernacular.—Arab.—Athalaka, Fanjangasht, Zûkham-satil. Bomb.—Katari. Burm.—Kiyou-bhân-bin. Can.—Lakki-gidâ. Cing.—Sudu-nikka. Duk—Shumbâli. Eng.—Fine-leaved chaste tree. Guz.—Nagoda, Shamalu. Beng., Hind.—Sanbhâlu, Nishinda, Nirgundi. Malyal—Ban-nuichi. Mar.—Nigudi Lingura. Panj.—Banna. Pers.—Panjangusht, Sishân. Sans.—Niragûndi shveta-surasa-vrikshaha Sindhuvâra, Sendhuka-Sephalika-Sveta pushpi Pushpanilika. Tam.—Vellai-Noch-chi. Tel.—Tella-vôvili.

Characters.—Shrub generally of an ash colour; leaves digitate, opposite, from 3 to 5 foliolate, on longish slender petioles; leaflets, lanceolate, entire, 3 larger, petioled, 2 smaller, sessile; under surface white and tomentose, upper surface greenish, smooth and shining; flowers minute, and of a light blue colour; taste bitter and nauseous, odour feebly nauseous.

Constituents.—The leaves contain an essential oil and resin; the fruits contain an acid resin, an astringent organic acid, malic acid, an alkaloid and a colouring matter.

Preparations.—Medicated baths, decoction of the leaves (1 in 10). Dose, ½ to 1 fld. oz.

Actions and uses.—Alterative, aromatic bitter and anodyne. The decoction is used in colic, dyspepsia, rheumatism and worms; locally the leaves, bruised, are applied to the temples in headache, and as varalians, over contusions, sprained limbs, rheumatic painful joints, leech bites, and also over the swollen testicles due to suppressed gonorrhœa. It is largely used as a vapour bath in febrile conditions. The fruit is resolvent and emmenagogue, and used in enlargement of spleen and in dropsy. The leaves are used to preserve rice and clothes from the ravages of insects. It is placed between the leaves of books to preserve them from insects.

Vitex Trifolia.

Habitat.—Coromandel, Concan, Deccan.

Parts used.—The leaves.

Vernacular.—Arab.—Aslage-âbi. Burm.—Kiyubhan-bin. Can.—Nira-lakki-gidda. Cing.—Valuru. Beng., Duk.—Pani-ki. Shumbala. Eng.—Indian wild pepper. Hind.—Nichînda Siduari, Sambhâlu. Malyal.—Nir-noschi, Lagondi. Pers.—Panj-angushte-âbi. Sans.—Jela-nirgundi, Sindhuka, Surasa, Vrikshaha, Jalnirgundi. Tam.—Shirunoch-chi. Tel.—Niru-vâvilli.

Characters.—Leaves ternate, leaflets ovate, acute, entire, hoary beneath ; flowers terminal, violet, and racemose.

Preparations.—Infusion of leaves. Dose, ½ to 1 fld. oz.

Actions and uses.—Alterative, diuretic, anodyne and demulcent ; used as dry hot fomentation in sprains, contusions and rheumatism. The infusion is given in intermittent fevers with scanty urine, rheumatism, enlargement of the spleen, &c.

Atropaceæ or the Deadly Night-shade family.

Characters.—This order agrees with solanaceæ in most respects, but differs from it in the æstivation of their corolla, being imbricated instead of valvate. In one or more of the stamens being sterile, anthers being dehiscent longitudinally.

Habitat.—Native of tropical regions.

Properties.—Many species are powerful narcotics. Some produce dilatation of the pupil.

Atropa Belladonna, B. P.

Atropa from Atropos, one of the three Fates which cuts the thread of life, in allusion to its poisonous property. Belladonna from bella, beautiful, donna, a lady. The berries were used by Italian ladies as a cosmetic and to dilate their pupils to give a handsome appearance.

Habitat.—W. Himalaya, Persia, hedges in mountainous districts of Central and S. Europe, United States.

Parts used.—The root.—Belladonna radix, B. P., and the fresh leaves and branches. Belladonnæ Folia, B. P., fresh juice of the leaves and young branches.

Vernacular.—Beng.—Belladonna. Eng.—Deadly nightshade, black cherry. Hind.—Suchi. Pers.—Inab-eth-thalib.

Characters.—A perennial herb, stems thick and smooth ; leaves smooth, alternate, 3 to 6 inches in length, stalked, ovate, tapering or acuminate, entire and unequal ; pubescent when young, of a greyish green colour, of a feebly bitterish and subacid taste and disagreeable odour. Flowers solitary, pendulous, dark purple, bell-shaped and glossy ; berries black, large and shining, of the size of cherries, of a fœtid odour and nauseous, bitter taste. The root is large, fleshy, cylindrical and tapering; about an inch thick, covered over with a thick light brown bark which is wrinkled longitudinally. Fracture transverse and short; internally whitish and starchy; taste bitter and acrid, without any odour. Dose, powdered leaves 1 gr., powdered root 1 gr.

Constituents.—The root contains hyoscyamine, atropine, belladonine, atropamine, atrosin, a colouring principle, malic acid and starch. The leaves contain, in addition, choline, albumen, gum, asparagin or althein, crysatropic and succinic acids, nitrates and ash, 14 p. c.

Atropina, Atropine, B. P., an alkaloid obtained from leaves or root of Atropa Belladonna. To obtain it, agitate the alcoholic tincture of the root with slaked lime, remove resin and fat, add sulphuric acid to precipitate the dissolved lime and filter. The filtrate contains atropine sulphate. To this add potassium carbonate in excess to precipate atropine. It occurs as colourless acicular crystals or powder without any odour and bitter acrid taste. It has an alkaline reaction, becoming yellow on exposure to air; soluble in water (1 in 300), in alcohol (1 in 3), chloroform (1 in 1), oleic acid and ether (1 in 36), and olive oil (1 in 40); very soluble in glycerin. It decomposes with caustic alkalies into tropin and tropic acid. Dose, $\frac{1}{200}$ to $\frac{1}{100}$ gr.

Atropinæ sulphas, B. P.—atropine sulphate—occurs as colourless, or white crystals without any odour, and of bitter nauseous taste, and of a neutral reaction; soluble in water (1 in 1), alcohol (1 in 10), insoluble in ether and chloroform. Dose $\frac{1}{200}$ to $\frac{1}{100}$ gr. Oleatum Atropinæ (1 in 40) used as local anodyne. Linimentum Atropinæ (1 in 100) also used as local anodyne. Unguentum atropinæ, B. P. (1 in 50). Injectio atropinæ Hypodermica, 4 grains of sulphate to 1 ounce. Dose, 1 to 2 ms.; for morphine poisoning and to check hæmoptysis. Injectio Morphinæ et atropinæ Hypodermica. 3 minims contains $\frac{1}{2}$ grain of acetate of morphia and $\frac{1}{80}$ grain of sulphates of atropine. Lamellæ Atropinæ, B.P., containing $\frac{1}{5000}$ gr. of atropine sulphate. Hypodermic tablets containing $\frac{1}{100}$ grain alone, or with morphine sulphate. Liquor Atropinæ Sulphatis, B. P.; gr. 1 in 110 ms. Dose, $\frac{1}{2}$ to 1 ms. Pilulæ Atropinæ $\frac{1}{80}$ gr. of atropine given to check night sweats. Pilulæ Atropinæ Arsenici et Quininæ—contains quinine sulphate 18 grs., solution of arsenic 12 ms., solution of Atropine sulphate 1 m, Extract Gentian 20 grs. made into 12 pills, used for catarrh. Vaselinum Atropinæ (1 in 120 of vaseline); Atropinæ salicylas, soluble in water (1 in 20); Liquor atropinæ salicylas, Atropine $\frac{1}{2}$ gr.; Salicylic acid $\frac{3}{4}$ gr.; water 1 oz.

Homatropine—a derivative alkaloid obtained by the action of baryta water, or dilute hydrochloric acid upon amygdalate of tropin. It occurs as white crystals or powder, soluble in oils, sparingly soluble in water. Dose $\frac{1}{180}$ to $\frac{1}{20}$ gr. Oleum Homatropinæ 2 p.c. in castor oil, and with 2 p. c. cocaine for the eyes. Homatropinæ Hydrobromidum B.P.—Colourless crystals, freely soluble in water (1 in 6), and absolute alcohol (1 in 133). Dose $\frac{1}{80}$ to $\frac{1}{20}$ gr. Lamellæ Homatropinæ, B.P.—contain $\frac{1}{100}$ gr. in each. Homatropinæ Hydrochloridum, similar to above. Homatropinæ Salicylas, similar to Hydrobromide. Guttæ Homatropinæ 4 grs. of the Hydrobromide to

1 oz. Injectio Homatropinæ Hypodermica (1 in 120.) Dose, 1 to 6 ms. Mydrine—a mixture of Ephedrine (an active principle of a Japanese Gentian) and Homatropine (1 in 100).

Preparations.—Of the fresh leaves and young branches. Extractum Belladonnæ Viride, B.P., green extract of Belladonna. Dose, $\frac{1}{4}$ to 1 gr. Chloroform Belladonnæ, 1 of root in $1\frac{1}{2}$ of chloroform; mixed with olive oil (1 to 3) used as an application to painful rheumatic affections. Collodium Belladonnæ or Emplastrum Belladonnæ Fluidum,—contains collodion, belladonna and camphor, used as application to painful affections of the breast. Emplastrum Belladonnæ, B.P.—contains 4 oz. of the liquid extract with resin plaster 5 ozs. Porous plaster and Plaster Mulls—contain 30 p.c. of Belladonna. Extractum Belladonnæ Alcoholicum B.P.—Prepared from the liquid extract, containing 1 p.c. of the alkaloids of the root. Dose, $\frac{1}{4}$ to 1 gr. Extractum Belladonnæ Liquidum, B.P.—liquid extract of Belladonna root, standardized to contain $\frac{3}{4}$ of a grain of the alkaloids in 110 ms. Glycerinum Belladonnæ (1 in 2), applied to boils to reduce pain and inflammation, and to the breasts to suppress milk. Linimentum Belladonnæ B. P. 1 of liquid extract of the root in 2. Linimentum Belladonnæ Compositum—1 Chloroform Belladonnæ to 7 Linimentum Belladonnæ. Linimentum Belladonnæ Æthereum—erthereal tincture of belladonna 1, of the root in $1\frac{1}{2}$, more readily absorbed than the emplastrum.

Pilulæ Aloin Belladonnæ et Strychiniæ, Tonic Laxative granules, containing aloin, $\frac{1}{5}$ gr.; extract of Belladonna, $\frac{1}{2}$ gr.; strychnine, $\frac{1}{16}$ gr. For habitual constipation. Pilulæ Ipecacuanhæ Belladonnæ et nucis vomici; belladonna cough granules—ipecacuanha, $\frac{1}{3}$ gr.; extract of nux vomica, $\frac{1}{3}$ gr.; extract of belladonna, $\frac{1}{12}$ gr. For cough. Pilulæ Podophylli Belladonnæ et Strychninæ "Tonic Liver granules." podophyllin, $\frac{1}{4}$ gr., extract of belladonna $\frac{1}{8}$ gr., strychnine $\frac{1}{30}$ gr.; given in hepatic disorders. Succus Belladonnæ, B. P. Dose, 5 to 15 ms. Suppositoria Belladonnæ, each containing $\frac{1}{60}$ gr. of the alkaloids. Tinctura Belladonnæ, B. P. (1 of liquid extract in 15). Dose, 5 to 15 ms. Unguentum Belladonnæ, B. P.—contains liquid extract of belladonna 2 oz. to $2\frac{1}{4}$ ozs. of benzoated lard.

Actions and uses.—Belladonna is mydriatic, antispasmodic, anodyne, diuretic and lactifuge. In small doses, it is a cardiac, respiratory and spinal stimulant. In large doses it depresses the respiratory centre in the medulla and causes contraction of the systemic arterioles through the sympathetic. The gastric and intestinal secretions are diminished at first, but are soon reproduced in larger quantities. There is disturbed vision (even by a very small dose of atropine). Dilatation of the pupils occurs if the drug is locally applied or taken internally. It paralyses motor oculi, increases the power of radiating fibres of the iris and lessens that of the circular fibre. An erythematous rash resembling the eruption of scarlatina appears on the skin and fauces, with desquamation of the epidermis and sometimes sore throat. In poisonous doses the heart becomes depressed, and the congestion of the brain leads to headache. The spinal cord being affected, there is complete motor paralysis, the sensation being unimpaired, ending in delirium, coma, convulsions and death. Internally atropine is used largely in poisoning by opium, physostigmine, hyoscyamine and in mercurial and idiopathic salivation. Belladonna is given in congestion of the brain and spinal cord, in congestion and inflammation of the lungs, bladder, kidneys, breast, pharynx and tonsils, and of the nasal and other respiratory passages. It is a good remedy in superficial erysipelas. It is given in excessive expectoration, profuse sweating of phthisis or that due to other causes and in spermatorrhœa and seminal weakness ; also to check incontinence of urine in children and in constipation due to atony of the bowels and in paralytic affections. It is also used as an adjunct to other purgatives. It is used as an antispasmodic in epilepsy, chorea, spasmodic asthma, whooping cough, puerperal convulsions, colic, spasms of the sphincter ani and urethra and bladder. As a sedative and anodyne it is given to relieve pain of rheumatism, gout, neuralgia, sciatica, tetanus, hydrophobia, dysmenorrhœa, cancerous and pelvic affections, &c. Locally it is applied to deaden pain in neuralgia, inflammatory condition of the tissues beneath the skin and of palpitation of the heart. It is applied over the breasts in women to dry up milk, and on boils and carbuncles to prevent suppuration. Atropine is hypodermically used in sweats of phthisis and in sudden failure of the heart from ether or chloroform inhalation. In lead poisoning, it is given in combination with potassium iodide with great success. Its chief use is, however, in ophthalmic practice, where atropine or homatropine, and its salts are largely used to produce mydriasis for ophthalmoscopic examination. It is used to lessen pain, to paralyze accommodation, and to diminish intra-ocular tension and in iritis, ulcers of the cornea and glaucoma, it is also used with success as an antidote to pilocarpine. It is given as an hæmostatic in profuse uterine hæmorrhage, and in hæmoptysis with marked relief. There is perfect physiological antagonism within certain limits between atropine on the one hand and opium, physostimine, ergotine, muscarine, aconite, bromal and prussic acid on the other. Atropine and its salts have the property of checking night sweats, uterine discharges, milk, saliva &c.

Atropa Mandragora, A. Acuminata, Mandragora Officinalis, M. Autumnalis, M. Vernalis.

Habitat.—Levant, South of Europe, Central Asia, North of India.

Parts used.—The root.

Vernacular.—Arab.—Astrang-Dastam harysh. Eng.—Mandrake. Hind.—Lakmuni, Lakhshmana, Putrada, Rakta Vindu, Bhagner, Luffat. Indian Bazaar.—Lebruj, Malay.—Lufahat. Pers.—Mardami, Giatya bruz. Tam.—Katav jati.

Dastam Harysh, perfuming the hand ; Lukshamana, possessed of lucky signs or marks ; Putrada, child-giver ; Raktavinda, a drop of blood ; Bhagner, co-heiress.

Characters.—Perennial plant ; root thick, fusiform, of a light brown colour, often bifurcating ; leaves radical, petioled, broad, acute, with undulating edges ; flowers numerous, on pedicles, shorter than the leaves. Fruit, a berry, yellow, round, of the size of a crabapple. Taste nauseous, odour acrid.

Constituents.—A basic substance, isomeric with hyoscyamine, known as mandragorine.

Actions and uses.—Sedative, narcotic and cholagogue. The root bark and leaves are local anæsthetic and applied to painful swellings. In actions it resembles belladonna, but weaker. Like datura, it is said to increase the sexual excitement in both sexes. Mandragorin is very drastic. The chief interest lies in the various myths connected with the fancied resemblance of the root to the human form.

Labiatæ—The Labiate or Tulasi family.

General Characters.—Herbs or shrubs, usually with square stems ; leaves strong, scented, opposite, exstipulate and generally serrated; odour strong and aromatic ; taste bitter and pungent ; flowers, axillary cymes in vertical clusters, generally irregular ; fruits contain from 1 to 4 achenes ; seeds erect, oblong and generally angular, with little or no albumen, each seed has a small scar at its attachment.

Habitat.—Natives of temperate climates.

Properties.—They are free from any deleterious properties. They abound in aromatic volatile oil and bitter extractive matter, and are therefore carminative, aromatic and stimulant. Many contain bitter and astringent principles, and possess tonic and stomachic properties. Several species have an agreeable odour and are used as perfumery. some are used for flavouring dishes as lemon, garden thyme, and marjoram ; some are edible.

Anisochilus Carnosus, Lavandula Carnosa, Coleus Spicatus.

Habitat.—W. Himalaya, Central and S. India, Mysore, Malabar.

Parts used.—The leaves and essential oil.

Vernacular.—Can.—Dodda-patri. Hind., Duk.—Sitaki Pangeri. Eng.—Thick-leaved lavender. Guz.—Ajmun. Malyal.—Kattu-kurkka chômara. Mar.—Kâpurli. Tam.—Karpura-walli. Tel.—Rôjâchettu, Omannelâku.

Characters.—Small plant; stem, erect and tetragonal; leaves petioled, ovate, obtuse, crenate, thick, fleshy, hoary and tomentosely villous on both surfaces.

Constituents.—A volatile oil.

Preparations.—The juice of leaves. Dose, ½ to 2 fld. drs.

Actions and uses.—Stimulant, diaphoretic and expectorant ; given to children in coughs and colds, and in tympanitis. Locally the juice mixed with sugar and gingelly oil is applied to the head in headache.

Anisomeles Malabarica, A. Ovata, Nepeta Malabarica. Ajuga Fruticosa.

Habitat.—Travancore, Southern India, Ceylon.

Parts used.—The herb, leaves and essential oil.

Vernacular.—Bomb.—Gaozaban. Duk.—Mogbirâ-kâspatta. Eng.—Malabar cat mint. Malyal.—Peyi-Meratti. Sans.—Bootan Koosham. Tam.—Iratta-i-pey maruttee. Tel.—Moga-bira.

Characters.—Shrub with branches, tomentose; leaves ovate, lanceolate, crenately serrated above, entire below; calyx covered with viscid pubescence; corolla white, anthers purple, whorls in racemes.

Preparations.—Infusion of leaves (1 in 10). Dose, ½ to 1 fld. oz. Decoction of the whole plant (1 in 10). Dose, ½ to 1 fld. oz. The essential oil. Dose, 2 to 5 ms.

Actions and uses.—Stomachic, carminative, diaphoretic and astringent; used in colic, dyspepsia, catarrhal affections and fevers due to teething in children; also in dysentery. As vapour bath it is used in fevers and rheumatism. The essential oil is used as an external application in rheumatism and as an emmenagogue in uterine affections.

Coleus Carnosus, Coleus Aromaticus, C. Amboinicus.

Habitat.—Moluccas, cultivated throughout India, Ceylon.

Parts used.—The leaves.

Vernacular.—Beng.—Patherchur. Eng.—Country Borage. Hind.—Pathar chur. Mal.—Ová pána, Sans.—Pashanabhedi. Tam.—Karpura valli.

Characters.—Leaves broadly ovate, very thick, and crenate at their margins, from 2 to 3 inches in length; both surfaces sprinkled with minute glandular bodies which resemble dew drops as if clothed with white villi and hairs; under surface highly reticulated, glandular hairs numerous, giving it a frosted appearance; odour and taste aromatic and pungent and resembling those of ovâ.

Preparations.—Juice of leaves. Dose, ½ to 1 fld. dr.

Actions and uses.—Antispasmodic, stimulant and stomachic; used in colic in children, asthma and dyspepsia; also as a local application to the head in headache and to relieve the pain and irritation caused by the stings of centipedes. It is also given in chronic cough, fever, asthma, epilepsy and other convulsive affections. The true ova is ptychotis ajowan; this is called ová pána from the taste and odour of its leaves resembling those of ova.

Collinsonia Canadensis.

Syn.—Stone root, ox balm, knot root, rich weed, horse weed, healall.

Habitat.—North America.

Parts used.—The rhizome.

Characters.—Rhizome 4 inches long, with short knotty branches, white within, without odour, and with a bitter nauseous taste. Dose, powdered root 5 to 30 grs.

Constituents.—Resin.

Preparations.—Tincture (1 in 10). Dose, ½ to 2 fld. drs. Liquid extract, miscible with water. Dose, 15 to 60 ms. Solid Extract. Dose, 2 to 5 grs. Infusion (1 to 20). Dose, 1 to 2 fld. ozs.

Actions and uses.—Alterative, antispasmodic and diuretic; given in genito-urinary affections, such as gravel. It relaxes spasms of the ureter and urethra and facilitates the expulsion of small calculi. In acute cystitis, it is combined with morphia and aconite. It is also used in prostatorrhœa, leucorrhœa, chronic gonorrhœa or gleet, when copaiba, cubebs and sandal oil have failed; in flatulent colic, in gastro-intestinal catarrh and catarrhal gastritis due to beer and alcohol drinking, it is used with benefit. In biliary calculi it is usually given in warm infusion. It is also given as an alterative in relaxed conditions of tissues as in relaxation of the throat, uvula, in chronic pharyngitis and affections of the vocal organs. As a general tonic it is given in dyspepsia, anæmia, and chlorosis. Ascarides are destroyed by rectal injection of fluid extract 1 to 4 of water. Suppositories are used in tenesmus and piles.

Hedeoma Pulegioides (Pennyroyal.)

Habitat.—North America, New England.

Part used.—The leaves and tops.

Characters.—Leaves opposite, short petioled, ½ inch long, oblong, serrated, glandular beneath; branches quadrangular and hairy; odour strong and mint-like but repulsive to insects, fleas and mosquitoes; taste warm and pungent. Dose, 15 to 60 grs.

Constituents.—Volatile oil, bitter principle and tannin. Oleum Hedeomæ (oil of pennyroyal). It is a yellowish, limpid liquid, odour and taste characteristic, soluble in alcohol and glacial acetic acid. It contains hedeomol 33 p.c.; pulegone, formic, acetic and isoheptoic acids. Dose, 2 to 10 ms.

Preparations.—Infusion (1 in 10). Dose, 1 to 2 ounces. Spiritus Hedeomæ (1 of oil to 9 alcohol), used externally or as a spray.

Actions and uses.—Stimulant, carminative, emmenagogue and aromatic. The infusion is given in flatulent colic, indigestion, and sickness. The hot infusion is useful to check diarrhœa. In amenorrhœa the leaves are taken with hip and foot baths. The spirit is applied to hands and face to keep away mosquitoes. As an abortifacient it is sometimes given in poisonous doses, often causing death by narcosis.

Hyssopus Officinalis, H. Parviflora.

Habitat.—Persia, S. Europe, Sind.

Parts used.—The flowering plant and husks of the seeds.

Vernacular.—Zupho. Arab.—Zûphâ-ê-yâbis. Hind., Bomb.—Juphá. Pers.—Ush-naz-daoud.

Characters.—A small plant from 6 to 10 inches in height, of a reddish or brownish purple colour, odour aromatic, like that of sweet hay, taste bitter and somewhat acrid ; stem square, very slender and thin, obtusely 4-angled, smooth and mottled with a purplish tint; young parts covered with small whitish hairs ; root woody, brownish externally and white within; flowers numerous and disposed in oblong spikes of a brownish or bluish purple colour ; seeds oblong, three-angled and of a dark brown or grey colour, mottled with a red tint; leaves opposite, linear, punctate on both sides, half folded and hairy. Dose, 15 to 30 grs.

Constituents.—Volatile oil, bitter principle, tannin, resin, fat, sugar, and mucilage. The oil is a pale yellow greenish liquid, freely soluble in alcohol.

Preparations.—Infusion (1 in 10). Dose, ½ to 1 fld. oz. Essential oil. Dose, 1 to 3 ms. compound syrup containing Zupho drs. 2, Tukhm-i-khitmi 4 drs., Khubázi 4 drs., Jethi madha 1½ drs., Anjir No. 5, Khaskas 6 drs., Anisun 6 drs., Gule banafshâ 3 drs., Râj Hansa, 2 drs. Kàkdâsin 2 drs., Kâle drâkh 2 ozs., Sopisatân No. 40, Unâb No. 40, Boiling water 80 ozs. Macerate the whole for 12 hours, then boil down to half the quantity of water and strain. Add 2 lbs. of sakara and prepare a syrup. Dose, drs. ½ to 1 fld. ozs.

Actions and uses.—Stimulant, carminative, diaphoretic and emmenagogue; given in dyspepsia, flatulence, asthma, chronic bronchitis in old people and fever complicated with cough ; also in amenorrhœa, rheumatism and sore throat ; the syrup is given in influenza, chronic cough, and catarrh of the lungs.

Lallemantia Royleana, Dracocephalum Royleanum.

Habitat.—Persia, Trans-Indus.

Parts used.—The seeds.

Vernacular.—Arab.—Bazarula-balank. Duk.—Balanka. Hind.—Balangu. Pers.—Tukhm-e-balangu.

Characters.—Nutlets, black in colour and resembling shâjira, shape oblong, smooth, or rugous, and 3-angled ; angles, rather sharp ; each seed arched on one side and tapering towards the umbilicus, where it is marked with a white scar ; surface slightly pitted, marked with three nerves on its back ; taste rather acrid and mucilaginous; when moistened they become coated with tenacious opaque grey mucilage.

Preparations.—Infusion (1 in 10). Dose, 1 to 2 fld. ozs.

Actions and uses.—Expectorant and demulcent ; used in cough, irritation of the throat and in gonorrhœa.

Remarks.—The seeds are sold for those of Mishk-i-taramashi.

Lanium Album, Urtica Mortua.

Habitat.—Europe.

Parts used.—The flowers—Flores urticæ mortuæ.

Preparations.—Infusion (1 in 10). Dose, 2 to 6 drs. Extract. Dose, 1 to 3 grs. Tincture (1 in 8). Dose, ½ to 1 dr. Succus. Dose, ½ to 1 dr.

Actions and uses.—Astringent, mucilaginous and hæmostatic; given in metrorrhagia, diarrhœa, dysentery and hæmoptysis. Locally, cotton dipped in an alcoholic solution arrests local hæmorrhages, like perchloride of iron.

Lavandula Stæchas.

Habitat.—Mediterranean Coast, Asia Minor, Arabia.

Parts used.—The flower spikes, and a volatile oil distilled from flowers.

Vernacular.—Arab.—Ustukhudus. Bomb.—Ustikhudus. Eng.—Arabian Lavender, the oil—false oil of spike. Guz.—Lavandara naphula. Hind.—Alaphajana, Dharu.

Characters.—The drug consists of flowering spikes, elongated and hairy, and of stalks slender and covered all over. The bracts are of a bluish colour and reticulated with distinct nerves, broad towards the apex and cuneate towards the base; flowers irregular, and longer than the calyx; calyx tubular, dentate and inserted with the bracts. The whole drug has a bluish brown colour, agreeable odour, resembling that of lavender, taste bitterish and aromatic. The oil is of a pale yellow colour, fragrant odour and bitter taste; soluble in alcohol.

Constituents.—Volatile oil, resin and tannin.

Preparations.—Tincture (1 in 8). Dose, ½ to 1 fld. drs. Spirit (1 in 10). Dose, 5 to 20 ms. Essential oil. Dose, 1 to 3 ms.

Actions and uses.—Stimulant, nervine tonic, carminative and antispasmodic; given in nausea, flatulence, gastralgia, colic and chest affections, and to relieve nervous headache, hysteria, hypochondriasis and bilious vomiting; also given to disguise the taste and smell of nauseating medicines. A fomentation of its flowers relieves local rheumatic or neuralgic pains. The oil is used locally to relieve nervous headache.

Lavandula Vera, B. P., Common Lavender.

Habitat.—South Europe, England.

Parts used.—A volatile oil distilled from flowers—Oleum Lavandulæ, B. P.

Characters.—A small shrub, spikes elongated and hairy; stalks, slender, and covered with white hairs; flowers irregular, calyx tubular and inserted with the bracts; of a fragrant odour and aromatic, camphoraceous taste.

Constituents.—A camphor, volatile oil 3 p.c., resin and tannin.

Preparations.—Oleum Lavandulæ, B. P., distilled from flowers and stalks. A pale yellowish liquid; odour fragrant and pungent; taste bitter; soluble in alcohol and in glacial acetic acid. Dose, ½ to 3 ms. The oil is sometimes adulterated with oil of spike. French oil of lavender is of a less agreeable odour than English oil of lavender. Lavender water—prepared from lavender flowers with oil of Bergamot and ambergis. Spiritus Lavandulæ, B. P. (1 in 10). Dose, 5 to 20 ms., used as a perfume and as a flavouring agent. Tinctura Lavandulæ Composita, B. P.—oil of lavender 45 ms., oil of rosemary 5 ms., cinnamon bark, nutmeg, ā ā 75 grs., red sanders wood 150 grs., alcohol (90 p.c.) to make 1 pint. Dose, ½ to 1 fld. dr.—a constituent of liquor arsenicalis.

Actions and uses.—Similar to Lavandula stæchas. The tincture is carminative, and given in flatulence, colic, gastralgia, nervous headache, and in bilious vomiting to arrest nausea. Flowers are employed as sternutatory.

Leonotis Nepetœfolia.

Habitat.—Throughout hotter parts of India.

Parts used.—The plant.

Vernacular.—Beng.—Hejur-chei. Guz.—Mâtisul, Mâtijer. Mar. —Dipmal.

Characters.—Flowers, orange coloured; flower head, globular and spinous; stem straight, four-sided; leaves opposite, spreading and long, cordate, serrate and downy.

Preparations.—Decoction of leaves (1 in 10). Dose, ½ to 1 fld. dr. and ash.

Actions and uses.—The ashes of the flower heads with curd is applied to ring-worm and to allay itching in skin affections. The decoction is a tonic and febrifuge, and given in intermittent fevers and during convalescence from acute diseases.

Leucas Cephalotes, Leucas Aspera, L. Linifolia.

Habitat.—Himalaya, Bengal, N. India, Deccan.

Parts used.—The herb.

Vernacular.—Beng.—Halkasa chato. Can.—Tigadi. Guz.—Kulmânu phul, Kubo. Hind.—Kubo, Goma, Madh apati, chatra. Malyal.—Tumba. Mar.—Tumba, Kumbha, Bahûphûl. Punj.—Guldora. Sans.—Drona pushpi, Kurumba chitra pattrika, chitrak shupa. Sind.—Kubo. Tel.—Tumini. Tam.—Thumbay keera.

Characters.—Herbaceous, hairy plant; leaves erect, slightly pubescent or tomentose, ovate, oblong serrated, linear, and entire; bracts linear, hoary. The plant contains large globose verticels of numerous white flowers.

Constituents.—A small quantity of essential oil and an alkaloid.

Preparations.—The juice. Dose, 5 to 15 ms.

Actions and uses.—Stimulant, expectorant and aperient; given in jaundice, cough, nasal and intestinal catarrh. It is also externally applied in skin eruptions.

Melissa Officinalis. Melissa Umbrosa.

Habitat.—S. Europe, Central Asia, Persia.

Parts used.—The whole plant, the leaves and tops.

Vernacular.—Arab.—Baklut-ul-Faristum. Bomb.—Badaranj. Duk.—Mekka-Sabzah. Eng.—Melissa, common balm, mountain balm, lemon balm, citronelle, dropsy plant, balm mint. Hind.—Ram-Tulsi. Pers.—Badrunj buyeh.

Characters.—The drug is much broken and consists of stems and fruit; stem hairy, quadrangular and of a purplish tint; leaves two inches long, petiolate, ovate, heart-shaped, and crenate at the base, margins serrated, upper surface marked with scattered hairs, under surface with glands on the axils of the nerves; calyx striated, hairy, five-toothed, each having a strong nerve; corolla not so hairy as the calices, rose coloured or brownish purple and rugous; seeds four, naked, brown, 3-angled, with a white patch on each side of the hilum and attached to the bottom of the calices, erect, angular and of a darkish brown colour, in size resembling Málunga; flowers axillary, in clusters of six and short peduncle. The whole drug has a light brown colour, and a peculiar aromatic odour or fragrance, resembling that of Banaphashâ or lemon; taste, astringent and bitter, similar to that of Nimbádá.

Preparation.—Aqua of leaves (1 in 10). Infusion (1 in 10). Dose, 1 to 2 fld. ozs.; compound spirit—to obtain it take citronelle 10, lemon peel 12, nutmeg 6, cinnamon 3, cloves 3, and spirit 150, and distil. Dose, $\frac{1}{2}$ to 1 dr.

Actions and uses.—Carminative, stimulant, diaphoretic and emmenagogue; chiefly given along with other diaphoretics and as a refreshing drink in febrile affections. It is also given in defective menstruation.

Mentha Arvensis, B. P., Vars. Piperascens et Glabrata, M. Piperita, B. P.

Habitat.—China and Japan.

Parts used.—The essential oil distilled from the leaves, flowering tops and stems, and a stearopten known as menthol or peppermint camphor.

Vernacular.—Arab.—Nannaul-Habagul Hindi, Chin.—The oil, Lintsas. Japanese.—The oil, Hakans, Aburo, Hatsea. Mar., Beng., Duk.—Pudnah. Malay—Putiyiana, Jiamanis. Tam.—Iech-chak, Karai, Widda. Tel.—Iga engili kura.

Characters.—Plant shrubby, with square stems; leaves opposite, exstipulate and strong scented. Flowers in cymes, axillary, arranged in a whorled manner. Calyx tubular, 5 to 10 toothed and regular; corolla bilateral ; ovary, seated on a fleshy disk, fruit achenia ; seed erect with or without albumen. The plant abounds in a volatile oil.

Constituents.—The leaves, stems and flowering tops contain a volatile oil, also bitter extractive matter and an astringent principle ; the oil is high coloured, very pungent and of a bitter after taste, and contains the stearopten, menthol, to which it owes its peculiar odour.

Preparation.—Infusion of leaves (1 in 10). Dose, 4 to 12 drs.

Actions and uses.—Stems and leaves are carminative, antispasmodic and stomachic. The infusion is given as a cooling drink in fever and dyspepsia.

Menthol, B. P., Menthylic Alcohol, Menthyl Propylphenol Hexahydride, Peppermint Camphor.

Vernacular.—Baisar.—Phudina-kâ-phul. Chin.—Pohoyo. Eng.—Menthol. Guz.—Ajmanâ-phul. Jap.—Halsea.

A crystalline stearopten obtained by cooling the oil distilled from Mentha arvensis, M. piperascens, M. glabrata and M. piperita and freezing the distillate by means of ice and salt.

Characters.— It occurs in permanent prismatic or colourless acicular crystals resembling sulphate of magnesium, very slightly soluble in water, giving it the odour and taste of peppermint, soluble in alcohol (5 in 1), freely soluble in glycerin, ether, chloroform, glacial acetic acid and volatile oils. Entirely volatilized by the heat of boiling water. Met with also in pencils or cones. The odour is strong like that of peppermint. It has a warm aromatic taste and produces a sensation of cold when the air is drawn into the mouth. An American variety is known as pipmenthol. Among the natives it is known as peppermint-na-phula, or flowers of peppermint. Dose, ½ to 2 grs.

Preparations.—Emplastrum menthol, B.P., (3 in 20) of yellow wax and resin. Menthol cones or pencils ; menthol lotion 20 p.c., Gossypium menthol or menthol wool 10 p.c ; used to stuff nostrils in catarrh. Menth-Iodol, a combination of menthol and iodol, used for neuralgia. Linimentum menthol consists of menthol 3, chloroform 4, and olive oil to 16, used in neuralgia, lumbago, sciatica, &c. Menthol cum aconitina (1 in 500), made in cones, 60 grs. each. Menthol Valerianas —"Validolum" contains 30 p.c. of free menthol. Dose, 10 to 15 ms. Menth-oleate—solution of menthol in oleic acid. Menthol Ointment containing menthol 1 dr., zinc oxide 1 dr., carbolic acid ½ dr., almond oil 10 dr., cerate 10 dr., applied to the mucous membrane of the nose in nasal catarrh. A liquid combination of menthol 2 drs., chloral hydrate 3 drs,. camphor 2 oz., oil of cinnamon 40 ms., ol-caryophilli 40 ms. alcohol 1 oz. is applied with a brush on forehead and temple, in cephalagia and migraine. Menthol snuff containing menthol 1, boric acid 2, ammonium chloride 3, used as a local stimulant in nasal catarrh. A compound liquid preparation triturated with equal weights of menthol, thymol, phenol, camphor, chloral and croton chloral, is applied on cotton wool and used for allaying toothache in decayed teeth. Tinctura Menthol Etherea (1 in 8), Pigmentum Menthol 1 to 4 of olive oil. Menthen, a hydrocarbon obtained from menthol—a clear fluid which dissolves in alcohol, ether and benzin.

Actions and uses.—Analgesic, anodyne, antiseptic, general and cardiac stimulant and antispasmodic; given internally in ten drops of 20 p. c., solution in vomiting of pregnancy, in low states of the system, in colic, gastralgia, flatulence and other stomach and bowel complaints. Externally as an antiseptic and local anæsthetic it is applied to the surface and menthol cones are rubbed to relieve pain, heat, itching and smarting. A saturated alcoholic solution is painted over the affected nerve in neuralgic affections, such as sciatica, toothache, headache, tic douloureux, rheumatic pains, pleurodynea, &c. Its application is also used in parasitic skin diseases. A spray or vapour containing 20 p.c. of menthol, is used in nasal catarrh and in violent sneezing, influenza and in tubercular laryngitis.

Mentha Piperita, B.P., M. Hirsuta, M. Crispa, M. Canadense, Mentha Incana, Micromeria Capitallata.

Habitat.—Asia, Europe, North America, Northern India, Thibet, Himalaya.

Parts used.—The leaves, tops and an essential oil.

Vernacular.—Bomb.—Peparaminta. Eng.—Persian Peppermint. Hind.—Piparaminta.

Characters.—A perennial herb with the root stalks creeping with long suckers, by which it multiplies; stem square and purplish; flowers 5-toothed, purplish, in terminal conical spikes; leaves oval, lanceolate, sharply serrated, and glandular; odour of the plant very powerful and aromatic, but refreshing; when put upon the tongue it produces a pungent and cooling sensation, followed by numbness; when swallowed it gives diffusible warmth in the abdomen.

Constituents.—A volatile oil, 1 to 1½ p.c., menthol, resin, tannin and gum. Volatile oil—oleum menthæ piperitiæ, B. P. Prepared from the leaves by distillation with water or steam—a colourless or yellowish green, thick and viscid liquid, on exposure becoming brown; odour peculiar and pungent, taste hot, camphoraceous and bitterish followed by a sensation of coldness when air is drawn into the mouth; it is soluble in alcohol (1 in 4). It contains chiefly a crystalline stearopten known as menthol, or mint camphor, and a liquid turpene; also glacial acetic acid, and carbon bisulphide. Dose, ½ to 3 ms.; the stearopten is obtained by cooling the oil.

Preparations.—Spiritus Menthæ Piperitæ B.P. (1 in 10). Dose, 5 to 20 ms. Aqua Menthæ Piperitæ, B. P.—peppermint water, 77 ms. of the oil in one and a half gallons of water and distilled to ⅔. Dose, ½ to 2 oz. Pilula Rhei Composita, B. P. Dose, 4 to 8 grs. Infusum menthæ (1 in 10). Dose, ½ to 2 fld. ozs.

Actions and uses.—The leaves are aromatic, stimulant, carminative and antispasmodic, and given in vomiting, gastric colic, cholera, dysentery and diarrhœa. In flatulence, it removes the flatus at first by its stimulant action and then exerts a sedative action on the bowels; it is also given in dysmenorrhœa with tea, in weak digestion, palpitation of the heart and in hiccough; as a corrigent, it is given with purgative medicine to prevent griping. Oleum menthæ piperitæ possesses the action of peppermint in a very high degree. As a powerful local anodyne, anæsthetic, antiseptic and germicide, it is superior to carbolic acid, iodoform and iodine, and is used as an antiseptic inhalation in phthisis and diphtheria; as an anodyne, it relieves the pain of superficial neuralgia, and is also used used locally as a counter-irritant in rheumatism. A lotion of the oil 5 ms. with borax 60 grs. and water 16 ozs. is used in pruritis caused by irritating discharges; it also allays the pain of herpes zoster. The solution (1 in 2,000) is given as germicide in cholera.

Mentha Sylvestris.

Habitat.—Cashmere, Temperate Himalaya, Pesria.

Parts used.—The herb, leaves, flower tops and oil.

Vernacular.—Arab.—Tudanaj. Bomb.—Pudina. Can.—Chetin maragu. Eng.—Wild mint, wild spearmint, crisped or curled mint. Guz.—Phudino. Mar.—Vatalau. Pers.—Pudang.

Characters.—Leaves oblong, obovate, lanceolate, subacute, serrate and hoary beneath; whorls in terminal spikes; calyx toothed, triangular or lanceolate; corolla hairy, glabrous within; nutlets pale, smooth and brown; odour fragrant; taste mild, hot and somewhat pungent. Dose, 30 to 60 grs.

Constituents.—A volatile oil similar in composition to peppermint, but differing from it in odour and flavour; resin, gum, and tannin.

Preparations.—Infusion (1 in 10). Dose, ½ to 2 fld. ozs.

Actions and uses.—Stimulant, carminative and stomachic; given in hiccough, vomiting, etc. A vapour of the leaves is largely inhaled with olen chaha in catarrh and fevers.

Remarks.—Fudina is a generic name, used for the plants of the mentha species.

Mentha Viridis, B.P.

Habitat.—Europe, the Canaries, the Cape of Good Hope, N. America, Cashmere, United States.

Parts used.—The leaves and flower tops; also an essential oil. Oleum Menthæ Viridis, B. P.

Vernacular.—Eng.—Spear mint. Hind.—Pahadi phudina. Pers. —Phudina kohi.

Characters.—Leaves 2 to 3 inches long, sessile, serrate, glandular, nearly smooth; branches square; herb is mostly green, of an aromatic odour and pungent taste. On drying it loses about 75 p. c. of its aroma. Dose, 30 to 60 grs.

Constituents.—Volatile oil $\frac{1}{2}$ p.c., resin, gum, tannin.

Oleum Menthæ Viridis, B. P., oil of spear mint. It is a volatile oil obtained by distillation.

Colourless, pale yellow, or greenish yellow oil, becoming darker by age. The odour is characteristic of the plant ; taste hot and aromatic. It is soluble in alcohol (1 in 1) but becoming turbid when diluted; soluble in glacial acetic acid and carbon bisulphide. It contains terpene, limonene and carvol. Dose, $\frac{1}{2}$ to 3 ms.

Preparations.—Of the leaves and flower tops. Spiritus Menthæ Viridis—essence of spear mint, an alcoholic solution containing the oil 10 p.c. and the herb 1 p.c. Dose, 10 to 40 ms. Aqua Menthæ Viridis 77 ms. in $1\frac{1}{2}$ gallons of water distilled to two-thirds. Dose, $\frac{1}{2}$ to 1 oz. Infusion of the leaves and tops. Dose, 1 to 2 ozs.

Actions and uses.—Carminative and stimulant, similar to mentha piperitæ, but less powerful ; given in cholera, bilious vomiting, colicky pain and for the relief of flatulence.

Marrubium Vulgare, M. Hamatum, M. Germanicum.

Habitat.—Europe (waste places), Western Temperate Himalaya, Cashmere.

Parts used.—The herb.

Vernacular.—Eng.—Common or white horehound, East Indian Peppermint. Ind. Bazar—Farásiyun, Hashishat-el-kalb (dog's herb).

Characters.—Stem branching, quadrangular and covered with a white felt; leaves opposite, petiolate, somewhat heart-shaped, pale green and downy above, and hoary beneath ; flowers axillary, with woolly whorls ; achenes four, dark brown ; odour somewhat aromatic and musky, taste pungent and bitter.

Constituents.—Volatile oil, a bitter glucoside called marrubiin resin, tannin and fat; marrubiin occurs in tibular crystals, of a bitter acrid taste. To obtain it treat aqueous extract with alcohol, distil, and treat the residue with ether.

Preparations.—Infusion (1 in 20). Dose, 1 to 2 fld. ozs. Juice or succus. Dose, 1 to 2 fld. drs.

Actions and uses.—Stimulant, expectorant, deobstruent, resolvent, and anthelmintic; in large doses, diaphoretic and diuretic ; given as a domestic remedy in coughs, in chronic bronchitis with copious expectoration and in dyspepsia. As an alterative, it is given in chronic rheumatism jaundice, chronic hepatitis, phthisis, amenorrhœa cachectic conditions, &c.

Monarda Punctata—Horsemint.

Habitat.—United States.

Parts used.—Leaves and tops.

Characters.—Stems branched and downy. Leaves, 1 to 2 inches long, lanceolate, serrate, punctate; flowers yellow, spotted, red or brown, and downy; calyx 5-toothed; odour aromatic and pungent; taste bitter. Dose, 15 to 60 grs.

Constituents—Volatile oil.—Oleum Monardeæ. It is a yellow or red oil, and contains terpenes, 50 p.c., thymol (monardin) 24 p.c., alcohol, acetic, butyric and formic esters.

Preparations.—Infusion. Decoction (1 in 10). Dose, 2 to 6 drs.

Actions and uses.—Carminative, stimulant, emmenagogue, diaphoretic, and diuretic; given in flatulent colic, neuralgia, diarrhœa rheumatism, &c.

Nepeta Cataria—Cutnep or Catnip.

Cats eat the herb ravenously, being, it is believed, fond of it for its aphrodisiac effects.

Habitat.—Europe, Asia.

Parts used.—The leaves and tops.

Characters.—Perennial herb; stem quadrangular, branching and hoary; leaves hairy, 2 inches long, triangular, ovate, cordate, and serrate; flowers whitish, purple, and dotted; calyx 5-toothed, 2-lipped; stamens 4, didynamous; odour, mint-like; taste bitter, aromatic, camphoraceous. Dose, 15 to 60 grs.

Constituents.—Volatile oil, bitter principle and tannin.

Preparations.—Infusion and Decoction (1 in 10). Dose, 2 to 4 drs.

Actions and uses.—Carminative, tonic, stimulant, emmenagogue, and antispasmodic; given in hysteria, chlorosis, colic, amenorrhœa, and toothache.

Ocimum Album, O. Canum, O. Americanum.

Habitat.—Brazil, East India, China, India.

Parts used.—The juice of leaves.

Vernacular.—Arab.—Badrûge-abiaz. Beng.—Sâdâ-tulshi. Eng.—Hoary Basil, wild mint. Duk., Guz., Hind.—Jangli tulsi, Ujli-tulasi. Malyal.—Vella-tolasi, Nâkkanni. Pers.—Raihâne-kohi. Sans.—Visva tulasi. Tam.—Cunjâm Koray. Tel.—Kukka tulasi.

Characters.—A shrub; flowers white; leaves very pleasant and aromatic in taste and smell.

Preparations.—Succus. Dose, ½ to 2 drs.

Actions and uses.—Stimulant, diaphoretic and carminative; given to children in cold and catarrh.

Ocimum Basilicum, O. Anisatum, Basilicum Citratum.

Habitat.—Persia, Punjab, Bengal, Oude, and Travancore.

Parts used.—The herb and seeds.

Vernacular.—Arab.—Raihân, Shâbasfaram. Burm.—Kala-pinzain. Can.—Kam-kasture. Eng.—Common Basil, sweet Basil. Beng., Duk., Guz., Mar., Hind.—Subzâ, nazbo, Babi tulsi. Malyal.—Tirunitru rach-châ. Pers.—Habak-i-kermani, Dabân-shab. Sans.—Vishva-tulasi. Tirunitru-pach-pach-ch-ai. Tel.—Vibudi-patri.

Characters.—Herb erect and glabrous; leaves petiolate, ovate, oblong, narrowed at the base, slightly toothed; pedicle ciliated; flowers small and white, in simple racemes; seeds of a brown colour or black; no odour; taste oily and slightly pungent. When moistened with water they become coated with semi-opaque mucilage.

Constituents.—The leaves contain a yellowish green oil, which, if kept for a time, crystallizes, and is then known as Basil camphor.

Preparations.—Cold infusion (1 in 10). Dose, ½ to 1 fld. oz.

Actions and uses.—Diaphoretic, mucilaginous, carminative and stimulant; given in intestinal fluxes, gonorrhœa, catarrh and to relieve after-pains in parturition; also given during the cold stage of intermittent fever and to allay vomiting. It is dropped into the ear in earache.

Ocimum Gratissimum, C. Zeylanicum.

Habitat.—Bengal, Nepaul, Chittagong, Deccan Peninsula (cultivated near temples.)

Parts used.—The leaves and seeds.

Vernacular.—Arab.—Faraujmishk. Can.—Kâda Tulasi. Beng., Duk. and Hind.—Rámatulasi, Banjari. Malyal.—Kattiv-tuttuva. Pers.—Raihâne-Qaranfuli; Palang-mishk, Bâlanki-khurd (the seed). Sans.—Râmatulsi. Tam.—Elumich-cham. Tel.—Nimma-Tulasi.

Characters.—Plant from 4 to 6 feet high; leaves drooping, opposite, oblong, serrated and smooth on both surfaces with a long petiole; flowers terminal, in racemes with the verticels of six pretty closely arranged flowers; seeds dark brown, larger than those of Tukhameria, somewhat pitted and three-angled; taste mucilaginous.

Preparations.—Cold infusion (1 in 10). Dose, 2 to 8 drs.; baths and fumigations.

Actions and uses.—Demulcent and carminative; generally combined with other expectorants, in cough mixtures; also used in urinary disorders, such as gonorrhœa, scanty and scalding urine, &c. Locally, the juice mixed with Gul-i-armâni is used as an application to swollen hands or feet. Baths and fumigations of tulasi are used in rheumatism.

Ocimum Sanctum, O. Hirsutum, O. Tomentosum.

Habitat.—Throughout India.

Parts used.—The leaves and seeds.

Vernacular.—Arab.— Badruj. Beng.— Krishna tulsi. Guz., Duk., Mar., Hind., Bom.— Kâlâ Tulasil, Barandâ. Burm.—Lun-Punzang-zee. Can.— Tulashi-gida. Cing.—Maduru-talla. Eng.—Holy Basil, purple stalked Basil. Malyal.—Nallatulluva tulasi. Sans.—Tulasi, Paranasa, Vrandi Sarasa, sitah vaya. Tam.—Kuli mitan. Tel.—Tulasi.

Characters.—Leaves opposite, petiolate, oblong or oval, serrated, pubescent, entire at the base, minutely dotted and hairy near the nerves; flowers verticelled, small, irregular and of a pink or purple colour; corolla inserted into a hairy toothed calyx; calyx shorter than pedicels, five partite, upper segment curiously revoluted and reniform in shape; ovary, four-seeded; seeds when fresh white, but becoming black or ripening, oblong, blunt pointed and somewhat arched; the smell of the leaves peculiarly aromatic, the aroma being chiefly due to the presence of oil cells on their surface; the smell of the flowers and seeds very fragrant, sweet and aromatic; taste pungent.

Preparations.—Medicated oil; decoction of seeds (1 in 10). Dose, ½ to 1 fld. oz. The medicated oil contains tulasi pana, bhuiringani, danti mula vaja, segata chhala, trikatu; equal parts make a paste; add gora tela and boil; used as drops into the nose in ozæna and into the ears in purulent discharges.

Actions and uses.—Demulcent, expectorant and antiperiodic; with kalamiri it is given in catarrhal affections of the lungs and cough. The powder of dry leaves is used by the natives as snuff in ozæna and for destroying maggots. The paste of the leaves with suntha and sapheda miri is given in intermittent and remittent fevers. The medicated oil is used as drops into the ears in earache and in purulent discharges and into the nose in ozæna. With lime juice the leaves are rubbed over ringworm. The seeds are mucilaginous and used as a diuretic in scanty urine and in cough.

Ocimum Pilosum, O. Hispidum, Basilicum Indicum.

Habitat.—Persia, India.

Parts used.—The seeds.

Vernacular.—Arab—Habak.Bomb.—Tukamerian. Hind.—Babui-tul. Pers.—Tukhm-i-rihana. Eng.—Nimb loke, Garden Basil.

The word Tuka-merian is a corruption of the Persian Tukhm-i-rihána which means the seeds of Rihana or ocimum. The specific name is derived from the condition of their inflorescence which is very pilose.

Characters.—Seeds small, black, slightly arched on one side and flattened on the other, oblong, and somewhat angular; each seed is marked with a small white scar at one end; surface very minutely pitted; odour pleasant and lemon-like; taste mucilaginous, oily and slightly pungent.

Preparations.—Mucilage.

Actions and uses.—Demulcent and nutrient; given in gonorrhœa, strangury and kidney diseases; also in dysentery and cough. The jelly is given in spermatorrhæa.

Origanum Marjorana, Marjorana Hortensis.

Habitat.—Portugal to Western Asia, Panjab, Himalaya.

Parts used.—The plant.

Vernacular.—Pers.—Mirzan gush. Bomb.—Kame phatusa. Eng. —Sweet Marjoram. Tam.—Marru. Tel.—Maruvamu. Ind. Bazar.—Marwa. Marzangush is derived from marzan, a mouse, and gush, ear. It means mouse ear; in allusion to the greyish downy character of the leaves resembling a mouse's ear.

Characters.—Stems slender, slightly quadrangular and covered with stellate, whitish hairs; leaves small, thick, obovate, or cuneate at the base, and covered all over with starry hairs; odour very agreeable; taste bitter at first, becoming after a time camphoraceous. Dose, 15 to 60 grs.

Constituents.—A volatile oil, soluble in alcohol, consisting mainly of terpene. Dose, 2 to 6 ms.

Preparations.—Infusum (1 in 10). Dose, ½ to 1 fld. oz.

Actions and uses.—Carminative, stimulant, diaphoretic, emmenagogue and tonic; given in colic, dyspepsia and dysmenorrhœa. The oil like oleum mentha is used as an application to the abdomen in colic, to the joints in rheumatism, and to the temples in hemicrania. The oil is given internally in flatulence.

Origanum Vulgare, common or wild marjoram.

Habitat.—Europe, N. Africa, N. America.

It is a perennial herb, containing a volatile oil, tannin, resin and a bitter principle.

Properties.—The dried leaves are employed as a substitute for China Tea; the red volatile oil, known as oleum origani, is now superseded by oil of thyme or that obtained from Thymus Vulgaris. It is used as a tonic, carminative, emmenagogue and stimulant.

Orthosiphon Staminens.

Habitat.—India, Java and E. Indian Islands and Australia.

Parts used.—The leaves.

Vernacular.—Eng.—Javatea. Malyal.—Koemis koetjing.

Koemis koetjing, meaning cat's moustache. In allusion to the lengthy stamens of flowers like a cat's moustache.

Characters.—Leaves in distant pairs, cuneately narrowed into the petiole, petiolate, ovate or ovato-lanceolate, often acuminate, one to two inches long, irregularly and coarsely toothed.

Constituents.—A glucoside—orthosiphonin, in fine crystals, very soluble in water, sparingly so in alcohol, very slightly in chloroform and insoluble in ether.

Preparations.—Fluid extract, 10 to 30 ms. Infusion (1 in 10). Dose, 2 to 6 drs.

Actions and uses.—Diuretic and uric acid solvent; under its use the urine, which for a long time has remained turbid and thick, becomes clear; given as a remedy in gravel, chronic cystitis and pyonephrosis.

Pogostemon Parviflorus P. Purpurascens, P. Plectranthoides, P. Purpuricaulis.

Habitat.—Deccan Peninsula, Ratnagiri.

Parts used.—The root, and leaves.

Vernacular.—Mar.—Phanglâ, Pangrâ.

Characters.—Plant about 6 feet high. stem smooth and of a purple colour; leaves 6 inches long, broad, ovate, and acuminate; seeds very small, black, and shining, of a strong black currant odour, and a slightly pungent taste. Root woody; knotted and bark, light brown and scabrous. The whole plant has a strong black currant odour.

Constituents.—An alkaloid—Pogostemonine, a yellow varnish of a slightly bitter taste and mouse-like odour, more soluble in chloroform than in ether; trimethylamine, a volatile principle of the odour like that of cedar wood, resin, and an astringent matter.

Actions and uses.—Stimulant; the fresh leaves are used as a poultice to clean wounds and to stimulate granulations. The root is used in India as a remedy for the bite of Phursa snake (Echis Carinata); the fresh root, about the size of an almond, is given internally three times a day and the paste of the root or poultice of the leaves is applied on the bites.

Pogostemon Patchouli.

Habitat.—Sub-tropical Himalaya, Deccan Peninsula, Penang.

Parts used.—The leaves, flowering spikes, or dried tops and root.

Vernacular.—Bomb.—Phangla. Beng.—Patcha, Patchauli. Guz.—Pácha, Nadadá. Malyal.—Kottam. Tam.—Kattam.

Characters.—The drug consists of broken stem and leaves; stem ascending, quadrangular, hairy and of a dark brown or reddish colour, slender and pithy; leaves thick, hairy, obtuse, ovate, cordate, crenate, serrated, and of a dark brown colour; spikes terminal and axillary and densely crowded with flowers; aroma fragrant and agreeable, more powerful than that derived from many other plants; when pure the odour is musty like that of Lycopodium, or of old clothes; taste camphoraceous.

Constituents.—The dried tops yield by distillation a strong scented volatile oil called oil of Patchouli.

Preparations.—Infusion (1 in 10). Dose, ½ to 1 fld. oz.

Actions and uses.—Diuretic and carminative; generally given along with tulasi bija in scanty urine and in biliousness. As an insectifuge the herb is kept in the wardrobe to drive away flees, ants, moths, gnats, and mosquitoes; also used as a perfume to prevent ravages of moths and insects in shawls and woollen clothes.

Rosmarinus Officinalis, B.P.

Habitat.—Mediterranean Basin, Asia Minor.

Parts used.—A volatile oil distilled from the flowering tops.—Oleum Rosmarini, B. P.

Vernacular.—Arab.—Aklil-ul-Jabbi. Eng.—Common Rosemary, Garden Rosemary.

Characters.—A shrub; leaves, ever green, very long, linear, blunt at both ends, margins resolute, dark green, shining above and woolly, with white stellate hairs beneath; odour pungently aromatic and camphor-like; taste bitter; flowers large, bilabiate and bright blue.

Constituents.—The flowering tops contain a volatile oil, resin, tannin and a bitter principle. Oleum Rosmarini is a colourless, pale yellow liquid with odour of the plant and warm camphoraceous taste, readily soluble in alcohol (1 in 2). It consists of a terpene isomeric with turpentine and a body allied to camphor. It is an ingredient of Linimentum Saponis. Dose, ½ to 3 ms.

Preparations.—Spiritus Rosmarini, B.P. (1 in 10). Dose, 10 to 30 ms.

Actions and uses.—Carminative, stimulant and diuretic; also emmenagogue and diaphoretic; given in hysteria, headache, neuralgias and other nervous disorders; also in flatulence, menstrual disorders; chiefly used as a stimulant liniment for sprains, bruises and rheumatism and as a lotion combined with cantharides in alopecia; it stimulates the growth of hair.

Salvia Hæmatodes.

Habitat.—Throughout India.

Parts used.—The root.

Vernacular.—Arab.—Behen. Beng.—Lal Behaman. Bomb.—Lála Bahamana. Eng.—Blood veined sage. Hind.—Lála Bahamana. Pers.—Bahaman-i-surkha.

Characters.—The root which closely resembles that of Pæony is shrivelled, and of the shape of quills; each piece from 2 to 3 inches long, about the size of a little finger, and of a reddish brown colour; bark soft and can easily be scratched; surface marked with scars of fallen rootlets; substance very compact and of a brownish red colour; smell like that of salama; taste slightly bitter and resembling musali.

Constituents.—Fat, tannic acid, and a bitter crystalline alkaloid, Bahmanine.

Actions and uses.—Tonic, astringent, and aphrodisiac. It is one of the ingredients of various compound astringent decoctions and aphrodisiac confections. Largely used among the natives for seminal debility, chlorosis, anæmia, amenorrhœa, &c.

Salvia Officinalis—Garden sage.

Habitat.—S. Europe.

Parts used.—The leaves.

Vernacular.—Eng.—Common or garden sage. Hind.—Salbia. Tam.—Sefa-kas.

Characters.—Perennial plant; leaves petiolate, ovate, oblong, obtuse at apex, rounded and heart-shaped at base; finely crenulate, thick and wrinkled, of a greyish green colour, hairy, soft and glandular beneath, of a strong fragrant or aromatic odour and bitter astringent taste. Dose, 20 to 30 grs.

Constituents.—Volatile oil, bitter principle, tannin, resin, extractive and albumen. The volatile oil is greenish or yellowish fluid, soluble in alcohol, and it is composed of terpene, pinene, cineol and salvial (thujone).

Preparations.—Infusion (1 in 20). Dose, 1 to 2 fld. ozs.

Actions and uses.—Stimulant, tonic, anti-emetic, carminative and astringent; used in fevers, dyspepsia, to check sweatings and colloquative sweats of phthisis, in flatulence, as a gargle in sore throat, ulcers in the mouth and relaxed uvula.

Salvia Plebeia, S. Brachiata and S. Ægyptica.

Habitat.—Many parts of India, Bengal, Oude, Khandalla, Sind, Beluchistan.

Parts used.—The seeds.

Vernacular.—Chin.—Chin-khing-kai. Guz.—Kammor kasa, Bijabuda. Panj.—Sammudar saka, sathi.

Kamarkasa, from kummar, which means waist or loins, and Kasa, to bind. It gives tone to the weak loins.

Characters.—Seeds very small, ellipsoid, smooth and of a brown colour, smaller than tukhmaria, oblong and angular at their attachment to the umbilicus with a very small white scar; surface rugous; those of S. Egyptica are larger; taste oily and mucilaginous.

Constituents.—Albuminoid 12 p.c.; oil 18·6 p.c.; gum, fibre 44 p c.; and ash 15 p. c. No alkaloid.

Actions and uses.—Demulcent and nutritive; used in gonorrhœa, and menorrhagia. They are also given to promote sexual powers like many other demulcent and nutritive drugs, and also used in leucorrhœa and seminal weakness.

Scutellaria Lateriflora.

Habitat.—Moist places and along ditches, N. America.

Parts used.—The herb.

Syn.—Blue skull cap, helmet flowers, hooded willow herb, mad weed.

Characters.—Perennial herb; stems erect and smooth; leaves ovate, acuminate, opposite, serrate and petiolate; flowers in racemes, one-sided and leafy; corolla pale blue, bilabiate; calyx closed, upper lip helmet-shaped; odour slight and taste bitter.

Constituents.—A bitter principle, volatile oil, fat, tannin, sugar and ash. The bitter principle is a crystalline glucoside, soluble in ether.

Preparations.—Fluid extract. Dose, ½ to 1 fld. dr. Decoction (1 in 20). Dose, 1 to 2 fld. ozs.

Actions and uses.—Nervine tonic and antispasmodic; given to calm the nervous system as in restlessness, tremors, spasms, twitching of muscles, hyperæsthesia, and in nervous exhaustion, due to fatigue or over excitement; also in epilepsy, hysteria, chorea, insomnia, delirium tremens, neuralgias, hydrophobia, convulsions, tetanus and hiccough.

Thymus Serpyllum, T. Vulgaris.

Habitat.—W. Temperate Himalaya, France, Persia, S.-W. Europe.

Parts used.—A volatile oil, oleum thymi, distilled from the leaves and flowering tops.

Vernacular.—Eng.—Wild thyme, common garden thyme—mother of thyme. Hind.—Ipar. Indian Bazaar.—Hâshâ. Panj.—Masho. Pers.—Hâsha.

Characters.—Small common shrub; stems and branches quadrangular; bark pale brown; leaves ½ inch long, oval, blunt, entire, margin revolute, thick and smooth; flowers in cymes, pale purple; odour aromatic.

Constituents.—A volatile oil, tannin and gum. The oil of thyme, also known as oleum origani, or oleum thymi, is a yellowish liquid, odour strong, of thyme; taste, aromatic, cooling and pungent; of a neutral reaction; on exposure, it darkens and thickens with age; soluble in alcohol (1 in 2), carbon sulphide, and in glacial acetic acid. It contains thymol, carvacrol, cymene and thymene.

Thymol, B.P., Thymylic alcohol, Thymic acid. It is a stearopten obtained from the oil of garden thyme, horse mint, Bishop's weed, &c. To obtain it saponify the oil with caustic soda; add hot water to the solution to separate the sodium thymol from thymene, and the oil will float on the top. Treat the oil with hydrochloric acid, or expose the oil to spontaneous evaporation when thymol will be set free. Thymol so prepared is next subjected to freezing to purify it and then recrystallised. When prepared from ptychotis ajowan, it is known as ajmana phul (Indian Bazaar). It occurs in oblique, large, colourless crystals of the strong odour of mint; taste pungent and aromatic; almost insoluble in cold water (1 in 1,200), freely soluble in alcohol, ether, chloroform, olive oil, glacial acetic acid and alkalies. It forms a liquid combination with chloral, camphor or carbolic acid. Dose, ½ to 2 grs. Carvacrol—Cymenol, is a liquid constituent of the oils of origanum, thymol, &c. Dose, 2 to 8 grs. used in pills. Carvacrol Iodide or Iodocrol—an iodine compound of carvacrol; it is a yellowish white powder without any odour. Dose, 2 to 8 grs. used as pills—as an antiseptic, given in gout Cymine and thymene are hydrocarbons and very volatile.

Preparations.—Of Thymol; ointment (10 to 30 grs. to an oz.) is used to keep off mosquitoes; and in eczema, ring worm, &c. Vapour or inhalation of Thymol 6 grs. to an oz. with light carbonate of magnesia. Dose, a teaspoonful in a pint of hot water; used for pharyngitis, laryngitis. The dusting powder Thymolite is a combination of silicate of alumina and thymol. Liquor Thymol (1 in 800), used for burns—Thymol gauze and wool 3 p.c., Pastillus Thymol, $\frac{1}{32}$ gr. each. Spiritus Thymol (1 in 10). Dose, 3 to 15 ms. Antiseptic fluid contains Thymol 1, alcohol 10, glycerin 20 and water 100.

Actions and uses.—The oil is stimulant, tonic, emmenagogue and antispasmodic and given in inveterate cough, combined with vinegar and salt, to facilitate expectoration. As a nervine sedative, it is given in epilepsy, difficulty of breathing, and asthma, in diarrhœa, gleet, gonorrhœa, leucorrhœa, vesical catarrh and in dyspepsia with flatulence. As a local stimulating liniment it is applied with vinegar, to remove callosities and warts; with olive oil, in diseases of the joints, in sprains and bruises. The seeds are used as vermifuge. Fresh Thyme is used as a condiment to aid digestion of fat pork, also to flavour insipid dishes. As an antiseptic it is superior to, but as a disinfectant it is equal to carbolic acid; for other actions it ranks between carbolic acid and oil turpentine. It is also anæsthetic and local irritant to the skin and mucous membranes. Internally in large doses it paralyses the end organs of sensory nerves and the nerve centres in the spinal cord and in the medulla. In poisonous doses, it produces a sensation of heat in the epigastrum, ringing in the ears, deafness, profuse sweating, irritation of the kidneys, leading to increased secretion of urine which assumes dark green colour, and of the respiratory mucous membrane, leading to extreme prostration, coma and death. It it given in typhoid and other specific fevers, diabetes, diphtheria, whooping cough, phthisis, intestinal affections, vesical catarrh, in tuberculosis, in chyluria, worms, in gastric fermentation and in rheumatism. Locally as an antiseptic it is used like carbolic acid in surgical dressings, and as an ointment. It keeps off mosquitoes; also used in psoriasis, ringworm, eczema &c.; as a spray or inhalation it is used in whooping cough, diphtheria, coryza, inflammation of the pharynx and larynx, and sometimes even in bronchitis and phthisis; as a gargle in sore throat, and bronchiectasis; as a mouth wash it removes the odour of tobacco from the breath. As an injection it is used in ozæna, otorrhœa, gonorrhœa ; also in uterine leucorrhœa ; as a wash for wounds, ulcers, skin diseases. Thymacetin is a derivative to thymol, as phenacetin is to phenol. It is a white crystalline powder, slightly soluble in water ; used in neuralgia, headache, like phenacetin. Dose, 5 to 15 grs.

Zataria Multiflora.

Habitat.—Europe, N. America, Arabia, Persia.

Parts used.—The herb in flower, stems and leaves.

Vernacular.—Hind. Bomb.—Sathara. Ind. Bazars.—Satar. Arab.—Baklat-ul Jazal. Pers.—Onsh neh. Tam.—Mridu-marur vamu.

Characters.—Stems very slender ; bark whitish and covered with hairs; leaves thick, oblong, ovate, rounded and studded with numerous pits on both their surfaces, each pit containing granules of red essential oil; flowers very small, of a light brown colour and studded with hairs ; calyx marked with numerous pits, colour lightish brown ; odour agreeable and aromatic ; taste lemon-like, pungent at first, but after a time giving a kind of burning sensation to the tongue, resembling the taste of Ajmo or lemon Thyme.

Constituents.—The leaves contain resin, tannin, an aromatic essential oil, of a minty odour and an alkaloid bitter principle.

Preparations.—Infusion (1 in 10). Dose, ½ to 1 fld. oz.

Actions and uses.—Stimulant, aromatic and diaphoretic. Like Thyme, it is given in biliousness, gastric irritation, fevers, &c.

Ziziphora Tennior.

Habitat.—Persia, Baluchistan.

Parts used.—The flowering plant.

Vernacular.—Eng.—Wild thyme. Ind. Bazaar.—Mishk-i-taramashia. Pers.—Ranga Shiraz.

Characters.—Stems quadrangular, slightly furrowed, of a greenish brown colour and covered with small hairs, about 1 to 3 or 4 inches long; leaves thick, of a brown colour, thickly studded with hairs and marked with numerous pits ; smell rather aromatic, taste like that of dried phudino, but sweeter ; ovaries 4, distinct, lobes erect, attached to one another at their base and separated a little below the middle, the lobes appearing as if they were 4 distinct fruits, placed around one another. Each lobe of a lightish brown colour, tapering below and marked with 8 to 12 strong nerves. Between the nerves are pale white hairs. At the margin of the apex of each lobe there are from 8 to 12 teeth lying horizontally and within which there is a circle of long hairs. In the middle of the hairs there is a hole from which the seeds escape ; seeds angular and of a darkish brown colour.

Preparations.—Infusion (1 in 20). Dose, ½ to 1 fld. oz.

Actions and uses.—Stimulant, carminative, lithontriptic, emmenagogue and expectorant ; similar to Phudina, and Badaranboye ; large doses cause hæmaturia ; given in cough and other chest affections, and in uterine diseases such as amenorrhœa, dysmenorrhœa, &c.

Phytolaccaceæ—The Virginian Poke-weed family.

Herbs or under shrubs, leaves alternate, exstipulate, entire ; flowers perfect, racemose ; calyx 4 to 5 partite ; stamens hypogynous ; anthers 2-celled ; ovary, superior, several celled ; carpels many, united in a ring, each forming a berry ; fruit dry or succulent ; seed, ascending ; embryo, curved, mealy and albuminous.

Habitat.—Native of temperate climate and tropics, India, Africa.

Properties.—Emetic, purgative. The acrid principle is destroyed by boiling in water.

Phytolacca Decandra.

Habitat.—N. America, W. Indies, S. Europe.

Parts used.—The fruit and root.

Characters—A perennial plant ; leaves alternate, entire, exstipulate ; flowers perfect, racemose ; fruit a berry, purplish black, globular, depressed, compound, berry composed of 10 carpels, each $\frac{1}{3}$ inch in diameter with one lenticular black seed. The juice is purplish red, without any odour and sweet acrid taste ; the clusters when dried resemble grapes or raisins. The root is large, conical and branched ; fleshy, thick, in transverse or longitudinal slices, wrinkled, of a greyish colour and of a fibrous texture. It is without any odour ; taste sweet and acrid. The wood is in several distinct concentric circles. Dose of the fruit, 10 to 30 grs. Dose of the root as an emetic, 10 to 30 grs., as an alterative, 1 to 5 grs.

Constituents.—The fruit contains phytolaccic acid, colouring matter, starch, sugar, gum. The root contains resin, glucoside, starch, tannin, mucilage, volatile oil, waxy matter, sugar, and ash containing mostly calcium malate.

Preparations.—Of the fruit. Infusion (1 in 10). Dose, 4 to 6 drs., Tincture (1 in 10). Dose, 10 to 30 ms. Decoction (4 in 10). Dose, 4 to 6 drs.

Actions and uses—Emetic and cathartic. Its action is slow but persistent, causing nausea and great depression. It depresses the heart and respiration, paralyses the spinal cord and the medulla, leading to tetanic convulsions and death. It is antagonistic to motor excitants, such as alcohol, ether, opium, digitalis, &c. As an alterative it is given in scrofula, syphilis, malignant tumours, varicose ulcers eczema, sycosis and chronic rheumatism. The root is antisyphilitic, hepatic stimulant, narcotic and resolvent, and given in orchitis, mastitis and epididymitis. Locally a powdered extract with extract of belladonna is used as an inunction over painful testes and mammæ. In tonsillitis, diphtheria and chronic pharyngitis, it is given internally and painted locally. In glandular enlargements, hæmorrhoids, fissures of the rectum and prolapsus ani, its application is similar in action to those of dulcamara and veratrum. The berries are sudorific and given in chronic rheumatism and syphilis.

Plantaginaceæ—The Rib wort or Ispaghula family.

Herbs generally without aerial stems ; leaves radical and ribbed ; flowers usually small, perfect ; spikes rarely solitary, sometimes unisexual; calyx 4 partite; corolla 4 partite, membranous; ovary simple, 2 to 4 celled ; fruit capsular, dehiscent ; seeds one or many, mucilaginous ; embryo, fleshy and albuminous.

Habitat.—Native of cold and temperate climates.

Properties.—The seeds of some species are demulcent and used like those of linseed. The roots of some are bitter and astringent.

Plantago Ispaghula, P. Ovata, P. Amplexicaulis.

Habitat.—Punjab, Sind, Persia, cultivated in India.

Parts used.—The seeds.

Vernacular.—Arab.—Bazre-katunâ. Beng.—Eshopghôl. Can.—Isabakolu. Eng.—Spage seeds. Bom., Guz., Mar., Duk., Hind.—Uthamu Jirun, Ispaghol. Pers.—Ispazah, Shikam-daridah. Tam.—Iskôl-virai. Tel.—Isapagala.

Characters.—Seeds ovate, elliptical, concave, half an inch long, boat-shaped, translucent, and of a pale brown colour with a pinkish tinge. On their convex side is a ridge which commences at one end of the seed and disappears about its middle in an oblong scar. On their concave surface is a deep channel which is widest in the middle and becomes narrower as it approaches the end. In the centre is a scar of a brown colour, and somewhat bifid. It resembles in appearance the foot mark of a calf's hoof on a soft clay. They are mucilaginous to taste and free from odour.

Preparations.—Decoction (1 in 10). Dose, 2 to 4 ozs.

Actions and uses.—Demulcent, emollient and diuretic ; used in inflammatory and other derangements of the stomach and intestines, as in gastric catarrh, dysentery, gonorrhœa and affections of the kidneys. Made into a poultice with vinegar and gora tela they are applied to rheumatic and gouty swellings; they are also useful in coughs and colds. When roasted, they are used with sâkara in protracted irritation of the bowels in children. Dose, of the seeds, 1 to 2 drs.

P. amplexicaulis is found in Punjab and Sind. It furnishes brown Ispaghul known as ejaj-pipli (Hind).

Plantago Lanceolata.

Habitat.—Europe and United States.

Parts used.—The leaves.

Preparations.—Fluid extract. Dose, 5 to 15 ms. The juice preserved in alcohol or glycerin. Dose, 20 to 50 ms. The paste of pounded leaves with glycerin. The dried leaves powdered.

Actions and uses.—The juice in large doses is used to check internal hæmorrhages or hæmorrhagical fluxes, menorrhagia, leucorrhœa, &c. The leaves are astringent and styptic. Its styptic properties are partly mechanical and partly physiological ; it causes stasis in the capillaries. The leaves when chewed relieve toothache. A poultice of the leaves is used in painful affections as mastitis, erysipelas, burns, scalds, bruises and wounds.

Plantago Major, Plantago Psyllium.

Habitat.—Persia, Temperate India, Panjab.

Parts used.—The seeds.

Vernacular.—Arab.—Lásána-el-hamala. Hind., Bomb.—Baratunga. Eng.—Greater plantain, cart track plant, way bread. Indian Bazaars—Bartang. Pers.—Tukhm-i-baratunga, Tukhm-e-bárhanga.

Characters.—Seeds small, oblong, or irregularly angled, of a darkish brown colour, and marked with longitudinal convolute lines, in size resembling asali, but somewhat smaller ; taste insipid and mucilaginous, like ispaghula ; smell oily when crushed. Soaked in water they become coated with mucilage. Dose, 30 to 90 grs.

Constituents.—Chlorophyll, resin, wax, albumen, pectin, sugar and a large quantity of mucilage.

Preparations.—Cold infusion (1 in 5). Dose 2 to 4 fld. ozs.

Actions and uses.—Demulcent ; used like ispaghula. With cardamoms and sugar candy it is given in urinary disorders and dysentery ; also used in arresting fluxes and griping pain in the bowels.

Nyctaginaceæ—The Marvel of Peru or Gulabasa family.

Herbs, shrubs, or trees ; stems tumid at the joints ; leaves opposite : flowers showy and with an involucre ; calyx tubular, funnel-shaped ; stamens one or many, hypogynous ; ovary, superior ; ovule solitary, stigma 1 ; fruit a utricle, enclosed by a hard calyx ; seed solitary, containing mealy albumen.

Habitat.—Native of warm regions.

Properties.—The roots of some species are purgative, some are expectorant, alterative and astringent.

Boerhavia Diffusa, B. Erecta, B. Procumbens, B. Repens.

Habitat.—Throughout India, Coromandel, Travancore.

Parts used.—The herb and root.

Vernacular.—Beng.—Swhet-poorna, Puneranabha. Cing.—Jantops. Can.—Bileganjali. Eng.—Spreading hog-weed. Guz.—Vakhakhapara ; Sadodi. Duk., Hind.—Besha-khapara, Thikri, Sant. Mar.—Punanava, Kalivasu, Ghetuli. Malyal.—Taludama. San.—Visha Khara-para, Sothaghni, Puna-ranava. Tam.—Mukku-rattai-kiray. Tel.—Atika-inâmidi.

Sothaghni sotha, or soja, a general swelling, and ghni, to kill. It means a killer or curer of swellings or dropsy. Punaranava Punaha, again, and Nava, new or fresh. The plant has a perennial habit; it develops afresh or becomes new again every year. It grows during the rains from the old and the same root.

Characters.—Two varieties; the red and the white. Creeping plant with diffuse stalks. Flowers, pale rose coloured and scattered in long branches; root of a light brown colour, as thick as a man's finger, and from 6 to 18 inches long; root bark longitudinally furrowed and marked with knotty scars of fallen rootlets; seeds brown, oblong, striated and rough; root tough, white and starchy when cut, smell somewhat aromatic; taste corky and somewhat acrid, also bitter and nauseous.

Preparations.—Decoction (1 in 20). Dose, 1 to 2 fld. ozs.

Actions and uses.—Stomachic, laxative, diuretic, expectorant, and emetic; given in asthma, gonorrhœa, dropsy, jaundice, enlargement of the liver and spleen, ascites, anasarca, scanty urine, and internal inflammations. As a remedy for scorpion bites, it is applied externally and given internally. Pounded leaves are applied over œdematous swellings.

Mirabilis Jalapa.

Habitat.—West Indies.

Parts used.—The leaves and root.

Vernacular.—Arab.—Shab-el-bili. Beng.—Krishna-keli. Burm.—Mizu-bin. Can.—Chandra-mallige. Cing.—Sindrika-gahâ. Mar., Guz., Hind., Duk.—Gulâ-bâsh. Malyal.—Anti-mantâram. Eng.—Marvel of Peru, four-o'clock plant. Pers.—Gule-a-abbâsa. Sans.—Sandhyakeli, Krishna-keli. Tam.—Anthinarlu. Tel.—Chandra-kanta.

Mirabilis means wonderful. It is in allusion to the flowers being of variegated or wonderful colours. The root was formerly supposed to be the true jalap plant, and hence the specific name M. Jalapa.

Characters.—Plant perennial, herbaceous, dichotomous; leaves thick, ovate, acuminate, smooth and of a dark green colour; flowers red, white or yellow, opening at sunset, and hence called four-o'clock plant; seeds black, muricated and of the size of pepper; tuber cylindrical above and tapering below and starchy; externally dark brown with circular rings, internally dirty white or greyish; transverse section, presenting concentric rings. The seeds are used to adulterate black pepper.

Constituents.—The root contains an alkaloid, and ash 6 p.c. free from manganese.

Preparations.—Infusion of the root (1 in 10). Dose, 1 to 2 fld. ozs.

Actions and uses.—The juice of the leaves is applied to wounds and bruises. The leaves boiled are applied as stimulating poultice to boils and buboes to hasten suppuration. The tuber is used as a poultice on carbuncles. The root has mildly purgative properties similar to those of Jalap.

Amaranthaceæ—The Amaranth, Cholai bhaji or Aghada family.

Characters.—Herbs or shrubs; stems striated, green or red coloured; leaves entire, wrinkled, simple, exstipulate, opposite, or alternate, generally oval, oblong, rhomboid shaped, and green or variously coloured; flowers small spiked, panicled, crowded or capitated, bracteated, occasionally unisexual, often having distinct sexes; clayx 3-5; stamens 5, hypogynous; ovary free, 1-celled; fruit an utricle, caryopsis, or berry; seed one or more, black, pendulous, and affixed to a central receptacle; albumen, mealy.

Habitat.—Tropical regions.

Properties.—Several species are mucilaginous, diuretic and astringent; some of them contain a large quantity of khâra or ashes.

Achyranthes Aspera, A. Obtusifolia, A Indica, A. Spicatus.

Habitat.—India.

Parts used.—The herb.

Vernacular.—Arab.—Atkumah. Beng.—Apang. Duk., Bomb. —Aghada. Burm.—Apang. Can.—Utrâni. Cing.—Gaskaral-Lebbo. Eng.—Prickly chaff flower. Guz.—Jhinjarwat. Hind.—Chirchira, Latchiræ, Agareh. Mar.—Pandhra-Aghada utrani. Malyal.—Katalâti. Pers.—Khâre-Vâzhgûnâh. Sans.—Apâamragaha, Khara-manjare, Ash-Agada-khâra. Tam.—Nâ-yurivi. Tel—Antisâ-Apâmargamu.

The word Apámarga is from Apá or Ab, water, and Marga, a washerman. This is in allusion to a large quantity of alkaline ashes the fruits contain, and which is used by washermen, along with water for cleaning clothes.

Characters.—Plant herbaceous, erect; root angular and longitudinally furrowed, colour greenish or reddish; leaves opposite and obovate; margins wavy; surface covered with whitish hairs, spikes terminal, long, and generally curved about the middle; flowers small and of a reddish colour; bracts green, old bracts tough, rigid, prickly, and adhering to the clothes; fruits conical, covered with sharp pointed bracts, and containing numerous seeds; seeds oblong and of a shining pale brown colour; taste like that of Bájari grams. The drug sold in the bazaar under the name of Aghada bija is the whole fruit.

Constituents.—The fruit contains a large percentage of alkaline ash containing potash.

Preparations.—Decoction and infusion of leaves (1 in 10). Dose, 1 to 2 fld. ozs. Khâr prepared by incineration of the plant. It is used in preparing alkaline preparations. Juice from the fresh herb. Paste and medicated oil.

Actions and uses.—Astringent, diuretic and alterative; given in menorrhagia, diarrhœa and dysentery Khar is largely used in anasarca, ascites and dropsy. It is also given in cutaneous affections and enlargements of glands, and to loosen expectoration in cough. It has a great reputation in dog-bites, and bites of snakes and other venomous reptiles, for which purpose it is given internally and also applied externally. The juice is sometimes applied in toothache and the paste as eye-salve (ânjan) in opacity of the cornea. A medicated oil is dropped into the ear in deafness and noises in the ears.

Ærva Javanica, Æ. Lanata, Achyranthes Lanata, A. Villosa, Illecebrum Lanatum.

Habitat.—Plains of India.

Parts used.—The herb.

Vernacular.—Duk.—Khul. Beng., Hind.—Chaya. Malyal.—Sherupala. Mar.—Kumra pendi, kapur-madhura. Ind. Bazar., Panj.—Bhui, kallan. Tam.—Sirru pulai. Tel.—Pendi conda.

Characters.—Leaves woolly, silvery-looking; flowers minute, white, in dense terminal spikes; calyx 5, hairy; sepals 5; stamens united into a cup at their base. Fruit roundish and an utricle.

Preparation.—Decoction (1 in 10). Dose, 1 to 2 fld. ozs.

Actions and uses.—Demulcent and diuretic; used in the treatment of lithiasis, strangury, gonorrhœa, &c. Also used by the natives as an antidote against poisoning by arsenic.

Amarantus Spinosus.

Habitat.—Southern India, Burma.

Parts used.—The leaves and roots.

Vernacular.—Beng.—Kântâ-nutia. Burm.—Hinkanœ-sûbâ Can.—Mulla-dantu. Bomb., Duk.—Kânterimât. Eng.—Thorny amaranth. Guz.—Kântalo-dâmbho. Hind.—Cholai. Malyal.—Mallan-chira. Sans—Tan-dulbija. Tam.—Mulluk-kire. Tel.—Erra-mulu, goranta.

Characters.—Plant erect, from 1 to 3 feet in height; root tapering and of a pinkish colour, here and there giving off a few fibres; taste somewhat sweetish and astringent; stem striated and of a green or reddish colour, surface rugous; leaves long, petioled, rhombo-ovate or lanceolate, oblong, and with sharp spines on the axes of the leaves, which are channelled. Flowers axillary and terminal, males above and females beneath.

Preparations.—Infusion and decoction (1 in 10). Dose, 1 to 2 fld. ozs.

Actions and uses.—Demulcent, astringent and diuretic. A poultice of the leaves is used as an application over unhealthy sores. The root is given in combination with other astringents in menorrhagia and in gonorrhœa. Its ashes are used for the same purposes as the ashes of Aghada, a paste of which is applied in eczema.

Celosia Argentea, C. Crestata, Amaranthus Polygamus, A. Hypochondriacus.

Habitat.—Throughout India, Tropical Asia.

Parts used.—The seeds, leaves and root.

Vernacular. — Beng. — Svet-murga. Can. — Goraji. Eng. — Prince's feathers, cock's comb. Guz.—Lapadi, safed murgha, Sarwari. Hind.—Sarwari, Deokoti. Mur.—Koordoo. Tel.—Gurugu.

Characters.—Seeds lenticular, brown, roundish, smooth, shining, convex, on both surfaces, in form resembling a curry dish ; colour black, testa hard ; taste slightly bitter and pea-like ; root of a pinkish red colour ; leaves roundish or variously shaped, margin red.

Constituents.—The seeds contain an oil, resin, starch, extractive, an alkaloid and ash.

Preparations.—Decoction or infusion (1 in 10). Dose, 1 to 2 fld. ozs., poultice of leaves.

Actions and uses.—Astringent and nervine tonic ; given in diarrhœa, seminal debility, leucorrhœa, and menorrhagia ; a poultice of the leaves with rarwanti and besmeared with honey is used as a cooling anodyne application to inflamed and painful parts.

Chenopodiaceæ.—The Palaka, Goose-foot or Spinach family.

General Characters.—Herbs or under shrubs ; leaves alternate, rarely opposite, exstipulate, and polygamous ; calyx persistent, stamens hypogynous, ovary superior, 1-celled ; fruit an utricle, achœnium or sometimes baccate ; seed solitary.

Habitat.—Universal, saline places.

Properties.—Many plants of this order are succulent, as the beet-root ; some of them are used as pot herbs ; seeds of some are nutritious. Several contain a volatile oil which renders them anthelmintic, antispasmodic, aromatic, carminative and stimulant. Several of them inhabit salt marshes and yield on combustion an ash called Barilla, known to the Greeks as salt-wort. The Arabs called it elkali, arkali, or ushnar, sujikhâra (Hind.)—a mixture of potash and soda.

Chenopodium Ambrosioides, C. Anthelminticum—American worm-seed.

Wild worm-seed, stinking weed, Jesuit tea, goose-foot.

Habitat.—West Indies (waste places), United States, Europe, Africa.

Part used.—The fruit.

Characters.—Fruit of the size of a pin's head, depressed, globular, and greenish yellow, containing an obtusely edged lenticular black seed ; seed glossy, odour terebinthinate, taste bitter and pungent. Dose, 10 to 30 grs.

Constituents.—Oleum chenopodii, a volatile oil, 3 p.c., obtained by distilling the fruit with water or steam. It is a thin yellowish liquid, of a highly camphoraceous odour and pungent bitter taste. It consists of a hydrocarbon and a liquid oxygenated oil. Dose, 4 to 10 ms.

Preparations.—Expressed juice. Dose, 2 to 4 fld. drs. Decoction (1 in 10). Dose, 1 to 2 fld. ozs. Fluid extract. Dose, 10 to 40 ms.

Actions and uses.—Anthelmintic; used chiefly for round worms. As an antispasmodic and stimulant, the oil is given in hysteria, chorea, flatulent dyspepsia, and malarial and intermittent fevers. It increases the action of the heart and promotes the secretion of the skin, kidneys and bronchi.

Beta Vulgaris—Common Beet, Garden Beet, Sugar Beet.

Habitat.—Europe, Africa, Asia.

Parts used.—The root.

Characters.—The roots are tapering, colour dark red, very tender, and of a sweet taste; cultivated as a source of sugar.

Constituents.—An active principle betin. Dose, 3 to 8 grs.

Preparations.—Infusion; decoction (1 in 10) Dose, 2 to 6 drs.

Actions and uses.—Aperient, resolvent, and emmenagogue; given in disordered secretions of the stomach and intestines, in atonic dyspepsia, constipation, and in hæmorrhoids.

Spinacea Oleracea—S. Setrandra.

Habitat.—Persia, India.

Parts used.—The herb and fruit.

Vernacular.—Arab.—Ispanaj. Eng.—Spinach. Beng., Bomb., Hind.—Sag, Pâluk, Chular, Ispanak. Pers.—Burhân-palak. Tam.—Vusoyley-keeray.

Characters.—Leaves thick, succulent, deep green, of a triangular form; stem erect, large, round and hollow; fruit prickly, of a brown colour, containing one seed, triangular, each angle terminating in two or more channelled tapering points or spines, darkish red, ovate, flat, and slightly pointed at the apex; surface rugous and wrinkled; taste acidulous.

Constituents.—A large quantity of mucilage, alkaline nitrates, fat and sugar.

Preparations.—Infusion and decoction (1 in 10). Dose, 1 to 2 fld. ozs.

Actions and uses.—Demulcent, diuretic, and astringent; used in fever, inflammation of the lungs and bowels, hurried breathing, biliary derangements, and as a lithontriptic in urinary calculi. The juice of the leaves is used as a gargle in sore throat.

Walsura Piscidia, Trichilia Emetica, Trichilia Trifoliata.

Habitat.—Malabar, W. Peninsula, Ceylon, Travancore.

Parts used.—The bark, and fruit.

Vernacular.—Arab.—Jauz-el-kai. Eng.—Emetic nut. Tam., Tel.—Walurosi.

Characters.—Bark $\frac{1}{4}$ inch thick, suber thick, brown, fissured longitudinally, generally in flakes ; liber hard, compact, and of a cinnamon colour ; taste bitter and astringent.

Constituents.—The bark contains resin, saponin and tannin.

Perparations.—Decoction (1 in 10). Dose, 2 to 4 drs.

Actions and uses.—The bark is stimulant and expectorant. It acts as a fish poison ; the fish so caught is not unwholesome to eat. The fruit is used in hair washes to kill lice, remove freckles, and to cure itch.

Polygonaceæ.—The Gul-i-hamaza or Buckwheat family.

General Characters.—Herbs or rarely shrubs ; leaves alternate, with a long petiole, attached to the stem by a sheath ; stem consisting of many swollen joints ; flowers sometimes unisexual ; calyx, persistent ; stamens, hypogynous ; ovary, superior, ovule, solitary ; fruit a nut, usually triangular ; seeds solitary and erect, embryo with starchy albumen.

Habitat.—Universal, temperate regions.

Properties.—Most plants are acidulous, astringent and purgative. The fruits and roots of some are more or less nutritious. The acidulous character is due to its containing oxalic and malic acids. The root of Rheum contains an abundance of oxalate of lime crystals.

Emex Sp. ?

Habitat.—Persia.

Parts used.—The herb.

Vernacular.—Arab.—Afsharniki. Shankat-el-baida. Bomb.—Shukai. Guz., Hind.—Shukai. Pers.—Kangara khára.

Characters.—Drug of a light brown or yellowish colour, consisting of pieces of stems, branchlets, portions of the roots, leaves and fruits. Stems round or triangular, furrowed and channelled, rugous externally ; epidermis thin ; interior full of soft pith. Branchlets and spines are channelled. Spines broad at the base and needle-pointed at the apex. Root knotty, and here and there marked with scars of leaf sheaths. Leaves toothed, lobed, thick, downy and leathery, each lobe ending in a spine. Fruits small, erect, and supported on a short stalk. From base of the fruit project 6 to 7 very small segments of the calyx, within which is the ovary surrounded by 7 or 8 erect, tooth-like processes. Seeds oblong, or triangular, of a brownish colour, and tough ; odour rather pungent and oily. The whole drug is aromatic and of a gummy or corky taste.

Constituents.—Resin and an alkaloid.

Preparations.—Decoction (1 in 10). Dose, 1 to 2 fld. ozs.

Actions and uses.—The whole plant is astringent, demulcent, and deobstruent. It is used in coughs and ague. The hakims generally use it for the same purposes as Bádávarda (Fagonia Arabica). Shukáyi is also a Marathi name for Tricholepis procumbens of the N. O. Compositæ, the spiny fruits of which resemble those of Shukayi.

Polygonum Aviculare, P. Bistorta.

Habitat.—Universal.

Parts used.—The root and seeds.

Vernacular.—Arab.—Asár-râi, Anjubar. Eng.—Knot grass. Hind.—Kuwar, Machoti, Nisomali, Bijband. Pers.—Hozâr bandak. Sans.—Miromati. Sind.—Endrâni.

Characters.—P. Aviculare. Root fibrous, very tough and somewhat woody. Stems several and spreading, leafy at the numerous knots or joints; seeds acutely triangular and black, and of a shining lustre.

P. Bistorta: Rhizome, S-shaped, bistorted, 2 inches long, and flattened, upper side striate, under surface marked with root scars.

Constituents.—Polygonic acid, tannic and gallic acids, starch and calcium oxalate.

Preparations.—Succus or juice. Decoction (1 in 10). Dose, 1 to 2 fld. ozs.

Actions and uses.—Expectorant, diuretic, tonic, astringent, and antiperiodic; given in malarial fevers, chronic diarrhœa and lithiasis; also used in capillary bronchitis, whooping cough, and other lung affections.

Polygonum Hydropiperoides—Smart Weed, Water Pepper.

Habitat.—United States.

Parts used.—The weed.

Characters.—Leaves, narrow, lanceolate. Flowers white, with slender spikes. The weed has a pungent, and acrid taste.

Constituents.—Tannin, a pungent volatile principle, polygonic acid, having acrid properties. Polygonic acid is crystallizable, soluble in alcohol, ether and chloroform, but insoluble in water.

Preparations.—Liquid extract. Dose, 10 to 40 ms. Solid extract. Dose, 1 to 5 grs.

Actions and uses.—Diuretic, emmenagogue, and aphrodisiac. The weed is acrid and produces a sensation of heat and tingling in the stomach. It stimulates the heart, increases the arterial tension, and the body temperature, promotes the secretions of the bronchi, skin and uterus. The juice excites inflammation and even vesication of the skin. It is highly extolled as an emmenagogue in amenorrhœa.

Half drachm dose of the extract a week before the expected period is given with benefit. In functional impotence, in diarrhœa, dysentery, and gravel, it gives marked relief. As a gargle it is given in sore mouth and in mercurial salivation.

Rheum Officinale, B. P., R. Palmatum, B. P., R. Emodi, R. Moorcroftianum, R. Webbianum.

Habitat.—South-Eastern Thibet, Turkey, Shanghai, Canton, China, Himalaya, cultivated in Europe, their leaf stalks being used as a fruit.

Parts used.—The erect rhizome or so-called root, Rhei Radix, B.P., Rhubarb root.

Vernacular.—Râvande-hindi. Beng.—Revan-chini. Burm.—Ta-rak-tsha. Can.—Nal-rèvâ-chini. Chines.—Huang-hâng. Duk.—Nat-ki-rêvan-chini. Eng—Rhubarb root. Hind., Guz., Ind. Bazaar.—Rewand-chini Lakri. Mar.—Reval-chini. Panj.—Riwas. Pers.—Chukri, Rewash. Tam.—Nattu-manjat-chinak. Tel.—Nattu, reval-chinni.

Characters.—An herbaceous perennial plant; stem slender, one or two; bark pubescent, externally the upper portion is purplish and the lower one green; internally it is white, soft and juicy; taste sour and somewhat astringent. The root, deprived of the corky layer, is the rhubarb. Good rhubarb should be moderately heavy, compact, and brittle, cylindrical or in conical or flattish segments, generally smooth or wrinkled, covered with yellowish or reddish brown powder and marked with whitish meshes, in which are found white spongy tissue. Internally it is white, with many red medullary rays; the odour is aromatic and peculiar. Taste bitter and astringent; the root is gritty when chewed between the teeth and colours the saliva yellow. It imparts its virtues to water and alcohol. Chinese rhubarb is the best. It is of a saffron colour, has a fractured surface, and is friable. Dose, as a stomachic, 3 to 10 grs.; as a purgative, 15 to 30 grs.

Constituents.—Resins as phœoretin, aporetin and erythroretin; chrysophan 0·14 p.c., chrysophanic acid 5 p c.; emodin 2 p.c.; rheumic acid; rheotannic acid, mucilage; malic acid, fat, sugar, starch, albuminoids, calcium oxalate and ash 12 p.c. Chrysophan—to obtain it exhaust rhubarb with water and treat the residue with benzene. It is in golden yellow needles, or powder, soluble in water, alcohol and ether; on the addition of ferments or dilute acids it splits up into sugar and chrysophanic acid. It is without any odour or taste. It becomes deep red with alkalies. Emodin is obtained by treating chrysophanic acid with benzene as a decomposition product. It is of an orange yellow colour insoluble in water; emodin is also found in frangula.

Phœoretin: To obtain it wash the extract with water, dissolve the residue in alcohol, and add ether. The precipitate contains phœoretin, and the concentrated liquid contains chrysophanic acid; a brown resin without any taste, soluble in alcohol. Rheo-tannic acid—on the addition of dilute acids, it is decomposed into sugar and rheumic acid. Calcium oxalate is the cause of grittiness.

Preparations.—Liquor Rhei Concentratus, B. P. (1 in 2). Dose, ½ to 1 fld. dr., Extractum Rhei, B.P. Dose, 2 to 8 grs. Infusum Rhei, B. P. (1 in 20). Dose. ½ to 1 fld. oz. Pilula Rhei Composita. B. P. contains rhubarb root in powder 3 ozs., socotrine aloes 2¼ ozs., myrrh in powder 1½ ozs., hard soap 1½ oz., oil of peppermint 1½ fld. drs., syrup of glucose, 2¾ oz. Dose, 4 to 8 grs. Pulvis, Rhei Compositus, B. P. contains rhubarb root 2 ozs., light magnesia 6 ozs., ginger in powder 1 oz. Dose, 20 to 60 grs. Syrupus Rhei, B. P.—Rhubarb root 2 ozs., coriander fruit 2 ozs., refined sugar 24 ozs., alcohol 8 fld. ozs., distilled water 24 fld. ozs., to produce 2½ lbs. Dose ½ to 2 fld. drs. Tinctura Rhei Aromatica—contains Rhubarb 20 p.c., cinnamon 4, cloves 4, nutmeg 2, percolate with glycerin 10, alcohol to make 100. Dose, 1 to 2 drs. Tinctura Rhei Dulcis—contains rhubarb 10 p.c., glycyrrhiza 4, anise 4, cardamom 1, percolate with glycerin 10, alcohol 50 and water 40. Dose, 4 to 6 drs. Tinctura Rhei Composita, B. P.—rhubarb root 2 ozs., cardamom seeds ¼ oz., coriander fruit. ¼ oz., glycerin 2 fld. ozs., alcohol to 20 ozs. (1 in 10). Dose, ½ to 1 fld. dr.; 2 to 4 fld. drs. for a single dose.

Actions and uses.—Aperient, stomachic tonic and slightly astringent. The cathartic effect is due to phœoretina, a resin, and the subsequent astringency to Rheo tannic acid and bitter principle. Both act on the duodenum. Rhubarb stimulates the muscular layer of the bowels and the intestinal glands. In small doses it is a gastric tonic and intestinal astringent. In large doses it is a cathartic, producing several copious yellow stools with some amount of griping as an after-effect. It generally leads to constipation as a cholagogue. It stimulates the liver. The yellow colour of the stools is due to the excess of bile, to the rhubarb pigment and probably to the resin phæoretin. It is eliminated by the skin, kidneys and breasts, and its pigment stains the urine, sweat and the milk. The milk becomes bitter and purges the child. Rhubarb, if applied as poultice to abraded skin or if used as a dusting powder for ulcers causes purgation. As an astringent following its cathartic effect, it is given in diarrhœa due to the presence of irritants in the bowel, in dyspepsia, chronic dysentery, hæmorrhoids and even thread worms. In bilious fevers it is combined with calomel, and with magnesia in stomach and bowel disorders. The tincture is a stomachic, tonic and digestive. It promotes the action of the liver without any catharsis.

Rumex Crispus, Yellow Dock—R. Vesicarius, Sour Dock—Rumex Acetosa, Common Sorrel.

Habitat.—Europe, Ajmere, Madras, grassy places, road-sides.

Parts used.—The root.

Vernacular.—Arab.—Hummaz. Hind., Duk., Beng.—Chukkah. Burm.—Kalâ khen-boun. Cing.—Suri. Pers.—Turshah. Sans.—

Shuta-vedhi-chukra. Sind.—Bijband, Endranee. Tam.—Sukh-gukire. Tel.—Shukku, Kûraku.

Characters.—Common weed, growing along road-sides; root embedded deep into the ground, fusiform, yellow, fleshy and highly wrinkled; externally of a rusty brown colour; internally whitish; bark thick with a short fracture; odour peculiar; taste bitter, and astringent. Leaves lanceolate, smooth, margins wavy, curled, acute, sub-cordate at the base. Fruit reddish brown, having 3 fringed leaf-like expansions each with a glandular body; seed dark brown, triangular and polished, often confounded with Bijband. Dose, 15 to 45 grs.

Constituents.—The root contains 2 principles—Rumicin and Lapathin, identical with chrysophanic acid; tannin, calcium oxalate. mucilage, and starch.

Preparations.—Fluid extract. Dose, ½ to 1 fld. dr. Decoction (1 in 10) of the herb. Dose ½ to 1 fld. oz. Tincture (1 in 10) of the root. Dose, 1 to 10 ms.

Actions and uses.—Astringent and sedative, like rhubarb and sarsaparilla; given in disorders of the lymphatic and glandular system; in scurvy it is of great benefit as it contains large quantities of oxalic acid; also given in chronic skin eruptions, dyspepsia, syphilis, scrofula hepatic disorders, in laryngeal irritation and catarrh. The root is used as a dentifrice for spongy gums. The juice is astringent and is given to allay pain of toothache. The seeds are astringent and used in chronic dysentery, in checking nausea and in promoting appetite.

Aristolochiaceæ, the Birth-wort, Sapasana or Kida Mara family.

Characters.—Herbs or shrubby climbers. Wood of the stem arranged in separate wedges; leaves alternate, cordate or entire, and of a brown or greenish colour; flowers axillary, perfect, dull coloured; calyx tubular, superior; fruit 3 to 6 celled, capsular or succulent; seeds numerous and albuminous.

Habitat.—Tropical climate, South America.

Properties.—The plants abound in a bitter principle and a volatile oil. They are generally tonic, stimulant and acrid; some species are regarded as useful in snake bites.

Aristolochia Bracteata.

Habitat.—Deccan, Travancore, Coromandel, Sind, Ceylon.

Parts used.—The herb.

Vernacular.—Bomb.. Duk., Guz, Hind.—Gadhatee, Kirâ Mâra. Can.—Sanajali pullu. Eng.—Worm killer, Birth wort. Malyal.—Atu-tin-tap. Mar.—Gandhani, gaval. Sans.—Pattra Bangha, Dhumra pattra, Gridhrani. Tam.—Adu-tinna pâlai. Tel.—Gadide.

Characters.—Plant trailing. Roots perennial and fibrous; stems striated, wavy, slender and of a pale brown colour; leaves very obtuse, kidney-shaped, curled at the margins and of a pale glaucous, green or darkish brown colour below; surface wrinkled or tubercled; flowers solitary, axillary, peduncled, and drooping; fruit oblong, about an inch long, depressed at the top, and with a rather curved stalk at the base. From the apex 12 prominent ridges spread out longitudinally and run down into the stalk, where they gradually disappear; surface of the fruit smooth and of a brownish colour; seeds small, deltoid or triangular, of a dark colour on one side, and brown on the other; upper surface dark coloured, minutely tubercled and rough. The other side has two brown smooth lobular projections. Dose, 30 to 90 grs.

Constituents.—A nauseous, volatile substance, an alkaloid and salts, especially potassium chloride.

Preparations.—Infusion (1 in 10). Dose, ½ to 1 fld. oz.

Actions and uses.—Purgative, emmenagogue, alterative. antiperiodic, and anthelmintic; given with castor oil in colic and tormina, amenorrhœa, dysmenorrhœa, tedious labour, intermittent fever and worms; also given in syphilis, gonorrhœa, and skin diseases. The juice of fresh leaves or the powder of dried leaves is applied to sores, obstinate itch, psora, and to destroy maggots; hence the vernacular name.

Aristolochia Indica.

Habitat.—Travancore, Coromandel, Bengal, throughout low country of India.

Parts used.—The root and rhizome.

Vernacular.—Arab.—Zarâvande-hindi. Bomb., Beng., Hind., Mar.—Soposan Ishora-mula, Rudrajata. Can.—Ishwai-bâru. Cing.—Satasanda. Duk.,—Sapsum, Isrivel. Eng.—Indian Birth wort. Goa.—Sapusa. Guz.—Iswari, Sapsand. Malay—Karalekam. Pers.—Izaravânde hindi. Sans.—Irka mula, Sunanda, Sudhi-upâsaya, Tam.—Ich-churamuli. Tel.—Ishvararvêru.

Sâpasana or sapasuna is derived from sâpa, a serpent, and sana or suna, senseless; in allusion to the belief that the root makes the part where the snake has bitten insensible to the ill effects of its poison.

Characters.—A twining shrub. The drug consists of roots and stems, often obtained in separate pieces; root bark brownish dark, brittle, fibrous, tough, marked with longitudinal furrows, and breaking with a transverse fracture; epidermis, smooth, and here and there marked with scars of rootlets and numerous small warty projections: within the epidermis is another layer of a greyish brown colour; wood of a white colour porous and composed of longitudinal bundles; taste nauseous bitter and camphoraceous; odour aromatic and agreeable, resembling fresh ginger.

Preparations.—Decoction (1 in 10). Dose, ½ to 1 fld. oz. Tincture (1 in 8). Dose, ½ to 1 fld. dr.

Actions and uses.—Tonic, stimulant, and emmenagogue; given in intermittent fever, bowel affections of children due to teething, also in cholera ; as an emetic the juice of the leaves is given to children in croup. It has a great reputation as an antidote to snake poison. With agara it is applied externally to the abdomen in colic and to the chest in bronchitis in children.

Aristolochia Longa.

Habitat.—Kashmere.

Parts used.—The root.

Vernacular.—Arab.—Zerawand Taweel ; Zerawand daraz.

Characters.—Root in whitish, twisted, cylindrical pieces of the size of a finger and nearly tasteless ; leaves petioled ; flowers yellowish brown.

Preparations.—Powdered root. Dose, 10 to 30 grs. Infusion Dose, 1 to 2 fld. ozs.

Actions and uses.—Nervine tonic and emmenagogue ; given in headache and diseases of the brain. The natives give it in dysmenorrhœa. Locally it is applied to ulcers and affections of the gums.

Aristolochia Rotunda.

Habitat.—South of Europe, Cashmere.

Parts used.—The plant.

Vernacular.—Arab.—Nukhund-i-alavandi. Bomb., Ind. Bazaars—Zaravand-i-gird. Pers.—Zaravand-i-gird.

Characters.—Roots tuberous, externally brownish or grey coloured, slightly conical or roundish in shape ; base compressed and broad ; top, narrow ; surface rugous, also slightly wrinkled, and here and there marked with pit-like scars, the remains of fallen stems ; on section they are hard, horny, starchy, and heavy, and have a ring-like brim in the middle of which a scaly mass is seen ; colour pale white, taste somewhat acrid, odour slightly acrid.

Preparation.—Decoction (1 in 10). Dose, $\frac{1}{2}$ to 1 fld. oz.

Actions and uses.—Tonic, diuretic, emmenagogue and vermifuge ; given in gout, jaundice, and intestinal worms, and for promoting the renal and menstrual secretion ; also given in itch, leprosy, and for drying up sores.

Aristolochia Serpentaria, B.P., A. Reticulata, B.P.

Habitat.—Virginia, United States.

Parts used.—Rhizome and roots—Serpentaria rhizoma, B.P.

Characters.—Herbaceous plants. Rhizomes tortuous and slender, upper surface marked with remains of aerial stems, under surface with numerous wiry interlacing roots ; colour yellowish brown, odour camphoraceous, taste strong, bitter and aromatic ; the root de teriorate by keeping and hence should be used fresh. The Rhizome of A. Reticulata is longer and thicker and the roots straighter.

Constituents.—Volatile oil, 1 p.c.: resin, and a bitter principle, aristolochine, tannin, starch, sugar, gum, albuminoids and ash 11 p.c.; Volatile oil—obtained by distilling the infusion—contains terpene (pinene) and borneol ester. Aristolochine—to obtain it precipitate the decoction with acetate of lead, exhaust the precipitate with alcohol and evaporate. It occurs as yellow amorphous mass or needles, soluble in water and alcohol.

Preparations.—Infusum serpentariæ B. P., (1 in 20). Dose, ½ to 1 fld. oz. Liquor serpentariæ concentratus, B. P. (1 in 2). Dose, ½ to 2 fld. drs. Tinctura serpentariæ, B. P. (1 in 5). Dose, ½ to 1 fld. dr.

Actions and uses.—Gastric, cardiac, and nervine stimulant. In small doses it improves digestion and stimulates appetite, increases the secretions of the bronchi and intestines; it also stimulates the heart and excites the brain; in large doses it is a gastric and intestinal irritant, causing nausea, vomiting, colicky pain, rectal tenesmus, distended abdomen, diarrhœa, and even headache, vertigo, &c. It often gives rise to hæmorrhoids and even to pruritis. As an alterative and emmenagogue it is used in gout, chronic rheumatism, amenorrhœa, chlorosis and bilious vomiting; also in atonic dyspepsia and low states of the system. As a vehicle for cinchona in fevers (intermittent) and in exanthemata. As a stimulant combined with ammonium carbonate it is given in typhoid fever, pneumonia, capillary bronchitis, cough, &c. In functional impotence it is given to restore the lost virile power.

Piperaceæ—The Pepper, Pana, or Pipali family.

Habitat.—Tropics.

Characters.—Herbs or shrubs, jointed, creeping or trailing and giving off small rootlets; woody matter in the stem arranged in wedges; leaves entire usually opposite or verticelled, and marked with strong nerves; flowers in spikes, perfect and bractioled; stamens 2 or more; ovary, simple, one-celled; fruit fleshy, small, globular; berries, 1-celled, 1-seeded; embryo erect; albumen, fleshy and abundant.

Properties.—Acrid, pungent, aromatic and stimulant. These qualities are principally found in their fruits, and are essentially due to the presence of an acrid volatile oil and resin; some are narcotic, others astringent and febrifuge.

Chavica Betel—Piper betel.

Habitat.—Hotter parts of India, Ceylon, Malay Islands.

Parts used.—The leaves.

Vernacular.—Arab.—Tanbôl. Duk., Hind., Bomb., Beng.—Pân. Burm.—Kinoyol. Can.—Viledele. Cing.—Balât. Eng.—Betel leaf. Malyal.—Vetrila. Mar.—Nagarvela. Pers.—Barge tanbôl. Sans.—Tamula, nâgavalli. Tam.—Vettilai. Tel.—Tamala pakoo.

Characters.—Fresh leaves membranous, adult ones coriaceous, shining above, glabrous on both sides; 3 to 5 inches in length, and

2 to 4 inches in breadth, cordate, petioled, acuminate; nerves from 5 to 7, prominent on their under-surface; both surfaces smooth, green, darkish, or of a faint yellow colour; taste burning, aromatic and bitter.

Constituents.—The leaves yield on distillation, a light aromatic and volatile oil known as betel oil and chavicol a very volatile pale essential oil. Betel oil contains terpene, betel phenol and sesquiterpene.

Chavicol or para-allyl-phenol.—It is obtained by treating betel oil with caustic alkali, separating phenol from alkaline solution, and precipitating it with dilute acid. It is a colourless liquid, soluble in alcohol, fixed oils, either and chloroform, very sparingly soluble in water. Dose, ½ to 2 ms.

Preparations.—Succus. Dose, ½ to 1 fld. dr.

Actions and uses.—Stimulant, carminative and antiseptic; given in flatulence, fœtor of the mouth, dyspepsia, colic, &c., mostly used as a masticatory by the natives of India. Chavicol is a powerful antiseptic, 5 times stronger than carbolic acid, and twice as strong as eugenol; the juice is also antiseptic and used in catarrhal affections and inflammation of the throat and bronchi in diphtheria, &c.

Piper Angustifolium, Artanthe Elongata.

Habitat.—Peru, Cuba, Brazil, Tropical America.

Parts used.—The leaves.

Characters.—A shrub; leaves long, petiolate, apex pointed, base unequally heart-shaped, crenulate, tessellate above and reticulate beneath, of an aromatic spicy odour, and spicy and bitterish taste.

Constituents.—A volatile oil, artanthic acid, (crystalline); resin, a bitter principle, tannin and mucilage.

Preparations.—Fluid extract. Dose, ½ to 2 drs. Tincture 10 p.c. Dose, 1 to 2 drs. Infusion (1 in 20). Dose, 1 to 4 fld. ozs.

Actions and uses.—Alterative, stimulant of the mucous membrane, and diuretic; like cubebs, it acts on the uninary passages It constringes the capillaries, hence controls mucous fluxes or catarrhs and hæmorrhages from the lungs, stomach, bowels, kidneys, and rectum. It is given in bronchitis, gonorrhœa, leucorrhœa, hæmorrhoids, menorrhagia, hæmaturia, vesical catarrh, and in incontinence of urine. Locally the powder is used as hæmostatic in all kinds of cuts and wounds. The under surface of the leaf, if applied to a bleeding surface, promotes coagulation of blood.

Chavica Officinarum, Piper Chaba.

Habitat.—India, Java, Ceylon, Malay Islands, Bengal, Philippine Islands.

Parts used.—The immature fruit and stem.

Vernaculars.—Beng.—Chai. Bomb., Hind.—Chavikâ, Châb, Gajphal.

Characters.—The aments consist of minute baccate fruits, closely packed round a common axis. Fruits ovoid, with a nipple-like point, and peltate, bract beneath ; stem or spikes jointed, as thick as the ring finger, bark covering them brittle, smooth, slightly rugous and of a dirty brown colour and easily removable ; wood arranged in numerous wedges ; colour the same as that of the bark ; taste slightly pungent and acrid and smell somewhat aromatic.

Preparations.—Decoction (1 in 20). Dose, 2 to 6 drs.

Actions and uses.—Carminative and stimulant ; given in colic, tympanitis and in renal disease.

Piper Cubeba, B. P., Cubeba Officinalis.

Habitat.—Java, Sumatra, Borneo, Ceylon.

Parts used.—The dried full grown unripe fruits—Cubebæ Fructus, B. P.

Vernacular.—Arab.—Kâbabah chini. Can.—Bâla-Menasa. Cing.—Vâtmologu. Duk—Dumki-mirchi. Eng.—Tailed pepper or cubebs. Guz.—Toda-miri, Kâbâb-chini. Bomb., Beng., Hind.—Kabab-chini, Kankola. Malyal.—Lada-barekor. Mar.—Kombonkoos and kabab-chini. Himsi mirie. Pers.—Hab-el-ams Sans.—Sugandha Marichi. Tam.—Valmalaku. Tel.—Salava Mirialia. Tailed Cubeb. The dried fruit is so called from having a short stalk attached to it.

Characters.—Fruit in form and colour resembling kâlâ miri but smaller in size ; pericarp highly wrinkled and brownish red coloured, enclosing a nut ; within the nut is a pale brown coloured oily homogeneous and highly aromatic albumen ; the smell is aromatic and resembling that of Jaephala ; taste spicy, aromatic and camphoraceous. Dose, 30 to 60 grs.

Constituents.—An active principle 3 p.c., a volatile oil, 5 to 15 p.c. oleo resin 3 p.c.; cubebin 2 p.c.; cubebic acid, fatty matter, wax starch, oil-gum and ash 5 p.c.

Oleum Cubebæ, B.P., a volatile oil, obtained by distilling cubebs with water or steam. A greenish, yellowish or often colourless thick fluid, of a faint odour and aromatic, camphoraceous taste and neutral reaction ; soluble in equal volume of alcohol. It contains cubeben (a liquid), depentene, sesqueterpene and cardinene. If long kept it deposits a stearopten or cubeb camphor. Dose, 5 to 20 ms. Oleo resin is extracted from cubebs by ether. It is an amorphous mass, soluble in alkalies and alcohol. It contains a volatile oil and cubebic acid ; on evaporation it deposits cubebin and wax. Dose, 5 to 20 ms.

Preparations.—Fluid extract. Dose, 5 to 30 ms. Tinctura Cubebæ B. P. (1 in 5). Dose, ½ to 1 dr. Infusion, 1 to 2 ozs. Trochisci—containing oleo resin 4, oil of sassafras 1, extract glycyrrhizæ 25, acacia 12, syrup of tolu to make 100. Dose, 1 to 2.

Actions and uses.—Stimulant and diuretic. In large doses it irritates the stomach, intestines, uterus and urino-genital passages. It disinfects the urine, perspiration and bronchial mucus. Applied to the skin it gives rise to urticaria and vesicular eruptions. The seeds kept in the mouth and chewed relieve troublesome cough ; as a stimulant and diuretic it is given in gonorrhœa, urethritis, cystitis, chronic bronchial catarrh, in affections of the genito-urinary organs, and in inflammation of the urinary passages. The powder is dusted or blown by an insufflator into the nose and pharynx in chronic nasal catarrh, follicular pharyngitis, &c., with benefit. It is smoked in cigarettes in acute nasal catarrh. Trochisci are kept in the mouth in chronic irritability of the air passages, by singers and public speakers, to prevent hoarseness. As a local irritant, the oil with rose water is applied to the head in headache and to syphilitic sores on the penis. The oil increases the quantity of urine, imparting to it a peculiar odour.

Piper Methysticum.

Habitat.—South Sea Islands, Samoa, Sandwich Islands, Polynesian Islands.

Parts used.—The rhizome and root, Kava Kava.

Characters.—A shrub, rhizomes fleshy, and pale yellow. Dose of the powdered root, 30 to 60 grs.

Constituents.—An essential oil, 2 resins (which are believed to be the active principles), a neutral crystalline principle 1 p.c. named kavalin or lewinin or methysticin, analogous to piperin, kawin or kavaine, an alkaloid, and an oleo resin of a semi-solid consistence; taste aromatic, pungent, and hot, like that of pepper at first, later on it causes local numbness.

Preparations.—Liquid extract. Dose, 15 to 60 ms. Solid extract. Dose, 3 to 8 grs. Tincture (1 in 8). Dose, $\frac{1}{2}$ to 1 fld. dr.

Actions and uses.—In small doses it is a mild intoxicant, producing pleasant dreams of an erotic character ; as a tonic and stimulant it lessens the sense of fatigue and sharpens the mental faculties and produces a sensation of peace and comfort ; in large doses it produces drowsiness followed by headache, and in still larger doses sweet and frequent sleep. Under its use there is great and frequent desire to pass urine. Used in chronic, rheumatism, blenorrhagia, urethritis, gonorrhœa, gout, leucorrhœa, cystitis, catarrh of the bladder and dysuria.

Chavica Roxburghii, Piper Longum, P. Officinarum.

Habitat.—Java, India, Ceylon, Bengal, banks of water courses, Circar mountains and South Concans.

Parts used.—The immature berries, dried in the sun, and stems.

Vernacular.—Arab.—Dar-phil. Bur.—Peik Khyen. Cing.—Tippli. Duk.—Pipaliana. Eng.—Long pepper. Beng., Guz., Hind.—Pipal, Pipali, Can.—Yippali. Mar.—Bengali pipali, pimple. Malyal.—Cutta, Terpali, chaba-jawa. Pers.—Magz pipal, filfila-daraz. Sans.—Pippali, chapalâ. Tam.—Pippili. Tel.—Pipallu.

Characters.—Pipali mula—stem cylindrical, joints swollen and irrigularly knotty. Each piece from ¼ to 1 or 2 inches long; irregularly thick, hard, and of a brownish colour; interior starchy, smell heating; taste pungent and biting.

Pipal—these are immature fruits, dried in the sun, or the dry catkins made up of a number of small berries spirally crowded together round a common axil; each is crowned with a style remnant; spikes varying in length, generally thick, cylindrical, uneven, dusty, and tapering slightly towards the apex; colour brownish dark; smell like that of miri; taste more pungent than that of pipali mula.

Constituents.—Resin, volatile oil, starch, gum, fatty oil, inorganic matter and an alkaloid.

Preparations.—Compound Tincture (1 in 5): containing black pepper, ginger, each 1, long pepper 4, spirit 20. Dose, ½ to 1 fld. dr. Infusion (1 in 10). Dose, ½ to 1 fld. oz. Decoction (1 in 10). Dose, ½ to 1 fld. oz. Compound powders, viz. Chaturushana: the four heating or biting agents—a compound preparation containing equal parts of pipali, miri, suntha, and pipali mula; used in colic and flatulence; also for cough and coryza. Pancha Kola: the five pungents, a compound powder containing equal parts of pipal, pipali mula, suntha, chavaka and chitraka. It is a good appetizer and is used in dyspepsia, cough, flatulence and enlarged spleen. Shadushana: the six acrids. These are pancha kola and miri, used as an appetizing agent in flatulence.

Actions and uses.—Stimulant, carminative, laxative, and alterative; given in chest affections, dyspepsia, chronic cough, enlargement of the spleen and other abdominal viscera, gout, lumbago, &c.; as a resolvent they are useful in relieving the symptoms due to obstructions of the liver and spleen. With pakhanabheda a paste of them is applied to the breasts as a lactagogue.

Piper Nigrum, B.P.

Habitat.—S. India, Malabar forests, Sumatra, Java, Singapore, Bornea, Siam, Travancore, N. Circars, Tellicherry, Penang, Batavia.

Parts used.—The dried unripe fruit—Piper nigrum, black pepper, B. P.

Syn.—Pepper corn, pepper vine, African black pepper.

Vernacular.—Arab.—Phil-phile-aswad. Beng.—Kalâ-morich. Bur.—Nagayok-konng. Can.—Menasu. Cing.—Kalu-miris. Duk.—Choca. Mar., Guz., Bomb., Hind.—Kâli-mirich, choca-mirich. Eng. —Black pepper. Malyal.—Kuru-mulaka. Pers.—Philphil-i-siyah. Sans.—Mareecha. Tam.—Milaguvally. Tel.—Kodi Miriyalu.

Characters.—Perennial plant. Fruits black, sessile, shape globular, pericarp thick, reticulated and wrinkled; the epidermis is thin and capable of being easily scratched; the interior is hard, containing a whitish yellow oily albumen, the innermost portion is soft and starchy or hollow ; smell very acrid, aromatic and heating ; taste pungent and spicy.

Piper Album—White pepper. These are dried ripened fruits of Piper nigrum ; black fruits are immersed in water and the epicarp and sarcocarp removed by rubbing them with hand ; they resemble in size vavading ; they swell in water and hence are somewhat larger than kala miri ; they are smooth, yellowish, hard, or horny, and mealy within ; the taste, owing to the process of ripening, is less acrid and less pungent than that of black pepper. Dose, 5 to 20 grs.

Constituents.—A volatile alkaloid Piperina 2 to 8 p.c., piperidin 5 p c., a balsamic volatile oil 1 to 2 p.c., fat 7 p.c., Mesocarp contains chavicin, a green acrid concrete oil, a balsamic volatile oil, starch, lignin, gum, fat1 p.c., proteids 7 p.c., and ash containing inorganic matter 5 p.c.

Chavicin is an acrid or pungent concrete resin, of a dark green colour, soluble in alkalies, water, ether and alcohol ; it contains very little piperine and no volatile oil. The medicinal virtues and pungency of pepper are due to this constituent. Pepperina, Piperin, Piperinum, a proximate or neutral principle, a feeble alkaloid in a state of powder. To obtain it treat the alcoholic extract of the pepper with solution of potash, which dissolves resin and forms soap or fat; wash the residue with cold water and treat with alcohol, piperine crystallizes in rhombic prisms, colourless or pale yellow or white at first, but become yellow on keeping; almost tasteless without any odour and a neutral reaction : insoluble in water, slightly soluble in ether (1 in 60), soluble in alcohol (1 in 30), soluble in volatile oils, in acetic acid, chloroform, benzole and benzin. It melts like wax into a yellowish oily liquid and congeals into a mass of resinous substance. Heated with an alkali it forms piperidine. Dose, 2 to 8 grs. as antiperiodic ; ¼ to 2 grs. as stomachic.

Piperidine, Peperidinum.—To obtain it mix piperin with soda or lime and distil or boil with alcoholic solution of piperine when it will resolve into picric acid and piperidine. It may be snythetically obtained by reducing piperin with nascent hydrogen. A colourless, limpid liquid, of an ammoniacal or pepper-like odour. Taste bitter, combined with tartaric acid it forms piperidine tartrate—crystalline powder of a pleasant taste, readily soluble in water. Dose, 5 to 15 grs.

Volatile oil : Distil pepper powder with water or steam. It is colourless and without any pungency. The commercial oil of black pepper contains a volatile oil, a fixed oil, and resin, a by-product in the preparation of piperin.

Preparations.—Fuid extract of black pepper, obtained by percolating pepper with ether. It is a mixture of volatile and fixed oils, holding in solution pungent resin and peperin. Dose, ½ to 2 ms. Confection (1 in 10). Dose, 60 to 120 grs. Infusion (1 in 10). Dose, 2 to 4 fld. ozs.

Trikatu or katutrika (three acrids) is a compound preparation of equal parts of pipali, miri and suntha. Dose, 5 to 12 grs. Given in indigestion, cold in the head, cough, hurried breathing and hoarseness of voice. Pipali Asava—contains pipali, miri, chavaka, halada, chitraka, motha, vávadinga, sopári, lodhra, venivela-nu-mula, amalá patola, válo, Ratnájali, kutha, lavanga, tagara, jatámanasi, taja, elachi, tamálapatra, nága kesara, each 1. Make a paste with water ; then add jaggary 10, dháuri phula 10, Drákhsha 60, and subject the whole to fermentation. Dose, 1 to 2 drs. Used in chronic, dyspepsia, enlarged liver and spleen, general debility, anorexia, &c.

Prânada Gudica.—A compound confection containing black pepper 32, ginger 24, long pepper 16, piper chaba 8, leaves of taxus baccata 8, flowers of mesua ferrea 4, long pepper root 16, cinnamon 1, cardamoms 2, root of andropogon muricatus 2, treacle 420, mix together. Dose, 2 drs. for piles.

Marichadi Tel—a medicated oil, containing, kála miri 10, bachanága 6, haratela 5, manasila 4, akada-nu-duda 5, vanera-nu-mula 5, nishota-nu-mula 4, indrayani-nu mula 6, upaleta 6, haloda 8, daru halada 6, devadaranu-lakadun 5, rakta chandana 4, raitela 100, water 400, boil and prepare in oil. Used in chronic skin diseases, and over paralytic limbs.

Action and uses.—It is a local irritant, causing intense burning on the skin. In medicinal doses it stimulates the heart, the kidneys, and the mucous membrane of the urinary and intestinal tracts. It is eliminated in the urine and fœces. In large doses it causes abdominal pain, vomiting, irritation of the bladder and urethra and urticaria on the skin. As a gastric stimulant it is chiefly used in flatulence, dyspepsia and atony of the stomach ; like cubebs, it is given in gonorrhœa, gleet, and hæmorrhoids and other rectal disorders. Peperin acts as an antiperiodic and antipyretic. It relieves intermittent fevers, by causing perspiration ; in neurosis and in congestion of the spleen, it is of benefit. Piperidine Tartrate has a high solvent power, like peperazine, lysidin or urotropin and is a fine solvent for gouty deposits, uric acid gravel, and calculi, and used as an application in paralytic affections. In toothache a paste of it is applied with benefit. The infusion is used as a gargle in relaxed uvula, sore throat, &c. ; with vinegar, the powder is applied over the bites of venomous reptiles. Mixed with onions and salt, it is rubbed over bald head in alopecia. The oil is applied to muscular rheumatic pains, headache and to pain of hæmorrhoids.

Piper Trioicum.

Habitat.—S. India.

Parts used.—The dried fruit.

Vernacular.—Eng.—Canarese Pepper, abortive pepper-corns. Hind., Mar.—Pokala mari. Tel.—Murial tiga.

Characters.—Fruit succulent when fresh, dried ones round and red, and excessively pungent.

Preparations.—Paste ; powder. Dose, 5 to 20 grs.

Actions and uses.—Pungent, stomachic, carminative, and stimulant; used like kala miri. They are locally used to relieve toothache and as an internal remedy for cholera.

Monimiaceæ—The Monimia Order.

Trees or shrubs; leaves opposite, exstipulate; flowers axillary, declinous, unisexual; anthers longitudinally dehiscent; seeds pendulous.

Habitat.—Native of South America, Australia, Java, New Zealand.

Properties.—Aromatic, and fragrant.

Boldoa Fragrans, Peumus Boldus.

Habitat.—Chili and Bolivia.

Parts used.—The leaves.

Characters.—An evergreen shrub. Leaves large, oval shaped, broader at the base than at the apex, 1 to 1½ inches long; when dry, the colour is ashy and greyish; odour aromatic and agreeable; taste slightly bitter and spearmint-like.

Constituents.—Boldine or boldoin—a glucoside obtained from the leaves 1 to 5 p.c. and a volatile oil 2 p.c.

Preparations.—Liquid extract. Dose, 1 to 4 ms. Tincture (1 to 5). Dose, 1 to 20 ms. Boldoin. Dose, 1 to 4 grs. in capsules.

Actions and uses.—In small doses, mild tonic and stimulant of the stomach, intestines, bladder and urethra. In large doses irritant and emetic; also somewhat narcotic; indicated in atonic dyspepsia, chronic cystitis, anæmia, rheumatism, general debility and catarrh of the genitals; also as a tonic in chronic hepatic diseases. It is a good substitute for quinine; also used as an alterative in syphilis and gonorrhœa. Boldoin is a safe hypnotic, superior to chloral hydrate, opium, cannabis and other preparations. It is also a local anæsthetic like cocaine.

Myristicaceæ—The Nutmeg or Jaephala family.

General Characters.—Trees with alternate, entire, exstipulate, thick, dotted leathery leaves; flowers declinate; calyx leathery, 3 to 4 cleft; male flower with 3 to 12 stamens, filaments distinct; female flowers of 1 or many carpels; fruits succulent; seed arillate, with copious oily fleshy ruminated albumen; embryo small.

Habitat.—Tropics, Cochin China, Ceylon, Java, Moluccas, Peninsula of India, America.

Properties.—The aromatic properties are contained generally in their seeds and arillus. The bark and pericarp are frequently acrid.

Myristica Malabarica, M. Tomentosa.

Habitat.—Forests of Travancore, Concan, N. Malabar, S. India, S. Canara.

Parts used.—The seed and arillus.

Vernacular.—Can.—Kanagi. Eng.—Malabar nutmeg. Guz.—The mace, Rampatri (arillus). Mal.—Panam-palka. Mar.—Râmphal, Rànjâphal. Bomb—Raiphal, Jangli jaephal.

Characters.—Seed larger and softer than, but inferior to nutmeg in oiliness and fragrance and other properties ; fruit hairy, oblong and tawny ; aril lucumose, lobes twisted and folded into a cone at the top, longer and thinner than the true mace ; colour dark brown or red ; shell hard and brittle ; kernel elongated and of reticulated structure ; odour fruity, on bruising and boiling it yields a yellowish concrete oil.

Preparations.—The oil. Dose, 1 to 2 ms.

Actions and uses.—Local stimulant ; used as an embrocation in rheumatism and for headache. The mace is used as a spice. The oil is a good application to indolent ulcers to allay pain and to give a healthy action. Internally it is used like true nutmeg.

Myristica Fragrans, B. P., M. Moschata, M. Officinalis.

Habitat.—India, Ceylon, Sumatra, Java, Philippine Islands, Malabar, Mauritius, Penang, Molucca Islands.

Parts used.—The dried seed (deprived of testa). Myristica-Nutmeg, B.P., the arillus-mace, and wood.

Vernacular.—(The nut).—Arab.—Jour-ut-tib, Jauz-buvâ.—Guz Mar., Duk., Beng., Hind.—Jaephal. Burm.—Za-te-pho. Can.—Jàji-Kâye. Cing.—Jâdikâ. Eng.—Nutmeg. Malay.—Buwahpala, Pers.—Jowz bôyah. Sans.—Jat bowwa Jâjiphulam, Jati-kosha, Jati-sâra, Shâluka. Tam. & Tel.—Jaji-kâya, Jati-phallmu (the mace). Arab.—Buzbâs. Beng.—Jotri. Burm.—Zadiphu-apoen. Can.—Jâpatri. Cing.—Vadu-vâshu. Mar., Duk., Hind., Guz.—Jâvantari, Jâptari. Malyal.—Banà pala. Pers.—Bazbâz. Sans.—Jajipatri. Tam., Tel.—Jâpatri. Jouz-i-buya—Fragrant nut.

Characters.—Fruit, a pendulous drupe, smooth, yellow, pear-shaped, of the size of a small walnut or peach. The fruit when mature splits along the furrow into two separate pieces. It consists of four layers : (1) the pericarp ; (2) the arillus mace, which is folliaceous, fleshy, thick, here and there lobed, and very aromatic. When fresh the mace is brilliant, scarlet and remains adherent to the nut. When dry becoming brittle, in narrow bands of yellow colour, which peel off. Generally the bands are lobed above and united into broader bands below, and contain many oil cells. They are fatty when pressed, and have a fragrant odour and warm aromatic taste. Dose, 3 to 20 grs. ; (3) Hard shell or testa, surface marked with impressions corresponding to the lobes of the fleshy and irregularly cut arillus, one side is of a paler colour than the other ; paler side flattened and marked with a line or raphe. It is bony, hard, thick and woody, and reticulated with a circular scar at the broad end ; (4) a thin membranous coat. The seed known as official nutmeg, is of oblong shape, end obliquely compressed at both ends ; surface wrinkled and marked with impressions ; the cut surface is reticulated and consists of abundant endosperm which is soft but firm, and marble like in appearance, due to a white albumen and numerous reddish brown vein-like partitions or lobes, which can readily be scratched with the nail ; on pricking it with a pin, the oil floats on its surface. Heavy specimens are superior. The odour is agreeably aromatic, taste acrid and spicy ; wood in thin slices of a brownish red colour, extremely light and soft ; substance porous and here and there sprinkled with a granular matter which on scratching emits an aroma similar to that of the seed. Dose, 10 to 20 grs.

Constituents.—The kernel contains a volatile oil, 2 to 8 p.c., a fixed oil, proteids, fat, starch, mucilage and ash ; concrete oil, called oil of mace, 20 p.c. The mace contains a volatile oil (by distillation) identical with the volatile oil from the kernel, a fixed oil (by pressure), resin, fat, sugar, dextrine and mucilage.

The concrete oil exists in two layers. The volatile portion is known as myristicine, and the oxygenated portion—myristicol or myristicin or nutmeg camphor.

Volatile oil—Oleum Myristicæ, B.P., is a colourless or pale yellow oil, soluble in alcohol (1 in 1). Dose, ½ to 3 ms. The fixed oil known as oil of nutmeg, or nutmeg butter, contains volatile oil 6 p.c., fat 24 p.c., and a brown yellowish resinous matter. Nutmeg butter is erroneously called oil of mace (Jawantri-katela) and occurs in oblong cakes like bricks. When discolored and hardened it is called Banda soap.

Preparations.—Spiritus Myristicæ, B.P., spirit of nutmeg (1 in 10). Dose, 5 to 20 ms. Decoction of wood (1 in 10). Dose, 4 to 8 drs.

Actions and uses.—Aromatic, stomachic and stumulant. In small doses it stimulates digestion, increases appetite, relieves flatulence, dyspepsia and colic. In large doses it causes stupor and delirium. As a carminative, anodyne and astringent, it is given in diarrhœa and dysentery, to allay nausea and vomiting. Small doses frequently given relieves strangury. A paste of it is used as an external application to the head in headache, palsy, cramps, &c. The wood is used as an astringent to check diarrhœa. The oil is stimulant and carminative, and in large doses, narcotic and is given in atonic dyspepsia, diarrhœa, and as an adjunct to other stimulant medicines. Locally, diluted with bland oil, it is applied in rheumatism, paralysis, sprains, &c. Butter of nutmeg is externally applied in rheumatism, contusions, sprains, &c. Mace is used for the same purposes as the kernel.

Lauraceæ, The Laurel, Taja or Dalachini family.

General Characters.—Trees or shrubs. Leaves exstipulate, usually alternate, sometimes dotted, generally smooth above and glaucous beneath; flowers perfect or imperfectly unisexual; calyx inferior, 4 to 6 cleft, in two whorls ; ovary, superior, 1-celled ; fruit a berry, or drupe ; seeds exalbuminous, embryo with large cotyledons.

Habitat.—Native of Tropics and Europe.

Properties.—The plants are almost universally remarkable for their stimulant and aromatic properties, due to the presence of volatile oils. Many of the species are narcotic, sudorific, astringent, tonic and febrifuge.

Cassytha Filiformis.

Habitat.—Peninsula, Bengal and Cochin.

Parts used.—The herb.

Vernacular.—Beng.—Akash-bullee. Duk.—Kotan-ka-patt. Hind. —Amarbelli. Malyal.—Acatajá-bulli. Mar.—Akasvela. Sans.—Akasavalli. Tam.—Cottan. Tel.—Nillootiga.

Characters.—Leafless, thread-like parasite ; spikes ascending on bushes or twisting round the branches of trees ; calyx 3-leaved, petals 3 ; flowers small and white ; stems tough and dark green ; the largest of the size of a crow-quill ; branches provided with small round suckers like those of the common dodder ; fruit a drupe, one-seeded, nut round of the size of a pea.

Constituents.—An alkaloid.

Actions and uses.—Alterative ; given in bilious affections, for piles, urethritis, &c. Locally it is used as a wash for the head to destroy vermin. Mixed with gingelly oil it is applied to strengthen the roots of the hair ; with ginger and butter it is used for healing ulcers.

Cinnamomum Camphora, B. P., Camphora Officinarum.

Habitat.—China, Japan, Formosa.

Parts used.—A stearopten (concrete volatile oil) purified by sublimation.

Vernacular.—Arab.—Kâfûr. Burm.—Payo, Paronk. Can.—Karpura. Cing.—Kapuru. Duk., Beng., Guz., Hind., Mar.—Kapur, Kaphur. Eng.—Camphor. Malyal.—Karppûram. Pers.—Kafur. Sans. —Karpûroh, Pákva and Apakva. Tam.—Shûdan Karuppuram. Tel. —Karpuram.

Characters.—Camphor, a stearopten, having the nature of a ketone, chiefly distilled from the root trunk and branches of cinnamomum camphora ; also obtained by heating comminuted plant or chips of branches, &c., in water, when camphor volatilizes, and it is purified by sublimation and condensed into balls, tablets, or sublimed powder, known as flowers of camphor. It is imported from Japan in a crude form and is mixed with lime and resublimed into the camphor cakes. Crude camphor possesses considerrable hygroscopic properties. Met with in solid colourless transparent crystalline pieces. The odour is powerful, taste pungent and bitter, followed by a sensation of cold ; it burns with a smoky flame ; soluble in water (1 in 700), alcohol (1 in 1), chloroform (4 in 1), and olive oil (1 in 4) ;

very soluble in ether, benzin and oil. It forms a liquid when triturated with chloral hydrate, menthol, phenol and thymol. Dose, 2 to 5 grs. Borneo camphor bears the same chemical relation to Japanese camphor as alcohol bears to aldehyde. It is also heavier than water.

Constituents.—Camphor, when heated with chloride of zinc and distilled, yields cymol or cymene; with nitric acid it is more or less oxidised, thus forming camphoric and camphoretic acids. Camphoric acid, a dibasic acid, occurs in acicular crystals, without any odour, and of an acid taste; soluble in alcohol, ether and fatty oils, in boiling water (1 in 10), and in cold water (1 in 100); insoluble in carbon sulphide. Dose, 5 to 15 grs.

Preparations.—Aqua Camphoræ, B. P., (70 grs. in 1 gallon) Dose, ¼ to 1 fld. oz. Linimentum Camphoræ, B.P., of camphor in 4 of olive oil. Linimentum Camphoræ Ammoniatum, B. P., compound liniment of camphor (1 in 8). Spiritus Camphoræ, B.P., (1 in 10). Dose, 5 to 20 ms. Camphora Salicylata contains camphor 14 and Salicylic acid 11. Dose, 1 to 5 grs. Tinctura camphoræ composita, B.P.. (paregoric elixir), contains one grain of opium in 4 fld. drs. of tincture. Dose, ½ to 1 fld. dr. Eau sedative contains ammonia water 2 ozs., sodii chloridum 2 ozs., camphorated spirit of wine 3 drs., water 40 ozs. For local application. Camphor chloral—camphor and chloral equal parts; useful as a paint in neuralgia and over the larynx in spasmodic cough. Camphorated chalk and camphorated myrrh, used as dentifrices. Essential oil of camphor--a bye-product in the manufacture of camphor—contains camphor in solution with a yellow-brown volatile oil; used as a rubefacient. Elixir camphor (1 in 15), miscible in water. Dose, ½ to 1 dr. Camphoid—pyroxylin 1, camphor and alcohol, 20 each. A good substitute for collodion. Camphora Monobromata —monobromide of camphor, bromo-camphor, prepared by heating together bromine and camphor. It occurs in prismatic, quite colourless needles or scales. It has a mild camphoraceous odour and taste, neutral reaction; soluble in spirit, ether and chloroform and fixed oils; sparingly soluble in water and glycerin. Dose, 2 to 10 grs. Camphor Naphthol—a mixture of melted beta naphtol 1 part, with camphor 2 parts. An oily fluid, soluble in alcohol, ether, and oils, insoluble in water. It dissolves iodine, cocaine, and cinchona alkaloids, &c., used as a local antiseptic and antiparasitic. Camphora Phenolata, a solution of camphor in carbolic acid. A clear oily liquid; taste and odour camphoraceous; insoluble in water, soluble in vegetable oils and in petroleum jelly. It dissolves salicylic acid, cocaine and iodoform. Dose, 5 to 10 ms. An oily solution 50 p.c. is used as an antiseptic, local anæsthetic, carminative and antipruritic. Camphor salol—contains melted camphor 2, and salol 3. It is light yellow oily fluid, freely soluble in ether, alcohol and oils, insoluble in water. Freely dissolves iodine and alkaloids. As an antiseptic it is locally used in epithelioma, lupus phagedenic and syphilitic sores.

Actions and uses.—Camphor is locally rubefacient and resolvent. In medicinal doses it stimulates the heart, respiration, and the vasomator ganglia ; and stimulates and increases the sexual appetite ; after a time it depresses the generative function. It stimulates the uterus and increases the menstrual flow. On the skin it produces increased diaphoresis. As an anodyne it allays pain, relieves sexual excitement as chordee and other neurotic affections. It is eliminated by the skin, kidneys and bronchi ; often causes dysuria. In large doses it produces gastro-enteritis and symptoms of irritant poison. It depresses the heart, gives rise to cold sweats, cold hands and feet, coma, convulsions, and death. In comparatively large doses it is given in puerperal mania. An enema of camphoris given to expel worms (ascarides). Externally it is used as a wash for ulcers. In toothache, camphor dissolved in alcohol and applied to the cavites of carious teeth gives relief ; used as snuff it checks coryza. The liniment is useful for sprains, bruises, for rheumatic pains of joints, also in spasmodic pains in muscles.

Monobromated camphor resembles bromides in action and is a nervous sedative, gastric irritant and hypnotic. It is used in insomnia, delirium tremens, convulsions and spermatorrhœa. Camphoric acid solution 5 p.c. is used in abrasions and ulcerations of the mucous membranes. As a spray 1 p.c. solution is used in severe catarrhal affections as trachitis, laryngitis and bronchitis. As a plug soaked in solution 2½ p.c. or the solution itself applied to the nasal surface, stops severe catarrh. In eczema and erysipelas, an ointment of the acid or 4 p.c. solution is used. In catarrhal cystitis with ammonical fermentation, a 2 p.c. aqueous solution with alcohol, injected into the bladder and given internally, relieves strangury and renders the urine a clear normal liquid.

Cinnamomum Zeylanicum, B.P. (Ceylon cinnamon), C. Saigonicum (Saigon cinnamon), C. Cassia (Cassia cinnamon) C. Aromaticum, Laurus cinnamomum, Cassia Laurus.

Habitat.—China, Assam, Cochin China, Ceylon, Southern India.

Parts used.—The dried inner bark of the shoots from truncated stocks, cinnamomi cortex, B.P., and essential oil, oleum cinnamomi, B.P.

Vernacular. — Arab. — Darasini. Bomb., Beng.—Dalachini, Taja, Burm.—Theet Kyabah, Chin.—Yuh or Juh—kwei Can.—Lavanga pattee. Cin.—Kurundu. Duk.—Qualami. Malyal.—Katu Karua. Hind.—Moti dârchini, Tvak, Guda tvach, Tvaksâra, Tvaksvadvi. Malyal.—Kulitmanis. Kana Manis Pers.—Saila Myah. Sans.—Darashita, Kalphah, Kira phah, Gudât vaka. Tam.—Karuvappattai, Lawunga. Tel.—Sanna—Lavanga-patta.

Tvacha.—Bark ; Guda tvach, a sweet bark or sugar bark ; Tvaksara, having excellent bark ; Tvaksvadvi, having sweet bark.

Characters.—The bark occurs in light yellowish brown quills consisting of several pieces rolled together, each very thin. Chinese variety—each piece in a single quill, rarely double, of irregular from and of a rough texture. Each quill is of the size of a lady's finger. When deprived of corky layer it has a light yellowish-brown colour. It is generally mixed with broad pieces of an ash colour, the remains of the external bark ; very brittle, breaking with a crackling noise. Odour agreeable, fragrant and aromatic; taste sweetish, aromatic and pungent. The aroma is due to its containing large quantities of an essential oil. Dose of the powder, 10 to 30 grs.

Constituents.—Volatile oil, 2 p.c., cinnamic acid, resin, tannin sugar, mannit, starch, mucilage, ash, &c.

The volatile oil, oleum cinnamomi, B.P., is distilled from the cortex and consists chiefly of cinnamic aldehyde, oxidizing into resin and cinnamic acid ; also cinnamyl acetate and hydrocarbons. It is a brownish liquid, becomes thicker and darker by age ; has a characteristic odour, sweet spicy taste, soluble in alcohol and glacial acetic acid. Fresh oil contains no cinnamic acid, but after keeping cinnamic acid is formed, which by further oxidation becomes converted into benzoic acid.

Cinnamic acid—cinnamylic acid—occurs in transparent crystals, sparingly soluble in water, used as an injection in phthisis. A 5 p.c. oily emulsion with yolk of egg injected in lupus.

Preparations.—Of the bark.—Aqua Cinnamomi B.P. (1 in 10); or oil 2, precipitated calcium phosphate 4, distilled water to 1,000. Dose, 1 to 2 fld. ozs. Tinctura Cardamomi Composita B.P. 2 p.c. Dose, 1 to 2 drs. Tinctura Catechu. Dose, ½ to 1 fld. dr. Tinctura Lavandulæ Composita. Dose, ½ to 1 dr. Pulvis aromaticus contains Ceylon cinnamon 35, ginger 35, cardamoms 15, nutmeg 15 ; mix and triturate. Doses, 10 to 30 grs. Tinctura cinnamomi, B.P. (1 in 5). Dose, ½ to fld. dr. Pulvis Cinnamomi Compositus, B.P., containing the bark, cardamoms and ginger in equal parts. Dose, 10 to 40 grs. Spiritus Cinnamomi, B.P., (1 in 10). Dose, 5 to 20 ms.

Actions and uses.—The bark is an agreeable, carminative, antispasmodic, aromatic, stimulant, astringent and germicide, and is used as adjunct to other medicines. The oil has no astringency. It is a vascular and nervine stimulant. In large doses the oil is an irritant and a narcotic poison. In medicinal doses it is a good remedy for flatulence, paralysis of the tongue, enteralgia and cramps in the stomach ; also to check nausea and vomiting. As an antiseptic it is used as an injection in gonorrhœa. As a germicide, it destroys the pathogenic bacilli and is used internally in typhoid fever. The bark is hæmostatic, and has a specific action on the uterus and is given with other uterine stimulants to promote parturition and to check uterine hæmorrhages ; also given in flatulence, nausea, vomiting, and to check diarrhœa and the gripes caused by other medicines. Cinnamic acid is antitubercular and is used as an injection in phthisis. The emulsion is injected in lupus.

Cinnamomum Iners, C. Nitidum, C. Eucalyptoides.

Habitat.—Peninsula, Malabar, Konkans.

Parts used.—The leaves and bark.

Vernacular.—Arab.—Tarnaly. Bur.—Sikeyabo. Bomb.—Tamalpatra. Can.—Adavi Lavanga patti. Duk., Hind.—Jangli Darachini, Talispatra (leaves). Mah.—Ranâcha dal, Tejpat. Mal.—Karunatoli. Tam.—Kattu, Kurrnap.

Characters.—Flat or slightly quilled pieces, thicker than the Chinese bark, and of a deeper colour, of a strong odour and taste, but less sweet ; an oil is distilled from these barks—tejpatra; the leaves of a brownish colour, from 4 to 6 inches long, and 1½ to 2 inches broad ; upper surface shining and smooth, under surface glaucous, oblong, ovate, coriaceous and obtusely pointed ; three to five longitudinal nerves extending from the base to the apex, most marked on their under surface. They have a pleasant odour, like that of cloves and cinnamon, and an aromatic taste.

Constituents.—The leaves contain an essential oil, eugenol, terpene, and cinnamic aldehyde. The bark contains an oil similar to cinnamon oil. The root contains an oil containing eugenol, saffrol, benzaldehyde and terpene.

Preparations.—A compound powder—Trijataka, containing taj and three other aromatics—elachi, tamala patra, and kâla nâga kesara Compound pill—Trijatakadi Goli, containing trijataka 1, pipali 4. sakara, drakhsha, jethi madha, each 8 parts. Dose, 3 to 5 grs. Used in cough, flatulence and dyspepsia. The pill is to be kept in. the mouth till it is completely dissolved.

Actions and uses.—Carminative, stimulant, diuretic, diaphoretic and lactagogue. The powder is used in many aromatic and carminative compound preparations and given in fevers, flatulence, dyspepsia, and urinary diseases. The bark is used like cassia bark.

Laurus Nobilis.

Habitat.—Southern Europe.

Parts used.—The berries and leaves.

Vernacular.—Eng.—The sweet bay laurels; Victor's laurels. Pers.—Hab-el-ghara.

Characters.—Leaves 2 to 4 inches long, pellucid, punctate and smooth ; berries oval or subglobular, about ½ inch long, greenish black or blackish brown ; when dry, slightly wrinkled and fragile ; seed oval, lying loose in the integument ; cotyledons two, plano-convex ; taste aromatic, oily and bitter.

Constituents.—The fruit and leaves contain a volatile oil, a fixed oil (oil of bay berries), and a resin.

Actions and uses.—Astringent, stomachic and stimulant. The leaves are used for flavouring medicines. The decoction is used in leucorrhœa, diseases of the urinary organs, and dropsy. The oil is used locally in relieving rheumatic pains and as a nervine stimulant in hysteria, epilepsy, &c.

Litsœa Sebifera, Tetranthera Roxburghii, T. Laurifolia.

Habitat.—Throughout the hotter parts of India.

Parts used.—The bark.

Vernacular.—Arab.—Maghath-i-Hindi. Beng.—Kukur Chita. Cing.—Boommeegass. Guz., Mar., Hind.—Maeda lakari. Pers.—Kilza. Tam.—Mushaippeyetty. Tel.—Naramamide.

Characters.—Bark hard, thick, and of a brown colour, sometimes soft and smooth ; external surface rugous and easily scratched, fragile and readily powdered ; section corky and composed of several layers of a soft granular matter ; when placed in water it affords a large quantity of mucilage ; taste feebly balsamic, bitter and mucilaginous.

Constituents.—The bark contains mucilage, taurotetanine, an alkaloid producing tetanic spasms in animals.

Preparations.—Decoction and infusion (1 in 10). Dose, $\frac{1}{2}$ to 1 fld. oz

Actions and uses.—Demulcent, and emollient ; given in diarrhœa and dysentery. Externally a paste of it is used as an emollient application to sprains, bruises, and rheumatic and gouty joints. The bark is generally given in combination with other alterative drugs.

Litsœa Stocksii, Tetranthera Lancifolia, Actinodaphne Lanceolata.

Habitat.—Concan, Canara, Matheran, Mahableshwar.

Parts used.—The leaves and oil.

Vernaculars.—Bomb.—Pisá. Goa.—Gino.

Characters.—Leaves ovate, lanceolate, long, pointed, coriaceous smooth, shining, and greenish above with impressed nerves and glaucous beneath, finely reticulated on both surfaces, and also minutely pellucid and dotted ; smell slightly aromatic ; taste bitterish, pungent and mucilaginous ; berries scarlet, of the size of a small acorn, pulp yellow, seed brown and polished ; kernel, oily and white, on exposure to the air becoming red ; taste aromatic like that of cubeb.

Constituents.—The fruit contains resin and fat, and an alkaloid allied to Laurotetanine ; the leaves contain mucilage.

Preparations.—Infusion (cold), (1 in 10). Dose, 1 to 2 ozs.; and oil.

Actions and uses.—Demulcent ; used in gonorrhœa, leucorrhœa, irritation of the bladder, other urinary disorders, and diabetes. The oil is used as an external application to sprains bruises and itch.

Nectandra Rodiæi, Bebeeru or Green-Heart Tree (Eng.)

Habitat.—South America.

Parts used.—The bark.

Characters.—Tree large ; leaves long, coriacious, and shining ; flowers yellow, of jasmine odour ; fruit pyriform and long ; taste bitter ; bark in flat pieces with many longitudinal depressions, coarsely striated with granular fracture; internally the colour is cinnamon brown. Dose, 20 to 60 grs.

Constituents.—The bark contains bebeerine (identical with buxine and pelosine) and sipirine; Bebeerine is a yellowish brown amorphous powder without any odour and of a bitter taste; soluble in alcohol and ether, insoluble in water. Dose, 1 to 10 grs.

Bebeerine sulphas—probably a mixture of sulphate of bebeerine, nectandrin and other alkaloids met with in dark brown scales, of a bitter taste, freely soluble in water, sparingly so in alcohol. Dose, 1 to 10 grs.

Preparations.—Decoction and infusion (1 in 10). Dose, $\frac{1}{2}$ to 1 fld. oz.

Actions and uses.—The bark is febrifuge, tonic and antiperiodic, and given like quinine, though inferior to it in every way. It is given in intermittents, dyspepsia and neuralgias; also as astringent in leucorrhœa and menorrhagia. Bebeerine is antipyretic and tonic.

Sassafras Officinale, B.P., S. Variifolium.

Habitat.—S. America.

Parts used.—The dried root, sassafras radix, B.P., oil, and pith of the branches—sassafras medulla.

Vernacular.—Eng.—Sassafras, ague tree, cinnamon wood.

Characters.—Root, deprived of grey corky layer, in irregular fragments, colour rust brown: internally corky and smooth; odour fragrant and taste sweet, aromatic and astringent—the pith of branches, otherwise called sassafras medulla, in slender cylindrical pieces, curved or coiled, and of a white colour, light and spongy, without any odour. With water it forms a mucilaginous liquid, which does not precipitate with alcohol.

Constituents.—The bark contains a volatile oil, oleum sassafras 5 p.c., sassafrid 9 p.c., tannin 6 p.c., starch gum, resin, wax—the pith contains mucilage.

Oleum sassafras—to obtain it, distil the bark with water or steam. It is a yellowish red liquid, of a characteristic odour, warm and aromatic taste, and neutral reaction; becoming dark and thick by age; soluble in alcohol, glacial acetic acid and bisulphide of carbon. With nitric acid it becomes dark red and is finally converted into a red resin. It contains eugenol, safrene (pinene), also safrol, sassafras camphor. Dose, $\frac{1}{2}$ to 3 ms. Sassafrid is the oxidation product of tannin. Safrol is the liquid stearopten of oil of sassafras, used in headache and sciatica and to disguise the odour of fatty bases. Dose, 20 to 30 ms.

Preparations.—Of the bark.—Infusum sassafras. Dose, 1 to 4 ozs. Concentrated compound solution of sarsaparilla, B. P. Dose, 2 to 8 fld. drs.

Actions and uses.—The hot infusion of the bark is alterative, diaphoretic, stimulant and emmenagogue, and is given to purify the blood. It is given in combination with guaiacum and sarsaparilla in cutaneous diseases, syphilis and rheumatism. The pith is demulcent and emollient and used in gastritis, enteritis and also throat troubles; as collyrium for conjunctivitis, and as an antidote in irritant, or corrosive poisons. The oil is anodyne, stimulant, alterative, diuretic, and tonic. It possesses violent toxic properties, and produces abortion ; often given in neuralgia and applied locally to dispel insects. Safrol is, like menthol, an anodyne, and also stimulant, and is given in neuralgia, headache, sciatica, &c.

Thymelaceæ—The Mezereon family.

General Characters.—Trees, shrubs or rarely herbs ; leaves entire and exstipulate ; flowers perfect, tubular or top-shaped ; ovary, superior ; calyx petaloid, 4-5 imbricated ; stamens perigynous; ovary one-celled ; fruits dry, nut-like drupes, capsular, bivalved, sometimes succulent and indehiscent ; seeds abortive and exalbuminous.

Habitat.—Australia, Cape of Good Hope.

Properties.—The plants are chiefly remarkable for the toughness and acridity of their bark. The fruits of some are dangerously narcotic and poisonous. The bark of some is used as a vesicatory, also as an alterative, diaphoretic, and stimulant. It contains an acrid resin and an acrid volatile oil—some yield a fragrant stimulant resin.

Daphne Laureola, B.P., D. Gnidium, B.P., D. Mezereum, B.P.

Habitat.—Europe, mountainous regions.

Parts used.—The dried bark.

Vernacular.—Arab.—Mâzeriun, Adoda. Eng.—Spurge, wild pepper. Hind.—Mazeriyuna. Pers.—Iskhes mazerun.

Characters.—Each piece is in thin bands of various lengths, and of the thickness of a black-lead pencil, often folded or rolled into disks ; surface smooth or scabrous, colour darkish or yellowish brown, covered with transverse scars or minute dots, very tough and thin ; internal surface light, of a white colour, or soft and silky ; taste acrid ; smell somewhat aromatic, like that of taggara ganthoda. There are two varieties, the white and the brown. Dose, 1 to 6 grs.

Constituents—Daphnin—a bitter glucoside and an acrid resin mezerein (an anhydride of a resinous acid) named mezereinic acid. Umbelliferin is obtained by dry distillation of the acrid volatile oil. To obtain daphnin add to the decoction of alcoholic extract, acetate of lead, filter the deposit, decompose the filtrate with sulphuretted hydrogen, refilter, evaporate, treat the residue with alcohol and crystallize. In fine crystals, soluble in alkalies, the solution giving it a yellow colour, and insoluble in ether. Mezerein, an acrid resin—to obtain it distil the solution of alcoholic extract and treat the residue with water. Hard brittle mass, colour blackish green, taste acrid.

Preparations.—Fluid extract, 1 to 5 ms. ; also used in the preparation of Liquor Sarsæ Compositus concentratus.

Actions and uses.—The white variety is to be preferred, as it is the least acrid. In small doses it is alterative, stimulant, diuretic, laxative and diaphoretic; in large doses sialogogue and intensely acrid and irritant, producing salivation, vomiting and purging. Locally the bark is highly irritant and produces vesication. As an alterative it is given combined with sarsaparilla in syphilis, scrofula, chronic rheumatism, and chronic skin diseases. It is seldom used alone. Externally as a local irritant its ointment is used like cantharides to excite vesication and to promote suppuration, or maintain discharges of indolent ulcers, and those caused by setons or flying blisters; also used in toothache and as a masticactory in paralysis of the tongue.

Lasiosiphon Speciosus.

Habitat.—Deccan Peninsula, Ceylon.

Parts used.—The bark.

Vernacular.—Bomb., Hind., Mar.—Rametha.

Characters.—A shrub 5 to 6 feet high ; bark of a brownish colour, very tough, and very acrid ; leaves like willow, linear, oblong, and of a whitish colour; flower heads horny and terminal.

Constituents.—A green resinous matter—the vesicating principle of the bark.

Preparations.—Powdered bark.

Actions and uses.—It is used as a powerful vesicant. The natives use the stem to procure abortion.

Loranthaceæ—The Mistletoe family.

Parasitic shrubby plants ; leaves opposite, exstipulate, greenish ; flowers perfect, diœcious ; calyx superior 3-8; ovary, inferior, 1-celled; ovules 1-3, erect, or suspended ; fruit succulent, 1-celled; seed solitary, embryo in fleshy albumen.

Habitat.—Natives of hotter parts of America and Asia.

Properties.—Some are astringent.

Viscum Sp.

Habitat.—Temperate Himalaya, Persia.

Parts used.—The berries.

Vernacular.—Arab.—Kishmish-i-kawaliyân. Eng.—Mistletoe. Hind.—Banda, Bhangra. Ind. Bazaar.—Kismish-kawali. Kawali, or kawli is the name of gipsy tribe in Persia.

Characters.—A plant, parasitic on many trees as willows, thorns, lime, elms, firs and apple-tree; fruit like a chickpea when fresh, succulent, containing a viscid pulp, rounded, smooth, soft and of a green colour externally ; when dry shrivelled and of a brown colour. The berries when crushed are highly sticky and contain a small seed of the size of poppy seed. Dose, 10 to 60 grs.

Constituents.—Viscin, resembling vegetable, wax, very elastic, of the consistence of honey and, like caoutchouc, capable of being drawn into long threads.

Preparations.—Tincture (1 in 10). Dose, ½ to 2 fld. drs. Decoction, (1 in 10). Dose, ½ to 2 fld. ozs.

Actions and uses.—Tonic, antispasmodic, narcotic and oxytoccic; also emetic and purgative ; given to reduce splenic and hepatic enlargements, to disperse swellings and in menorrhagia and hæmorrhages. Like digitalis, it may be given in palpitation or tumultuous action of the heart. As an antispasmodic it is given in hysteria and epilepsy. Locally it is used to mature abscesses.

Aquilariaceæ—The Agar family.

Trees; leaves entire, exstipulate ; calyx tubular or top-shaped, 4-5 lobed, persistent; ovary superior, 2-celled ; fruit capsular, 2-valved, sometimes succulent and indehiscent ; seeds, 1 or 2, exalbuminous.

Habitat.—Native of Tropical Asia.

Properties.—Some species yield stimulant, fragrant resin.

Aquilaria Agallocha, A. Ovata.

Habitat.—Malay Islands, Assam, E. Himalaya.

Parts used.—The wood.

Vernacular.—Arab.—Ud-el-juj, Ayalodgi. Burm.—Akyan. Beng., Hind.—Agara. Eng.—Aloes wood, Eaglewood. Malyal.—Kaya-gahru. Pers.—Belanjirj. Sans.—Agaru, Rajarâh kalijya, Jishva-rupa. Tel.—Krishna Agaru. Chinese—Chin heang.

Characters.—Wood in irregular pieces, of a grey or dark brown or black colour and marked with longitudinal dark veins, hard, heavy, and not fibrous when powdered ; taste astringent, bitter, and odour fragrant; when burnt they diffuse an agreeable odour. Only the diseased part is found infiltrated with odoriferous resinous secretion ; secretion obtained by tapping the trunk is known as lign-aloes, or wood aloes. The decayed wood is generally heavy, oily and black.

Constituents.—A volatile oil.

Preparations.—Decoction (1 in 10). Dose, 4 to 12 drs. Incense, known as vadanâ rokshognair dhupalli :—It contains agaru, gugala (shorea robusta), acorus calamus, râi, nim leaves, and salt equal parts. As an anodyne fumigation, used to relieve pain in gout, and in surgical wounds and ulcers.

Confection known as java-rasa-uda, contains agar 5, elachi 8, post-e-turanj 6, lavang 8, tabâshir 12, mastaki 6, kesar 4, golâb kali 8, salem misri 6, sumak 6, sâkar 10, sumbul tib 4, zirishk 3, rupâ leaves 1, sonâ leaves 1, taj, sunth, peppermint leaves each 1, mix, add sâkara sufficient to make a confection to be given with arak-e-kevarâ. Dcse, 20 to 60 grs.; given as a nervine tonic in seminal debility, giddiness, faintness, and leucorrhœa.

Actions and uses.—Used as perfume and as stimulant cholagogue, also deobstruent. It is an ingredient in various nervine tonic, carminative, and stimulant preparations. It is used in gout and rheumatism, also to check vomiting. A paste of agara and sápasandà, with brandy, is applied to the chest in bronchitis of children and to the head in headache.

Remarks.—It is a chief ingredient in incense sticks known as agara batti. The sticks are ignited, like candles, and hence the name. There are two kinds of agara batti, black and white. Taggar wood is heavy and dark coloured, oily and resinous. It comes from Zanzibar. To water it gives a greenish yellow colour. It yields an oil of a yellow colour. The odour resembles that of sandalwood oil and is used in the preparation of attar by the natives.

Aquifoliaceæ—The Holly order.

Evergreen trees or shrubs ; leaves coriaceous, simple, exstipulate ; flowers small, axillary, unisexual ; sepals distinct, 4-6 ; corolla imbricated ; fruit flesy, indehiscent ; seeds suspended ; embryo small, albumen, fleshy.

Habitat.—Native of Europe.

Propersies.—They are bitter, tonic, and astringent; some are emetic and purgative. Some are used as substitutes for China tea.

Ilex Paraguayensis—The Brazilian, or Paraguay Holly.

Habitat.—Brazil and Argentine Republic.

Parts used.—The dried leaves and young twigs—called maté or Paraguay tea ; bark and berries.

Characters.—A small evergreen tree, exstipulate, coriaceous.

Constituents.—Contains theine or caffeine, 1 to 2 p.c. like China tea; also theobromine, but a larger proportion of mineral salts than either tea or coffee. It also contains a volatile oil, tannin and a glucoside.

Preparations.—Decoction of leaves. Fluid extract. Dose, 30 to 60 ms.

Actions and uses.—The berries are diuretic and exhilarant, and in large doses emetic and cathartic. The decoction when taken to excess produces a kind of intoxication. In moderate doses it promotes digestion and augments appetite ; but its continued and immoderate use produces dyspeptic symptoms. It sustains the system when undergoing hunger or great fatigue. The leaves and bark are very beneficial in intermittent fever. Used in South America as tea, and known as Matê or Paraguay tea.

Santalaceæ—The Sandalwood or Chandana family.

Herbs, shrubs or trees; leaves entire, alternate ; flowers perfect, calyx small, superior, 4 or 5 cleft ; stamens perigynous; ovary one-celled, inferior ; ovules 1-4 ; fruits indehiscent, one-seeded ; seed with fleshy albumen.

Habitat.—Native of temperate climate and tropics.

Properties.—some of the species are astringent, others are well known for their wood, which is highly fragrant and contains an essential oil. The seeds are oily. Fruit edible.

Santalum Album, B.P. Sirium Myrtifolium.

Habitat.—South of India, E. Indian Islands, Malabar.

Parts used.—The wood and a volatile oil (Oleum Santali) B.P.

Vernacular.—Arab.—Sandale-abyaz. Beng.—Sâdâchondan. Bur.—Sandakû. Can.—Gandhadâ-chekke. Cing.—Handun. Duk.—Sandal. Eng.—White sandal wood, white-saunders. Guz.—Sukhada. Hind.—Safed-chondana. Malyal.—Chanduna-mutti. Mar.—Gandhâ-châ-kodâ. Pers.—Sandale-supêd. Sans.—Pitachandana—yellow sandal (or darker heart wood). Shrikhanda—white sandal (the lighter heart wood). Tam.—Shandanak. Tel.—Gandhapu-chekka.'

Characters.—Wood yellow inside and white outside; trunk in long pieces of various shapes and sizes and covered over with a brownish scabrous bark, firmly adherent to the wood. Central portion or heart wood, when rasped or rubbed, highly fragrant; colour varying from pale white externally (sapwood) to pale yellow or dark red within (heart wood); central portion of a deep dark brown colour; the fragrance depends on the presence of an essential oil, chiefly found in the dark central wood. Fruits known as chandana bija are of the size of káka mári, of a dark brown colour and spherical in form with a small stalk at the bottom; apex crowned by a circular brimmed rim, in the centre of which is a conical protuberance. The interior of the fruit contains one single seed. The seed is globular, and of a brownish red or cinnamon colour; surface tubercled; at the centre of the apex are four projecting ridges which run divergently and disappear about the middle; testa, brittle and easily separable; kernel semi-opaque, oily, resinous, and of a brownish colour; odour balsamic; taste acrid and oily.

Constituents.—The wood contains a volatile oil 2 to 2 5 p.c., a dark resin, and tannic acid. Oleum Santali, B.P., obtained from the wood by distillation. A pale yellowish and thickish liquid, of a strong, peculiar, balsamic and aromatic odour; taste pungent and spicy, acid reaction, soluble in alcohol (1 in 6). Dose, 5 to 30 ms., given in emulsion, pills or capsules.

Actions and uses.—The wood is bitter, cooling, sedative and astringent. The oil is an astringent to the mucous membrane. It causes dryness in the fauces, great thirst, colicky pains and fulness in the loins; a paste of it is applied to the body in pains in the limbs during high fever; with rose water and camphor or with sarcocolla, to the head in headache, to inflammatory swellings, or to the skin in skin affections. The oil is astringent, diuretic, expectorant and stimulant; given internally with cardamoms and bamboo manna in gonorrhœa, bronchitis, in inflammation of the mucous membranes as cystitis, pyelitis and chronic diarrhœa. The seeds are used as pessaries by native women to procure abortion. A preparation known as khamire chandana (confection) is of common use among the natives; it consists of safed chandana 2 parts, gulegolâb 4, kâsani 4, elachi 1, tabâshira 3, âmlâ (without seeds) 3, sakara 45 ; given in headache.

Euphorbiaceæ, The Spurge wort, Erandi or Thuvara Family.

Characters.—Shrubs or herbs, generally with an acrid, milky, poisonous juice ; leaves alternate, mostly opposite, simple or compound, and stipulate or exstipulate. Flowers unisexual, axillary, and terminal with bracts ; calyx wanting ; corolla none ; sometimes males and females are on the same plant and sometimes on separate plants; ovary, superior, 3-celled; ovules 2 from each cell ; fruit tricoccous ; 3 to 6 seeded capsule, dry, and opening with elasticity ; or succulent and indehiscent ; seed one or more in each cell, embryo in fleshy albumen, radicle superior.

Habitat.—Natives of temperate climate, tropics.

Properties.—They generally contain an acrid milky juice. Poisonous properties are common in most of the plants. In proper doses it is emetic, nauseous, purgative, diuretic and rubefacient. Pure starchy food is obtained from some edible roots, other contain caoutchouc. The wood of some of the species is very fragrant ; embryo of the seeds is mostlyviolently emetic or purgative.

Acalypha Indica, A. Paniculata.

Habitat.—Hotter parts of India, Bengal, Deccan Peninsula.

Parts used.—The herb.

Vernacular.—Beng.—Shvet busanta. Can.—Chalmari. Duk.—Koop-pie Khokali. Eng.—Malabar cupa mani, Indian acalypha. Guz.—Dâdaro. Bomb., Hind., Duk.—Koop-pie, Khokali. Mal. Tam.—Cheti Kuppanvani. Tel.—Harita Manjari.

Khokali means cough. The plant has a reputation of being a good expectorant.

Characters.—The plant is 1 to 2 feet high, with many branched stems, rounded, erect, and smooth ; leaves, on long petioles, ovate, serrated, of a green or dark green colour above, and pale beneath ; minutely dotted ; spikes axillary and hairy, long as the leaves ; flowers small, greenish; male uppermost, enclosed in a cup shaped involucre, opening on the inner side ; stamens 8 to 16, styles 3, capsules tricoccous, 3-celled, one-seeded; fruits small, three-lobed, covered with bristly hairs, and seated on a finely dentate calyx ; smell of the plant disagreeable. Dose of the powdered herb, 10 to 30 grs.

Constituents.—An alkaloid, acalyphine.

Preparations.—Succus, expressed juice. Dose, ½ to 1 teaspoonful. Infusion of root, (1 in 10). Dose, 1 to 2 fld. ozs ; Cataplasm of the leaves. Decoction of leaves (1 in 20). Dose, ½ to 1 fld. oz. Tincture (1 in 8). Dose, ½ to 1 fld. dr. Liquid Extract. Dose, 10 to 60 ms.

Actions and uses.—Cathartic, emetic, expectorant and vermifuge. The infusion with a little garlic is used to expel worms in children. The decoction is a safe, speedy and sure laxative and emetic like senega or ipecacuanha. It increases the pulmonary secretions but does not cause any depression of the vital powers; given in pulmonary tuberculosis, croup, asthma and bronchitis of children. Externally the decoction is used in earache. The juice made into liniment with oil is used in rheumatism, and venereal pains; with lime (chunam) it is used as an application in skin diseases. Cataplasm of leaves relieves pain attendant on bites of venomous insects; also recommended for syphilitic ulcers; suppository of bruised leaves relieves constipation in children.

Aleurites Moluccana, A. Triloba.

Habitat.—Pacific Islands, India.

Parts used.—The nuts and oil called kakui or kekune.

Vernacular.—Arab.—Jouze-barri. Beng.—Banglâ-akrôt. Burm.—Tosikiya-si. Can.—Nat-akrodu. Cing.—Kakkuna. Eng.—Filberts, candle nut, berry or Belgaum walnut. Guz., Hind.—Hindi-akhrot-hijjle-badam. Malyal.—Kamari, Kamira. Mar—Rânakhrot, Japhal. Pers.—Girda-gâne-hindi. Tam.—Woodooga. Tel.—Akrotu-vittu.

Characters.—The oil expressed from the nuts is used as a drying oil for paint and resembles castor oil. Nuts vary in size from a small sopári to a big sopári; very hard, ovate, and slightly acuminate. At the base is a large brownish scar, like that found in arithá; apex pointed; except at the scar, the surface is smooth, somewhat shining, and of a darkish red or brownish red colour. The shell is thick and contains a thin reddish testa within, which is oily and resinous looking; whitish seeds, very rancid. Kernel on being lighted burns like a wax candle. Dose of the oil, 1 to 2 ozs.

Constituents.—The almond contains cellulose, fat, organic matter, mineral matter, and ash containing lime, magnesia, phosphoric anhydride, &c.

The oil contains oleine, myristin, palmitin, stearin and an acrid resin in which resides the purgative principle.

Actions and uses.—The nuts are used for their aphrodisiac properties; the oil is used as an aperient like castor oil.

Baliospermum Montanum, B. Axillare, Croton Polyandrum, Croton Roxburghii, Jetropha Montana.

Habitat.—Tropical Himalaya, Deccan Peninsula, Bengal, Circars.

Parts used.—The root and seeds.

Vernacular.—Burm.—Tha-du-wa. Guz.—Dante-mul. Hind.—Hakni. Sans.—Danti-nânâ, dante upachitra, dânte vija, maku laka. Tel.—Konda-amadum. Tam.—Nâga-dante.

Characters.—Root nearly straight, seldom branched; pieces about 2 or 3 inches in length, and as thick as the little finger; bark smooth, of a light yellow or brown colour and tubercled or scabrous;

taste bitter and pungent with a little aroma; wood very light, of a yellowish white colour, soft, less fibrous than the bark, somewhat coarsely tough, and loaded with starch; smell disagreeable; seeds like those of eranda, but smaller ; sometimes sold as croton seeds.

Constituents.—The root contain resin and starch.

Actions and uses.—The root is purgative, often used with aromatics in constipation with flatulence, and in anasacra and jaundice. The seeds are drastic purgative, and given with trikatu and tankana khára, &c. Dose, 1 seed of 1 to 3 grs.

Bridelia Retusa, B. Spinosa, B. Crenulata, B. Montana.

Habitat.—Throughout the hotter parts of India.

Parts used.—The bark.

Vernacular.—Cing.—Kattakaala-gas. Can.—Asânâ. Hind.—Khâja-kharaka. Malyal.—Mullic-vangay. Mar.—Phattar-phoda-kánte-hasan. Tam.—Adamaruthu. Tel.—Kora-maddi.

Characters.—Trees with or without thorns ; branches numerous, spreading ; thorns large but few ; bark scabrous yielding a blood-red juice, very astringent ; dry bark light brown externally with fungous protuberances, internally smooth and fibrous and of a cinnamon colour. It is one of the most astringent barks in India.

Constituents.—Tannic acid, in very large quantities.

Preparations.—Decoction (1 in 20). Dose, 2 to 6 fld. drs.

Actions and uses.—The bark is astringent. In general use for tanning leather. It is also used as lithontriptic.

Breynia Rhamnoides.

Habitat.—Tropical India.

Parts used.—The leaves and bark.

Characters.—Shrub with young angular shoots; leaves alternate, short petioled and spreading, broad or oval.

Preparations.—Decoction (1 in 20). Dose, 2 to 6 fld. drs.

Actions and uses.—The bark is astringent. The leaves are smoked like tobacco in cases of enlarged uvula and tonsils.

Cicca Disticha, Phyllanthus Distichus, Phyllanthus Longifolius, Averrhoa Acida.

Habitat.—India.

Parts used.—The fruit, seeds and leaves.

Vernacular.—Beng.—Nubâree, Hurriphal. Burm.—Them-ban-h'soke-gyee. Cing.—Ratanelli. Eng.—Country gooseberry. Mar., Guz.—Kantha avala. Bomb., Hind.—Chelmeri, Haraphálevadi. Malyal.—Chirimi. Port.—Chirambola. Sind.—Kâkadana. Tam.—Arunelli. Tel.—Racha-usherihe.

Kantha avala, from kantha, trunk or stem, and avala, the tree of emblic myrabolams. The fruits of Cicca Disticha are apparently seen to grow on the kantha or stem of avala, and hence the name.

Characters.—Leaves long, pinnate ; leaflets many, small. alternate stalked orbicular, 3 inches long, and with short small petioles ; petioles round or oblong, or rather acute, smooth, ending in a raceme of male flowers. Racemes numerous, terminal or axillary ; flowers numerous small, reddish in globular heads ; fresh fruits yellow, fleshy, and marked with from 6 to 8 deep grooves ; in size they resemble small fanduka, or gooseberry ; dried fruits of a greyish or dark brown colour ; surface highly wrinkled. Pulp thick, brittle and rather fibrous ; nut very hard, of a pale brown colour, containing 6 seeds, 3-celled and marked with 6 striæ; seeds reddish brown and resembling Káládáná in shape.

Preparation.—Decoction of leaves (1 in 20). Dose, ½ to 1 fld. oz.

Actions and uses.—The decoction of the leaves is a good diaphoretic. The leaves are mucilaginous and demulcent, and given in gonorrhœa. The ripe fruits are used as adjuncts to cough mixtures. They are also pickled and preserved as Amalá. Seeds are cathartic.

Croton Eluteria, B. P.,

Habitat.—Bahamas, Cuba.

Parts used.—The dried bark, cascarilla, B. P.

Characters.—Bark in quills or curved pieces, long, thick of a greyish colour, and fissured : surface, covered with whitish lichen. Inside it is smooth and resinous ; odour agreeable and aromatic ; taste warm, bitter and aromatic. Dose, 10 to 30 grs.

Constituents—Aromatic volatile oil, 1 p.c.; cascarillin a bitter crystalline principle, resin 15 p.c., tannin, pectin, gum, starch.

Cascarillin—Precipitate the infusion with acetate of lead, remove lead by sulphuretted hydrogen, evaporate the filtrate and crystallize ; soluble in alcohol, ether and hot water.

Preparations.—Tinctura cascarillæ, B. P. (1 in 5). Dose, ½ to 1 fld. dr. Infusum cascarillæ, B.P. (1 in 20). Dose, ½ to 1 fld. oz.

Actions and uses.—Aromatic bitter, stimulant, expectorant, stomachic, tonic and febrifuge; in large doses it causes nausea, vomiting and even diarrhœa. It stimulates the secretion of the stomach, salivary glands and intestines. It acts as an astringent owing to its containing tannin ; chiefly used in flatulence, dyspepsia, chronic diarrhœa, dysentery, colic, general debility and intermittent fever ; also in chronic bronchitis with excessive expectoration.

Croton Oblongifolium.

Habitat.—Bengal, Behar, S India. Deccan, Burma, Ceylon.

Parts used.—The root bark, leaves and fruit.

Vernacular.—Beng.—Barâgach. Goa.—Gonsurong. Hind.—Arjuna. Malyal.—Kote, Putol. Mar.—Ganasura. Sans.—Bhutam, Kusam, Bhutala-bhairi.

Characters.—Root twisted, often flattened; bark thick, scaly, pretty smooth, and ash coloured externally; internally yellowish and mottled with brown, substance compact and resinous; odour, highly aromatic, taste like that of miri; leaves, petioled, alternate, oblong, obtuse, pointed, smooth on both sides; capsulse globular, fleshy, six-furrowed and tricoccous.

Constituents.—An alkaloid and various acid principles.

Preparations.—Infusion of the bark (1 in 20), and decoction of the leaves (1 in 20). Dose, ½ to 1 fld. oz.

Actions and uses.—The bark and root are alterative and cholagogue. The seeds are purgative. The bark is used in reducing chronic enlargement of the liver and in remittent fever. It is applied externally to the hepatic region and in chronic hepatitis and also to sprains, bruises and rheumatic swellings.

Croton Tiglium, B.P.,

Habitat.—India, China, Japan, Eastern Bengal.

Parts used.—The seeds and fixed oil from the seed—oleum crotonis B.P.

Vernacular.—Arab.—Habbel-salatin. Beng.—Rechuk. Burm.—Kanakoh. Can.—Japâlada. Cing.—Nepalam. Eng.—Cathay castor seeds, croton seeds, purging croton, the oil, croton oil, nepala oil. Duk., Hind., Mar., Guz.—Jamâlagota, nipâlo, jaypala. Malyal.—Kadelavanaku. Panj.—Juphlota. Pers.—Bedanjire. Sans.—Dunti, Napal, Jayâpalâ Tittiriphal, Kanaka-phala. Tam.—Nêrvalam. Tel.—Nepalam.

Characters.—A small tree. Fruit a capsule, of the size of a hazel nut, externally smooth and brownish yellow, tricoccous, dehiscent, each cell containing one seed; seeds oblong or ovoid, heavy, mucilaginous and about half an inch in length; upper surface convex, the dorsal and ventral surfaces arched; testa thin, brittle, brownish, red and shining or mottled. On scratching the scurf is easily removed and the surface then presents a black appearance; old seeds generally deprived of the scurf are black. The surface is marked with four ridges. The kernel consists of an abundant oily albumen, of a lightish yellow colour, enclosed in a delicate white membrane adherent to the testa. Dose, 1 to 2 seeds.

Constituents.—The entire seed contains expressed or fixed oil—oleum crotonis, 30 to 40 p.c., and the kernel alone contains the oil 50 to 70 p.c.; proteids albumin, &c.

The oil obtained by expression is transparent, colour brownish yellow to dark, reddish brown, viscid, slightly fluorescent of a slightly fatty rancid smell, and of an acrid burning taste, of a slightly acid reaction; applied to the skin it produces pustular eruptions; entirely soluble in absolute alcohol, freely soluble in ether, chloroform, carbon disulphide, and fixed and volatile oils. It contains glycerides of acetic, butyric, formic, lauric, myristic, palmitic, stearic, and other fatty acids, also tiglinic acid, which is isomeric with angelic acid; the purgative principle crotonol ; the vesicating principle crotonoleic acid, insoluble in alcohol.

Preparations.—Linimentum crotonis B. P. (1 in 8) with oil of cajuput ; a compound pill largely used by the natives called Maha narakha rasa, which means drastic purgative. It contains:—chebulic myrobalans, pulp of cassia fistula, emblic myrobalans, baliospermium axillare, picorrhiza kurrooa, milky juice of euphorbia nerii folia, root of ipomea turpethum, tubers of cyperus rotundus each one part ; mix together and make decoction. Then add husked croton seeds 1 part and boil till reduced to the consistence of an extract. To this next add croton seeds 8 parts, ginger, black pepper 2 ; parakajali and sulphur 1, rub together and make a pill mass. Dose, 2 grs. given in tympanitis, colic, ascites &c.

Actions and uses.—The seeds are never used until the testa and embryo are removed, and the kernel boiled in milk. It is a powerful drastic cathartic and rubefacient. The oil is highly irritant. Applied to the skin, it pustulates, leaving an unsightly scab. In small doses as a powerful cathartic it acts promptly, producing copious watery stools. In large doses it causes vomiting and produce gastritis; it also irritates the intestinal glands as well as setting up inflammation of the intestinal mucous membrane and giving rise to increased peristalsis. The addition of an alkali increases hypercatharsis where prompt derivative action is desired, with speedy discharge of alvine evacuations and lowering of the blood pressure. It is given in apoplexy, mania, coma, intestinal obstruction, paralysis, dropsy, and constipation. It should not be given in inflammation of the stomach or intestines or if any organic obstruction exists. It may be used where bulky doses cannot be taken. In persons who refuse to take purgatives, the oil may be dropped upon the tongue with benefit. The seeds and the oil are especially used in fever, constipation, intestinal worms, anasarca, ascites, dropsy, enlargement of the abdominal viscera, tympanitis,colic,calculous affections and gout. Externally as a vesicant it is applied to the scalp in acute cerebral diseases, to the cord in spinal meningitis, to the chest in chronic bronchitis, and to the throat in laryngitis. Its liniment is used as a powerful counter-irritant in neuralgia, sciatica, ovaritis, gout, glandular swellings, chronic articular rheumatism, pulmonary diseases, as bronchitis, pleurisy and tinea tonsurans of the scalp.

Euphorbia Antiquorum.

Habitat.—The hotter parts of India, Ceylon.

Parts used.—The juice.

Vernacular.—Arab.—Lakkûme-hindi. Beng.—Narasij. Burm.—Shâzâvangi. Can.—Mudu-mula-kalli. Cing.—Dalûk. Duk.—Tindhari-send. Eng.—Triangular spurge. Hind., Guz.—Tandhâri Thohar Narsij. Malyal.—Shadi-dakalli. Mar.—Tridhari-nevadunga, naraseja. Pers.—Lakuniyâl-hindi. Sans.—Sunhi sehunda mahataru, Vajra tundi, gandera. Tam.—Shadre-kalli. Tel.—Boutache-mudu.

Characters.—Stems erect, ramous, 3 or 4 pointed, angles furnished with stipulary spines; joints straight; peduncles, solitary or in pairs, usually 3 flowered; flowers greenish yellow.

Constituents.—The dried juice contains euphorbon 35 p.c. two resins one 25 p.c. soluble in ether; another 13·7 p.c. insoluble in ether; caoutchouc 1·5 p.c. and gum.

Preparations.—Succus. Dose, 2 to 5 ms.

Actions and uses.—Purgative, alterative, rubefacient and vesicant. The juice is corrosive, used externally in rheumatism and in toothache. Internally the bark or the juice is used as a purgative in obstinate constipation.

Euphorbia Corollata—Large Flowering Spurge.

Habitat.—United States.

Parts used.—The root.

Characters.—Root many headed, 8 inches long and 1 inch thick; externally brown and fissured; bark, thick and white internally; taste sweet and bitter acrid. It yields milky juice when punctured. Dose, 2 to 10 grs.

Constituents.—A glucoside, resin and euphorbon.

Preparations.—Infusion and decoction (1 in 20). Dose, ½ to 1 oz.

Actions and uses.—Diaphoretic, cathartic, emetic, expectorant and vesicant. Given in obstinate constipation and in cough, intermittent fever, jaundice and rheumatism. As a vesicant it is applied to warts, corns, &c.

Euphorbia Neriifolia, E. Nivulia.

Habitat.—Deccan Peninsula, Beluchistan, Ajmir.

Parts used.—The juice and root.

Vernacular.—Arab.—Dehu. Beng.—Hydaona pâtâsij. Burm.—Shazavn-mina. Can.—Yale kalli. Duk.—Kuttê-ki-gibh. Eng.—The common milk hedge. Guz.—Thohara kantâro. Hind.—Sehund, thohar, pattonki send. Malyal.—Elak-kalli. Mar.—Nivadunga, mingût. Sans.—Sunahi, pattakari. Tam.—Elle kalli. Tel.—Akuje-mudu.

Characters.—Prickly milky tree or shrub; stem ash coloured; branches round and jointed stipular, covered with short and sharp thorns; leaves tongue-shaped, entire, smooth and thick, flowers greenish yellow; root thick and woody; root bark pale white. Every part of the shrub when cut exudes a pure white milky juice which is acrid, very sticky and becomes thick on drying. Dose of the powdered root, 2 to 4 grs.

Constituents.—Euphorbon, resin, gum, caoutchouc, malate of calcium &c.

Preparations.—Succus. Dose, 2 to 5 ms. Compound powder. To obtain it steep mudâr flowers, aghâdâ root, gokarna root equal parts in the milky juice of thoar and add harade $\frac{1}{3}$ of the weight of the whole and dry. Dose, 2 to 4 grs.; mixed with honey it is given in asthma.

Actions and uses.—The juice is a purgative and expectorant, locally rubefacient and a popular application to warts, when it acts as a blister. Heated with common salt it is used as a remedy for whooping cough, asthma, dropsy, enlarged liver and spleen, dyspepsia, jaundice, colic, flatulence, &c. In small doses it promotes the expectoration and is often given with the juice of adulasâ. By mixing with other purgatives its purgative properties become increased. It is given in visceral obstructions, in dropsical affections consequent on long continued intermittent fever, in jaundice and in rheumatism. Externally it is mixed with margosa oil and applied to stiff limbs in rheumatism; and also used in killing maggots in wounds. The root is used for snake-bites.

Euphorbia Pilulifera, E. Hirta, E. Parviflora.

Syn.—Australian asthma weed, snake weed and cats hair.

Habitat.—Bombay, on gravel rocks and waste grounds, seen after the rains.

Parts used.—The herb.

Vernacular.—Beng.—Barakeru. Guz., Hind., Bomb.—Mothi dudhi, Dudheli. Can.—Barasu. Mar.—Goverdhan, mothi dudhi Nayeti. Sans.—Rakta vinduchada. Tam.—Amum patchai aressi. Tel.—Bidari. Nayati—signifies ringworm.

Characters.—A hairy weed, obliquely erect and with apices recurved; branches, coloured, hairy and pressing flat on the earth; flowers small, numerous in clusters; seeds papillose or ovoid. Easily recognised by acute leaves, globular, hispid hairiness and small fruits.

Constituents.—Active principle, wax, caoutchouc, chlorophyll, resin, tannin, sugar, mucilage, calcium oxalate, carbohydrates and albuminoids. The active principle is a gum resin, soluble in water and weak spirit, insoluble in ether, alcohol, chloroform, bisulphide of carbon and turpentine.

Preparations.—Solid extract. Dose, $\frac{1}{2}$ to 2 grs. Fluid extract. Dose, 10 to 30 ms. Decoction (1 in 20). Dose, 1 to 2 fld. ozs. Tincture (1 in 5). Dose, 10 to 30 ms.

Actions and uses.—Demulcent, anthelmintic, antispasmodic and local parasiticide. It is a popular remedy for cough, bronchial affections and diseases of the respiratory passages generally; also given for worms, bowel complaints, gonorrhœa, &c. In dyspnœa due to asthma, emphysema and pulmonary cardiac disease it is very beneficial. In spasmodic asthma the fluid extract is very usefulc. It is a very useful remedy in acute and chronic dysentery, in coryza where arsenic and iodide of potassium have failed. In should be given after meals. Its action is chiefly exerted through the pneumogastric, paralysing the heart and respiration.

Euphorbia Resinifera.

Habitat.—Morocco.

Parts used.—The dried juice or concrete gum (Euphorbium) and resin.

Vernacular.—Arab.—Farfiyun. Burm.—Shia-dzaon. Cing.—Daluk-gahek-kiry. Hind.—Saynd-kâ-dudh. Bomb., Ind. Bazaar.—Afarbiyun, farfiyun. Malyal.—Sudu-sadu, Vajrak-shira. Sans.—Vautaka.

Characters.—The gum resembles rich Hinga ; colour yellow brown ; met with in pieces of irregular shape as if excavated or scooped out ; taste bitterish acrid and rather burning ; odour peculiar, acrid, and resembling that of wax. The gum is also found in Euphorbia canarienses of Arabia and Africa, Euphorbia antiquorum of Arabia and India, and in E. Tetragonia.

Constituents.—The juice contains resin, euphorbon, mucilage, malates of calcium and sodium and other mineral compounds.

Actions and uses.—Euphorbium is a powerful irritant ; a paste of it is applied in sciatica and lumbago. Made into pessaries it is applied to the os to procure abortion ; diluted with some inert powder, it is blown into the ear in deafness.

Euphorbia Thymifolia.

Habitat.—Throughout India, Ceylon, Central Asia.

Parts used.—The plant.

Vernacular.—(Beng).—Raktakeru. Hind.—Nigachuni. Mar.—Lahan nayeti. Punj.—Hazardana. Sans.—Rakta-vinda-chhada. Tam.—Sittra-paladi. Tel.—Reddi-vari.

Characters.—Small milky prostrate plant ; stems slender, reddish leaves opposite, obliquely oval, serrate, slightly aromatic and astringent flowers axillary, on short peduncles, small and greenish ; capsule erect, or obtusely keeled, pubescent ; seeds with 5 or 6 shallow transverse furrows.

Constituents.—A crystalline alkaloid principle allied to quercitrin.

Preparations.—Decoction (1 in 40). Dose, 1 to 2 ozs. milky juice. Dose, 1 to 2 drs.

Actions and uses. Vermifuge, demulcent, stimulant and laxative ; chiefly used in bowel complaints in children, worms, gonorrhœa and amenorrhœa. Locally the juice is applied in ringworm.

Euphorbia Tirucalli.

Habitat.—Africa, India, Asia.

Parts used.—The milky juice.

Vernacular.—Arab.—Azfur, sukkum. Beng.—Lankâ shij. Bomb.—Netario Thoar. Cing.—Nava hanadi. Can.—Bonta Kalli. Hind., Duk.—Kârki send. Barkisend. Eng.—Milk hedge, Indian tree purge, milk bush. Guz.—Ranashira, Netruo-thora, Khurassani-thora, Thora dana dalio. Javanese—Kayoo-oorb. Mar.—Vajra duhû. Malyal. —Kolkalli. Pers.—Taqunâi-yâl-hindi. Tam—Tiru Kalli. Tel.—Kâda chemudu.

Characters.—Smooth green milky bush; branchlets slender jointed, long and blunt : colour green or greenish dark; leaves very small; juice acrid.

Constituents.—Euphorbon, resin gum, caoutchouc, malate of calcium, &c.

Preparations.—Succus. Dose, 1 to 3 ms.

Actions and uses.—In small doses the juice is used as a purgative. It is applied as a vesicant to painful joints in rheumatism and neuralgia. The milky juice mixed with flour is considered very useful as a blister in syphilitic nodes.

Execaria Agallocha, Arbor Execans, Execaria Camettia.

Habitat.—Forests of India, Rangoon, Ceylon, salt swamps near the sea, Cochin, Travancore.

Parts used.—The juice and cork.

Vernacular.—Beng—Ugaru, Burm.—Ka yau. Cing.—Tella keeriya gass. Eng.—Tiger's milk tree, blinding tree. Hind.—Gengiva, Tejbala. Mal.—Kametti. Can.—Karo. Mar.—Phungali Hura. Tam.—Tillae cheddi. Tel.—Tella Chetu.

Characters.—Wood knotty, grey or blackish, soft, spongy and smooth. All parts abound in acrid resinous milky juice which when dried hardens into a kind of caoutchouc. From the lower part of the trunk and roots is obtained a soft light suber. It occurs in irregular shaped pieces from which the epidermis has been removed by scraping and resembles in structure a coarse cork.

Actions and uses.—The juice is highly irritating, the caoutchouc in 1 to 2 gr. doses is used as a purgative and alterative in epilepsy. It is locally applied to inveterate ulcers, leprous sores, &c. Tejbala is reputed among the natives as an aphrodisiac.

Hevea Brasiliensis, B.P., H. Guyanensis, Siphonia Elastica. Hevea Elastica.

Habitat.—India, Tropics, S. America.

Parts used.—The prepared milky juice.

Vernacular.—India rubber, caoutchouc, para rubber.

Characters.—Large trees ; leaves trifoliate ; leaflets, obovate, long, dark green above and lighter below, flowers in racemes—Caoutchouc is a prepared milky juice met with in clusters. It is elastic, in masses of varying thickness, brownish black externally and mottled and pale internally; odour peculiar and empyreumatic, without any taste; soluble in chloroform, oil of turpentine, carbon bisulphide, benzol, and benzin, insoluble in water, ethylic alcohol, diluted acids and diluted alkaline solutions. Combined with sulphur and heated, it is converted into hard rubber. Caoutchouc is also obtained from ficus elastica, jatropha elastica, artocarpus integrifolia and urceola elastica.

Constituents.—Resin 32 p.c. volatile oil, fat, albumen, and colouring matter. The resin, a solid hydrocarbon—is the elastic principle known as caoutchouc.

Preparations.—Liquor caoutchouc, B.P., solution of India-rubber; contains India-rubber 1 oz., benzol 10 fld. ozs., carbon bisulphide 10 fld. ozs., Charta Sinapis, B.P.

Actions and uses.—Woven into fabrics to reduce varicose veins, hydrocele and hernia ; also used for the preparation of bougies, pessaries, &c.

Jatropha Curcas, Curcas Purgans, J. Multifidus, Curcas Multifidus.

Habitat.—Throughout India, Ceylon, Coromandel and Travancore.

Parts used.—Seeds, juice, leaves and oil.

Vernacular.—Arab.—Dunde-birri. Beng.—Bagbha-randa, Ratanojota. Bomb.—Moglai erandi. Burm.—Them-ban-kyst-hsoo. Can.—Mara narulle. Chin.—Tung-shu. Cing.—Ratendaru. Eng.—Angular leaved physic nut, paraguya nut, purging nuts. Goa.—Galamark. Guz., Duk., Mar., Hind.—Bâghbheranda, Mogalai eranda. Malyal.—Kat-avanakoo. Sans.—Kânona eranda, nepala, Parvata yeranda. Tam.—Kata-manak. Tel.—Adivi amida.

Characters.—Large wooded evergreen shrub, abounding in milky juice with young stems which are rounded ; leaves quite smooth and green on long and round petioles, 3 to 5 angled or lobed, middle lobe rather large and more acute. The fruits resembling âmalâ in appearance and walnuts in size. They are greenish, glaucous, obtusely 3 angled and marked with 6 striæ, 3 seeded and 3 celled ; seeds oblong, ovate, compressed, dark coloured, resembling in shape but are larger than erandi ; testa dark. The whole plant abounds in a viscid pus-like juice. The oil, pulza oil or seed oil or purging oil, expressed from the seeds is a fixed oil, slightly yellow or of a paler colour than the linseed oil, without disagreeble odour of castor oil and of a pleasant almond like taste, and differing from castor oil in being slightly soluble in alcohol. Dose of the oil, 4 to 15 drops.

Constituents.—The seeds contain a fixed oil 30 p.c., sugar, starch albumen, caseine and inorganic matter. The oil contains an active principle, jatrophic acid.

Preparations.—Decoction of leaves (1 in 10). Dose, ½ to 1 fld. oz.; succus, embrocation, cataplasm of the leaves.

Actions and uses.—The seeds are acrid and emetic and even poisonous ; the oil is purgative, parasiticide, and insecticide ; the milky juice is hæmostatic, rubefacient and galactagogue ; the oil is applied in chronic skin diseases such as itch, eczema, ringworm, herpes, &c.; also used as a stimulant embrocation in chronic rheumatism. Internally like croton oil it is used as a purgative and given in paralysis and constipation and as a vermifuge, and is useful in constipation, dropsy, worms &c. The decoction of the leaves is said to excite the secretion of milk in women. As a discutient, the juice or the oil, rubbed with castor oil, is applied to buboes and abscesses to promote suppuration. As hæmostatic and styptic, the viscid milky juice when applied has the property of healing cuts and wounds like collodion ; it forms a thin film and thus checks hæmorrhages from bleeding surfaces and wounds and from hæmorrhoids ; as a styptic it is superior to turpentine, alum or the perchloride of iron. If injected into a varicose vein or aneurism (about a drachm) it coagulates the blood with good result.

Jatropha Glandulifera.

Habitat.—Northern Circars, Deccan Peninsula, Bengal, Panderpore, Bunds of Tanks.

Parts used.—The juice, fruits, leaves and oil.

Vernacular.—Bomb.—Velaty-erand, Hind., Beng.—Lâl Bheranda Mar.—Underbibi, Tadki Erandi. Sans.—Nikumba. Tam.—Udalai Tel.—Dundigapu.

Characters.—Shrub small, erect, and pubescent ; young branches and leaves red and studded with green, succulent, glandular or capitate. hairs; leaves 3 lobed, serrated, smooth, glaucous, almost veinless and. on long villose petioles ; upper surface covered with glands ; lower surface smooth and shining ; margins finely ciliated with small glandular hairs ; fruits six, striated, smooth, shining, of a greenish colour and here and there sprinkled with simple white hairs ; in form they resemble erandi or hazel nut, 3 seeds in each fruit ; seeds of a brown colour, of the size of a pea ; surface marked with 4 ridges; back rather flat and marked with two broad, black, longitudinal stripes. Between these a brown coloured ridge passes lengthwise. At the hilum there is a caruncule of a brownish yellow colour, on both sides of the caruncule two black lines extend downwards and outwards forming side ridges ; from the bottom of the hilum another central ridge extends and occupies the middle of the front surface ; cotyledon albuminous, white and oily, thus resembling kapura. The whole plant abounds in an acrid, greenish and viscid juice ; the oil is yellow. Dose, of the root, 2 to 5 grs.

Constituents.—Similar to those of jatropha curcas.

Actions and uses.—Purgative, counter-irritant and stimulant. The root brayed in water is given to children suffering from enlargement of the abdomen due to diseases of the liver and spleen ; it purges and reduces glandular swellings. The juice is escharotic, acrid, counter irritant, and is used by the natives to remove opacity of the cornea or thickening of the conjunctivæ ; the oil is applied to joints in chronic rheumatism, chronic ulcerations, sinuses, ringworm and paralysis.

Jatropha Macrorhiza.

Habitat.—Northern Mexico and Southern States adjoining.

Parts used.—The root.

Characters.—Root very thick, short, tuberous, with an erect herbaceous stem.

Preparations.—Fluid extract. Dose, ½ to 2 fld. drs.

Actions and uses.—Alterative, cholagogue, hydragogue, and cathartic; resembling in action calomel and vegetable purgatives such as leptandra podophyllum, and euonymin.

Jatropha Manihot, Manihot Utilissima.

Habitat.—Brazil, West Indies.

Parts used.—The fecula of root or rhizome.

Vernacular.—Eng.—Tapioca plant, cassava meal.

Characters.—A shrub; stems jointed; leaves glaucous and petiolate; root fleshy white, tuberous and very heavy, containing poisonous milky juice. To remove the acridity or the poison from the cassava meal, the juice is expressed by pressure, the meal is next washed, and the starch finally heated and dried, and the fecula or the starch is then known as cassava starch, tapioca meal, or Brazilian arrowroot. There are two varieties, sweet and bitter. The bitter variety contains prussic acid.

Constituents.—Starch and glutin.

Actions and uses.—Nutrient and demulcent; given during convalescence, debility, and low state of the system. Dose, ½ to 1 oz.

Mallotus Philippinensis, Croton Philippinensis, Rottlera Tinctoria.

Habitat.—Throughout tropical India, Philippine Islands, Arabia, China, Abyssinia.

Parts used.—The glands and hairs from the capsules.

Vernacular.—Arab.—Quinbil. Beng.—Kamela-tung. Burm.—Memasho. Can.—Chandrahittu. Cing.—Hamparandella. Eng.—Monkey faced tree, Dyers Rotlera. Guz., Hind.—Kamela, Kapilo, Kamud, Kembal. Mar.—Shendri, Kapila, Kamila. Malyal. Poonagam Pers.—Kampila, Konbela. Sans.—Kampilla Rocha nika, kambha, lohita rakla, rochanarakta, keshoor, punnaga, kambha. Tam.—Kopilla podi. Tel.—Bendu rupu.

Characters.—Kamal—a granular mobile brick red powder, chiefly consisting of small glands covering the ripe capsule or fruit. When collected the powder is generally mixed with pieces of capsules, stalk and hairs; other parts of the plant contain it in small quantities and of a lighter colour. In appearance it is resinous and shining, nearly tasteless and inodorous, partly soluble in alcohol and in ether. It is inflammable. Dose, 30 to 120 grs.

Constituents.—Resins 80 p.c. tannic acid, gum ; volatile oil, rottlerin, albuminous matter 7 p.c. ; colouring matter, cellulose 7 p.c. and ash 4 p.c.

Resins—These contain the colouring matter; to obtain them digest the root with ether, alcohol, glacial acetic acid or carbon sulphide ; one of them is soluble in cold alcohol and the other hot alcohol. Rottlerin, is an extract obtained by digesting the root with ether or carbon sulphide ; occurs as yellowish needles, soluble in hot alcohol, ether, benzene and carbon bisulphide.

Preparations.—Tincture (3 in 10). Dose, 1 to 3 drs.

Actions and uses.—Cathartic and anthelmintic ; given with treacle it kills and expels round and thread worms ; as a purgative it causes nausea but does not cause vomiting ; it relieves colicky pain and removes bile. It is a local remedy for ringworm, pityriasis, freckles and scabies.

Phyllanthus Emblica, Emblica Officinalis.

Habitat.—Throughout tropical India.

Parts used.—The dried fruit without nut—Emblicæ Fructus, bark and flowers.

Vernacular.—Arab.—Amlaj. Beng.—Amritphala, amlaki. Bomb. —Aavalakâthi. Burm.—Ziphiyu-si. Can.—Nelli-kayi. Cing.—Nellika. Eng.—Emblic myrobolans. Guz.—Ambala. Hind.—Aolâ âmlâ. Amvurâh. Malyal.—Amalakam. Pers.—Amelah. Sans.—Sriphala Amritphala. Tam.—Toppu nelli. Tel.—Amalakam.

Characters.—Fresh fruit globular with fleshy pulp, six striated, rather compressed, succulent, smooth and of a greenish yellow colour, as large as a walnut with a thick acidulous pulp enclosing a nut, which is triangular, obovate, 3 celled ; each cell has 2 triangular seeds ; taste sweetish, astringent, acid and somewhat acrid. Amalâ are of two kinds: true and false. True ones, phyllanthus emblica, are subhexagonal, and break upon pressure into 6 fragments and are of darkish colour. Each fragment consists of a section of a pulp and nut and contains one triangular or brown seed which is wrinkled and generally curved in at both ends. The false âmalâ are the fruits of cicca disticha, and are smaller than true âmalâ and of a pale brown colour.

Constituents.—Gallic acid tannic acid, gum, sugar, albumen, cellulose and mineral matter.

Preparations.—Decoction of the root (1 in 10). Dose, ½ to 1 fld. oz. Confection. Dose, 1 to 2 teaspoonfuls. Crystallized fruit. Dose, 1 to 2, and paste

Actions and uses.—The fresh fruit is refrigerant, diuretic, and laxative, and is used in chronic constipation. The dried fruit is cooling, stomachic and astringent; a powder of the fruit, nilotphar, kesara and rose water is used as a paste to the forehead in cephalalgia. It is also applied to the pubes in irritability of the bladder and in retention of urine. With grapes and honey it is a favourite cooling drink for fever and diarrhœa. An extract, prepared from the wood, is astringent like kátho. Its branches put into muddy water render the latter clear. It is one of the ingredients in the preparation known as triphalâ.

Phyllanthus Madraspatensis.

Habitat.—Tropical India.

Parts used.—The seeds.

Vernacular.—Kanocha Kanochhá (Hind. and Bom.).—The word kanochá is similar to the English word concha, which means the larger cavity of the external ear. Kanochhá seeds resemble in appearance concha, and hence the name.

Characters.—Seeds smaller than those of bhánga, triangular, highly polished, and of a grey colour; surface reticulated or marked with fan-like, delicate dark lines, like basket work. One side of the seed is arched and the other presents two sloping surfaces united so as to form a longitudinal ridge. At the pointed end is a small scar; the kernel is oily, with a sweet nutty taste.

Preparations.—Mucilage and decoction (1 in 20). Dose, ½ to 2 ozs.

Actions and uses.—The seeds are demulcent. With other demulcent decoctions, they are used in urinary affections such as gonorrhœa and internal inflammations on account of the mucilage they contain.

Phyllanthus Reticulatus.

Habitat.—Throughout tropical India.

Parts used.—The leaves and bark.

Vernacular.—Beng.—Pankûshi. Guz.—Dotwan. Hind.—Pânjoli. Malyal.—Katunirure. Mar.—Pavana. Sans—Krishna-kamboji. Sind.—Kunohi. Tam.—Pulavayr. Tel.—Pulaguda.

Characters.—Bark in pieces, about a foot long, thick as the wrist and dark brown externally; taste somewhat sweet; leaves oval, obtuse, and bifarious.

Constituents.—Tannic acid, gum and a crystalline principle.

Preparations.—Decoction of bark (1 in 20). Dose, 1 to 2 fld. ozs. Infusion of leaves (1 in 10). Dose, 1 to 2 fld. ozs.

Actions and uses.—Astringent, diuretic and alterative; a pill made of its juice mixed with camphor and cubebs is dissolved in the mouth as a remedy for spongy and bleeding gums.

Phyllanthus Niruri, P. Urinaria.

Habitat.—Deccan Peninsula, Bengal, Travancore.

Parts used.—The plant (herb).

Vernacular.—Beng.—Sadahajur-muni. Mar., Hind., Bomb.—Bhui ânmalâ. Bur.—Mi-ziphiyu. Can.—Kiranelligidâ. Duk.—Dheen ounlah. Malyal.—Kizkhaylnelli. Sans.—Bhûmy amalaki, Tamra velli, bahu patra. Tam.—Kilanelly. Tel.—Neela ooshirika.

Bahu patra means having many leaves.

Characters.—Plant from 6 to 10 in. long, annual, erect and ramous; stem angular, smooth and wiry; leaves like those of âmali, elliptical, mucronate, entire, glabrous, 3 in. long and one inch broad, divided into 6 or 7 leaflets, oblong and very short petioled and arranged alternately; flowers, axillary, sessile; fruits very small; capsules globose, 3-celled; seeds in each cell two, smooth and triangular; smell rather disagreeable; taste astringent and acidulous. Dose of the powdered plant, 30 to 60 grs.

Constituents.—A bitter principle, pseudo chiratin, an alkaloid, fat and colouring matter.

Preparations.—Infusion, (1 in 10). Dose, ½ to 1 fld. oz. tincture (1 in 8). Dose, ½ to 1 fld. dr.

Actions and uses.—Antiperiodic, diuretic, stomachic and demulcent. It is used in intermittent fevers, to prevent paroxysms; also given in diseases of the spleen and liver, in dropsy, gonorrhœa, acid urine and in jaundice. A poultice of the leaves mixed with salt is used for itch and scaly affections of the skin. The infusion, mixed with methi, is used as a stomachic, bitter and astringent, and also given as a remedy in chronic dysentery.

Ricinus Communis. B. P.

Habitat.—Throughout India, United States, Italy.

Parts used.—The oil, expressed from the seeds, Oleum Ricini—Castor oil, B. P.; leaves and seed.

Vernacular.—Arab.—Dhun-ul-kerwa. Beng.—Bharanda. Burm. Kyethsu. Chin.—Psuna. Can.—Haralu. Cing—Endaru. Duk.—Yarandî-kâ-jhar. Guz.—Erando. Hind.—Arandi-ka-per. Malyal.—Sit avanakka. Pers.—Bed-i-anjir. Sans.—Eranda, vâtâri, ruvuka, uruvuka. Tam.—Amanak-kan-chedi. Tel.—Amudupu-chettu, chittamin drak.

Characters.—Roots long and tapering, light, soft and of an acrid taste; stem hollow, smooth and glaucous, and generally marked with transverse rings; leaves large, smooth, green, or glaucous and from 7 to 10 lobed, lanceolate, acute, pointed and dentate. There are two jointed small glands, one at the attachment of the petiole to the blade; the other gland is seen a little above the insertion of the petiole to the stem. Fruits tricocous, obtusely triangular, six striated and marked with bristles; when fresh of a glaucous green colour; dry ones dark brown. On section each fruit is 3-celled; each cell containing 1 seed; seeds large of the size of coffee grains, oblong or ovate and compressed; dorsal surface more arched than the ventral; apex carunculated, caruncule, of a brownish colour; whole surface mottled with white, brown or dark patches. On the convex side, the blotches spread in a fan-like manner from the base of the caruncule; kernel, white and oily; seeds of two kinds, large and red seeded, and small, and grey seeded; the small ones containing superior oil. The oil separates if water be brought in intimate contact with the powdered kernel ; taste of the kernel oily and nauseous. The oil is drawn in two ways : by heat (decoction) and without heat (expression). This latter is the official variety and is known as cold drawn oil. Dose of the seeds, 10 seeds; of the oil, 1 to 8 drs.

Constituents.—Fixed oil, 45 p.c. an inert alkaloid, ricinin, proteids, 20 p.c.; starch, mucilage, sugar, ash 10 p.c.; also a poisonous aluminoid principle called ricin. The oil—oleum ricini—castor oil, contains recinolein, ricinoleic acid, palmitin, stearin and myristin and an acrid principle. The oil is a yellowish or pale coloured slightly viscid or oily, transparent liquid, of an acrid offensive and mawkish taste, mild nauseating odour, and neutral reaction ; soluble in absolute alcohol (1 in 1) in alcohol (1 in 5).

Preparations.—Decoction of roots (1 in 10). Dose, ½ to 1 fld. oz., mistura olei ricini B.P. (3 in 8). Dose, 1 to 2 fld. oz. Medicated oil : to erandi tela 10, add a watery paste of majitha 5, triphla 5, halad 4, sunth 4, daruhalad 3, boil, strain and evaporate.

Actions and uses.—All the constituents of the seeds except the oil are drastic, generally given with ginger tea or with decoction of deshmula dikvâth. The oil is non-irritant; when it reaches the duodenum it is decomposed by the pancreatic juice into recinoleic acid which irritates the bowels, stimulates the intestinal glands and the muscular coat and cause purgation ; it does not stimulate the liver. It acts in 4 or 5 hours, causing liquid stools without pain or griping and has a sedative effect on the intestines. With glycerine the effects of the oil are increased. Recinoleic acid is absorbed into the blood and tissues and is excreted with the human milk which when sucked imparts to the child its purgative action. Ricin, a toxic ferment, is a violent irritant of the intestines, kidneys and bladder. It gives rise to inflammation of the bile duct and very often to jaundice and to dysuria. The oil is best given in flatulence, costiveness, fever, rheumatism and in inflammation of the genito-urinary organs as nephritis, cystitis, gonorrhœa, calculi, stricture of rectum or urethra. In diarrhœa due to the presence of irritating substances in the intestines leading to congestion or to excessive secretions it acts without exhausting the strength. It is used after operations on the abdominal or pelvic viscera. It overcomes constipation of typhoid fever, during pregnancy and before labour and in post-partem conditions. In intestinal or renal colic it is given with the juice of fresh ginger with prompt relief. It expels lumbrici. In enteritis, peritonitis and dysentery it is given with laudanum. If depression exists, oil of turpentine 5 to 10 ms. may be added. A poultice of the crushed seeds is used to promote suppuration, to mature boils and to reduce gouty and rheumatic swellings ; as a galactagogue, varalians or poultices of the leaves are applied to inflamed breasts in women during lactation. Hot leaves are applied to the hypogastrium to increase the flow of menses. The root bark is an alterative and given in chronic visceral enlargements and in chronic skin diseases.

The medicated oil is used as an embrocation to the abdomen in colic, to the back in lumbago, to the thigh in sciatica, &c., and as an inunction to the whole body in fevers. A small seeded variety o erandi, with red seeds and big leaves, is known as erando or eddo. Its long tubular petiole is used as a tube to inhale medicated vapours in cough and chest diseases. Castor oil as obtained in capsules is sometimes an admixture of castor oil with croton oil.

Stillingia Sylvatica.

Syn.—Queen's delight, silver leaf, Queen's root, cock-up-hat, yaw root.

Habitat.—United States (sandy soil).

Parts used.—The fresh root.

Characters.—A perennial plant; root long, thick, subcylindrica and branched; also compact, wrinkled and tough; wood porous; bark thick; inner bark studded with many brown resin cells; odour peculiar and unpleasant; taste pungent, bitter and acrid. Dose, powdered root, 15 to 30 grs.

Constituents.—Sylvacrol, a volatile oil, a glucoside, resin, fixed oil, tannin, gum, starch, ash 6 p.c. Sylvacrol is an acrid resin to which the pungency of the root is due; soluble in alcohol, chloroform, benzene.

Preparations.—Fluid extract miscible with water. Dose, 15 to 60 ms. Decoction (1 in 20). Dose, 1 to 2 ozs. Tincture (1 in 8), ½ to 1 fld. dr.

McDade's "succus alterans" also known as "compound antisyphilitic mixture" or "mistura smilacis composita" contains fluid extract of stillingia 4, sarsaparilla 4, lappa minor 4, phytolacca decandra 4, and xanthoxylum carolinianum 4. Dose, 1 to 4 fld. drs.

Stillingin—The dried extractive, a brown powder. Dose, 1 to 2 grs.

Actions and uses.—In small doses expectorant, alterative, antisyphilitic, diaphoretic, diuretic, sialagogue and cholagogue; in large doses, emetic and purgative. As an alterative it is given in secondary and tertiary syphilis where mercurials and iodides may have been given in excess and without relief. It is given in scrofulous and cutaneous affections, in bronchitis, pneumonia and rheumatism; also in incontinence of urine, impotence and sterility; in ascites and in cirrhosis due to hepatic diseases or torpid liver, in portal congestion and in jaundice following malarial intermittents it is given with quinine and arsenic. A decoction of it is given to ward off an attack of ague; it is of benefit if given in hæmorrhoids due to hepatic congestion, or in habitual constipation.

Tragia Involucrata, T. Cannabina.

Habitat.—Throughout India.

Parts used.—The root.

Vernacular.—Beng.—Bichhuti. Burm.—Bet-ya. Duk., Bomb.—Kancha-kuri. Can.—Haligilu. Hind.—Canchorre, Bichhute. Mar.—Khâjkotti-kanchkuri. Malyal.—Shariganam. Sans.—Kásághinnie, Dustparisha. Tam.—Kanchuri. Tel.—Dula-gondi, revati.

Characters.—A twining shrub, growing in hedges, perennial, from 3 to 4 feet high, and common in dry barren grounds; leaves hairy, three-lobed, alternate, petioled and serrated; stem erect; branches numerous, smooth and woody; small ones hairy and twining; root succulent and of a pleasant odour. The hair stings like common nettle.

Preparations.—Decoction (1 in 10). Dose, ½ to 1 fld. oz. Infusion (1 in 20). Dose, 1 to 2 fld. ozs.

Actions and uses.—Diaphoretic, diuretic and alterative; given in biliousness and liver diseases, fever, cachexia, and secondary syphilis; a paste is applied for the extraction of guinea-worms.

Trewia Nudiflora, Rottlera Indica, Rottlera Hooperiana, Trewia Macrophylla.

Habitat.—India.

Parts used.—The root.

Vernacular.—Bomb.—Pittori. Can.—Kât-kamba. Hind.—Pindâra. Mar.—Pitari, sivani. Malyal.—Kanchi. Sans.—Pindara, karahâta, kurangaka.

Characters.—Root thick, of a light brown colour, internally studded with a few cuticular corky warts. The bark is tough and fibrous, subaromatic and of a bitter astringent taste.

Constituents.—Resinous matter, and fat.

Preparations.—Decoction of root (1 in 10). Dose, ½ to 1 fld. oz.

Actions and uses.—Stomachic, and alterative; used in rheumatism, gout and to relieve flatulence; a paste of the root is applied locally to reduce swellings.

Urticaciæ—The Vada, Pipal or Nettle family.

Herbs, shrubs or trees with watery juice; leaves stipulate, lobed and alternate, with stinging glands containing an acrid juice; flowers unisexual, in small flower heads or catkins; fruit indehiscent, one-seeded, surrounded by persistent calyx; embryo, straight and albuminous. Radicle superior.

Habitat.—Found universally.

Properties.—The plants of this order possess acrid stinging juice which is contained in the glands.

Antiaris Saccidora.

Habitat.—Deccan Peninsula, Java, Ceylon.

Part used.—The nuts.

Vernacular.—Can.—Jajhugri. Malyal.—Arayaangeli. Mar.—Chândul, sapsundi. Tam.—Nettavil, maram. Borneo—Bina. Java—Anticar, anchar.

Characters.—Nuts subglobular, of a light brown colour, of the size of a marble and enclosed in a sweet yellow pulp, forming a small, one-seeded fig ; shell thin and fragile ; kernel loose inside the shell. Dose of the powdered seed, $\frac{1}{3}$ to $\frac{1}{2}$ gr.

Constituents.—The seeds contain a nitrogenous principle, very bitter and poisonous.

Actions and uses.—The seeds are used as febrifuge and as a remedy in dysentery, colic and diarrhœa.

Ficus Asperrima.

Habitat.— Central India, Ceylon, Deccan, Peninsula.

Parts used.—The leaves and bark.

Vernacular.—Bomb., Mar.— Kharoti, Kharvat. Can.—Khargas. Guz.—Sariro. Hind.—Sheoda, Kalumar. Portuguese.—Folasda raopa. Sans.—Shakhataka. Tel.—Pindi chettu.

Characters.—The bark is wrinkled and of a lightish brown colour externally ; internally fibrous, rather tough and greenish brown or pale in colour ; leaves from 2 to 4 inches long, oblong or oval, slightly dentate, scabrous and hard ; colour greenish dark ; surface very rough, and hence used as sand papers. The roughness is due to the presence of calcareous hairs.

Constituents.—A crystalline principle, soluble in alcohol an inorganic acid, white calcareous matter and ash 18 p.c.

Preparations.—Infusion of leaves (1 in 10). Dose, 2 to 6 drs.

Actions and uses.—Alterative ; used in glandular enlargement of the liver and spleen. The juice is applied to cracks and fissures on the palms of hands and soles of feet. The leaves are used to polish ivory. The bark, which is mildly acrid, is used as a tooth brush to remove the tartar or to cleanse the teeth.

Ficus Bengalensis, F. Indica, Urostigma Bengalensis.

Habitat.—East Indies.

Parts used.—Milky juice and bark.

Vernacular.—Arab.—Tinê barry. Burm.—Nan-kidâv. Can.—Ahlada mara. Cing.—Kiripelle. Duk.—Jangli guller, Kakudu-mara. Eng.—Indian fig tree, common Banyan tree. Beng., Guz., Mar., Hind.—Bargat, vad, Kadugh. Malyal.—Perâlin pâla. Pers.—Anjire dasht. Sans.—Vata, sriksha, Nya grodha, Skandaja Veta-kshiram, Bahu pada, Sikhandun. Tam.—Alamaram. Tel.—Marri-pâllu.

Characters.—Fruits large, resembling cherries; bark milky, lightish brown or ash coloured, and scabrous ; external surface generally smooth, epidermis often broken and here and there fissured ; internally the bark is very fibrous and tough, the fibres are white and cottony.

Between the fibres and the epidermis are numerous, soft, greyish, granules which give the bark a reddish colour ; taste astringent and nauseous ; odour nauseous.

Constituents.—The bark contains tannin, wax and caoutchouc.

Preparations.—Infusion (1 in 10). Dose, ½ to 1 fld. oz.

Actions and uses.—Tonic and astringent ; given in diabetes, dysentery and hæmorrhagic fluxes, and in gonorrhœa and seminal weakness. Locally the juice is applied as a remedy for toothache and to the soles of the feet and palms of the hands when cracked.

Ficus Carica, B. P.

Habitat.—W. Asia, Subtropics, Persia, India, Asia Minor, Shores of Levant.

Parts used.—The dried fleshy receptacles—Ficus—figs, B. P.

Vernacular.—Arab.—Tin-teen. Beng.—Doomoor. Hind., Mar., Duk., Bomb.—Anjira. Burm.—Saphansi. Chin.—Wu-hwa-kwo. Cing.—Rata-attika. Eng.—Fig. Can., Malyal., Tam.—Shima-atti. Pers.—Anjira, Ravi, Jamir. Sans.—Udeunbara. Tel.—Tene-atti.

Characters.—Male and female flowers are in hollow receptacles, walls covering them is thick and fleshy. The fleshy receptacle or the fig bears fruit upon its inner surface. The fig is funnel-shaped generally compressed, irregular, and slightly gibbous at the top and tapering at the bottom to which a small stalk is attached. Immature figs are green or greenish yellow, tough and leathery ; when cut or when pricked a milky juice escapes. Mature figs are soft, juicy, fleshy, yellowish or brownish red externally and deep red within, covered with sugar instead of the milky juice. The pulp is very mucilaginous, sweet, with a fruity odour and palatable. Figs may dry on trees or are dried by ovens or sun and are known as natural figs. They contain numerous seeds which are hard and of a whitish yellow colour.

Constituents.—The receptacle contains grape sugar 62 p.c.; gum, fat and salts. The milky juice (latex) contains a peptonizing ferment, the effects of which on fibrin and milk are similar to those of papaine ; it converts starch into sugar. Fig is a constituent of confectio sennæ, B. P.

Preparations.—Syrup. Dose, 1 to 2 drs.

Actions and uses.—Laxative, demulcent and nutritious. Fresh fruits are sweet, wholesome and delicious ; taken in moderation they are digestive ; in excess they lead to flatulence, enteralgia and diarrhœa. Both these and the dried figs are laxative and pectoral and are used in catarrh of the respiratory passages. The saccharine and mucilaginous constituents render them nutritious and laxative, hence used to remove habitual costiveness. The seed and tough skin if taken internally cause indigestion and flatulence. A poultice made of figs is used over gum boils and abscesses on the anus and vulva to hasten suppuration.

Ficus Glomerata.

Habitat.—India.

Parts used.—The root bark, fruit, milky juice and galls.

Vernacular.—Arab.—Jammaiz. Burm.—Saphânti. Can.—Kithmara. Cing.—Atteekkâ-gass. Eng.—Glomerous fig tree. Beng.,—Jagnodumar. Hind.,Duk., Bomb.,Guz.—Gullar-umbro. Mar.—Chaphal. Malyal.—Atti-yalum. Pers.—Samare-pash-shah. Panj.—Rumbal, palah. Sans.—Udumbara zajmiya, (sacrificial) Parvitraka (purifier). Tam.—Atti-payham. Tel.—Bodâ-mamidi.

Characters.—Root bark externally ash coloured and smooth to the touch, here and there studded with brownish scars; internally tough, fibrous, and of a lightish brown or red colour, containing a milky juice which is sticky; smell somewhat aromatic, taste sweet and astringent; fruit a pedicel, as large as common fig, covered with soft down; when ripe, purple; leaves alternate, oblong, tapering at each end and entire and studded with glands; they issue from the trunk or large branches; the galls are like blister.

Constituents.—Tannin, wax and caoutchouc.

Preparations.—A medicated oil; decoction of the bark (1 in 8). Dose, ½ to 1 fld. oz. and milky juice. Dose, 1 to 4 drs.

Actions and uses.—Astringent, carminative and stomachic; given in hæmaturia, menorrhagia and hæmoptysis. The juice is used as a vehicle by the natives (anupana) for metallic preparations. With cumin and sugar, the juice from the root is given in gonorrhœa; a decoction of the root bark with nimado is used as a gargle in salivation, as a wash for ulcers and as an injection in leucorrhœa. The milky juice is given internally as an alterative, tonic and also applied as a lepa to the chest, abdomen, and to rheumatic joints, mumps and other glandular enlargements. The application is covered with a pad of cotton.

Ficus Hispida, F. Oppositifolia, F. Dæmona.

Habitat.—Bengal, Coromandel, India.

Parts used.—The fruit and bark.

Vernacular.—Arab.—Tine-barri. Beng.—Kako-dumur. Bomb.—Bokhera, Dhed-umbro. Can.—Adavi atti. Duk., Guz.—Jangli oombro. Hind.—Kâtgular. Madras.—Pe-attis. Mayal.—Pârakh-pazam. Mar.—Vèda umde. Pers.—Anjirê-dashti. Sans.—Ummetto-dumbara. Tam.—Pê-attip-pazam. Tel.—Versi-atti-pandlu and Kako dumbara, crow's fig.

Characters.—Fruit like a small fig and very downy, growing from the stem near or beneath the ground.

Constituents.—Tannin, wax, a caoutchouc-like substance and a glucosidal principle having the properties of saponin.

Preparations.—Decoction (1 in 10). Dose, ½ to 1 fld. oz.; and poultice.

Actions and uses.—Emetic and laxative ; given in hepatic obstruction. A poultice is applied to buboes to disperse it or bring it to maturity.

Ficus Religiosa, Urostigma Religiosa.

Habitat.—India.

Parts used.—The root bark.

Vernacular.—Arab.—Medah. Beng.—Ashwuth. Can.—Rangi-basri. Cing.—Bo-gass. Duk.—Ani-pipal. Eng.—Poplar leaved fig tree, Pipal-tree. Guz.—Pipalo. Hind.—Pipal. Mah.—Pipal, pipar, munga. Malyal.—Ari-alu. Sans.—Ashwatha, sikhandin. Budhidru, yajnika, shrimana, seuya, vipra. Tam.—Arosa-maram. Tel.—Raya manu.

Characters.—Bark tough and lightish brown ; outer surface smooth or slightly scabrous, brittle and soft; internal bark fibrous, very tough and studded here and there with soft granules ; odour slightly nauseous; taste astringent, but disagreeable.

Constituents.—The bark contains tannin, caoutchouc and wax.

Preparations.—Decoction (1 in 10). Dose, ½ to 1 fld. oz. a medicated oil containing twigs boiled in gora tela. *Pancha Valakal Kasheya.*—Compound decoction of five barks, containing besides Ficus religiosa, Ficus Indica, F. Glomerata, Mangifera Indica, Mimusops, Elengi and Mulsari, equal parts. Dose, 4 to 8 drs.

Actions and uses.—With honey it is locally applied to aphthæ and sore mouth. The powder is given internally in asthma. The medicated oil is used as an astringent injection in leucorrhœa, into the rectum in dysentery, as a wash for unhealthy ulcers and as a gargle in salivation.

Geronniera Reticulata.

Habitat.—Sikkim, Himalaya, Assam, Burma, Ceylon, Deccan, Peninsula.

Parts used.—The wood.

Vernacular.—Cing.—Urenne. Eng. Hellish incense. Ind. Bazar—Narakiyaood. Nilgiri—Kho-miang. Portuguese—Pao sugo. Tam.—Koditâni.

Characters.—Stems thick, branches many, odour disgusting and resembling human ordure ; wood, light brown in irregularly shaped pieces.

Constituents.—A solid crystalline picrate ; skatole, a crystalline substance of a fœcal odour, similar to naphthylamine. Obtained from the putrefaction products of animal proteids (human fæces). Synthetically prepared by fusing potash with albumen, also from propylidine phenyl hydrazine.

Preparations.—Decoction of the wood (1 in 10). Dose, 2 to 4 fld. drs.

Actions and uses.—Alterative ; mixed with lime juice, the decoction is used in itch and chronic skin diseases ; also given internally. It is burnt under the superstition that it drives away evil spirts.

Ulmus Fulva (Slippery elm), U. Campestris.

Syn.—Indian elm, sweet or American elm, British tea (the leaves).

Habitat.—N. America, New England, S. Carolina.

Parts used.—The inner bark, Ulmi cortex.

Characters.—The bark in thick flat pieces of a pale brownish white colour ; inner surface finely ridged, having a mealy fibrous fracture ; odour peculiar, slight and fenugreek-like ; taste mucilaginous.

Constituents.—Mucilage starch, tannin and a bitter principle. Alcohol separates from its solution a gelatinous liquid.

Preparations.—Mucilage. Dose, 4 to 8 drs. poultices and suppositories.

Actions and uses.—Demulcent, and emollient ; used in diseases of the urinary passages, dysentery, diarrhœa and in bronchitis ; locally a poultice is applied over the abdomen and chest in bronchitis, and also used as vaginal and urethral suppositories, and as tents to dilate the uterus and other strictures and fistula.

Moraceæ—The Shetur or Mulberry family.

Trees or shrubs with milky juice ; leaves with large stipules ; flowers very minute, unisexual, in heads, spikes or catkins ; fruits sorosis or syconus; seeds solitary and pendulous ; albumen, fleshy ; embryo hooked.

Habitat.—Natives of temperate and tropical climates,

Properties.—The milky juice of some species possesses acrid and poisonous properties ; others are bland and contain beverage ; some species are stimulant, sudorific, tonic and astringent ; fruits of some are refrigerant, fleshy and agreeable in taste.

Morus Nigra, M. Rubra, M. Indica.

Habitat.--India, N. America.

Parts used.—The fruit.

Vernacular.—Arab.—Tut. Beng.—Tut. Burm.—Posa. Can.—Hippal. Cing.—Rata-ombilla. Eng.—Indian Mulberry. Bomb., Duk., Hind., Mar., Guz.—Shetura. Kashmir.—Tukhlu. Malyal.—Babi-saram. Pers.—Tut. Sans.—Shâlmah-vrikshaha. Tam.—Mushi-kattai, cheddi. Tel.—Kambeli-buchi.

Characters.—Fruit in dense spikes, perianths coalesced, sorosis, fleshy cylindrical and of a dark purple colour ; smell disagreeable ; taste sweet ; shining in appearance and moist when touched.

Constituents.—Sugar, pectin, citrates, malates, &c.,

Preparations.—Syrup (1 in 3). Dose, 1 to 2 drs. and drink (or juice). Dose, 2 to 6 drs.

Actions and uses.—The fruits are cooling, refreshing, flavouring and slightly laxative. The juice and jelly are used in fever, sore throat and catarrhal inflammation of the air passages.

Juglandaceæ—The Walnut Family.

Trees ; leaves pinnate, alternate and exstipulate ; flowers unisexual monœcious, sterile in catkins and fertile in spikes. Calyx 3 to 5 lobed irregular, ovary, 2-4 celled, inferior; ovule, solitary, and erect; fruit dry drupe with crustaceous or bony nut shell, containing 4 lobed seed, without albumen; embryo with sinuous oily cotyledons.

Habitat.—Temperate Climate, Persia, Caucasus.

Properties.—Generally cathartic. The seeds of some are oily and edible.

Juglans nigra, Juglans alba or Cinerea.

Habitat.—N. America, Canada, United States.

Parts used.—The inner bark of the root, and volatile oil.

Characters.—Bark dark grey, in flat or curved pieces ; internally striated and smooth ; fracture short, of a feeble odour and bitter acrid taste. Dose, 20 to 60 grs.

Constituents.—Nucin or juglandic acid, resembling chrysophanic acid. Fixed oil, 14 p.c., volatile oil, resin, no tannin. Nucin is an acrid volatile substance, occurs in orange yellow needles or crystals, becomes purple with alkaline solutions, and decomposes by long keeping. Dose, to 3 grs.

Preparations.—Extract. Dose, 5 to 15 grs. Decoction, 1 in 10. Dose, 4 to 8 drs. Spirit made by distilling fresh walnuts with alcohol. Dose, ½ to 1 dr.

Actions and uses.—Rubefacient, cholagogue, like rhubarb a mild cathartic, diuretic and tonic ; it is not an irritant, and does not gripe; given in chronic constipation, also in dysentery. In intermittent fever it is mixed with calomel and administered with benefit. Locally the bark is a rubefacient and may cause a blister. Country, wild Indian or Belgaum walnut is the fruit of aleuritis triloba.

Juglans Regia.

Habitat.—Persia, Himalaya, Cashmere, China, and cultivated in Europe.

Parts used.—The oil leaves and bark.

Vernacular.—Arab.—Jouz. Burm.—Siskhya-si. Chin.—Hu-t'au, King-t'au. Can.—Akrôdu. Duk.—Akharot. Eng.—Candle berry tree, Indian or English walnut. The oil—nut oil, or Artists' oil Beng., Mar., Hind., Guz.—Akharota. Pers.—Chârmaghz. Tam.—Akrôttu. Tel.—Akrotu.

Characters.—A handsome tree; leaves long, imparipinnate; leaflets in pairs, sessile and oblong, round at the base, acuminate, and serrate; bark flat or in curved pieces, dark grey, inside smooth; fruit fleshy, a drupe, oblong in form and when immature of an olive green colour; in size it resembles a small apple-nut, ovoid and somewhat flattened; shell hard and thick; kernel thick, white and oily.

Constituents.—Nucin or Juglandic acid. Resin, fixed oil of a drying nature like linseed oil. The oil is palatable. Dose, 1 to 2 drs.

Preparations.—Spirit. Dose, ½ to 2 drs. Decoction of leaves and bark (1 in 10). Dose, 4 to 12 drs. and oil.

Actions and uses.—The leaves are alterative and given in scrofula, rickets, and leucorrhœa. The oil is a sure and mild laxative, and cholagogue, and given in torpid liver. It does not cause nausea nor any other distressing symptoms. The decoction of the bark is galactafuge and used to stop mammary secretions. As an astringent it is given to check diarrhœa, and menorrhagia; and as a gargle in sore throat. The spirit is used as an antispasmodic for checking vomiting of pregnancy. The kernel is supposed to possess aphrodisiac and vermifuge properties, and given in general debility and in children for worms. It is also used as an article of food when dried. When stuck on a reed, it is a good substitute for candles like fanduka. The oil is used as a drying agent for paints.

Remarks.—The nut has no resemblance to fanduka.

Corylaceæ or Cupuliferæ, the Majuphala or the Oak family.

Trees or shrubs; leaves alternate, usually feather-veined, simple with deciduous stipules; flowers unisexual, monœcious; male flowers clustered; stamens 5–20 inserted into the base of membranous calyx; female flowers solitary or clustered, surrounded by an involucre of bracts which form a cupule round the ovary or fruit; ovary inferior; fruit a gland or a nut; seed one or two without albumen.

Habitat.—Native of forests of temperate regions.

Propertieis.—The bark and capsules are highly astringent; some species are tonic and febrifuge; the gall of some is astringent.

Castanea Dentata.

Habitat.—N. America, S. Europe, W. Asia.

Parts used.—The leaves.

Vernacular.—Burm. —Theel-khya Hind.—Ni-keri. Eng.—European chestnut, sardian nut.

Characters.—The leaves are long, wide, lanceolate, acuminate and mucronate, sinuate, or serrate at the margin, feather veined and smooth, with a slight odour and astringent taste. Dose, 30 to 60 grs.

Constituents.—Gallic acid, tannic acid 9 p.c., resin, fat, gum, albumen, ash 6 p.c.; mainly salts of magnesium, potassium, lime, iron, their carbonates, chlorides and phosphates. The fruit contains starch 35 p.c., fat 2 p.c., proteids 4 p. c. and sugar 2 p. c.

Preparations.—Fluid extract. Dose, 30 to 90 ms. Infusion (1 in 40). Dose, ½ to 1 fld. oz.

Actions and uses.—Tonic, sedative and astringent; used in whooping cough to control paroxysms and in dysentery. The nuts are edible.

Quercus Alba—White Oak.

Habitat.—America, Mississipi, Texas, Florida.

Parts used.—The bark.

Characters.—Tree stately; branches many and spreading; leaves long, oval, tapering at the base; lobes pinnatifid, smooth, rounded, and entire; colour green, glaucous, with prominent veins; flowers monœcious; nut one-seeded, capsular at the base, the cup formed by scaly involucre; fruit ovoid and long; bark in nearly flat pieces of a pale brown colour without any corky layer; internally tough, covered with sharp, short, longitudinal ridges, and breaking with a tough fibrous fracture; odour faint, taste astringent. Dose, 15 to 60 grs.

Constituents.—Quercitannic acid, 10 p.c.; oak red, quercin, resin, and pectin. Quercitannic acid is a yellowish or reddish brown, amorphous mass. To obtain it wash the bark with ether, precipitate with lead acetate. Quercin is a bitter principle; to obtain it boil the bark in acidulated water, add milk of lime to neutralize, then add solution of potassium carbonate, dissolve the precipitate in alcohol and evaporate; occurs in yellow needles.

Preparations.—Pessaries. Decoction (1 in 20). Dose, ½ to 1 oz. Fluid extract. Dose, 15 to 60 ms.

Actions and uses.—Astringent and tonic, similar to tannin; given in scrofula, chronic diarrhœa, intermittent fevers, dysentery, hæmoptysis, uterine hæmorrhages and bronchial fluxes; the decoction is used in gonorrhœa and leucorrhœa; as a wash in prolapsus ani, ulcers and hæmorrhoids; as a gargle for relaxed uvula; as a lotion for flabby ulcers and suppurating wounds. The bark powder is used as a dentifrice in tooth powders. A poultice of the bark is used as an application in gangrene.

Remarks.—Persons working in tan vats seldom suffer from intermittent fevers or phthisis.

Quercus Infectoria, B. P.

Habitat.—Asia Minor, Persia, Greece, Syria, Turkey, Mediterranean Basin.

Parts used.—The excrescences—Galla, galls, B. P.

Vernacular.—Arab.—Ajees-aafs. Burm.—Pajeen-le-garneethu. Beng., Duk., Bomb., Ind., Guz.—Maephala, majuphal. Can.—Mashi, kâyi. Cing.—Mâsaka. Eng.—Galls, the dyer's oak, gall oak, mad apple, Dead Sea apple. Mar.—Maiphala, mashika. Malyal.—Majakanee. Pers.—Mazoo. Sans.—Mayin mayeka, Mjâuhu. Tam., Tel. —Mâshik-kay.

Characters.—Galls are of two kinds, hard and soft. The soft is blind. The hard white gall is used in commerce. The insect cynips gallæ tinctoriæ produces hard galls of commerce. The soft variety is produced by diplolepis gallæ tinctoriæ. They puncture, or sting, the buds and tender bark and deposit ova (eggs) in the puncture. This deposit sets up irritation and the surcharged sap oozes out, which on evaporation leaves solid constituents forming the excrescence. Those galls which contain the insect are heavy and of a blackish colour and highly astringent; those without the insect are angular with a round central cavity and less astringent. Both varieties are globular or pyriform and have their surface studded with numerous tubercles. In some, the tubercles are scattered. In others the lower half is smooth and without turbercles. At the base each gall has a scar of a grey brown colour projecting and corresponding to the attachment of the gall on the tree; the cut portion is whitish brown except in the centre, where it is deep brown, resinous looking and sprinkled all over with sparkling white granules. In the interior there are 2 or 3 cavities ; taste astringent.

Constituents.—Tannin 50 p.c , Gallic acid 2 to 3 p.c., Ellagic acid, mucilage, sugar, resin and starch in the nucleus. Tannic acid often splits up into digallic acid and glucose by fermentation.

Acidum Gallium, B. P., Tri-hydroxy-benzoic acid, dioxy-salicylic acid. To prepare it make a paste of powdered galls, boil it repeatedly with water, add diluted sulphuric acid and ferment, and finally purify with charcoal, filter and crystallise.

Characters.—Acicular crystals, triclinic prisms or silky needles, nearly white, generally of a slight brownish tinge without any odour and of a faintly acid astringent taste ; soluble in cold water (1 in 100), in boiling water (1 in 3), in alcohol (1 in 5), in ether (1 in 40), glycerin (1 in 12). Dose, 5 to 15 grs.

Acidum Tannicum, B.P. Tannic acid, tannin, gallotannic acid or digallic acid. To prepare it expose gall powder to a damp atmosphere for a few days, then add sufficient ether and water to dissolve the acid, press and dry. A light brownish powder or thin glistening scales of a characteristic odour and strong astringent taste ; becoming dark by age and acid in reaction ; soluble in water (1 in 1), alcohol (1 in 1). hot glycerin (1 in 1), insoluble in absolute ether, chloroform, benzene or benzol. Dose, 2 to 5 grs. In wafer, pill or capsule.

Ellagic acid, a white crystalline powder, almost insoluble in water, alcohol and ether ; it also exists in many vegetables and forms the sole constituents of the intestinal concretions known as bezoar. It exists in herbivarous animals eating those vegetables.

Preparations.—Galls—unguentum gallæ, B. P. (1 in 5) ; unguentum gallæ cum opio B. P. (7½ p. c. of opium). Tinctura gallæ, tincture of nut gall, 20 p. c. Dose, 1 to 2 drs.

Of Tannic acid—trochiscus acidi tannici B. P. ½ gr. in each, collodium stypticum, styptic collodion contains tannin 20, alcohol 5, ether 25, and collodion 50. Glycerinum acidi tannici, B. P., glycerin of tannic acid (1 in 5).

Glycerinum aluminis et acidi tannici, contains potassium alum 1, glycerine 6, and tannic acid 1. Suppositoria acidi tannici, B. P., with cocao butter, each contains 3 grs.

Actions and uses.—The galls are astringent and tonic. They constringe the muscular tissue in the walls of the minute vessels, check hæmorrhage and cut short local inflammations. The natives use galls combined with pomegranate bark and barâs kapur to check hæmorrhage and use it locally as a gargle for relaxed throat and as an injection for relaxed vagina and rectum.

Tannic acid is a powerful astringent. When taken into the stomach it precipitates albumen and coagulates the intestinal mucous secretions; also coagulates albumen and gelatine of tissues, lessens peristalsis and leads to constipation. From the stomach it is excreted mixed with albumen and pepsin. It is thus a valuable antidote in poisoning by alkaloids and by tartar emetic. If given for a long time it disorders digestion, sets up irritation of the mucous membranes and leads to emaciation. It is preferred to gallic acid as a local and intestinal astringent. In the intestines, it is converted into gallic acid, hence largely used in epistaxis, anal fissures, hæmorrhoids, and hæmorrhage from the lower bowels. It is of benefit in chronic discharges, as diarrhœa, leucorrhœa, gleet and vesical catarrh. Externally it is applied to the fauces in sore throat, to aphthæ, to chapped nipples, to ulcers and piles; also in otorrhœa, certain skin diseases as eczema, intertrigo and impetigo; as a styptic colloid it is used to check bleeding and to unite wounds. Gallic acid does not coagulate albumen and gelatin, hence its topical astringent effects are less marked. It is useful for internal hæmorrhages as from the lungs, kidneys, &c.; also in profuse excretions as in diabetes, bronchorrhœa, night sweats, chronic diarrhœa, &c. Internally, however, it is more powerful and less prone to disturb digestion or cause stomach irritation than tannic acid.

Betulaceæ—The Birch family.

Trees or shrubs; leaves simple, alternate with deciduous stipules; bark astringent and resinous; flowers unisexual or amentaceous, no calyx, but having small scaly bracts arranged in a whorled manner; flowers male, opposite the bracts, with 2 or 3 stamens and with 2-celled ovaries; fruit dry, indehiscent, 1 celled, 1 seeded; seed pendulous, exalbuminous.

Habitat.—Temperate climate and colder regions.

Properties.—Astringent, tonic, and febrifugal.

Betula lenta.

Cherry birch, spice birch, mountain mahogany.

Habitat.—N. America, Indiana.

Part used.—Volatile oil from the bark.

Characters.—Bark dark brown, separable into layers; taste sweet and aromatic, when wounded cambium exudes sweet, acid, edible juice.

Constituents.—Volatile oil, tannin 3·5 p.c., Betulin, a camphoraceous principle.

Oleum Betulæ volatile, a volatile oil. Prepared from the bark by distillation. It is identical with methyl salicylate and nearly identical with oil of gaultheria procumbens, the latter having an additional terpene. It does not pre-exist in dried bark but is formed by reaction between water and gaultherin. Dose, 1 to 5 ms.

Actions and uses.—Stimulant, diuretic and emmenagogue ; used in rheumatism, gout, scrofula, in irritable bladder and skin diseases ; also in amenorrhœa and intermittent fevers.

Remarks.—Often sold as oil of Teaberry or winter green oil.

Gnetaceæ—The Jointed Fir family.

Small trees or shrubs ; stems and branches pointed ; leaves opposite, entire, net veined ; flowers in catkins or heads, unisexual ; calyx 1 leaved ; anthers 1 celled ; ovules 1-2, naked ; seeds succulent, embryo dicotyledonous, in the axis of fleshy albumen.

Habitat.—Native of tropical and temperate regions.

Properties.—Some are astringent and alterative. The seeds of several species are eaten as food.

Ephedra Vulgaris, E. Pachyclada.

Habitat.—Western Himalaya, Afghanistan, Central Asia.

Parts used.—Dried branches and root.

Vernacular.—Bom., Pers.—Huma. Japan.—Ma-oh. Punj.—Butshur. Sutlej.—Phok.

Characters.—Shrub rigid and tufted ; branches striate, nearly smooth and green ; bracts connate, spikelets $\frac{1}{4}$ to $\frac{1}{2}$ inch, often whorled ; fruit fleshy, succulent 1-2 seeded ; seeds biconvex ; odour terebinthinate and taste astringent.

Constituents.—Ephiderine, an alkaloid. By oxidation it splits up into benzoic acid, monomethylamine and oxalic acid.

Preparations.—Decoction of the root (1 in 40). Dose, $\frac{1}{2}$ to 1 fld. oz.

Actions and uses.—Alterative, diuretic, stomachic, and tonic. Ephederine, like atropine, has the property of dilating the pupil of the eye. The decoction is alterative and used for rheumatism and syphilis, especially for acute muscular and articular rheumatism. It is given in cases where antipyrine, salol, antifebrine, and salicylate of soda have failed to give relief. As a stomachic it improves digestion and gives tone to intestines.

Salicaceæ—The Willow family.

Trees or shrubs ; leaves simple, alternate, and stipulate ; flowers unisexual, amentaceous, naked or with a cup-like or membranous calyx ; both kinds are found in catkins one in each bract ; fruit one-celled 2 to 4 valved ; pod many seeded, each seed having long silky hairs at one end ; ovary 1 celled, superior ; embryo erect and exalbuminous.

Habitat.—Native of temperate climates.

Properties.—The bark of some species is tonic, astringent, and febrifuge. The hairs which invest the seeds are used for cushions. The timber is used for basket making and for the manufacture of charcoal. The buds of some secrete an oleo-resin of a stimulant character.

Salix and Populus, B. P., various Species.

Habitat.—N. America, Europe.

Parts used.—A neutral principle (glucoside), salicinum, salicin, B.P.

Salicin: To obtain it treat the decoction of the bark with litharge and filter; the residue contains tannin, gum, extractive and colouring matter. The filtrate contains salicin and lead; separate the lead by sulphuretted hydrogen and sulphide of barium, filter, evaporate and crystallize. Another method—boil the bark with milk of lime to remove tannin, evaporate and filter and digest with alcohol. Occurs in colourless shining crystals with very bitter taste, soluble in cold water (1 in 28), alcohol (1 in 60), insoluble in ether or chloroform. Dose, 5 to 20 grs.

Salicin, by boiling it with dilute sulphuric acid, is converted into saligenin and sugar (glucose) and by further boiling into saliretin, a resinous body.

Actions and uses.—Bitter, tonic, antiperiodic, antipyretic, and antiseptic; used in rheumatism, fevers, coryza, influenza and neuralgia; externally in solution with borax it is used in eczema, burns and fœtid perspiration. It is, however, not so depressing in its action as salicylic acid.

Salix Caprea, Salix Tetrasperma.

Habitat.—Persia, Europe, N. W. India.

Parts used.—The bark, leaves, seeds, flowers and a watery essence distilled from the plant.

Vernacular.—Arab.—Khilaph-ula-balakhi. Beng.—Pani-jurna. Burm.—Moma-kha. Duk.—Bêde-mushk. Eng.—Goat's sallow, round leaved sallow. Hind.—Bed, Laila safeda Bhainsa. Pers.—Bêda-mushk.

Characters—Flowers unisexual, naked or with a membranous calyx; bark purplish brown, externally white, internally tough and fibrous; catkins long, thick, cylindrical, bright yellow and fragrant; bracts oblong, in small scales, obovate, blackish and hairy; leaves long, pointed, entire.

Constituents.—Salicin, wax, fat, gum and tannin.

Preparations.—Infusion (1 in 10). Dose, $\frac{1}{2}$ to 1 fld. oz., and distilled watery essence.

Actions and uses.—Tonic and febrifuge, used in ague and during convalescence from malarial fever and cachexia.

Salix Nigra—Black Willow or Pussy Willow.

Habitat.—Southern States of America.

Parts used.—The bark and buds or catkins.

Characters.—Leaves narrow, pointed and tapering at each end, serrate, smooth and green; stipules small and deciduous, covered with short rounded and woolly glands; catkins pedunculated, long and loose; filaments hairy below; ovary stalked and glabrous; bark of a brown colour, light, soft and close grained.

Preparations.—Of the buds, fluid extract. Dose, ½ to 1 dr., as a sexual sedative. Of the bark, solid extract. Dose, 3 to 8 grs., as a tonic and antiperiodic.

Actions and uses.—Antiperiodic and febrifuge; sexual and general sedative and anaphrodisiac; used in sexual and urinary disorders, in ovarian hyperæsthesia and spermatorrhœa, gonorrhœa, hysteria, epilepsy and neurosis. Its action is similar to that of hydrastis, conium and potassium bromide, but not so depressant.

Cannabinaceæ, the Hemp or Ganja Family.

Herbs rough, with a watery juice; leaves alternate, stipulate and lobed; flowers small, unisexual, diœcious; male flowers in racemes or panicles; calyx scaly; stamens 5; female flowers in spikes or strobiles; ovary, superior, 1-celled; ovule 1, solitary, pendulous; fruit indehiscent; seed solitary, exalbuminous; embryo hooked.

Habitat.—Temperate parts of northern hemisphere, Europe or Asia.

Properties.—Some species possess narcotic, stomachic and tonic properties; some yield fibres.

Cannabis Indica, B. P., Indian Hemp.

Habitat.—Cultivated in India, Asia, Persia, N. India. Found within N.-W. Himalaya and Kashmir.

Parts used.—The dried flowering or fruiting tops. The leaves, seeds and resinous exudation.

Vernacular.—Large leaves, capsules or fruits with stalks. Arab.—Nabâtul. Ben.—Bhâng. Burm.—Bin-segâv. Can.—Bangi. Cing.—Mat Kansa. Hind., Duk.—Bhâng, siddhi, sabji. Eng.—Indian hemp. Guz.—Bhang. Malyal.—Lacki. Mar.—Bhangâ-châ-pana. Pers.—Bang. Sans.—Vajàya, vriga patta, Ananda, Harasini Bhanga Chapola. Indràsana, Dnayana Vardhani, urjiya, vajradin, matulam, Mahini, sidhu. Tam.—Bangi-elai. The dried flowering tops of the female plants containing the resin of the cannabis sativa. Arab.—Kunnab Haschisch. Beng.—Gânjâ. Burm.—Segiyav. Can.—Bangi. Cing.—Kansâ. Guz.—Gânjâ. Malyal.—Kanchá. Hind., Mar., Duk., Pers.—Kinnah shadanah. Tam.—Kalpamá. The resinous concrete exudation from flowers, stems and leaves. Bomb.—Guz., Beng., Hind., Duk.—Charas. Burm.—Segiyav-asi. Can.—Banji-gondu. Cing.—Kansakiri. Malyal—Chetip-pasha. Sans.—Charma. Tam.—Ganjapal. Tel.—Ganji palu.

Siddhi, Siddhu means perfect. Hindu mythology applies the term Siddhu to Jogis or monks in allusion to their having gained a perfect knowledge of the way to one true God; they then spend the rest of their days in this one belief. The Jogis generally use Bhánga to concentrate their idea upon one God. This drug is, therefore, known as Siddhi, *i.e.* used by Siddha (Saddhu).

Dnyána Vardhani : Dayána, knowledge, and Vardhani, promoter. Bhánga taken is exhilarating and promotes knowledge of things It is said of jewellers that they take Bhanga when testing the true value of jewels to sharpen their intellect. Vajayá, victorious or unbeaten. The drink of bhang drives from the fighting Hindu the haunting spirits of fear and weariness. It means giver of success. The drink gives success in all undertakings. Vrijapáta means a strong nerved; Châpola, the cause of reeling gait; Ananda, causing laughter or involuntary movements; and Harasini the excitor of virile passions; Indrasana, a favourite drink of Indra, the king of gods.

Charas is derived from Sanscrit, Charma, Chamra, a skin. It signifies a leather bag, charas being stored in leather bags by cultivators. Hemp seeds are termed Shâ dânâh (Pers.), meaning Royal seeds.

Characters.—An annual herb; stems angular and tomentose; leaves palmate with compound leaflets, lanceolate, serrate and linear; flowers diœcious, yellow; flowering tops generally compressed and brittle, often mixed with leaves, leaflets, bracts and sometimes with nearly ripe fruits; seeds achenes, of a roundish shape, shining, reticulated, also angular and hard; taste acrid, narcotic and oily. Different parts of the plant bear different names. Bhang, subjee or sidhi is of a deep green colour. It consists usually of broken leaves in coarse powder, fruit and seeds without stalks. Ganja is the flowering and fruiting tops of female plants from which the resin has not been removed. It consists of compressed brittle spikes with leaves, leaflets, bracts, and small pistillate flowers and sometimes nearly ripe fruits, the whole is more or less agglutinated with resinous exudation, colour brownish green, odour powerful and peculiarly narcotic. Charas, or churrus, is a resinous exudation spontaneously oozing from the entire plant or from the leaves and flowering tops. It is mixed with the hairs and fragments of the leaf, and is of a darkish green or brown colour and has a peculiar odour. In consistence and appearance it resembles Afima.

Constituents.—A volatile oil and resin, which is the most active principle, and contains an alkaloid cannabine; tetano cannabine and cannabinon; gum, sugar and potassium nitrate. Cannabine is a dark brown syrupy resin in a semiliquid state. It is a powerful sedative, and is given in mania and sleeplessness. It is more soporific than cannabin tannas. Dose, 1 to 4 grs.

Cannabinon.—A dark brown resin, semi-liquid. Dose, $\frac{1}{4}$ to 1 gr. as a sedative, given in mania, insomnia &c.

Cannabinol.—A toxic red oil a constituent ,of cannabinon, charas ganjah and haschisch.

Tetano Cannabine is a crystalline alkaloid; its action is similar to that of strychnine.

Garado or hemp paste contains bhang, miri, and ganja made into a paste in water. Majum, majoon (Calcutta), Mapanchari (Cairo),

Dawames (Arab) a confection or electuary. It contains bhang, ganja, churus, opium, poppy seeds, dhatura leaves, and seeds, cloves, mastic, aniseeds, cinnamon, cumin, cardamoms, tabashir, milk, ghee, sugar and flour. Dose, 1 dr.

Subjee, otherwise known as sidhu or gutado. It is a liquid paste containing bhanga, miri, goláb̈a kali, khasa-khasa, the five cucurbitaceæ seeds, badàma and elachi equal parts, to which sugar and water is added. If milk is added the intoxicating effects become more marked. Dose, 2 drs.

Cannabin Tannas—cannabin tannate, a brown powder, insoluble in water or ether, slightly soluble in alcohol, freely soluble in water. It is free from the irritating volatile oils present in the drug. Dose, 2 to 10 grs.

Preparations.—Extractum cannabis Indicæ, B. P. Dose, ¼ to 1 gr. Tinctura cannabis Indicæ, B. P. (1 of extract in 20). Dose, 5 to 15 ms. It is not miscible with plain water.

Actions and uses.—Anodyne, hypnotic, antispasmodic, sudorific, aphrodisiac, and appetizing; in large doses narcotic. In medicinal doses and taken for the first time it acts as an agreeable intoxicant, as a result of which, time, distance and sound are magnified. It exhilarates the spirit, excites the imagination and increases the appetite; medicinally it acts as an anodyne and antispasmodic, but is inferior to opium. It has, however, the advantage of not producing constipation, loss of appetite, nor the unpleasant after effects peculiar to opium. It is largely used in headache of a continuous or chronic character, asthma, whooping cough, chronic bronchitis, tetanus, hydrophobia and other spasmodic affections as hysteria, chorea, &c. It is also used in nervous vomiting, mental depression, delirium tremens &c. It is sometimes used in place of opium as a hypnotic where opium cannot be borne; and largely used in menorrhagia and dysmenorrhœa; also used in chronic rheumatism.

Among the natives it is largely used as an aphrodisiac and as an intoxicant like opium and alcohol. In large doses, or if habitually taken, or its use persevered in, it produces a bloated face, congested eyes, tremulous and weak limbs, imbecility, weakness or loss of memory. They use bhang in gonorrhœa and dyspepsia. Locally a decoction of the leaves is applied to erysipelas and neuralgic painful parts. Its application to the anus is used to relieve the pain of hæmorrhoids. A paste applied to the head relieves dandruff and vermin.

Ganja is smoked through chillum, an improvised hooka, in arsenical poisoning; also the smoke is passed into the rectum to relieve tenesmus and tormina of dysentery. Locally as an anæsthetic it relieves the itching of eczema, pruritus &c.

Charas.—It is a powerful stimulant and narcotic, and used for the same purposes as ganja. Majam is used as an excitant and aphrodisiac. Subjee is used as intoxicating and cooling. Cannabin Tannas is hypnotic, especially in nervous sleeplessness and acute mania. Cannabinon is given in acute mania and sleeplessness, more certain than cannabin tannas.

Humulus Lupulus, B. P.

Habitat.—N. America, Europe, Central Asia, Australia, Dera Dhun.

Parts used.—The dried strobiles, Lupulus, the hops or Humulus, B.P.

Characters.—Strobiles ovate, long, and consisting of thin hairy undilated axis and many greenish ovate and obliquely membranous scales; upper portion reticulately veined toward the base, glandular and surrounding sub-globular achene, which is covered with yellowish numerous aromatic glands; these are the most active parts of the hops. The odour is aromatic and taste bitter and astringent.

Constituents.—A volatile oil, resin, asparagin, choline, tannin and ash, an aromatic and a bitter principle reside in the glands. The bracts contain lupuline; the volatile oil contains a hydrocarbon and valerol.

Lupulinium—Lupulin, B. P. Glandulæ Lupuli. A granular brownish yellow powder composed of glands obtained from the strobiles of the hop. Each gland consists of a single hemispherical layer of cells of strong beef-like odour and bitter aromatic taste. Dose, 2 to 5 grs.

Preparations.—Oleo-resin extracted by means of ether. Dose, 2 to 5 grs. Tinctura Lupuli, B. P. (1 in 5). Dose ½ to 1 dr. Infusum Lupuli (1 in 20). Dose, 1 to 2 fld. ozs. Extract obtained by ether. Dose, 2 to 5 grs.

Actions and uses.—Tonic, stomachic, hypnotic, narcotic, somewhat diaphoretic, diuretic, astringent and aphrodisiac. It increases the action of the heart, skin and circulation. It is used in insomnia, alcoholism, delirium tremens, seminal debility, priapism, incontinence of urine and irritable bladder. Locally hops are used as poultice to sprains, bruises, abscesses and over the abdomen in colic. Pillows filled with hops are, on account of the narcotic odorous vapour from them, employed to induce sleep.

Myricaceæ.—The Gale Bog Myrtle or Kataphala family.

Shrubs with alternate, simple resinous and dotted leaves; flowers unisexual, amentaceous; fruits drupaceous, 1-seeded; embryo without albumen.

Habitat.—Native of temperate parts of Europe, India and Cape of Good Hope.

Properties.—The plants of this order are remarkable for their aromatic and astringent properties; the berries of myrica cerifera contain a beautiful green wax which burns like spermaceti or candles.

Myrica Sapida, M. Nagi, M. Cerifera.

Syn.—Wax Myrtle, Wax berry, Candle berry.

Habitat.—Himalaya, Nepaul.

Parts used.—The bark of the root and seeds.

Vernacular.—Eng—Bay berry. Arab.—Azûri, Aûdul-barg. Beng., Mas., Duk.—Kâiphala. Hind.—Kâtaphala. Malyal.—Maru tam toli. Pers.—Kandula, Darshishaan. Can.—Kirishivani. Sans.—Kataphala Kumuda, kumbli, pâki. Tam.—Marudam-pattai. Tel.—Kaidaryamu.

Characters.—The bark in quills or thick pieces, about 1 to 2 inches long, and from ¼ to ½ inch in thickness; epidermis of a brownish colour and scaly, soft, and easily separable from the true bark by scratching; true bark soft, is of a reddish colour and brittle; cut surface here and there studded with a red or dark red gummy or resin-like substance; smell like that of camphor; taste astringent and somewhat pungent; seeds larger, softer and longer than jaephala, of a taja colour; interior of a deeper colour and resembling jaephala; in structure, lighter, softer, and much inferior in oiliness to jaephala; odour fruity and somewhat less acrid and aromatic; cut portion sticking to the fingers when touched; arillus thick, of a darkish brown colour, twisted, as if folded into a cone, and adherent to the seed; aroma very faint.

Constituents.—The bark contains tannin, saccharine matter and salts.

Preparations.—Decoction (1 in 10). Dose, ½ to 1 fld. oz. Medicated oil. Compound powder, katphaladi churana, containing katphalchhal, mustaka, curcuma, zedoaria, karkatshringi, kushta, equal parts given with ginger and honey. Dose, ½ to 1 dr.

Actions and uses.—Stimulant, alterative, aromatic, diaphoretic and astringent; given in fevers, catarrh of the intestinal mucous membrane, diarrhœa, dysentery, scrofula, chronic gonorrhœa, catarrh of the lungs, asthma &c. The powdered bark is used as a sternutatory. The seeds—a paste of them with stimulant balsams is mixed with ginger and externally used as a rubefacient and as a stimulant application to the fore-arms, calves and extremities during the collapse stage of cholera. Its powder is locally applied to strengthen the gums; also as a lep for bruises, sprains and fractures. With catechu, asafetida and camphor, a paste of it is applied over piles with benefit. The arillus is used as an ingredient in numerous carminative mixtures. The powder or the lotion of the bark is applied to putrid sores. Pessaries made of it are given to promote secretion of menses. The bark when chewed acts as a sialogogue and relieves toothache. An oil prepared from it is dropped into the ear in earache to allay pain. Fruits when boiled yield a kind of wax, called wax myrtle, which is used as a healing application to ulcers.

Remarks.—Kataphala is the bark, and not the fruit, as the name implies. It should not be mistaken for kakaphala which is the name of the fruit of kâkamâri.

Coniferæ or Pinaceæ—The Gandhabiroja or Devadara or Pine family.

Trees very large, resinous; shrubs evergreen; stems branched and continuous; leaves linear, needle-shaped or lanceolate, parallel veined, imbricate, fascicled; flowers unisexual, naked, monœcious; no perianth;

male flowers in catkins; stamens 1 or many, monadelphous; anthers 2 or many celled; female flowers in cones; ovules, naked, two or more; fruits woody and cone-like; seeds naked with hard custaceous testa, albuminous; cotyledons 2 or many.

Habitat.—Native of temperate climates,

Proberties.—Several species abound in an oleo-resinous juice or turpentine; some contain a volatile oil and resin; they are generally stimulant, diuretic, emmenagogue; also anthelmintic and expectorant. Many produce good timber.

Abies Balsamea, B.P.

Habitat.—Canada, N. United States.

Parts used.—An oleo-resin, Terebinthina canadensis, Canada turpentine, Canada Balsam, B.P.

Syn.—Fir balsam, the silver fir or balm of gilead fir, balsam spruce, hemlock fir, balsam poplar.

Characters.—Transparent, viscid liquid; colour yellowish or faintly greenish; odour agreeable and terebinthinate; taste slightly acrid and bitter. On exposure to the air, it dries up slowly into a hard transparent mass; soluble in ether, chloroform or benzol. Dose, 20 to 30 grs.

Constituents.—Volatile oil, 20 to 30 p.c. resin or rosin, a bitter principle.

Preparations.—Collodion Flexile, B.P., Flexible collodion, contains collodion 48, Canada balsam 2, and castor oil. 1 Does not contract on drying. It is better than contractile collodion.

Actions and uses.—Local stimulant and protective, similar to oil of turpentine. It dries up into a varnish, thus acting as a protective. As a stimulant it acts chiefly on the mucous surfaces. Seldom used internally.

Abies Canadensis—Pinus Canadensis, Tsuga Canadensis,

Syn.—Hemlock spruce fir. Canadian fir tree, hemlock pitch.

Habitat.—N. America.

Parts used.—The bark and the prepared oleo-resinous exudation known as Canada pitch.

Character.—A tree of damp, mountainous swamps; branches numerous, giving the tree a pyramidal shape, smooth, reddish grey, full of reservoirs containing the balsam; leaves long, linear and silvery beneath; flowers in catkins or cones: pollen bright yellow; seeds with large wings; oleo-resin is obtained by exudation, or by incision in vesicles of the bark, or by evaporation of the wood tar. It is a faintly greenish, reddish brown or translucent, yellow or opaque liquid. On exposure it gradually dries up into a hard, brittle mass; fracture shining and conchoidal; odour mild and balsamic; taste bitter, terebinthinate; soluble in ether, chloroform, benzene. Dose, 20 to 60 grs.

Constituents.—Volatile oil 20 or 30 p. c., oleo-resin.

Preparations.—Of the bark. Liquid extract. Dose, 15 to 60 ms. Glycerinum abietis 1 in 4, readily miscible in water. Dose, 1 to 2 drs.; of the oleo-resin. Plaster.

Actions and uses.—The oleresin, like Burgundy pitch, is non-irritant, astringent, and stimulant, of the mucous membranes of the stomach, intestines, uterus, vagina, bronchi, lungs &c. The oil is used as abortifacient ; the liquid extract well diluted is non-irritant and astringent ; used as injection in leucorrhœa, catarrh &c.; as a gargle in mouth affections and as lotion in sores and hæmorrhoids. Internally it is given in dysentery, hæmoptysis, night sweats, diarrhœa &c.

Picea Excelsa, B. P., Abies Excelsa, Pinus Picea.

Habitat.—Europe, North and South Asia, Burgundy Province.

Parts used.—The resinous exudation from the stems. Pix Burgundica, Burgundy Pitch, B P.

Characters.—Exudation yellowish brown, opaque, hard and brittle, of a conchoidal fracture ; odour aromatic ; taste sweet and aromatic, without bitterness; entirely soluble in glacial acetic acid, very fusible and becomes soft and adhesive at the ordinary temperature or by body heat.

Constituents.—Volatile oil, resin (to which the odour is due), and pimaric acid.

Preparations.—Emplastrum Picis, pitch plaster, B.P., contains Burgundy pitch 26, frankincense 13, resin $4\frac{1}{2}$, yellow bees-wax $4\frac{1}{2}$, olive oil 2, distilled water 2.

Actions and uses.—Stimulant and rubefacient ; mainly used as a plaster in rheumatism, joint affections, chest troubles, liver affections, to the chest in chronic coughs and other pulmonary affections and to the loins in lumbago &c.

Juniperus Communis, B.P.

Habitat.—Europe and North America.

Parts used.—The berries (Juniperi Fructus) and the volatile oil, oleum juniperi, B. P.

Vernacular.—Arab.—Habul hurer, Shâmrat-ul-arar. Bomb.—Hanbera. Duk.—Abbal. Eng.—Juniper. Hind.—Aaraar-kâ-phal. Ind. Bazaar—Padma, kanawar, Bilhar. Pers.—Abhala. Port.—Zembro. Sans.—Hapusha.

Characters.—Evergreen shrub ; fruit roundish, berries of a darkish brown colour, size of black currants, or somewhat bigger than kâla miri; surface gibbous and wrinkled. At the base of each fruit are small pointed bracts arranged in whorls of three. The top of the fruit is marked with three lines which diverge from a central point. They are broad at their point of attachment and become narrow as they extend outwards; the pulp is reddish brown, with oil glands and sticky; the seeds are three, angular and of a reddish colour; odour of the berries aromatic and balsamic ; taste slightly bitter, sweetish, terebinthinate and acrid.

Constituents.—A volatile oil 1·2 p.c., grape sugar 30 p.c., resin 10 p.c.; a non-crystallizable principle (Juniperin), fat, wax, proteids 4 p.c., malates, formic and acetic acids.

Oleum juniperi, oil of juniper, B.P., obtained from the full-grown unripe green fruit by distillation, is a colourless, or pale greenish yellow liquid, rapidly becoming thick and paste-like, having the characteristic odour of juniper and a warm aromatic terebinthinate and sweetish taste; soluble in alcohol (1 in 4), in carbon sulphide (1 to 1). It contains pinene and cadinene and an ester to which the odour and taste are due; it fulminates with iodine. Dose, ½ to 3 ms. It is contained in spirituous drinks as Hollands and gin.

Preparations.—Spiritus Juniperi, B. P., spirit of juniper (1 in 20). Dose, 20 to 60 ms. Infusion, (1 in 20). Dose, ½ to 1 fld. oz. Spiritus Juniperi Compositus :—compound spirit of juniper, contains oil of juniper 8, oil of carraway 1, oil of fennel 1, alcohol 1,400. It is allied to gin. Dose, 1 to 4 drs.

Actions and uses.—The oil is a stimulant of the skin and kidneys. In large doses it irritates the kidneys and sets up strangury, priapism, hæmaturia, suppression of urine and even uræmic convulsion ; taken for some time it gives violet colour and terebinthinate odour to the urine ; when inhaled it produces diuresis ; used also as a vehicle for less irritant diuretics. Like oil of turpentine it is given in renal dropsy, chronic catarrh of the urinary passages, seminal debility, in pyelitis, gleet, flatulent colic ; also in chronic gonorrhœa and leucorrhœa ; locally the powder is rubbed on rheumatic and painful swellings. It should not be given in acute nephritis.

Juniperus Oxycedrus, B. P., and other Species—Prickly Cedar.

Habitat.—South of Europe and Spain.

Parts used.—The oil, known as Oleum Cadinum B. P., oil of Cade, juniper tar oil, oleum juniperi pyroligneum or oleum juniperi empyreumaticum. Obtained by the destructive distillation of the wood.

Characters.—Shrub ; branches spreading and drooping ; leaves pointed, awl-shaped ; fruit reddish, shining, thick, with two white lines on the apex. The oil is an empyreumatic, dark, reddish brown or black viscid liquid of a pleasant tarry odour and aromatic bitter and acrid taste; soluble in oils, fats, carbon bisulphide and also in ether and chloroform ; partially soluble in cold and almost wholly in hot alcohol, very slightly soluble in water. Dose, 3 to 5 ms.

Constituents.—Phenols and sesquiterpene-cadinene.

Preparations.—Unguentum olei cadini (1 in 1) of yellow wax.

Actions and uses.—Oil of cade is anthelmintic and externally stimulant and parasiticide; used like the oil of tar, in psoriasis, chronic eczema, pityriasis rubra, prurigo, psora, and favus.

Remarks.—Often substituted for coal tar, ordinary tar, or oleum picis liquidum.

Juniperus Sabina—The Common Savine.

Habitat.—Siberia, Northern Europe, Asia, Canada.

Parts used.—The tops and the oil.

Characters.—Small evergreen shrub, compact, spreading; top, short, thin, yellowish green, sub-quadrangular; branchlets or twigs covered with minute leaves. The leaves are dark green, opposite, lanceolate, scaly, pale reddish brown; flowers in catkins or small cones; fruit berry like, size of a pea, bluish purple, soft and enclosing seeds 1 to 3; odour peculiar and terebinthinate; taste nauseous, acrid, bitter and resinous. Savin grows at very high elevation and closely resembles red cedar (J. Virginiana), but the latter has large size and small fruits. Dose, 5 to 10 grs.

Constituents.—Volatile oil, 2 p.c. acrid resin, tannin, extractive matter, chlorophyll. The volatile oil, distilled from savine, is a limpid colourless liquid, of a pale yellow colour, isomeric with oil of turpentine; taste bitter, acrid and camphoraceous; odour peculiar and terebinthinate, reaction neutral; soluble in alcohol (1 to 1). It contains pinene and cadinene. Used as emulsion, pill or alcoholic solution. Dose, 1 to 4 ms.

Preparations.—A paste containing powdered tops with burnt alum and acetate of lead is used as a caustic. Tincture (1 in 8). Dose, $\frac{1}{2}$ to 1 dr. Fluid extract 2 to 5 ms. unguentum sabinæ (1 in $3\frac{1}{2}$); cerate contains fluid extract 1 in 4 of cerate.

Actions and uses.—Locally irritant; internally it is a diuretic, emmenagogue and vermifuge. In medicinal doses it causes a sensation of heat in the body, gives rise to nausea, eructations and flatulence. It increases the action of the heart, kidneys, skin, bronchi, uterus and ovaries. It also increases the flow of menses. The oil is excreted in the breath, perspiration and urine. In large doses, it is a gastro-intestinal irritant and causes violent vomiting and purging, severe pain and rupture of gall bladder. In poisonous doses the symptoms are those of narcotic poison. It produces uterine contraction, and leads to abortion. As an emmenagogue it is given in amenorrhœa, hæmorrhage after abortion, leucorrhœa, dysmenorrhœa, when not due to mechanical causes or to other menstrual derangements. The paste is used as a local caustic to syphilitic warts, condylomatas, polypi and to other excrescences; also to dental caries, tinea capitis, &c. The ointment is used to prolong discharges from blistered surfaces, setons, or issues; and as a stimulant application for healing indolent ulcers.

Picea Succinifera.

Habitat.—Shores of the Baltic and Adriatic Sea, Prussia, Coal mines Bohemia, Sicily.

Parts used.—A fossil oleo-resin.

Vernacular.—Arab.—Inkitrum, Kuru-ul-bahr, Misha hareruma. Burm.—Ambeng. Chin—Hu-peh. Eng.—Amber, electrum. Guz.—Kerabo. Duk.—Kehruba. Pers.—Kahruba.

Some coniferæ species which are submerged under sea-water from time to time yield by natural exudation this oleo-resin, which when submitted to the destructive distillation and purified yield the oil of amber.

Characters.—As gum of this or other coniferous plants, it is met with in irregular sized pieces of a yellowish colour, hard and brittle; polished externally, semi-transparent, yellowish or opaque and resembling copal gum ; usually associated with lignite ; sometimes insects or parts of vegetable are found imbedded in its interior. It is lighter than sea water and friable in cold weather, having a waxy or resinous appearance ; electrical, as when forcibly rubbed with linen it acquires the power of attracting pieces of paper from a short distance, and the pieces remain stuck to it for a few seconds. When ground or heated it emits a pleasant odour.

Constituents.—Empyreumatic oil, a bituminous principle, a yellow resin, succinic acid, several resins. Oleum Succini, an empyreumatic oil, is a volatile, colourless or pale yellow and thin liquid, becoming darker by exposure to the air. It has a balsamic odour and warm, acrid taste, neutral or faintly acid reaction, and is soluble in alcohol. Dose of the oil, 5 to 15 ms. Succinic acid. It is met with in the form of scales or prisms, having a slightly acid taste and without smell.

Actions and uses.—Antispasmodic, stimulant, and diuretic, also rubefacient ; given in whooping cough, amenorrhœa, epilepsy, hysteria, &c. It has a specific action on the generative organs and is given in amenorrhœa, dysmenorrhœa. It is also given in low fevers. It is locally applied as liniments over painful swellings, paralyzed limbs and rheumatic joints. It is rubbed over the spine to relieve convulsions and mixed with olive oil it is rubbed to the chest in whooping cough.

There are two varieties : Kerabo Manakans is in the form of court beads and ornaments and of a superior quality. Kerabo chhodans is in irregular flat pieces resembling slices of wood (chhodan).

Pinus Deodara, Abies Devadara, Cedrus Libani.

Habitat.—N.-W. Himalaya.

Parts used.—The wood and turpentine,

Vernacular.—Arab.—Shajrat-ul devadar. Guz., Duk., Beng.—Debadâru. Can.—Dêvadâri. Hind.—Kilân devdâr. Mar.—Dêvadaru-chà-jhâd, Devatârm. Pers.—Sanobar-i-Hind. Sans.—Suradaru Sura-ruma.—Devadaru, vrikashapa, sneha—viddha. Tam.—Dêvadri. Tel.—Dêvâdâri.

Characters.—Wood somewhat heavy; colour lightish yellow or brown, consisting of layers of coarse fluid resin arranged longitudinally, resin thick towards the middle, and becoming less so as it approaches the bark; odour balsamic and slightly aromatic; taste oily and resinous. Near the heart wood the oleo-resin when touched feels sticky to the fingers. It is one of the ingredients of Rasna-di-kvath and Chandra Prabha Gotika.

Constituents.—An acid resin.

Preparations.—Tar and compound decoction—Devdari Kvatha: contains devadára, vaja, motha, kariatun, dhamáso, gokharu, kali jiri, kutha, kutaki, ativisha, dhana, gula vela, suntha, harade, pipali, ringani, gaja pipli, kakará singi, all in equal parts. Dose, ½ to 1 oz. A powerful alterative, given in general debility especially after delivery, rheumatism, syphilis, fever, vomiting, constipation, dry cough, and headache. The tar is prepared by the destructive distillation of wood. Dose, 10 to 40 ms.

Actions and uses.—The wood is carminative, diaphoretic, and diuretic; given in fever, flatulence, dropsy and urinary diseases as gravel. In ascites it is given in combination with shegata chhála and aghádo. In gonorrhœa, syphilis, gout and rheumatism, the decoction is given as a powerful alterative. With halada and gugala its paste is applied to indolent swellings. The tar is used as a favourite alterative, and given in chronic skin diseases and in large doses, given in leprosy and also applied externally to ulcers.

Pinus Gerardiana.

Habitat.—N. W. Himalaya, Afghanistan, Persia.

Parts used.—The pine nuts.

Vernacular.—Afghan.—Chilgoza. Arab.—Sanobara el-ki bâr. Eng.—Neozapine—Edible pine. Guz., Mah.—Chilgozâh. Hind.—Gunobar, rhee, neoza. Panj—Miiri, gogojal. Pers.—Tukhm-i-Sanobara, (seeds).

Characters.—Seeds about an inch long, roundish at the base, and tapering towards the apex, somewhat arched towards the upper part where the apex is drawn to one side like the beak of a bird; testa brittle, rugous, brownish red, or yellow externally, and greyish white within; kernel covered over with a thin, lightish brown, membranous layer. Within the layer the kernel is albuminous and oily, and resembles the kernel of badâm; smell somewhat acrid, oleaginous and terebinthinate; taste heating, oily and slightly acrid; embryo, of a yellowish colour, occupying the whole length of the seed; radicle seen towards the apex of the seed.

Constituents.—Albuminoids, starch, oil and ash.

Preparations.—Confection. Dose, 1 to 2 drs.

Actions and uses.—Stimulant, nutritive, tonic, and aphrodisiac; similar to those of badâm, pisatan, charole, &c., and used in chronic rheumatism, seminal debility, leucorrhœa, and gleet.

Pinus Longifolia.

Habitat.—Himalaya ranges.

Parts used.—The wood and turpentine (oleo resin), and oil.

Vernacular.—Arab.—Aâlakus. Guz., Duk.—Chirkà-jhâr., samghus gandah birozah (resin). Hind.—Chirkâ-pêr, saral (wood). Birji goond (gum) sanâbar. Nepal.—Dhup-salsei dup. Panj.—Nashtar. Pers.—Sanôbar-e-hindi. Tam.—Shurul Dèvadâri. Tel.—Dêvadari-chettu.

Characters.—The oleo resin is a white, opaque, sticky mass, of a paste-like consistence, often found mixed with pieces of broken leaves; odour strong and agreeable, more aromatic than that of commercial turpentine. The oil, a limpid sherry coloured fluid, is obtained by distilling the oleo resin. The residual resin is dark brown and a fair substitute for Burgundy Pitch. Dose of the oil, 1 to 3 ms.

Preparations.—Plaster.

Actions and uses.—Stimulant and antiseptic; the oleo-resin is used as fumigation. It is highly recommended as a plaster for painful chest and enlarged liver. The oil is in much repute, internally, in gleet and long-standing gonorrhœa. Ganda Biroza is the name also applied to olibanum, the produce of boswellia floribunda.

Pinus Pumilio, B.P.—The Mugho or Mountain Pine.

Habitat.—Hungary.

Parts used.—Volatile oil distilled from fresh leaves—Oleum Pini B.P., oil of pine, pinol, pumiline.

Characters.—A pure, essential, colourless oily liquid, of a pleasant, permanent, exquisite, refreshing aromatic odour and pungent taste, more agreeable than other fir oils. Dose, ½ to 3 ms.

Preparations.—Extract. A thick semi-liquid mass, very soluble in water; Pumilio Pine soap; wood wool wadding, sanitary wood wool, also used as inhalation, gargle or lotion (10 minims, in 10 ounces of water), as embrocation, poultices, baths and plasters.

Pinus Sylvestris, B. P., Wild pine, Scotch pine, Scotch fir, and other Species of Pinus.

Habitat.—America and Europe.

Parts used.—The wood, concrete oleo-resin and oil distilled from fresh leaves Oleum Pini Sylvestris and the oil distilled from the oleo-resin, oleum terebinthinæ, oil of turpentine B. P.

Characters.—The wood is hard and resinous and contains the concrete oleo-resin known as terebinthina; the oleo-resin occurs in yellowish opaque tough mass, highly brittle when cold, interiorly crystalline; taste and odour terebinthinate. Dose, 5 to 30 grs. By the distillation of the fresh leaves an oil is obtained known as Oleum Pini Sylvestris, Firwood oil, or Scotch fir oil. It is a colourless, thin liquid of an agreeable thyme-like or terebinthinate odour and aromatic, terebinthinate taste ; slightly soluble in water, and soluble in alcohol and glacial acetic acid (1 to 7) ; used as liniment to the chest or as an inhalation in chronic laryngitis or as vapour containing Oleo Pini Sylvestris 40 ms., in a pint of hot water, the air passed through the mixture and inhaled.

Preparations.—Fir wood extract, readily soluble in water ; bath—2 or 3 ozs. of the oil in 30 gallons of hot water as a bath for rheumatism. Fir Wool wadding. Fir wool, made of the fibres and hairs of pinus sylvestris or of cotton wool, impregnated with the oil used for rheumatism. Pine Wool Felt, made like fir wood and used as chest protectors (belts) &c.

Pinus Palustris. B. P., Tæda, B. P.

Habitat.—N. America.

Parts used.—The concrete oleo-resin, Thus Americanum, frankincense, B. P., and turpentine.

Characters.—A large tree, growing in dry sandy soil ; bark thin, scaled and furrowed ; wood hard and resinous ; leaves many, very narrow and sharp pointed in clusters, surrounded by a sheath ; flower sterile, of a violet colour ; fruit oblong, large, scales armed with short spines ; young trees resembling brooms.

Constituents.—Volatile oil, 20 to 30 p.c. ; also resin 50 to 60 p.c., bitter principle and formic, succinic, pinic and sylvic acids.

The oleo resin is obtained by scraping the trunk. It is a soft pale yellow; opaque, tough, solid resin ; odour terebinthinate, an alcoholic solution having acid reaction. On keeping it becomes dry, translucent and of a fainter odour. Dose, 15 to 30 grs. Resina, B. P. rosin is the residue left after distilling off the turpentine from the oleo-resin. It is clear, amber coloured, solid, hard, brittle and of a glassy conchoidal fracture. It can easily be reduced to powder ; the odour and taste are terebinthinate. It is soluble in alcohol, ether, fixed and volatile oil and alkaline solution. It contains anhydride of abietic acid, pinic and sylvic acids, The volatile oil, oleum terebinthinæ, oil of turpentine, B. P., obtained by the distillation of the oleo-resin by the aid of steam and then rectified, is a thin, clear and colourless neutral liquid, very inflammable, of a strong peculiar odour, and hot, pungent taste ; sparingly soluble in water, moderately so in alcohol (1 in 3) and glacial acetic acid (1 in 1) readily mixing with ether and other volatile and fixed oils. It dissolves resin, wax, sulphur, phosphorus, fats and caoutchouc. On exposure to the air it absorbs oxygen and becomes yellow or somewhat denser; with hydrochloric acid it forms crystalline camphor. It is a mixture of several hydrocarbons. Dose, as a stimulant, 2 to 10 ms. ; as an anthelmintic and purgative, 3 to 4 drs.

Preparations.—Of Resin: Ceratum Resinæ, Resin cerate, Basilicon ointment—resin, yellow wax, lard. Emplastrum Resinæ, B. P. resin plaster, adhesive plaster ; resin, lead plaster and yellow wax. Of turpentine: Linimentum Terebinthinæ, B.P. (13 in 20).

Linimentum Terebinthinæ aceticum B., P., liniment of turpentine and acetic acid, contains oil of turpentine 4, glacial acetic acid 1, ; linimentum camphora 4 ; Emulsio terebinthinæ. Inhalation or vapour 40 ms. to 1 ounce with light carbonate of magnesia. Dose, 1 dr. in a pint of hot water.

Derivatives of turpentine.—These are terebene, turpin hydrate and turpinol. Terebenum B.P., Terebena Pura or pure. Terebene, a liquid consisting of pinene and small proportions of dipentene, and turpinene. It is obtained by the oxidation of the oil of turpentine or by agitating it successively with sulphuric acid and then distilling it in a current of steam. It is a clear, colourless liquid, odour thyme-like ; taste terebinthinate ; soluble in alcohol (1 in 1), glacial acetic acid (1 in 1), slightly soluble in water. Dose, 5 to 15 ms. ; used as vapour terebinæ 40 ms. to 1 oz. with light magnesia, 1 dr. in a pint of hot water ; also is used as inhalation.

Terpinum hydratum—Terpin hydrate, terpini hydras, hydrate of oil of turpentine, also known as turpentine camphor. To obtain it mix together rectified oil of turpentine, nitric acid and alcohol. Distil and crystallize : in rhombic prismatic crystals resembling those of chloral hydrate, of the odour of terebene and of aromatic bitter taste; soluble in water (1 in 200), alcohol (1 in 10), boiling water (1 in 2), ether (1 in 100) and oil (1 in 6), sometimes deposited from oil of turpentine when the latter contains water. Dose, 2 to 6 gr., useful in neuralgia ; in bronchitis and chest affections, it loosens the expectoration.

Terpinol—an oily body obtained by the action of sulphuric acid on terpini hydras. A colourless oily aromatic liquid. Dose, 2 grs., used as a sedative and antiseptic, given in chest affections.

Actions and uses.—Oleum Terebinthinæ—the volatile oil, is a cardiac stimulant, antispasmodic, expectorant, anthelmintic, diuretic and hæmostatic ; also laxative and intestinal and vesical irritant ; locally rubefacient or counter-irritant ; inhalation of its vapours, antiseptic and sedative.

In small doses it causes salivation, burning in the mouth and at the pit of the stomach ; in large doses, it sets up gastro-enteritis with vomiting, diarrhœa, suppression of urine, severe scalding, burning in the urethra and bloody urine. Inhalation of the vapour gives rise to nasal and renal irritation with frontal headache, bloody urine, &c. If long continued and in toxic doses it is a narcotic poison, causing muscular and sensory paralysis, profound insensibility, abolished reflexes, cyanosis, dilated pupils, laboured respiration and death. It is supposed to dissolve gall stone. Its power of absorbing oxygen from the air renders it a powerful antidote to phosphorus poisoning. It converts phosphorus into an insoluble substance.

As a cardiac stimulant, it is given in typhoid and typhus fevers, puerperal fever, in erysipelas, pneumonia, and capillary bronchitis ; also in chronic bronchitis, chronic cystitis, &c. ; as an astringent it is given in passive hæmorrhages from the lungs, stomach, intestines, kidneys and uterine and intestinal ulceration, and hæmorrhoidal fluxes. It should not be given in hæmaturia. As an antispasmodic, combined with ether, it is given in hysteria, epilepsy, lead and biliary colic, biliary concretions, ileus, convulsions and tetanus; as a vermifuge, given with castor oil to expel lumbrici and tænia.

The vapour is antiseptic like eucalyptus oil and is inhaled in cough, chronic bronchitis, winter cough, emphysema, phthisis and bronchorrhœa; or used as an atomizer either alone or in combination with eucalyptus oil or oil of sandalwood and cubebs, &c. Locally, as a rubefacient and counter-irritant, it is used as turpentine stupes; it relieves the pain of chronic rheumatism, neuralgia, sciatica, lumbago, peritonitis, pleurisy, tympanitis and renal colic. As a hæmostatic its application to the bleeding tooth or to the nose in epistaxis is of benefit. Terpine hydrate is antiseptic, expectorant and diuretic, and used in bronchitis, whooping cough, night cough of phthisis; also in chronic nephritis, cystitis and gonorrhœa. Terebene is a stimulant disinfectant. Its vapour is inhaled in phthisis, winter cough, emphysema of the lungs. Its emulsion is given in dysentery, flatulence, dyspepsia, cystitis and gleet. As a spray it is used in nasal catarrh, coryza, and in bronchorrhœa. Terpinol—Its actions and uses are similar to those of terpin.

Pix Liquida, B. P., Tar.

A bituminous liquid, obtained from the destructive distillation of the wood of Pinus palustris, P. Tæda, P. Sylvestris, &c.

Vernacular.—Arab.—Quir. Burm.—Kattra-asi. Cing.—Kel. Duk.—Kil. Eng.—Tar, Stockholm tar. Hind.—Kil. Pers.—Quil. Tam.—Kil-tar. Tel.—Taru-kilu.

Characters.—Tar, an empyreumatic oleo-resin, is a thick viscid liquid, granular in appearance owing to the crystals of pyrocatechin, of a brown-black colour; odour peculiar and aromatic; taste sharp, and empyreumatic; slightly soluble in water, soluble in alcohol (1 in 10), fixed and volatile oils, and in alkaline solutions. By keeping it separates into crystalline pyrocatechin.

Constituents.—Methylic alcohol, acetic acid, acetone, trace of formic, propionic and capronic acids, mesit, pyroliginous acid, oily bodies, toluene, zyline, cumine, methylene and other hydrocarbons, naphthalin pyrene, chrysene, paraffin, phenols, creasote 25 p.c., pyrocatechin, and empyreumatic resin.

Preparations.—Of Pix Liquida, Unguentum Picis Liquidæ, B. P., tar ointment (5 in 7), used in psoriasis and ringworm. Pixol—a disinfectant made from tar, made soluble by the aid of caustic potash and potash soap. Aqua Picis—Tar water, Eau-de-Goudron (1 in 200). Dose, 2 to 5 ozs. Capsules de Goudron—Tar capsules 2½ grs. in each. Dose, 1 to 2. Liquor Picis Ligni, prepared with tincture of quillaia. Pilula Picis Liquidæ. Dose, 2 to 5 grs. Syrupus Picis Liquidæ 6 p.c. syrup of tar. Dose, 1 to 4 drs. Oleum Picis Rectificatum—light oil of tar, a volatile oil distilled from tar—dark reddish brown or colourless liquid, of a tarry odour and taste, acid reaction ; soluble in alcohol. It contains a variety of hydrocarbons, phenols, creosote, carbolic acid, paraffin, &c.

Pix Carbonis Liquida Præparata or commercial coal tar. Prepared from coal tar, a mixture of resins and hydrocarbons, obtained by heating coal tar for one hour ; used as pills. Liquor Picis Carbonis, B. P.—A mixture of prepared coal tar with tincture of quillaia and alcohol digested for two days. Liquor carbonis detergens—An alcoholic solution of coal tar. A dark coloured fluid, used as lotion (1 in 20) ; emulsion and ointment (1 in 8).

Actions and uses.—Irritant like creosote or carbolic acid ; if applied to the skin it is a gentle rubefacient. It sometimes produces vesicles or pustules ; it stimulates the lymphatics and promotes absorption. Internally as a stimulant it is very beneficial in chronic bronchitis, typhoid fever, vesical catarrh, phthisis and hæmorrhoids ; it disturbs digestion. In large doses it is a gastro-intestinal irritant, leading to vomiting, colicky pain, headache, dark urine, giddiness, &c. As an antiseptic it acts like turpentine. The ointment is used in chronic skin eruptions, as eczema, scabies, prurigo, psoriasis, ringworm, fissured nipples and hæmorrhoids. Its fumes destroy foul odour and it is inhaled in phthisis, pharyngitis, laryngitis, winter cough and other chronic pulmonary diseases. As a surgical dressing it is used in the form of oakum or as marine lint ; oakum is an old tarry rope carded ; marine lint is a tow impregnated with fresh tar.

Taxus Baccata.

Habitat.—Temperate Himalaya.

Parts used.—The leaves.

Vernacular.—Arab.—Zaranab. Bomb.—Barami. Eng.—Himalayan Yew. Ind. Bazars. Beng, Hind.—Thuneer. Zurnub, Talisapatra, Barambhi, Sapani. Jehlum.—Burin. Sans.—Talisa-patra, Manduparami, Barahmi.

Characters.—Drug of a brown colour, and of an aromatic and somewhat acrid odour ; taste acrid and somewhat bitter ; pieces of stems from one to three inches long, and about 2 to 3 lines in thickness; bark brittle, and marked here and there with cracks ; surface shining as if varnished ; wood of a lightish white colour ; leaves 1 to 2 inches long, and about 2 to 3 lines in breadth, linear, flat, mucronate, and rigid ; upper surface shining as if varnished. and slightly rugous ; under surface marked with a prominent midrib ; margins curved towards the under surface, thus giving the upper surface a convex appearance towards the edges; a concave channel-like depression is seen on their upper surface, situated between the margins and the midrib on each side. Dose, of the powder, 2 to 5 grs.

Constituents.—A crystalline alkaloid known as taxine.

Preparations.—Tincture (1 in 8). Dose, ½ to 1 dr. Infusion (1 in 20). Dose, 4 to 12 drs.

Actions and uses.—Antispasmodic, given in asthma, hæmoptysis, epilepsy and other spasmodic affections.

Thuja Occidentalis—Arbor Vitæ.

Habitat.—Canada, United States.

Parts used.—The fresh tops.

Characters.—Tree, very high; trunk, crooked; bark pale and shreddy; wood soft and light; leaves ovate, pointed with glands on the back, in four rows; odour balsamic and terebinthinate, taste camphoraceous, pungent and bitter; twigs flat. Dose, 15 to 60 grs.

Constituents.—Volatile oil 1 p c., resin, tanin pinipicrin, thujin and thujigenin.

Preparations.—Infusion. Decoction 1 in 10. Dose, 2 to 6 drs.

Actions and uses.—Stimulant, diuretic and irritant; given in fevers, coughs, rheumatism, dropsy, pulmonary catarrh and scurvy.

Cycadaceæ—The Cycas Family.

Small, palm-like unbranched trees or shrubs; leaves clustered at the summit, pinnate, parallel veined, hard and woody; flowers quite naked, unisexual; male flowers in cones, consisting of scales with one-celled anther; female flowers naked ovules, seeds hard or succulent, embryo one or several; albumen, fleshy or mealy.

Habitat.—Temperate and tropical countries.

Properties.—Stems and seeds contain mucilage and starch.

Cycas Circinalis, C. Inermes.

Habitat.—Malabar Coast, Madras.

Parts used.—Male bracts and flour of the nuts.

Vernacular.—Bomb.—Buzoorbutu. Burm.—Mudang. Cing.—Madoo guss. Duk.—Pahari madan mastaka. Mar.—Malabari supari. Malyal.—Rin badam. Tam.—Madana Kamapu. Tel.—Ranaguvva, Kamakshi.

Characters.—Bracts or scales, spear-head shaped and covered at the back with much down. Dose of the powder 10 to 30 grs.

Constituents.—The bracts or scales contain albuminous and mucilaginous matter, but no alkaloid that would account for its narcotic action. It yields a gum resembling tragacanth; also a kind of sago, or flour made from the nuts and stems called Indapadi.

Actions and uses.—Stimulant, aphrodisiac, and narcotic; given in hiccough and seminal weakness. Flour is used as food like sago. The fruit-bearing cones reduced to poultice are applied to the loins for the removal of nephritic pain.

Smilaceæ—The Choba Chini, or Sarsaparilla family.

Herbs or shrubs, more or less climbing; leaves petiolate, net-veined and articulated; flowers small, regular, hermaphrodite or unisexual and diœcious; perianth inferior, 6 parted; stamens 6, perigynous; ovary superior, 3-celled; stigma 3; fruit baccate; seeds few or many embryo minute, albuminous; root tuberous, abounding in fecula.

Habitat.—Tropics, temperate climates.

Properties.—The plants of this order generally possess alterative properties. The roots of some are nutritive, tonic, diaphoretic and invigorating.

Smilax Chinensis, S. Glabra, S. Aspera, S. Pseudo China.

Habitat.—China, Sylhet, Southern United States.

Parts used.—The root and rhizome.

Vernacular.—Arab.—Khashabus sini. Beng.—Shook China. Burm.—Tsein apho-ta-roup. Chin.—Tu-fu-ling. Eng—China root bamboo, briar root. Hind., Guz. Mar.,—Chopa Chinni. Malyal—China-pagu. Pers.—Chuba-chini. Sans.—Dvipâta, vacha, rasna, suganda mula. Tam.—Poringay. Tel.—Pirangi chakka.

Choba chini—choba means a stick or wood, and, chini Chinese. The rhizomes are in sticks or pieces imported from China.

Characters—Rhizomes $\frac{1}{5}$ of an inch thick, very long, cylindrical, longitudinally wrinkled, rosy and heavy, free from large knots; tubers irregular, found upon the fibrous roots of the plant, somewhat flattened and covered with a dark brown or rusty coloured bark; interior homogeneous, rose-coloured, white and starchy and sprinkled with white, silvery and shining granules; tubers in slices or in masses, heavy and often hard from 2 to 4 or more inches in length and from 1 to 2 inches in breadth; irregularly flat and resembling an elongated potato. The taste is mucilaginous, bitterish and acrid, without any odour. The slices are sold under the name of choba khatai. What is sold is usually peeled and trimmed and hence it presents a very irregular form.

Constituents.—Fat, sugar, a glucoside, colouring matter, gum and starch.

Preparations.—Decoction (1 in 10). Dose, 4 to 12 drs.

Actions and uses.—Diaphoretic, stimulant, alterative and resolvent; given with ananta mula in long-standing headache. Chobchini, with masataki, elachi and taja boiled with milk, is given in rheumatism, gout, and epilipsy; also in general cachexia, scrofula, seminal weakness and constitutional tertiary syphilis. The rhizome is made into a paste and applied to swelled hands and feet in general obesity.

Smilax Ovalifolia.

Habitat.—Concans.

Parts used.—The root.

Vernacular.—Beng.—Kumarika. Bomb.—Gutavela. Burm.—Kuku. Eng.—Wild sarsaparilla. Guz., Hind.—Guti, Jangali-ushabah. Malyal.—Kuri vilandi. Tam.—Krin koddy-nar. Tel.—Konda-tamara.

Characters.—A climbing shrub; roots numerous, resembling sarsaparilla; bark dry, tuberous and of a brown colour; in the centre soft and starchy.

Preparations.—Decoction (1 in 10). Dose, 4 to 12 drs.

Actions and uses.—It is the country sarsaparilla of the Portuguese, and used as a good alterative in syphilis, scrofula, &c.

Smilax Ornata, B. P., S. Officinalis, S. Medica, S. Papyracea.

Habitat.—Mexico to Brazil.

Parts used.—The dried root, sarcæ radix, sarsaparilla. B. P.

Vernacular.—Arab.—Ushbah. Beng.—Chabal chaba, salasá. Cing.—Retai, rissu. Guz., Duk., Hind.—Ushbah, salsa, magrabi. Malyal.—Narotensi. Pers.—Maghrabi.—Tam.—Sharasha-vera. Tel.—Sima, sugundhi pâlâ.

Characters.—Dried root, long, cylindrical, tough, flexible, greyish brown or dark reddish brown, folded together and bound with a root stalk; roots deeply wrinkled longitudinally. On section the cortex is reddish brown; wood yellowish white, without odour; taste slightly bitter.

There are several varieties of smilax, classified according to the physical properties and the amount of starch contained in the roots. Hence the roots are known as non-mealy and mealy. In the non-mealy variety the starch is pasty, rarely in granules, and more horny; root stalks with longitudinal and irregular folds; found in Jamaica Sarsaparilla, smilax ornata (red); Lima sarsaparilla, S. officinalis; true Vera Cruz sarsaparilla, in the similax medica. In the mealy variety starch is in granules, root stalks with outer surface uniform or in shallow wrinkles; found in Honduras. Sarsaparilla (Smilax officinalis), Lisbon sarsaparilla or Brazilian Sarsaparilla (Smilax papyracea and similax officinalis), Caraccas or gouty Vera Cruz (Smilax syphilitica).

Constituents.—Parillin, saponin, sarsa saponin, volatile oil, resin, starch, colouring matter, calcium oxalate and other salts; also smilacin, parillic acid, pariglin, salseparin, parillinic acid.

Parillin, to obtain it exhaust the root with warm alcohol, and distil; occurs as a white glucoside resembling saponin, of a bitter taste; soluble in water and alcohol.

Preparations.—Liquor sarsæ compositus concentratus. B. P. (1 in 1). Dose, 2 to 8 dr.; extractum sarsæ liquidum, B. P. (1 in 1). Dose, 2 to 4 drs. Decoctum sarsaparilla compositum. Dose, 1 to 2 ozs.

Actions and uses.—Alterative, diaphoretic, tonic, diuretic and resolvent; mostly given with iodide of potassium, in scrofula, skin diseases, tertiary syphilis, gout, rheumatism, &c.

Orchidaceæ—The Orchis or Salama Misari family.

Herbs or shrubs, terrestrial or epiphytical; roots fibrous or tuberculated; no true stems but a pseudo bulb; leaves entire, generally thick and sheathing; flowers irregular, reptile shaped, solitary or numerous, with a single bract, hermaphrodite, showy, and of various colours; perianth superior, petaloid, arranged in two whorls; pollen powdery, more or less collected into grains or in waxy or mealy masses; fruit capsular, 3 valved, rarely fleshy and indehiscent; seeds many, minute; testa loose netted, exalbuminous; embryo fleshy.

Habitat.—Found in every region of the globe.

Properties.—Some of the plants are aromatic, antispasmodic and fragrant; others nutrient and aphrodisiac.

Cypripedium Pubescens, C. Parviflorum.

Syn.—Yellow ladies' slipper, Indian or Venus shoe, nerve root, Venus cup, monkey flower, bleeding heart, yellow umbel, Noah's ark, American valerian.

Cypripedium, from Cypris, Venus, and pes, pedis, the foot—Venus' foot, or slipper. The flower's lid is of the form of a slipper.

Habitat.—N. America, Canada.

Parts used.—The rhizome and roots.

Characters.—Rhizome, horizontal, long, thick, and studded with cup-shaped scars, closely covered with wiry rootlets; roots from 4 to 10 inches long, brittle, of a dark brown colour, and of short fracture; odour peculiar. Taste sweet and bitter. Dose, 5 to 15 grs.

Constituents.—Volatile oil, resin, fixed oil, volatile acid, tannin, starch, sugar, ash 6 p. c.

Preparations.—Fluid extract. Dose, 10 to 30 ms. Tincture (1 in 10). Dose, ½ to 1 dr. Alcoholic Extract—Cyprepedin, 1 to 2 grs.

Actions and uses.—Tonic, antispasmodic, stimulant and diaphoretic; used as a substitute for valerian but inferior; given in hysteria, chorea, epilepsy, nervousness, hypochondriasis, insomnia, neuralgia, nervous headache, tic douloureux, and low fevers. It quiets the system without producing the stupefying effect of opium or of other narcotics. Under its influence the patient wakes up after a pleasant dream. It does not produce constipation.

Dendrobium Macraei.

Habitat.—Sikkim, Tenasserim Coast, Concan, Nilgiri Hill, Khasia mountains.

Parts used.—The plant, roots and stems.

Vernacular.—Beng.—Jibanti. Chin.—Shih hup. Hwang-taau. Mar., Hind., Guz.—Jiba sâg. Sans.—Jeva jevaniya, saka shreshtha, yasasvini, jiva bhadra.

Characters.—An air plant, growing on jâmbul tree, much branching, stems long, pendulous, and knotty, with many oblong pseudo bulbs, leaf one, red, sessile and long ; flowers white, with a yellow lip 3 or 4 inches in diameter and exquisitely fragrant.

Constituents.—Two resinous principles termed alpha and beta jibantic acids and an alkaloid called jebantine.

Preparation.—Decoction (1 in 20). Dose, ½ to 1 fld. oz.

Actions and uses.—As a tonic, given in debility, due to seminal discharges.

Eulophia Vera, E. Campestris, E. Nuda.

Habitat.—Bengal, Deccan Peninsula, Plains of India, Punjab, Oudh.

Parts used.—The tubers.

Vernacular.—Beng.—Budbara. Eng.—Whitton root. Hind—Goruma. Malyal.—Kanta katon. Mar.—Ambarkand mankand. Tel. —Goru chettu, unani turphylla, Saturyun orkis. Mânkand from mân, the neck, and kand, the tubers. The tubers resemble in appearance scrofulous glands in the neck ; mân in Marathi means scrofulous disease in the neck.

Characters.—The tubers, conical or pyriform, externally surrounded with circular marks, the remains of leaflets, yellowish white or of a green colour. Dose, 10 to 20 grs.

Constituents.—Large quantities of white mucilage and ash 3·6 p.c.

Actions and uses.—Anthelmintic and tonic. It is a fair substitute for salap. The natives use it in scrofulous disease in the neck both externally and internally.

Orchis Latifolia, O. Laxiflora, O. Mascula.

Habitat.—Persia and Afghanistan, Nepal, Cashmere, O. Mascula, S. Europe.

Parts used.—The tubers and the fecula of the root.

Vernacular.—Arab.—Salab-misri. Beng.—Chhâle michhari. Bur.—Sala-misri. Cing.—Salama-misiri Eng.—Oriental salep. Duk., Mar., Hind., Guz.—Salob-misri. Malyal.—Sala-mishri. Pers.—Saalab-misri. Tam., Tel.—Shala-mishiri.

Characters.—Orchis mascula. Root (tubers) consists of 2 fleshy tubers, one inch long, deprived of epidermis by scalding in water, yellowish brown, hard, horny and insipid, tuberous hard and horny, amber coloured, often whitish, opaque and somewhat translucent; taste mucilaginous or gum-like. When boiled with milk it emits an odour resembling that of semen hominis.

Constituents.—Starch, 27 p.c., mucilage 48 p.c., sugar, albumen, a trace of a volatile oil, and ash consisting chiefly of phosphates and chlorides of potassium and lime. The starch is obtained by grinding the root under water and straining.

Preparation.—Confection—Kattana Batrisana, contains Sálama 5, Dholi mulsali 5, Káli musali 4, Ekhará-ná-bija 1, Gokharu 2, Balabija 2, Kavacha 1, Satávari 2, Kamarakasa 2, Trikatu 1, Kulaphá-ná-bija 1, Niragundi 1, Vansalochana 1; Asana 2, Sakakula misari 2, Behaman-i-sapheda 1, Behaman-i-surkha 1, Ajamo 2, Suvá 2, Taja 3, Elachi 2, Jáephala 1, Jávantri 1, Vávdinga 2, Akalakaro 1, Asálio 1, 2 Pipalia mula 2, Ispaghula 4, Khasakhasa, 4, Bávaliogonda 4, Lendi pipali 2, Singodan 2, Kesara 1, Pobadi 2, Sàkara 15. Dose, 2 to 5 drs.

Unani hakeems omit from the confection Ispaghula, Niragundi, Sakákula misari, and Behaman-i-surkha, and add Nága kesara, Tamálapatra, Madanamasta, Mocharasa, Máephala, Methi, Kháraka, Lavanga, Safed Kapur, Panini-jar. Used in seminal debility, chronic diarrhœa, and general weakness in debilitated women after delivery.

Actions and uses.—Nervine tonic, demulcent, and nutritive; given in seminal debility, paralytic affection, &c. It is also nutritive and astringent; hence useful in chronic diarrhœa, cholera, and tubercular diarrhœa. Dose of the powder, 5 to 20 grs.

Remarks.—Three kinds of salama are generally met with. Panjab-i-salaba. The word Punjah, means a palm. The tuber is palmate or handshaped; this name is converted into Punjabi. The ordinary Abushaheri, also called lasanio (garlic-like). It is either branched or with one large bulb. Badashai or Basarai-salem. All these roots are decorticated before being dried. An imitation of these tubers made of pounded potatoes, gum, and wheat flour is sold under the name of Banavati (artificial) salema.

Vanda Roxburghii.

Habitat.—Bengal, Gujerat, Behar, Coacum.

Parts used.—The root—Rasnâ.

Vernacular.—Hind., Beng., Bomb.—Rasana.

Saccolabium Papillosum.

Habitat.—Bengal, Lower Himalaya, Assam, Circars, and Burmah.

Parts used.—The root.

Vernacular.—Kanbher.

Characters.—Leaves coriaceous, in two rows, oblique at the apex; flowers axillary, racemose or solitary; stem climbing; roots in thin quills, long branching, same as sarsaparilla; colour dark greyish brown; bark thin, marked by longitudinal furrows; without odour, and of a starchy, bitterish, astringent taste.

Constituents.—2 resinous acids, a neutral resin, an alkaloid, white neutral principle, and a neutral fluorescing principle.

Preparations.—Confection. Dose, 10 to 40 grs. Rasna Panchaka—Decoction of five roots—containing Rasna, Tinospora Cordifolia, Cedrus devdar, ginger and ricinus communis, equal parts. Dose, 4 to 6 drs. in rheumatism.

Actions and uses.—Bitter tonic and alterative; given in rheumatism, sciatica and neuralgia. Another kind of rasna called Khadaki Rasna is the root of tylophora asthmatica.

Vanilla Planifolia.

Habitat.—Tropics, Mexico, West Indies, cultivated in Java.

Parts used.—The fruit.

Characters.—A perennial climbing plant, which can be planted in a mixture of leaf mould and sand and trained to climb stone pillars to form a lattice work; fruit long, thick, linear and narrow; bent at the base; and oblique at apex; wrinkled, warty, of a dark brown colour and leathery, 1-celled, containing blackish brown pulp with many minute seeds and acicular crystals; odour fragrant and taste peculiar.

Constituents.—Vanillin or vanillic acid 2 p c., fixed oil 11 p.c.; resin, sugar, mucilage, and ash 5 p.c. Vanillin—a crystalline odourous principle, an aldehyde of methyl-proto-catechuic acid, is obtained by exhausting vanilla with alcohol. It is artificially prepared from coniferin, carbolic acid, eugenol, and guaiacol—occurs as colourless needles, oxidises slowly in damp air, soluble in alcohol, ether and volatile oils, and insoluble in water.

Preparations.—Tincture (1 in 10). Dose, $\frac{1}{2}$ to 1 dr.

Actions and uses.—Carminative, stimulant, aphrodisiac and anti-spasmodic; used in hysteria, low fevers, atonic dyspepsia; chiefly used as a flavouring agent. Those working in it get pruriginous eruptions.

Scitaminaceæ Zingiberaceæ—Ginger, suntha or halad family.

Herbs aromatic, rhizomes creeping; leaves broad, simple, stalked and sheathing, with parallel curved veins springing from the midribs arising from membranous bracts; perianth superior, arranged in whorls; stamens 3, anthers 2-celled, ovary inferior, 3-celled; flowers fragrant, in racemes and in spikes; fruits from 1 to 3 celled, capsular or baccate; seeds many, arillate, albuminous and enclosed in a vitellus.

Habitat.—Native of the tropics.

Properties.—The rhizomes of some are stimulant, aromatic and stomachic. These properties are due to the presence of resin and volatile oil. Some species are used as food, as they contain starch in large quantities.

Alpinia Galanga, Maranta Galanga, Amomum Galanga.

Habitat.—Java, Sumatra, S. India, Bengal.

Parts used.—The rhizome and fruit.

Vernacular.—Arab.—Khulanjâne-kabira. Duk., Beng., Bomb., Hind.—Sapheda-pana-ki jara; Bara kalanjana, Kochthe-kalanjan. Burm.—Podagoji. Chin.—Hung-tau-kau. Can.—Dumpa-râsmi. Cing.—Kaluwala. Eng.—Java galangal, grand or greater galangal, Galanga cordamoms. Malyal.—Chitta-ratta. Pers —Khusarava-dâru-ê-kalân. Sans.—Dharnula tikshra mula, Sugandha vacha, Mahabhara vacha Kulanjana. Tam.—Perre-arete. Tel.—Pedda-dumpa.

Characters.—Rhizome resembling in many respects the lesser galangal, but larger in size and irregularly knotty; externally brownish black, like lesser galangal; homogeneous and fibrous; colour dirty white; odour and taste feebler than that of small galangal and resembling those of kusht, and hence it is also known as kushta kalinjana; fruit when fresh of the size of small cherries, obovate, soft, of a deep orange red colour; dried fruit ½ inch in length, oblong, somewhat constricted about the middle; some of them are three-sided.

Preparations.—Powder. Dose, 5 to 10 grs. Tincture (1 in 10), ½ to 1 dr.

Actions and uses.—Aromatic, stimulant and bitter; used in fevers, catarrhal affections, rheumatism, incontinence of urine &c.

Alpinia Officinarum.

Habitat.—China.

Parts used.—The rhizome.

Vernacular.—Arab.—Khulanjana. Hind., Bomb., Beng.—Chini Kalanjana, kulijana, chhota or kala pana-ki-jara. Can.—Sauna rasmi. Cing.—Sitta Ratai. Chinese.—Kuon-cang-keang. Eng.—The lesser or the Chinese Galangal. Sans.—Rastama. Sind.—Kunjara kathi. Tam.—Shitta Ratio.

Characters.—Dried rhizomes, cylindrical, as thick as the little finger, about two inches long; colour rust-brown like that of taja; in shape long and irregularly bent, thus resembling ginger; surface marked with circular rings which are the remnants of radical leaves, and here and there presenting traces of rootlets on branches; fracture, short, fibrous; interior homogeneous, of a reddish brown or yellow colour and containing fibres, many brownish resin cells and fecula; odour peculiar and aromatic; taste hot and spicy, resembling that of Pipali mula. Dose of the root, 20 to 30 grs.

Constituents.—Volatile oil, ½ p.c. resin, fat, glucose, a neutral tasteless, odourless, yellowish, crystalline body, kœmpferide, galangalu galangin, and alpinin; the essential oil is the odorous principle. Kœmpferide is slightly soluble in water, ether and benzene, freely soluble in alcohol and soluble in alkalies. Galangalu occurs in yellowish white needles; alpinin in yellowish needles.

Preparations.—Powder; infusion. (1 in 20). Dose, 4 to 12 drs.

Actions and uses.—Aromatic, stomachic, stimulant and carminative; given internally to relieve flatulence, promote digestion, allay vomiting of indigestible food and to check fever. It is given to young children under the idea that it makes them speak early. A paste of the drug made by rubbing it with oil or water and applied to the face removes freckles. It is useful in reducing the quantity of urine in diabetes. It corrects foul breath when chewed.

Canna Edulis

Habitat.—Peru, Brazil.

Parts used.—The fecula of rhizome—Canna starch.

Characters.—Rhizome creeping, fleshy, with thick joints. Starch, a white satiny powder, granules, large, long, flat, ovate, hilum at narrow end. The fecula is obtained by grinding the rhizome under water, kneading, straining and allowing to subside. Dose, 10 to 30 grs.

Actions and uses.—Demulcent, nutritive and dietetic. Given in urinary and bowel complants and during convalescence from acute or chronic diseases.

Canna Indica, Canna Orientales.

Habitat.—Throughout India.

Parts used.—The rhizome and fruit.

Vernacular.—Beng Swebajaya. Can.—Sugundaraju. Duk.—Akalbarki, Manker. Hind.—Sabbajaya, Akalbar. Malyal.—Kattu-Bula. Mar.—Deokele, Kàmàkshi. Sans.—Sarvajaya, Kâmâkshi, Eng.—Indian bread or Indian shot. Tam.—Kanda-mani. Tel.—Krishna Tamara.

Characters.—Fruit, capsule, bristly, 3-celled, many seeded; seeds round, black, hard and shining, of the size of a pea or buck-shot; rhizome, thick, fleshy.

Constituents.—Fat, traces of an alkaloid, gum and starch.

Preparations.—Decoction (i in 20). Dose, 1 to 2 fld. ozs.

Actions and uses.—Diaphoretic, diuretic and stimulant; used in fevers, dropsy and dyspepsia.

Curcuma Amada.

Habitat.—Bengal.

Parts used.—The rhizome.

Vernacular.—Beng.—Amada. Duk.—Am-kî-bô-kî-adrak. Eng.—Mango ginger. Mar., Hind.—Am-hal-di. Malyal.—Toman munga. Tam.—Arukam laka. Tel.—Shadgrandika.

Characters.—Tubers lateral, colour pale yellow and peculiar; smell resembling that of the rind of green mango; taste acrid and astringent.

Preparations.—Paste—containing amba halad, revanchino siro, and white of egg.

Actions and uses.—Carminative, stomachic and cooling; other properties similar to those of zinger and it is used as such. The paste is applied, like turmeric, externally to bruises, sprains, contusions, rheumatic pains and black eye.

Curcuma Aromatica.

Habitat.—Throughout India.

Parts used.—The tuber or rhizome.

Vernacular.—Beng., Guz., Bomb., Beng.—Bân-halodi. Burm.—Kiyâsanoin. Can.—Castûri-arishinâ. Eng.—Wild turmeric, Cochin-turmeric, round zedoary, yellow zedoary. Hind.—Jangali-haladi. Mar.—Vedi-halad. Malyal.—Anakûva. Sans.—Vana haridra, shati. Tam.—Kastûri-arishina. Tel.—Kattu manal.

Characters.—Rhizome, very hard, oblong, rather ovate, 2 to 3 inches long, and 1½ to 2 inches in diameter; surface wrinkled and hairy, and marked with circular disks or rings which are marks of fallen leaflets, and scars of fallen rootlets, with other slender rootlets attached. It exhales a camphoraceous and jambula-like fragrant odour; taste oily and balsamic.

Constituents.—A volatile oil, resin, starch, mucilage, sugar, gum, albuminoids and curcumin, a yellow colouring matter.

Preparations.—Powder, 3 to 6 grs.

Actions and uses.—Stomachic, stimulant, carminative and tonic; given to promote eruptions in exanthematous fevers and in skin diseases; its chief use is as a dyeing agent.

Curcuma Angustifolia, Indian Arrowroot.

Arrowroot, is so called from its bruised rhizomes or roots being employed by the Indians as an application to poisoned wounds inflicted by arrows.

Habitat.—Tropical Himalaya, Oudh.

Parts used.—The tubers.

Vernacular.—Ben.—Tikhura. Chin.—Bheshanio. Duk., Hind.—Tavakhir, tikor. Malyal.—Kughai, kusy, kaking. Eng.—Indian or Curcuma Arrowroot, Curcuma Starch. Sans.—Tavak sphiryeka pattrika. Tam.—Kûvâ marû.

Indian arrowroot is obtained from the following plants. Curcuma Angustifolia C. Leucorhiza, C. Montana, C. Aromatica, C. Longa, C. Rubescens, Hitchenia caulina.

Characters.—Bulb oblong, pendulous, of a pale colour and containing starch ; when dried and powdered it is the chief source of arrowroot in India. Milkmen add this powder to milk in order to make it appear less watery.

Constituents.—Starch, sugar, gum, and fat.

Actions and uses.—Nutritive, demulcent and restorative; used as food for infants in diarrhœa and dyspepsia ; locally it is mixed with katha and applied over cracked or sore tongue and in sore throat.

Curcuma Cæsia.

Habitat.—Bengal.

Parts used.—The tubers.

Vernacular.—Hind., Bomb., Mar., Beng.—Nila kantha, kâli halad, Nara kachura. Tel.—Manapasupu.

Characters.—Tubers of the size of halada ; colour lightish brown externally and greyish black within ; surface wrinkled, hard and marked with irregular longitidinal furrows and with traces of scars of rootlets and of fallen leaves ; section homogeneously greyish black, and marked with a circular ring ; odour camphoraceous ; taste peculiar, like that of ambá halada.

Constituents.—An essential oil, resin, sugar, gum, starch, albuminoide and ash 7 p.c.

Actions and uses.—Stimulants and carminative ; uses similar to those of karchura ; chiefly used as a cosmetic.

Curcuma Longa B. P., Amomum Curcuma.

Habitat.—Behar, India S. Asia, Indian Ocean Islands.

Parts used.—The tubers.

Vernacular.—Arab.—Zirsud, urukus safé. Beng.—Holodi. Burm.—Tanin.—Can.—Arisinâ. Cing.—Kahâ, Haradul. Eng.—Turmeric Hind.—Haldar, Haldi. Guz., Mar., Malay.—Kunhet. Malyal.—Monjella kua. Pers.—Zard Chobah, karkum. Sans.—Haridra petta, rajani, nisha, gauri, varnavát, kamal. Tam.—Manjal. Tel.—Pasupu.

Characters.—Rhizome, hard and thick, 1 to 2 or 2½ inches long, and 4 to 6 or 8 lines in breadth; more or less arched; in shape ovoid and elongated and narrowed at both ends ; from the body project laterally small, knotty tubercles of a roundish form ; surface wrinkled, hard, rough, dark, brownish or yellow grey and marked with scars of rootlets and rings of fallen leaves ; cut portion resinous, with a distinct ring separating the outer from the central portion ; interior of a deep orange red colour; smell peculiar and aromatic ; taste ginger-like, acrid and rather oily. The powder is deep yellow. Dose, ½ to 1 dr. of the powder.

Constituents.—An essential oil 1 p.c. ; resin, curcumin, the yellow colouring matter ; turmeric oil or turmerol. Turmeric oil is a thick yellow viscid oil. The curry powder owes its aromatic taste and smell to this oil.

Curcumin—to obtain it, grind turmeric root with light petroleum when the turmeric oil is removed. To the paste add ether, which dissolves curcumin and large quantity of resin—purify and crystallize ; met with as needle-shaped crystals, arranged in radiate groups ; colour orange or yellow ; without any odour ; insoluble in water, soluble in hot alcohol, more in glacial acetic acid, less in ether, slightly in benzene and carbon bisulphide.

Preparations.—Tincture (1 in 6) B. P., used for the preparation of turmeric paper ; a medicated oil, and kunkun used for colouring ointment, solutions &c.

Actions and uses.—Stimulant, tonic, and aromatic ; given in jaundice, and in chronic bronchitis. When mixed with tila tela, it is applied to the whole body to prevent skin eruptions. With kali chuno, the powder of it is applied to bruises, sprains, contused wounds, black eye, with relief. A paste of it stops bleeding from leech bites. A decoction of it is used as a cooling lotion in conjunctivitis. Boiled in milk and sweetened with sákara, turmeric is a popular remedy for cold. The fumes of burning turmeric passed into the nostrils relieve coryza. Internally halada is given in affections of the liver and jaundice. On account of its yellow colour, cloth dipped in its paste is employed as an eye-shade. It is used in urinary diseases, and with sáji-khára as an external application to reduce indolent swellings. The powder mixed with Ghee and Kumár-no-rasa, or with milk, is given to relieve cough and cold.

Curcuma Zedoaria, C Zerumbet, Amomum Zerumbet.

Habitat.—Eastern Himalaya, throughout India.

Parts used.—The tubers.

Vernacular.—Arab.—Zarambad, Maha firfeen. Beng.—Suthi, Kar-chur-amu, Banhaldi. Burm.—Tha-nu-wen. Can.—Kachôrâ, Nirbishi. Cing.—Hinhurh, wal-kaha. Eng.—Long Zedoary. Hind., Mar., Guz.—Kâchura, Malyal.—Katon-inshi-kua kezhanna. Malay.—Toman, Pers.—Jadvar khata, Kazhur. Sans.—Sate Ganda masli, Krachura. kasturi manjal. Tam.—Pulân kizhanga. Tel.—Kushthuri pasupu.

Characters.—Rhizome oblong, pearl coloured, and solid; met with in circular slices of a greyish brown colour ; margin presenting traces of rootlets and of the epidermis ; surface concave and marked with a ring which is nearer the margin than towards the centre ; fracture, short and mealy ; taste camphoraceous, bitter and tingling ; odour highly camphoraceous. Dose, 10 to 30 grs.

Constituents.—A volatile oil 1 p.c., a bitter soft resin, bitter extractive matter, gum, starch, curcumin and albuminoids. The oil is turbid, yellowish white and viscid, of a camphoraceous taste and smell.

Actions and uses.—Carminative, rubefacient, diuretic and stimulant like ginger; given in gonorrhœa, menorrhagia and nephritic complaints. It is an ingredient of various alterative decoctions.

Elettaria Cardamomum, B. P., E. Repens, Amomum Cardamomum

Habitat.—Malabar, W. and S. India mountains.

Parts used.—The dried ripe seeds—Cardamomi semina, cardamom seeds, B. P.

Vernacular.—Arab.—Kakula ebil, Hêl-bavâ. Bomb., Guz., Beng. —Ilachi. Burm.—Palah, Bala. Can.—Yalakki. Cing.—Ensal, enasal. Hind., Duk.—Chhoti eelachie. Eng.—Nepaul cardamoms. Lesser cardamoms. Malay.—Kapulaga pinvar. Mar.—Veldoda. Pers.—Kakelah-seghar. Malyal.—Yalum. Sans.—Truti, Kapeta, Varni, Karangi, Dravidi, Upa-kunchika, Ela. Tam.—Ella-cheddie. Tel.—Elakichettu.

Varieties: Ammomum amarum—bitter seeded cardamom; cardamomum repens; A. grana paradisi—grains of paradise or Mala guetta pepper; A. aromaticum, Bengal cardamom; A. Maximum—Java winged cardamom, 9 to 12 winged from base to apex. A. Globosum,—Elachi dáná; the seeds of a species of Amomum xanthioides, bastard wild or Nepal cardamom. A. Subulatum—Bada ilachi, (Hind.) Kakulah, (Mar.) nara elachi. The fruit is very large and of a dark colour; capsules coarsely striated; seeds more numerous, less aromatic and less camphoraceous than that of kagadi, kaghazi or Malabari elachi.

Kardruna, nutmeg cardamom or cardamomum magnus; (Pers.) Hilbawa—conical fruit, in size and shape like a small fig reversed. The seeds are roundish and angular; odour agreeable, and aromatic, devoid of pungency of elachi; used by Arabs as rosaries. Each fruit has a hole in it due to the habit of hanging each fruit on a cord to dry.

Characters.—Capsules ovate or bluntly triangular, with tufts of fibres at its smaller end, 1 inch in length, 1½ inches in circumference, ribbed, coriacious and reddish brown; three-sided, oblong or somewhat roundish, of a yellowish brown or dirty white colour, with a small curved stalk at the base; stalk curved on the same side with the capsule; surface rugous, slightly wrinkled, and marked with longitudinal striæ; seeds small, round or bluntly angular and brown; closely packed and surrounded with membranous arillus in three rows, each row being separated by a thin membrane of a rich brown colour; membrane about two lines in length and transversely rugous; each row with generally five seeds; seeds with a depressed hilum; surface deeply channelled, resembling in shape, those of convolvulaceæ; odour pungent, camphoraceous and agreeable; taste pungent and leaving a sensation of cold upon the tongue when chewed.

Constituents.—Fixed oil 10 p.c., volatile oil—the active principle, 5 p.c., potassium salts 3 p.c., starch 3 p.c., nitrogenous mucilage

2 p.c., yellow colouring matter, ligneous fibre 77 p.c., and ash 6 to 10 p.c., containing manganese.

The essential oil is isomeric with oil of turpentine and is obtained by distillation or extraction with ether; found mostly in the testa; odour and taste camphoraceous; it contains terpinene, acetic and formic acids.

Preparations.—Tinctura cardamomi composita. B. P. (1 in 80). Dose, ½ to 1 dr. Extractum Colocynthidis compositum, B. P. Dose, 2 to 8 grs. Pulvis aromaticus, B. P. Dose, 10 to 40 grs. Tinctura Gentianæ composita, B. P. Dose, ½ to 1 dr. Tinctura Rhei composita, B. P. Dose, ½ to 1 dr.

Actions and uses.—Carminative, stomachic, stimulant, aromatic and masticatory; used for the same purposes as other carminatives. As a corrective it is given in flatulence, griping of purgative and other medicines.

Hedychium Spicatum.

Habitat.—China, Himalaya.

Parts used.—The tubers.

Vernacular.—Duk.—Vilayati-kachur. Guz., Mar.—Kâpur-kachri, kachur, seer, rutti. Hind.—Sidhoul. Sans.—Kapur kachli, shedwu. Tam.—Kizhangu. Tel.—Sima-kich-chilik.

Characters.—Circular slices from ¼ to ½ inch in diameter; margin rugous, wrinkled, of a brownish red colour and marked with white rings and traces of rootlets, some of the rootlets being also present; slightly convex on both surfaces; white internally, homogeneous and full of starch; starch powdery, granular and containing sparkling globules; smell peculiar, agreeable and aromatic; taste fragrant, mucilaginous, warm and aromatic, but not peppery or pungent, leaving a tingling sensation behind. It is called Vilayeti kachur, as its smell, taste and colour resemble those of zedoary.

Constituents.—Starch, cellulose, mucilage, albumen, oils, saccharine matter, acid resin, fixed oil, and an odorous body.

Preparations.—Paste, powder and decoction (1 in 20). Dose, 1 to 2 fld. ozs.

Actions and uses.—Stomachic and carminative; given in dyspepsia. It is also used in the preparation of cosmetic powders to promote the growth of hair. The sliced root is an ingredient in scented powder known as abira.

Kæmpferia Galanga.

Habitat.—Throughout India.

Parts used.—The tubers.

Vernacular.—Burm—khaminig. Beng., Hind.—Chandra mûla, Humula. Mar.—Chandra mûlâ, utnen. Malyal.—Kats julum. Sans.—Chandra mulika. Tam.—Kats julam. Tel.—Kachoram.

Characters.—Leaves radicle, petioled, ovate, and cordate ; margins membranous and waved ; upper surface smooth and green ; under surface pale and woolly ; roots branched ; tubers resembling ginger, giving off fleshy fibre ; odour agreeable and camphoraceous ; taste acrid and peppery.

Constituents.—An alkaloid, starch, gum, fatty matters containing a fragrant liquid oil and a solid white crystalline substance.

Actions and uses.—Stimulant and expectorant; the aromatic leaves and roots are used as perfume. With honey the root is given in cough and pectoral affections ; used also as a masticatory with betel leaves and areca nut. Boiled in oil it is used to promote nasal secretions.

Kæmpferia Rotunda, K. Longa.

Habitat.—Throughout India.

Parts used.—The tubers and the whole plant.

Vernacular.—Burm. Myoban touk. Beng., Guz., Hind., Mar.—Bhui champa. Cing.—Kahasan-kanda. Malyal.—Milankua. Sans.—Bhume champaka. Tel.—Konda-ka-lava.

Characters.—Leaves oblong and coloured ; spikes radicle ; flowers fragrant, purplish white ; root consisting of several globular rhizomes from which spring numerous fleshy rootlets ; taste bitter and camphoraceous like that of zedoary.

Actions and uses.—The small globular tubers are used as local application to tumours and glandular swellings of all kinds, as mumps, &c., the natives use the whole plant bruised as an application to anasarcous swellings ; an ointment of the whole plant is applied to fresh wounds. It is given internally in cases of pyæmia with the idea of removing blood or pus from the body.

Musa Paradisiaca, M. Sapientum.

Habitat.—Throughout India, tropical regions.

Parts used.—The fruit, leaves and stems.

Vernacular.—Arab.— Maoz. Beng.—Kachkula. Burm.—Huget-pyan. Can.—Bale. Cing.—Anawallu-Kesul. Duk.—Mouz. Eng.—Plantain, banana. Guz., Hind.—Kelâ, kel. Java.—Godang. Malay.—Pessang. Malyal.—Vella. Pers.—Mong. Sans.—Aramakadale, rambha, bhampso-labha, Rajishta, Van Luksham, autikadali. Tam.—Vallipalavu. Tel.—Kommu ariti.

Characters.—Stem simple, thickly closed with the sheathing petioles of the leaves ; leaves forming a tuft on the apex of the stem ; flowers compound, yellowish white in a spathe ; fruit oblong and fleshy ; seeds numerous, buried in the pulp.

Constituents.—The ash contains potash and soda salts, phosphoric acid and magnesia. The ripe fruit contains starch, sugar, gum, fat, albuminoids and non-nitrogenous extractives.

Actions and uses.—Demulcent, nutritive and astringent ; the fruit is used in soreness of the throat, dry cough and in irritability of the bladder. The root is used as an anthelmintic. The meal prepared from the fruits is nutritive ; the starch prepared from the unripe fruits is astringent and used in bowel complaints. A syrup of banana is given in chronic bronchitis with benefit. In hæmoptysis and hæmorrhagic fluxes, the juice of the stem obtained by incisions is very beneficial. The young leaves are a good substitute for gutta percha tissue in dressing wounds and as cooling dressing for blistered surfaces.

Remarks.—The natives use the leaves as a shade protector in eye diseases.

Maranta Arundinacea.

Habitat.—West Indies, Bermuda, Brazil.

Parts used.—The fecula of the rhizome.—Arrowroot.

Vernacular.—Burm.—Penbwa.

Characters.—The rhizome, tuberous and fleshy. To prepare arrowroot, the rhizome is dug, washed, deprived of scales, ground under water, kneaded and strained and the solution allowed to subside ; met with in powder or lumps, thick, white and opaque. It produces the West India arrowroot or maranta starch.

Constituents.—The root contains starch 27 p.c. and fat.

Actions and uses.—Demulcent and nutritive ; the most palatable and digestive of the starches known and used as food for infants and during convalescence from bowel and urinary troubles. The jelly is more tenacious than that from any other starch except canna starch.

Samadera Penatpetala, Niota Tetrapetala, S. Indica.

Habitat.—Cochin, Konkan, Travancore, South of Ceylon.

Parts used.—The bark root, fruit and oil.

Vernacular.—Cing.—Samadara-gass. Eng.—Neepa bark. Malyal.—Karin gota. Tam.—Neepa.

Characters.—Bark in quills, ½ to 1 inch in diameter, fissured externally; colour dark brown, dotted here and there with white patches; inner surface yellowish white ; fracture short and fibrous ; taste bitter ; the wood has properties resembling those of quassia. Dose, 30 to 60 grs.

Constituents.—A fixed oil of a light yellow colour and bitter taste, a bitter principle samaderin, also called quassin.

Preparation.—Infusion of bark (1 in 80). Dose, 1 to 2 ozs.

Actions and uses.—Intensely bitter and febrifuge like quassia ; given with myrobolans in fevers and dyspepsia. The oil is used as an external application in rheumatism. The seeds are superstitiously strung together in a wreath and tied round children's necks as a preventive against asthma and other affections of the chest.

Remarks.—The plant belongs to n. o. simarubaceæ.

Zingiber Cassumunar, Z. Purpureum, Z. Cliffordii.

Habitat.—India.

Parts used.—The rhizomes.

Vernacular.—Beng.—Ban-âda. Mar.—Nisa Malabari halad· Sans —Vana adrakam. Tel.—Kurapashupu, Karu-allamu, Van Adrak· Van, wild, and adrak, ginger—wild ginger.

Characters.—Fresh rhizomes jointed, 1 to 2 inches in diameter and compressed ; surface wrinkled and marked with numerous fleshy radicles, to some of which white tubers are attached externally ; epidermis scaly and dark brown ; interior of a golden yellow colour ; odour fragrant and nutmeg or kapura like ; taste hot, burning, and kapura like. It resembles amba halada in other peculiarities.

Constituents.—Resin, essential oil, fat, sugar, gum, starch, albuminoids and ash.

Actions and uses.—Stomachic, carminative and stimulant ; used in diarrhœa and colic. Other uses are similar to those of turmeric.

Zingiber Officinale, B. P.

Habitat.—Throughout India, W. Indies, Africa. Cultivated in Jamaica, Sierra Leone.

Zingiber from gingas gringa, or Shringa, means a horn, and ber or ver, a body. The body of the root is horn-shaped.

Parts used.—The scraped and dried rhizome Zingeberis, ginger, B. P.

Vernacular.—The fresh rhizome. Arab.—Zengabil. Bomb.—Alen, adu. Burm.—Gin-sin, Khen-seing. Can.—Hasisunthe. Chin—Kan-Kiang. Cing.—Ammuingurn. Eng.—Green ginger. Guz.—Adu. Beng., Duk., Hind.—Adraka, ada. Malayal.—Alia.Maleal.—Ischia.Mar.—Alen. Ala. Pers.—Zinjabile. Sans.—Katubadra. Tam.—Inji. Tel —Allam- The dry rhizome. Arab.—Zanjabile yâbis. Beng,—Duk., Guz., Mar.—Sont, Sunth. Burm.—Ghinsi—khiâb. Eng—Dry ginger. Hind.—Sontha Sindhi. Pers.—Zanjabile khushak. Sans.—Suntheka, Mahaushadha, Vishva-cheshajam. Malyal—Chukka. Tam.—Shukku. Tel.—Sonte.

Characters.—A plant with dingy yellow flowers on a leafless flower stalk and long lanceolate leaves on a separate stem ; rhizomes, 2 to 4 inches long ; tubers branched, knotty, and somewhat compressed, on one side lobed and clavately branched without a wrinkled and corky epidermis, buff coloured, and striate ; on section, fracture mealy and fibrous, showing many scattered resin cells and fibro vascular bundles ; odour agreeable, aromatic and penetrating ; taste acrid and pungent. The pungency is due to their containing an essential oil and resin ; soluble in alcohol or ether, partially in boiling water. Dose, 5 to 30 grs.

Varieties are named after their nativity. Jamaica ginger deprived of epidermis sometimes steeped in milk of lime and covered with calcium carbonate yields 5 p.c. of oleo resin. African dried ginger covered with light brown suberous tissue. Other varieties are East Indian and Chinese or Cochin.

Constituents.—A volatile oil 2 p.c., fat, a crude liquid oleo resin, gingerol or gingerin, mucilage, resin, starch 20 p.c.; ash 4 p.c. The volatile oil contains camphene and phellandrene. Gingerol, an active principle extracted from ginger, is a viscid, inodourous pungent liquid, of the colour and consistence of treacle, and aromatic hot taste; soluble in alcohol, ether, volatile oil and fat, slightly soluble in benzene ; it contains all the virtues of the root. The resin yields protocatechuic acid.

Preparations.—Fluid extract. Dose, 10 to 20 ms. Tinctura Zingbieris, B.P. (1 in 10). Dose, ½ to 1 dr. Syrup Zingiberis, B.P. (1 in 40). Dose, ½ to 1 dr. Trochisci each contains 3 ms. of the tincture. Tinctura Carminativa—contains cardamoms 10 drs., essence of ginger 10 drs., oil of cinnamon 1½ dr., oil of carraway 1½ dr., oil of cloves 1½ drs., macerate and dissolve, add rectified spirit to make 20 ozs. Dose, 2 to 10 ms.

Actions and uses.—Dried ginger is aromatic, stimulant and carminative, produces a sensation of warmth at the epigastrium and expels flatus ; as a carminative it is given in colic ; as a masticatory in relaxed throat and to increase the saliva. Locally it is rubefacient, anodyne and sialogogue. When chewed, fresh ginger is stomachic and digestive. The dry rhizome powdered and made into a paste with warm water is used as cataplasm or fomentations to the forehead in headaches, neuralgia, colic, and toothache ; also given in atonic dyspepsia, loss of appetite, to correct flatulence in colic, diarrhœa, chronic bronchial cough, palpitation of the heart, dropsy, cholera and tympanitis, and as a corrective to nauseous medicines and to check griping of purgatives. It is also used as a flavouring adjuvant to bitters.

The juice is given as an adjuvant to laxatives, as castor oil ; with garlic and honey it is used for cough and asthma.

Iridaceæ—the Kesar, Cornflag or Iris family.

Herbaceous plants, usually with bulbs, corms or rhizomes ; leaves with parallel and straight veins ; flowers regular or irregular, spathaceous ; perianth superior in 2 whorls ; stamens 3 ; ovary inferior, three-celled ; style 1 ; stigmas 3, petaloid ; fruit capsular, dehiscent, three-celled, three-valved ; seeds numerous ; albumen hard and horny.

Habitat.—Tropics and temperate climates, Cape of Good Hope.

Properties.—The rhizomes of several species are acrid, and hence used as a purgative, emetic, &c.; some tubers are in addition carminative and antispasmodic ; others are used as colouring agents, and many contain starch.

Crocus Sativus B. P.

Habitat.—W. Asia, France, Greece, Asia Minor, Persia. Cultivated in Europe.

Parts used.—The dried stigmas with tops of the styles—Crocus saffron, B. P.

Vernacular.—Arab.—Zafran. Burm.—Than-wen. Can.—Kum-kuma, Kesari-kumkamada, Huvû, Kesari. Chin.—Fan-hung-hwa. Cing.—Kohoon, Kunga mamal. Cash.—Konga. Eng.—Crow saffron, Hay saffron. Guz., Duk., Beng., Hind.—Kangan-mundi, Kesara, Zaffran. Malyal—Piwva Konger. Mar.—Kesarê. Pers.—Karkum, abir. Sans.—Kuna kûma, Saurapha kêsara. Tam.—Kaon goomapu. Tel. —Kum-kuma puvoo.

Characters.—Stigmas of a brilliant yellow or orange-red colour, like that of the rising sun ; style ½ to 1 inch long, and of a yellowish colour. Upon the style three long and rather twisted stigmas rest ; stigmas thread-like, narrow towards the base, and broad and partite or crenate at the apex ; colour deep orange red ; odour highly aromatic, strong and peculiar ; taste, mucilaginous, slightly bitterish and pungent ; one pound of saffron contains 60,000 stigmas. Dose, 5 to 30 grs.

Constituents.—A volatile oil, crocin—a glucoside, also called poly chroit (many colours), which is the colouring matter, picrocrocin—bitter principle, wax, proteids, fixed oil, mucilage, sugar, ash 5 p.c., moisture 12 p.c. The volatile oil is obtained by distillation and by heat. Crocin —To obtain it exhaust saffron with ether, then with water ; add alcohol to aqueous tincture when gum will be precipitated, filter and add ether. Met with in amorphous, yellowish brown mass ; taste sweetish ; soluble in alcohol and water. It splits up into sugar (crocose) and red crocetin. Picrocrocin, or saffron bitter, the bitter principle, occurs as colourless needles, soluble in water. With alkalies it yield crocose and volatile oil.

Preparation.—Tinctura Croci, tincture of saffron, B. P. (1 in 20). Dose, 5 to 15 ms. *Infusion* (saffron tea) (1 in 80). Dose, 1 to 4 ozs.

Actions and uses.—Stimulant, aromatic, and antispasmodic, also used as a colouring agent ; given in amenorrhœa, chlorosis, seminal weakness, leucorrhœa, dysmenorrhœa, in flatulent colic, spasmodic asthma and cough. Owing to its containing the volatile oil, it is used in rheumatism and neuralgic pains. It is given to children with ghee in looseness of the bowels. It is reputed to promote exanthematous eruptions in specific fevers, as measles. Externally a paste of it is used in removing bruises and superficial sores and in headache. Pessaries of saffron are used in painful affections of the uterus. It gives the urine a yellow colour.

Remarks.—American saffron—safflower, is from carthamus tinctorius.

Iris Germanica, I. Pallida, I. Florentina.

Habitat.—N. Italy, Germany, France, N. India, S. Europe, Persia.

Parts used.—The rhizome and roots.

Vernacular.—Arab.—Sosan, Kusht-el-hali, Aersa Arastan. Bomb.—Balva-ekhanda. Chin.—Pehchi. Eng.— Orris root, violet root. Ind. Bazaar, Guz.—Kevara-nu-mula, Bikh-i-banafsa. Pers.—

Padma pushkara, Sus-an-i-asman guni. Sans.—Bikh-i-sostana, Pushkara mula.

Characters.—Root in pieces, of a greyish brown, or violet colour, hard and compressed; bark wrinkled externally, where it is marked with scars of fallen rootlets; cut surface, resembling in appearance and colour darunaj-i-akrabi; smell violet-like or resembling that of Tagara ganthoda; taste acrid and slightly bitter, also starchy.

Constituents.—Volatile oil (orris camphor), starch, resin, and tannin.

Preparations.—Decoction (1 in 10). Dose, 1 to 2 fld. ozs.

Actions and uses.—Cathartic, stimulant, alterative and diuretic; used in bronchitis, dropsy and liver complaints; also externally as an application to sores and pimples. As a masticatory for perfuming breath and in teething of infants.

Iris Versicolor.

Habitat.—N. America, moist meadows and swamps.

Parts used—The rhizome and roots.

Syn.—Poison or water-flag, snake-lily, blue-flag, liver-lily.

Characters.—A perennial herb; flowers large blue; rhizome in circular pieces, about half an inch to an inch in length and of a dark brown colour; bark easily separable, scaly, wrinkled, and here and there marked with scars of fallen rootlets. Wood, hard, granular and resinous looking; in colour and appearance resembling choba chini; taste somewhat acrid and astringent; odour slightly aromatic. Dose, 5 to 20 grs.

Constituents.—An acrid resin 25 p.c., a camphoraceous body, an alkaloid, fat, sugar, gum and tannin.

Preparations.—Decoction (1 in 10). Dose, ½ to 1 fld. oz. Extract, Dose, 1 to 5 grs. Fluid extract. Dose, 5 to 60 ms. Iridin or Irisin, a powdered extractive. Dose, 1 to 5 grs.

Actions and uses.—The fresh root is cathartic, but it produces nausea and great prostration. As a cholagogue it is given in hepatic disorders as jaundice, due to duodenal catarrh and obstruction of the bile ducts. In malarial jaundice and in malarial and bilious remittents, also in scrofula and syphilis, it is given with benefit. As a diuretic it is given in dropsy, glandular swellings and skin affections. It is also given in drop doses, in vomiting of pregnancy and in supra-orbital headache, chiefly of hepatic origin; also in round and tape worms. Iridin is freely used combined with henbane and euonymin as a mild aperient, cholagogue, alterative and diuretic. It is a special stimulant of the secretion of bile and is used in enlarged liver combined with oxgall and other cathartics. It is gentler than podophyllin and more reliable and more purgative than euonymin. It is also given in intestinal troubles and in vomiting of pregnancy and in malarial jaundice. Generally given with euonymin (4 to 1), when it does not irritate the rectum, and produces bilious stools. It has no subsequent astringency.

Amaryllidaceæ. The Amaryllis or Sukadarsan family.

Plant, bulbous or fibrous rooted without any aerial stem ; leaves with parallel and straight venation, linear ensiform ; flowers on scapes and spathaceous ; fruit capsular, 3-celled, 3-valved, dehiscent or berry ; seeds numerous ; albumen fleshy or horny ; embryo with a radicle next to hilum.

Habitat.—Native of warm parts of the globe, Cape of Good Hope.

Properties.—Several are emetic, purgative or poisonous ; the juice of a few species is saccharine, from which fermented liquors are obtained ; others contain starch.

Crinum Asiaticum, C. Toxicarium, C. Bracteatum.

Habitat.—Throughout India, Concan.

Parts used.—The leaves and the fresh bulb.

Vernaculars.—Beng., Guz., Mar., Hind.—Barâ kanwâr, Nâgdowna, Gaer-hônâr-pata, Sukhdursan. Burm.—Koyanji. Cing.—Mahabtobalis. Duk.—Nâgina. Eng.—Poison bulb. Malyal.—Visha-mûla, Beluta-patalah. Sans.—Visha-mandala. Tam.—Visha-munge-elle. Tel.—Kêsara-chetu.

Characters.—The fresh root is bulbous, brownish white, terminal and of varying size ; odour narcotic, acrid and disagreeable. It can readily be powdered after desiccation ; leaves long, thick, fleshy, linear, lanceolate, smooth and striated, green, or greenish yellow.

Preparations.—Of the juice of fresh bulb. Succus.—Dose, 2 to 4 drs. Syrup (1 in 3). Dose, 2 drs. as an emetic for children.

Actions and uses.—Emetic, nauseant and diaphoretic. It acts without causing griping, purging or any other distressing symptoms and is a good substitute for ipecacuanha and squill. It is given in croup, whooping cough, asthma, and chronic bronchitis. The leaves bruised, made warm and besmeared with a little castor oil are applied over inflamed whitlows and as fomentations to inflamed joints and sprains. The juice of leaves is dropped into the ear in earache. The dried roots are emetic, but require double the dose.

Crinum Zeylanicum, which is plentiful in most parts of India, has the properties of squills. The root is bulbous, of varying size and somewhat acrid. The toasted bulb is applied to tumours, buboes, and to piles to promote suppuration. The bulb roasted is used as a rubefacient in rheumatism.

Hypoxidaceæ,—The Hypoxis or Kali musali family.

Herbaceous plant; leaves dry, harsh, with parallel, straight, generally linear and ensiform venation ; seeds carunculate; radicle of the embryo, remote from the hilum.

Habitat.—Native of warm parts of the globe.

Properties.—Some are bitter and aromatic; roots of some are fleshy and mucilaginous.

Curculigo Orchioides.

Habitat.—Hotter regions of India, Ceylon.

Parts used.—The tuberous root.

Vernacular.—Beng.—Sada mushli, tamuli. Bomb.—Musali-kânda Cing.—Hinbintal. Can.—Nela-tâti-gadde. Guz., Hind., Duk.—Kâli musli, Shea-musli. Malyal.—Nilapana-kizanna. Sans.—Tâla-mûlikâ, Hema-pushpi. Tam.—Nila panay kalangu. Tel.—Nalla tade.

Characters.—Dried root, translucent, in pieces about ½ to 1 inch in length and from 4 to 5 lines in thickness, cylindrical and of a brownish dark colour, surface wrinkled and here and there marked with scars of fallen rootlets; cut portion studded with soft fibrous bundles and granular matter; taste mucilaginous and slightly bitter; smell rather disagreeable. Dose of the powdered root, 1 to 2 drs.

Constituents.—Resin, tannin, mucilage, starch and ash containing oxalate of calcium, &c.

Preparations—Confection.

Actions and uses.—Bitter, aromatic, tonic and demulcent; used in general debility, in affections of the urino-genital system as impotence; also in asthma, piles, jaundice, dysuria, diarrhœa, menorrhagia, and gonorrhœa. As a tonic it is generally mixed with aromatic bitters and aphrodisiac medicines.

Hæmodoraceæ—The Blood-root family.

Herbs, rarely shrubs; roots fibrous; leaves ensiform, usually equitant; perianth superior, tubular, six parted; stamens 3; ovary, inferior, three-celled; fruit dehiscent or indehiscent; seeds few or many; albumen cartilaginous.

Habitat.—Native of America, Cape of Good Hope, Australia.

Properties.—Roots are bitter, astringent, tonic and stomachic.

Aletris Farinosa, True Unicorn Colic root or Star wort.

Habitat—United States.

Parts used.—Rhizome or rootlets.

Characters.—Fibrous, of a dark brown colour externally, taste amylaceous and bitter.

Constituents.—Starch, and an active bitter principle.

Preparations.—Powder. Dose, 5 to 10 grs. Aletrin. Dose, ½ to 2 grs. Decoction (1 in 20). Dose, 2 to 4 drs. Dried extract. Dose, 2 to 5 grs. Fluid extract. Dose, 10 to 30 ms. Tincture (1 in 8). Dose, ½ to 1 dr.

Actions and uses.—Tonic, diuretic, in large doses emetic and cathartic. It has a specific influence upon the uterus in amenorrhœa, dysmenorrhœa, prolapsus uteri, and sterility. It gives tone and vigour to the reproductive organs, and is chiefly indicated to prevent miscarriage. It should be given during the whole period of gestation.

Liliaceæ—The Lily, Eliyo or Kanda family.

Trees, shrubs, or herbs, with bulbs, rhizomes, tuberous or fibrous roots ; stem generally simple, rarely branched ; leaves sessile or sheathing, with parallel veins ; flowers regular ; perianth green, petaloid, or inferior, 6-parted ; stamens 6 ; ovary, superior, 3-celled ; style 1 ; stigma simple ; fruit loculicidal, capsule, pod or berry, or succulent and indehiscent, 3-celled ; seeds numerous with fleshy albumen.

Habitat.—Temperate climates or tropics.

Properties.—The properties vary : some plants are purgative, others emetic, diaphoretic, diuretic, stimulant and acrid, several are astringent. The bulbs of Kanda, Lasana, young shoots, roots, and seeds of many species are used as articles of food and condiment.

Allium Cepa—Onion, A. Porrum—the Leek, A. Ascalonicum—the Shallot.

Habitat.—India.

Parts used.—The bulb and seed.

Vernacular.—Arab.—Basal. Beng.—Pulantu. Bur.—Kyet-thwon-ni. Can.—Kunbatti. Chin.—Tsung. Cing.—Luno. Hind., Duk., Guz.—Dungali, Kânda, Pyaz. Malyal.—Ira-venyayam. Mah. —Kandê. Pers.—Goondina. Sind.—Dungari. Sans.—Platandu. Tam.—Vengâyam. Tel.—Erra-vulli.

Characters.—Bulb varying in size from a walnut to a large orange, colour varying between red and white; other characters similar to those of the Bana Kanda ; taste very acrid and pungent ; odour very pungent ; when cut into thin slices, the oil volatizes and irritates the eyes, giving rise to secretion of tears.

Constituents.—An acrid volatile oil containing sulphur.

Action and uses.—Onions are stimulant, expectorant, and diuretic. The juice of the bulb and conserve of the white variety are used in colic. With salt Kándá is held to the nose in fainting. Its juice is dropped into the ear to relieve ear-ache ; when roasted its poultice is applied to inflamed and indolent boils. The seeds are demulcent and given in gonorrhœa. With navaságara; the juice is given in retention of urine.

Allium Macleani.

Habitat.—Persia, Badghis.

Parts used.—The bulbs, scalded and dried.

Vernacular.—Eng.—Royal salep. Ind. Bazar.—Bâdshahi or Padshahi Sâlap.

Characters.—Dried bulbs, nearly spherical, sometimes ovoid, pointed at the upper extremity, with a depressed cicatrix or a white elevated scar at the lower end; surface striated longitudinally, translucent, of a purplish brown or yellow colour, dense and horny; taste bitter. They readily absorb moisture from the air. Dose, ½ to 2 drs.

Constituents.—Mucilage, cellulose, mineral matter and ash containing manganese.

Actions and uses.—Tonic and demulcent; given in general debility, nervous exhaustion and seminal weakness.

Allium Sativum.

Habitat.—Central Asia, S. Europe (Italy, Sicily), and America.

Parts used.—The bulb.

Vernacular.—Arab.—Sôm, Sum. Burm.—Kesûn-phiû. Can.—Beluli. Cing.—Sudu, Lûlû. Chin.—Swan, Livan. Eng.—Clove garlic or common garlic. Guz., Hind., Mar., Duk., Beng.—Lashuna. Pers.—Sir. Sans.—Ugra-gandha, Bhutaghna, Lasuna, Mahu Shuda. Tam.—Vellai-pundu. Tel.—Tella-gidda.

Characters.—The bulbs which are called cloves of garlic are subglobular, surrounded by dry membranous scales, and contain from 5 to 8 small bulblets arranged in a circle round the stem, projecting from the base of the tuber. The bulb is round externally, wedge-shaped towards the stem, and compressed at both sides. It has a peculiar, pungent and disagreeable odour, and an acrid burning taste. Dose, ½ to 2 drs.

Constituents.—An acrid volatile oil, starch, mucilage 35 p.c., albumen, sugar, &c.

Oil of garlic—a volatile oil, obtained by distillation; it contains allyl, propyl disulphide, diallyl disulphide, and other sulphur compounds. It is a clear limpid liquid of a dark brown or yellow colour; odour very repulsive; taste repugnant. The medicinal properties are due to this oil. Dose, ¼ to 2 ms.

Preparations.—A compound garlic powder, Sval Parasona Pinda, containing garlic, sonachala, cumin, asafetida, rock salt, trikatu, ginger, long pepper, black pepper, jirun saphed, equal parts. Given in rheumatism, facial paralysis, sciatica, convulsions, tetanus, epilepsy, &c. Dose, 10 to 20 grs. Syrup (1 in 5 of sugar and acetic acid). Dose, ½ to 2 drs. Poultice; extract (inspissated juice) 4 to 10 grs.; Succus. Dose, ½ dr. and Liniment.

Actions and uses.—As a gastric stimulant, it aids digestion, and is given in flatulence; as an expectorant it has a special influence over the bronchial and pulmonary secretions; as an emmenagogue it promotes the flow of menses. It is a tonic, carminative and stimulant of the skin and kidneys. In large doses it is an irritant and produces flatulence, headache, nausea, vomiting, diarrhœa, &c. As a local stimulant and irritant, it reddens the skin and causes vesication.

Like Kanda, it is applied to the nose of hysterical girls when in a state of swooning. Given with common salt it relieves colic and nervous headache. As a vermifuge it expels round worms. Like onion, it causes copious diuresis and is hence used in dropsy or anasarca. Locally in bronchitis and in cold or catarrh in children, bruised garlic and onions are applied to the chest as a poultice or liniment. Applied to the perineum it relieves strangury. It is also applied to the bites of venomous reptiles. Mustard powder is added to promote its rubefacient effects. It is rubbed over ringworm with relief. Garlic juice slightly warmed, or the bulb is boiled with salad oil and the oil when cool, is dropped into the ear for the relief of earache.

Aloe Vera, B. P., A. Chinensis, B. P., and other species.

Habitat.--India, Dutch West India Islands, Barbadoes, Curacoa.

Parts used.—The juice flowing from the transversely cut leaves, and evaporated to dryness. Aloe Barbadensis—Barbados aloes, B.P., sometimes found adulterated with akakia and babul gum.

Vernacular.—Arab.—Nabâ tussibr, sabar or sibar. Burm.—Sha-zavu-le-pa. Can.—Lola sarâ. Cing.—Komarika. Duk.—Kalbanda. Eng.—Hepatic Aloes. Hind., Guz.—Kumâr-Kuvâra. Malyal.—Katru-vazha. Bomb., Mar.—Kora-kánda. Pers.—Darakhte sibr. Sans.—Kumari. Tam.—Shotu katraz lai. Tel.—Kaiabanda.

Aloes Indica, A. Abyssinica, A. Perfoliata.

Habitat.—Africa, India, Abyssinia.

Parts used.—The expressed inspissated and dried juice of the leaves.

Vernacular.—Arab.—Sibar, Sahar, musabbar. Beng.—Ghertokumari. Burm.—Mok. Can.—Kumarika. Chin.—Chin-hiang Cing.—Kumarilla. Duk.—Kanwar. Eng.—Bitter aloes, Indian aloes. Guz.,—Aba Elva. Hind.—Ban-ushtaki. Malyal.—Alivah. Pers.—Bol Shiah. Tam.—Karia bulan. Tel.—Mussambram.

Aloes Perryi, B.P., and other species.

Habitat.—Isle of Socotra, Eastern coast of Africa, near the Red Sea.

Parts used.—The juice flowing from transversely cut leaves, inspissated by heat or solidified without the aid of heat—Aloe socotrina B. P., soctrine aloes, Zanzibar aloes, Bombay aloes.

Vernacular.—Hind.—Ban-ushtaki, Ghi-kumar. Panj.—Kwar Gondal, masti. Tam.—Sirru kattalay.

Varieties.—Aloes Litoralis—Sea-side aloe, known as Kumari (Beng.), Chota Kamvar (Duk.).

Arabian aloes—Ya mani, or Moka, or Aden aloes, yielded by Aloes Indica ; it is of a blackish colour, shining on the surface, porous and translucent ; when held before the sunlight the colour changes to red. It is also known as Bandhano Eliyo and Petino Eliyo. The former is mixed with stone, clay, &c., and is wrapped up in mats. The latter is clean and is packed in boxes. Cape aloes is yielded by Aloes Spicata.

Characters.—The plant has orange coloured flowers, and resembles the century plant, or Agave Americana. Leaves succulent, thick, flat, and fleshy, broad at the base, tapering at the apex, and spiny at their margins; colour generally greenish yellow. The juice when fresh is thick, mucilaginous, transparent or yellow ; generally found in central part of leaves, in ducts near the margins or from parallel brownish green vessels found beneath the epidermis of the leaves. Aloes (or dry inspissated juice) is met with in opaque brown powder or in masses or in translucent thin slices; sometimes soft, of a bright golden yellow colour, and breaking with a smooth waxy or glassy fracture, not conchoidal ; when scraped and powdered, of a bright golden yellow colour ; odour peculiar, disagreeable and saffron like ; taste nauseous, very bitter, slightly aromatic and very persistent ; entirely soluble in alcohol, diluted with half its volume of water, in water (1 in 2 or 3). Dose, 2 to 5 grs.

Constituents.—Aloin ; resins 30 to 50 p.c., volatile oil and ash 1 p.c., also aloetic and chrysammic acids. The odour is due to the volatile oil. Aloin, B. P.,—a neutral active principle : to obtain it digest aloes in alcohol, boil, filter and crystallize. Occurs in tufts of yellow acicular crystals without any odour ; the taste is like that of aloes; sparingly soluble in cold water, and acetic ether, more soluble in alcohol, freely so in hot liquids, nearly insoluble in ether. Dose, $\frac{1}{2}$ to 2 grs. Aloin is named as Socaloin, Barbaloin, Natаloin and Zanaloin, according as it is obtained from Socotrina, Barbadoes, Natal and Zanzibar.

The purgative properties of aloes are due to this principle. The activity of aloin is increased by giving it with an alkali, presumably to decompse it. Aloin in itself is not an active purgative, but becomes decomposed in the intestines into a more active body, hence its slowness of action.

Preparations.—Of aloin—Pilula Aloin Composita—contains aloin, extract of nux vomica, sulphate of iron, myrrh and soap, of each $\frac{1}{2}$ gr.; also with ipecacuanha $\frac{1}{16}$ gr. and of extract of belladonna $\frac{1}{8}$ gr. for constipation. Dose, 2 to 4 grs ; Pilula Aloin Strychninæ et Belladonnæ contains aloin $\frac{1}{5}$ gr., strychnine $\frac{1}{16}$ gr. extract belladonna $\frac{1}{2}$ gr. in each, make 1 pill. Formaloin, a compound of aloin with formaldehyde. In yellow amorphous powder without any taste, insoluble in water. Of Aloes Extractum Aloes Barbadensis, B. P. Dose 1 to 4 grs. Pilula aloes Barbadensis, B. P. Dose, 4 to 8 grs. Pilula Aloes et Myrrhæ B. P.(4 in 9). Socotrine aloes 2, myrrh 1, syrup of glucose $1\frac{1}{2}$. Dose, 4 to 8 grs. Pilula Aloes et Asafetidæ B. P. (1 in 4). Dose, 4 to 8 grs. Wine. Dose, 1 to 2 fld. drs. Tinctura Aloes, B. P. (1 of extract in 40). Dose, 1 to 2 fld. drs. Enema. Tinctura Benzoini Composita, Friars' Balsam, (1 in 60). Dose, $\frac{1}{2}$ to 1 dr. Pilula Rhei Composita B. P.—Rhubarb 48, aloes 36, myrrh 24, hard soap 24, oil of peppermint 3, syrup of glucose 44, contains aloes $\frac{1}{5}$ of its weight. Dose, 4 to 8 grs. Extractum Colocynthidis compositum. P. B. Dose, 2 to 8 grs. Decoctum aloes compositum, B. P., Compound decoction, contains extract of Barbadoes aloes $\frac{1}{2}$ ounce, myrrh, saffron and potassium carbonate, each $\frac{1}{4}$ oz.; extract of liquorice 2 ozs., compound tincture of cardamoms 15 ozs.; distilled water to make 50 ozs. Dose, $\frac{1}{2}$ to 2 fld. ozs. Pilula aloes et ferri, B. P. (2 in 9). Dose, 4 to 8 grs. Pilula Colcynthidis Composita, B. P., contains Barbadoes aloes $\frac{1}{3}$ weight. Dose, 4 to 8 grs. Pilula Colocynthidis et Hyoscyami, B. P. Dose, 4 to 8 grs. Pilula Cambogiæ Composita B. P. (1 in 6). Gamboge 1, Barbados aloes 1, compound powder of cinnamon 1, hard soap 2, syrup of glucose 1. Dose, 4 to 8 grs.

Vinum aloes compositum—Kumari Asava. To prepare it, to the decoction containing kumara juice 100, jaggary 20, bhânga 5, and water 50, add madha 1, dhâuriphula 6, jàephala, lavanga, kankola, kabâba chini, jatâmânasi, chavaka, chitraka, jâvantri, kakadâ singi, behedân, pokara mula, each 1, trâmbâ bhashma, loha bhashma each $\frac{1}{2}$, mix, keep for about a month, and allow it to ferment.

Actions and uses.—Hepatic stimulant, cathartic, emmenagogue and vermifuge ; in small doses stomachic, hepatic tonic and astringent. It stimulates the mammæ, liver and the pelvic organs. giving rise to abortion, hæmorrhoids, and priapism in the male ; and the milk in the female assumes a purgative quality ; in large doses it is an indirect emmenagogue and cathartic. It acts chiefly on the lower half of the large intestines, and especially on the rectum, producing copious soft stools with some griping and pain. It diffuses into the blood and is eliminated by the mucous membranes of the colon. It is chiefly given in fevers and in enlarged glands, as the liver, spleen, &c. It is rubbed round the navel to open the bowels in young children. It is commonly given with honey to children (newly born) to hasten expulsion of the meconium. It has a slow but certain action in constipation, dependent upon the atony of the intestinal muscular coat, which supervenes upon fever and debilitating diseases, due to old age, to sedentary habits and to repeated pregnancies. In hæmorrhoids with mucous discharges it is very useful. As an enema it is used to expel ascarides. Aloes with myrrh, nux vomica, and iron is useful in amenorrhœa, hypochondriasis, atonic dyspepsia and constipation. As a local stimulant it acts favourably in skin diseases.

Asagræa Officinalis, Schœnocaulon Officinale, B. P.

Habitat.—Mexico.

Parts used.—The dried ripe seeds, sabadilla, cevadilla ; and an alkaloid, veratrina, B. P.

Characters.—A bulbous herb ; bulb ovoid with numerous black scales ; leaves linear and grass-like, long, smooth, entire, with strong midrib ; flowers numerous, lower ones hermaphrodite, upper ones male ; fruit composed of 3 follicles : pericarp, pale brown, and papery ; seeds 2 to 5 ; testa in each follicle, thin, dark brown, fusiform, compressed and wrinkled ; albumen whitish and oily ; without any odour and bitter acrid taste.

Constituents.—The seeds contain veratrine or cevadine, cevadilline, sabadine, sabadinine, angelic acid, methyl crotonic acid, cevadic acid, veratric acid, fixed oil, and ash. Veratrina or veratrine, B. P., is a poisonous alkaloid or a mixture of alkaloids. To obtain it express the seeds with alcohol, evaporate, add water to remove resin and oil, and filter. It occurs in grey amorphous mass, highly acrid and bitter, irritating to the nostrils and causing tingling and numbness to the tongue ; insoluble in water, soluble in glycerin (1 in 96), alcohol (1 in 3), chloroform (1 in 3), olive oil (1 in 56), ether (1 in 6), completely soluble in acids. Dose, $\frac{1}{60}$ to $\frac{1}{16}$ gr. in a pill with milk sugar and gum tragacanth.

Preparations.—Oleate (1 in 50) of oleic acid—used locally. Unguentum Veratrinæ, B. P., contains veratrine 10, oleic acid 40, lard 450 ; anodyne amyl colloid.

Actions and uses.—Veratrine is an antipyretic and may be used in fevers and acute inflammations. Like aconite it is a powerful irritant, causing sneezing, a sensation of pricking and twitching of the muscles. In large doses it leads to vomiting and purging. Locally the ointment is used in pruritis, pediculi, over stiff joints, sprains, &c. It should not be applied on an abraded surface. Cevadilla seeds may be given as an anthelmintic. Powdered seeds are used locally to destroy lice or vermin.

Asparagus Ascendens.

Habitat.—Rohilkhand, Gujerat, C. India.

Parts used.—The tuberous root, decorticated.

Vernacular.—Arab.—Shaqa-q-ul-e hindi. Bomb., Hind., Mar., Guz.—Safèd musli ; Malyal.—Shada veli, Tam.—Tannir vittang. Tel.—Tsalla gadda.

Characters.—Tubers shrivelled, decorticated, 2 to 3 inches long, and about 3 to 4 lines in thickness, of an ivory white colour, rather pointed at both ends, and twisted, brittle, hard, homogeneous and thorny ; also longitudinally shrivelled or fissured at their lower end ; taste like that of salema misari.

Constituents.—Albuminous matter, mucilage and cellulose.

Preparations.—A compound powder containing sapheda musali 6, kali musali 5, talma khana 3, beja banda 3, gokharu 5, kavacha 2, mocharasa 2, kikara no-gunda 5, samurda sosha, 5, dudheli 3, satavari 3, gilo 5, kakada singi 5, bahuphali 3, sankhahuli 3, akalakara 3, meda lakadi 5, salepa 5, nagakesara 2, taja 5, tamala patra 5, elchi 5, nishota 3, sakara 10. Mix and make a powder. Dose, 5 to 30 grs. in milk. A nuitritive tonic used in seminal weakness and impotence.

Actions and uses.—Nutritive, tonic and demulcent; boiled in milk and sakara they are used in spermatorrhœa, gleet, and chronic leucorrhœa; also in diarrhœa.

Asparagus Officinalis.

Parts used.—The plant, root and ripe fruits (seeds).

Habitat.—Europe, Turkey, Russia, Persia, N. India.

Vernacular.—Arab.—Isferaj, Halyun. Eng.—Common asparagus. Hind.—Nakdoun, Margiyeh. Ind. Bazaar.—Halyun. Malyal.—Akar parsi. Pers.—Marchubeh.

Characters.—Root consisting of short horizontal succulunt shoots or rhizomes; upper side scaly and marked with stem scars; below it gives off numerous whitish simple roots which become wrinkled on drying. It has no odour, but a mawkish and sweet taste; berries, 3-celled, scarlet, of the size of a pea, containing 1 to 2 seeds in each cell; embryo transverse and albumen horny.

Constituents.—The root contains asparagin, a yellow resin, sugar, gum, albumen, chlorides, phosphates, malates, &c. The berries contain grape sugar and spargancin, a colouring matter; the seeds contain a fixed oil, aromatic resin, sugar and a bitter principle spargin.

Asparagin or althein is met with in colourless, transparent, hard crystals or right rhombic prisms, of acid reaction, without odour or taste, soluble in cold water (1 in 50), insoluble in alcohol. An aqueous solution dissolves yellow oxide of mercury and hence used as a vehicle for hypodermic injection. Dose, 1 to 2 grs.

Asparagin is also found in the roots of marsh mallow, liquorice, belladonna, &c.

Preparations.—Infusion (1 in 10). Dose, 1 to 2 fld. ozs.

Actions and uses.—A mild aperient, diuretic and sedative; given in flatulency, in calculous affections, in cardiac dropsy and chronic gout; roasted seeds are used as a substitute for coffee; young shoots when boiled are used as vegetable. Asparagin is recommended as a diuretic in 1 to 2 grains doses in cardiac dropsy and chronic gout, combined with potassium bromide.

Asparagopsis Sarmentosus, Asparagus Racemosus.

Habitat.—Throughout India, Concan, Deccan.

Parts used.—The roots.

Vernacular.—Arab.—Shakakula. Beng.—Sutamuli. Burm.—Kanyomi. Cashm.—Sejpana. Can.—Shipari. Cing.—Hata vari. Duk.—Shaka-kule. Guz.—Satavari. Hind.—Sadabori, Bozidan. Jehlum.—Sabuni. Malyal.—Satavali. Mar.—Satvari. Panj.—Satavar. Patna Bazaar.—Utees. Pers.—Shakkula. Sans.—Suta muli. Tam.—Tamur. Tel.—Challa, Phillitaga.

Satamul, from sata, a hundred, and muli, roots; in allusion to the numerous fisiform roots.

Characters.—Root brownish white in colour, in length from 6 to 8 inches, and in breadth resembling a slender quill. Deeply furrowed and rugous ; on section tough, resinous, or starchy ; in the centre a thin, slender and wiry wood, minutely furrowed and porous ; smell like that of burnt sugar ; taste mucilaginous.

Constituents.—Contains large amount of saccharine matter and mucilage.

Preparations.—Confection ; decoction (1 in 20). Dose, 1 to 2 fld. ozs. A medicated oil, the Narayen-tel.

Actions and uses.—Nutritive, tonic, demulcent, and galactagogue ; given in biliousness, rheumatism, dyspepsia and diarrhœa. In combination with other diuretics it is given in scanty urine ; as a tonic, it is used in seminal debility, and pulmonary complaints.

Convallaria Majalis—Lily of the Valley.

Habitat.—Europe, N. Asia and United States.

Parts used.—The rhizome, roots and flowers.

Characters.—Stemless, perennial plant ; flowers bell-shaped, white, sweet-scented ; leaves smooth and elliptical ; rhizome horizontal, thick, with internodes ; surface wrinkled and marked with few circular scars, joints annulate ; odour peculiar, and pleasant ; taste, sweet, bitter, and acrid. Dose, 2 to 8 grs.

Constituents.—Convallarin, convallamarin resin and a principle contained in the flowers only. Convallarin, a glucoside, in colourless prisms, taste bitter and acrid ; colour pale brown ; soluble in alcohol, insoluble in water, foaming like saponin. With dilute acids when boiled it splits up into sugar and convallaretin. Dose, 3 to 4 grs. It acts as a purgative. Convallamarin—a bitter glucoside. To obtain it, precipitate the alcoholic tincture with acetate of lead, filter and evaporate ; neutralize the precipitate with sodium carbonate, then precipitate with tannin, dissolve with alcohol, decolorize with charcoal, and decompose with zinc oxide, filter and evaporate. A white powder of a bitter-sweet taste, soluble in water and alcohol. Dose, $\frac{1}{4}$ to 1 gr. It contains active properties of the drug.

Preparations.—An aqueous extract from the root and leaves. Dose, 1 to 6 grs. Fluid extract from the flowers. Dose, 2 to 10 ms. Tincture from flowers (1 in 8). Dose, 5 to 20 ms.

Actions and uses.—Convallaria is a heart tonic ; it acts on the heart more slowly than digitalis, and its effect is persistent. The root is sternutatory ; freed from resin, it is a gastric tonic, increasing peristalsis of the intestines without producing catharsis. Its action lasts for several days even after the use has been suspended. Convallaria is free from any deleterious effects, and has no cumulative action. As a diuretic it is given in senile hypertrophy, chronic pericarditis, valvular disease with cardiac dropsy, in mitral stenosis, dilatation of the heart, palpitation and in weak heart. It is also given in pneumonia, typhoid fever, and renal dropsy.

Dracœna Cinnabari, D. Schizantha D. Draco.

Habitat.—Socotra.

Parts used.—The resinous substance.

Vernacular.—Arab.—Katira ad-dam, Dama-le-tinnin, Dam-ul-akhwain, Chin.—Ki-lin-keep, Lung-sin-hiang. Bomb.—Heraadkhan. Duk.—Indarume. Eng.—Dragon's blood. Hind.—Hiradukhi, jaida rumi. Malyal.—Jarnang. Socotra.—Damkhoheil. Sans.—Catga-muruga-rakta. Tam. Kanda-moorga. Tel.—Khadga, murgam.

Characters.—It is a spontaneous resinous exudation from the ripening fruits and occurs in irregular tears or globular pieces of a dark red colour ; fracture dull and irregular ; surface shining and covered over with a reddish powdery substance ; cut surface resembling black varnish ; very brittle and capable of being easily reduced to a coarse powder when pressed between the fingers ; powder red and rather sticky ; taste sweetish and resinous, and resembling that of Râjana ; odour perceptible only when heated, when it is aromatic like benzoin. Dose, 10 to 30 grs.

Constituents.—Red resin and cinnamic acid.

Preparations.— Compound decoction (1 in 8). Dose, 2 to 4 drs.

Actions and uses.—A mild stimulant and astringent. It is given in diarrhœa, dysentery, bleeding from piles, and in internal hæmorrhages as hæmaturia, hæmoptysis, &c. The powder is used in the preparation of tooth paste.

Remarks.— What is sold in China is the product of Pterocarpus draco, and of calamus draco.

Gloriosa Superba, Curculigo Superba.

Habitat.—In low jungles throughout India, Travancore, Ajmere, Ceylon, Malacca.

Parts used.—The tubers.

Vernacular.—Beng.—Ulat chandal. Burm.—Sunnu-dav. Can.—Radagari. Duk.—Nat-kâ-bachanag. Eng.—Superb-lily. Guz.—Khadya-naga. Hind.—Kalahari, languli, kariari. Mar.—Nagakaria, nagamodia. Malyal.—Mavdoni. Sans.—Langalika, agnishikha, kalikari, gorbha-ghatini. Tam.—Katijan. Tel.—Agui-shekka.

Characters.—Root tuberous, oblong, or flattened, and covered with a brown epidermis ; on section white and starchy ; odour faintly acrid ; taste mucilaginous, slightly bitter and acrid ; starch pure white and of a bitter taste. Dose of the root, 5 to 10 grs. ; of the starch 10 to 15 grs.

Constituents.—Two resins, tannin and a bitter principle, superbine, allied to the bitter principle of squill. The white farinaceous starch is obtained from the root by repeated washings and grindings, throwing away the supernatent liquid and washing the residue carefully for half a dozen times.

Actions and uses.—Tonic, alterative and purgative. It increases the secretion of bile and used in colic, intestinal worms and leprosy. The starch is given internally with honey in gonorrhœa. The Natives apply a paste of it to the navel or over the hypogastrium, to promote labour pains or for expulsion of the placenta. With chitraka chhala it is applied to painful piles with relief.

Remarks.—Before being used the root is soaked in butter milk and salt to remove its poisonous properties. It is one of the seven nim or poisons mentioned in the Hindu system of medicine.

Ledebouria Hyacinthoides, L. Maculata, Erythronium Indicum.

Habitat.—Hydrabad, Bundelkund, sandy plains of India.

Parts used.—The bulb.

Vernacular.—Bomb.—Pàhadi-kandá. Eng.—Small wild squill. Guz., Mar, Duk.—Chhôtî-jangli-piyaz. Tam.—Shiru-nari vengâyam. Tel.—Cheru-adavi-vulli-gadda.

Characters.—A small bulb with smooth and fleshy scales; external scales dry and brownish; internal ones fleshy and cream coloured; in size resembling a large jaephala; odour nauseous; taste very bitter.

Preparations.—Tincture (1 in 10). Dose, 10 to 30 ms.; syrup ½ to 1 dr.

Actions and uses.—Stimulant, expectorant and diuretic; used in relieving strangury, in fevers, dysuria, cough, dropsy, &c, generally given for the same purposes as the official variety.

Polyanthus Tuberosa.

Habitat.—Concan, Bombay.

Parts used.—The bulb.

Vernacular.—Beng.—Pajuni-gundha. Hind.—Gulcheri. Malyal.—Andi-malleri. Sans.—Sandhy-araga. Tel.—Undi mandare.

Characters.—The bulb resembles dried onion, and has the fragrant odour.

Preparations.—Tincture (1 in 10). Dose. ½ to 1 dr. Paste.

Actions and uses.—Diuretic; chiefly used in gonorrhœa; locally rubbed with turmeric and butter over small red pimples which trouble new-born infants; also applied to buboes. It sometimes emits phosphorescent light in the dark.

Urginea Scilla B. P., Urginea Martiima, Urginea Indica.

Habitat.—France, Spain, Italy and Southern Coast of Europe, Indian Peninsula, Mediterranean, Coromandel Coast.

Parts used.—The bulb divested of its dry membranous outer scales, cut into slices and dried, the central portion being rejected. Scilla—squill B. P.

Vernacular.—Arab.—Basal-el-unasala. Guz., Bomb., Beng.—Banpiyâz, Jangli kanda. Burm.—Tankast-tva. Can.—Adavi-irulli. Cing.—Val-lûnû. Duk.—Kandra. Eng.—Squill, sea onion. Hind.—Kocudree. Mar.—Kochinda. Malyal.—Kâttulli. Pers.—Piyaze-dâshte, Hindi, Sans.—Vana-palândam. Tam.—Nâri-vengayam. Tel.—Adavi-tella.

Characters.—Bulb round and white, conical or pear-shaped and of the size of common onion, consisting of many fleshy scales like coats of a browish white colour; each coat separating from the other like flakes of abraka. At the bottom of the bulb small fibre-like rootlets of a dirty brown colour are given off. The dried slices are yellowish white, scentless, slightly translucent, brittle, easily pulverizable, and occur in the form of curved stripes, and are of a bitter, disagreeable taste; on exposure to the air they readily become flexible and moist. Dose, powdered pulp as an expectorant 1 to 3 grs.; emetic 10 to 15 grs.

Constituents.—Scillapicrine soluble in water and alcohol, scillamarine soluble in alcohol and chloroform, and scillinine soluble in alcohol but insoluble in water and chloroform; a peculiar carbo-hydrate, sinistrin, sugar, mucilage and citrate of calcium, ash 3 p.c.

Preparations.—Pilula Ipecacuanhæ cum Scilla B. P. (contains 5 p.c. of opium). Dose, 4 to 8 grs. Oxymel Scillæ B. P. (1 in 15). Dose, ½ to 1 dr. Pilula Scillæ Composita B. P. Contains squills 1¼, ginger 1, ammoniacum 1, hard soap 1, syrup of glucose 1, as an expectorant. Dose, 4 to 8 grs. Syrupus Scillæ B. P. (1 pint of acetum scillæ in 3lb. and 100zs. of the syrup). Dose, ½ to 1 dr. Syrupus Scillæ Compositus, fluid extract of squill 8, fluid extract of senega 8, tartar emetic 1, Calcium phosphate ⅕, sugar 75, water to 100, contains tartar emetic 1 gr. to 1 oz. Dose, as an emetic, 5 to 60 ms. For adults as an expectorant 20 to 30 ms. Tinctura Scillœ B. P. (1 in 5). Dose, 5 to 15 ms. Acetum Scillæ B. P. (1 in 8). Dose, 10 to 30 ms.

Actions and uses.—In small doses, stimulant expectorant and diuretic. It slows heart beat and increases the flow of urine. It is excreted by the bronchial, genito-urinary and gasto-intestinal secretions. In large doses, it is emetic and cathartic, and in excessive doses a narcotic acrid poison, causing nausea, strangury or bloody urine, often suppression of urine, gastro enteritis followed by convulsion and paralysis of heart and death. As an expectorant it is given in chronic bronchitis, whooping cough, asthma, croup and catarrhal affections; generally combined with ammonia, ipecacuanha, asafetida and benzoin. In croup it is generally given with tartar emetic. It should never be given in the acute stage of inflammation of the lungs. As a diuretic, it is given with digitalis and salines, in asthenic form of cardiac dropsy when there is no fever, in rheumatism, calculous affections and skin diseases. In these it is generally mixed with figs, anise, grape juice and honey. Syrup of squills is of great value in acute bronchitis where the sputum is tenaceous and scanty; also in chronic bronchitis, associated with emphysema and in spasmodic croup.

Veratrum Viride—American or Green Hellebore.

Syn.—Swamp Hellebore, Devil's bite, Indian poke root, tickle weed or itchweed, bug bane.

Habitat.—N. America.

Parts used.—The dried rhizome and rootlets.

Characters.—Rhizome upright, conical, simple or divided and thick ; tufted above and truncate below; section presenting many short, irregular wood bundles ; roots numerous, from all sides of the rhizome, shrivelled and of a yellow brown colour ; without any odour and of a bitter acrid taste.

Constituents.—Several alkaloids, veratroidine, jervine, pseudo jervine, rubi jervine, cevadine, resin, starch. Jervine—a crystalline substance, not sternutatory is without any taste; soluble in alcohol and chloroform ; with hydrochloric acid, it becomes red and on cooling changes to yellow ; with sulphuric acid, it gets yellow green. Pseudo jervine resembles jervine. Veratroidine—a non-crystalline substance, probably a mixture of rubi jervine and toxic resin, soluble in ether, chloroform and benzene. With sulphuric acid it becomes yellow and then red ; with hydrochloric acid pale red ; it is sternutatory, emetic and cathartic, depresses the cord and paralyses respiration.

Preparations.—Fluid extract—Dose, 1 to 4 ms. Tincture (1 in 5) Dose, 5 to 20 ms.

Actions and uses.—Emetic and errhine ; similar to aconite. In small doses as a cardiac and nervous depressant and spinal paralyzant it lowers the respiration, and the temperature of the body and reduces the pulse force, but does not affect its rate. In large doses the pulse becomes frequent and feeble, skin cold and clammy. There is vomiting, giddiness, impaired vision and partial unconsciousness. Jervine is a depressant of the heart and respiration and causes death by asphyxia. Veratroidine is emetic and cathartic, depresses the cord and paralyzes respiration.

Veratrum is used in acute rheumatism, gout, in the beginning of inflammatory affections as in heart disease, spinal spasms, pneumonia, typhoid fever, nervous palpitation, tetanus, chorea, diphtheria and in puerperal convulsions. It requires to be used with caution. Externally it is used as an errhine and to destroy vermin.

Melanthaceæ or Colchicacecæ.—The Colchicum or Surinjana family.

Herbs with bulbs, corms, tuberous or fibrous roots ; flowers regular, usually hermaphrodite, rarely unisexual ; perianth inferior, white, green or purple and petaloid; stamens 6; ovary, superior, 3-celled; fruit three-celled and three-valved, septicidal, dehiscent ; seeds with membranous septa ; embryo minute, albumen fleshy.

Habitat,—Europe, Northern parts of Asia, America.

Properties.—The plants are usually poisonous, owing to their containing a poisonous alkaloid. Some are purgative, emetic, diuretic, acrid and narcotic.

Colchicum Autumnale. B. P.—Meadow saffron.

Habitat.—Europe, N. Africa, moist pastures.

Parts used.—The corm and dried ripe seeds—Colchici Semina B.P. and Colchici Cormus B.P.

Characters.—Bulbous, perennial plant, a corm ; the drug consists of fresh ones stripped of their coats, cut transversely and dried ; the slices are thick, an inch long, ovoid, convex on one side, flattish and grooved or concave on the other and of about the size of a walnut ; it occurs in transverse reniform pieces, having a short and mealy fracture ; composed of starch granules, parenchyma and spiral ducts. The taste is bitter and it has no odour. Dose, 2 to 5 grs. The fresh bulb is solid and fleshy; externally it is brown and whitish within, yielding on section a milky juice. The dried and ripe seeds are sub-globular, thick and pointed at the hilum, very small, hard, and tough, reddish brown and pitted ; endosperm oily ; taste bitter, acrid, without any odour. Dose, 1 to 5 grs.

Constituents.—Colchicine, colchico-resin, beta colchico resin, a trace of veratrine, fat, gum, starch, sugar, tannin and gallic acid. Colchicine, an alkaloid, is intensely bitter and poisonous and is a weak base. Its salts are decomposed by water. It is the methylic ether of colchicein obtained by the action of mineral acids or acetic acid on colchicum. A white amorphous or yellowish micro-crystalline powder, darkening on exposure to light; odour saffron-like, and taste bitter ; soluble in water, alcohol, and chloroform; insoluble in ether. Dose, $\frac{1}{120}$ to $\frac{1}{60}$ gr., used hypodermically. Colchico resin—a brown powder, soluble in choloroform and alcohol, insoluble in ether, sparingly soluble in water.

Preparations.—Of the corm. Extractum colchici B. P.—Dose, $\frac{1}{4}$ to 1 gr. Fluid extract—Dose, 1 to 5 ms. Vini colchici B. P. Colchicum Wine (1 in 5) Dose, 10 to 30 ms. Of the seeds. Fluid extract—Dose, 1 to 5 ms. Tinctura colchici Seminum B. P. (1 in 5) Dose, 5 to 15 ms.

Colchicine Salicylate, Colchi-sal contains colchicine $\frac{1}{240}$ gr. and oil of winter green (Methyl salicylate) 3 grs. Dose, $\frac{1}{60}$ grs. In capsules. Dose, 1 to 2.

Actions and uses.—Colchicum is emetic, diaphoretic, diuretic, gastro-intestinal irritant, drastic purgative and cardiac depressant. It increases the secretions of the skin, liver and kidneys, and also the flow of bile. In large doses, it is a gastro-intestinal irritant, producing vomiting, purging and extreme prostration. It depresses the heart, produces convulsions, collapse and death. It is given in gout with an alkali ; in ascitis due to liver disease it is a very efficacious remedy. In cerebral and hepatic congestions it acts as a purgative with benefit. Good results follow its use in gonorrhœa and chordee. In rheumatic diathesis, the capsules of colchicine salicylate are used with relief.

Cochicine is a powerful poison, paralysing the brain and spinal cord and is given with caution in acute gout, rheumatic gout, asthma, cerebral congestion, and uræmea.

Colchicum Luteum.

Habitat.—Afghanistan, Punjab, Cashmere, and Northern India.

Parts used.—Solid extract prepared from the corm called Haran-Tuttha or Harantutiya.

Vernacular.—Indian Bazaar.—Haran Tutiya. Sans.—Tutham Tutthanjana. Tutthamjana means collyria made of sulphate of copper or of this plant with yellow flowers.

Characters.—Corms are dark brown when dry.

Preparations.—Extract—Dose, ¼ to 1 gr.

Actions and uses.—Alterative; chiefly used in rheumatism, gout, &c.

Colchicum Variegatum. Oriental Hermodactyl.

Hermodactyl means finger of hermes. The plant resembles garden tulips. Marandera Persica is probably the source of sweet or inert variety.

Habitat.—S. Europe, Asia Minor, N. Africa.

Parts used.—The corm and seed.

Vernacular.—Surinjan.

Varieties—white or sweet, yellow or bitter, and black; the black is poisonous.

The white variety—tuber or corm thick, ovoid, convex on one side, flattened with a groove on the other; outside brownish or dirty yellow, starchy and wrinkled; inside white and solid; breaking readily with a short mealy fracture, and is generally found as if worm eaten; taste sweetish, bitter and acrid.

The bitter variety—a good substitute for English colchicum, having bitter taste and smaller size; the corm occurs in pieces from 1 to 1½ inches long, 1 to 2 inches broad, colour dirty brown; each piece resembles a shell, presenting two surfaces, one convex, scaly, striped or reticulated; the other concave and rugous; on section, pale yellow or brownish white and starchy; starch in silvery and shining granules of an acrid odour; seeds thick, slightly pointed at hilum, of a reddish brown colour; inside the albumen is heavy, hard and tough, of a bitter acrid taste, and without any odour. Dose of the corm, 2 to 8 grs., of the seeds 1 to 5 grs.

Constituents.—Resin, an organic acid allied to malic acid, colchicina.

Preparations.—The corm. Extract—Dose, ¼ to 1 gr. Wine. Dose, 10 to 30 ms. Of the seeds: Tincture (1 in 5). Dose, 5 to 15 ms.

Actions and uses.—Alterative, diuretic, cathartic, emetic and sedative. It is useful in gout and rheumatism. With eliyo it is given in chronic gout with torpid liver ; also in dropsy and enlarged spleen. In gout and rheumatism it increases the quantity of uric acid in the urine. It is given with trikatu in seminal weakness. Like ipecacuanha it is given to relieve catarrh in congestion of the throat and in dysentery.

Bromeliaceæ—The Pineapple or Bromelia family.

Characters.—Herbs or woody plants generally epiphytical; leaves persistent, crowded, channelled, rigid, sheathing at the base, generally scurfy, margins spiny ; flowers showy, perianth arranged in 2 whorls, the outer of which is united into a tube, the inner one imbricated ; ovary, 3-celled ; fruit capsular or indehiscent, 3-celled ; seeds numerous ; embryo minute ; albumen mealy ; radicle next the hilum.

Habitat.—Tropical regions, America, East Indies.

Properties.—Some yield edible fruits, other fibrous materials, some are anthelmintic.

Ananas Sativa, Bromelia Ananas.

Habitat.—America, throughout the East.

Parts used.—The unripe fruit.

Vernacular.—Arab., Duk.—Ananas. Burm.—Nanas. Guz.-Hind., Mar., Beng.—Ananas, anaras. Cing.—Anassi. Can.—Ana nasu-hannu. Eng.—Pine-apple, European jack fruit. Malyal.—Purithi. Tam.—Anâsa-pazham. Tel.—Anasa-pandu.

Characters.—Leaves of a hard fibrous texture, with numerous short sharp spines on the edges ; fruit growing on a short stem which rises from the centre of the plant ; bearing a scaly conical spike surmounted by small spiny leaves ; fruit succulent, of an orange yellow colour.

Constituents.—The juice contains a proteid digestive ferment, which acts equally well in acid gastric or alkaline intestinal secretions. It also contains a milk curdling ferment. The ash contains phosphoric and sulphuric acids, lime, magnesea, silica, iron, chlorides of potassium, and sodium.

Preparations.—Essence of the juice. The essence is also artificially prepared by mixing butyrate of ethyl with 8 or 10 parts of spirit of wine.

Actions and uses.—Abortifacient ; also given to relieve flatulent distension of the abdomen. Under its use the uterus contracts within 12 hours followed by hæmorrhage and the ovum is expelled. The fruit is rendered unwholesome on account of its strong fibre which acts as an irritant on the bowels for abortifacient purpose, a whole unripe fruit decorticated being required.

Palmaceæ.—The Palm or Sopari family.

Trees or shrubs; trunk straight, slender, simple or rarely branched; leaves large, with sheathing stalks feather like and terminal; flowers unisexual, perfect, arranged generally on a branched spadix, enclosed by a large boat-shaped spathe; perianth inferior, in 2 whorls; stamens 3 or numerous, hypogynous or perigynous; ovary, superior, 1-3 celled; fruit drupaceous, baccate or nut-like; seeds with minute embryo; albumen, fleshy or horny, often ruminated.

Habitat.—Temperate and tropical regions.

Properties.—Highly useful both for dietetic and economical purposes. Several species yield sugar, oil, starch, wax, resin, astrigent matters, and wine; also edible fruits and seeds; terminal leaf buds when boiled are eaten as vegetable.

Areca Catechu.

Habitat.—E. Indies, Cochin China, tropical India.

Parts used.—The seed or kernel and extract.

Vernacular.—Arab—Fufil. Beng.—Shupari, Kunthi, Gua. Burm.—Kwun. Can.—Adike. Cing—Puivak. Chin.—Pinlang-taze. Eng.—Areca catechu, peper betel, nut palm. Hind., Duk., Mar., Guz.—Sopâri, Hopâri. Jav.—Jambi. Malay, Pinang—Kachu. Malyal—Adaka, kavaghu. Pers.—Girda choba, papal. Sans.—Fûgi-phallain, kramuka, Guvâka, kuvara. Tam.—Pakumaram kotâi pakku. Tel.—Paka-vakka.

Characters.—Nut orange colored, of the size of a hen's egg and containing one seed of the shape of a short rounded cone, depressed at the centre of the base, brown, thick and horny inside; on section it presents white ruminated albumen, traversed by a network of veins resembling nutmeg. It has a very faint odour and very astringent taste. The extract known as betel nut catechu or kassu, occurs in round flat cakes, 2 or 3 inches in diameter, ½ inch thick, blackish brown internally, without odour and of an astringent bitter taste. Dose, as an astringent, 15 to 25 grs.; as an anthelmintic, 2 to 4 drs.

Constituents.—The kernels contain catechu, tannic and gallic acids, oily matter, gum, arecoline, arecaine, and guvacine.

Arecoline, an anthelmintic principle, is a liquid which forms a white crystalline hydrobromide.

Preparations.—Areca nut charcoal tooth powder. Fluid extract. Dose, 2 drs.

Actions and uses.—Fresh nuts are intoxicating and produce giddiness. Dried ones are gentle stimulant, astringent and tænifuge; they increase the flow of saliva, lessen perspiration, sweeten the breath, strengthen the gums, remove bad taste from the mouth, and produce mild exhilaration. It is recommended in worms, diarrhœa, dysentery, and as an ingredient in the preparation of a masticatory of great antiquity known as betel. The powder obtained by calcining the nut is known as areca charcoal and used as a tooth powder. The dried expanded leaf stalks are used as splints. The extract is used for the same purpose as that obtained from acacia catechu. Arecoline—its action resembles that of pelletierine, muscarine or pilocarpine; internally it causes vomiting and diarrhœa. It is a sialogogue and diaphoretic; as a myotic it resembles physostigmine.

Borassus Flabelliformis.

Habitat.—India.

Parts used.—The root, juice and fruit.

Vernacular.—Arab.—Dom, tafi. Beng.—Talgachh. Bomb.—Tar, the seeds; galali, taragola. Burm.—Thanbin. Can.—Panemarâ. Eng.—Palmyra-brab-tree. Mar., Hind., Duk.—Tar. Cing.—Tâlgahâ. Malyal.—Pana, ampana. Malay.—Lontar. Pers.—Darakhte-tar. Sans.—Tad, Tala. Tam.—Panam maram. Tel.—Potu-tadi.

Characters.—Fruit of a globular form and consisting of a husk containing three seeds, known as galeli. Each seed reniform, compressed, and containing a jelly like albumen, which is edible, refreshing, delicious and sweet. The juice obtained from the spathe and known as Tada-ni-todi, is a dirty white fluid, of a pleasant and delicious saccharine taste, somewhat intoxicating. When fermented it gives arâk.

Constituents.—Gum, like tragacanth, fat, albuminoid.

Actions and uses.—Demulcent, refrigerant, and diuretic; the root is cooling and restorative; the juice is cooling and diuretic when fresh; the pulp obtained from the upripe fruit is diuretic, demulcent, and nuitritive; given in gonorrhœa, leucorrhœa, &c.; the toddy, when fermented, is converted into Tada-no-daru (Arrak), a country drink. It is used as a diuretic in gonorrhœa. The terminal bud of the tree and embryo of the germinating seed are used as vegetable, and are nutritive and diuretic. The ash of the spathe is used by the natives in the treatment of enlarged spleen.

Caryota Urens.

Habitat.—Assam, India.

Parts used.—The juice and spirit.

Vernacular.—Beng.—Bankhjur. Can.—Yels-kae. Cing.—Nepara. Duk.—Marikâ—jhad. Eng.—Jagari palm, Malabar sagopalm, Ghat palm, Bastard sago. Guz.—Ardhi sopari. Malyal—Irampana. Mar.—Berali-mada. Tam.—Konda-pan. Tel.—Kondaa-jiligu. Hind.—Ram guoah.

Characters.—Fruit consisting of two nuts joined together so as to form one whole sopari; when separated, each nut resembles in shape a common sopari cut into two pieces. It is of a chestnut colour, shining and smooth ; externally marked with reticulations or ribs, which proceed from an attachment at the base and join at the top.

Constituents.—Palm sugar.

Preparations.—Palm juice and palm wine. Confection, sago,—from the trunk.

Actions and uses.—The natives use it as a paste to apply to the forehead in hemicrania. As an aphordisiac the confection is used in seminal weakness and urinary disorders The juice is used as palm toddy. Khoti aradhi sopari (fictitious) is nothing more than a common severadhani sopari cleverly glazed so as to resemble Bhirali mada.

Cocos Nucifera, Palma Indica Major.

Habitat.—The Tropics, Indian Archipelago, coasts of India.

Parts used.—The flowers, root, fruit, oil, and ash ; the fruit contains shell, juice and kernel.

Vernacular.—Arab.—Jouz-i-hindi, shajratun, narjil, dhonun. Beng.—Narikal. Burm.—Onsipin. Can.—Theinghana. Cin.—Tambili, polnawasi. Chin.—Ye-taze. Eng.—Cocoanut. Hind., Duk. Guz., Mar.—Koperu, Nariel. Malay.—Kalapa Nur. Maleal.—Tenga. Pers.—Drakhte-bading Sans.—Narikela, Punga, Trinaraja, Skandhataru Dur-arasha, dridhaphal, rasaphal, Narikela, Narekera, kurcha sekharu. Tam.—Tenan cheddi. Tel.—Gujju-Narekadum.

The dry kernel—Hind., Guz., Bomb., Kepparun. Can.—Koharu Malyal—Kapera. Tam.—Kobharait tengay. Tel.—Kohera tanquaia

The juice—Eng.—Cocoanut toddy, palm wine. Arab.—Ganje. narjilli Duk.—Narilli-ka-pani. Guz.—Nariel-nu-pani. Tam.—Tennaur-kallu. Tel—Tenkayia.

Characters.—Cocoanut (formerly written coconut) is the name derived from the Portuguese coco, a mask ; in allusion to its having three holes which make it resemble the head and face of a cat. The fruit consists of a husk or fibrous portion of the pericarp ; coir or cocoanut fibres are obtained from the husk, which is thick, tough and fibrous ; shell oval or ovate, very hard or ivory-like, and of a dirty red colour. On exposure to the air it becomes dark brown ; cocoanut or kopurùn, is fleshy, albuminous, and oily, of a globular, oval, or ovate form, epidermis brownish red ; interior of a pure white colour. Juice within the albumen is a liquid portion known as cocoanut milk. The fruits are of 3 kinds : (1) Nalier ; (2) The miniature sized khakhota ; (3) The immature ones known as shiala or kakro. In the third variety the shell is less hard. Kernel soft, jelly-like, and very sweet, and contains a clear fluid known as cocoanut milk (kakara-nu-pani), of a sweetish taste and without any odour. In one variety of cocoanut, the milky juice solidifies and is known as pushpa. Jaggary is an impure sugar obtained from the juice which oozes out when the spathes, stems, or the neighbouring parts of the tree are injured. The fresh juice is known as Naliera-ni-taddy which, when fermented, produces vinegar and a kind of spirit known as arrack.

Constituents.—The fresh kernel contains nitrogenous substance, fat, lignin, ash, palm sugar, and inorganic substances.

Preparations.—The oil from the shell and kernel ; juice, paste and confection.

Oleum cocos—It is a fixed oil expressed from palm seed. It is a white, watery liquid, semisolid or of the consistence of butter ; the oil from shell (Katlinutel), is prepared by burning the shells over a fire and the oil collected. The oil so obtained is of a dark colour and has a smell resembling that of dammar. The concrete oil is extensively employed for making candles, soap and pomatum. It congeals at a low temperature into a white, buttery, concrete mass. The odour is unplesant and it soon becomes rancid. The oleine obtained by pressure from the crude oil and purified is used in place of cod liver oil.

Actions and uses.—Cocoanut milk—refrigerant, nutrient, aperient, diuretic and anthelmintic. Nariela-nu-pani is cooling, refrigerant, demulcent and in large doses aperient. The oil is used as a substitute for cod liver oil in debility and phthisis, but is not so very digestible. An inunction of it to the whole body is used in fevers, and to the chest in lung diseases. It is used as an application for the growth of hair and to prevent them from turning grey. Katalinu-tela is applied in chronic skin diseases, such as ringworm, psoriasis, pityriases, &c. The fresh kernel or the tender pulp is nourishing, cooling, diuretic and refrigerating. The pulp of the ripe fruit is hard and indigestible. The terminal buds are nourishing, agreeable and digestive, and are used as vegetable. The root is a diuretic. The fresh juice of the tree (toddy) is refrigerant and diuretic. Naliera-nu-dudha, juice of the kernel, with kali jiri is locally applied to freckles with reliet. Koparâ-ni-vati—old and dried kernel is cut into thin slices and used as an aphrodisiac ingredient in confection ; also as an anthelmintic, it is used in removing tapeworms.

Lodoicea Seychellarum, Nux Medica, Cocos Maldivisa.

Habitat.—Seychelles, Indian Ocean.

Parts used.—The kernel.

Vernacular.—Arab., Pers.—Narajile-bahri. Bomb.—Jahari-nári-al. Burm.—Peule-on-si. Guz., Hind., Duk.—Daryâ-kâ-nârel. Cing.—Mudu-pâl. Eng.—Marine cocoanut, double cocoanut. Malyal.—Katal-tenna. Port.—Cocos-de Maldives. Sans.—Ubdil nari kaylam. Tam.—Kaddet-taynga. Tel.—Samudrapu-tenkaya.

Characters.—Fruit covered externally with thick fibrous husk and containing one or two or sometimes 3 kernels or nuts, with hard thick black shells, each nut divided half-way down into two lobes ; nut; in broken pieces, each hard and horny ; external surface brownish red ; covering albumen white or yellowish, homogeneous, and externally tough, resembling ivory ; smell resembling that of cocoanut ; no taste. Dose, 2 grs.

Actions and uses.—Tonic and stomachic; with lignum colubrinum, it is given in indigestion, diarrhœa, and for the relief of colic. A paste of it with sábarasinga and kuchalâ (strychnos nux vomica) is a popular local application to swollen glands.

Remarks.—The shell is often used by jogis as a vessel for holding water.

Metroxylon Sagu, Sagus Farinifera, S. Spinosus, Sagus Rumphii, Pearl Sago.

Habitat.—East India Islands, Borneo, Muluccas and Eastern Archipelago.

Parts used.—Prepared fecula.

Vernacular.—Beng., Hind.—Sagu chaval. Chin.—So-muh-mien. Guz.—Sabu-chokha. Java.—Sagu. Malyal.—Sagu, rambiya. Tam. —Showarisi. Tel.—Zow-bium.

Characters.—A small palm; stems thick and covered with remains of leaf stalks; leaves many, pinnate at the apex; fruit a round nut, covered with an imbricate coat, 1-seeded; seeds abortive. It propagates by suckers from the root of the old trees. The stem before maturity consists of a thin hard wall and in the centre contain tissue commonly termed medulla or pith from which before maturity or previous to it, farina or sago is obtained by splitting the tree trunk. Starch is extracted from the pith, which when powdered form sago meal, or granulated sago; pearl sago occurs in pearl-like grains, the granules are oblong, truncate, hilum rounded; common sago is larger grained. When the fruit forms, the medulla disappears and the stem is no more than a hollow shell.

Actions and uses.—Demulcent, and nutrient; used for weak digestion and fevers. Fictitious sago is made from potato and other starch.

Phœnix Dactylifera, P. Sylvestris.

Habitat.—Africa, Arabia.

Parts used.—The fruit and juice obtained from the trunk (toddy).

Vernacular.—Arab.—Khurmae-yabis, Tamr-na-khal. Hind., Bomb., Beng.—Khur-ma, khâjur, chuhara. Burm.—Swon-pa, iwon. Can.—Khurjura. Cing.—Indi. Duk.—Paynd, khanjur, sandole. Eng.—Date palm. Guz.—Khajur, dried fruit khârak. Malyal.—Kattinla. Panj.—Khaj. Pers.—Khur-mâ, kurjan. Sans.—Khar juraha. Tam.—Perch chankay. Tel.—Kharjurapu chettu.

Characters.—Dried fruit, cylindrical, drupaceous, and covered with thin brown pedicle; external surface much wrinkled and containing a rich succulent sugary pulp. Within it is imbedded a bony seed; taste sweet and mucilaginous; no odour; undried fruit is ripe, lumpy and sticky; pulp juicy. The juice of the wild date palm, boiled down, yield gur or jagary, from which sugar is obtained. It also yields shenda or palm wine, commonly known as toddy. This juice is either drunk fresh from the tree or boiled down into sugar or fermented for distillation, when it gives out a kind of spirit called arak. The inner wood furnishes by boiling a kind of catechu, which is formed into square cakes of a uniform texture and of a dark red colour. It contains tannin, extractive matter and mucilage.

Constituents.—Tannin, extractive, mucilage, insoluble matters and lime.

Preparations.—Confection.

Actions and uses.—Khajur is nutritive, tonic and diuretic; used as dessert. Kharaka is used as an ingredient in various aphrodisiac and tonic confections. Boiled with milk it is given during convalescence from fevers and small-pox. The juice or toddy obtained from the stem is a good diuretic. A spirit known as kajura-no-daru (lagbi) is obtaind by distillation of the fruits.

Serenoa Serrulata—Saw Palmetto berry.

Habitat.—Sandy soil, South America, Georgia, Florida.

Parts used.—The herb.

Characters.—Stem creeping, branching; leaves circular, fan-shaped, bright green, erect; with more or less spiney-edged petiole (15 to 30) divisions, slightly cleft at the apex; spadix densely tomentose, much shorter than the leaves; petals scarcely united; style slender; drupe, ovoid, oblong; berries about the size of the olive, dark purple in colour and containing a large quantity of juice. The berries are at first exceedingly sweet but soon become acrid, giving a pungent sensation in the mouth that spreads to the fauces, nasal mucous membrane, and larynx and then succeeded by butyraceous oil-like taste. The sweet taste increases with the age of the fruit. The seeds are enveloped in tough, fibrous membranes; they are very hard, like ivory, and when cut open present a white, oily, glistening substance which burns readily with a blue flame and gives off the odour of roasted coffee. Flowers yield a kind of honey known as palmetto honey.

Constituents.—A volatile oil, soluble in alcohol; and a fixed oil; both obtained from the expressed juice. By evaporation the juice yields a rich, golden, syrupy extract.

Preparations.—Extract; solution for inhalation. The oil—Dose, ½ to 1 dr.

Actions and uses.—Nutritive tonic and stimulant, having fat producing property. By its soothing power it relieves troublesome coughs, promotes expectoration, improves digestion and increases fat, flesh and strength. As a sedative and diuretic it is given in cardiac asthma, phthisis (especially laryngeal phthisis), chronic bronchitis, and dilation of the bronchial tubes, and is a good substitute for cod-liver oil. As inhalation, it has been found useful in chronic ozæna. Like copaiba sandalwood oil, cubebs and kavakava, it is given in sexual debility, in enlarged prostate, in irritation of the bladder and urethra, &c.

Acoraceæ or Orontiaceæ, The Vekhanda, Vaja or The Sweet Flag family.

Herbs ; leaves broad or sometimes ensiform ; flowers hermaphrodite, perfect or arranged on a spadix with or without a spathe ; perianth absent or composed of scales which are inferior ; stamens 4 to 8, hypogynous or perigynous ; ovary superior, 1 or more celled ; fruit succulent, baccate ; juice acrid and pungent ; seed with an exile embryo ; albumen fleshy or mealy, rarely exalbuminous.

Habitat.—Cold, temperate, and tropical regions.

Properties.—Acrid, but the acridity may be usually got rid of by drying or by heat. Rhizomes of some are aromatic and stimulant ; of a few others, antispasmodic, expectorant and diaphoretic ; some contain starch ; others are used as food.

Acorus Calamus, A. Odoratus.

Habitat.—Europe, Western Asia, swampy places throughout India.

Parts used.—The dried rhizome.

Vernacular.—Arab.—Ighir, Ikaroon, Ud-ul-vajja. Beng.—Swetbach, Gora-bach. Burm.—Linhsy. Chin.—Shai-chang-pu. Cing.—Wadda-kaha. Can.—Bajê Duk.—Gand-ki-lakri. Eng.—Sweet flag, sweet or grass myrtle, myrtle flag. Guz., Hind.—Gora-vach, Dydya-vaj, Bâlâ-vaj. Malyal.—Vashambu. Mar.—Vekand, Bâl-vekhand. Pers.—Vuj, Ugir-turki. Sans.—Vacha-golomi, Shad-grandtra Ugragantha, Jatila. Tam.—Vasambu. Tel.—Vasa, vudya.

Goravaj—Gora, or ghoda, means a horse; and vaj, a corruption of Sanscrit word vajâ, or vacha, which means talking in allusion to its fiery or biting properties when tasted. Bàla-vaj—Bâlâ, children —the drug used for children is, however, not so fiery. Shad-grantha, from shad, six, and granth, gondha, knotted, the root being six knotted, Ugragantha, strong smelling root. Jatila, having entangled hairs. Another variety of vaja is known as Hima vate or khorasani vaja. It is useful in relieving flatulence.

Characters —Rhizomes tortuous, sub-cylindrical or flattened pieces of varying lengths, usually rough, and shrunken ; colour varying from dark brown to pale brown ; one side marked with numerous broad and transverse triangular leaf scars—the remains of leaflets ; other side tubercled, or marked with remains of fallen rootlets ; interior pale brown or of a pink colour, and very minutely porous or corky. It breaks easily with a short corky fracture and emits a very sweet, aromatic, and agreeable, but heating odour ; taste bitterish and very pungent. Dose, powdered rhizome, 20 to 40 grs.

Constituents.—A volatile oil, acorin—a bitter principle, acoretin (choline), calamine, starch, mucilage, &c., the volatile oil is a yellowish brown fluid, of aromatic odour, and contains pinene, sesquiterpene and a small quantity of phenol. Acorin—a glucoside, is a honey-like liquid, very bitter and aromatic; soluble in alcohol, chloroform, ether; splitting into sugar and volatile oil. Acoretin is a resin like body, yielding by reduction ethereal oil and sugar. Calamine is a crystalline alkaloid, soluble in alcohol and chloroform.

Preparations.—Infusion (1 in 10). Dose, 1 to 2 ozs. Extract—Dose 2 to 8 grs. fluid extract 15 to 60 ms. Tincture (1 in 5), ½ to 1 dr. A compound decoction—contains vekhand, asafetida, trikatu, chebulic myrobolans, sanchal salt, tubers of aconitum heterophyllum equal parts ; water ten times the quantity of the whole. Dose, 2 to 4 drs. A compound powder containing vekhand, sagargota, chiretta and bitters is used in fevers.

Actions and uses.—Bitter aromatic, stimulant, tonic, and a carminative; usually combined with vegetable bitter tonics and aromatics, and given in ague, habitual constipation, atonic dyspepsia, colic, flatulence, and paralytic and nervous affections; as a stimulant it is given in low fevers, epilepsy and as a deobstruent and depurative in parotitis, dropsy and other glandular diseases. It is an ingredient of various approdisiac confections. As a poultice it is applied to paralysed limbs and rheumatic swellings. Powdered rhizome, rubbed with cashew spirit, is used in chronic rheumatism; a watery solution is dropped into the ears in noises in the ears. Bálávacha is given to children to bite to promote teething. Its action is similar to that of soothing syrup. It is also given in capillary bronchitis and cough. It acts by setting up emesis. Gora-vaja is used as a diuretic in calculous affections, and as an anthelmintic in worms in children. As an astringent, the drug is given in dysentery and diarrhœa. Like neem it is also burnt as an incense. It is regarded as an insectifuge and insecticide for fleas, &c. The volatile oil is used for scenting snuff and preparation of aromatic vinegar.

Alocasia Indica. A. Montana.

Habitat.—Indigenous in India.

Parts used.—Root stock.

Vernacular.—Beng.—Man-kacha. Hind.—Mankand-kâchu. Mar.—Kas-alu.

Characters.—Root of a very large size, 6 to 8 inches in length, and as thick as a man's leg. When dry, it is in round pieces, brown externally, wrinkled and marked with remains of leaf petioles and their sheaths. Internally it is white, opaque, and starchy ; petioles and root stocks acrid. It contains a large quantity of starch.

Constituents.—Contains acicular crystals of oxalate of lime, to which its acridity is due.

Preparations.—Ash, juice and poultices.

Actions and uses.—The juice of the petioles is styptic and astringent as is dropped into the ears of children in otorrhœa. Tubers made hot are locally applied to painful parts in rheumatism. In anasarca, canjee made of the root stock is given with benefit. It is a mild laxative and diuretic, and is given in piles and habitual constipation. The ash is used as a local application for aphthæ in the mouth.

Araceæ, Aroideæ.—The Madanmasta, Arum or Surana family.

Herbs or shrubs, with an acrid juice and subterranean tubers corms, or rhizomes ; leaves sheathing, usually net veined, simple or rarely compound ; flowers monœcious, small, either males or females, and arranged on a spadix or within a spathe ; perianth none ; stamens few or numerous ; anthers upon very short filaments ; ovary, 1-3 celled ; fruit succulent ; seeds pulpy ; albumen mealy or fleshy ; rarely exalbuminous.

Habitat.—Tropical countries, and cold and temperate regions.

Properties.—More or less acrid : often highly poisonous ; the acrid principle is frequently volatile or decomposed by heat ; hence commonly got rid of by boiling the corm in water ; starch is usually associated with the acrid principle, but when extracted it may be used like other starchy substance. Under-ground stems when cooked are eaten.

Amorphophallus Campanulatus. A. Sylvaticus. Arum Companulatus.

Habitat.—India.

Parts used.—The corm or tubers.

Vernacular.—Burm.—Wa. Beng.—Ol. Burm.—Wa. Can.—Mulen-shina. Eng.—Teluga potato. Bomb., Mar., Hind.—Jangli suran, ol, Madana masta, Jamkund. Malyal.—Kizhanna. Sans.—Arsaghna. Tam.—Karuna. Tel.—Manchi kanda—gadda.

Characters.—The tubers when peeled and cut into segments are known by the name of Madana masta. They are of a reddish brown colour, wrinkled, and shrunken. Each segment is from 2 to 3 inches long and about an inch broad. It is hard and homogeneous, also brittle. The taste is mucilaginous and acrid, resembling that of sálma.

Preparations.—Powder. Dose, 5 to 10 grs. Confection—known as Laghu surana madaka or vrihat suran madaka, contains madan mast, treacle, trikatu and plumbago root, equal parts. Dose, ½ to 2 drs. in dyspepsia.

Actions and uses.—Stomachic and tonic ; used in piles and given as a restorative in dyspepsia, debility, &c. Pieces of the tubers are generally threaded upon a string and hung in shops.

Arisæma Triphyllum—Indian Turnip. A. Atrorubens—Dragon root.

Habitat.—N. America.

Parts used.—The corm.

Characters.—The corm is broad, of a brownish grey colour, white and mealy within and of a burning acrid taste. Dose 5 to 15 grs.

Constituents.—A volatile acrid principle, starch, calcium oxalate, &c.

Preparations.—Syrup (1 in 4). Dose, 20 to 60 ms.

Actions and uses.—Stimulant, expectorant, and diaphoretic ; used in flatulent colic, chronic bronchial catarrh, whooping cough and rheumatism. Locally it is applied to aphthæ in children.

Pistia Stratiotes.

Habitat.—Tanks and ponds of India.

Parts used.—The whole plant.

Vernacular.—Duk.—Unter ghunga. Hind.—Jal-kumbhi. Malyal.—Kodda pail. Mar.—Gondâla, sherval. Sans.—Jalad-bhuta, Jalasaya, Guccha bodhra, Paniya prêshthajà. Tam.—Agasatamaray. Tel.—Nerubudiki.

Characters.—An aquatic plant ; leaves found floating on stagnant pools, obcordate, waved on the margins ; nerves spreading like a fan, united in a truncate arc at the base.

Constituents.—It contains salts of potassium, sodium, magnesium and lime. Also iron aluminum and silicic acid.

Preparations.—Powder. Dose, 30 to 120 grs. and ash.

Actions and uses.—Demulcent and sedative, given in dysuria. The ashes are applied as a paste with rose water to ringworm of the scalp. A poultice of the leaves is applied to painful piles.

Scindapsus Officinalis. Pothos Officinalis.

Habitat.—Bengal.

Parts used.—The fruit.

Vernacular.—Beng.—Gaja-pipal. Can.—Dadda-hipulli. Malyal.—Ounatipili. Hind., Guz., Mar.—Gaja-pipali, Bari-pipli, Thora-pimpali. Sans.—Kari-pippali, Kafee-pippali, Kotu-valli, Shreyasi, Vashira. Tam.—Atti-tipili. Tel.—Gaja-pippali.

Gajâ pipali is derived from Gaja, an elephant ; and pipali, long pepper. The fructification resembles in appearance pipali ; gaja-pipli is of a huge size, and hence the comparison with an elephant.

Characters.—A fungoid-looking plant, gall-like in appearance, and of a dark or brown colour, parasitic in its nature, and selecting plants of the vitaceæ order for its growth. The fruit, cut into transverse pieces and dried, occurs in slices of a greyish colour and without any odour. Each slice has a central core surrounded by seeds, enclosed in a dry pulp of the arils. The pulp contains needle-shaped crystals of oxalate of lime ; seeds larger than hemp seed, kidney shaped and containing oily kernel ; smell acrid and disagreeable ; taste acrid.

Constituents.—An alkaloid (a trace) gum and ash.

Preparations.—Decoction (1 in 10). Dose, 2 to 6 drs.

Actions and uses.—Aromatic, carminative, and stimulant ; generally used as an adjunct to various alterative and astringent preparations ; given in fevers, chronic coughs, diarrhœa and asthma.

Synantherias Sylvatica—Wild Suran—(Eng.)

Habitat.—India.

Parts used.—The seeds.

Characters.—Fruit yellow, of the shape and size of a grain of maize, closely set round the upper part of the spike ; skin tough; pulp, scanty and yellow, enclosing 2 seeds ; seeds placed with flat surfaces in apposition ; testa soft and greenish brown ; kernel white and adherent to the testa ; fresh kernel soft and juicy ; when dry hard ; taste acrid, causing burning on the tongue, much salivation and facial numbness.

Actions and uses.—The crushed seeds are used to cure toothache. It acts by rapidly benumbing the nerves. It is also applied externally to bruises on account of its benumbing effects. The paste of seed is locally applied to reduce glandular swellings.

Tacca Aspera, T. Lavis, T. Pinnatifida.

Habitat—Tropical India.

Parts used.—The tubers.

Vernacular.—Beng.—Vârâhi-kand. Burm.—Pân-khade, Toukta. Can.—Handi-gedde. Duk.—Barâ-kandâ. Hind.—Vârâhi-kand Mar.—Dukar-kand, Sakara-kand. Malyal.—Chaney-kizhama. Malay.—Laka-liker. Sans.—Surana. Tam.—Kara. Tel.—Kunda-gadda.

Characters.—Root oblong and curved, tuber with wiry fibres from its sides. Externally dark brown or black and yellowish white within. Taste bitter and nauseous. It contains starch resembling arrowroot.

Preparations.—Confection, 1 to 2 drs.

Actions and uses.—Alterative, nutrient and tonic, given in cachexia, leprosy, scrofula, &c.

Cyperaceæ.—The Sedge or Nagaramotha family.

Rush-like or grass-like herbs ; stems solid, without joints or partitions, frequently angular ; leaves with closed tubular sheaths surrounding the stem; flowers spiked, unisexual, perfect and imbricated ; each arising from the axil of 1 to 3 bracts ; stamens hypogynous; anthers 2-celled ; ovary, one-celled, superior ; embryo lenticular; fruit, one-seeded and indehiscent ; seeds with fleshy or mealy albumen.

Habitat.—Marshy ditches, running streams all over the world.

Properties.—Closely allied to graminaceæ, but deficient in nutritive qualities. Some of the plants are aromatic, stomachic and diaphoretic ; others demulcent and alterative ; underground stems of some are edible when roasted or boiled.

Cyperus Pertenuis C. Scariosus. C. Hexastachyus.

Habitat.—Damp places in Bengal.

Parts used.—The tubers.

Vernacular.—Arab.—Soade-kufi. Bomb.—Musta. Burm.—Vomoungie Can.—Konnâri-gadde. Cing.—Jata-makutu. Eng. Indian Cypress. Hind., Beng., Duk.—Nâgara-Motâh. Malyal.—Kôra kizanna. Mar.—Lavâla. Pers.—Muske Zamin. Sans.—Mustâka. Tam.—Mutta-kâch. Tel.—Kala-tunga, muste.

Characters.—An aquatic plant growing in ponds and ditches; tubers aromatic, of a brown colour, 1 to 2 inches long, resembling finger in thickness, and marked with transverse rings ; root blunt at the lower end with a projecting acute point, rings on its lower half distinctly marked with the remains of leaf sheaths. Between the rings the scars of fallen rootlets or the traces of fibril-like rootlets are seen ; upper half, densely covered or imbricated with striated and scale like leaf sheaths ; interior of a pale brown colour, and sprinkled with a red powdery substance. An irregular thread like ring separates the central portion from the margin ; odour strongly aromatic like that of kutha or godávaja, and somewhat terebinthinate.

Preparations.—Decoction (1 in 20). Dose, 1 to 2 fld ozs.

Actions and uses.—Refrigerant, aromatic and stomachic; also alterative ; given in torpid liver, chronic fevers, dyspepsia and derangements of the bowels. In chronic fevers it relieves thirst and heat of the body. It is also useful in ascitis, and as anthelmintic in lumbrici.

Cyperus Rotundus, C. Communis.

Habitat.—Throughout India.

Parts used.—The tubers.

Vernacular.—Arab.—Sab. Beng.—Moothoo. Chin.—Tsau-san-ling. Cing.—Kalandura. Duk.—Kôre-ki-jar, Mushtaka. Hind., Guz.—Motha, Barânâga-moth. Mar.—Bimbal. Malyal.—Kora. Pers —Suod. Sans.—Bhadramuste. Tam.—Kôrau, kore. Tel.—Bhadra-muste, Kaiwartaka-musta.

Characters.—Root tuberous, sweet smelling, round, black and hard like a knot ; culms erect, triangular, with rounded angles ; tubers often crowded together, each of the size of filberts, black externally, white internally ; odour like that of acorus.

Preparations.—Infusion (1 in 10). Dose, $\frac{1}{2}$ to 1 fld. oz.

Actions and uses.—Diaphoretic, diuretic, demulcent, stimulant and galactagogue ; given in fevers, dyspepsia, diarrhœa and cholera ; also in urinary calculi and amenorrhœa. As a galactagogue the fresh tubers are applied to the breasts.

Kyllingia Triceps, K. Monocephala.

Habitat.—Throughout the Peninsula of India.

Parts used.—The root and oil distilled from the roots.

Vernacular.—Beng.—Sveta-gothubi. Hind.—Nirbishi, Malyal.—Motheuga, Peemottenga. Mar.—Musta.

Characters.—Roots creeping; culms erect, triangular and leafy at the base; leaves membranous, flat, ciliated; margins covered with bristles; flower heads solitary, globose and white..

Preparations.—Decoction (1 in 10). Dose, 1 to 2 fld. ozs. oil distilled from the root.

Actions and uses.—Refrigerant, demulcent and tonic. A decoction of the root is given to relieve thirst in fevers and in diabetes. Locally the oil is used to relieve pruritis of the skin. Internally the oil is given in torpor of the liver. Other properties are similar to those of Cyperus rotundus.

Pandanaceæ—The Kevada, or Screw Pine Family.

Palm like trees or shrubs; leaves simple or pinnate, sheathing and imbricated, spirally arranged in three rows; flowers unisexual or polygamous, numerous, and arranged on a spadix with numerous spathaceous bracts; perianth absent or scaly; stamens numerous; anthers 2·4 celled; fruits consisting of a number of one-seeded, fibrous, drupes or many celled, many seeded berries; embryo, minute, solid, with fleshy albumen.

Habitat.—Tropics.

Properties.—Some are edible; the juice of some is used to produce a kind of wine. From the male inflorescence of Pandanus odoratissimus, a highly odorous Aarka is prepared and used as medicine.

Pandanus Odoratissimus, P. Sativa, Anthrodactylis Spinosa.

Habitat.—India, Persia, Arabia.

Parts used.—The stem, seed and male inflorescence.

Vernacular.—Arab.—Kâdhi, keder. Beng.—Keori, keakaida. Burm.—H'sat-ta-phu. Bomb., Guz., Mar.—Kevada. Burm.—Vettakayâ. Cing.—Woti kayiya. Can.—Kyâ dage-gidâ. Duk.—Katagi. Hind.—Kevarah, Gaganphula. Eng.—Screw pine, Caldera bush. Malyal.—Thala kaida, Pandaing. Pers.—Gul-i-kivea, kavondi. Sans.—Keteka, Dhuli push pika. Tam.—Talam Talay. Tel.—Gojjanji, mogali.

Dhuli pushpika, means Dust flower.

Characters.—Kevado—the male flowering spike with bracts of a whitish colour, linear, oblong, concave and pointed. In the axils of these bracts are highly odorous bunches of small whitish yellow anthers; fruit of the kevada oblong and as large as a cocoanut or pine apple.

Preparations.—Aqua prepared by distilling flowering tops in water (1 in 20). Dose, 30 to 60 ms.; perfumed oil.

Actions and uses.—Stimulant, diaphoretic and antispasmodic; given in general debility, faintness, giddiness, often with javarasha. Locally it is used for the relief of long-standing headache. The oil is dropped into the ear in earache and in otorrhœa; the root brayed in milk is given in cases of threatened abortion.

Lycopodiaceæ—The Club Moss family.

From Lukos Lykos, a wolf and Podos foot; in allusion to the likeness of the shoot to a wolf's foot.

Characters.—Herbaceous plants resembling mosses, terrestrial or aquatic; terrestrial plants with creeping stems and forked ramification; aquatic with corm-like stems; leaves small, sessile, usually imbricated, tufted or linear, and cylindrical; sporangia or fructification in axils of leaves or immersed in their substance often spicated; scales reniform, 1-3 celled, 2 valved, containing many yellow spores.

Habitat.—Universal—cold, temperate and warm climates.

Properties.—Many contain an acrid principle, in moderate doses emetic, purgative, and aphrodisiac; in large doses poisonous; the spores of some are inflammable.

Lycopodium Clavatum.

Syn.—Club moss, vegetable sulphur, wolf claw, stag horn.

Habitat.—Europe, United States, Asia.

Parts used.—The spores.

Lycopodium is collected by cutting off tops when fruit spikes or cones are nearly ripe. The spores are shaken out of the sporangia. They resemble moss; they are 4-sided, reticulated with short projections on the edges. The sporules known as vegetable sulphur are $\frac{1}{800}$ of an inch in diameter, forming a pale yellow fine powder, mobile, repellent of water, without any odour or taste; when thrown over a flame it burns quickly with a hissing noise, giving a yellowish white light.

Constituents.—A bland fixed oil 48 p.c., cane sugar 2 p.c., volatile base (methylamine) and ash 4 p.c.

Preparations.—Tincture (1 in 10). Lycopodium being first treated with ether. Dose, 15 to 60 ms, dusting powder.

Actions and uses.—Antispasmodic and diuretic; given in rheumatism, epilepsy, and pulmonary disorders. In irritability of the bladder, frequent micturition, and in incontinence of urine, it is very beneficial; also in nocturnal micturition in children or adults; externally as a protective and absorbent powder, it is used in erysipelas, eczema, herpes, between the thighs and armpits of infants; also used as a pill excipient in coating pills to render them tasteless and as a powder for hygroscopic pills to prevent them from adhering together.

Graminaceæ, The Ghas or Grass family.

Herbs, shrubs, or arborescent plants with round, commonly hollow jointed stems, marked with irregular knots from each of which proceeds a sheathing leaf; leaves with split sheaths and a ligule with parallel veins; fruits caryopsis; seed with mealy albumen; embryo lenticular; flowers perfect, unisexual, arranged in spikes, panicles, or racemes or solitary and no perianth; stamens 1—6 or more; ovary superior, 1-celled, ovule solitary, stigma feathery or hairy.

Habitat.—Universal; in temperate and cold climates they are herbaceous; in tropics they are shrubby.

Properties.—Most of them afford fruits known as cereals or nutritive grains. The pericarp of some grains, as wheat grains, is demulcent; that of barley is astringent. Some grasses are purgative, others narcotic and poisonous; some are used as fodder; culms and stems of some contain sugar and starch. Some of the species yield sugar, and others yield a volatile oil. A powder made of seeds and their envelope is known as flour. The pericarp when separately collected is known as chaff or husk. By incineration a kind of ash is produced which contains iron, silica, alumina, lime, magnesia, &c. Silica is the most abundant of all. The existence of silica accounts for the slow decomposition of seeds under water, and for the use of their ashes for polishing wood and marble.

Andropogon Citrarum, A. Schœnanthus, Cymbopogon Schœnanthus.

Habitat.—Eastern Archipelago, Ceylon, throughout India, Western Ghauts.

Part used.—The essential oil, the herb.

Vernaculars.—Beng.—Agiyâ-ghâs. Burm.—Mikkothu. Can.—Parimalada-ganjani. Cing.—Pengiri-mang. Duk.—Masaleh-kâ-air. Eng.—Sweet rush, lemon grass, ginger grass, oil of verbena, oil of Indian Melissa, Rosa oil. Hind., Guz.—Ghandabela. Java.—Sirch. Malyal.—Sambhara-pulla. Mar.—Sugundhi. Pers—Gourgia, Rohishe-gavat, Sans.—Devajugdhaka; Malatrina Kang. Gandha Kheda; Sugandha Rohisha, Bhustrina. Tam.—Sakanaru Tel.—Chippa-gaddi.

Characters.—Leaves green or glaucous, linear, lanceolate and very long; in breadth from ½ inch to 2 inches, keeled or channelled and striated; margins sharply ciliated; under surface markedly scabrous, due to very small, minute white hairs, which are slantingly arranged, their tops being directed upwards; upper surface of the leaf, from below upwards smooth to the touch, and scabrous from above downwards; taste pungent, smell, agreeable and lemon-like, due to the presence of volatile oil. The oil is obtained by macerating the grass in sweet oil and exposing to the sun.

Constituents.—The volatile oil—lemon grass oil, oil of verbena, Indian Melissa oil, contains citrol and is obtained by distillation from the fresh plant. The oil is of a pale sherry colour, and of a pungent and agreeable taste, approaching that of ginger. Dose, 2 to 6 ms.

Preparations.—Infusion of the leaves (1 in 20). Dose, 2 to 6 drs.

Actions and uses.—Stimulant, diaphoretic, antispasmodic and carminative. The infusion of the leaves with phudino, mire and suntha is much used by the natives in colic, fever, flatulent affections of the bowels, gastric irritability, catarrh, and in dysmenorrhœa. It is also used as a fumigatory. The oil is used as a carminative and stimulant in cholera to arrest vomiting ; externally as an embrocation in chronic rheumatism, neuralgias, sprains and other affections.

Andropogon, Laniger.

Habitat.—N. India, Arabia, S. Africa, Tibet.

Parts used.—The plant.

Vernacular.—Arab.—Kilal-el-Marmun, Iz khir. Beng.—Karankush. Hind.—Ushirbhed, Asha, khara. Guz., Mar.—Jvara-nakusha, Pivala-vala. Pers.—Karanch-i-dashti. Sans.—Ushira, Lamajjak, Dirgha mulaka.

Characters.—Roots hidden in the ground, slender, brown, and knotty, and like válo giving off many long fibrillæ ; surface rugous and marked with traces or rings of fallen leaf sheaths ; cut portion of a deep brown colour; odour resembling that of caraway ; leaves, linear, lanceolate and of a pale brown colour, smooth on both surfaces, striated, but not channelled at their insertion to the stem ; leaf sheath slightly hairy ; odour when rubbed between the hands is like rose or like that of the root ; taste aromatic, bitter and acrid.

Constituents.—The grass contains an essential oil.

Preparations.—Infusion (1 in 40). Dose, 1 to 2 fld. ozs.

Actions and uses.—Tonic, stimulant, diaphoretic and carminative; given in fever, in enlarged glands, dyspepsia, hysteria, and cough. A paste of the roots is used as an inunction to the body in fevers.

Andropogon Martini, A. Calamus Aromaticus, A. Pachnodes.

Habitat.—Indian Peninsula, Ceylon, Burma, Western Ghats.

Parts used.—The essential oil.

Vernacular.—Beng —Gandha-bêna. Burm.—Mik-ko-thu. Cing. —Pengiri-mana. Duk.—Rousâ-ka-attar. Eng.—Grass oil of Nemaur, roosa grass oil, geramol, Turkish essence of geranium. Hind.—Merchya-gandh kubel, ganjni. Malyal.—Sireku. Mar.—Rasâ-sugandhi, rohishe. Pers.—Gour-gia. Sans.—Rhustrina, Mula trina kang, Bhustrina. Tam.—Kamak-sha-pillu. Chor-pillu. Tel.—Kamachi —kassuvu.

Characters.—Essential oil of a pale sherry colour; odour agreeable, pungent, resembling that of ginger. Dose, 1 to 4 ms.

Constituents.—Geraniol.

Actions and uses.—Carminative and stimulant; used internally in bilious affections for neuralgia and rheumatic pains. The grass is used as medicated baths in fevers to cause diaphoresis. Internally its tea is used as a stimulant and carminative in colic, bilious vomiting and dyspepsia; other uses are similar to those of kájaputa oil. It also prevents hair from falling after acute fevers, confinement or prolonged lactation.

Andropogon Muricatus.

Habitat.—Coromandel, Mysore, Bengal, N. India, E. India.

Parts used.—The fibrous wiry roots from the rhizome (Khuskhus grass).

Vernacular.—Arab.—Usir. Assam.—Khor. Beng.—Khaskhas. Burm.—Pen-yen, Miya-môe. Can.—Lâvanchâ. Cing.—Savandra mûl. Duk.—Bâlâ. Eng.—Cuscus vetivert, vetiviera. Guz.—Vâlo-khaskhas. Hind.—Bala, Bena-ushir, Malyal.—Ramach-cham-vêr. Mar.—Vârêlu. Pers.—Izkhir-i-jami; Bikh-i-wola-khas. Sans.—Jalasayah-ushiram, Venimulaka, Lamajjakamu, Sugundhi mulaka, Viratara. Tam.—Viranam. Tel.—Veda-vali-veru.

Characters.—Culm sweet, compressed, with smooth nodes; roots fibrous and slender, giving off numerous very minute fibrillæ and of a pale yellowish brown colour; surface hairy, with a peculiarly agreeable aroma, somewhat like myrrh; taste slightly camphoraceous; distilled with water, the roots yield a fragrant oil which is used as a perfume.

Constituents.—A volatile oil, a resinous substance of a deep red brown colour, a coloring matter, a salt of lime, oxide of iron and woody matters. Dose, powdered root, 5 to 20 grs.

Preparations.—Infusion (1 in 40). Dose, 1 to 2 fld. ozs.

Actions and uses.—Tonic stimulant, antispasmodic, diaphoretic, diuretic, and emmenagogue; given in flatulence, fevers, deranged menstruation, hysteria, convulsions, rheumatism, gout, &c.; also used in perfumery.

Andropogon Nardus, Citronelle grass (Eng.).

Habitat.—Madras, Peninsula, Ceylon, Travancore, Singapore.

Part used.—The essential oil.

Vernacular.—Beng.—Kâmâ-kher. Burm.—Sinug-on-mea-si. Can.—Khaddi yaune. Cing.—Manna. Duk.—Gandbel. Eng.—Citronelle oil. Hind—Ganjni-ka-atra. Malay.—Kâmâkashi-pulla. Sans.—Guchcha. Tam.—Wassa-na-pillu. Tel—Allapu-kommu.

Characters.—Herb with acrid rhizomes, branched, with scars of leaf sheaths ; stem very high, erect, cylindrical and shining and concealed by the leaf sheaths ; leaves large and long odour ; fragrant, taste somewhat acrid. The oil obtained by distillation is similar to lemon grass oil and is volatile.

Constituents.—The oil contains an aldehyde, a terpene, an isomer of borneol named citro-nel-lol and acetic and valeric acids.

Actions and uses.—Antispasmodic, carminative and stimulant ; given in flatulence, spasmodic affections of the bowels and in cholera. Dose, 1 to 4 ms.

Remarks.—It is considered a wild form of lemon grass.

Andropogon Odoratus.

Habitat.—W. Ghauts.

Parts used.—The grass.

Vernacular.—Mar.—Vaidi gavat-usadhana.

Characters.—Culm erect, branching from lower part, glabrous and long; rachis, bearded; spikes and pedicles covered with silky hairs.

Constituents.—A volatile oil of a deep sherry colour.

Preparations.—Infusion (1 in 10). Dose, 1 to 2 fld. ozs.

Actions and uses.—The grass is used as a stimulant carminative in bowel complaints of children.

Bambusa Arundinacea.

Habitat.—Throughout India.

Parts used.—The siliceous concretions, young shoots, articulations and seeds.

Vernacular.—Arab.—Tabâshira. Beng., Duk., Hind.—Bansa-kapûra, Bans-lôchan. Burm.—Vadegâsâ. Cing.—Una-maku, Unali, Can.—Tava-kshira. Chin.—Chuh-hwang-chukan. Eng.—Bamboo-sugar, Tabashir. Guz.—Vans-kapura, Vans-nû-mith. Malyal.—Mole-uppa. Mar.—Bansa-lochana. Pers.—Tabashira-nai. Sans.—Tvaka-kshiri, Vanas-kapura, Vans-sarkara, Vonu-lavanam. Tam.—Mungi-luppu. Tel.—Veduru-uppu.

Characters.—Stems erect, bending at the summit and pointed hollow between the joints ; branches alternate; thorns 2 or 3, alternate on the joints ; leaves sheathing, linear, lanceolate; sheaths downy ; seeds the size of oats. Tabashira is a white siliceous concrete crystalline substance, irregularly shaped, light, soft and brittle; pieces of an opaque white or greyish white colour; larger pieces an inch in diameter, concavo-convex, and resembling in appearance the joints of the female bamboo, within whose hollows these deposits take place ; taste sweet adn cooling. It readily imbibes volatile and fat oils, which produce an opacity; with oils tinted with acetate of copper, sulphuric or malic acid, tabashir assumes the colours of emeral, ruby, topaz &c.

Constituents.—Tabashir contains silica 70 or silicium as hydrate of silicic acid, per oxide of iron, potash, lime and alumina.

Preparations.—Decoction of leaves and of bamboo joints (1 in 20). Dose, 1 to 2 fld. ozs.—a compound powder. Sitopaladi Churana, containing tabashir 8 parts, long pepper 4 parts, cardamoms 2, cinnamon 1, sugar 16. Dose, 1 dr., as an alterative in phthisis and cachexia.

Actions and uses.—The leaves are emmenagogue. Tabashir is stimulant, tonic, cooling and pectoral, and used in cough, consumption, asthma and fever. In combination with other astringent medicines, it is given in chronic dysentery and internal hæmorrhages. The young shoots are used as vegetable and made into pickles. A decoction of bamboo joints is said to increase the flow of lochia after delivery. The juice of leaves with aromatics is given in hæmatemesis. Older and dried stems of bamboo are used as splints in fracture.

Coix Lachryma.

Habitat.—Plains of India, Khassya Hill slopes.

Parts used.—The seeds.

Vernacular.—Assam.—Damu Ayab. Beng.—Gargur-kunch Burm.—Kalethee, kalinsi, kyeit. Chin.—J'yi-jin. Guz.—Kassai-bija. Hind.—Sankhlu, Gargari-dhan. Eng.—Job's tears. Mar.—Ran-makai. Sans.—Gave dhuka, Damu. Arab.—Dand, Damu Ayab.

Characters.—The seeds resemble those of Karadi; shell large, highly polished and very hard, larger and coarser than pearl barley; colour greyish white, in shape resembling drops of tears and hence the name Job's tears; silicious involucre of this grass containing the seed is sold in shops like cowrie shell, which are shining white and very hard; kernel sweet.

Constituents.—The seeds contain albuminoids 1-7 fatty oil 5, resin, sugar, starch 58, fibre 1·5, ash 2·5.

Preparations.—Emulsion. Dose, 1 to 2 drs.

Actions and uses.—The seeds are strengthening and used as food in the form of canji or gruel. As a diuretic they are given in cystitis, dysuria, &c.

Cynodon Dactylon, Panicum Dactylon, Agrostis Liniaris.

Habitat.—Plains of India.

Parts used.—The herb.

Vernacular.—Mar., Hind., Beng., Duk.—Hariali, Durva, Doorba, Doob. Eng.—Creeping dog's tooth grass. Panj.—Khabal, khabbar. Sans.—Granthi, sveta ruha, durva. Tam.—Arugam pilu. Tel.—Garika kasuvu, tella gariki.

Characters.—Roots slender, wiry, and trailing or creeping, giving off fibres below. Plants from ½ to 1 foot in length, ascending; leaves small, linear, lanceolate, and sheathing; mouth of the sheath withered and studded with white hairs. The white variety, which is only a diseased state of the plant, is used in medicine. Other characters are similar to those of Olen cha. At the top of the plant, digitate linear spikes are given off, on the lower surface of which several small pale yellow stamens (the rest being shaken off by the wind) and the purple serrated stigmas are seen ; taste aciduous.

Preparations.—Infusion (1 in 20), ½ to 2 fld. oz.

Actions and uses.—Demulcent, astringent and acid ; used in checking vomiting. As a diuretic it is given in dysuria, and as an astringent in epistaxis and to stop bleeding from wounds. It is used as a substitute for triticum repens.

Poa-cynosurioides.

Habitat.—Plains of India, Punjab.

Parts used.—The herb.

Vernacular.—Bomb.—Dudu. Mar., Hind., Beng.—Kusha Panj.—Chinka, kuri ; mirukar. Bomb.—Darbha. Sans.—Durbha Bharhis, Suchy-agra, Yejna blushana, Durga-pattra, vijna, punya-trina, Suchi-mukha.

Characters.—Root creeping ; culms straight, rigid and smooth ; leaves numerous, long, chiefly about the base of the culms ; margins rigid, panicle erect, linear, oblong, often conical and composed of horizontal verticelled ramifications.

Preparations.—Infusion (1 in 20). Dose, 4 to 6 drs.

Actions and uses.—Diuretic and astringent ; it is an usual ingredient in the native prescription for dysentery and menorrhagia.

Hordeum Distichon (English Barley).

Habitat.—Java.

Parts used.—The decorticated seeds and malt.

The Malt is prepared from barley by a process of germination started by artificial means. The grain after having undergone germination, by soaking in water, is allowed to remain for a few days until the germ (acrospire) is ⅓rd length of grain or develops the maximum amount of diastase-ferment by which the starch of the grain is converted into glucose.

Constituents.—Vegetable albumen, phosphate of lime, diastase, dextrin, sugar, starch, mucilage, gluten, fibrous or ligneous matter. Diastase a ferment, it converts starch into dextrin and maltose. This property renders it useful for digesting starchy food.

Preparations.—Extractum Malti, extractum Bynes, malt extract, an aqueous extract containing all the soluble principles of malt as dextrine, diastase, glucose &c.; given in wasting diseases, weak digestion, general debility. Dose, 1 to 4 drs. Extractum malti liquidum, liquid extract. Dose, 1 to 4 fld. drs. Infusum Malti (3 in 7). Dose, 2 to 4 drs. It is generally combined with cod liver oil 30 p.c., iron hypophosphite, pepsine, chemical food, citrate of iron and quinine, phosphorus, &c.

Vinegar—it is an acid liquid, obtained from malt and from unmalted grain or any liquid susceptible of vinous fermentation, or undergoing acetous fermentation. In India it is prepared from toddy, the juice of various palms ; also from the juice of sugar cane and from all the sweet and delicious fruits, rice, sugar, honey &c. It is a brown or colourless liquid, of a fruity odour and acid taste.—Dose, 1 to 2 drs.

Marrol—A proprietary preparation containing besides malt extract, ox marrow, and hop extract; given in wasting diseases.

Taka Diastase—An enzyme extracted from aspergillus oryza, a variety of malt. Given in cases of disturbed and deficient secretion of saliva or in hyperacidity of the stomach. Dose, 1 to 5 grs.

Actions and uses.—Malt extract contains food elements, and is nutritive and restorative ; given with milk and cod-liver oil, it aids digestion and assimilation in wasting diseases, weak digestion and debility of all kinds. It converts its own weight of starch into sugar and dextrine in 15 minutes.

Vinegar is refrigerant, sedative and antiseptic ; like dilute acetic acid, it is chiefly used to sponge the body in high fevers and in recent inflammation and other local affections. It is sometimes applied to burns, scalds, bruises, and sprains. It is used in the preparation known as aceta. It is a direct antidote to poisoning by alkalies. In tonsillitis and in sore throat its vapour is inhaled with benefit.

Hordeum Hexastichon, H. Distichon, Hordeum Vulgare, Scotch bere or bigg.

Habitat.—N. W. Provinces of India, Temperate Asia, Great Britain.

Parts used.—The dried decorticated seed or grain (with husks, and integument removed), pearl barley.

Vernacular.—Arab.—Shair. Hind., Mar., Beng.—Jab. Burm.—Muyau. Eng.—Barley, raw barley, winter or common barley. Duk.—Satu. Sind.—Jao. Pers.—Gao. Tam.—Bâraley-arishi. Tel.—Baraley biyyam.

Characters.—Seeds straw or of a greyish yellow colour, elliptical, long, flat, back angled ; sides grooved, front smooth and greyish yellow from adherent paleæ ; husk when removed dark brown ; interior white and hard, taste very sweet.

Constituents.—Fixed oil or fat 2 p.c., starch 60 to 80 p.c.; proteid compounds (gluten albumin) 12 to 15 p.c., cellulose, other nitrogenous principles, ash, containing silicic acid, phosphoric acid, iron and lime. Fixed oil or fat 2 p.c. contains glycerin mixed with palmitic and lauric acid.

Preparations.—Decoction (1 in 15). Dose, 1 to 2 fld. ozs.

Actions and uses.—Java is nutritious and used as food by the poorer classes, and as canji in the dietary of the sick. The seeds are demulcent in the same way as Tukhm-i-balango, and used in diseases of the lungs, bronchial affections, sore throat and urinary disorders ; also in fevers.

Hordeum.

Habitat.—Asia, Europe, N. Africa.

Parts used.—The weed.

Vernacular.—Arab.—Zuvân, shailam. Eng.—Bearded darnel. Hind.—Muchhni. Pers.—Gandum-i-diwâheh. Gandum-i-diwâheh means fool's wheat.

Characters.—A noxious weed, growing among wheat ; roots with downy fibres ; stems annulated, smooth, often branched ; leaves large, sheathed, smooth, dark green, linear and tapering ; spikelets large ; flowers sessile.

Constituents.—Seeds contain gluten 50 p.c., starch, albuminoids and a thick concrete green oil. The oil is partly saponifiable, insoluble in water and soluble in alcohol and ether.

Actions and uses.—Used locally with salt and radishes on ulcers, With sulphur and vinegar for skin eruptions. With linseed to disperse glandular swellings ; the seeds are narcotic and cause cerebro spinal and gastro intestinal irritation.

Oryza Sativa.

Habitat.—Throughout India.

Parts used.—The grain, spirit and vinegar.

Vernacular.—Arab.—Ruz. Beng., Hind.—Dhan, Pusnee(husked). Burm.—Sa-ba. Can.—Akki-bhatta, (husked). Chin.—Tak, Kang-mi, (husked). Duk.—Chawal. Eng.—Rice. Beng., Mar., Hind., Guz.—Chokha, tandul, bhat, chawal. Malay.—Paddy (in straw), Gábah (in husk), Bras (husked). Malyal—Paijera. Pers.—Birinji shali. Sans.—Grihi. Tam.—Arishi, nellu. Tel.—Blum-uri.

Constituents.—It contains more starch than any other starchy grains. It contains no fat and a very small quantity of proteids. Nitrogenous matter 7·5 ; carbohydrates 9·75 ; fat 8 ; mineral matter 9.

Actions and uses.—Nutrient ; it requires some oil and albuminoids to make it a suitable diet.

Saccharum Officinarum.

Habitat.—Tropics, India, S. Asia, Cuba.

Parts used.—The juice from sugercane and a crystallized sugar obtained from the juice—Saccharum Purificatum, B. P.

Vernacular.—Arab.—Kufseh-us, Sukr. Beng.—Uk, Ik, Aka'h, ukyo. Burm.—Kyàn. Can.—Khabbu. Cing.—Uk. Chin.—Kanchi. Duk.—Gândâ. Eng.—Sugar cane. Hind.—U'ch Ghanna, Khulea, Kajuli. Mar., Guz.—Sheradi, Nai-sâkara, uss. Malyal.—Karimba. Panj.—Paunda. Pers.—Nai-sukr. Sans.—Itchu-tunda, karkara, rusala, gudatrina. Tam.—Karimbu. Tel.—Cheruku, aru, tella.

The extract prepared from the juice, when crystalline. Arab., Guz., Hind.—Sakkara. Burm —Saghia. Beng.—Bhurra-chini. Bomb. —Pithi-sakara. Burm.—Kyan. Can.—Sakkare. Cing.—Sini, sakkere. Chin.—Shih-mih-sha-tang. Guz.—Sakkar chini, Buro. Hind.—Misari, khadi sakkara. Maleal.—Gula. Malyal.—Panjasâra, soola, sakar. Mar.—Sâkhar. Persian.—Shakkar. Sans.—Sûkâra panjasâram maluy-andica. Tam.—Shakkarai. Tel.—Pancha-dara.

The extract pasty or in granules—known as jaggery, prepared from several vegetable substances as sugar cane, palmyra, phœnix sylvestris, caryota urens, cocoanut, &c. Arab.—Land. Can.—Bella, Tale. Cing.—Akuru, Talakuru. Duk.—Gur, Tarka gur. Eng.—Jaggery. Hind.—Gur. Malyal.—Vella. Pers.—Kand. Tam.—Vellam. Tel.—Bellanim.

Characters.—A perennial plant; culm or rhizome thick, solid, containing white fibrous juicy pith; colour outside yellow, greenish yellow or purple, often striped and resembling Indian corn; cane annular or jointed, smooth and resembling bamboo; leaves sheathing, hairy, very long, narrow and lanceolate; from the juice a kind of residue or black extract is prepared; it is a brown fermentible syrup which when soft and sticky is called gûd, treacle, molasses, and when dry it is called gûda sarkara, or khand treacle. The careless evaporation of the juice causes the extract to be mixed with little of burned sugar, and hence the Indian gûr is very dark in colour, of a peculiar flavour, and slightly bitter after taste.

Saccharum purificatum, refined sugar, B.P., cane sugar, sucrose or sàkar, is in compact snow white crystals. permanent in the air, dry, scentless and purely sweet. soluble in water (1 in ½), alcohol (1 in 175), and boiling alcohol (1 in 28); insoluble in ether. It should be free from grape sugar (glucose) and from inverted sugar (glucose and lævulose). The uncrystallized residue of the refining sugar is known as treacle or theriaca, a thick fermentable syrup.

Barley sugar, a derivative product; it is cane sugar, melted carefully and suddenly cooled, and occurs in amorphous transparent mass, gradually becoming crystalline. Rock candy, saccharum crystallizatum, also a derivative product in large transparent crystals, very pure.

Caramel is cane sugar, burned for a short time; it is dark brown and bitter and contains caramelan and caramelene. Cane sugar is also obtained from various species of sorgham, such as S. Saccharatum (Broom corn), one or more varieties of Beta vulgaris, common or sugar beet, &c.; also from several grasses as zea mays, the maize, and from the juice of palm, birch, maple, &c.

Constituents.—The juice contains saccharine matter, water, mucilage, resin, fat, albumen, &c.

Preparations.—Syrupus, B.P. (2 in 3). Dose, *ad libitum.*

Actions and uses.—Preservative, demulcent, antiseptic, aperient and dietetic; sugar-cane increases the solubility of lime in water. It is used as food and nutrient to adipose tissue, hence sugar or sugar-forming food is needed in health; absence of it in dietary leads to rapid emaciation. It is also diuretic, cooling, demulcent and laxative. As a refrigerant drink, it is given in biliousness and jaundice. It is a good remedy in cough, hiccough, apthæ and hoarseness and locally in granulations of the eyelids and cornea As a snuff it is used in chronic ozœna ; as rectal injection, it is given in worms. Syrup is chiefly used as a vehicle to disguise the taste of various nauseous medicines and chiefly of medicines given to children. It is of little value for its independent effects. It is largely used as a preservative and antiseptic to protect active ingredient and certain iron preparations against oxidation and putrefaction, but not against fermentation.

Zea Mays, B.P.

Habitat.—Warm temperate climates, Indian Islands, S. America, India.

Parts used.—The styles and stigmas and the fecula of the seed—amylum, B.P., starch.

Vernaculars.—Arab.—Durah shami. Beng.—Bhuththâ Mokkâ. Bur.—Pysungboo. Can.—Bottah. Cing.—Munwairingu. Duk.—Mukkah juari. Eng.—Indian or Turkish corn, maize, corn starch, corn silk. Hind.—Makka, Buttah. Malyal.—Jagung. Mar.—Makai-bonda. Pers.—Khôshahe-makki. Sans.—Yavanala. Tam.—Makka Sholam. Tel.—Makkâ-zonnalu.

Characters.—Stiff, unbranched, grooved on one side ; generally smooth, externally solid and spongy within and jointed ; flowers simple ; male spiklets in pair bearing at the summit—the tassel, female spike—the ear ; rachis—the cob and pistils—the silk and bracts of the spathe—the husks. Kernels, or the seed grains, occur in 10 or 12 rows ; color may be white or yellow or red and purple. Styles and stigmas (corn silk) are thread-like, thick, yellowish or greenish and very soft, silky or hairy, delicately veined longitudinally; they are gathered when the tassels have shed their pollen. It has no odour ; kernels sweetish in taste.

The fecula of the seeds—starch, amylum B.P. occurs in irregular, angular, white, inodorous and tasteless masses of neutral reaction. It can easily be powdered ; insoluble in cold water, ether and alcohol ; with boiling water it forms mucilage which gelatinizes on cooling.

Constituents.—The stigma or corn silk contains maizenic acid 2 p.c., fixed oil (oleum maydis), resin, sugar, mucilage and salts. Maizenic acid is soluble in water, alcohol or ether.

The fixed oil is a viscid transparent liquid of a pale brown colour, non-drying, and does not become rancid ; taste bland ; odour of corn meal.

Starch is found in miaze, wheat, barley, rice, oats, arrowroot, sago, and tapioca, also in Cetraria Islandica (Lichen starch), in the liver of animals, animal starch or glycogen. It occurs as granules in many stems, fruits, seeds roots &c. It is formed by plants from inorganic materials under the influence of light and is stored up in their seeds.

Starch undergoes many chemical changes ; it is converted into glucose (or grape sugar) by the action of diastase, ptyalin, and pancreatin, or by boiling it with dilute mineral acids ; into oxalic acid by the action of hot nitric acid, or by cold fuming nitric acid, when it forms an explosive compound. Alcohol or carbon dioxide by the action of ferments. Dextrine by the action of dilute acids—an intermediate product in the conversion of starch into glucose.

Preparations.—Extractum maidis stigmatum liquidum, miscible with water. Dose, 1 to 2 drs. Decoction—Dose, 1 to 2 ozs. Aqueous extract—Dose, 5 to 10 grs.

Actions and uses.—Diuretic, demulcent, antiseptic and lithontriptic ; also anodyne and alterative. It is reputed to possess a specific alterative influence over the genito-urinary disorders. Its action on the kidneys is well marked ; it augments its secreting power, and has a tonic action on the secretory membranes. In diseases of the urethra, in vesical catarrh, acute and chronic cystitis, uric acid and phosphatic gravel, in hæmaturia, in gonorrhœa and in cardiac dropsy it is very beneficial. In renal colic it relieves the pain of gravel and vesical irritation. Starch is nutritive and also demulcent when taken internally. It is absorbed into the blood and is taken up by the animal organism. It undergoes digestion by the action of pancreatic and intestinal secretions, and is converted into soluble dextrine and into grape sugar. It is also used as a dusting powder in erythema, urticaria, erysipelas ; also as a vehicle for enemata. The seeds are roasted and used as an article of food by poor people, or ground into flour and made into cakes. Makkai is more nutritious than rice ; it is useful in consumption and in relaxed bowels ; also for invalids and children ; other actions are similar to those of sorghum vulgare.

Triticum Repens.

Habitat.—Europe, N. America, in meadows and cultivated grounds.

Parts used.—The rhizomes, deprived of roots.

Characters.—A perennial plant, rhizome thick, very long, creeping with internodes ; surface wrinkled, centre hollow, colour straw yellow ; taste sweet, but without odour. Dose, ½ to 1 dr.

Constituents.—Triticin 8 p.c. ; fruit sugar, 3 p.c. inosit, glucose, mucilage, malates and ash. As a result of fermentation lactic acid and mannit are formed. Triticin is a gum-like substance, resembling inulin and is convertible into levulose. To obtain it, exhaust the rhizome with water, neutralize with baryta, concentrate and precipitate with acetate of lead ; remove lead, treat with charcoal, neutralize and concentrate and precipitate with alcohol. A deliquescent, amorphous white powder without any odour, or taste.

Preparations.—Fluid extract. Dose, 1 to 4 fld. drs. Infusion and decoction. Dose, 1 to 2 ozs.

Actions and uses.—Diuretic, aperient, demulcent, and emollient; used in cystitis, irritable bladder, dysuria and gravel; also in jaundice and bronchitis; it is also given to allay thirst in fevers, in gout and skin diseases.

Triticum Sativum, B. P.

Habitat.—The Euphrates region, N.-W. India, Central Provinces, Bombay.

Parts used.—The grains and fecula—amylum, B. P. (starch).

Vernacular.—The grains.—Arab.—Hintah-burr. Bomb., Beng.—Ghaun, Godhama. Burm.—Gyung-sa-bâ. Can.—Godhi. Chin.—Sian-meh. Cing.—Tiringu. Duk.—Gehun. Eng.—Common wheat. Hind., Mar.—Ghavum Guz.—Ghaum-no-nisha'sto. Malyal.—Kâtanpan. Pers.—Gandam. Panj.—Kunuk. Sans.—Soomuna, yava, gadhuma. Tam.—Gôdumai. Tel.—Gôdhumulu.

Characters.—Wheat, a most important staple food of the upper classes of people, is met with in two kinds, soft and hard; soft used for bread making, the hard ones for preparing vermicelli. To prepare starch the grain is soaked in hot water, to which some alkali is added when the testa is softened. This is next ground under water and washed through sieves, the fecula or gahunuduh passes in that water, and after a time deposits; gluten remains on the sieve or floats in the supernatant liquid. Fecula or starch occurs in powder or masses of a white colour. Gluten is the proteid material of the grain, and occurs as milky yellowish gray, elastic and glutinous mass.

Constituents.—Wheaten flour contains all the constituents of wheat except cellulose, a part of starch, sugar and a large proportion of gluten, hence of less nutritive value than brown bread. It contains albuminoids 13·5 p.c., starch 68·4, oil 1·2, fibre 2·7, ash 1·7. free extractive 6·7, and saccharine matter. The ash contains phosphoric acid. The flour contains nitrogenated principles, chiefly gluten or vegetable fibrin, vegetable caseine and fat.

Preparations.—Glycerinum Amyli, B.P. (1 in 9). Dose, 1 to 2 dr.

Actions and uses.—Wheat starch is nutritive, restorative, demulcent, and emollient. It is used by women to check profuse menstruation and in leucorrhœa. As an emollient, it is dusted over the inflamed skin as in burns, scalds, &c. It also makes an excellent binding material in bandage. The bran is used for making poultices. Starches.—These are hydrocarbons found in vegetable food and represent fats in animal food. They are heat producing agents, and do not enter into the structure or into the repair of the waste of tissues; for the well being of human frame about 14 ozs. of hydrocarbon is necessary. In vegetable food, starch and sugar exists in four or five times the quantity of proteid material. Wheat contains starch in very large quantity. When taken in excess it delays tissue metamorphosis, deposits fat and increases the production of adipose tissue and often leads to flatulence and acidity. It often produces sugar in the urine. Given in disorders of the stomach and intestines as diarrhœa, dysentery, in hepatic disorders, in Bright's disease, alcoholism, gout and rheumatism. In fevers, these carbo-hydrates are very useful in supporting life and in preventing starvation and exhaustion due to want of fuel food. Toast bread, which contains soluble dextrine, also milk, sugar with beef-tea are very useful. Grape sugar, which is digested starch, may be given with benefit. Pure starch is medicinally inert, and is used as a vehicle for medicated enemas and in iodine or bromine poisoning.

Filices—The Hansaraja, or Fern family.

Plants, arborescent, flowerless, generally leafy ; stems cylindrical and rhizomatous ; leaves commonly called fronds, petiolate or coiled up when young, arising from the rhizome or placed in tufts at the apex of the stem, simple or divided into many segments, almost circinate in vernation ; reproductive organs consisting of small reticulated sporangia or capsules collected in heap and placed on the under surface of the fronds or along their margins. Sporangia may be stalked or sessile at last splitting, discharging many minute spores, circinate in the bud ; they are arranged like spikes on a simple or branched rachis.

Habitat.—Universal, moist temperate regions.

Properties.—Leaves of several species are bitter, tonic, astringent, pectoral, anthelmintic, and aromatic ; some are sweetish. The rhizomes and leaves of some are mucilaginous. The silky hairs on rhizomes and lower portions of caudex of some species are used for cushions ; these are known as capillary herbs. The ashes of most of the species being used as a wash to promote the growth of the hair. They generally grow near moist rocks and walls near the sea. Several species have farinacious rhizomes or stems which, when roasted and boiled, are edible.

Adiantum Venustum, A. Capillus Veneris, A. Caudatum, A. Lunulatum, A. Pedatum, Polypodium Vulgare, Osmunda Regalis, Flowering Fern.

Habitat.—Afghanistan, Himalaya, Persia.

Parts used.—The fronds.

Vernacular.—Arab.—Kuzburat-el-bir, Shuir-ul-jin, Sak-el-aswad. Bomb.—Hansaraja, mobarakha. Cashm.—Duur-lali. Eng.—Venus, or Fairies hair, Maiden hair. Hind.—Galmarium, Hansraj, Mubarakha. Ind. Bazar.—Râjahansa, Hansaraja, Mubârkh. Panj.—Parisosan. Pers.—Parosi-ava-shana, sans.—Hansa padi.

Hansapadi, Hansa, means geese, and Padi Pedi, the fool. The segment of the leaves resemble feet of geese.

Characters.—Raja hansa consists of stems and leaves ; stems very slender, black and highly polished as if varnished, one or more channelled. Channels deep, irregular, and on one side : leaves small, reniform, rugous and marked with fan-like veins, serrated at the top like coriander. of a brownish dark colour ; taste faintly astringent ; odour rather disagreeable.

Preparations.—Syrup of fronds.

Actions and uses.—Stimulant, tonic and demulcent ; given in pulmonary catarrh, asthma, and as a flavouring agent in expectorant mixtures. A plaster is used as an application to chronic, gouty and other swellings. Ashes mixed with olive oil and vinegar are used in alopecia and as an application for itch.

Asplenium Parasiticum, A. Falcatum.

Habitat.—India.

Parts used.—The rhizomes.

Vernacular.—Goa.—Kali-pândan. Mar.—Mâhâ-pâna. Malyal.—Kari-beli, pauna-maravara.

Characters.—Rhizome thick externally, to which is attached bases of fronds and numerous black radicles. It is parenchymatous within with bundles of vessels. It has an astringent and slightly bitter taste.

Preparations.—Decoction (1 in 10). Dose, ½ to 1 fld. oz.

Actions and uses.—Alterative and demulcent ; used in chronic, malarial fevers and cachexia. It has the property of reducing the size of spleen ; also given in incontinence of urine and jaundice. The fronds of Asplenium Leucidum is regarded by the New Zealanders as a sacred plant and the priests wave a frond over the head of the sick ; should it happen to break it is regarded as a fatal omen ; also used as a badge of mourning by the wife for her husband, by binding it round her head.

Aspidium, Filix Mas. B. P. Dryopteris Marginalis, D. Filix Mas.

Habitat.—Europe, N. America, N. Asia.

Parts used.—The rhizome. Filix Mas—male fern B.P.

Characters.—Rhizome, horizontal, long and thick, covered with stipe remnants ; when denuded of the stipes, the root is thick, brownish externally and greenish within, consisting of 8 to 12 scalariform ducts. The tuft simulates the form of animals ; odour is slight and disagreeable ; taste acrid, bitter and astringent. Dose, ½ to 1 dr.

Constituents.—Filicin, an active principle. Filicic acid, 6 p.c. ; filitannic acid, 10 p.c. ; gum, starch ; filix red, chlorophyll, a green fatty oil, a volatile oil, resin and salts.

Filicin (Filicic anhydride), is a non-poisonous crystalline substance, soluble in alcohol, ether and chloroform, and yielding, on fusing with potash, butyric acid and phloroglucin. Acidum Felicicum (Filicic acid) extracted from the oleo resin is a white amorphous powder, very poisonous ; soluble in alcohol, insoluble in water. Dose, 6 to 15 grs.

Preparations.—Oleo-resina Aspidii, oil of fern ; oleum filicis maris. Dose, 20 to 50 ms. Extractum Filicis Liquidum, B. P. Dose, 45 to 90 ms. Mistura Filicis—Extractum Filicis Liquidum, 1 dr. ; syrup of ginger, 1 dr.; tincture of quillaia, ½ dr.; water, 12 drs. In tape worms.

Actions and uses.—Tæniafuge ; used against tape worms, to be followed by castor oil or by calomel, jalap, gamboge, or epsom salt, or given with cusso or pomegranate or pumpkin seeds.

Cibotium Barometz.

Habitat.—Sumatra.

Parts used.—The silky hairs, covering the lower part of the caudex. Penavar or Penghawar Jambie.

Vernacular.—Chin.—Kan-tsih, Scythian or Tartarian-lamb.

Characters.—The hairs found on the rhizomes and lower portions of the caudex are silky, about two inches long, and of all shades between bright yellow to dark brown.

Actions and uses.—Astringent and styptic ; used as an absorbent hæmostatic. It is directly applied to the bleeding surface. About 5 or 10 grains will generally suffice to stop the bleeding from small vessels, either cut, torn or laid open by sloughing ; in some instances even from very extensive surfaces ; also used for plugging.

Polypodium Quercifolium, Oak-leaved Polypody.

Habitat.—India, Tenasserim.

Parts used.—The rhizome.

Vernacular.—Mar.—Bâsing, Vandar-basing, Ashvakátri. Bomb.—Kadik-pan, Kali-pandan.

Characters—Rhizome thick and silky, found closely adherent and overlapping branches of trees with its large oak-like leaves ; ferns do not partake of the properties of the tree they grow upon like other parasites, belonging to Lauranthaceæ. The fern growing upon Nux vomica is the best for medicinal purposes.

Preparations.—Decoction (1 in 20). Dose, 1 to 2 fld. ozs., compound decoction containing besides bâsing, nine other drugs, viz., Kakra Singi, chiretta, ghâs, pitpapra, baelphal, padmini, sonar-wel, Gokharu, and ringani mûla. Mix together, prepare decoction (1 in 8) of water. Dose, 2 ozs. twice a day. Largely used for phthisis, hectic fever, dyspepsia, cough, &c.

Polypodium Vulgare and other species.

Habitat.—Europe, Persia.

Parts used.—The rhizomes or caudex.

Vernacular.—Arab.—Kathir-el-riyl, Tha-kib-el-hajar. Eng.—Common polypody. Mar., Duk.,—Kalabichva, bisfaija. Hind.—Khankàli, khankli, Ind. Bazaars.—Kala bichva, Basfaija. Pers.—Tashtiwân Baspaik.

Characters.—Found growing in rocks or under trees; root fibrous, of a dark brown or grass green colour, hard and heavy; surface, rugous, longitudinally fissured, upper surface presenting several horn-like tubercles or scaly projections or suckers. Each projection is curved about ½ inch long and fissured—the remains of the stipes of the fronds; interior darkish or brownish red. starchy or resinous; each piece is flattened, more compressed on one side than on the other; aroma disagreeable, somewhat resembling that of opium; taste acrid or sweetish.

Actions and uses.—Aperient, alterative and deobstruent; locally used for the relief of rheumatic pains of the joints, for indolent tumours and acne. As a purgative combined with myrobolans, it is used in bilious disorders. The powder is snuffed into nostrils in polypus of the nose.

Lichenes—The Pathara-phulla, or Lichen family.

Plants perennial, cellular, flowerless, composed of hyphal tissue resembling that of fungi, fructified in the air, nourished through the medium in which they grow, often growing and spreading on the bark of trees or old paling, stones or walls or the surface of the earth or rocks or trees. They are composed of parenchymatous cells of a gray brown or blackish colour, and so arranged as to form a foliaceous, somewhat scaly, hard and crustaceous or leprous thallus, usually propagated by spores, epiphytic, or sometimes parasitic and commonly presenting a dry, more or less shrivelled and lifeless appearance. Reproduction vegetative by gonidia or by true fructification.

Habitat.—They are spread universally.

Properties.—Several plants are nutritious from containing starchy substances, which exist about 80 p.c., in Cetraria Islandica. They are also emollient and demulcent: many of them contain bitter principles and are therefore tonic and astringent. Some yield with ammoniacal solution a variety of colours, hence used as dye stufis. A few are aromatic, some contain a large amount of oxalate of lime; none are poisonous.

Cetraria Islandica.

Syn.—Iceland moss. Iceland lichen (Eng.)

Habitat.—Himalayas, Iceland. N. Hemisphere, mountains and sandy plains.

Parts used.—The dried Lichen.

Vernacular.—Bomb., Hind.—Lahana dagada phula, Kâla-chhadila.

Characters.—This lichen has a high, folliaceous thallus. It occurs in irregular thin strap-like pieces of a greyish brown colour; upper surface dark, under surface brownish red and marked with depressed spots; surface highly wrinkled, margin of the thallus irregularly cut or fringed; fructification on the upper surface presenting a cup-like elevation, black within and white externally; taste rather pungent, smell aromatic. When used as food, the bitterness should be removed by boiling in water or by digesting it with weak alkaline solution.

Constituents.—A gummy substance called lichenin, 70 p.c., a bitter principle called citrarin or citraric acid 2 p.c. Isolichenin, lichen stearic acid, sugar, cellulose 16 p.c., ash 2 p.c. Lichenine is a kind of starchy matter—lichen starch like inuulin. Acidum Citraricum, a crystalline white powder, soluble in alcohol, slightly so in water and ether, taste bitter. Dose, ½ to 2 grs.

Preparations.—Decoctum Cetrariæ (1 in 20). Dose, 1 to 4 fld. ozs.

Actions and uses.—Nutritive, tonic and demulcent. As a nutritious food and mucilaginous tonic cetrarin increases appetite, promotes digestion. It is given in chronic catarrh, chronic diarrhœa, in dyspepsia, consumption and other lung, bowel and stomach disorders. It has a good effect in relieving nocturnal discharges. It increases the formation of red and white blood corpuscles and is given in anæmia and chlorosis. In amenorrhœa it causes the flow of menses. When burnt the smoke is used to relieve headache. The starch is a good emollient. Its powder is applied to promote healing of wounds and used as food—its bitterness must be removed by heating it in water to a boiling point or by adding to it carbonate of potash.

Parmelia Kamtschadalis, P. Perlata, P. Parietina, P. Perforata Lichen Odoriferous.

Habitat.—Europe, Himalaya, Punjab, Persia, India.

Parts used.—The plant. The Lichen (Thallus).

Vernacular.—Arab.—Ushnâ, Hunna-i-Korisha. Burm.—Kéyar-Poen. Can.—Kallu Luvvu. Chin.—Shih-jui. Eng.—Stone flowers. Guz.—Chadila, Ghabilo, Pathara-ka-phula. Hind.—Charêla, char charela, Silâbâk, Motâ-dagada-phula, Patharake-phula. Himalaya.—Ausneh-chalchalira, charcharita. Pers.—Dowalah, Hazaz-el-sakkar. Sans.—Silâvalkâ.

Characters.—Thallus of a dirty white or greyish brown colour, about 2 to 4 inches long, and made up of numerous fibres spreading from a common stalk upon the trees, fibres flat, generally dichotomously, rarely trichotomously branched; surface of the thallus rugous and marked here and there with irregular depressions; fructification undeveloped, looking like punched tubercles on the fibres; smell rather aromatic; taste mucilaginous, bitterish, or rather saline. With water it becomes soft and cartilaginous. With boiling water it forms a jelly.

Constituents.—It contains yellow crystalline matter called chrysophanic acid—identical with the colouring matter of rhubarb, lichenin, cellulose, sugar, &c.

Preparations.—Infusion (1 in 20). Dose, 1 to 4 drs., decoction liniment.

Actions and uses.—Demulcent, tonic, febrifuge and diuretic; given in amenorrhœa, chlorosis, and leucorrhœa. As a soporific and sedative it is given to stop nocturnal emissions. The powder as a snuff is used to relieve headache. As a diuretic and emollient, a poultice placed over the lumbar and renal regions causes a copious flow of urine—as in dropsy As a liniment it is applied to the head in cases of headache. It is much used as an incense, and also in the preparation of a masálá used for washing the hair. It is administered in disorders of the stomach, dyspepsia, vomiting, pain in the liver or womb.

Fungi—The Phonasa Alamba, or Mushroom family.

Characters.—Several plants formed of parenchymators, cellular, or hyphal tissue. Fruitification produced in the air and consisting of congeries of cells having no flowers. Filaments found intermixed with cells, growing in or upon, decaying or living organic substances as parasites or saprophytes, nourished through their vegetative structure called the spawn or mycelium. They are without chlorophyll, variously coloured, soft, fibrous, gelatinous, fleshy or leathery.

Habitat.—Universal, except very cold regions.

Properties.—They have very variable properties; some are edible, growing solitary in dry airy places, generally white, do not change colour, have compact flesh; taste pleasant, contains watery juice; odour agreeable. Many species are rich in phosphorus, and are hence aphrodisiac; some are narcotic, tonic, astringent, emetic, purgative and styptic; poisonous mushrooms grow in clusters, and have bright colours; flesh, soft and watery, if kept for a time become brown, green or blue. The juice is often milky and odour very disagreeable; taste bitter and acrid.

Agaricus Albus, Polyporus Officinalis, Fungus Laricis, Boletus Laricis, White or purging Agaric (Eng.).

Habitat.—South Europe, Asia minor, Punjab.

Parts used.—The fungus on the larch, quercus, and fagus species.

Vernacular.—Bomb.—Ghâre-kûm. Cashm.—Jangli bulgar. Eng.—White agaric, agaricus, touchwood, agaric of the oak. Hind.—Ghârekûm, Chattri. Punj.—Kiain.

The fungus is of two kinds, male and female; female being the best and having a comb-like or horse's foot structure; male convolute, round and compact growing horizontally on the larch, on the stems of Larix Siberica, producing fructification in the air. Deprived of the outer rind, it is an irregular piece of a brownish, white colour, porous underneath; it is found of the size of a fist or larger; it is light, spongy and friable, but cannot easily be powdered. In shape and appearance it resembles Bhui-kohala; juice milky; odour faint and acrid; taste sweetish afterwards saltish bitter. Dose, 10 to 30 grs. in powder.

Constituents.—Resin, bitter extractive matter, gum, vegetable albumen and wax. The true active principle agaric, fungic or laricic acid ; also phosphoric acid, potash, lime, ammonia sulphur, &c. Agaric acid.—Agaricin or agaricinic acid. Agaricin the resin, an impure agaric acid, contains 97 p.c. of agaric acid and 3 p.c. of agaricol. Agaric acid occurs in minute white crystals, soluble in alcohol, chloroform and ether ; boiled with water it forms a gelatinos solution. Dose $\frac{1}{6}$ to 1 gr. given to check night sweats.

Preparations.—Extractum agarici. Dose 3 to 6 grs. Extractum Agarici Liquidum. It is not miscible with water. Dose, 3 to 20 ms. Tinctura Agarici (1 in 10). Dose 20 to 60 ms.

Actions and uses.—Astringent, cathartic and lactifuge. As a cathartic it is given in large doses with honey in eruptive fevers to promote the rising of the eruptions. It produces large watery motions. Agaracin in small doses is astringent and given to check diarrhœa. It is very useful in checking colliquative night sweats, bronchial secretion and hæmoptysis. Applied to the breasts as a galactafuge after weaning it stops the secretion of milk. It checks bleeding from leech bites. Agaric acid is specially useful in profuse sweating of pulmonary tuberculosis and other diseases.

Agaricus Muscarius. Amanita Muscaria. Fly Agaric.

Habitat.—Kamtschatka, Russia.

The mushroom acts as a poison to flies, hence its specific name.

Parts used.—An alkalod—Muscarina, muscarine.

Characters.—A poisonous mushroom, odour disagreeable ; taste burning and acrid.

Constituents —An alkaloid muscarine, obtained from the fungus. It is produced synthetically by the oxidation of choline and as a derivative from brain substance. It is a syrupy liquid, without any odour or taste, soluble in water and alcohol, readily so in water and in dilute acetic acid.

Muscarinæ Nitras, Muscarine nitrate, an uncrystallizable viscid yellowish brown hygroscopic liquid, soluble in water. Dose $\frac{1}{20}$ to $\frac{1}{4}$ grs. used hypodermically.

Actions and uses.—Narcotic and intoxicant. As an intoxicant it produces vertigo, delirium, paralysis of the respiratory centre and of the heart. As a vaso constrictor it contracts the pulmonary vessels and causes dyspnæa. It increases the secretion of the salivary and lachrymal glands, of the skin, intestines, liver and pancreas ; it diminishes the secretion of the kidneys. As an irritant of the gastro-intestinal tract it causes colic, vomiting, purging, profound stupor, coma and death. Muscarine, like gelsemium, contracts the pupils when given internally, but dilates them widely when locally applied. Its action is similar to that of pilocarpine, but it is almost completely antagonistic to atropine. Muscarine has been used hypodermically in night sweats of phthisis. In inflammatory affections with profuse exudation in eye, in catarrhal jaundice, acute bronchitis, pulmonary hæmorrhage, diabetes, torpid liver and constipation it is given with benefit. It produces salivation, profuse flow of tears and purgation. In chorea and chilblain the tincture of agaricus may by used with benefit.

Boletus Crocatus. Polyporus fomentarius. Agaricas Ostreatus. A. Palmatus.

The fungus growing on artocarpus integrifolia, jack tree.

Habitat.—India.

Parts used.—The fungus.

Vernacular.—Eng.—Agaric of the oak. Touchwood. Oyster mushroom. Mah.—Phanasa amba, phanasa alombê.

Characters.—The fungus grows on the stumps of jack tree and is very beautiful and edible. It resembles in shape oyster shells or hoof of a horse. It is tufted, sessile or marked with stalks or sub-lateral stipes. The stalks are from 4 to 5 inches long, and from 3 to 4 lines in thickness. The cap is shell like, smooth, and fleshy ; upper surface convex and of a pale bluish grey, or brown colour ; under surface concave and formed of several layers resembling the rib-bones or lamellæ. The lamellæ are of a whitish or pink colour, separate above and anastamosing with one another as they extend below.

Constituents.—Resin, organic acid and gelatine.

Actions and uses.—Astringent; a paste of it is applied to the gums in aphthæ ; it prevents excessive salivation. It is supposed to act as a good styptic and is given in diarrhœa and dysentery.

Polyporus gigantius. It sometimes grows in the same localities as agaricus, but is corky, hard, variable in size, and highly fœtid, and of a disagreeable smell. The juice flowing from them appears to resemble Iodine paint. They are poisonous. Many varieties of fungi grow on the waste ground in Bombay. These are known as *Kutarâ-ni-topi* (Guz.).

Claviceps Purpurea B. P.

Habitat.—Eastern Countries, Spain, France, Germany.

Parts used.—The sclerotium originating in the ovary of secale cereali—Ergota, ergot, B. P.

Syn.—*Smut* of rye, mother of rye, horn seed, cock spur rye.

Characters.—Ergot is fusiform, curved, obtusely triangular, three-furrowed. Externally purplish black and whitish within. It has a short fracture, the odour is peculiar and disagreeable. The taste is oily and disagreeable. It rapidly deteriorates ; the deterioration is due to the oxidation of the fixed oil contained in it and to the attack of insects. This can be avoided by dropping a little chloroform upon it from time to time. Dose of the powder, 20 to 60 grs.

Constituents.—Sclerotic, Sclerotinic or ergotic acid, 4 p. c.; Ecboline cornutine, the active principles ergotine and ergotinine. Fixed oil, 30 p.c.; proteids; cholesterine, ash 3 p.c. trimethylamine.

Acidum Scleroticum—An active constituent, is a yellow brown amorphous powder without any taste, very hygroscopic, soluble in water; one grain is equal in activity to 30 grains of ergot. Dose, $\frac{1}{2}$ to $\frac{3}{4}$ gr. Used as tablets $\frac{1}{2}$ to 1 gr. each; used as Injectio Acidi sclerotici Hypodermica—strength 1 gr. in 6 ms. Dose, 3 to 5 ms. This injection is preferable to ergotin, as it causes no pain at the seat of puncture. Ergotinina or Ergotinine, an alkaloid, occurs in small white crystals, insoluble in water, soluble in ether, chloroform and alcohol. Dose $\frac{1}{200}$ to $\frac{1}{60}$ gr.; used as tablets $\frac{1}{150}$ and $\frac{1}{300}$ gr.; used hypodermically, dissolved in lactic acid, for post-partem hæmorrhage. Ergotininæ citras, a soluble salt of ergotinine used for hypodermic injection. Dose, $\frac{1}{150}$ to $\frac{1}{30}$ gr. Spasmotin Spacelotoxin, a poisonous element of ergot, a yellow amorphous powder, insoluble in water, dilute acids and petroleum ether, soluble in ether and alcohol. With alkalies it forms salts. Dose, $\frac{1}{2}$ to 1 gr. Cornutine or ecboline, an alkaloid. Dose, $\frac{1}{6}$ gr. Hydrochloride of cornutine and citrate of cornutine are prepared.

Preparations.—Of Ergot. Tinctura Ergotæ, Ammoniata B. P. (1 in 4). Dose, $\frac{1}{2}$ to 1 fld. dr. Extractum Ergotæ commonly called Ergotin B.P., a purified solid or semi-solid extract of ergot. Dose, 2 to 8 grs. Injectio Ergotæ Hypodermica B.P. (110 ms. contain 33 grs. of ergotin). Dose, 3 to 10 ms., an injection (1 in 1,000) is recommended for gonorrhœa. Infusum Ergotæ (1 in 20). Dose, 1 to 2 ozs. Pilulæ Ergotini Compositæ—ergotin 1 gr., dried sulphate of iron, 1 gr.; extract of hellelbore, 1 gr.; extract of aloes, 1 gr.; oil of savin, $\frac{1}{2}$ ms., make one pill. Pilulæ Ergotini cum quinina,—ergotin $2\frac{1}{2}$ grs.; quinine $1\frac{1}{2}$ grs. in each.

Actions and uses.—Motor excitant, vascular constrictor, anhydrotic, emmenagogue, ecbolic, parturient, and hæmostatic. It stimulates the functions of the cord, the vasomotor centres, raises the blood pressure, produces contractions of unstriped muscular fibres, diminishes the calibre of the arterioles, depresses the heart, slows the pulse and increases the intestinal peristalsis. It acts as an irritant of the gastro intestinal tract, causing nausea, vomiting, great thirst, colic, painful micturition and purging; also headache, vertigo, continuous labour pain, contraction of the sphincter vesicæ and ani; if pushed further, there are tetanoid convulsions of the muscles of the flexsors, of the uterus, intestines and respiration, coldness of the limbs, formication of the whole body and skin, loss of sensibility, abolition of spinal sensatious, bullæ containing blood and dry gangrene of the lower extremities, convulsion ending in coma and death. It is given in hæmorrhages from the uterus, lungs, nose, stomach. It has the property of causing powerful continuous instead of natural intermittent contraction of the muscular coats of the arterioles and of the muscular wall of the uterus,hence dangerous in early labour, as it might rupture the uterus, cause laceration of the perineum, and paralyse the fœtal heart. It should only be given in labour cases when the os is fully dilated or the head is born; and generally after the child is born to guard against post-partem hæmorrhage and to promote expulsion of the placenta; given also in labours when the uterus is becoming exhausted. It is highly useful in chronic metritis, subinvolution, disordered menstruation as dysmenorrhœa, and menorrhagia, in fibroids of the uterus and in polypi; in which it contracts the uterus and promotes absorption of inflammatory products; in atonic spermatorrhœa, in incontinuence of urine, or where the spinctors are relaxed, it may be given with benefit. It may be given for about one week after delivery to prevent subinvolution. In inflammation of the mucous membranes, as conjunctivities, gonorrhœa, &c., it is useful both externally and internally. It is usefully given in mania, hemicrania, migraine in myelitis and in cerebral congestion. In cardiac hypertrophy it slows the action of the heart, and the blood current. In diabetes mellitus, it is a valuable remedy. With quinine, it causes contraction of the uterus and of the spleen if enlarged. In night sweats of phthisis it is very useful. In low state of the pulse it is largely given with digitalis in fever and acute diseases. In atonic hæmorrhages, as hæmoptysis, menorrhagia and hæmaturia; in acute and chronic fluxes, dysentery, chronic diarrhœa, &c., it is given with benefit. Hypodermically ergotine and ergotinine are used, in post-partem and other hæmorrhages, in prolapse of the rectum, chronic metritis, subinvolution of the uterus, in uterine fibroid and varicose veins.

Torula Saccharomyces, T. Cerevisæ, Ferment, Yeast (Eng.).

Parts used.—The plant.

Characters.—It is a peculiar insoluble product of the fermentation of malt liquors produced by aid of alcoholic fermentation of saccharine fluid by this fungus. It occurs in two forms, the top or surface yeast, a semi fluid, frothy mass and cellular, of a peculiar odour; the bottom or sediment yeast. Dose, ½ to 1 oz.

Actions and uses.—Tonic, stimulant and laxative, used in diabetes, diarrhœa, scurvy, typhoid fever, &c.; used also as antiseptic poultice on sores and bruises.

Ustilago Maydis, Corn Smutt, Corn Ergot, Maize Ergot.

Parts used.—The fungus or smut.

It is a fungus or parasite growing chiefly upon the stem, the grain, young ears, the pistils and the male inflorescence, of zea mays, or Indian corn. It occurs in irregular globose masses consisting of blackish gelatinous membrane enclosing many globular, nodular spores; the taste and odour are very disagreeable. Dose, 15 to 30 grs.

Constituents.—Fixed oil 2·5 p.c., an acid resembling sclerotic acid, a volatile crystalline principle, an alkaloid—secaline, isomeric with trimethylamine, resin, pectin, gluten volatile base, sugar, mucilage and ash 5 p.c.

Preparations.—Liquid extract. Dose, 20 to 60 ms.

Actions and uses.—Similar to those of ergot and nux vomica combined; *i.e.*, emmenagogue and hæmostatic. As a spinal excitant it increases the sensibility and the reflexes, and gives rise to convulsions. In large doses it stimulates the pneumo-gastric, dilates the pupils, causes paralysis of the muscular system and death by respiratory spasms. Its oxytoccic action is not well marked. If given in uterine fibroids, it causes contraction of the uterus. The contractions are clonic or intermittent instead of continuous as in ergot. It is used to check hæmorrhages and given in spermatorrhœa, psoriasis, eczema, &c.

Algæ—The Chinai-ghasa or Sea Weed family.

Characters.—The weeds are cellular. Like the lichens these are flowerless parenchymatous plants, nourished through their whole surface. They grow in fresh or salt water, or in moist places. The thallus has neither true woody fibre nor vessels. It is foliaceous, branched, filamentous or pulverulent. Many algæ are microscopic, others are of large size, usually greenish brown or rose-coloured.

Habitat.—Universal, growing in salt or fresh water or in moist situations; some are found in boiling springs, others in mineral springs, some in chemical solutions.

Properties.—Several species are employed as food. Their nutritious properties are due to the presence of starch, sugary matter (mannite), mucilage and albumen. Some species contain a principle called gelose, and to it to a great extent is due their nutritious property—one part of gelose dissolved in 500 parts of boiling water will on cooling leave a colourless transparent jelly behind. The edible bird's nests used by the natives for food owe this nutrient property to a species of algæ, and more especially to the secretion of the swallows, by which they are constructed. Some algæ are used medicinally as demulcent, emollient and alterative. Several species contain iodine, and are reputed as remedies in goitre and scrofulous diseases. Some species when burnt leave an ash known as kelp, once used in the preparation of carbonate of soda. Some species are reputed to possess verimifugal properties.

Chondrus Crispus, C. Mamillosus and Gigartina Mamillosa.

Habitat.—Atlantic Ocean, Irish coast, New England.

Syn.—Carrageen moss, pearl moss, salt rock moss, Irish moss.

Parts used.—The entire plant dried and bleached.

Characters.—It grows upon rocks under water, attached by a small disk. Fronds yellowish. Spore vessels or capsules imbedded in the frond. It is pale yellowish white, horny, translucent and forked; odour seaweed-like; taste mucilaginous and saline. It swells in cold water; boiled with water (1 to 30), it forms a gelatinous solution.

Constituents.—Water 19, albuminoids 9½, mucilage 55½, a kind of pectin called carageenin, cellulose or gelatin 2; and mineral matter 14, containing chlorides, sulphates and phosphates of potassium, sodium, calcium and magnesium, iodine, bromine—no starch.

Preparations.—Decoction (1 in 4). Dose, 1 to 2 fld. ozs., jelly 2 ozs. in a quart of water.

Actions and uses.—Nutrient, dietetic, emollient and demulcent. As nutrient it is given like tapioca, sago or barley in consumption and other bronchial catarrhal and pulmonary complaints; also in dysentery, diarrhœa, kidney and bladder complaints and scrofula.

Fucus Vesiculosus, F. Nodosus, F. Serratus.

Bladder wrack, Sea wrack, Common Sea Weed.

Habitat.—Muddy rocky shores of the Atlantic and Pacific Oceans.

Parts used.—The whole plant, the expressed juice of its vesicles or bladders.

Characters.—A perennial multi-cellular sea weed growing in salt water, forming a foliaceous or filamentous thallus, and of an olive green or olive brown colour. It is propagated by reproductive particles, called spores or sporules. It is flowerless and consequently seedless. It is 40 inches long, and about an inch broad. It has a flat leaf branched with a midrib, and small spherical vesicles filled with air in the leaf throughout its length; odour sea weed-like; taste mucilaginous and saline. Dose of the dried plant, 20 to 100 grs.

Constituents.—Iodine less than in other algæ. It also contains organic matters, including mucilage, fat, mannite &c., the ash is known as vegetable Ethiops—it is a kind of charcoal, procured by incineration in a close vessel; the ash contains soda in combination, as chlorides, bromides, iodides, phosphates and sulphates.

Preparations.—Extract—Dose, 3 to 8 grs. Liquid extract—Dose, 1 to 2 fld. drs. Decoction (1 to 20). Dose, 4 to 8 drs. Wine, Vegetable Ethiops. Dose, 2 to 4 drs.

Actions and uses.—An alterative and tonic; given for diminishing glandular swelling, goitre, and enlargements of joints. It produces absorption of fat in obese subjects without in other respects injuring the health. The first signs of its favourable action is the increase in the flow of urine, and the appearance of a black pellicle on its surface; also given in goitre and in scrofulous and glandular affections. The ash is used for similar purposes. The frictions of the plant have been employed externally in glandular and scrofulous affections.

Gelidium Cartilagineum; Sphœrococcus Compressus, Gelidium Corneum.

Habitat.—Indian Ocean, Java.

Parts used.—Gelatine.

Vernacular.—Thao or Japanese Isinglass. Indian Bazars.—Chinai Ghâs

Characters.—Met with in the form of compressed four-sided sticks composed of shrivelled semi-transparent yellowish-white membrane, very light, full of cavities, very flexible, easilys broken and without any taste or smell; combined with large quantitie of water, it forms jelly. This power is due to its containing a principle named gelose or parabin; also used in the manufacture of glue.

Constituents.—Gelose, a gelatinous principle containing no nitrogen. Sugary matter (Mannite), starch and albumen.

Actions and uses.—Nutrient and demulent like gracilaria or edible moss, and used like it. The nutritious properties are due to gelose.

Remarks.—A very good medium for cultivating germs for bacteriological investigations.

Gracilaria Lichenoides, G. Confervoides, Fucus Lichenoides.

Habitat.—Back water of Ceylon and Indian Ocean.

Parts used.—The dried plant (moss).

Vernacular.—Burm.—Kiyâv-poên. Bomb.—Chinai-ghasa. Ceylon.—Agar-agar. Duk.—Darya-ki-pachi, môs. Eng.—Edible seaweeds, Ceylon moss, Japanese isinglass. Malay.—Rumi yarwakar Sajar karang. Tel.—Samudrupu-pâchi.

Characters.—A small and delicate fiucus; fronds filiform, filaments much branched; colour light purple; occuring in bundles. Each, filament from 12 to 15 inches long, dry, quadrangular or cylindrical in form, nearly white in colour, and reticulated, resembling the pith-like substance, found in the interior of a quill, very light, rather flexible, but can easily be broken; odour resembling sea-weed; taste mucilaginous and saline, resembling that of rice canji.

Constituents.—Vegetable jelly (40 to 80 p.c.), albumen, iodine, true starch, ligneous matter, mucilage and salts, as sulphate and chloride of soda; sulphate and phosphate of lime, wax and iron.

Preparations.—Decoction (1 in 20). Dose, 1 to 2 fld. ozs. Jelly.—The moss is reduced to a fine powder. The powder is boiled with water and strained. The solution when cold is filtered and flavoured with Limbu-nl-chhála (lemon-peel) taja, &c.

Actions and uses.—Nutritive, emollient, demulcent and alterative; given to invalids in pectoral affections, and in phthisis; the jelly is also given in dysentery, diarrhœa, leucorrhœa and profuse menstrual flow. It contains iodine, and hence is useful as an alterative in goitre, scrofula, &c. As a demulcent and an emollient it is useful in chronic catarrh of the intestines (diarrhœa), and in irritation of the urinary passages.

Remarks.—It is a good substitute for isinglass. It requires a very large proportion of water to form a jelly.

Laminaria Saccharina—Sweet Tangle (Eng.), L. Digitata, L. Potatorium.

Habitat.—Throughout India, Salt lakes, Deep seas, Cashmere, Lahore.

Parts used.—The plant.

Vernacular.—Chin.—Seatape-hai-tai. Eng.—Sugar sea beet. Hind.—Gillur-ka-patta, Galhar-ká-pâtta.

Characters.—The plant is a sea-weed, obtained from salt lake in Tibet and consists of long ribbon-like pieces.

Constituents.—It contains 12 p.c. of mannite and iodine.

Actions and uses.—A syrup made of this plant combined with decoction of quince seeds is given for the cure of goitre (Bronchocele); also given in scrofulous and syphilitic affections. Young parts of L. Saccharina mixed with those of L. Digitata form a preparation known as tangle and used as an article of diet.

CLASSIFICATION OF DRUGS ACCORDING TO THEIR PHYSIOLOGICAL EFFECTS ON THE HUMAN SYSTEM.

Alteratives.

Alangium Lamarckii
Amoora Rohitika
Argemone Mexicana
Asclepias Incarnata
Baptisia
Bauhinea Variegata
Bassia Latifolia
Bavachee seeds
Berberis Aquifolium
Bharangi
Bryonia Epigœa
Cassia Tora
Calotropis Gigantea
Cascara Amarga
Celastrus Paniculatus
Cocculus Villosus
Condurango
Coptis Teeta
Cuscuta Reflexa
Cratæva Religiosa
Croton Oblongifolia
Cyperus Pertenuis
Dalbergia Sympathetica
Daphne Mezereum
Derris Uliginosa
Dipterocarpus Turbinatus
Echinops Echinatus
Franciscea Uniflora
Galium Aparine
Guaiacum Officinalis
Gynocardia Odorata
Hemidesmus Indicus
Hydrocotyle Asiatica, powdered leaves. Dose, 5 to 8 grs.
Indigofera Tinctoria
Ipomæa Pescapræ
Jadvar
Juglans Regia
Karanj leaves
Khodaki Rasna
Lepidium Sativum
Marrubium Vulgare
Michelia Champaca
Mimosa Pudica
Menispermum Canadense
Mercuro Vegetal
Nyctanthes Arbortristis
Olden Landia
Pæonia Officinalis
Pæderia Fetida
Pongamia Glabra
Plumbago Rosea
Psoralia Corylifolia
Physalis Alkekengi
Peganum Harmala
Phytolacca
Pitpâpra
Samudar Shokha
Sassafras
Sarsaparilla
Satvin
Siegesbeckia Orientalis
Spermacoce Hispida
Solanum Dulcamara
Sweet cloves
Tacca Aspera
Tenacetum Umbelliferum
Tinospora Cordifoli
Thespesia Populnea
Tragia Cannabina
Tryamân
Tylophora Asthmatica
Tribulus Terestris
Thespesia Populnea—the viscid juice of capsules
Vanjai
Vitex Negundo
Withania Somnifera

Formula.—Syrup Trifolium compound :—Contains trifolium pretense—4, burdock root 2, stillingia 2, phytolacca 2, *Berberis* aquifolia 2, cascara amarga 2, Xanthoxylon ½, potas iodid 1, and sugar 40. Dose, 1 to 2 drs. Alterative in scrofula, rheumatism, skin diseases, &c. (*See page 380, Vol. I.*)

Anodynes or Analgesics.

Aconite, Aconitine, used locally in neuralgia of the 5th nerve, in gout, and in restlessness
Aconite Tincture, in drops doses
Atropine, hypodermically in tic douloureux
Belladonna Ointment, in pains in the pelvic region
Camphor
Cannabis Indica
Chloroxylon Swietenia
Cimicifuga, in ovarian neuralgia or dysmenorrhœa
Cocaine, a 4 p.c. solution locally in toothache and for minor surgical operations
Codeine, to relieve abdominal and overian pain
Conium fluid extract in pain of cancer, of rheumatism, or overian pain
Duboisine, same as atropine
Heliotropium Indicum (local)
Hyoscyamus
Lupulus
Morphine $\frac{1}{4}$, atropine $\frac{1}{100}$ injected hypodermically in sciatica and neuralgia
Opium Liniment in pleurodynia and neuralgia
Piscidia Erythrina
Rhatany, to relieve pain of blisters, burns, and ulcers
Stramonium Ointment
Taberna Montana (locally)
Theine Injection, in neuralgic pains

(*See page 381, Vol. I.*)

Anæsthetics—Local Anæsthetics or Anodynes.

Acid Hydrocyanic—local anæsthetic
Aconite
Atropine
Belladonna
Boldoin, local anæsthetics like cocaine
Cocaine
Erythroxylum Coca
Erythrophlæum, local anæsthetic
Eugenia Caryophyllata
Gelsemium (general)
Guaiacol with olive oil injected hypodermically
Gymnema Sylvestris, Anæsthetic on the sense of taste
Kavaine (local)
Menthol (local)
Morphine and atropine injection after operation.
Morphine, injected hypodermically before Chloroform or Ether inhalation
Opium (local anodyne)
Quabain (local anæsthetic)
Veratrine (local anodyne)
Volatile oils (local anodyne)

Anhydrotics

These are agents which reduce sweats or perspirations. Atropine, jaborandi, Dover's powder, picrotoxine, strychnine, &c., are respiratory stimulants, and they act in reducing the sweats of phthisis. In severe cough the respiration becomes depressed and the circulation is interfered with, owing to the carbonic acid gas being accumulated in the blood; this accumulation stimulates the sweat centres and gives rise to profuse perspiration. (*See page 383, Vol. I.*)

Abies Canadensis
Acid acetic dilute (locally)
Acid Agaric, internally—checks sweats
Acid Camphoric, 10 grs. on the tongue to check night sweats
Acid Gallic, to check night sweats
Acid Sulphuric Aromatic, to check sweating, but is bad for digestion
Agarcine, 10 with atropine 1, and aromatic sulphuric acid 1,000, to check sweats of phthisis. Dose, 10 ms.
Atropine, a respiratony stimulant $\frac{1}{250}$ gr. hypodermically or $\frac{1}{50}$ to $\frac{1}{30}$ internally in pill to relieve sweating of phthisis and exhausting diseases.
Belladonna Liniment locally
Belladonna Tincture, internally in weakly children to check fœtid sweats
Camphoric acid
Duboisine sluphate, a good substitute for atropine
Diachylon ointment for fœtid sweats
Ergot, internally very useful
Gallic acid with belladonna, to diminish sweats of phthisis
Hamamelis fluid extract with iron chloride and glycerin for application
Hyoscyamus, acts on the sweat glands
Ice, locally over the abdomen relieves sweats

Anhydrotics.—(contd.)

Jaborandi, internally
Muscarine, to check sweats
Oils, to rub over the whole skin to prevent sweating
Opium with ipecacuanha to check colliquative sweats
Picrotoxin, internally
Pilocarpine, internally $\frac{1}{20}$ gr. to check perspiration
Potentilla sarmentosa, infusion of leaves and root internally in night sweats
Quinine preparations with sulphuric acid in general sweating or exhaustion
Quinine and alcohol (1 in 100), rubbing with a sponge over the body in general sweating
Quillaia Infusion, to dispel fœtor of feet and arms
Salvia tincture or infusion, internally, or locally to sponge the body
Sage tea infusion for night sweats of phthisis internally and locally to sponge the body
Soft soap as inunction
Stramonium, acts on the sweat glands
Strychnine in sweats of phthisis
Starch, locally as dusting powder
Tannin, to relieve sweating in axilla and groins
Vinegar, locally

Antiperiodics.

Alstonia constricta
Anthemis nobilis
Apocynum cannabinum
Azadirachta Indica
Berberis aristata
Cedrela Toona
Cinchona and its alkaloids
Clerodendron
Conessi bark
Coptis Teeta Tincture, ½ to 1 dr.
Cœsalpinia coriara
Eucalyptol
Eupatorium
Gardenia gummifera
Holarrhena antidysenterica
Nectandra Rodica
Oldenlandia Corymbosa
Picrorrhiza Kurroa
Quebracho
Quinine
Soymida febrifuga
Swertia Decussata
Toddalia aculiata
Trichosanthes Dioica

Antiphlogistics. (*See Vol. I, page 388.*)

Aconitum Napellus, tincture for the respiratory tract
Arnica
Digitalis
Ergot
Gelsemium
Ipecacuanha
Opium
Pilocarpine
Purgatives
Resinol
Veratrum Viride

Antipyretics. (*See Vol. I, page 388.*)

To reduce circulation.

Aconite tincture, 2 to 5 ms.
Arnica
Belladonna
Colchicum
Digitalis
Quebracho
Salicin
Veratrum

To produce perspiration.

Aspidospermin
Gelsimium
Ipecacuanha with opium
Nectandra
Piperin
Quinine and its salts

To diminish tissue changes.

Beberine
Benzoic acid
Berberine
Camphor
Chinolin
Cinchona and its salts
Essential oils
Eucalyptol
Eu Quinine
Galtheria oil
Hydroquinone
Pyrocatechin
Quillaja Saponaria
Quinine and its salts
Veratrum
Thymol

Antiscorbutics.

Averrhoa Carambola
Carissa Corundas
Feronia Elephantum
Tamarindus Indicus
Vitis Indica

Antiseptics. (*See Vol. I, page 389.*)

Ajowan (Ptychotis)
Aloes, as dusting powder
Anthrarobin
Artemisia sieversiana
Balsam of Peru
Baptisia Tinctoria
Benzoates
Cajuput oil
Camphor and its preparations
Caryophyllum oil
Chamomile

Antiseptics—(*contd.*)

Chavicol
Coal tar
Coffee
Coumarin
Echinacea
Eucalyptus oil, gauze and ointment
Eugenol
Gaultheria oleum
Inula
Liquid Amber
Lycopodium
Mentha oleum
Menthol
Mint essence
Myrtle
Nux Vomica
Oil of Cade
Oleum Pinus sylvestris
Petroleum
Pinus longifolia
Pix liquida
Quinine
Staphisagria seeds
Styrax Benzoin
Terebene
Thymol
Tobacco
Turpentine

Formula.—Antiseptic powder contains acid boric 1 dr., acid citric 2 gr., acid carbolic 30 ms., acid salicylic 10 grs., hydrargyri bichloridi 1 gr., sodii chloridi 6 grs., thymol 2 gr., zinci chloridi 1 gr., zinci sulpho carbolatis 1½ dr., in 20 ozs. of water, evaporate and dry.

Antisialagogues. (*See Vol. I, page 392.*)

Atropine, hypodermically to paralyse the ends of nerves of secretion
Belladonna
Cinchona with potassium salts
Ficus religiosa
Hamamelis
Hyoscine Hydrobromate
Krameria
Mimops Elengii
Myrrh gargle
Opium, to lessen, the secretion
Pellitory, to eliminate the poison
Pilocarpine, as injection
Tannic acid
Vegetable Astringents
Physostigma, to lessen the blood supply to the secreting glands

Antispasmodics. (*See Vol. I, page 392.*)

Acid hydrocyanic
Aconite
Ailanthus glandulosa
Ambergris
Amber electrum
Ammoniac
Andropogon
Asafetida
Aspidosperma
Balsamodendron
Belladonna
Blumea balsamifera
Camphor
Chamomile (cherry laurel)
Cimicifuga
Cloves (oil)
Coleus Carnasus
Conium maculatum
Curare
Gelsemium
Gynandropsis pantaphylla
Hyoscyamus
Ipecacuanha
Junde bidaster
Kevado
Lactucarium
Lobelia
Lycopodium
Menthol
Morphia
Opium
Pæonia officinalis
Pandamus odoratissimo
Physostigma
Pœderia Fetida
Ptychotis ajowan
Pulsatilla tincture, 2-10ms.
Randia Dumetorum
Stramonium
Sumbul
Symplocarpus fœtidus
Terebinthina
Thyme oil (garden Thyme)
Tobacco
Treak Ferook
Valerian
Viburnum Prunifolium
Viverra Zebetta—(secretion)
Viscum sp.—Wild jasmine

Astringents. (*See Vol. I, page 393,*)

Acacia catechu
Achyranthes aspera
Acid gallic
Acid tannic
Ægle marmelos, syrup of pulp, 1 oz.
Alocasia Indica
Alstonia
Alum root
Amoora rohitika
Areca catechu
Avalkanthi
Babul chhal
Bari mai
Berberis aquifolia, tincture, 10-40 ms.
Black alder
Blue berry
Bombax malabaricum
Butea frondosa
Burgundy pitch
Cantium parvifolium
Catechu
Celosia argentea
Chinai kath
Chote-mai
Cochlospermum gossypium

Astringents.—(*contd.*)

Cæsalpinia
Crane tree
Cyperus rotundus
Diospyros glutinosa
Dita bark
Dragon's blood
Ergot
Eucalyptus (gummi)
Eugenea Jambolana
Faronia Elephantum, (gum)
Flacourtia cataphracta
Galls
Garcinia mangostina (intestinal)
Gymnema sylvestris
Hamamelis
Holarrhena, antidysent·rica
Iron wood tree
Jussiæ suffruiticosa
Kaiphal
Kanchan-chhal
Katphal
Kino (intestinal)
Krameria (Rhatany)
Leea sambucina
Mango bark and stone
Matico
Mimusops elengia
Myristca
Myrtus communi
Oak bark
Odina wodier
Patanga
Pistacia
Poppy seeds
Pterocarpus santatinus
Punica granatum. decoction of the rind of the fruit, 1 to 2 ozs.
Quercus alba (oak bar.
Rhus
Rubia cordifolia
Rumex crispus
Spondias mangifera
Tamarix gallica
Terminalia
Thea bohea
Turpentine (chian)
Uncaria gambier
Urtica dioica
Uva ursi
Woodfordia floribunda
Yerba reunia
Zizyphus jujuba

Carminatives. (*See Vol. I page 394.*)

Acorus calamus (Rhizome)
Ajowan
Allspice
Andropogon
Anethum sowa, fruit
Anise oil
Anthemis nobilis
Apium graveolens
Asafetida
Cajuput oil
Camphor
Capsicum
Cardamom
Carraway fruit and oil
Carui
Caryophillus aromaticus—flower buds
Cascarilla
Chamomile
Citrus
Cinnamon oil
Coffee
Cichorium intybus
Coriander oil
Cuminum cyminum
Curcuma aromatica
Eucalyptus oil
Feniculum panmorium
Gaultheria
Ginger
Hedeomæ oil
Lavender
Lupinus albus
Mace
Menthol
Methi seeds
Mustard
Nigella sativa
Nutmeg oil
Orange peel
Origanum marjora
Parsley
Patchouli oil
Pavonia odorata
Pepper (long)
Peppermint oil
Pimenta oil
Rosemary
Rosa gallica
Ruta graveolens
Salix nigra
Salvia officinalis
Sambucus
Spearmint oil
Star anise
Tamal patra
Todalia aculeata
Valerian oil
Xanthoxylon
Ziziphora tenuor

CATHARTICS OR PURGATIVES.

(a) Aperients, Laxatives. (*See Vol. I, page 395.*)

Ægle marmelos, in habitual constipation
Aleurites triloba, the oil a substitute for castor oil. Dose ½ to 1 oz.
Allamanda cathartica
Argemone mexicana, oil of seeds. Dose, 20 to 60 ms.
Belladonna, to prevent habitual constipation
Cascara Sagrada, fluid extract 1 dr.
Cassia senna
Castor oil
Canoora decussata
Cocos Nucifera
Emblic myrabolans
Euphorbia
Figs
Frangula
Fraxinus
Hydrastis, in sluggish liver
Ipecacuanha
Indian walnut oil. Dose, 1 to 2 ozs
Leptandrin
Linseed
Liquorice powder compound
Manna
Nishot
Nux vomica tincture, before meals, to overcome torpor of the bowels
Olive oil
Oatmeal
Physostigma with nux vomica and belladonna, in intestinal torpor

Aperients—(*contd.*)

Prunes
Pharbitis nil
Rose buds
Rhubarb with capsicum
Saponaria trifoliatum (soap)
Sessamum oil
Stramonium suppository
Tamarind pulp with Cocculus indicus, and glaubers salt
Taraxacum
Treacle
Turpentine, in atony of the bowels with gaseous distension
Vitis venifera
Zizyphus Vulgaris

Formula.—Pathyadi Kvâth Decoction contains:—Myrabolans, emblic and chebulic (mature fruit), each 6, purging cassia 4, baliospermum axillare 3, picorrhiza karroa 6, euphorbia neriifolia 3, turpeth root 4, cyperus rotundus 5, senna 6. rhamnus palamatius 4. and water 10 to 1 of the whole powder. At first boil and evaporate to the consistence of an extract, then add croton seeds 1, ginger 5, sulphur 4, mix and make a pill mass. Dose, 2 grs., in constipation.

1. Podophyllin $\frac{1}{6}$, extract nux vomica $\frac{1}{4}$ gr., ferri sulph. $\frac{1}{3}$, gr.. capsici pulv. $\frac{1}{4}$, extract belladonna $\frac{1}{8}$ gr., extract hyoscyamus $\frac{1}{4}$ gr., aloin $\frac{1}{6}$ gr., mix Pil 1. Dose, 2 pills.

2. Extract cascara sagrada 2, extract nux vomica $\frac{1}{8}$ gr., extract belladonna $\frac{1}{8}$ gr., euonymus 2, xanthoxylon 2, capsicum resin $\frac{1}{6}$, mix, make pills 2. Dose 1 to 2 pills.

3. Croton oil $\frac{1}{2}$, extract elaterii $\frac{1}{24}$, calomel 1 gr., extract jalapæ 1, extract colocynth 2, gingerine $\frac{1}{12}$, mix, make pil 1. Dose, 1 pill.

4. Aloes 1 gr.; resin scammony $\frac{1}{2}$ gr., resin jalapæ $\frac{1}{2}$ gr., calomel $\frac{1}{2}$ gr., extract belladonna $\frac{1}{6}$ gr., extract stramonii $\frac{1}{6}$ gr., mix Pil 1.

5. Fel bovinum 1 gr.; pulv. ipecacuanha $\frac{1}{6}$ gr.; aloes 2 grs.; pilulæ asafetida compositæ 2 grs. mix. Dose, 2 pills.

Artificial Hunyadi water—Magnesii sulphatis 1 dr.; sodii sulphatis 1 dr.; Potassii sulphatis 5 gr.; sodii bicarbonatis 8 gr.; sodii chloridi 10 grs., aqua 1 oz. mix. Dose, a wine glassful.

(b) Simple Purgatives. (*See Vol. I, page 395.*)

Aloes with iron sulphate or Aloin
Carthamus tinctorius
Cassia Fistula (pulp or pods), 1 to 2 drs.
Castor oil
Clitorea ternata seeds, 1 dr. with pot. bicarb.
Colchicine
Colocynth Pulv, 2 to 8 grs., or extract 2 to 6 grs., with ainse oil and hyoscyamus
Confectio sennæ with sulphur
Cucumis Trigonus—(pulv of fruit)
Embelia ribes
Exogonum purga
Friedricshall waters
Glycerrhiza (compound powder)
Jalap
Luffa echinata
Pharbitis nil (seeds)
Podophyllum, gr. $\frac{1}{4}$, with essence of ginger $\frac{1}{12}$ gr., when the secretion is deficient, and accompanied with bilious headache
Rhamnus frangula, extract
Rhubarb
Stillingia fluid extract 15 ms. in habitual constipation
Terebenthina
Terminalia Chebula (fruit)
Victoria water

(c) Cholagogue-Cathartics. (*See Vol. I, page 395.*)

Aloes
Atropa mandragora
Biophytum sensitivum
Cosmostigma racemosum
Euonymin
Euphorbium
Iridin
Leptandrin
Podophyllin
Sangninaria
Scammony

(d) Drastic and Hydragogue Cathartics. *(See Vol. I, page 395.)*

Allamanda cathartica
Apocynum cannabinum
Bryonia alba
Camboge
Cathartic acid
Chelidonium majus, extract
Colocynth
Croton oil in impaction without inflammation. Dose 1 to 2 ms.
Elaterium
Gamboge
Garcinia
Jalap
Jatropha
Kâlâ dânâh
Myrobolans
Sumbucus nigra
Trichosanthes nerii-folia
Turpethum

Deliriants. *(See Vol. I, page 396.)*

Belladonna
Cannabis
Hyoscyamus
Lupulus
Opium
Stramoninm
Turpentine

Demulcents and Emollients. *(See Vol. I, page 396.)*

Abelmoschus esculentus (E)
Abutilon Indicum
Acacia Arabica
,, Farnesiana (E)
Almond oil (E)
Althœa officinalis
Arachis hypogœa (E)
Arrowroot
Asparagus
Astragalus gummifera
Balsamodendron
Barley
Bassia latifolia (E)
Bland oils
Blapheris edulis
Bombax Malabarica
Boswelia
Buchanania latifolia
Carrot seeds (E)
Cœsalpinia bonducella
Cetraria
Choclospermum gossypium
Clitoria ternata
Coccos nucifera
Corchorus elitórius
Cucumis
Curculigo orchioides
Curcuma Angustifolia
Figs
Flax seed
Fraxinu ornus
Guizotia olifera (E)
Glycerrhiza glabra
Gossypium herbaceum
Gracilaria lichinoides
Helecteris Isora
Hibiscus
Iron wood tree
Isinglass
Lactuca sativa
Lichen odoriferous
Linum usitatissimum
Liquorice
Malva sylvestris
Marsh mallow
Methi seeds
Momordica chinchinensis
Mussonda Frondosa
Nymphœa
Oatmeal
Ocimum
Olive oil
Oriza sativa
Papaver somniferum
Pedalium murex
Phyllanthus madraspatensis
Pistacia vera
Plantago ispaghula
Polygonun officinalis (E)
Pongamia glabra
Pulmonaria officinalis (E)
Pyrus cydonia
Quince seeds
Salep
Salvia officinalis
Saccharum officinarum
Sessamum orientale
Shorea robusta (D)
Spinacea oleracea
Starch
Sterculia fœtida
Strychnos potatorum
Theobroma cacao
Tinospora cordifolia
Tragacanth
Tribulus terrestris
Trigonella fœnum græcum
Triticum
Ulmus fulwa
Vateria indica (E)
Viola odorata (E)
Zea mays

Dental Anodynes. *(See Vol. I, page 396.)*

Aconite
Capsicum
Caryophillum
Cocaine salts
Eucalyptus
Gaultheria
Guaiac pulv
Hazeline
Opium
Thymol

Dentifrice. *(See Vol. I, page 396.)*

Acid benzoic
Cinchona cortex
Cinnamon
Cornus florida
Iris florentina
Myrrh, as disinfectant

Cinchonæ rubræ pulveris 2 drs., capsici pulveris 15 grs., potassii chloratis pulveris 1 dr., pulveris aromaticus 2 drs., magnesia carbonatis 4 drs., iridis florentino pulveris 8 drs., saponis castilensis pulveris 1 dr.—tooth paste.

Dentrifrice.—(*contd.*)

Cinchona cortex 2, myrrh pulv 1, caryophilli ½, ol. cinnamon ⅛, calcii carbonas præcipitatus 4, creta preparata 2—tooth powder.

Creta præcipitata 4 drs., iridis florentino pulv. 4 drs., os sepiæ pulv. 2 drs., ol. limonis 10 ms.—tooth powder.

Thymol 4, acid benzoic 90, eucalyptifolia 200, ol. gaultheris 20, ol. menthœpip 20. Dose, 1 dr. in 4 ounces of water. As an antiseptic application for the teeth.

Tinctura capsici compositæ 2 drs., spiritus vini gallici 2 ozs., tincturæ quillaja 12 drs., tinturæ gentianæ compositæ 8 drs., acidi acetici diluti 4 drs., acidi carbolici 5 ms., oleum gaultheriæ 10 ms., mix—to be used with a brush to the gums and teeth. To remove mucous deposits.

DEPRESSANTS. (*See Vol. I, page 398.*)

(a) Cerebral Depressants.

Aconite
Caffeine
Camphor
Opium

(b) Hepatic Depressants.

(1) Those which lessen the secretion of bile without producing purgative effects

Atropine, Castor oil, Gamboge

(2) Those which lessen the production of urea :

Codeine
Colchicum
Morphine
Opium
Quinine

Those which lessen the production of glycogen :

Codeine
Morphine
Opium

(c) Motor Depressants.

Aconite, indirect action to reduce the spinal circulation
Acid hydrocyanic
Ailanthus
Apomorphine hydrochlorate
Arnica
Atropine
Belladonna
Camphor, in large doses
Cannabis
Codeine
Conine
Curare
Digitalis, act indirectly by reducing the spinal circulation
Elaterium
Emetics
Eucalyptus
Gelsemium
Grindelia
Hyoscyamus
Lactuca
Lobelia
Morphine
Muscarine
Nauseants
Opium, in large doses
Phytotlacca
Physostigma
Pilocarpine
Pulsatilla
Quebracho
Quinine, in large doses act indirectly
Saponine
Spartene sulphas
Stramonium (smoke)
Tobacco (smoke)
Veratrine

(d) Renal Depressants.

These lower the function of the kidneys by lessening or suppressing the secretion of urine. They act through the circulation by stimulating the vasomotor centre and thereby contracting the renal vessels *e.g.*, opium, ergot, caffein, &c.

(e) Spinal Depressants or Sedatives.

Acid hydrocyanic
Atropine
Coniine hydrobromate
Curare
Ecballium elaterium
Eserine
Gelsemium
Hyoscine
Muscarine
Physostigimine
Quinine (in large doses)
Salix nigra
Sparteine sulphate
Viburnum
Pilocarpine

(f) Respiratory Depressants.

Aconite
Caffeine
Camphor
Conium
Gelsemium
Hydrocyanic acid
Lobeline
Muscarine
Nicotine
Opium
Physostigmine
Quinine
Saponin
Veratrine

(g) Uterine Depressants.

Acid hydrocyanic—vapour and internally
Aconite
Caffeine
Camphor
Cannabis
Conium
Emetics
Gelsemium
Lobeline
Muscarine
Nicotine
Opium
Piscidia
Quinine
Tobacco
Veratrine

Deobstruents.

Anthriscus cerefolium
Apium graveolens
Blumea balsamifera
Calotropis gigantea
Cheiranthus cheiri
Elæodendron glaucum
Rhamnus catharticus

Diaphoretics (a) Simple. (*See Vol. I, page 399.*)

Absinthium
Aconite tincture. Dose, 2 to 5 ms.
Acorus calamus (rhizome)
Agrimony tea
Andropogon citratum
Berberis lycium
Biophytum sensitivum
Calotropis gigantea
Camphor
Carthamus tinctorius
Carissa caronda
Celastrus paniculata
Chamomile
Chelidonium majus
Crinum asiaticum
Elder flowers
Guaiacum
Ichnocarpus
Ipecacuanha
Menispermine
Moringa pterygosperma, root
Nyctanthes arbortristis
Opium
Salvia officinalis
Sanguinaria
Serpentaria
Sida acutangula—root
Tea
Zingiber officinalis

(b) Refrigerant Diaphoretics.

Aconite
Capsicum
Eucalyptus
Guaiacum
Ipecacuanha
Jaborandi
Lappa
Lobelia
Opium
Origanum
Pilocarpine
Physostigma

(c) Nauseating Diaphoretics.

Ipecacuanha
Lobelia
Sassafras
Senega
Serpentaria
Stillingia
Sumbucus
Tenacetum
Tobacco
Ulmus
Xanthoxylum

Discutients, Resolvents or Sorbefacients. (*See Vol. I, page 400.*)

Apium graveolens, with linseed or barley meal, used as a poultice on swollen glands
Bryonia, to promote absorption of effusion in glands
Camphor
Cocao butter
Gundha biroza
Ichthyol
Moringa pterygosperma, poultice of the leaves to reduce glandular swellings
Phytolacca, locally
Papaw juice
Rumex crispus like sarsaparilla

Diuretics. (*See Vol. I, page 401.*)

Abelmoschus esculentus
Acanthodium hirtum, in high coloured urine
Acid benzoic, on the bladder
Actea racemosa—hydragogue, diuretic
Adonis vernalis, tincture, 10-30 ms. as a hydragogue diuretic
Ærva javanica, used in lithiasis and strangury
Agava americana
Althein
Arctium lappa
Asparagin, with potassium bromide as stimulant diuretic
Azema tetra cantha, in dropsy
Balsam peru on the bladder
Berberis aquifolium
Betula, extract or oil
Blatta orientalis, as stimulant diuretic
Boerhavia diffusa, in dropsy with scanty urine
Broom tops—hydragogue diuretic, in dropsy, due to renal disease
Buchu, as stimulant diuretic to act on the bladder
Cannabis, as stimulant diuretic
Capsicum, as a stimulant diuretic
Centaurea behen
Chelidonium majus—infusion in dropsy
Citrulus vulgaris
Convallaria, as a hydragogue diuretic
Crysanthemum coronarium
Cubebs, stimulant diuretic on the urethra
Cynodon dactylon
Damiana, on the urethra
Erythrophlœum, as a hydragogue diuretic
Eugenia jambolana
Fabiana imbricata
Fennel, stimulant diuretic
Galium aparine
Gaultheria oleum
Gaozaban
Geranium maculatum
Gokharu
Guaiacum, stimulant diuretic
Horse radish
Humulus lupulus
Hydrangea
Ichnocarpus fruitescens
Illicium verum
Iridin
Juglans nigra
Juniper oil, as a stimulant diuretic in dropsy
Lichen
Linum usitatissimum
Moringa pterigosperma
Myrtus chikan
Nymphœa edulis. Decoction
Pareira root
Parsley
Pedalium murex
Petrosilinum
Pakhan bhed
Pichi
Piper angustifolia
Polygonum
Pulsatilla tincture, 2-10 ms.
Quillaja saponaria
Rhus coriaria
Rosmary
Rubus chamemorus
Sambucus
Santalum album
Scopola carniolica
Sessamum orientale
Silajita
Solanum jacquini
Spartene, as a hydragogue diuretic
Squill, as hydragogue diuretic
Strychnine
Sugars of milk
Tamal patra
Theobromine, as a hydragogue diuretic
Tobacco, hydragogue diuretic
Trayaman
Triticum repens
Turpentine, stimulant diuretic
Urginia scilla
Uva ursi, stimulant diuretic
Viola odorata
Water
Zea mays, stimulant diuretic

Eliminants.

Medicinal agents excreted in the milk when taken by the nursing woman are :— The oils of anise, cumin, copaiba, cubebs, garlic, dill, turpentine, worm wood, castor oil. The active principles of rhubarb, senna, scammony, castor oil, opium, atropine, hyoscyamine, indigo, turpentine ; copaiba if given to the mother can be detected in the urine of the child. Opium given to the mother may narcotize the child; mercurials may salivate. Atropine and hyoscyamine have been found in the milk after their ingestion by the woman.

Emmenagogues. (*See Vol. I, page 402.*)

Actæa racemosa, to restore menses
Aletris farinosa
Aloes with iron (indirect), in torpor, a few days before the period
Andropogoan muricatus
Anthemis nobilis
Apium graveolens
Aristolochia
Asafetida (direct), with aloes in torpor
Bambusa arundinacea
Baptisia tinctoria
Betula oil
Cadaba Indica
Cambogia
Capparis trifoliata, with myrobolans and ginger
Carrot seeds
Caulophyllin (direct)
Cedreia toona
Chamomile
Cinnamon (indirect), causes the flow of blood to the uterus
Collinsonia
Common rue
Crocus sativus
Crotolaria juncea
Digitalis (direct)
Ergot (direct), to restrain hœmorrhage
Erythrina indica
Ferula persica
Fœniculum vulgare
Gossypum herbaceum, decoction of the root, extract 10—60 ms.
Guaiacum officinalis (direct), in torpor of the uterus
Hedeome oil (direct)
Hydrastine indirect
Hyssopus officinalis
Indigo, 1 dr. (direct)
Juniper
Lupinus albus
Myrrh, in torpor (direct)
Nardostychos jatam ansi
Nigella sativa
Nux vomica, with iron in hepatic torpor and anæmia
Origanum oil (direct)
Pœonia officinalis
Papaya juice and seeds
Parsley
Peganum harmala
Penny royal
Petroselinum sativum
Plumbago rosea
Polygonum alone ½ dr, or with iron (direct), in anæmia before the period
Quinine (indirect)
Ruta graveolens, atony of uterus, or ovary
Sabina oil (direct), 20 ms. in atony
Salvadora persica, the root bark
Sanguinaria
Santonin before the period
Strychnine (indirect)
Tansy (direct)
Thuja
Thyme (garden)
Trigonella fœnum grœcum
Viscum flavescens (direct)
Xanthoxylon
Yarron
Zende bedaster

External remedies.—Hot hipbath, leeching to the genitals, rubefacient to the thighs.

Emetics. (*See Vol. I, page 402.*)

Allamanda cathartica
Alangium lamarkii
Apomorphine hydrochloride
Aristolochia
Asclepias
Barrintonia acutangula—
Brassica campestris
Bryonia root
Calamus
Catotropis gigantea
Cerbera odollum
Codeine hydrochloride
Common salt and hot water
Condurango
Crinum asiaticum
Emetine
Erythrophlœum
Eupatorium
Ipecacuanha
Jatropha curcas
Lagenaria vulgaris
Luffa amara
Naregamia alata
Phytolacca
Pilocarpine
Pœderia fœtida
Quabain
Randia dumatorum
Sapindus trifoliatus
Sanguinaria canadensis
Sabadilla
Sedum acre
Thevetia nerii folia
Tobacco
Tylophora asthmatica, with tartar emetic
Viola odorata—nauseating
Walsuria piscida

Formula.—Compound emetic powder—contains ipecacuanha 2, lobelia 2, blood root 1, Dose, 30 to 90 grs,

Enemata and Injections.

Injections.—These are liquid preparations used for introduction into the cavities of the body by means of a syringe.

Enamata.—Enemas or clysters. The term is applied to preparations thrown into the rectum. The agents used may be demulcents, laxatives, nutrients, stimulants or vermifuges. They are incorporated with warm or tepid water.

Enemas.—Simple enema contains soap, common salt and warm water. Warm water enema contains gruel or warm water with soap, turpentineand castor oil.

Medicated enema contains aloes, asafetida, tobacco, opium, &c. Starch enema—starch boiled or rice boiled with laudanum, in extreme cases.

Nutrient enemata contains materials for artificial digestion ; it should not exceed 4 ounces, should be acid to secure osmosis, as rectum is not an organ of digestion, and to be repeated every 6 hours. It contains olive oil, opium, pepsine, soup, starch, brandy, &c. ; there are clysters enema containing glycerin or any similar fluid along with acetate of lead or dilute hydrochloric acid or yolk of eggs.

Errhines and sternutatories. (*See Vol. I, page* 403.)

Anacyclus pyrethrum
Arnica montana
Artemisia sternutatoria
Boldo, leaves
Calotropis gigantea (dried milk)
Camphor
Capsicum
Canscora decussata
Chamomile
Convallaria
Cubebs
Euphorbium
Ginger
Hellebore
Ipecacuanha
Lobelia
Menthol
Quillaja saponaria
Sanguinarine
Saponaria vaccaria
Sassybark
Thalictrum foliosum
Tobacco (snuff)
Veratrum
White hellebore

Expectorants. (*See Vol. I, page* 404.)

Abrus precatorius
Acacia arabica
Acid benzoic (stimulant)
,, camphoric
Adhatoda vesica
Agaricin
Althœa officinalis
Alhagi maurorum
Ammoniacum
Apocynum
Apomorphine hydrochloride (nauseating)
Asclepias
Balanitis roxburghii
Balsam tolu
,, peru
Balsamodendron gummifera
Buchanania latifolia
Boswelia carterii
Caparis spinosa
Chekan
Citrarin
Emetine (nauseating)
Euphorbium
Galbanum
Garlic (stimulant)
Glycerrhiza glabra
Grindelia
Guaiacum
Inula
Ipecacuanha and squill (nauseating)
Justicia adhatoda
Lactuca sativa
Liquid amber orientalis
Leucas cephalotes
Lobelia (nauseating)
Marrubium vulgare
Mastiche
Nelumbium speciosum
Nux vomica
Onion
Pinus sylvestris (stimulant)
Papaver rhœas, syrup. Dose, ½ to 1 dr.
Pilocarpine hydrochlorate (nauseating)
Polygonum aviculare
Prunus virginiania
Quebracho (nauseating)
Quillaja saponaria
Saccharine substances
Sanguinaria canadensis
Saponin (stimulant)
Senega (,,)
Solanum jacquini
Squills (stimulant) for catarrh
Strychnia (stimulant)
Tar (stimulant)
Terpentine
Tylophora asthmatica
Urgenia scilla
Veratrum album
Viola odorata, purple flowers
Wood tar (stimulant)
Zizyphus vulgaris

Febrifuges.

Ailanthus
Anthocephalus cadamba
Aralia guilfoylia
Artemisia
Alstonia scholaris
Berberis aristata
Bonducnuts
Calendula officinalis
Cedrela toona, bark, infusion
Cinchona
Clerodendron inerme
Desmodium gangeticum
Dichroa febrifuga
Embelia ribes
Eucalyptus oil
Gentian root
Hollarrhena antidysenterica, bark
Melia azadirachta. Decoction. Tincture
Nagar moth
Ophelia chiretta
Parsley
Picrœna excelsa
Picrorrhiza kurroa, rhizome
Pittosporum floribundum
Quinine
Quassia
Salix nigra
Samadera indica
Soymida febrifuga, bark
Strychnos calubrina
,, nux vomica, seeds
Swertia chirata
Tinospora cordifolia

Galactagogues. (*See Vol. I, page 405.*)

Alstonia scholaris
Anise
Asparagus racemosus
Black tea
Dill
Erythema Indica
Fennel
Galega purpurea
Gossypium. Decoction of the root or emulsion of seeds useful
Ipomæa digitata, given with wine
Jaborandi, objectionable as it causes profuse sweats and salivation
Jatropha curcas, milky juice
Nigella sativa, decoction of seeds
Peganum harmala
Paucidanum graveolens
Pilocarpus, very useful in nursing women to increase the milk
Physostigma
Pulsatilla
Ricinus, extract, or decoction internally, or infusion or leaves locally to the breasts
Sage
Vanilla

Attention to sore nipples. Give tonics. Correct anæmia, exposure to fresh air; hot infusion of fennels as fomentation to the breasts, succulent food.

Formula.—Ricini Fol., 1½ dr.; fœniculi, 1½ dr.; anise, 1½ dr.; extract gaultheria, 15 grs.; aquæ, 3 oz. Dose, 1 oz.

Galactafuge—Lactifuge. Antigalactics. (*See Vol. I, page 435.*)

These agents are opposed to galactagogues. They are measures which reduce or dry up the secretion of milk.

Agaricus with potassium iodide
Allium cepa
Anethi fructus
Apiol leaves, locally
Atropine internally and locally 4 grs. to 1 oz. of water round the breasts
Belladonna internally and locally
Bandaging the breasts to cause compression
Chavica, warm leaves
Camphor and Glycerin locally
Collodion
Conium used in enlargement of the breasts with profuse secretion of milk
Desmodium trifolium
Jasminium sambac, to arrest secretion in cases of milk abscess
Parsley, leaves applied hot to the breasts
Quinine
Sinapism

Hypnotics and Soporifics. (*See Vol. I, page 405.*)

Boldoa fragrans
Camphor monobromate
Cannabine tannate, 2 to 10 grs.
Cannabis indica
Codeine
Coninæ hydrobromate, amotor depressant
Digitalis
Duboisine
Ergot, as cardiac tonic
Gelsemium

Hypnotics.—(*contd.*)

Humulus lupulus
Hydrocyanic acid, as pulmonary sedative against cough
Hyoscine hydrobromate, hypodermically
Jamaica logwood
Lactuca
Opium and the alkaloid
Pellotine
Piscidia erythrina, extract
Stramonium

Hæmostatics and Styptics. (*See Vol. I, page 405.*)

Absorbent cotton (locally)
Acid sclerotic
„ gallic
Asclepias carrasavica
Astragalus sarcocolla (locally)
Camphor
Capsella bursa pastoris (locally)
Colocasia antiquorum
Digitalis
Erigeon
Ergot
Ergotine, hypodermically
Galium aparine
Hamamelis useful as it contains tannin
Hydrangea
Ipecacuanha
Kalanchoe (locally)
Kino
Lanium album
Matico
Opium in uterine hœmorrhages
Plantago
Punica granatum
Pterocarpus marsupium
Rhus aromaticus
Turpentine, useful in passive hœmorrhages or in hæmorrhagic transudation on the free mucous surface
Tannin
Vegetable astringents

Irritants and Counter-Irritants (a) Rubefacients. (*See Vol. I, page 406.*)

Ajwan oil
Alluim sativum
Ammoniacum as resolvent
Andropogan citratus, volatile oil
Anisomeles malabarica, oil of leaves
Anise oil
Anthrarobin
Argemone mexicana, seeds narcotics, acrid
Balispermum montanum, oil of seeds
Cajuput oil
Calophyllum minnophyllum
Camphor
Canada pitch
Capsicum oleo resin
Chaul moogra oil
Chavica Roxburghii, long pepper
Cinnamon oil
Coal tar
Eucalyptus oil
Eugenia caryophillata
Menthol
Myrtis commune
Mustard
Myristica officinalis, expressed oil
Picea succinifera
Piper nigrum
Pitch
Plumbago rosea
Pix burgundi
Pongamia oleum
Rhus toxicodendron
Sapindus trifoliatus
Semicarpus anacardium, acrid oil
Thapsia garganica
Turpentine
Tobaccum
Volatile oils
Zingiber

(b) Vesicants.

Adonis vernalis
Andira araroha
Agiya
Ammania vesicatoria
Anacardium occidentalis
Argyrea speciosa
Bhui champa
Bhilamo
Celastris paniculata
Chelidonium majus
Croton oil, (pustulant)
Cochlearia armoracea
Chrysarobin
Climatis triloba
Daphne mezereon
Drosera peltata
Euphorbium
Gynandropsis pentaphylla
Ipecacuanha (pustulant)
Juglans cineria
Moringa pterygosperma
Oil mustard (volatile)
Plumbago rosea, root bark
Polygonum acre
Ranasura
Salvadora wightiana, root bark
Sanguinaria canadensies (escharotic)

Lithontriptics.

Acid benzoic
Caffeine
Cretæva religiosa
Feronia elephantum
Hydrangea
Pareira roots
Raphanus sativus
Terminalia arjuna
Zea mays

Mydriatics.

These agents cause dilatation of the pupil of the eye. They act by causing temporary paralysis of the ciliary muscle leading to loss of accommodation. The tension within the organ is increased and thus focussed for distant objects only. The dilatation is due to stimulation of the end organs of the sympathetic nerve leading to increased power of the radiating muscular fibres of the iris. It is also due to paralysis of the third cranial nerve, the motoroculi lessening the power of the circular muscular fibres of the iris.

When given internally they act directly or locally on the conjunctiva or through the circulation.

Anemone pulsatilla
Aconitum napellus
Anæsthetics
Atropine
Duboisine
Daturine
Homatropine and its salts
Hydrastine
Henbane
Hyoscyamus
Mydrine
Muscarine
Piscidin
Stramonium

Myotics.

These agents act by producing contraction of the pupil, by stimulating the circular muscular fibres of the iris and causing temporary contraction of the ciliary muscle. They have an opposite action to mydriatics. Under their use the eye is accommodated for near objects and the tension (intra ocular) is diminished. Some of them act upon the end organs of the oculomotor nerve. The myotic action of others is of a central origin leading to paralysis of local reflex excitabliity.

Ericolin Hydrobramate
Eserine, internally or locally. It neutralizes the action of atropine
Gelsemine internally
Lobeline, internally
Morphine
Muscarine
Nicotine (locally)
Opium to paralyse local reflex excitability
Physostigmine
Pilocarpine (locally)

Narcotics. (*See Vol. I, page 407.*)

Absinthium
Atropine
Belladonna
Camphor monobrome, to subdue reflex excitability
Cannabis sativa
Chamomile, to relieve restlessness in children
Conium tincture, to soothe restlessness in delirium
Essential oils
Erythroxylum coca
Hops
Hydrocyanic acid
Hyoscyamus
Humulus luplulus
Ignatia, to allay excitability
Lettuce
Opium and its alkaloids
Papaver somniferum syrup
Solanine
Stramonium
Strychnine, to sooth restlessness
Sumbul tincture, with chloric ether in relieve restlessness
Tobacco
Turpentine
Valerian, to allay reflex excitability

Parasiticides. *(See Vol. I, page 407.)*

Anamirta paniculata, insecticide
Andira Araroba
Anona squamosa, insecticide
Balsam of Peru
Cassia alata
Cajuput oil
Cleome viscosa, to kill maggots
Dádmurdan
Delphinium staphisagria
Derris uliginosa
Euphorbia Pilulifera
Hydnocarpus
Jatropha curcas
Karanj tel
Myrtus communis
Oil of cade
Picrasma quassioides
Pangamia glabra
Picrotoxin
Rhinacanthus
Staphisagria seeds, oil or ointment
Stercospermum xylocarpum
Storax
Sagundus margioratus, pediouli
Ventilago madraspatana

Poultices.

These are local applications or baths supplying heat and moisture to the part thereby relaxing the tissues and relieving pain. They are useful agents in subduing inflammation and in promoting suppuration. They should be applied when hot, thick or thin according to the condition of the part. In case of the peritoneum poultices should be thin. They should be covered with oiled silk and frequently changed. In size, they should cover the inflamed area, they should be applied either direct over the inflamed tissues, or some sedative or anodyne first be smeared over the tissues and then applied.

When ready they should be medicated by ammonium chloride, opium or Gonlards extract—They are prepared of the following substances :—

Alum, bran, capsicum, carbolic acid and linseed, carrot, charcoal, flour and linseed, chlorinated soda, fucus crispus (cataplasm), hemlock, hops, iodide of starch linseed meal alone or with bran, linseed meal with olive oil, mustard with linseed oatmeal, potato, slippery elm, starch, wheat bread.

Refrigerants. *(See Vol. I, page 408.)*

Adansonia digitata (pulp) of fruit
Anthocephalus cadamba
Averrhœa bilimbi
,, carambola
Aurantii succus
Borassus flabelliformis, (saccharine juice)
Byophitum sensitivum
Carissa carunda
Cicer arietinum, (acid juice)
Cichorium imtybus
Citrus, bergamia (juice of fruit)
Cocos nucifera (saccharine juice)
Diaphoretics
Embilia ribes
Flacourtia catafracta
Fruit juices
Gmelina arborea (compound decoction)
Garuga pinnata
Grape juice
Hibiscus rosasinensis (petals)
Ionidium suffruticosum, locally to head
Lactuca
Mori syrup
Nymphœa alba, syrup of flowers
Oxalis corniculata
Pterocarpus santalinus
Prunus domesticus
Rosa damascus
Rubus idœus
Tamarindus indicus
Viola odorata, purple flowers
Vitis venifera
Vegetable acids

Restoratives.—Nutritives. (*See Vol. I, page 408.*)

Almonds
Apricot
Arrowroot
Asparagus
Bombax malabaricus
Bassia latifolia
Buchanalia latifolia
Benincasa
Citrullus vulgaris
Coffee
Cucumis sativus
Cucumis melo
Curcuma angustifolia
Ceropegia acuminata
Cetraria Islandica
Chinese pumpkin
Cocos nucifera
Euryale ferox, the seeds
Ficus
Hordeum
Mangifera indica
Malt extract
Milk
Nelumbium speciosum, the seeds
Ocymum pilosum
Oryza sativa
Panax pseudoginsing
Pistacia vera
Plantain
Prunus bokhariensis
Quince seeds
Saw palmetto
Serenoa
Theobroma cocao
Trapa bispinosa
Triticum sativum
Vicia faba

Sialagogues, Topical and General.

Armoracea
Capsicum (topical)
Chrysanthemum
Cubebs (topical)
Horse radish (topical)
Hydrangea
Ipecacuanha (general)
Jaborandi
Kava kava
Lobelia inflata
Mezereon
Muscarine (general)
Mustard (topical)
Myrica sapida
Pepper
Physostigma (general)
Pilocarpine (general)
Plumbago rosea
Pyrethrum (topical)
Rhubarb („)
Tobacco („)
Xanthoxylum fraxinum
Zingiber

SEDATIVES.

(*a*) Cardiac Sedatives.—(*See Vol. I, page 409.*)

Acid hydrocyanic dilute (direct)
Aconite, acts directly by depressing muscular fibres and the cardiac motor ganglia
Adonidin.
Cactus grandiflorus
Cold
Digitalis, to stimulate the vagus centre and the cardiac muscle. It slows the frequency and rhythm of the pulse

(*b*) General Sedatives—

Anæsthetics
Belladonna
Mandragora
Opium
Piscidia erythrina [10 ms.
Pulsatilla tincture, 2 to
Rumex crispus
Tobacco

(*c*) Local Sedatives.

Anagallis arvensis
Barringatonia racemosa
Lactuca sativa
Martynia diandra

(*d*) Gastric Sedatives.

Acid hydrocyan dil
Belladonna
Cocaine
Henbane
Ipecacuanha, small doses
Opium
Prunus laurocerasus

(*e*) Nerve Sedatives.

Aconitum napellus
Camphor monobromate
Cannabis
Cocaine
Cocculus indicus
Codeine
Conium
Duboisine sulphate
Hyoscine
Lactucarium
Lobelia
Morphine
Narceine
Salix Nigra
Stramonium
Tobacco
Valerianates
Wild jasmine

(f) Pulmonary Sedatives.

Acid hydrocyan dil
Belladonna
Emetics
Lobelia
Morphine
Turpentine
Veratrine

(g) Vascular Sedatives.

Aconite
Digitalis
Emetics
Tobacoo
Veratrine

(h) Vesical Sedatives.

Barley water (mucilaginous)
Belladonna, to relieve pain
Buchu, as astringent
Cannabis, to relieve pain
Copaiba as an antiseptic
Cubebs– antiseptic
Hyoscyamus, to relieve pain
Linseed tea (mucilaginous)
Opium, to relieve pain
Pareira as astringent
Stigmata maidis, to relieve pain
Uva ursi as astringent

STIMULANTS. (*See Vol. I, page 411.*)

(a) Cardiac Stimulants.

Adonis vernalis
Aromatic oils
Cactus grandiflorus
Guaiacum
Kava kava
Menthol
Pimpinella anisum
Sumbul
Terebinthinates

(b) Cerebral Stimulants or Excitants.

Ammonia
Aromatic, volatile oils
Asafetida
Camphor
Coca
Coccos
Coffee
Convallaria
Ergot
Guarana
Kola
Nux vomica
Opium
Strychnine
Tea
Theine
Valerian

(c) Diffusible Stimulants.

Ambergris
Camphor
Nardostachys jatamansi
Strychnos nux vomica
Valeriana officinalis
Xanthoxylon rhetsa

(d) Gastric or Stomachic Stimulants.

Aromatic bitters as gentian, orange, calumba, &c.
Aromatic volatile oils
Capsicums
Mustard
Vegetable, simple bitters

(e) Hepatic Stimulants.

Acid benzoic
Aloes
Cholagogues
Colocynth
Euonymin
Hydrastine hydrochlorate
Ipecacuanha
Iridin
Jalapin
Leptandrin
Phytolacca
Podophyllin
Rhubarb
Sanguinaria
Scammony

(f) Intestinal Stimulants or Tonics.

Colocynth
Elaterium
Jalap
Podophyllin
Scammony

(1) Those affecting glandular apparatus, muscular fibres and intestinal nerves :

Aloes
Belladonna
Cascara
Frangula
Nux vomica
Physostigma
Rhubarb
Senna

(g) Stimulants (local), Cutaneous or Rubefacients.

Allspice
Argemone mexicana, oil of seeds
Asafetida
Bavachee seeds
Cajuput oil
Camphor
Eucalyptus oil
Karanj tel (the oil)
Liquidamber
Mustard
Oil of cade
Petroleum fluid
Pix burgundica
Ruta graveolens (oil)
Turpentine
Volatile oils

(h) Motor or Spinal Excitants.

Absinthin
Atropine, in large doses affecting the respiratory centre
Calabarine
Camphor
Convallaria
Damiana
Digitalis
Ergot
Nicotine
Nux vomica
Opium
Rhus toxicodendron
Strychnine, affecting the respiratory centre
Thebaine, or paramorphine

(i) Vaso-Motor Stimulants.

Belladonna, local vascular dilator
Digitalis acting on vaso-motor centres
Squill acting on vaso-motor centres
Strychnine acting on vaso-motor centres
Volatile oils acting on local vascular dilators

(j) Respiratory Stimulants.

Apomorphine
Aspido spermine
Atropine
Belladonna
Brucine
Digitalis
Duboisine
Liquidamber
Opium
Strychnine
Thebaine
Tobacco

TONICS. (*See Vol. I, page 411.*)

(a) Bitter Aromatics.

Absinthin (bitter)
Azadirachta Indica
Canella alba
Capsella bursa pastores
Cascara amarga
Chicorium intybus
Citrus aurantium
Conessi bark
Hydracotyle asiatica
Limonia acidissima
Mesua ferrea
Myrtus chekan
Nagkesar
Origanum oil
Pepper methysticum
Rhus aromatica
Rumex crispus
Soymida Febrifuga
Tinospora cordifolia—rootstem
Xanthoxylon rhetsa

(b) Cardiac Tonics.

Caffeine
Cimicifuga
Convallaria
Digitalis
Erythrophlœin
Hellaborein
Sparteine
Strychnine
Strophanthus

(c) Gastric or Stomachic Tonics.

These excite the activity of nervo muscular apparatus of the stomach.

Ægle marmelos
Alum root
Anthemis nobilis
Aromatic bitters
Aromatic oils
Atees
Bitters, vegetable
Capsicum
Coptis teeta
Coriandrum sativum
Cratæva religiosa
Cuminum cyminum
Embelia ribes
Eugenia caryophellata
Fennel
Garden angelica
Gmelina arborea
Gentiana kurroa
Kava kava
Laurus nobilis
Melia azadirach
Mentha sylvestris
Myrtus chekan
Myristica moschata
Nux vomica
Ophelia chiratta
Picrasma quassioides

Gastric.—(*contd.*)

Pimenta
Ptychotis ajwan
Punica granatum
Pungent carminatives to stimulate the local circulation
Quassine
Quinine
Strychnine
Taraxacum officinalis
Trichosanthes dioica
Vakhma infusion
Volatile oils, to excite the activity of nervo-muscular apparatus of the stomach
Zingiber

(d) Nervine Tonics.

Arnica, 5 drops to relieve aching of limbs and muscles and nerve prostration
Cimicifuga, for headache when due to fatigue or overwork
Coca, in the weakly and convalescent, who are easily fatigued under exertion
Cocaine, if exhaustion is due to loss of blood, diarrhœa, and sunstroke
Cannabinum tannate
Coffee or Tea very reviving
Conium fluid extract.
Damiana
Erythroxylon cocoa
Food fattening, highly assimilable
Kola
Lupulin
Nux vomica
Opium tincture mixed with nux vomica Tr. in headache, flushing, dyspepsia from overwork
Scutellaria fluid extract, ½ to 1 dr.
Theobroma cacao
Turnera aphrodisiac

(e) Uterine Tonics.

Abroma augusta
Aleteris farinosa
Hydrastis
Paganum harmala
Pulsatilla
Sapindus emarginatus
Savine
Viburnum prunifolium

(f) Urinary Stimulants, Vesical Tonics.

Azadirachta Indica
Copaiba
Croton tiglium
Dipterocarpus turbinatus
Lasiosiphon speciosus
Rhus aromatica

Vascular Contractors.

Belladonna
Cocaine
Digitalis
Ergot
Hamamelis
Hydrastin
Opium
Squills
Strophanthus
Strychnine

THERAPEUTICS.

Abdominal Plethora; Obesity; Corpulency.

Abdominal massage
Antifat
Fucus vesiculosus, to reduce adipose tissue
Hydragogue cathartics in congestion of portal circulation
Grape cure if the liver is engorged and sluggish
Lemon juice
Pilocarpine
Vegetable acids
Vinegar with care as it causes anæmia

Diet.—Dry diet if obesity is due to dyspepsia, hepatic enlargement or to excessive beer drinking; avoid much bread, salted or highly cooked meats, sauces, solid vegetables and fruits. (*See Vol. I, page 417.*)

Abortion; Abortifacients; Ecbolics; Oxytocics; Uterine Excitants.

Acid tannic with opium and ipecacuanha in habitual abortion
Actæa racemosa, an uterine stimulant
Aleteris, to prevent miscarriage
Ananassa sativa, essence of the juice
Asafetida, 2 grs., to check habitual abortion
Cannabis indica, in impending abortion

Abortion.—(*contd.*)

Carica papaya seeds—locally
Cascara segrada. as a laxative
Caulophyllum thalectroides to prevent miscarriage
Cimicifuga, a prophylactic in irritable and prolapsed uterus
Cotton root bark
Crotolaria juncea, seeds
Daucus carota seeds, to cause abortion
Ergot, alone or with quinine to restrain hæmorrgage in threatened abortion
Hydrastis hydrochloride, to induce abortion
Mimusops hexandra, paste of the seeds—locally to procure abortion
Oil of rue, to procure abortion
Opium and ergot, to restrain uterine hæmorrhage
Pilocarpine as an ecbolic
Piscidia
Plumbago rosea, root introduced into the os.
Plumeria acuminata, the branches inserted into the os.
Production of irritation of abdomen and pelvic organs
Savine, powdered leaves, or tincture to check hæmorrhage in threatening abortion
Semicarpus anacardium, locally to the os.
Tamponade to the cervix uteri with cotton or sponge dipped in glycerin or vinegar
Ustilago maydis, as abortifacient
Viburnum prunifolium, in habitual and threatened abortion

Abscess; Boils; Suppuration. (*See Vol. I, page 417.*)

Aconite, to abort
Albizzia leaves, as poultice
Ammoniac and mercury plaster to abort
Anona squamosa, to hasten suppuration
Arnica tincture locally as lotion to abort
Atropine, 4 grs., rose water 1 oz or glycerin 4 oz., applied locally to relieve pain
Barleria prionitis, paste of the root to disperse swellings
Belladonna alone, internally to abort, or as paint round the areola to relieve pain; liniment or plaster is used to subdue preliminary inflammation
Blisters round the seat of abscess
Biophytum sensitivum, seeds powdered mixed with butter and applied to abscesses
Camphorated alcohol or camphor carbolated, applied locally to relieve pain
Cerevisine. Dose, 1 to 2 drs. before meals to relieve pain. The yeast is veryuseful. The boils soon subside and disappear
Cocaine solution, applied locally to allay pain
Dœmia extensa; the juice, mixed with lime is locally applied to boils and abscesses
Dhatura alba, as poultice
Ferula galbaniflua, locally as a stimulant to indolent boils
Gynandropsis pentaphylla, the oil or the bruised leaves are applied locally to the boils to promote suppuration
Heliotropium indicum, leaves locally applied to gumboils
Lippia nodiflora, paste of the herb is applied to promote suppuration
Menthol, ethereal solution 1 to 2, locally applied
Mirabilis jalapa, leaves locally as poultice to hasten suppuration
Morphine and mercury oleate, to diminish induration due to old abscesses and to prevent the formation of new ones
Poultices linseed or bran, medicated, or besmeared with opium or belladonna to assist maturation; to allay pain and inflammation
Sarsaparilla, in chronic abscess with profuse discharges
Symplocos racemosa, the plaster is used to promote maturation of boils
Veratrum viride, often aborts

External Remedies.—Drainage tube after free opening of a deep abscess and irrigation of the cavity. Pressure after opening; weaning of the child in mammary abscess.

Acne; Acne Rosacea; Seborrhœa. (*See Vol. I, page 419.*)

Acid tannic, used as solution or as dusting powder with starch
Belladonna, locally to check excessive secretion from the sebaceous follicles

Acne.—(*contd.*)

Berberis tincture, 5 ms. internally in the acne of girls at puberty
Camphor with chalk powder locally
Cajuput oil as local stimulant in acne rosacea
Chrysarobin
Coca
Hamamelis fld. extract, 1 to 20 of water, applied locally
Hydrastine hydrochlorate, locally ½ p.c. solution
Quinine

Adynamia; Anæmia; Chlorosis. (*See Vol. 1, page 420.*)

Bitters, vegetable bitters
Buchanania latifolia
Caffeine
Camphor
Capsicum tincture, 15 ms. with nux vomica tincture 5 ms. in adynamia of drunkards
Cinchona alkoloids and their salts
Digitalis
Hydrastine, a good substitute for quinine to promote digestion and to improve assimilation
Nux vomica with tincture capsici in adynamia of drunkards, in weak heart with strophanthus; it stimulates the blood-making organs and is an adjunct to restorative remedies
Quinine or cinchona with arsenic useful in badly fed subjects
Sanguinaria
Sarsaparilla in syphilitic cachexia
Turpentine
Valerian

Afterpains (Uterine). (*See Vol. 1, page 420.*)

Actæa racemosa, to relieve pain and to restore lochia if suppressed
Ailanthus excelia, the juice of the bark with cocoanut milk and aromatics to stop afterpains
Atropine sulphate, $\frac{1}{100}$ gr. to lessen pain
Belladonna ointment, application to the hypogastrium
Camphor 10 grs. and morphine $\frac{1}{6}$ gr. internally
Cimicifuga, to allay nervous excitement and to relieve pain
Ergot, to prevent accumulation of clots, to keep uterus contracted, and to relieve pain
Gelsimium to stop pain
Heroin
Mentha
Morphine, $\frac{1}{4}$ gr.; atropine, $\frac{1}{100}$ gr hypodermically
Ocymum basilicum—infusion of seeds, internally to relieve afterpains
Opium, certain in action
Poultices, warm to the hypogastrium
Pilocarpine, to lessen lacteal secretion
Quinine, 10 grs. internally every morning with chloroform liniment locally to the uterine region in neuralgic afterpains
Vaginal injections of soothing drugs
Viburnum prunifolium, internally

Albuminuria. (*See Vol. 1, page 420.*)

Acid gallic or tannic, 10 grs. in the acute form to restrain albumen and hæmaturia
Aconite, to lower high temperature in acute nephritis
Cantharis with cannabis indica, as diuretic after the acute symptoms have subsided to check bloody urine
Chimaphila, as diuretic
Copaiba, to restrain renal hæmorrhage, to lessen albumen when due to cardiac or chronic Bright's disease
Croton oil liniment to the loins
Digitalis or capsicum poultices to the loins in dropsy. Infusion digitalis internally in dropsy due to cardiac disease
Elaterium as hydragogue cathartic to relieve dropsy
Ergot, to lessen albumen
Fuchsin, 1 to 3 grs. to relieve albuminuria with œdema
Hydrastis, to lessen albumen
Jaborandi in uræmia, renal dropsy or in dropsy occurring in pregnancy
Juniper oil, a fine diuretic
Pilocarpine
Pulsatilla
Rhus aromaticus, the bark is useful
Turpentine internally, to increase the quantity of urine, to check bloody urine, to lessen dropsy in albuminuria with marked symptoms of Bright's disease

Alcoholism; Alcoholic Intoxication; Drunkenness. (*See Vol. I, page 421.*)

Actæa racemosa, given in dyspepsia due to alcoholism
Apomorphine hydrochloride, hypodermically
Capsicum tincture 10 ms. alone before meals or with bromides and arsenic, or with lupulin to overcome habit, to remove distress, to prevent morning sickness, to promote appetite and digestion, to relieve restlessness and to induce sleep
Cinchona rubra, to relieve gastric catarrh of drunkards
Cocaine, to remove the craving, to restore appetite, to induce sleep, to soothe the brain, and to induce a feeling of contentment
Gelsemium, same as bromides
Hydrastine hypodermically
Lupulin with capsicum, to quiet nervous system
Nux vomica tincture, 5 ms. with capsicum 15 ms. as tonic and stimulants, to aid digestion, to relieve tremors, and to diminish craving for spirits in chronic alcoholism
Opium with tonics is given before meals to relieve pain of gastritis and to produce sleep
Orange sucked
Picrotoxin, to relieve tremors, given in small doses
Piscidia, as a soporific to those addicted to alcohol
Quinine, a nervine sedative, and to restore digestion
Strophanthus tincture in dipsomania
Strychnine nitrate, hypodermically is useful in dipsomania, to cure chronic alcoholism and craving for spirits
Strychnine with atropine, cocaine and codeine as injection hypodermically to remove habit
Sumbul, to relieve headache of old drinkers

External remedies—Stomach pump, in acute cases, cold douche to the head, warmth to the feet and limbs, artificial respiration.

Formula.—Tamarind, dates, raisins, pomegranate seeds, oxalis corniculata, each 12 grs. given internally. Dose. 1 dr. to remove habit.

Alopecia, Tinea Decalvans. (*See Vol. I, page 422.*)

Capsicum tincture with cantharides, [locally
Eucalyptus
Frequent shaving
Jaborandi
Quillaja saponaria, to remove scurf and to renew the growth of hair
Quinine lotion externally
Nutgall
Pilocarpine, as subcutaneous injection
Rosemary, as lotion combined with cantharides
Savine oil, locally
Tannin, solution or ointment locally
Thymol, locally

Formula.—Almond oil, 8 drs.; oil of rosemary, 2 drs.; liquor ammonia, 2 drs.; spirit of wine, 12 drs.; and honey, 50 drs.; as lotion for the hair.

Amaurosis and Amblyopia.

Arnica
Digitalis
Emmenagogues
Guaiacum, to improve vision in persons with rheumatic diathesis
Nux vomica
Opium with brandy or whisky to relieve dimness due to tobacco
Pilocarpine, if due to tobacco or alcohol
Rue to relieve dimness of sight due to functional causes
Santonine
Seton in the back of the neck
Strychnine, hypodermically to relieve dimness due to excess of tobacco, lead or alcohol

Amenorrhœa. (*See Vol. I, page 422.*)

Aconite tincture 2 to 3 ms., to restore the discharge if suppressed from cold and from wet feet or chill
Actæa racemosa, to restore secretion to remove headache and lessen ovarian pain
Aloes, a good emmenagogue alone or with iron
Apiol—if due to functional activity of the pelvic organs to be preceded by iron and aloes
Arnica internally is useful

Amenorrhœa—(*contd.*)

Asafetida with aloes in chlorosis
Bapticin
Berberine carbonate
Cimicifuga at the onset of the flow to relieve pain in the head, pain in back and loins and in disordered menstruation
Colocynth in chlorotic cases, with constipation
Cocculus indicus, tincture to be given prior and during the period if menstruation is irregular, scanty and painful
Croton oil
Ergot in plethoric subjects
Eupatorium, hot infusion if due to cold
Guaiacum, as uterine stimulant
Ignatia, to restore the discharges if suppressed from hysteria
Mustard hipbath
Myrrh as a tonic and emmenagogue
Nux vomica with iron
Opium is useful to restore the suppressed discharge from violent mental emotions
Polygonum with iron a few days before menses are expected
Pulsatilla, useful when the discharge is scanty or delayed by fright or chill
Quinine
Rue in atonic condition
Sauguinaria like rue
Santonine before the expected period
Savine fld. extract in general atony as uterine tonic
Senecio aureus, useful in functional ammenhorrœa, inadmissible in cases of phthisis or of anæmia
Senega root as decoction is very useful, given during the preceding few days
Serpentaria in anæmia
Tansy
Turpentine

Formula Pil.—Pulv. rutœ, ¾ gr.; ergotine, 1 gr.; aloes, 1 gr.; ol. sabinæ, ½ mn. hellebore niger, 1 gr.; ferri sulph. 1 gr.; extract gossypii herbacii, 1 gr. Make a pill mass. Dose, one pill.

2. Aloes, 1 gr.; myrrhæ, 1 gr.; croci sativi, ½ gr.; glycerrhiza extract, 1 gr.; pulv. sabina, 1 gr. make 1 pill.

Anœsmia, loss of smell.

Cerebral depressants and agents which produce changes in the nasal mucous membrane, lessen the sense of smell

Nux vomica
Strychnine, alone internally or with sugar as snuff increases the sense of smell

Aneurism. (*See Vol. I, page 423*)

Acid gallic and iron internally in aortic cases
Aconite to slow the circulation
Ergot, in any form to favour coagulation of blood in sac
Eucalyptus
Lactucarium with hyoscyamus, to promote coagulation
Morphine with atropine and croton chloral, locally to lessen pain
Posture recumbent is absolutely necessary
Surgical treatment, ligature of the vessels, or introduction, of fine wire into the sac
Veratrum viride with opium to quiet the circulation

Anorexia.

Absinthin
Anthemidis, with rhubarb and zinger
Bitters, vegetable, as berberine carbonate, calumba, gentian, chiretta, quassia, cascarilla, &c., to promote appetite
Cannabis indica, produces ravenous appetite
Capsicum, in convalescence
Carissa caronda, as adjuvant to digestion
Celerina
Cetrarin
Cinchonine
Digestive ferments as papaine ingluvin, pepsin, &c.
Eupatorium
Ignatia, in hysterics
Nux vomica with quassia
Pine apple juice
Quassia
Rhubarb with anthemedis and ginger

Angina Pectoris. *(See Vol. I, page 423.)*

Aconite is useful, but uncertain if angina is due to cardiac disease
Atropine
Cactine, in pseudoangina or in hysterical cases
Camphor with opium or with hydrocyanic acid is useful
Chamomile, if hysterical
Convallaria
Cocaine, internally and topically is useful
Coniine hydrabromate
Digitalis
Morphine, hypodermically, strengthens the heart if there is cardiac dyspnœa
Quinine, when the pain is intermittent or when malarial taint is present
Strophanthus
Strychnine
Tobacco internally to be avoided, used locally as a preventive
Turpentine, stupes to the chest to relieve paroxysms in the aged

External remedies.—Avoid fatigue, sexual excesses, climbing hills, apply issue to the nape of the neck, warmth to the extremities. Dry air is essential.

Aphonia. *(See Vol. I, page 424.)*

Aconite, to allay pain in the throat
Atropine $\frac{1}{120}$ gr. in hysterical cases and when from fatigue of vocal cords
Balsam of tolu with ether sulphuric as inhalation in laryngeal catarrh
Belladonna
Benzoin vapour, from dusting it over live coal as inhalation in laryngial catarrh
Capsicum as gargle in relaxed vocal chords
Collinsonia canadensis
Electricity, locally in hysterical or nervous cases
Ginger, to chew in the mouth or essence of ginger with water for gargle
Glycerite of tannin—locally
Ignatia like atropine
Ipecacuanha wine, as spray if congestion of vocal cords
Nux vomica
Pyrethrum tincture internally
Rue oil as inhalation in chronic catarrh
Turpentine and tannin by inhalation

Aphthæ, Aphthous Stomatitis. *(See Vol. I, page 425.)*

Abietis cannadensis, extract as gargle
Acid tannic, locally
Alum root
Callicarpa lanata, decoction of the root bark as a wash
Indian liquorice
Quinine
Quercus bark as gargle
Rhubarb
Tamarind solution as gargle

Apoplexy and Cerebral Hyperæmia. *(See Vol. I, page 426.)*

Aconite or veratrum viride, if the pulse is full and strong, skin hot and dry. Given to lower blood pressure and to prevent hæmorrhage
Belladonna
Cactus in threatening cases
Croton oil with glycerin internally, or placed on the back of the tongue
Elaterium with colocynth internally, or with soap as a rectal suppository
Opium and calomel
Paulliniæ, fluid extract. If there is severe pain in the head
Strychnine, hypodermically if respiration fails

External remedies.—Avoid stimulating food or drink, avoid exposure to hot sun and heated rooms. Give tepid bath to the body, with cold water to the head, bleeding from the arms in sthenic cases, blister to the neck, capsicum with mustard as plaster to the neck and cardiac region, cupping to the nape of the neck, electricity, embrocation of turpentine to the feet, calves and thighs, enemata of turpentine, head to be kept higher than the body, ice to the head, leeches to the anus or to the temples if congestive or hæmorrhagic tendency, loosen the tight clothes use mustard footh bath.

Arthritis Rheumatoid. (*See Vol. I, page 565.*)

Aconite, internally or externally as liniment
Cimicifuga if due to uterine derangements, the joints stiff and enlarged, and pain worse at night
Colchicum with alkalies
Counter irrilation, small blisters
Guaiacum ammoniated tincture, internally
Viburnum extract with cimicifuga internally if joints are stiff and enlarged

ASTHMA. (*See Vol. I, page 427.*)

Aconite, in spasmodic cases and in asthma following coryza or sneezing
Ajowan seeds as paint to velum palati
Ammoniacum with squills and conium in spasmodic and hysterical cases
Apomorphine, $\frac{1}{10}$ gr. with ipecacuanha, $\frac{1}{12}$ gr. internally, or $\frac{1}{12}$ gr. alone hypodermically.
Asafetida, with antispasmodics and narcotics as opium and ether given as a palliative
Aspidosperma quebracho, $\frac{1}{3}$ gr., or aspidospermine extract $\frac{1}{2}$ dr. is given to relieve dyspnœa
Atropine or duboisine, as hypodermic injection gr. $\frac{1}{100}$ to abort paroxysms
Belladonna internally if the expectoration abundant, and skin cool and moist
Caffeine citras. Dose, 2 grs.
Camphor, 3 grs., with opium $\frac{1}{2}$ gr. in nervous and spasmodic form. It is often given with musk, castor, and asafetida
Cannabis Indica, tincture 5 ms. internally in nocturnal asthma
Cocaine leaves alone as cigarettes or the solution in water applied locally to the nostrils, or cocaine $\frac{1}{2}$ gr. and morphia $\frac{1}{8}$ gr., used as injection hypodermically
Euphorbia pilulifera, the dry extract or fluid extract or decoction in asthma
Grindelia, extract 3 grs., or fluid extract 30 ms. in spasmodic form to prevent the attack
Hyoscine hydrobromate, $\frac{1}{200}$ gr. with morphine sulphate $\frac{1}{8}$ gr. and strychnine sulphate $\frac{1}{60}$ gr. as combination in spasmodic form of cardiac or pulmonary asthma
Ipecacuanha wine, in nauseant and emetic doses, given in bronchial asthma as spray or internally
Lactucarium with potassium iodide and chloral is very useful
Lobelia tincture, 10 ms. every 15 minutes during the spasm is of benefit
Morphine and atropine, hypodermically cuts short the paroxysms
Nux vomica tincture every 5 minutes in cardiac and bronchial asthma
Pilocarpine hydrochlorate, $\frac{1}{8}$ gr. at bed-time, or hypodermically in spasmodic and bronchitic asthma
Sanguinaria tincture, 20 ms. in spasmodic form and repeated till vomiting occurs
Stramonium, internally alone or with tincture of tobacco, oleum anisi, and ipecacuanha
Veratrum viride; tincture mixed with morphia and ipecacuanha is given with water in nervous asthma

Cigarettes are made of any one or more of the following :—Belladonna, grindelia extract cannabis, coca leaves, datura, lobelia, stramonium, nitre and tobacco.

Fumigation.—Dhatura leaves, eucalyptus leaves, menthol, mullein leaves, pumuline, sanitas oil, yerba santa.

Inhalation.—Ailanthus glandulosa (oil), dhatura leaves, lobelia, stramonium, leaves or root, cannabis Indica herb.

Smoking.—Adhatoda vesica leaves, dhatura leaves, eucalyptus oil, stramonium, belladonna, tobacco.

Formula.—Internally. (1)—Tinct. sanguinariæ, 1 dr.; tinct lobeliæ, 1 dr.; tinct. polygalæ, $\frac{1}{2}$ dr.; ammoniæ iodidum, 1 dr.; syrup tolutani, 6 drs. Dose, 1 dr.

(2) Extract thebaine, 1 gr.; tinct. lobeliæ, $\frac{1}{2}$ dr.; pot iodid, $\frac{1}{2}$ dr.; extract grindeliæ fld., 1 dr.; ammon carbonatis, $\frac{1}{4}$ dr.; ammon bromidum, 2 drs.; aqua laurocerosi, 4 ozs. Dose, $\frac{1}{8}$ during the paroxysms.

(3)—*Cigarettes*:—Dhatura leaves, 6 drs.; stramonium leave, 6 drs.; cannabis herb, 6 drs.; lobelia herb, 6 drs.; potassium nitrate, 8 drs.; eucalyptus oil, 6 drs.; for smoking.

(4)—*Inhalation.*—Potassium nitrate, 2 ozs.; myrrh, 2 drs.; oilbanum, 2 drs.; belladonna, 15 grs.; stramonium, 15 grs.; digitalis, 15 grs.; mix and add this to a macerated white paste of a paper, then roll into sheets and dry, used for smoking.

Astigmatism.

Atropine solution, to dilate the pupil and to paralyze accommodation for examination

Duboisine, a good substitute for atropine, rapid in effects, but has a short duration; it causes less conjunctival irritation

Atheroma—Calcareous Degeneration.

Digitalis, in general atheroma of capillary vessels is of benefit

Lemon juice retards degeneration of the vessels and hence usefnl

Quinine, 3 to 5 grs. is useful

Balanitis. (*See Vol. I., page 429.*)

Acid tannic with alcohol as a dressing after washing the part with a solution of common salt

Cleanliness to be strictly observed

Oil or vaseline to be applied locally to the inflamed part beneath the foreskin

Bedsores, Preventive and Curative Remedies. (*See Vol. I., page 429.*)

Camphor with alum and white of eggs as paint to the sore

Catechu with acetate of lead locally applied to harden the skin

Charcoal over the black slough followed by poultices

Echinacea angustifolia, the root is locally applied to the reddened skin

Lemon juice is useful locally

Styptic collodion is a nice protective

Thymol ointment is useful

Beriberi. (*See Vol. I., page 430.*)

Anodyne liniments, to allay cramps and muscular hyperæsthesia

Digitalis in small doses if beriberi is due to cardiac disease

Morphine, internally to overcome palpitation

Pilocarpine hydrochloride, subcutaneously as diuretic or diaphoretic

Strophanthus in small doses in cardiac cases

Strychnine, internally as tonic, for nervous or muscular complication

Biliousness; Dyspepsia; Duodenal Catarrh. (*See Vol. I., page 430.*)

Acid hydrocyanic dilute, to relieve irritability of the stomach

Aconite, to improve the effect of podophyllin should be given occasionally

Allamanda cathartica, as a hydragogue cathartic is useful

Aloes, extract with ipecacuanha in duodenal dyspepsia with constipation

Angustura bark, in worst forms of bilious fevers

Asafctida to remove flatulence

Berberis aristata, alone or with euonymin as an alterative

Bryonia, in bilious headache, with sluggish liver and vomiting

Buttered milk or skimmed milk is of benefit

Gynandropsis pentaphylla decoction as a carminative is useful

Hydrastis, 5 to 15 ms. of the fluid extract before meals in inspissation of bile and in gallstones with chronic gastric catarrh and dyspepsia

Mustard plaster to the stomach

Podophyllin $\frac{1}{20}$ gr. alone or with nux vomica $\frac{1}{6}$ gr. as a cathartic in children; given in hepatic torpor, to correct deficient secretion of bile

Rhubarb as a cholagogue is very useful

Stillingea with nux vomica in place of mercury is given in deficient biliary secretion; also in jaundice, cirrhosis of the liver and ascites

Bites and Stings of Insects. (*See Vol. I, page 430.*)

Achyranthes aspera, the flowering spikes, locally against stings of reptiles

Argemone mexicana, fresh root, locally to scorpion bites

Boerhavia diffusa, against scorpion bites

Calotropis gigantia, the root applied locally relieves pain and burning

Coleus carnosus, locally to relieve pain and irritation caused by stings of centipedes

Dâdmardan, locally to poisoned bites

Eucalyptus, for mosquito bites

Eupatorium (ayapana) the leaves applied to bites of poisonous insects

Bites and Stings of Insects.—(*contd.*)

Feronia elephantum, the pulp or powdered rind applied locally to bites of venomous insects
Heliotropium indicum, the juice boiled with castor oil to allay pain of scorpion bites
Ipecacuanha as poultices, or paste to allay pain or irritation caused by mosquitoes or scorpions
Krameria, locally to bites of venomous reptiles
Lime water, locally for bees and wasps
Martynia diandra, against scorpion bites
Melissa oil, against insect bites
Menthol, locally for insect bites
Onion, or tobacco poultices for scorpion bites
Penny royal, essence locally for mosquitoes
Piper longum, against the stings of reptiles
Pogostimon patchouli against the bites of gnats, mosquitoes and as insecticide
Quassia infusion, as a wash for floors infected with fleas
Sapindus trifoliatus locally to bites of venomous reptiles
Sugar pounded and applied to stings of wasps
Thymol, locally as an antiseptic, to keep off mosquitoes
Underkani, against rat bites
Veta, against rat bites
Vitex negundo, the leaves are used to preserve clothes from ravages of insect

Formula.—Paste against bites of animals, contains butea superba root nyctanthes root, woodfordia floribunda root, cassia tora seeds, vernonia anthelmintica seeds, trichosanthes palmata stem juice, mix and apply locally.

Bites—Snake bites. (*See Vol. I, page 431.*)

Acanthus illicifolius—varalians, of shoots and leaves
Aristolaochia indica, as an autidote
Baptisia tinctoria, against rattle snake
Bragantia wallichii, the juice of leaves for cobra [bites
Calmettes—anti-venous serum for snake
Calycopteris root, made into paste with that of croton oblongifolium is used for bites of phoorsa snake
Euphorbia neriifolia and E. prostrata, locally for rattle snake
Gymnema sylvestris, the root with castor oil, locally applied to snake bites
Ipecacuanha and capsicum as poultice for snake bites
Nagchampa for snake bites
Pittospermum floribundum, as antidote to snake poison
Rhinacanthus roots and leaves are regarded as antidotes
Violet, internally for rattle snake

Formula.—Eau-de-luce, mastich, 3 drs.; alcohol, 1 oz.; ol. lavand, 14 ms.; ol. succinii 4 ms.; spt. ammon. aromat., 20 ozs. mix. Dose, 10 to 50 ms. internally.

Bladder, Irritability of. (*See Vol. I, page 431.*)

Acid benzoic, to remove fœtor of urine, to render phosphatic or alkaline urine acid when due to enlarged prostate
Aqua puncture is very useful
Belladonna, 5 to 20 ms. of the tincture to relieve irritation or relaxation of the sphinctor leading to incontinence of urine
Cannabis indica, in irritation or spasm of the bladder
Cubebs, a good substitution for cantharidis, useful in vesical catarrh [useful
Eucalyptol, 2 to 5 grs. on sugar is very
Gelsemium, in hysterical women with frequent desire to urinate
Strychnine, to lessen irritability

Formula.—Internally extract jaborandi, 1 dr.; extract belladonna fluid, 1 dr. extract tritici repentis fluid, 4 drs.; extract ergotæ fluid, 6 drs.; extract rhois arom.; 6 drs.; aqua 8 drs. mix. Dose, 1 dr.

Bladder, Paralysis of.

Arnica, as a curative is very useful
Cannabis indica, in retention of urine and paralysis due to spinal disease or in spasm of the bladder
Catheterisation
Ergot, in incontinence of urine due to paralysis of the sphinctor or from overdistension; also in paralytic dysuria
Galvanism, the electro-magnetic current from the bladder to the spine
Nicotine, 4 p. c. solution, for injection
Strychnine, $\frac{1}{30}$ to $\frac{1}{20}$ gr. is of benefit

Blepharitis. (*See Vol. I, page 432.*)

Acid tannic powder or as solution, 10 grs. to 1 oz., as application locally is useful
Ergot fluid extract, locally
Hydrastis, as lotion
Pulsatilla, internally and locally

Bone Diseases. (*See Vol. I, page 433.*)

Cratæva religiosa, leaves smoked in caries of the nasal bones
Mezerion, in rheumatic and scrofulous [periostitis
Morphia and oleate of mercury, locally in nodes and periostitis
Sarsaparilla, in caries
Staphisagria, in periostitis
Stramonium leaves, locally in nodes

Breath fœtid or foul. (*See Vol. I, page 433.*)

Camphor as a corrective
Myrrh as gargle
Myrica sapida
Thymol, in solution as a mouth wash—to remove fœtor of tobacco from the breath

Bright's Disease (Acute). (*See Vol. I, page 434.*)

Aconite, as a diuretic. to lower the temperature, immediately on the appearance of nephritis, also useful in scarlatina
Chimaphila, extract 10 to 30 ms. to diminish albumen and to increase the quantity of urine
Digitalis infusion alone, or with squills and spt. ether nitrosi, given internally as diuretic, in dropsy, due to acute nephritis
Diuretics, simple as water; stimulant diuretics to be avoided
Hyoscyamus, is useful in irritable kidney
Jalap powder, if uræmic symptoms supervene to relieve the kidneys
Juniper oil, as diuretic to increase the quantity of urine
Oil of turpentine, in drop doses, controls dropsy. Turpentine stupe is useful to increase the action of the kidneys
Pilocarpine fluid extract, 5 ms., with tincture of digitalis to produce sweating

Bright's Disease (Chronic). (*See Vol. I, page 435.*)

Acid benzoic, during uræmic attacks
Apocynum cannabinum, in dropsy, ascites and anasarca
Buchu and corrosive sublimate, internally
Caffeine hydrobromate with digitalis internally
Elaterium, as a derivative, or as cathartic, to remove dropsy and tendency to uræmia
Eucalyptus in chronic desquamative nephritis
Jaborandi, 20 ms. of the fluid extract if the urine is very scanty; in uræmia 1 dr. very useful
Oleum erigerontis to lessen albumen, to lower vascular tension, to improve general condition, and to relieve uræmic symptoms
Scoparius infusion, as a diuretic
Scarifications over the kidney region

Bronchitis (Acute). (*See Vol. I, page 435.*)

Acid benzoic as stimulant expectorant or as inhalation
Aconite root, or tincture with belladonna in bronchial catarrh
Ammoniacum useful in old people
Anemone pulsatilla root mixed with milk and taken internally
Apomorphine hydrochlorate, $\frac{1}{30}$ gr., hypodermically or internally with senega infusion as an expectorant
Asafetida, useful in wheezing in old people; in bronchitis, it acts as a respiratory stimulant when the capillaries are clogged with inflammatory products and suffocation is imminent
Camphor in oil as hypodermic injection in bronchitis from cold. To be avoided in bronchitis with emphysema
Cimicifuga, extract with opium (tincture) and syrup of tolu as an expectorant after the acute symptoms have subsided
Copaiba as a nauseant expectorant after subsidence of fever
Cubebs, if secretion is copious and system relaxed
Guaiacum officinalis, in bronchorrhœa
Ipecacuanha wine in profuse expectoration, difficult to expel
Lobelia, with opium if expectoration is profuse, in paroxysmal dyspnœa

Brouchitis (Acute).—(*contd.*)

Morphine, alone hypodermicaly or with quinine internally to check excessive secretion and violent cough ; also useful to abort the attack
Muscarine, $\frac{1}{8}$ gr. with digitalis in the beginning is very useful
Opium in full doses, given with expectorants, to avert the attack, to allay cough, to check excessive secretion ; as a soporific it is very useful
Sanguinaria, in advanced stage a good expectorant
Squill syrup with paregoric elixir, in advanced stage when the secretion is copious but difficult to expel
Turpentine oil as inhalation or the stupe if expectoration is profuse
Urginea scilla
Veratrum viride, useful in the early stage

External remedies.—Ægle marmalos leaves, as poultice; croton oil liniment, or dry cupping to the chest; herpestris monieria the herb applied hot to the chest ; inhalation of steam, amber oil locally to the chest, mustard plaster, garlic poultices.

Bronchitis (Chronic), Chronic Cough ; Emphysema. (*See Vol. I, page 436.*)

Althœa officinalis
Ammoniacum, with ammonium chloride, or with ammonium carbonate; in old people with wheezing and with abundant secretion
Angelica, in catarrh of old people
Anthemidis oleum, 2 ms. ; in tenaceous expectoration
Apomorphine, alone or with morphine as an expectorant by the mouth
Asafetida, in spasmodic cough
Balsam of Peru, as inhalation, or vapour when there is copious expectoration of [pus
Balsam of tolu, internally
Benzoin, compound tincture, poured on boiling water as inhalation eases cough and lessens expectoration
Chekan, fluid extract of leaves, very useful
Cimicifuga, useful in cough of old people
Copaiba, to check purulent secretion
Eucalyptus, useful in chronic bronchopulmonary catarrh
Euphorbia pilulifera fluid extract $\frac{1}{2}$ dr., useful in asthma of chronic bronchitis
Grindelia, as expectorant in troublesome cough
Hydrastis, locally and internally in chronic coryza
Ipecacuanha, a nice expectorant, used in cough with dyspnœa as a spray ; also internally and as an inhalation
Larix europea, to check profuse bronchial [secretion
Liquorice, a useful expectorant
Lobelia inflata, in paroxysmal dyspnœa
Marubium vulgare as expectorant—a domestic remedy
Morphine, $\frac{1}{4}$ gr., with Dover's powder 5 grs , at bed time
Myrtol, in chronic bronchial catarrh, to remove fœtid expectoration
Oleum anthemidis, in bronchial catarrh with excessive secretion, but difficult to expectorate
Opium, with expectorants to allay cough when violent and frequent, and to check excessive secretion
Pix liquida, in bronchial catarrh
Poultices, linseed meal to the chest
Prunus virginiana, a nice sedative, softens secretion
Sanguinaria with lobelia and ipecacuanha, or with ammonium chloride internally or as a spray
Senega, in the aged
Squill syrup, with ammonium carbonate, in mild catarrhal cases, difficult to expectorate
Stramonium tincture, 10 ms. in the aged with dyspnœa
Strychnia, as a respiratory stimulant given with iron in the aged, to relieve dyspnœa and dry secretion
Tar, 2 gr. in pill to diminish secretion when profuse, and to allay cough
Terebene, suspended in magnesium carbonate is very useful
Terpin hydrate, 3 grs., with glycerin and syrup of Lactucarium, in chronic and obstinate cases of bronchitis
Urginia scilla, internally
Yerba sancta, fluid extract with syrup of prunes as an expectorant very useful

Bronchitis (Capillary). (*See Vol. I, page 437.*)

Camphor, to promote expectoration and to allay cough
Hydrocyanic acid, to allay spasm and cough
Ipecacuanha, as emetic if profuse expectoration but difficult to expel
Lobelia, if dyspnœa paroxysmal
Mustard poultices to the chest or as foot [bath
Oil of amber with olive oil (1 to 3), locally applied to the chest and back
Serpentaria, as a stimulant expectorant, in capillary bronchitis in children
Squill syrup, as expectorant is useful
Turpentine, as a stimulant when vital powers are depressed and circulation imperfect

Bronchocle; Exophthalmic Goitre. *(See Vol. I, page 438.)*

Convallaria, relieves painful palpitation of the heart
Digitalis in the young, raises arterial tension and slows the heart, hence very useful. It should be avoided if there is gastric irritation or irritable heart
Ergotin, internally, or as hypodermic injection into the tumour
Strophanthus tincture, 5ms., to quiet the heart's action
Stramonium with nitre to be burnt in the room to relieve dyspnœa

Bruises, Contusions, Sprains. *(See Vol. I, page 439.)*

Aconite liniment, locally to relieve pain
Ambâ halad with rivanchino siro, locally
Arnica infusion, internally or locally for bruises, and blows
Calandula officinalis, tincture as embrocation for sprains and bruises
Camphor liniment, for sprains
Capsicum tincture with gum acacia locally applied to sprains to remove discoloration
Cocaine hydrochlorate with glycerin (1 to 4), locally
Curcuma powder locally and also internally to remove black eye
Hydrastis tincture, or solution locally applied to the abraded os and cervix
Myrabilis jalapæ, the bruised leaves applied locally
Myristica oil, used locally
Odina wodier, (gum) beaten up with brandy applied to bruises and sprains
Opium with soap liniment applied or rubbed to relieve pain
Oil of bay. locally as, stimulating liniment to the contused part
Oleum menthæ piperitæ with glycerin, locally
Rosemary, as a stimulating application
Turpentine liniment for sprains

Formula—Paste containing juice of marking nut, 1 oz.; garlic, 2 oz.; tamarind (juice of leaves), 2 oz.; cocoanut oil, 2 oz.; sugar, 2 oz.; used locally in sprains, contusions

Lep or Native plaster—contains aloes, berberis, galbanum, gandha biroza, gugal, frankincense, hirabol, isus, lobân, maidâ lâkri, râl, raswanti, and rosin

Cachexia due to Anæma; Scorfula and Syphilis. *(See Vol. I, page 441.)*

Arnica, internally in bad cases, acts as an excitant of the nervous system
Cocos nucifera oil, internally and as inunction generally
Eucalyptus, a nice tonic and stimulant
Grape cure is very serviceable
Hydrastis, in malarial and splenic cachexia, very useful
Sarsaparilla of benefit
Smilax chinensis

Calculi, Biliary or Hepatic Gallstones. *(See Vol. I, page 442.)*

Cratæva religiosa, as lithontriptic, to increase the secretion of bile
Linseed or mustard poultices to the hypochondrium
Morphine, $\frac{1}{3}$ gr. with atropine $\frac{1}{100}$ gr. hypodermically as an anodyne to relieve paroxysmal spasm and vomiting
Olive oil with brandy and menthol as a prophylactic and solvent, given internally followed by a saline purgative
Sapo animalis, castile soap, very useful for their solution and breaking up
Turpentine oil and ether, to relieve pain and also acts as a prophylactic

Formula—As solvent of gallstones—chloroform, 4 drs.; ether sulphuric, 4 drs.; mucilæ acacia, 16 drs.; olei terebenthinæ, 2 drs.; sacchari albi, 2 drs. Dose, 1 dr.

Calculi, Renal and Vesical. *(See Vol. I, page 442.)*

Acid benzoic, in impacted stone
Belladonna, internally; or as suppository or as plaster or as liniment, to relieve pain of the passage of stone
Cotton root, decoction as a demulcent given internally to relieve strangury
Erigeron to relieve irritability of the bladder
Eupatorium, in uric acid diathesis
Hot fomentations, or mustard poultices to alleviate spasm and pain
Morphine, hypodermically as an anodyne and to relieve vomiting
Olive oil is very useful
Orthosiphon staminens, as uric acid solvent
Pareira, to relieve irritation due to gravel

Calculi.—(*contd.*)

Pichy, to disintegrate the calculi
Tribulus terrestris
Triticum repens, as antilithic
Uva ursi, in antilithic, in urinary gravel

Diet.—Use freely fresh green vegetables, milk, mineral waters, lemon juice—avoid sugar, fats, animal food, alcoholic beverages

Avoid the use of such substances as contain oxalic acid. Avoid black tea, cocoa, chocolate, chicory, pepper, coffee, parsley, white beans, celery, radishes, potatos, crust, crumb, barley, Indian corn, wheat, sorrel, spinach, rhubarb, cabbage, beet root, green peas, beans, tomatos, carrots, endives, dried figs, currants, plums, gooseberries, raspberries, oranges, lemons, cherries, strawberries. Avoid hard waters, tea, coffee, wines and beer.

Cancer. (*See Vol. I, page 443.*)

Acid tannic as injection into the growth
Belladonna, locally to relieve pain and internally 5 to 10 ms. as palliative
Berberis aristata, internally to relieve pain
Cannabis Indica tincture, internally to relieve pain
Chian turpentine, combined with resorcin
Codeine, as hypnotic and sedative
Condurango extract in cancer of the stomach
Conium, as poultices, and internally to relieve pain—a nice palliative
Coffee, as disinfectant; locally in fine powder
Hæmatoxylon, extract to the fungous growth
Hydrastis, as palliative, locally very useful
Hyoscyamus, leaves bruised and applied locally
Morphine salts, hypodermically or morphine dissolved in glycerin and applied locally
Opium as a palliative, locally and internally to relieve irritation and pain
Poultices of starch
Phytolacca fluid extract internally, the juice of the leaves with chloride of zinc and opium applied externally
Rumex acetosa very useful to relieve the pain and to cut short the growth
Terebinthina chia, with sulphur internally in pill

Carbuncle, Anthrax. (*See Vol. I, page 445.*)

Arnica, extract as strapping and internally
Belladonna or opium, extract with glycerin locally to relieve pain
Borassus flabiliformis as poultices
Boswelia floribunda, locally as *lep*
Echinacea angustifolia, as anti-suppurative, applied locally
Galbanum and opium plaster, to relieve pain
Ipecacuanha alone as poultice or with morphia internally
Poultices, linseed
Turpentine or terebene, as antiseptic locally
Withania somnifera, leaves and root bruised and applied locally

Catarrh Nasal (Acute). (*See Vol. I. page 446.*)

Abies canadensis, with glycerin as injection (1 to 4), into the nose
Acid hydrocyanic dilute, in bronchial catarrh
Aconite Tincture, ½, to 1 m., alone is useful in commencing cold in the head or in severe cold in the head, or in severe cold with headache, chilliness, aching of limbs; also given in catarrh accompanying measles. Given internally with belladonna (1 to 2) in high fever, sore throat, and as a liniment it is applied to the nose
Belladonna tincture, 5 to 10 ms., internally or 1 in 5,000 as a spray in acute catarrh with profuse watery secretion
Camphor spirit, as vapour for inhalation or with opium and ammonium carbonate in powder as snuff to break off or modify cold
Codeine, as palliative in common cold
Conii extract, as a spray (1 in 50)
Cimicifuga, as expectorant in rheumatic cold, pain in bones, headache
Cocaine sulphate solution, 5 p.c., locally or the powder 5 to 10 grs. to 1 oz. of cosminol as spray into the nose. It causes contraction of the venoussinuses of the nasal mucous membrane

Catarrh.—(*contd.*)

Cubebs tincture, internally with infusion and of linseed. or as confection, in cold, headache or as cigarettes to smoke as palliative in the dry and congestive stage of cold in the head, or as insufflation

Cold powder, against cold containing camphor 5, dissolved in ether, ammon carb 4, and opii 1. Dose, 3 to 10 grs. as a prophylactic

Coptis teeta, with berberis asiatica used as a snuff

Datura, dry leaves as smoke

Eclipta alba, the juice of leaves with ajowan seeds internally in catarrh

Eucalyptol, contains acid saliyclic 6, acid carbolic 1, eucalyptus 1, alcohol 10. Dose, 1 to 3 ms. internally, or 5 to 10 ms. to 1 oz. of cosminol as spray

Eupatorium perfoliatum, infusion internally in general cold

Euphrasia useful in coryza

Ipecacuanha wine, as spray to the fauces, or with opium internally for acute nasal and bronchial catarrh and cold.

Jaborandi, fluid extract 10 ms. internally or $\frac{1}{8}$ gr. of pilocarpine hydrochlorate, aa hypodermic injection for abating a cold and as a diaphoretic

Menthol alone 2 to 10 grs. with 1 oz. of cosminol as spray or menthol with chloroform (1 to 10), to inhale through the mouth and nose alternately. It relieves cold in the early stage or arrests its progress

Nux vomica in dry cold in the head is very useful

Oil as inunction, to the whole body will prevent susceptibility to cold in the head

Opium, with whisky toddy, and belladonna at night will abort the attack

Pilocarpine hydrochlorate, $\frac{1}{16}$ gr. gives relief

Pulsatilla, a good substitute for aconite, useful as lotion (1 in 20) to syringe the nasal passages in coryza with muco puruent secretion To be avoided if there is gastro-intestinal irritation

Quinine 10, with morphiæ $\frac{1}{8}$ gr., to abort acute coryza

Rhatany with gelatine, as Bougies for the nose

Sugar finely powdered as a snuff, in catarrh due to potassim iodide

Thymol, 5 to 10 grs. to 1 oz. of cosminol as a spray

Thalictrum foliosum, as a snuff in coryza

Terebene, 30 grs. to 1 oz. of cosminol as a spray

Turmeric, burnt and fumes used for inhalation or as a spray

Catarrh (Chronic Nasal.) (*See Vol. I, page 447.*)

Acid tannic solution, with rectified spirit as nasal injection or tannin with glycerin or with acid salicylic, bismuth, calomel, and white sugar as snuff or as insufflation

Agati grandiflora, the juice of leaves and flowers is blown up the nostrils with relief

Ammoniacum with ipecacuanha and ammonium carbonate internally to lessen the secretion

Asafetida, as stimulant expectorant.

Benzoin and opium over a piece of hot iron as fumigation, useful in chronic rhinitis

Cocaine is useful with tobacco snuff and astringent powders for chronic catarrh

Cubebs powder, blown into the nose or as insufflation, or smoked or given internally, is useful in follcular, nose and pharyngeal disease

Hamamelis is used as snuff

Hydrastis, tincture internally, or with water injected by syringe in coryza with ulceration of the septum nasi

Pulsatilla, 1 in 20 as a wash in subacute inflammation of the nose with fœtid discharge of mucus and pus

Sanguinaria, tincture 10 ms. internally, or as dusting powder locally to the nose in nasal catarrh

Turpentine oil, as liniment to the chest

Formula.—(1) Menthol, 2 ; coffee powder, 50 ; cocaine hydrochlorate, 1; acid boric, 100 ; as snuff, in nasal catarrh.

(2) Sodii chloridi, 120 ; pot. chlorate, 50 ; ammon. iodide, 2 ; acid carbolic, 8 ; camphor pulv., 8 ; hydrastis rad. pulv., 20 ; mix as a snuff, in nasal catarrh.

Catarrh (Bronchial) Bronchorrhœa. (*See Vol I, page 439.*)

Agaricin
Ammoniac
Asafetida, very useful
Copaiba as stimulant expectorant, but is nauseant, to lessen copious secretion of pus
Cubeb, in chronic bronchitis with profuse secretion
Eucalyptus oil, 2 ms. on sugar internally
Grindelia, as a respiratory stimulant, very useful
Myrtol, eliminated by the lungs, as stimulant and antiseptic, useful to remove fœtor and check profuse secretion
Pinus sylvestris oil, as inhalation
Terpin hydrate, or turpentine oil, as stimulant, expectorant for inhalation by an atomizer or internally

Catarrh of the Bladder or Urethra.

Betol
Hydrastis tincture
Juniper
Pareira brava
Pix carbonis liquida
Quercus infectorius
Saccharum officinarum
Tinospora cordifolia
Zea mays

Catalepsy. (*See Vol. I, page 446.*)

Apomorphine during the paroxysm ; it causes nausea, the spasm ceases and consciousness returns
Cold douche
External stimulation to arouse consciousness
Faradization
Restoratives
Tonics
Turpentine, as enemas or embrocation along the spine, to stop the paroxysms

Cerebral Anæmia. (*See Vol. I, page 448.*)

Asafetida, as cerebral excitant
Caffeine, in hypochondriasis
Guarano, as a restorative after acute disease
Mustard liniment, in spinal anæmia
Serpentaria, as cerebral excitant
Strychnine, with iron to stimulate the circulation and as a tonic
Valerian, as cerebral excitant

Cerebral Concussion.

Arnica, if due to a fall is very useful with warmth to the extremities and rest;
Remedies which are useful to recover from collapse and insensibility, to prevent inflammation, and to restore impaired faculties

Cerebral Congestion. (*See Vol. I, page 448.*)

Aconite, a good remedy in the active form
Belladonna, in hyperæma of the brain or cord
Cathartics, as colocynth to lessen the blood pressure
Colchicum, in plethoric and gouty subjects
Croton oil or scammony or elaterium, as cholagogue
Ergot fluid extract with sodium bromide internally
Mustard, foot bath
Venesection is good to prevent injury to the brain ; it should be avoided in anæmia, aortic disease, or in cases commencing with syncope

Chapped, Sore and Fissured Hands, Feet, Lips and Nipples.

(*See Vol I, page 449.*)

Balsam of Peru or Tolu with almond oil, gum arabic and rose water locally
Benzoin. compound tincture with glycerin locally applied
Hydrastis, as lotion used as a compress
Menthol, with salol, locally applied to relieve pain
Rhatany powder with glycerin and water as a wash, or with cerate locally in fissures of the nipples
Starch with glycerin and rose water locally

Chest Pain.

Belladonna, as ointment applied in hyperæsthesia of the skin of the chest

Bryonia, useful in painful chest with catching of breath

Cimicifuga, in pain under the breasts and for intercostal pains

Strychnine gives relief to wandering neuralgic pains due to nervous irritability

Chilblains. (See Vol. I, page 450.)

Acid tannic with iodine made hot and applied to the body

Avoid application of vaseline and other fatty substances to the body

Balsam of Peru ointment to separate sloughs

Benzoin, compound tincture with glycerin applied after thoroughly washing and drying

Brassica, cabbage leaves as varâlians

Cajuput oil, locally applied

Capsicum tincture, with gum arabic locally applied in unbroken skin relieves itching and pain

Camphor cream or camphor with eau-de-cologne locally with friction

Digitalis, infusion or tincture, internally to improve circulation, to relieve arterial tension and peripheral vaso-dilatation

Galls with opium, turpentine and spirit of wine locally

Opium tincture locally

Thiol powder, locally applied

Turpentine alone as a wash or with basilicon ointment used as a local application

Cholera Asiatica. (See Vol. I, page 451.)

Acid tannic, by enemata

Aloes or castor oil as evacuant in the early stage

Argemone Mexicana oil, as laxative, combining the action of castor oil and cannabis

Atropine hypodermically, $\frac{1}{100}$ to $\frac{1}{60}$ gr. in collapse

Caffeine citras, as a diuretic

Camphor spirit with opium tincture, capsicum tincture and chloroforn in water

Caryophylli oil, as rubefacient to the epigastrium

Cholera toxin, for hypodermic injection

Ginger with myrica sapida, locally to rub on calves

Ipecacuanha, if greenish stools with mucus and blood

Morphine, hypodermically in the early diarrhœa or in collapse to relieve cramps. To be avoided if kidneys are diseased

Musk root, as a substitute for musk

Myristica fragrans, against cramps

Opium, hypodermically to prevent collapse to check preliminary diarrhœa; to be avoided if kidneys are implicated; enema of opium with starch is very useful

Piper nigrum with asafetida, capsicum and camphor internally

Podophyllin, if stools are pasty

Poultices to the abdomen containing cloves, ginger, cinnamon mixed with brandy or whisky

Quinine hydrochloride or quinine sulphate or quinine carbamide as hypodermic injection

Starch and opium as rectal injection

Strychnine, as prophylactic, in the early diarrhœa as stimulant to prevent collapse

Turpentine oil, 10 to 20 ms. as stimulant

External Remedies.—Saline injection of table salt is used alone or as saline intravenous injection in collapse; saline injection contains sodium chloride, 1 dr., sodium carbonate, 1 dr.; warm water, 8 pints; milk by transfusion during collapse; irrigation of intestines with soap and hot water; absolute rest, recumbent posture; mustard to the heart or to the neck; warm milk by enema; fresh air; heat to the abdomen, legs and feet; Ajowan, made hot, or cajuput oil to rub over the skin during collapse.

Formula.—In the early stage acid carbolic, 2 ms.; capsicum tincture, 2 ms.; asafetida, 2 grs.; piper nigrum, 2 grs.; spiritus vini gallici, 1 dr.; aqua, 1 oz. for a dose.

Extract cannabis indica, 1 gr.; camphora, 2 gr.; chloroformi, 8 ms.; olei terebinthinæ, 4 oz.; mucilage, 2 dr. Dose, 10 to 20 ms.

Chloroformi, 30 ms.; spiritus ætheris sulphurici, 90 ms.; olei menthæ piperitæ, 8 ms.; oleum caryophylli, 5 ms.; oleo resini capsici, 2 ms.; extract cannabis indica, 6 grs.; morphiæ muriatis, 6 grs.; acidi hydrocyanic diluti, 16 ms.; acid hydrochloric, dilute, 60 ms.; glycerini, 4 oz. Dose, 15 to 25 drops.

Cholera Infantum. (*See Vol. I, pge 452.*)

Camphor spirit in milk for choleraic diarrhœa
Coto bark tincture, 1 to 5 ms. is useful
Ipecacuanha, if stools are greenish with mucus and blood
Morphine with ether hypodermically
Mustard foot bath or mustard plaster over the heart
Poultices of cloves, ginger, cinnamon mixed with brandy and linseed
Tea, weak solution to be drunk freely to keep vessels filled and prevent paralysis of the heart

Cholera Simplex. (*See Vol. I, page 453.*)

Atropine, hypodermically
Cajuput oil locally is very useful
Castor oil with opium internally
Ginger wine, internally
Ipecacuanha, internally used with benefit
Morphine, hypodermically internally
Mustard internally as an emetic in collapse and as a cardiac stimulant
Salol, internally very efficient
Sumbul, very serviceable
Veratrum album, to check vomiting

Chordee. (*See Vol. I, page 453.*)

Aconite, 1 mn. of the tincture gives relief to chordee
Belladonna, with camphor and opium internally
Bromides internally
Camphor monobromate, with lactucaria internally
Cannabis Indica tincture internally
Cocaine hydrochlorate, 4 p. c. solution locally to the glans penis or injected into the urethra to destroy erectile power
Colchicum wine, in gouty subjects
Hyoscyamus with camphor internally
Linseed tea internally
Lupuline, very useful
Morphine, hypodermically injected into the perineum
Stramonium
Tobacco, very useful

Chorea. (*See Vol. I, page 453.*)

Camphor monobromate
Cannabis Indica, internally
Cimicifuga, fluid extract in chorea due to menstrual derangements or to rheumatism
Conii succus, 1 dr. as palliative to quiet muscular agitation
Duboisine, for nervous and debilitated children
Eserine, hypodermically or internally
Hyoscyamine, hypodermicallyvery useful
Morphine with chloral, in large doses to procure sleep
Physostigmine, hypodermically is useful
Quinine, as stimulant to the inhibitory centres which control motor discharges from the spinal cells and which are weakened in chorea
Scutellaria, to calm the nervous system
Stramonium tincture, internally
Strychnine, in chorea due to fright or commencing puberty
Valerian if due to worms, to restrain undue movements

Colic Intestinal, Renal, Hepatic and Lead. (*See Vol. I, page 455.*)

Ajowan, internally or as poultice
Allamanda cathartica,in lead or painter's colic
Argemone Mexicana, the oil to relieve pain
Atropine, with potassium iodide, relieves colicky pain and assists in removing lead poison
Asafetida emulsion, in flatulent, intestinal colic, in children and in hysterics
Belladonna, in children to relieve intestinal spasmodic colic
Blumea balsamifera, powder of the leaves as antispasmodic in intestinal colic
Cajuput oil, locally to the abdomen followed by poppy seeds fomentation
Calotropis gigantea, the leaves besmeared with oil are used as varâliâns
Camphor oil

Colic.—(*contd.*)

Carminatives as allspice, anise oil, anethum, cardamoms, rue, ginger, cloves, cinnamon, capsicum, &c., useful in flatulut colic
Castor oil and turpentine ennema. or castor oil with opium internally gives relief
Caryophyllum, infusion, or volatile oil
Chamomile oil, with sugar in intestinal colic in hysterical women
Cocculus villosus, of great value, in intestinal colic during pregnancy
Coleus aromaticus, used as antispasmodic
Croton oil with opium is very effectual when other remedies fail in lead colic
Counter irritation, as flying blisters for renal colic
Essential oils, to relieve flatulence
Ipomæa pescapræ, the leaves applied as varalians to the abdomen
Linseed, tea or poultices
Matricaria infusion during bathing
Mentha piperita, oil, internally
Morphine, hypodermically, or internally in all forms of colic
Mustard plaster
Myristica officinalis oil internally
Nux vomica, with nitrate of silver and hops internally, to subdue abdominal cramps and spasms
Olive oil duiing the attack gives relief in renal and hepatic colic
Oil of turpentine, is useful in ileus, colica pictonum, flatulence, decomposed bile ; in renal colic it stops spasms of the ureters
Opium, with morphia or with chloroform, useful internally in flatulent colic and in hepatic colic
Opium tincture with alum internally is of benefit. (Alum converts the poisonous salts of lead in the system into innocuous sulphate of lead.) To be followed by a dose of castor oil to relieve the pain
Tobacco by the mouth may control colic but is dangerous if given by the rectum
Turpentine is useful in biliary colic

Climacteric Disorders. (*See Vol. 1, page 454.*)

Aconite tincture, 1 mn. for nervous palpitation and restlessness
Belladonna with opium and nux vomica if the heart is fluttering, if there is fulness of the head and flushing
Camphor alone internally for drowsiness and headache, or with eau-de-cologne locally to the head in headache
Cimicifuga internally for distressing headache
Cannabis Indica, if there is much headache
Ergot with cannabis indica internally if much flooding
Nux vomica, in flushing, fulness of head, with hot or cold prespiration
Opium internally
Physostigma extract, for sensation of fluttering at the pit of the stomach and in flatulence

Chyluria. (*See Vol. 1, page 454.*)

Gallic acid in large doses gives relief
Thymol, 1 gr. internally is useful, it filaria in the blood

Collapse ; Exhaustion ; Shock ; Coldness. (*See Vol. 1, page 450.*)

Bath, with friction for cold feet
Caffeine citras and brandy internally
Camphor, solution in oil, hypodermically injected into the fore arm in collapse of pneumonia
Cocaine or atropine injection to raise the body temperature
Digitalis, with ammonia or brandy internally as cardiac stimulant
Electricity to the phrenic nerve
Friction to the limbs
Ginger powder with kantol powder for friction to cold hands and feet
Liniment terebinthinæ, locally
Morphia, hypodermically
Mustard baths
Oleum cajuputi locally [internally
Stimulants, as brandy and ammonia
Strychnine, with ether and digitalis hypodermically if failure of heart
Turpentine with cannabis, internally
Valerian internally

Conjunctivitis—Catarhal, Diptheritic, Gonorrhœal, Granular; Phtyctenular, Purulent or Strumous Ophthalmia (*See Vol. I, page 456.*)

Akakia, as a wash

Atropine, solution locally and internally very useful, as cornea is liable to slough and become hazy as in granular lids

Belladonna, locally and internally in strumous ophthalmia to relieve pain

Castor oil, as drops into the eye to relieve pain and photophobia

Cocaine hydrochlorate, solution or oleate applied to the palpebral conjunctiva as a palliative

Ergot fluid extract, in catarrhal and phtyctenular conjunctivitis

Euphrasia, as a mild astringent locally

Hydrastine hydrochlorate, as lotion if lids adhere

Jaquirity, to produce purulent conjunctivitis and thus cure granular conjunctivitis

Morphine, with zinc salts or alum, as collyria

Opium, fluid extract or wine, as drops into the eye to relieve pain and improve the condition of the conjunctiva

Physostigmine, locally in phlyctenular conjunctivitis to reduce the pupil and shut out the light

Pulsatilla tincture, in water as a wash, and internally

Rhubarb, to remove gastric disorder

Staphisagria, in tarsal ophthalmia to destroy vermin

Tannin with glycerin (1 to 8), as application in granular lids; the powder dusted over the lids in chronic catarrhal conjunctivitis with injection of vessels and œdema.

Convalescence. (*See Vol. I, page 458.*)

Achillœa millefolium, as a bitter tonic

Alstonia scholaris, compound decoction as a bitter tonic

Anthemis nobilis, as a gastric stimulant

Berberis aristata, the bark and stem as a tonic and aperient

Bitters, vegetable

Bixa orellana, as a stomachic tonic

Calumba

Cetraria islandica

Clerodendron, bitter tonic

Coca fluid extract

Cocos nucifera, internally and as an inunction

Coptis teeta tincture, bitter gastric tonic

Coscinium fenestratum bitter tonic

Guarana, highly useful

Hydrastis, to promote digestion

Opium as a rectal enema in insomnia

Picræna excelsa, a pure bitter tonic during convalescence from fever with biliousness

Portulacca compound tincture, with citrate of iron, as bitter tonic

Premna integrifolia, infusion of leaves as a stomachic tonic

Roborans syrup, containing quinine, strychnine, manganese and hypophosphites as a tonic and constructive agent

Quinine and its preparation, to promote digestion and appetite

Toddalia aculeata, as a bitter stomachic

Vegetable bitters

Convulsions—Epileptic, Hysterical, Infantile. (*See Vol. I, page 458.*)

Asafetida, given as an enema, is very useful to mitigate convulsions due to teething

Belladonna, for infants if due to teething or to whooping cough

Gynandropsis pentaphylla, as antispasmodic

Ignatia for children if due to intestinal irritation without cerebral congestion

Ipecacuanha, as an emetic

Opium is dangerous in young children efficient in adults

Valerian in children if due to worms

Convulsions Puerperal—Eclampsia of Pregnancy.

Acid benzoic, as a prophylactic and to hasten convalescence

Aconite tincture, internally to reduce the arterial pressure

Atropine, hypodermically

Belladonna tincture, internally

Caffeine citras, internally or hypodermically

Cannabis tincture, internally

Jaborandi extract. as rectal injection

Morphine, with chloral internally or alone hypodermically to relieve uræmic convulsions

Mustard poultice to the calves

Opium tincture, as enema with starch, should be preceded by free purgation

Pilocarpine nitrate, $\frac{1}{8}$ gr. to $\frac{1}{4}$ gr. hypodermically is very useful

Veratrum viride extract, internally or hypodermically, or by enema

Corns; Warts; Condylotmata. (See Vol. I, page 459.)

Anacardium occidentale, juice locally
Argemone Mexicana, the oil as a soothing application
Belladonna plaster
Chelidonium majus, as an irritant locally
Chrysarobin solution, 10 p. c., in ether or gutta percha locally for warts after they are pared down
Cocaine hydrochlorate, as a local anæsthetic
Conium, externally and internally
Papaine, locally applied
Plaster of soft material with hole in the centre over the corn
Rue, the oil with honey, locally
Savine 1, with alum 2, as caustic
Thuja tincture, internally, and also locally for warts about the anus or pudenda

Cough. (See Vol. I, page 460.)

Acid hydrocyanic dilute, in irritable cough, in cough of phthisis, and in simple nervous cough due to irritable state of the system
Anemonin is useful in irritative cough of phthisis, and in asthma
Aconite, in short dry tickling cough in the asthmatics with anxious look and in throat cough
Apomorphine hydrochlorate, in hacking cough without expectoration or with difficult expectoration
Aspidosperma quebracho, in spasmodic cough of asthma
Asafetida, owing to its containing sulphur, is useful in habitual cough
Belladonna, internally or externally as plaster to the chest in spasmodic and nervous cough
Burgundy pitch plaster to the chest to allay cough of bronchitis and of phthisis
Camphor and chloral, allays spasmodic cough if painted over the larynx
Chamomile oil, 2 ms., useful in cough in hysterical women
Codeine, ½ to ¾ grs., a mild expectorant; also laxative. It does not cause vomiting and is used to relieve the cough of phthisis
Conium, useful in highly spasmodic cough
Cubeb kept in the mouth and chewed or with linseed tea, taken internally to relieve cough of chronic catarrh, of emphysema or of influenza
Crescentia cujete (calabash), as poultice to the chest
Drosera, fluid extract, in spasmodic or phthisical cough
Euphorbia pilulifera, in spasmodic cough
Emplastrum picis as rubefacient and counter irritant to the chest in winter cough
Gelsemium, to relieve excessive irritability of the respiratory centre. It relieves convulsive nervous spasmodic cough
Grindelia, useful in habitual cough and in spasmodic cough
Gaultheria oil, useful in spasmodic tickling night cough
Herpestis monniera, the plant made hot and applied to the chest in cough and in bronchitis in children
Hyoscyamus, internally in spasmodic tickling night cough
Ipecacuanha, in winter cough with whizzing; in troublesome night cough the wine is used as a spray to the fauces; also internally as an expectorant in coughs in children
Lactucarium, useful as a vehicle for cough mixtures
Laurocerasus, useful in spasmodic cough
Linseed poultices to the throat in troublesome hacking cough
Lobelia, useful in dry spasmodic cough with tickling sensation
Marrubium vulgare, a domestic remedy in cough
Morphia acetas, alone or with glycerin as application to the fauces to relieve cough and irritation of the air passages
Morphine, with chloroform and molasses internally in paroxysmal dry cough
Nux vomica tincture, has a very quieting action in laryngeal cough of neurotic origin; also in nervous and periodic cough. It has a prompt action on the pneumogastric, hence an efficient remedy in bronchitis, pneumonia, phthisis and emphysema
Opium, internally, to allay irritation and to lessen hypersecretion. To be avoided if the secretion is copious and expulsory power feeble. Highly useful in bronchial congestion, in violent cough with little rhonchus, and in cough due to inflamed and ulcerated throat
Picis liquida or tar water, internally in winter spasmodic cough, and in cough of bronchitis and of phthisis.
Pinus longifolia, as a plaster to the chest in chronic coughs
Prunal, a stimulating expectorant to relieve cough
Prunus virginiana, contains hydrocyanic acid and hence useful in irritative cough

Cough.—(*contd.*)

Sanguinaria, with hyoscyamus in nervous spasmodic cough

Senega, as stimulant expectorant given in chronic bronchitis and in subacute chest affections

Squill syrup or as acetum, or oxymel scillæ for catarrhal cough and tickling in the throat

Tannin, with glycerin, locally to chronically inflamed throat producing cough

Terpene hydrate, in bronchial cough and in night cough

Terebene pure as inhalation or as spray

Thuja occidentalis, tincture internally in chronic cough

Tobacco smoking to relieve cough

Valerian, in asthmatical and hysterical coughs

Formula.—Mixture :—Tinct. sanguinariæ, 2 drs ; tinct. lobeliæ, 3 drs.; vin ipecac 8 drs. ; tinct. opii camphorata, 12 drs. ; syrup scillæ, 12 drs. ; aqua cinnamon, 6 ozs. Dose, 4 drs., in harrassing cough.

Formula.—(For winter cough)—Syrup picis liquidæ, 1 dr., syrup of virginian prunes, 2 drs. ; apomorphine, 2 p. c. solution. ½ dr. Dose 6 ms.

Decoction.—Viola odorata, 6 drs. ; althœa officinalis 10 drs. ; zizyphus, fruit, No. 25 ; ficus, No. 5 ; cordia laltifolia fruit, No. 10 ; glycerrhiza radix, 3 drs.; water 20 ozs. Make decoction. Dose, 1 oz.

Emulsion.—Buchanania latifolia, cucumber, dates, almonds, sessamum, as emulsion for cough.

Prunal, a stimulating expectorant, contains ammonium chloride, scillæ, senega, glycerrhiza, prunes, eucalyptus, balsams of peru and tolu, each 1 dr. ; pix liquida, pini sylvestris, heroin hydrochloride, $\frac{1}{12}$ gr. in each dram given in coughs due to bronchial and laryngeal irritation.

Croup Catarrhal, Membranous or Laryngeal; Diphtheria.

(*See Vol. I, page 465.*)

Acid tannic, as spray

Aconite, ½ mn. every hour till fever subsides

Apomorphine, as an-emetic very effective but highly depressant

Ipecacuanha, as an emetic at the outset

Mustard plaster locally to the chest

Quinine, in large doses with ammonii carbonas and senega in membranous croup

Sanguinaria, as emetic, very useful in membranous croup

Senega, as an auxilliary to emetics

Turpentine oil with almond oil internally

Cystitis (Acute and Chronic); Compare; Irritable Bladder ; Dysuria ; Eneuresis. (*See Vol. I, page 465.*)

Acid benzoic, with soda biboras, internally in chronic cystitis with enlarged prostate; it removes fœtor from the urine, and also renders the alkaline urine acid

Acid camphoric, ½ to 3 p. c. solution in hot water is used as vesical injection to prevent decomposition of urine

Buchu either alone or as infusion or the fluid extract, 10 to 30 ms. with tincture conii and morphine sulphate is given internally in chronic cystitis, in cystic catarrh complicating the ureters or the kidneys leading to muco-purulent discharge

Belladonna, extract locally as suppositories or internally as tincture, 5 ms. acts as a sedative to relieve any form of vesical irritation. It is useful in vesical catarrh due to chill attended with pain ; in nocturnal incontinence due to relaxed sphinctor of the bladder it is very useful

Benzoate, of alkalies with glycerin, useful when the urine is alkaline

Chimaphilla is given internally as a more active diuretic in chronic cystitis than pareira or uva ursi

Cystitis, &c.—(*contd.*)

Cannabis Indica, an excellent anodyne in cases of dysuria with irritability of the bladder and spasm of the neck

Cantharides, internally in dysuria, vesical catarrh, enlarged prostate, and in chronic cystitis—large doses cause inflammation of the urinary tract

Cessampelos pareira, in chronic cystitis

Cocaine solution, 5 p. c, injection into the bladder to relieve dysuria

Colchicum, internally with pareira brava or buchu, in cystitis with alkaline urine

Collinsonia canadenses, with morphia and aconite useful in acute cystitis

Cotton root, decoetion, useful to relieve strangury

Copaiba, alone or with cubebs ; is useful for its local action on the mucous membrane, but its use is objectionable for its nauseous taste and producing gastric disturbance

Cubebs, internally, as a stimulant of the mucous membrane, useful in cystorrhæa and in chronic cystitis

Enema (rectal) of atropine, 1 gr. to 8 ozs. of water useful in dysuria

Erigeron canadense, the oil, useful to relieve irritability of the bladder

Ergotine hypodermically increases the contractile power of the bladder and enables it to empty itself more perfectly

Eucalyptus, the oxygenated oil is beneficially given, internally 2 ms. with sugar, in chronic catarrh of the bladder

Gelsemii tincture, 1 dr. with sodii benzoas 1 dr. and water 50 drs. as a wash in hysterical women, to relieve irritability of the bladder with frequent micturition

Gokhru, useful in dysuria, resembles in action buchu and uva ursi

Hyoscyamus, to relieve dysuria and vesical irritation

Juniper oil is useful in cystitis due to urethral irritation

Linseed infusion, useful in dysuria

Morphia, hypodermically, relieves strangury

Mucilaginous drinks useful in cystitis

Oleum santal, internally very useful in ordinary cystitis

Opium and hyoscyamus, as rectal suppository or opium tincture with starch as rectal, enema is useful to relieve pain of strangury caused by blisters, or to prevent frequent micturition. Its use is to be avoided if the kidneys are diseased

Orthiosyphon useful as uric acid solvent

Oryza sativa, decoction, a useful drink to relieve dysuria

Pareira infusion given internally in chronic irritability of the bladder with ropy mucus in the urine. It is superior to uva ursi

Pichi, fluid extract, 20 mn., internally useful if the urine is alkaline, ropy, ammoniacal and purulent

Quinine, internally is useful in acute vesical catarrh, or the solution 1 in 500 as an injection into the bladder containing pus in the urine

Stigmata maides (1 to 10) infusion, is given internally in chronic cystitis with benefit

Triticum (rhizomes), decoction (1 in 10), is given internally, in chronic cystitis

Turpentine oil, internally and as an epithem is useful in cystitis due to urethral irritation or prostatic disease

Uva ursi, infusion given internally is useful in chronic cases, but less powerful than buchu

Injections to wash out the bladder—Lead acetate, 10 grs. to 4 ozs. of warm water ; acid nitric dilute, 2 mns. to 1 oz. of water ; acid tannic, 1 gr. to 1 oz. of warm water ; borax, 1 dr. with glycerin 2 drs., and warm water 4 drs.

External Remedies.—Foot bath, fomentation or poultices to the hypogastrium. Avoid coffee, salt, lime juice, &c.

Deafness. (*See Vol. I, page 161.*)

Achyranthes aspera. the medicated oil used as drops into the ear

Blister behind the ear and followed by morphine, dusted over the denuded blistered skin

Cajuput oil with olive oil (1 to 4) as drops

Capsicum tincture—with borax and nitre as gargle in deafness of a nervous origin

Colchicum internally in deafness due to gout

Gelsemium tincture, useful in nervous deafness

Pilocarpine, hypodermically, in deafness due to affections of the labyrinth

Quinine, iron and strychnine, internally, cures some cases. It often causes deafness

Tannin with glycerin, a local application useful for deafness due to throat affection

Turpentine with glycerin (1 to 6), to be dropped into the meatus in deafness due to defective secretion of cerumen

Delirium. (*See Vol. I., page 464.*)

Belladonna, in delirium of severe form in typhus and other fevers

Camphor, or camphor monobromate in low muttering delirium of fevers

Hyoscyamus in delirium of typhus of a mild form with hallucinations due to nervous excitement and slight cerebral congestion

Opium with tartar emetic internally in delirium of fevers. In traumatic cases opium should be used as rectal injection

Stramonium, in wild and furions delirium in puerperal mania with restlessness and suicidal tendency

Valerian in delirium of low fevers

Delirium Tremens; Chronic Alcoholism; Dipsomania; Inebriety.—(*See Vol. I, page 465.*)

Aconite with opium, in violent delirium

Apomorphine, to set up vomiting and thus lessen delirium

Arnica tincture is useful in delirium tremens with depression

Belladonna is useful in congestion of the brain, in insomnia with coma vigil in cyanosis and cold surface

Caffeine hydrobromate to lessen delirium

Cannabis Indica extract, $\frac{1}{3}$ to $\frac{1}{2}$ gr., a useful hypnotic in nocturnal delirium

Capsicum, with honey, or as tincture to induce sleep in the early stage of delirium tremens due to dyspepsia of chronic alcoholism

Cimicifuga or cimicifugin, an excellent brain tonic, relieves delirium

Digitalis tincture, or infusion alone, or with bromides useful to lessen delirium due to cerebral anæmia with effusion

Duboisine, a sedative and hypnotic given in delirium tremens with benefit

Gelsemium useful to lessen irritability

Hyoscyamus, or hyoscine, useful in delirium tremens, and to relieve tremors due to other diseases

Lupuline tincture or oleo resin, as cerebral sedative checks delirium

Morphia subcutaneously is useful

Mustard, as an emetic relieves delirium

Nux vomica or strychnine is very useful

Opium, as rectal or hypodermic injection, is useful in boisterous delirium in sthenic cases

Picrotoxine, useful to relieve tremors

Quinine, with mineral acids is useful in horrors and adynamic states

Spiritus ammoniæ aromatic with capsicum is of benefit

Strychnia, in delirium tremens, hypodermically used with benefit

Sumbul, is very useful in insomnia of alcoholism

Formula.—In insomnia and extreme nervousness:—Tinct. capsicum, 4 drs., potass. bromide. 4 drs.; liq. potas. arsen. 1 dr.; tinct. nux vom, 2 drs.; spt. ammon. aromat., 24 drs.; syr. tolutau, 16 drs. Mix. Dose, 4 drs. to overcome habit.

Dentition in Children. (*See Vol. I, page 465.*)

Belladonna tincture, or aconite tincture with chloroform and water (1 to 3), of this 2 to 3 drops rubbed on the gums, to relieve convulsions or other complication of dentition in painful dentition

Calumba or dulcamara infusion, to check diarrhœa and vomiting accompanying dentition

Cannabis, hyoscyamus, and chloral with bromide of potassium known as bromidia causes tranquillity and rest

Castor oil useful to check diarrhœa of dentition to be followed by chalk, catechu, or zinc oxide to reduce peristalsis

Chamomile tincture, as a sedative internally is useful

Hyoscyamus, is useful to relieve pain and subdue irritation

Rhubarb with soda is given internally to relieve aphthæ

Dhobee's Itch.

The parasites attacking the axilla or any other part of the skin leading to ringwormlike affection attended with itching. The parasites are the trichophytons or ordinary body ringworms, microsporon minutissimum, and diplococcus.

Cassia alata, infusion locally

Chrysarobin is useful

Diabetes Insipidus; Polyuria. (*See Vol. 1, page 466.*)

Acid gallic. Dose, 15 grs. internally
Anacardium occidentalis, the bark as infusion internally
Avoid tomato, asparagus, beans
Belladonna internally is very useful
Dry diet
Ergot, fluid extract, $\frac{1}{2}$ to 1 dr., is useful
Galvanism, constant current, is useful
Jaborandi, is useful to reduce the quantity of urine
Krameria, to lessen the quantity of urine
Muscarine, often successful to lessen the quantity of urine
Opium, alone or with gallic acid, is useful in large doses
Pilocarpine, $\frac{1}{30}$ to $\frac{1}{25}$ gr. internally causes diaphoresis and lessens the quantity of urine
Strychnine and iron as tonic is very useful
Valerian is useful ; given in large doses it restrains the increased flow of urine

Diabetes Mellitus. (*See Vol. I, page 466.*)

Almond bread
Aloin, to relieve constipation
Codeine, $\frac{1}{4}$ to $\frac{1}{2}$ gr., is useful to allay thirst and control appetite
Dulcin like saccharine is of benefit
Ergot, is useful to decrease the quantity of sugar and the volume of urine
Helicteris isora, the root bark as decoction internally, useful in lessening the quantity of sugar
Jambul pulp, or the bark, given after meals with saccharine gives favourable results
Levulose or diabetin, a saccharine food, a carbo hydrate, well assimilated and oxidized is very useful
Nux vomica, is very useful
Pea nuts, as food, rich in albumen, fat, and non-nitrogenous extractive matters &c. is of benefit
Quabain, lessens the quantity of sugar
Tabashir is of benefit
Thymol is useful

External remedies.—Regular living, fresh air, moderate exercise, free bowels, avoid alcohol.

Diarrhœa. (*See Vol. I, page 467.*)

Acacia catechu, extract of the wood is useful
Aconite, in diarrhœa due to exposure to chill with high fever and cutting pains in the abdomen
Acorus calamus, in atonic diarrhœa
Alstonia scholaris, in chronic diarrhœa
Arnica, to check exhausting diarrhœa
Atees, as a tonic in atonic diarrhœa
Balsam of peru, an excellent remedy in diarrhœa with tenesmus
Berberine phosphate, internally in intestinal catarrh
Calumba, useful in relaxed state of intestinal mucous membrane, but to be avoided if inflammation exists
Capsicum, in diarrhœa due to putrid injesta
Castor oil, in large doses with opium in diarrhœa due to indigestion or to irritating materials in the intestinal canal
Catechu compound powder, in atonic diarrhœa or that following withdrawal of morphia or opium habit. In children, catechu is given with chalk mixture with benefit
Chamomile oil, or infusion, is useful in summer diarrhœa and in that due to dentition
Cinnamon with chalk and opium in atonic cases
Coto bark, fluid extract, or cotoin is useful in atonic diarrhœa
Creosote with spirit ammon aromat, capsicum and opium is very useful
Dulcamara, in diarrhœa of children if due to dentition
Gall and opium, as rectal suppository
Ginger, with opium, in diarrhœa with flatulence
Helenin, useful in diarrhœa of phthisis
Hæmatoxylon being quite non-irritant, is given internally in advanced cases of diarrhœa in children
Ipecacuanha wine, in drop doses if vomiting is due to food irritation, or the powder in diarrhœa with greenish motions
Kino powder, or tincture, is useful in atonic diarrhœa, or that resulting from withdrawal of opium habit
Kola, useful in atonic diarrhœa
Krameria, very useful in atonic form
Mustard plaster to the abdomen is useful
Nux vomica, in atonic and epidemic diarrhœa, useful as an adjunct to other remedies
Opium is very useful when the motions are watery ; to be given with mineral acids or with acetate of lead or used as rectal injection with starch

Diarrhœa.—(*contd.*)

Podophyllin, $\frac{1}{30}$ to $\frac{1}{8}$ gr., alone or with aconite in violent form of bilious diarrhœa with vomiting; very useful in gastro-entiritis with cutting pains and in prolapsus of the anus
Pulsatilla, in mucous and dyspeptic diarrhœa or in diarrhœa due to piles
Quinine sulphate or quinine carbolate, in periodic diarrhœa with dysentery and jaundice
Resorcine solution, 1 gr. in 1 dr. of castor oil, useful in diarrhœa in children
Rhubarb tincture or powder, in the early stage to remove irritants and to check diarrhœa
Rumex, to check morning diarrhœa
Tannin suppositories or internally with opium, in atonic, chronic or profuse diarrhœa
Turpentine, very useful
Thymol, as an internal antiseptic in diarrhœa of phthisis and in chronic diarrhœa
Veratrum album, in diarrhœa with vomiting

Formula.—Kataja arishta or astringent wine:—contains—Kudâ chhal, 500; raisins, 250; flowersof bassia latifolia, bark of gmelina arborea, àà 320; water, 10,000; boil together to 2,500, then add flowers of woodfordia floribunda, 100; and treacle, 400. Mix and set aside to ferment for one month usually buried under ground. The wine has an agreeable flavour. Used in chronic diarrhœa.

Diphtheria (*See Vol. I, page 469.*)

Acid benzoic, in solution as gargle
Acid boric or with glycerin as a gargle (1 in 20) as a swab (1 in 1,000)
Balsam tolutani with ether and iodoform locally
Belladonna is useful if throat and tonsils are inflamed and swollen. It is given early to abort the exudation, given later on to support the heart
Chinolin, 5 p. c. solution as a swab
Camphor phenique, with almond oil as a paint to the throat
Capsicum tincture, as gargle or a local stimulant application
Cubebs in large doses in the early stage in the catarrhal form is very useful
Eucalyptus oil with alcohol as a spray with an atomizer
Papaine solution as inhalation by a steam atomizer to dissolve the membrane and to remove the exudation
Pilocarpine hydrochlorate, internally, to loosen the membrane; it produces free salivation, but depresses the heart
Pineapple juice, if sipped, is highly beneficial
Sanguinaria, as emetic, very useful
Strychnine and atropine, hypodermically, as a prophylactic against subsequent paralysis
Tannin, 5 p. c. as a spray is useful
Turpentine, internally or as fumigation alone or with tar and vapour prepared by burning coal tar burnt in a room
Thymol and glycerin as gargle—fresh thyme as spray or as inhalation

Dropsy (Hepatic, Renal, Cardiac). (*See Vol. I, page 479.*)

Acetum scillæ in cardiac dropsy
Aconite tincture, 2 to 5 ms., in dropsy due to scarlet fever
Apocynum cannabinum, an active hydragogue diuretic, very useful in dropsy
Argemone mexicana oil. in dropsy
Bryonia, as a drastic purgative and diuretic. Its infusion with aconite is useful in renal dropsy
Cactus, in cardiac dropsy, and in Bright's disease
Caffeine citrate or iodide, as a hydragogue diuretic, to eliminate waste products; useful in cardiac and renal dropsies; should be avoided if urethritis is present
Chimaphila, extract, useful in renal dropsy, a fine substitute for scoparius
Cimicifuga, in hepatic and cardiac dropsy
Colchicum as hydragogue diuretic given in dropsy, supervening on scarlet fever or heart disease
Copaiba, as stimulant diuretic; useful in ascites due to hepatic cirrhosis
Delphinium zalil. Decoction in cardiac and renal dropsies

Dropsy.—(*contd.*)

Digitalis Infusion is useful in dropsy due to acute desquamative nephritis, tricuspid regurgitation, scanty urine, and if there is general venous engorgement

Digitalis, with squill and mercury is useful in cardiac or renal disease; to be avoided in aortic regurgitation and in cardiac hypertrophy

Elaterium, $\frac{1}{8}$ gr., with hyoscyamus, 1 gr., useful as a derivative in renal dropsy. It is contra-indicated if there is gastro-intestinal irritation

Grapes, very useful in cardiac dropsy

Hellebore, fluid extract, or tincture, in anasarca, or dropsy with general effusion after scarlatina

Jaborandi, useful in renal dropsy

Jalap, with podophyllin or with potassium bitartrate and ginger as a hydragogue, is useful in dropsy from Bright's disease

Juniper is useful in dropsy after scarlatina, and in asthenic, cardiac or renal dropsy

Kâlâdânâ, useful in renal dropsy

Luffa amara, useful in dropsy with enlarged liver or spleen

Paracentesis (abdominal), if excessive effusion

Pilocarpine hydrochlorate, in renal dropsy where the secretion of urine is scanty or suppressed

Raphanus sativus, useful in cardiac dropsy

Scoparius, infusion with diluents, as a hydragogue diuretic, is useful in cardiac dropsy

Senega, useful in dropsy, due to renal disease

Squill alone is useful in cardiac dropsy or with iron if anæmia co-exists ; to be avoided if renal disease is present

Stillingia as a hydragogue cathartic, useful in ascites due to liver affections

Strophanthus, useful in cardiac dropsy

Taraxacum, as a diuretic, is used in cardiac dropsy

Turpentine oil, is useful in dropsy due to non-desquamative renal disease with albumen in the urine

Formula—(1) Azima tetracantha, 10 ozs.; tribulus terrestris (fruit), 1 dr.; trianthema monogyma root, 1 dr.; cephalandra indica, 1 dr.; belleric myrobolans, $\frac{1}{2}$ dr.; chebulic myrobolans, $\frac{1}{2}$ dr.; iron dross, 10 oz.; water, 12 oz. as decoction. Dose, 1 oz. in dropsy.

(2). Tinct. digitalis, $\frac{1}{2}$ dr.; extract ergotæ liquidi, $\frac{1}{2}$ dr.; acidi gallici, 20 grs.; potasii bromidi, 120 grs.; oxymel scillæ, 4 oz.; syrup, 3 oz.; aqua laurocerasi, 2 ozs. Mix. Dose, 4 to 6 drs.

(3). Vâhni rasa: The word Vâhni means "fire." It signifies an agent which drives away water from the abdomen just as fire causes water to evaporate when brought in contact with it. Hence a specific for dropsy. It contains pârâkajali, 4; gandhaka, halada, triphalâ, each 2 ; nishota, jamâlagotâ, seed, chitraka, each 3 parts ; suntha, miri, pipali, dântimula, jirun, each 8 ; triturate, the powder in the juice of arani and bhângro, and then add erandi-tela sufficient to make a pill mass. Dose, 5 to 10 grs. in dropsy.

Duodenal Catarrh. (*See Vol. I, page 472.*)

Hydrastis, in catarrh with gallstones

Ipecacuanha, very useful

Podophyllin, in catarrhal and malarial duodenitis

Rhubarb

Sanguinaria tincture

Water melon juice as a drink

Formula—Methi Modak or Confection of Fenugreek:—contains Fenugreek, 20; triphla, 1; trikatu, 1; cyperus rotundus, 1; black cumin., 1, carraway, 1; coriander, 1; myrica nagi, 1; pistachio nut, 1; Bishop's weed, 2; rock salt, 2; bid lavana, 1; mesua ferea, $\frac{1}{2}$; cassia leaves, 1; cinnamon, 2; cardamoms, 3; nutmegs, 2; mace, 2; cloves, 2; camphor, 1; sandalwood, 1; sugar, 40. Mix, and make a confection. Dose, 1 dr. in chronic indigestion, atonic diarrhœa, pregnancy, and in wasting disease.

Dysentery (Acute, and Chronic). (*See Vol I, page 472.*)

Aconite tincture, 2 ms., internaly when there is fever and griping pains

Ægle marmelos, internally in atonic cases as astringent and soothing

Ailanthus glandulosa, infusion, with cinnamon, is useful in chronic dysentery

Balsam of peru, 3, alcohol, 60, with syrup of lemons, 240, and water 1,000, an excellent drink in dysentery

Belladonna, externally and internally in chronic cases

Berberis aristata, internally in chronic cases

Benzoin, with opium, catechu, and hæmatoxylon, in obstinate cases with benefit

Calumba in chronic cases in the advanced stage with ulceration of the colon

Cannabis Indica of benefit

Castor oil, 1 oz. as a mild cathartic, with tincture opium, 10 ms. in catarrhal cases. Mixed with sugar and gum or with milk given for children in dysenteric diarrhœa

Chebulic myrobolans, with ginger and sweet fennel, internally very useful

Chochlospermum gos-ypium (gum), with curd or whey internally in chronic cases

Ergot, with opium and nux vomica in acute and chronic cases in anæmia

Garcinia mangostina, in the advanced stage

Geranium, useful as a rectal injection

Grape cure, is useful in chronic cases

Holarrhæna antidysenterica, bark and seeds in chronic cases

Hydrastis, a good stomachic tonic and cholagogue ; it promotes intestinal secretions

Ipecacuanha, as enema in acute cases. In ordinary cases internally in large doses; 25 grs. with milk, very useful in greenish motions with mucous and blood. In dysenteric diarrhæa with vomiting ipecac wine is used in drop doses. Ipecacuanha with opium as Dover's powder, is given in chronic cases.

Lanium album. Infusion 4 drs., or Succus ½ dr., internally in chronic cases

Lemon juice, with cinchona, very useful

Linseed infusion, with glycerin (4 to 1) to allay tenesmus

Matico infusion, by the mouth or by the rectum in hæmorrhagic dysentery

Mesua ferrea, flower buds. internally

Myrobolans chebulic (himaj), fried in butter Dose, 5 to 10 grs. ; very useful

Nux vomica pulv, in epidemic dysentery when stools are attended with much depression

Opium given internally in dysentery in every stage and in every form, or as an enema with starch and milk; in chronic cases it is given internally to allay pain, moderate peristalsis moderate vascular excitement, and to promote the action of the skin. It should be used after the canal is emptied by salines.

Plantago ispaghula, as demulcent, very useful

Punica granatum, decoction useful in advanced stage

Poppy seeds with cardamoms burnt or fried in butter, internally very useful

Quinine alone or with morphia internally in dysentery due to malaria and in periodic cases like fever. It is also used as a rectal injection (1 in 1,000)

Turpentine oil, internally useful in chronic cases

Diet.—Avoid animal food and stimulants. *External remedies.*—Leeches to the anus, turpentine stupes to the abdomen.

Formula.—Pancha mulâ di kavâth. Decoction containing, ægle marmelos, cissampelos pareira, abutilon indicum, gmelina arborea, holarrhæna antidysenterica, and water, to make a decoction. When ready add picrorhiza kurroa, kudâchhâl, ginger and tinospora cordifolia. Dose, 1 oz. in bilious dysentery.

(2). Terminalia chebula, acorus calamus, cedrus deodâra, aconitum heterophyllum, cessampelos pareia, embelia ribes, cyperus rotundus, piper nigrum, holarrhæna antidysenterica, add water to make decoction. Dose 1 oz. in dysentery.

(3) Compound powder.—Dhânya panchaka churana (powder of 5 drugs), coriandrum sativum, cyperus rotundus, andropogon muricatus, ægle marmelos, and ginger. Make powder. Dose, ½ dr.

(4) Inderjav, moth, dhâoriphul, vâlo, lodhra, mocharas, sunth. Mix and add jaggery. Dose ½ dr. in chronic dysentery.

(5) Mâhâ Gangâdhar Churna:—dhâoriphul, âmlâ, moth, pahadmul, jethi madh, jambulbij, âmbâgope, kudâ chhâl, sunth, ativisa, lodhra, vâlo, inder jav. Dose, ½ dr. in chronic dysentery.

Dysmenorrhœa.—(*See Vol. I, page 473.*)

Aconite, given early is useful in congestive form and in plethoric subjects
Aletris, cordial internally is of great benfit
Apiol 3 to 5 ms. as emmenagogue is useful in neuralgic cases ; should be given for several days before the period
Belladonna, as mild injection or as pessary is useful in neuralgic or spasmoic forms if the discharge is dark and fœtid with severe crampy pains attended with chills ; or in $\frac{1}{6}$ gr. dose given internally gives relief
Cajuput oil, locally is useful to relieve the pain
Camphor internally, or as enema with opium or as liniment locally is very useful
Cannabis indica, is useful as a palliative in dysmenorrhœa
Caulophyllum, extract given in the interval is a good curative in spasmodic cases
Cimicifuga tincture, with stramonium tincture and colchicum wine, given internally to relieve pain in the congestive variety
Cicer arietinum, as vapour or steam locally to the pubes is useful
Cocculus indicus tincture, given two days before the term is very useful
Codeine, $\frac{1}{4}$ gr., is useful where morphine cannot be well borne
Crocus sativus with camphor and opium as poultice to the pubes
Ergot, in the congestive form and during the molimen is very useful
Gelsemium, the fluid extract, relieves pain in neuralgic cases
Gossypium, 10 with ergot 10 and tinct. hellebori nigri 5, given internally is useful
Guaiacum ammoniated tincture, 1 dr., with potassii iodidi 10 gr., is useful in the rheumatic and the neuralgic form of dysmenorrhœa
Morphine, hypodermically injected at each period; or morphine with belladonna as suppository if pain is severe is of benefit
Mustard foot bath is of high value
Opium internally to relieve the pain or as a paint to the os, or with linseed as poultice or as an enema is very useful
Pulsatilla tincture, or extract internally only in the functional form if the discharge is scanty, and in clots. It should be avoided in the membranous, obstructive or neuralgic form
Tea, hot, with ginger internally is useful
Turpentine oil in membranous variety is of benefit
Valerian with opium, as rectal enema
Viburnum, the fluid extract, with bromides and cannabis indica is useful in spasmodic and in neuralgic cases

Dyspepsia ; Hyperacidity ; Flatulence ; Gastralgia ; Pyrosis.

(*See Vol. I, page 474.*)

Allspice
Asafetida, useful in the hypochondriac, to improve flatulence
Alium sativum tincture internally is useful
Aurantii tincture, or infusion, very useful
Belladonna, $\frac{1}{8}$ gr. of the extract internally to lessen gastric pain and to relieve constipation
Bitters, as calumba gentian and quassia good vehicles for acids and alkalies in dyspepsia
Bryonia, is useful in hepatic disorders, in bilious vomiting and in bilious headache
Cannabis indica is very useful in indigestion
Capsicum with compound rhubarb pill and ipecacuanha is of benefit internaly
Carminatives, internally, is useful to promote expulsion of gas from the stomach and intestines
Chamomile, 2 ms. of the oil in atonic dyspepsia is useful
Colocynth, with pilulæ rhei compositus, and olei caryophilli internally is very useful
Coca wine of great benefit
Eucalyptus, in atonic cases due to presence of sarcinæ in the stomach
Euonymin and pepsin, in hepatic dyspepsia
Ginger, as an adjunct
Ignatia, useful in nervous dyspepsia
Ipecacuanha, $\frac{1}{2}$ to 1 gr., with rhubarb or the wine in 5 ms. is useful in atonic and catarrhal cases to relieve depression or the constipation when the food is like a heavy weight
Kino with opium and cinnamon is useful in pyrosis
Lipidium iberis, as confection, of benefit internally
Malt extract is useful
Milk cure—koumyss and butter milk is of benefit
Morphia, subcutaneously, in irritability of the stomach is useful

Dyspepsia.—(*contd.*)

Nux vomica, before meals as a stomachic tonic is useful to relieve flatulence, heartburn, heavy head; also useful to relieve dyspepsia of drunkards

Opium with nux vomica, in cases of irritability of the stomach

Papayotin (papain), useful in various forms of dyspepsia with benefit; it has a marked action over acid, alkaline or neutral solution and in the presence of antiseptic chemicals and therapeutic agents

Pepsin, with diluted hydrochloric acid is of benefit in gastric indigestion

Physostigma, to relieve flatulence in women at climacteric period

Pine apple juice, a digestive of proteid and albuminous matters, being an active ferment in the presence of acids or alkaline carbonates or neutral solutions

Podophyllin with euonymin, leptandrin chiretta and creosote is of great benefit

Pulsatilla, 5 ms. when the tongue is coated and white, taste greasy, feeling of nausea, flatulence, heartburn, and depression

Quinine preparations, useful to check excessive fermentation in the alimentary canal

Rhamnus purshiana, useful in torpid liver with constipation

Sanguinaria, the tincture, or the alkaloid given in atonic dyspepsia to promote gastric secretion and increases appetite

Sugar of milk, useful in dyspepsia with flatulence

Turpentine on sugar relieves flatulence

Taraxacum, in simple atonic dyspepsia is very useful

Valerian, relieves flatulence in hypochondriasis

Vegetable diastase

Vegetable ptyalin

Xanthoxylum, fluid extract is useful as a stomachic tonic in atonic cases

External remedies.—Diet—Avoid tea, use hot water as drink, sufficient mastica tion, well performed massage.

(2). *Formula.*—Magnesii sulphatis, 1 oz.; magnesii carbonatis, 90 grs.; vinaloes, 6 drs.; tinctura humuli, 2 drs.; acidi hydrocyanic dilute, 15 ms.; and infusion cascarillæ, 6 oz.; Mix. Dose. 1 oz.

(3). Confection—Jecrâ-no-pâkh:—Carium nigrum, 15; black pepper, 5; ginger (dried), 5; long pepper, 5; satap, 5; peppermint, 5; apium graveolens, 5; myrobolans, 5; sonchal salt, 5; eagle wood, 5; honey, 20. Mix. Dose, 1 to 2 drs., used in deranged digestion, biliousness, &c.

(4). Amrita Haritaki.—Compound powder—Chebulic myrobolans, full size and ripe. Boil it in milk and remove the seeds. Stuff this seedless myrobolans with a compound powder containing trikatu, cinnamon, plumbago rosea, bishop's weed, chavak root and the three salts—Potas. bicarb., soda bicarb. and ammonium chloride; also asafetida, cloves, each 4 parts. This is soaked in tamarind juice and lime juice. then dried in the sun and used in dyspepsia. Dose, ½ to 1 dr.

Dysphagia. (*See Vol. I, page 476.*)

Cajuput oil, in the nervous form

Cocaine hydrochlorate, 20 p. c. solution by swab, or as spray to relieve dysphagia in phthisis

Strychnine, iron and quinine as tonic are useful

Dyspnœa, a symptom due to Cardiac, Pulmonary, Pharyngeal, Laryngeal or Tracheal Disease. (*See Vol. I, page 476.*)

Asafetida, with antispasmodics in dyspnœa due to chronic bronchitis

Cimicifuga, relieves cardiac dyspnœa

Croton oil, liniment to the chest is of benefit

Dhatura useful in dyspnœa of phthisis

Grindelia, useful in dyspnœa with cough occurring in pulmonary emphysema

Morphine, used hypodermically. relieves cardiac dyspnœa. It should be avoided if urine is albuminous. It is very energetic, giving power to breathe

Prunus virginiana, very useful in cardiac dyspnœa

Quebracho extract. Dose, ½ to 1 dr. in dyspnœa of pulmonary asthma, palpitation, &c.

Spigelia anthelmia, in dyspnœa accompanied with palpitation

Strophanthus tincture, in cardiac dyspnœa

Strychnine, as a respiratory stimulant, useful in dyspnœa due to lung mischief or to palpitation of heart in the hysteric

Terebene capsules, useful in dyspnœa of chronic emphysema and other lung affections

Terpini hydrate, is useful in asthmatic dyspnœa

Valerian, in nervous dyspnœa is very useful

Ecchymosis.

Amba halad, made into paste with white of egg and brandy is very useful

Arnica tincture, with water locally applied disperses ecchymosis, due to injury

Capsicum tincture, or strong infusion mixed with glycerin and mucilage, is used as a paint to relieve black eye or a bruised surface

Hamamelis tincture, 1 in 5 of water as lotion is useful when there is much discoloration

Turmeric, locally to the chemosed portion is useful

Ecthyma. *(See Vol. I, page 477.)*

Chrysarobin, internally, is useful

Grape cure is very effective

Quinine is useful when ecthyma is due to malnutrition

Eczema. *(See Vol. I, page 477.)*

Anacardium occidentale oil, ointment (1 to 8 of lard) is useful in chronic cases

Belladonna extract, $\frac{1}{4}$ gr. with quinine 3 gr. internally, or externally with bismuth subcarbonate as a dusting powder is useful in eczema of the hand and feet

Benzoin. The paint of tincture benzoin compound is useful to allay itching

Buck wheat flour as dressing is useful

Chaulmugra oil, as an ointment is useful

Conium tincture with olive oil, 1 to 8 as antipruritic is of benefit

Croton tiglium, seeds bruised in brandy used as liniment. The oil is used as a basis of stimulating applications in the chronic form

Graphite, containing lycopodium, calcium phosphate, &c., locally applied is very useful

Hamamelis, locally is useful as antipruritic and in chronic cases

Iris versicolor, tincture is useful as a hepatic stimulant in eczema in gouty subjects

Oleum cadini with simple ointment (1 in 8) is very useful

Phytolacca, is useful in obstinate cases

Rhus toxicodendron tincture, given internally in acute cases; also applied externally to subdue burning and itching

Tar or pix liquida, internally where arsenic fails. Locally used in the chronic form only

Viola tricolor, infusion with senna, is very useful in chronic form; should be avoided in acute cases

Elephantiasis.

Calotropis gigantea, root bark as paste locally applied to the legs or scrotum

Dhatura, paste with gul-e-armani, locally to legs or scrotum

Electrolysis

Eclipta alba, the paste is locally applied

Ionidum parviflorum, a good remedy in elephantiasis

Limnophila gratioloides, locally applied to legs or scrotum

Massage is of benefit

Moringa pterygosperma, root as a paste is useful

Nux vomica, with chaulmoogra oil, locally applied

Piper nigrum with nigella sativa, locally applied in brandy and belladonna with benefit

Pressure over the affected part

Formula.—Nigella sativa, 2; acorus calamus, 1; piper nigrum, 1; gingiber, 1; and fresh juice of dhatura alba as a paste, to paint over the scrotum.

Bole armenean, 4; barringtonia, 4; acorus calamus, 2; nux vomica, 1; piper nigrum, 1; and brandy as a paste for legs and scrotum.

Emphysema. *(See Vol. I, page 480.)*

Digitalis is useful

Grindelia, useful in emphysema with asthmatic breathing

Lobelia, to allay dyspnœa accompanying capillary bronchitis in emphysema

Morphine, $\frac{1}{6}$ gr. and atropine $\frac{1}{100}$ gr. hypodermically is useful as a palliative for the asthmatic attacks

Stramonium leaves, as smoke to relieve dyspnœa and asthma

Strychnine, a valuable respiratory stimulant, is useful to relieve dyspnœa with prolonged expiration

Terebene, to relieve dyspnœa

Endocarditis. *(See Vol. I, page 481.)*

Aconite powder or the tincture, useful in inflammation of serous membranes
Digitalis, useful to regulate the heart's action
Opium, to relieve inflammation of serous membranes
Quinine, to check inflammation
Spigelia anthelmia, in endocarditis due to rheumatism
Veratrum viride, to give tone to the pulse

Enteritis. *(See Vol. I, page 481.)*

Aconite, useful in acute sthenic cases of enteritis with high temperature
Castor oil is useful
Opium tincture, to control intestinal inflammation and to quiet the peristalsis
Podophyllin with aconite, to allay vomiting and diarrhœa
Turpentine stupes, hot, over the abdomen, gives relief

Enuresis. *(See Vol. I, page 482.)*

Atropine
Belladonna, 10 ms. of the tincture
Ergot, is useful in paralysis of the sphinctor vesicæ to relieve a feeling or sensation of the bladder being imperfectly emptied
Lupulin, is useful
Quinine, in enuresis accompanied with chorea
Rhus aromatic, fluid extract, with glycerin is useful
Santonine, useful in enuresis, due to worms
Scutellaria, fluid extract, is very useful
Strychnine, is useful in enuresis in old people with paralysis of the bladder
Turpentine, in small doses is useful to relieve enuresis

Formula.—Extract jaborandi fluidi, 1 dr.; extract belladonni fluidi, 1 dr.; extract tritici repentis fluidi, 4 drs.; extract ergotæ fluidi, 8 drs.; extract rhois aromatici, 6 ds.; and aquæ, 4 ozs. Dose, $\frac{1}{12}$ part.

Epilepsy. *(See Vol. I, page 482.)*

Atropine sulphate, 1 p. c. solution 1 mu. with brandy is useful
Belladonna, with bromides is useful in nocturnal epilepsy occurring in anæmic subjects and when due to fright
Cannabis indica, alone or with strychnine, belladonna or picrotoxin, in anæmia with depression in nocturnal cases
Digitalis tincture, 10 ms. given with bromides 20 grs. as a cardiac tonic, in paroxysms occurring at night
Hydrastine hydrochloride, internally is useful
Ignatia amara in epilepsy, free from cerebral congestion
Opium is a useful adjunct to potassium bromide
Picrotoxin hypodermically or internally is useful in anæmic subjects, if it occurs at night, or due to aneurism
Quinine useful in epilepsy if of malarial origin and having an intermittent character
Rue, in epilepsy accompanied with seminal emission
Solanum as tincture internally is very useful
Strychnine, $\frac{1}{30}$ gr. is useful in idiopathic epilepsy in anæmic subjects where bromides fail. It is injurious if given in symptomatic form
Turpentine is very useful if due to worms

Epistaxis. *(See Vol. I, page 484.)*

Aconite is useful in children and in plethoric subjects
Arnica locally is useful where epistaxis is due to injury or mechanical violence
Belladonna, when bleeding is due to congestion of the nasal vessels
Digitalis infusion internally is of great benefit
Ergot, of the powder, or of the liquid extract is useful
Hamamelis is useful if the hæmorrhage is of a venous character
Ipecacuanha is very useful, as it acts upon the vessels

Epistaxis.—(contd.)

Tannin powder, is used as insufflation into the nose or the solution 2 drs. to 4 ozs. of water injected into the nose with advantage

Turpentine, useful if given internally in epistaxis occuring in the debilitated

External remedies.—Compression of facial arteries. Feet and hands to be kept warm. Head to be kept elevated and cool. Ice to the nose. Vinegar as tampon into the nostrils.

Eruptions produced by Drugs.

Aconite produces vesicular exanthemata

Atropine, erythema like rash of scarlet fever

Belladonna, erythematous rash

Castor oil, urticaria

Chinchona, erythema

Codliver oil, acne

Copaiba urticaria, erythema, eczema pemphigus, copaiba rash has preference for the ankles and wrists

Croton oil, papules or pustules

Digitalis erythema

Opium and morphine erythema, papular eruptions, squamation and itching

Quinine erythema, purpura, pemphigus prurigo papular eruptions, itching' generally ephemeral, first appearing on the face and neck and then over the body. In some, indistinct spots like measles appear

Rhus toxicodendron, visicles and pustules with redness and itching.

Santonine pemphigus, vesicles

Stramonium, erythematous rash

Strychnine erythema, papular eruptions, itching

Tar, acne

Turpentine, similar to copaiba

Eruptions produced by articles of food:—

Apples, acne about the mouth

Fish and oatmeal, acne eruptions

Fruits, and acid fruits, acute eczema

Roast turkey or shell fish, urticaria;

Strawberries, urticaria

Walnuts, inflammation of the buccal gland

Erysipelas. (See Vol. I, page 484.)

Aconite is useful in the beginning with high fever, and in erysipelas following vaccination

Belladonna tincture, internally or locally, is useful in superficial and non-vesicular form; if there is much fever, combine it with digitalis or aconite; if much depression add quinine.

Cotton wool sprinkled with starch and zinc oxide or with flour as an application is useful

Jaborandi, fluid extract, causes diaphoresis and the disease is checked. To be avoided in anæmic subjects, and those with a weak heart

Pilocarpine, $\frac{1}{8}$ gr. in the beginning used hypodermically to abort the disease

Quinine, with iron, if the pulse is soft and tremulous, and there is low muttering delirium. It sustains vital powers and prevents cerebral embolism

Rhux toxicodendron, useful in vesicular form

Turpentine is useful as a paint over the surface as a stimulant in traumatic cases, more serviceable than alcohol

Erythema. (See Vol I, page 485.)

Belladonna, in obstinate cases

Quinine, in erythema nodosum

Rhus toxicodendron is very useful

Thiol, as a dusting powder

Esophageal Affections. (See Vol. I, page 486.)

Belladonna liniment, applied with friction to the sternum, is a nice palliative in stricture of the esophagus

Conium, is useful to relieve spasms and cramps of the stomach, in flatulence and in globus hystericus

Hyoscyamus, if there is great irritability of the esophagus

Leeches to the esophagus to relieve pain, tenderness and spasms

Eye Diseases. (*See Vol. I, page 487.*)

Atropine, as drops locally in iritis, injected hypodermically in glaucoma

Belladonna, locally and internally in conjunctivitis, iritis, and other inflammations

Cocaine, 4 p.c. solution as a local anæsthetic and mydriatic, injected into the muscle for squint operations

Ergot as a myotic, is very useful in disturbances of accommodation

Morphine with mercury oleate applied outside the lids in syphilitic iritis, palpebral conjunctivitis and stye

Physostigmine, applied locally to contract the pupils

Pilocarpine, in amblyopia, from alcohol or tobacco; also useful in iritis, keratitis, hæmorrhage of the retina, atrophy of the optic nerve, &c.

Ruta, useful in amaurosis and dimness of vision

Santonine, useful in inflammation and atrophy of the retina, in inflammation of the optic nerve and to relieve inflammatory effusion

Eyelids. (*See Vol. I, page 487.*)

Capsicum tincture, or infusion, locally for the black eye

Ergot, as collyrium, to relieve ptosis and paralysis of the eyelids

Morphine and oleate of mercury, 20 p.c. locally for stye

Pulsatilla, internally and as a wash externally to abort the stye

Tannin, as lotion or ointment, or as powder is employed with benefit

Veratrine, locally in solution, to brush overlids in painful spasm of the orbicularis

FEVERS (*See Vol. I, page 488.*)

Ephemeral Fever, Dengue Fever.

Acetum or vinegar, diluted, used locally as a refrigerant

Acid drinks, as syrup of raspberry, citric acid, lemons with water are useful as refrigerants

Aconite, alone or with salines in dengue fever, useful in hyperpyrexia in the early stage of simple inflammatory fevers, in pneumonia, acute congestions and in sthenic fever; it reduces the temperature and induces perspration

Arnica tincture useful as an antipyretic, in asthenic cases and in rheumatic and typhoid fevers

Aristolochia serpentaria, in advanced stage and in adynamic form

Atropine, hypodermically, during the cold stage aborts the fever

Baptisia tincture, in common continued and typhoid fevers

Belladonna tincture as a prophylactic, to relieve delirium, and insomnia in febricula, eruptive fevers, dengue and typhus fever; it relieves the head symptoms

Berberis bark as decoction is useful in intermittent, ague and remittent fevers

Bitter tonics, in advanced cases

Bonducella seeds, as antiperiodic, very useful

Camphor, useful to subdue reflex excitability, to relieve delirium, and as a stimulant in adynamic fevers

Chinolin as antipyretic and diaphoretic useful to moderate the intensity of fever as in pneumonia, typhoid fever, &c.

Cicer arietium, as a refrigerant drink

Cimicifuga, a substitute for digitalis, is useful in hectic fever and in fever with high temperature and quick pulse

Cinchona and its alkaloids, a good prophylactic against ague

Climatis triloba, infusion useful in chronic fevers

Emetics, every morning useful to prevent the attack

Guaiacol, locally with olive oil as an inunction to the surface of the skin, is a nice antipyretic

Guarana, given as a palliative

Hellebore. rhizome powder, is useful

Humulus lupulus, is useful in intermittent fever

Lemon, decoction or the juice in ague useful as diaphoretic and to check recurrence of paroxysms

Nimb, as a bitter tonic useful in advanced cases

Opium acts as a diaphoretic to relieve pain and restlessness, useful in dengue

Picrœna excelsa, useful in paroxysmal ague

Pilocarpine hydrochlorate, hypodermically in the cold stage, excites profuse sweats and thus lessens the attack

Fevers—(*contd.*)

Piper nigrum, useful in intermittent fever.
Quinine as an antiseptic and antiphlogistic, given by the stomach or as an injection by rectum or hypodermically, is of great value in septicæmia, hectic fever, eruptive fevers, malarial, remittent and intermittent fevers, and in paroxysmal pyrexial stage. As antipyretic it is less favourable than baths; it is useless in typhus and typhoid fever
Rhus toxicodendron, in rheumatic or scarlet fever with typhoid symptoms
Stillingia, with quinine and arsenic in malarial cachexia
Strychnine with arsenic is very efficient, is equal to 1 gr. of quinine
Strychnos colubrina, in malarial cachexia
Sumbul radix, is useful in fevers with typhoid symptoms
Thevetia neriifolia tincture, as anti-periodic is of benefit
Thuja occidentalis, or arbor vitæ tincture, is useful
Turpentine, internally as stimulant to vasomotor nervous sytem, useful in typhoid, yellow, and puerperal fevers; it is given as an enema with starch and opium in typhoid fever to check intestinal hæmorrhage with tympanitis
Viola odorata syrup.
Valerian, useful in fevers to relieve nervous excitability
Veratrum viridic is useful as antipyretic in febricula and rheumatic fever; also useful to relieve delirium of fever in pneumonia

Formulæ.—Panch Vakatra Rasa—the five fever cures or remedies. They include parakajali, sulphur, each, 1; black pepper, long pepper, and ammonium chloride, each 5. Dose, 2 to 5 grs. in fever.

Shadnaj paneya naj contains:—Root of andropogon muricatus, cyperus, rotundus or C. pertensis, red sandal wood, herb of oldenlandia herbacea, root of pavonia odorata, and dry ginger; equal parts and water to make a decoction. Dose, 4 to 8 drs. as a cooling stomachic drink in fever.

Antifibrile Mixture contains:—Quinine sulphatis, 2 grs.; tinct. ferri chloridi, 2 ms.; liq. potassii arsenitii, 2 ms.; tinct opii, 2 ms.; strychine sulphatis, $\frac{1}{40}$ gr.; alcohol, $\frac{1}{2}$ dr.; and aquæ, 4 drs.

Compound powder for chronic fever or chronic malarial disease:—Dogwood bark, 3 grs.; calumbæ root, 3 grs.; clerodendron, 3 grs.; eupatorium, 2 grs.; and cayenne pepper, 2 grs.

Hay Fever.

Aconite, a good substitute for arsenic, is very useful
Belladonna, to restrain profuse nasal secretion
Cocaine, 5 to 10 p.c. solution dropped into the nose, or 5 to 10 grs. with an ounce of cosminol sprayed up the nostrils or applied as a palliative to the nasal mucous membrane with good results
Coffee, black, is very useful
Eucalyptus oil, 5 to 20 ms. to 1 oz. of cosminol used as a spray
Euphrasia, to relieve the catarrh.
Grindelia, useful in cases complicated with asthma
Ignatia tincture. is very useful
Ipecacuanha, is very useful
Lobelia, is very useful
Opium or morphine, given till the discharge abates is very useful
Quinine, given internally or injected to check catarrh, is useful after the acute symptoms have subsided, or as hydtrochlorate locally appl ed with a brush to the nasal mucous membrane to arrest the disease
Tobacco smoking, or internally is usefu

Fever Intermittent, Ague (*See Vol. I, page 488.*)

Acorus calamus in adynamic form
Apiol, before paroxysm, useful in mild caes where prejudice exists against quinine
Cascarilla with chamomile, very useful
Chinoidine and its salts, good substitutes for quinine, but requires larger doses
Cinchonine, cinchonidine, quinidine and their sulphates are useful
Eucalyptus tincture is useful in ague

Intermittent Ague.—(*contd.*)

Emetics as ipecacuanha to aid the action of quinine; inadmissible if there is gastric irritation

Ergot is useful if the spleen is enlarged

Hydrastis is useful like quinine if there is profuse sweating

Lemon juice, to prevent recurrence of paroxysms

Narcotine, as an antiperiodic, as good as quinine, cures intermittents quickly and surely

Nux vomica, as an antiperiodic given with quinine is of benefit

Opium internally, or morphine, hypodermically lessens the chill and aids the action of antiperiodics. It is generally given with quinine

Plumbago zeylanica, useful as an antiperiodic.

Purgatives, as jalap, scammony, podophyllin, useful during intermission before antiperiodics

Quinine sulphate, 5 to 10 grs., in coffee, in acute ague; or 10 to 15 grs. at first in the sweating stage and to be repeated 4 or 5 grs. two hours after or six hours before the next paroxysm. It may be given internally, or by the rectum or injected subcutaneously. Best plan is to give with morphine; very useful in uncomplicated cases and in those of recent growth; should not be given during the early stage of ague as it would increase headache and distress

Fever—Malarial—Chronic Malaria.

Capsicum, with black pepper, used as an adjunct to promote the action of quinine

Clerodendron, of much benefit

Eucalyptus, to reconstruct damages in the organs of assimilation

Quinine and its salts, or quinine salicylate, are useful in periodic affections due to malarial cachexia, better borne in recent malarial cases. It is a nice prophylactic, but should be given with care, the indiscriminate use of it often leads to the weakening of the heart

Tannin is useful in malarial fever resisting quinine

Vegetable bitters, useful in chronic malaria, and during convalescence from malarial fever

Formula.—Aragbadhadi qvâth contains:—Cassia fistula, picrorrhiza kurroa, chebulic myrobolans, long pepper root, cyperus rotundus áá 2 drs. water, 20 fld. oz. make decoction. Dose, 4 to 6 fld. drs. In fever and chronic malaria.

Fever—Remittent.

Aconite, in the hot stage with headache

Alcohol or brandy locally applied to the back, abdomen and chest

Gelsemium, is very beneficial in biliousness and to reduce the temperature

Morphine, hypodermically is useful to abort

Quinine, large doses without regard to exaserbations until the temperature is reduced; very useful in bilious, remittent and other forms of malarial fevers; it should be accompanied by an aperient dose of calomelo if vomiting is severe,

Vegetable tonics, as calumba and quassia with mineral acids during convalcsence very useful

Wurberg's tincture is very useful

Wet sheet packing is of benefit

Formula.—Pancha bhadra, containing five bitters—pârpata, mustâkâ, gulanchâ, chirettâ and ginger, equal parts in water (1 in 40) make decoction. Dose, 1 to 2 oz.

Fever—Scarlet.

Aconite, in the early stage to lower temperature and to develope eruption

Asclepias, to promote the eruption

Belladonna, extract, $\frac{1}{8}$ to $\frac{1}{6}$ gr. internally as a prophylactic when depression exists and to promote eruptions

Digitalis, with hyoscyamus and juniper to lower temperature and to maintain renal secretion free

Elaterium, with potassii bitartratis and scammony powder, is useful

Fever—Scarlet.—(*contd.*)

Juniper oil, as diuretic if dropsy exists
Mustard bath is of benefit
Oil inunctions, as cocoa butter in desquamative stage is very useful
Pilocarpine is useful
Quinine, internally or by enema if delirium and restlessness exist
Rhus toxicodendron to overcome typhoid or rheumatic symptoms
Veratrum viride in convulsions

Fever—Typhoid, Enteric leading to Intestinal Hæmorrhage; Rectal Ulceration, Tympanitis.

Arnica is useful in asthenic cases or when vital powers are greatly depressed
Aspidospermine sulphate hypodermically to lower the temperature
Bals tolu or tincture benzoin compound with guaiacol, useful in fever complicated with cough
Baptisia, in the early stage is very useful
Belladonna, to steady the pulse, to lower the temperature and to clean the tongue; also useful if pupils are contracted and there is low muttering delirium. Its effect is to counteract the poison of typhoid
Caffeine, with sodium benzoate subcutaneously is useful
Cinnamon oil is efficient to abort the fever
Digitalis with aconite, tinct. iodine and carbolic acid in drop doses is useful to lower the temperature and pulse rate and to sustain the heart's action; it is inadvisable in the later stages
Ergot fluid extract for intestinal hæmorrhage hypodermically if the symptoms are urgent
Eucalyptus oil, with spirit ammon. aromat. spt. chloroform and glycerin, is useful
Guaiacol, used as inunction in the axilla and groins to reduce the temperature when above 102 deg.
Guaiacol carbonate, a good non-poisonous, abortive; lessens the temperature and acts as an intestinal antiseptic
Hydrastine to relieve copious sweats
Hyoscyamus to relieve the brain symptoms as delirium, headache and to relieve constipation
Opium internally given at bed time or as injection or as suppository to relieve diarrhœa or intestinal perforation or to check delirium and wakefulness or to arouse vital powers when much depressed; useful in advanced stage of fever characterised by low muttering delirium, picking up of bed clothes, twitching of muscles, &c.
Quinine hydrobromate is useful in typho-malarial fever. To be avoided if the typhoid element predominates or in purely continued fever
Serpentaria, if much depression exists to be avoided if there is intestinal irritation
Turpentine oil, with tincture opii and oleum caryophylli is given at the end of the second week to check intestinal hæmorrhage, tympanitis, dry or red tongue and diarrhœa. It arouses the vital powers if coma or stupor supervenes
Veratrum viride tincture, one drop as a cardiac sedative to reduce temperature
Vinegar, aromatic, for sponging the body

External remedies.—Avoid solid food; use cold bath, cold packing if temperature above 102 deg., cold compresses or wet sheets or washing with cold water.

Observe cleanliness, free ventilation, perfect rest, milk diet, eggs, broth, coffee, stimulants if necessary.

Formula.—Acid carbolic, $\frac{1}{4}$ mn.; guaiacol, $\frac{1}{2}$ gr.; menthol, $\frac{1}{8}$ gr.; thymol, $\frac{1}{10}$ gr.; eucalyptol, 2 ms.; podophyllin, $\frac{1}{25}$ gr.; and ipecacuanha, $\frac{1}{8}$ gr.; make pil. Dose 1 pill.

Fever—Typhus.

Arnica is very useful
Belladonna, to reduce the temperature, to strengthen the pulse, to control delirium, moisten the tongue, and shorten the course of disease; useful if the pupils are contracted
Baptisia is very useful
Camphor of great benefit; to be avoided if the tongue is fleshy and red, abdomen tender or tympanitic
Coffee in adynamic state is very useful
Digitalis is useful in large doses

Fever-Typhus.—(*contd.*)

Hyoscyamus, to relieve brain symptoms
Podophyllin, as a laxative at the onset to relieve bilious headache, constipation, and hepatic derangements
Rhatany, a good tonic in advanced stages
Serpentaria, with ammonium carbonate, in delirium, wakefulness, and dry tongue. It excites diaphoresis and supports vital powers

External remedies—Isolation as the disease is contagious. Diet should be nutritious and supporting.

Fistula (*See Vol. I, page 489.*)

Calotropis gigantea, in combination with the juice of nateriothuhar and with the wood of berberis asiatica as a caustic
Capsicum infusion locally is useful as stimulant in fistulous ulcerations
Piper nigrum, confection, a nice stimulant in anal fistula
Sanguinaria, injection is very beneficial
Ulmus fulva, the bark is used as a lint into the fistula

Fractures and Dislocations (*See Vol. I, page 490.*)

Aconite, useful if fever sets in
Arnica tincture, internally or the infusion locally to neutralize the illeffects of mechanical injury
Benzoin compound tincture, in severe injuries locally as a dresssing for compound fracture. It leads to rapid healing
Opium internally or morphine hypodermically as anodyne, to relieve nervousness or muscular spasms

Formula—Astragalus Sarcocolla, 9 ; delphinium (jadwar), 1 ; aloes, 15; alum, 8 ; boswelia, 8; letsœa sebifera, 4; shorea robusta, 4; benzoin, 7 ; curcuma aromatica, 7; and gamboge, 12; mix, make lep (soft plaster) in spirit of wine. Application for dislocations, fractures, simple sprains, and contusions.

Freckles; Sun burn. (*See Vol. I, page 490.*)

Alpinia galangal
Amygdala amara, emulsion locally
Balanitis roxburghii
Benzoin compound tincture with water locally as cosmetic
Sagargota

Gangrene. (*See Vol. I, page 490.*)

Charcoal, as poultices
Cinchona or quinine is of benefit
Lemon juice is, sometimes, dropped into the wound and covered with chlorine solution
Myrtol, useful in gangrene of the lungs
Opium, to relieve pain and restlessness
Turpentine, is useful after the gangrenous part has been removed; it may be given internally or inhaled from warm water in pulmonary gangrene or applied locally in dry or chronic gangrene

Gastralgia, Gastrodynia.

Atropine, is very useful to relieve neuralgic pain of the abdominal viscera
Belladonna, to relieve gastric pain
Coca internally is of benefit
Cocaine, 5 p. c. solution, gastric sedative and anodyne ; it may be given internally with benefit
Codeine internally is useful
Ergot is useful in gastric and other visceral neuralgia
Hydrocyanic acid is useful to check vomiting, to relieve gastric pain and to cure gastralgia due to nervous derangements
Morphine internally in small doses given with bismuth or milk or injected hypodermically is very useful
Nux vomica, tincture is very useful as a stomachic in gastric disorders
Opium is useful to relieve pain
Pulsatilla is efficient in dyspepsia characterised with pain, coated tongue, headache, and nervous depression
Quinine is useful in gastric pain showing periodicity and a neuralgic character
Strychnine hypoderimically is very useful in gastrodynia and gastralgia

Gastric dilatation.

Nux vomica
Strychnine, internally or hypodermically
Stomach to be washed

Gastric ulcer. *(See Vol. I, page 493.)*

Acid gallic, 5 gr., internally for hæmorrhage
Atropine, to relieve pain and vomiting
Charcoal to ease the pain by preventing formation of acid products
Ergotine, hypodermically injected to check hæmorrhage
Morphine, to relieve pain and vomiting, to localize peritonitis ; in full doses if perforation occurs until adhesions take place
Turpentine, internally for hæmorrhage

Gastritis (Acute). *(See Vol. I, page 492.)*

Antidotes, in cases of irritant poisons
Morphine, hypodermically or opium internally to relieve pain
Mustard poultices to the stomach

Formula.—Tinct. veratrum viride 15 ms. ; liq. morphiæ sulphatis, 25 ms. ; acidi carbolici, 4 ms. ; and aquæ menthæ pip, 1 oz. Dose, 1 dr.

Gastritis (Chronic). *(See Vol. I, page 492.)*

Acid hydrocyanic dilute, with lime water very useful
Andropogon citratum, to relieve gastric irritability
Belladonna extract, locally to the pit of the stomach
Cinchona, infusion with mineral acids to promote healthy state of the mucous membrane in gastric catarrh of drunkards
Caffeine in gastric catarrh when associated with migraine is very useful
Calumba and other vegetable bitters
Caryophylli oleum, to allay irritation
Eucalyptus, as a stomachic very useful ; it should be avoided in inflammatory gastritis
Food, starchy, very useful
Hydrastis tincture, or the fluid extract, useful in gastric catarrh due to alcoholism
Ipecacuanha wine to check nausea and vomiting
Morphine, to check pain of gastric catarrh due to alcoholic excess
Nux vomica, tincture in gastric catarrh with sick headache or in gastric catarrh occurring in the course of chronic diseases
Opium, to quell pain of gastritis due to alcohol
Podophyllin, as a purge to act on the upper bowels
Pulsatilla to relieve gastric catarrh associated with heartburn, nausea, no taste, white tongue, flatulence &c.
Tannic acid, alone or with acetate of morphia is useful to check vomiting

Glaucoma. *(See Vol. I, page 494.)*

Atropine, hypodermically with care.
Physostigmine, alone or with quinine to lower intra-ocular tension, to abort threatened glaucoma
Pilocarpine is very useful

Glandular Affections as Buboes, Goitre, Parotitis, Tabes Mesenterica, Tonsilitis, &c.

Barleria prionitis, root as paste, applied locally
Belladonna, useful in tonsilitis
Cheiranthus cheiri, the seeds as a paste locally applied
Elæodendron glaucum, the bark as a paste
Ficus glomerata, the milky juice locally applied to mumps
Kæmpferia rotunda, the tubers applied locally to glandular swellings
Pilocarpine, in acute inflammation of parotids and of sub-maxillary glands
Valerian with guaiacum, internally in strumous enlargements

Gleet.

Asparagus adscendens, compound powder in milk
Balsam of tolu and peru
Buchu infusion or tincture internally
Canada balsam internally
Copaiba, locally to the urethral canal will stop gleet
Eucalyptol, useful in chronic catarrh of the urino genital tract
Pinus gerandiana as confection internally
Piper methysticum, internally useful in obstinate cases
Quercus infectorius as urethral injection
Sandal wood oil internally
Tannin with glycerin and olive oil for urethral injection
Turpentine, if gleet is due to relaxed condition of the urethra

Gonorrhœa. (*See Vol. I, page 494.*)

Aconite tincture, is useful in the acute stage
Allium cepa internally is useful
Boldoin, local anæsthetic like cocaine, useful as urethral injection
Borassus flabelliformis, the juice or toddy when fresh is of benefit
Chimaphilla, fluid extract, internally
Cannabis indica, tincture, is very useful to relieve pain and diminish discharge and it acts like copaiba or sandal oil
Chrysanthemum internally with kala miri, as infusion is very useful
Colchicum wine very useful
Copaiba, given with glycerrhiza, gaultheria oil and spirit of nitre is of benefit, it is injurious in the early state, should not be given until pain in urination and chordee is gone, and the discharge becomes yellow
Cubeb oleo resin, better than copaiba is non-irritant. In acute cases it gives good results
Dipterocarpus turbinatus balsam, useful like copaiba
Eregeron canadensis, (fleabane) oil, with santal oil and alcohol internally is useful
Garjan balsam, with star anise, internally
Gelsemium serviceable in the acute stage
Gmelina, internally as demulcent in gonorrhœa
Plantago ispaghula as demulcent is useful
Plumeria acuminata, as a useful demulcent
Pareira tincture is useful
Pulsatilla in sub-acute and gonorrhœal ophthalima
Saw palmetto fluid extract, internally very useful
Salvia plebia, as demulcent
Santal oil with cinnamon oil or with buchu and cubeb in subacute cases
Uva ursi, useful

Avoid injections in acute cases

External remedies.—Injections chiefly used are:—Lead acetate with acetic acid useful for urethral injection; cocaine, 2 p. c solution; gallabromol, 1 or 2 p. c. solution is useful; hydrastis root, infusion 1 dr. to 8 oz. of water or the fluid extract with bismuth and glycerin; quinine with diluted sulphuric acid or with lactic acid; hydnocarpus wrightiana infusion of seeds; opium with lead acetate and glycerin; matico; tannin, &c.

Formula.—Tinctura sanguinaria, 1 dr.; tinctura kino, 1 dr.; oleum santal 1 dr.; balsam copaiba, 1 dr.; spiritus etheris nitrosi, 1 dr.; olei gaultheriæ, 10 ms.; and liquor potassæ, 1 dr. Dose, 1 dr. internally.

(2) Copaiba oil, cubeb oil, santal oil, aà 5 drops; salol, 1 gr.; pepsin, 1 gr.; Mix. make a pill mass. Dose, 2 pills.

Gout. (*See Vol. I, page. 497.*)

Aconite, both internally and locally to relieve pain
Belladonna, internally, also externally to soothe the pain, useful in stomach gout
Cajuput oil, locally to the joints
Cascara sagrada, to promote elimination of uric acid
Caffeine is useful in eliminating the poison of gout from the system

Gout.—(*contd.*)

Colchicine salicylate, or colchicum wine, a good palliative to remove heat, pain and swelling of joints; useful in acute and rheumatic gout, in bronchitis. asthma, dyspepsia, and urticaria in gouty subjects

Menispermun canadense, like sarsaparilla is useful

Morphine, hypodermically injected close to the affected joint but outside of the red areola to relieve pain

Poultices linseed meal, with sodium carbonate, a useful application

Strychnine, is very useful in later stages of g ut or paralysis

Veratrine, ointment locally to relieve the inflammation from painful joints

Gums (Spongy). (*See Vol. I, page 499.*)

Benzoin tincture, locally

Catechu, with honey locally or catechu alone to dissolve in the mouth for spongy gums

Cocaine 5 p.c. solution applied locally to gums

Krameria, as gargle is useful

Myrrh with cinchona infusion as gargle or as a mouth wash, useful for spongy or ulcerated gums

Pomegranate bark infusion as gargle, usefnl in relaxed gums

Quercus bark, as gargle is useful

Rhatany, is used as a dentifrice

Tannin with glycerin locally applied, useful for spongy and bleeding gums

Headache—Congestive Headache ; Bilious, Dyspeptic or Sick headache Nervous Headache ; Hemicrania ; and Hysterical Headache. (*See Vol. I, page 509.*)

Allium or ginger paste applied locally to the forehead

Aconite, internally to lower the circulation, locally as ointment applied over the eyebrow in hemacrinia

Belladonna, 3 to 5 ms. of the tincture to relieve pain ; the extract applied over the eyebrows when headache is due to over fatigue or mental over work or to biliousness or to stomach or uterine disorders

Bryonia in bilious headache

Caffeine citras with lime juice or caffeine with antipyrine or with sodium bromide, given internally or used hypodermically is useful to relieve pain when headache is due to overwork

Cajuputi oleum, externally and internally is very useful

Camphor with hyoscyamus, internally or its saturated solution mixed with eau-de-cologne locally applied to the forehead is useful in uterine headache or in hysterical headache

Cannabis indica tincture, or the extract is of benefit in climacteric headache. It chiefly acts on the nervous centre whence the disorder arises

Cimicifuga useful in rheumatic headache and in that occurring at the menstrual period

Calocynth (pilulæ colocynthides compositus,) with silver nitrate, useful to relieve hysterical headache or that due to overwork

Digitatis, useful to relieve congestive hemicrania

Guarana, or the fluid extract as a palliative, useful to relieve periodical headaches

Gelsemium with hydrastis, internally useful if the headache is accompanied with constipation

Ignatia, useful to remove hysterical headache

Iris, useful to relieve headache with supra-orbital pain, accompanied with nausea and vomiting or due to hepatic derangement

Menthol, locally to the forehead is useful in frontal headache

Mustard foot bath or as plaster is useful

Nux vomica after meals. The extract with iron and quinine is useful in hysterical or chlorotic headache associated with gastric catarrh and nausea

Oleum menth. pip dissolved in alcohol, locally applied to the forehead and base of the occiput in bilious headache

Picrotoxin, for the stomach is useful in periodic headache

Purgatives as aloes, colocynth or podophyllin with capsicum and belladonna, act as derivatives to relieve headache occuring near the menstrual period accompanied with constipation or when due to suppression of hæmorrhoidal discharges

Quinine internally is of great benefit

Sanguinaria useful in headache due to gastric disorder

Headache.—(*contd.*)

Strychnine with belladonna and aloes is useful in bilious headache with constipation

Tea, strong, useful to relieve nervous headache

Valerian, in excitable, nervous or hysterical persons, given with either sulphuric, compound tincture of lavender or tincture of hyoscyamus

Zinc valerianate with belladonna often given with success

External remedies.—Liniments, of belladonna or veratria, or chloroform or aconite; hot foot bath or mustard footbath; mustard or capsicum plaster to the nape of the neck, or cajuput oil; camphor solution saturated with eau-de-cologne applied locally to the forehead; dry cupping; a paste to the forehead containing menthol dissolved in alcohol or ginger, or of cloves, sandal wood, black pepper, ajmânâ phul, nimb oil; poultices of nâgli, bâjri to the head.

Formula.—Extract belladonna, $\frac{1}{6}$ gr.; extract cannabis indica, $\frac{1}{6}$ gr.; pilulæ asafetidæ co 1 grs.; quininæ disulph, 1 gr.; acid carbolic, $\frac{1}{2}$m.; oil cajuputi, $\frac{1}{2}$ m.; mix; make pill. Dose, 1 pill.

Heart Affections—Functional, Dilated Heart, Fatty Heart, Heart Palpitation, Hypertrophied Heart. (*See Vol. I, page 512.*)

Acid hydrocyanic dilute or aqua laurocerasus to relieve palpitation if due to dyspepsia

Aconite tincture, to diminish cardiac excitement or irritability; useful in pericarditis, in fluttering heart, due to nervous palpitations and hypertrophy. It prevents heart complication if given in rheumatic fever

Adonis vernalis tincture or Adonidin as cardiac regulator to increase the heart beats; given in dropsy due to dilatation or to mitral regurgitation

Apocynum cannabinum, to diminish the frequency of pulse

Belladonna internally in irregular rhythm as a plaster over the cardiac region. In cardiac dyspnœa it is useful

Camphor monobromate, internally useful in tumultuous heart

Caffeine citrate, as a diuretic, an excellent heart stimulant, in cardiac pain, dyspnœa and weak heart

Cimicifuga safer than digitalis. It is stimulating and tonic in fatty heart to relieve dyspnœa and in dilated weak heart

Convallaria majalis, infusion acts like digitalis in functional and organic cardiac affections; also in aortic disease with œdema of tissues

Coronilla scorpioides tincture is useful

Dhatura useful in cardiac dyspnœa

Digitalis, infusion, acts as a stimulant tonic and sedative. Best given when the heart is weak, and irritable with irregular pulse; if the dilation is due to spermatorrhœa, it may be given with ergot

Eucalyptus, is useful in nervous palpitation with weak heart

Grindelia robusta, in cardiac dyspnœa and in cough due to cardiac hypertrophy

Hyoscyamine sulphate, hypodermically or hyoscyamus tincture in functional derangement from emotion or excited brain; in palpitation of the heart and other functional derangements in nervous persons it is useful

Jaborandi useful as a diaphoretic in cardiac dropsy

Morphine internally, or hypodermically in cardiac dyspnœa due to nervous emotion; also in mitral regurgitation, in angina, and insomnia

Nicotine useful for functional disturbance

Nux vomica, tincture every half hour, is very useful in cardiac hypertrophy or mitral insufficiency and sudden heart failure; in nervous palpitation it is given with benefit

Heart Affections.—(*contd.*)

Opium and belladonna, in cardiac dropsy
Prunus virginiana is useful in dyspnœa
Sparteine sulphate ; useful in mitral or aortic disease
Senega, with ammonia and hyoscyamus in hysterical heart irregularity
Strophanthus, like digitalis, a cardiac stimulant, useful in palpitation and valvular disease
Strychnine with iron and nourishing diet as a cardiac tonic, to strengthen the heart beats
Theobromine with sodium salicylate and valerian, useful in nervous palpitation with dyspnœa
Veratrum viride, as cardiac depressant, given in chronic heart disease with hypertrophy when digitalis is dangerous ; unguentum veratrinæ applied to the chest in palpitation with dyspnœa, lividity of the face, inability to lie down, irregular pulse and dropsy
Wild cherry, useful in cardiac dyspnœa

Heart (Valvular) Disease. (*See Vol. I, page 513.*)

Aconite tincture, useful to relieve palpitation; it diminishes the blood pressure in the arterioles. It is dangerous in hypertrophy due to organic disease
Cactus, in complicated aortic regurgitation and mitral insufficiency; it stimulates the heart's action
Convallaria in mitral disease
Digitalis infusion, or tincture, in aortic regurgitation, mitral insufficiency and in weak heart
Jaborandi in aortic insufficiency
Morphine, hypodermically to relieve dyspnœa due to mitral disease and in aortic insufficiency
Quebracho cortex to relieve cardiac dyspnœa
Veratrum viride tincture, with tinct aconite and tincture zingiber, as sedative.

Formula.—Infusum digitalis; 6 oz. ; caffeine citras, ½ dr. ; tincturæ strophanth 1 dr. ; liq potassii citratis, 2 ozs. ; ext., glycerrhizæ, 1½ dr. ; mix. Dose, ½ oz. in anasarca due to heart disease.

Heat, Stroke. (*See Vol. I, page 514.*)

Bleeding if the patient is plethoric, with high arterial tension
Digitalis tincture, hypodermically injected
Morphine, hypodermically, to control convulsions
Quinine hydrochlorate, hypodermically injected if malaria is suspected or germs discovered in the blood

Hectic Fever. (*See Vol. I, page 514.*)

Aconite tincture, to relieve irritative hectic fever of phthisis
Digitalis, with iron—to abate the fever and diminish sweats
Morphine, and other anodynes very useful.
Prunus virginiana, the bark is very useful to relieve irritable cough
Quinine, in large doses, to be given before the paroxysm

Hæmatemesis. (*See Vol. I, page 499.*)

Acid gallic, is useful in combination with dilute sulphuric acid to relieve hæmorrhage
Ergot hypodermically
Hæmostatics very useful
Hamamelis tincture, very useful
Ipecacuanha, useful in small doses if bleeding is due to vicarious menstruation
Krameria internally useful
Logwood very useful
Morphia hypodermically or opium as enema
Tannin, useful if bleeding is due to hepatic obstruction or to gastric ulcer
Turpentine oil, useful in passive hæmorrhage with debility ; and in hæmorrhagic transudation on the free mucous surface

Hæmatocele (Pelvic). (*See Vol. I, page 499.*)

Bandage to the abdomen
Cold application to the abdomen
Hæmostatics, as gallic acid, lead or turpentine to arrest hæmorrhage, or ergot and iron with mercury bichloride
Ice into the vagina
Opium or morphine, to relieve pain
Rest absolute
Tonics

Hæmaturia. (*See Vol. I, page 500.*)

Acid acetic or vinegar with ice water injected into the bladder to arrest alarming hæmorrhage
Acid gallic, 10 to 20 grs., is very useful
Camphor, removes renal hyperæmia with bloody coagulable urine caused by copaiba, cantharis, turpentine or oil of mustard
Cannabis indica, in dysuria, strangury and bloody urine is very useful
Chimaphilla, very useful to control hæmorrhage
Digitalis with krameria, internally is useful
Ergot, internally, alone, or combined with astringents as krameria, &c., or injected hypodermically is very useful
Hamamelis, useful in severe cases
Mustard to the spine or mustard with capsicum application to the extremities
Matico infusion, as an astringent, very useful
Quinine, when it is intermittent or due to malarial infection
Turpentine, in small doses with digitalis is very useful in hæmaturia associated with constitutional debility.

Hemiplegia. (*See Vol. I, page 503.*)

Aconite, if due to organic cerebral lesion
Cocculus, is useful in hysterical choreic and epileptic hemiplegia
Physostigma, to prevent wasting of muscles
Strychnine, internally and hypodermically when the paralysis is incomplete, and the muscles flaccid but not wasted

Hæmoptysis. (*See Vol. I, page 500.*)

Acid gallic, with ergotine and digitalis very useful
Acid tannic as inhalation
Aconite of benefit
Arnica is useful in cases due to violence
Atropine, hypodermically stops hæmorrhage of phthisis
Bursa pastoris is useful
Digitalis infusion or tincture is very useful
Dragon's blood internally is useful
Ergot, liquid extract, with ipecacuanha and opium internally or ergotin hypodermically is of benefit
Erigeron, useful when there is no fever or other signs of constitutional irritation
Hamamelis fluid extract or the tincture is very useful
Ipecacuanha is useful in large doses till nausea is produced
Laricis tincture is useful
Morphine, hypodermically, or opium internally to lessen the excitement
Turpentine oil is very useful after other hæmostatics have failed

Hæmorrhage; Hæmorrhagic Diathesis. (*See Vol. I, page 501.*)

Acid gallic, alone or combined with ergot and digitalis, is useful in passive hæmorrhages in relaxed and debilitated subjects
Aconite, to lower the circulation, useful in bleeding from the nose or lungs
Agaric or laricic acid locally, in leech bites
Arnica, in ecchymosis, due to mechanical violence
Atropine, hypodermically useful in internal hæmorrhages
Belladonna is useful in hæmorrhage from rectal ulcers
Cetratria islandica, soft filaments used like styptic cotton
Digitalis, alone or with restoratives, is very useful in uterine and other hæmorrhages and in hæmorrhagic diathesis
Ergot, internally or ergotin hypodermically, is useful in removing purpura and in checking uterine hæmorrhage of any kind
Hamamelis tincture very useful
Hæmatoxylon, least irritative, and hence useful to check intestinal and other hæmorrhages

Hæmorrhage—(*contd.*)

Ipecacuanha, beneficial in internal hæmorrhages, when given in moderate doses. In large doses it produces hæmorrhage

Myristica, burned and powdered, useful in hæmorrhagic diathesis

Nux vomica alone or with quinine, phosphates and iron, useful in anæmic subjects and in hæmorrhagic diathesis

Turpentine, internally and locally in passive hæmorrhages, in small doses useful in hæmorrhage of typhoid fever in hæmaturia, and hæmoptysis

Vinegar (apple vinegar) as injection in hæmorrhage from the bladder; locally to check hæmorrhage from leech and other insect bites, and from piles, cuts, &c.

Hæmorrhage (Intestinal). (*See Vol. I, page 502.*)

Acid gallic, or acid tannic with tincture of opium useful in hæmorrhage during typhoid fever

Belladonna, to relieve bleeding from irritable rectal ulcers

Ergotin, used hypodermically

Hamamelis, is useful as it contains tannin in large proportion

Opium as adjunct to astringents to allay nervous excitement

Saw palmetto very useful

Turpentine oil useful in hæmorrhage accompanying typhoid fever

Hæmorrhage (Uterine, Post Partem). (*See Vol. I, page 502.*)

Acid gallic

Achillea

Atropine, hypodermically is useful

Cimicifuga, is useful to check tediously prolonged hæmorrhage

Digitalis, infusion internally or injection hypodermically with ether is useful in urgent cases

Ergot extract, internally or ergotine injected deeply into the tissues of the arm is of benefit

Hamamelis in continuous oozing is very useful

Ipecacuanha, in emetic doses to check post partem hæmorrhage

Nux vomica tincture, with ergot extract liquid internally is very useful

Opium with brandy, if hæmorrhage is profuse

Tampon by iodized gauze, or absorbent cotton, useful to check hæmorrhage from abortion or placenta prævia. To be avoided in post partem hæmorrhage

Vinegar, astringent and antiseptic, used as a plug into the cavity of the uterus. It acts promptly by causing uterine contraction

External remedies.—Firm pressure on the uterus, compression of the abdominal aorta, intra-uterine injection of hot water most prompt and certain to check hæmorrhage, tamponade by absorbent cotton, enemata of hot water.

Hæmorrhoids (*See Vol. I, page 502.*)

Acid gallic and benzoin, or acid tannic with opium as suppository

Aloes, with hyoscyamus and ipecacuanha to relieve the bowels and thus to relieve pelvic congestion

Anal douche

Chrysarobin, 12; iodoform, 4; extract of belladonna, 8; vaseline, 60; as application or as suppositories

Cocaine solution, 5 p. c. locally

Datura alba, poultice to external piles

Ergot, liquid extract with or without nux vomica given internally in dilated hæmorrhoidal veins, or with acid carbolic used locally is very useful

Galls, as ointment or galls combined with acetate of lead and opium is very useful

Grape cure is used with benefit

Hamamelis tincture, internally or locally as enema or suppository or as lotion or ointment in bleeding piles

Hydrastis tincture, internally, and as lotion or ointment locally to external piles to relieve congestion

Hyoscyamus, the leaves bruised and applied locally to relieve pain

Krameria, with mucilage as injection into hæmorrhoids

Linseed oil boiled and given internally is of benefit

Menthol, with thymol and eucalyptol with chloroform locally

Hæmorrhoids.—(*contd.*)

Nux vomica, very useful
Piper nigrum confection.
Pitch ointment, locally
Podophyllin, as cathartic, is useful in recent piles and to check bleeding from stasis in portal circulation
Quercus bark decoction, as a wash or as injection
Senna, confection to procure soft evacuations
Stillingia, very useful if due to constipation; gives temporary relief if due to hepatic obstruction
Stramonium, leaves bruised or ointment locally to relieve pain

Formula —Acid tannic, 1 ; acid carbolic, 2, alcohol, 4 ; and glycerin, 8. Injection into the pile.

Ointment.—Galls, 1 ; chloroform, 1 ; extract ergotæ, ½ ; ext. stramonii, ¾ ; extract hamamelis, 1 ; oleum tar, ½ ; cerate, 20, locally.

Ointment.—Opium, 20 ; acid tannic, 20 ; acid carbolic, 10 ; extract ergotæ, 120 ; ungt. petrolei, 500. Extract belladonna, 15 gr. ; extract thebain, 15 gr. ; antipyrin, 30 grs. ; ungt. hydrargyri, 2 drs ; and lanolin, 18 drs. applications for inflamed hæmorrhoids.

Hepatic Diseases. (*See Vol. I, page .*)

Bitters, vegetable tonics as gentian, &c., useful in functional disorders
Bryonia, useful in various hepatic diseases chiefly hepatalgia
Chelidonium is useful
Euonymin, useful in torpid liver with accompanying headache
Ipecacuanha, to promote the flow of bile, useful in functional hepatic disorders
Malt liquors are to be avoided in fatty and other liver affections
Nux vomica, with podophyllin and mercury in small doses is useful
Podophyllin as an active cholagogue, very useful in a variety of liver diseases
Resinous cholagogues or purgatives as iris, euonymin, leptandrin and rhubarb
Quinine, useful only in malarial subjects
Sanguinaria, in hepatic engorgement in the hysteric without any organic lesion
Stillingia, useful in torpid liver. In jaundice following ague it is very useful ; also in ascites from hepatic changes and in the first stage of cirrhosis
Taraxacum, is useful in chronic liver affections

Hepatitis and Hepatic Abscess. (*See Vol. I. page 505.*)

Aconite, in the early stage
Chelidonium, useful in both acute and chronic hepatitis
Colchicum and alkalies when the subject is gouty
Ipecacuanha, in large doses if dysentery be present
Linseed alone or with opium as poultices over the hepatic region in acute hepatitis
Quinine, useful in acute parenchymatous inflammation; also in chronic suppurative hepatitis without abscess
Veratrum viride in the early stage

Hepatic Cirrhosis. (*See Vol. I, page 504.*)

Boldo
Coptis teeta
Menispermum
Rubus
Stillingia, is useful in the early stage

Hepatic Torpor, Hepatic Congestion. (*See Vol. I, page 503.*)

Avoid starch, fats and alcohol
Boldoa fragrans extract, in chronic cases
Colchicum, to relieve congestion associated with dropsy
Chelidonium majus, as a deobstruent to relieve congestion
Chevica leaves made warm and applied over the hepatic region are of benefit
Iris, useful if stools are clay coloured, and skin jaundiced ; a nice aperient
Quinine, alone or with morphia, in acute congestion due to malarial and climatic causes
Taraxacum, with aloes and ipecacuanha
Turpentine stupes to the hepatic region very useful

Hernia. (*See Vol. I, page 505.*)

Belladonna and ether locally
Castor oil or olive oil and turpentine as enema
Coffee, large doses, aids in reducing strangulated hernia
Ipecacuanha, as sternutatory or as snuff to cause sneezing ; it has often succeeded after taxis has failed to effect reduction. The patient should lie on his shoulders with elevated hips
Morphine, hypodermically for strangulation
Oak bark extract injected into the tissues to stimulate occlusion of the ring
Oil
Opium to narcotism sometimes obviates the necessity for an operation
Oil of cloves, used as injection into the tissues
Tobacco, as rectal enema
Sternutatories to cause sneezing

Herpes—Herpes Zoster. (*See Vol. I, page 505.*)

Acid tannic, locally
Aconite or opium, locally to relieve pain in herpes zoster
Belladonna, locally in herpes zoster
Cocaine solution, 2 p.c. locally
Dulcamara, in herpes zoster
Ergot oil, prepared by the action of benzin upon ergot, useful as a coating in herpes on the genitals and in other skin diseases
Grindelia, useful to relieve pain
Menthol locally, in herpes zoster
Morphine oleate, to relieve pain ; used locally or hypodermically
Myrtal, a nice remedy
Pix liquida, to relieve itching
Rhus toxicodendron, to relieve itching or burning in herpes zoster
Starch, bandage or dusted over the part gives relief
Veratrine ointment to relieve neuralgia following herpes zoster

Hiccough. (*See Vol. I, page 507.*)

Apomorphine is useful
Atropine and morphine, hypodermically useful to check hiccough
Camphor is very useful
Cannabis indica internally is useful
Capsicum tincture internally
Conium succus internally
Morphine, hypodermically alone or with atropine to arrest hiccough
Laurel water
Mentha piperitæ spirit, internally
Mustard with hot water taken internally is very useful
Nux vomica, with dilute nitric acid internally is very useful
Opium with chloroform is useful
Physostigma
Pilocarpine hydrochlorate, is very useful in obstinate cases
Pepper, 2 to 5 grs. useful to stop hiccough
Pressure over the phrenic nerve, hyoid bone or the epigastrium
Tobacco smoking
Valerian with zinc internally

Formula.—Oleum succini, 1 dr. ; spt. etheris nitrosi, 4 drs. ; olei menthæ pip, 1 dr. spt. ether comp, 3 drs. ; pot. bicarb, 2 drs. ; and mucilage, 4 ozs. Mix. Dose, 1 to 2 drs.

Hydrocephalus (Acute and Chronic). (*See Vol. I, page 507.*)

Croton oil liniment as derivative or as revulsive, applied locally to the scalp
Cod liver oil inunction or internally in the chronic form
Malt extract internally in chronic cases
Turpentine, as enema or internally, or with castor oil as inunction

Hydrophobia. (*See Vol. I, page 508.*)

Belladonna, in hyperæmic state of the brain and spinal cord
Calabar bean
Cannabis
Conine
Curare, hypodermically injected to antagonize convulsions, dispel symptoms and replace them by paralysis of the limbs
Excision of the bitten part
Garlic powder, locally and decoction internally
Hydrastine hydrochlorate, hypodermically
Morphine injected deep into the tetanized muscles is a good palliative
Nicotine
Pasteur's treatment
Stramonium

Hydrothorax. (*See Vol. I, page 508.*)

Apocynum cannabinum, a useful diuretic
Broomtops, internally
Copaiba resin is useful
Digitalis infusion as a diuretic is given to relieve the dropsical form, useful in pleuritic effusions
Elaterium, as a derivative is very useful
Jabcrandi is very useful
Sanguinaria, produces good effects

Hypochondriasis. (*See Vol. I, page 508.*)

Aloes, myrrh and nux vomica internally
Asafetida, to relieve flatulence and mental depression
Caffein citrate, as a cerebral stimulant is useful
Coca, fluid extract or wine, useful in cases marked by debility, nervousness and mental affections accompanied by depression
Cimicifuga, is useful in puerperal hypochondriasis and that accompanying spermatorrhœa
Hyoscyamus, in syphilophobia
Ignatia tincture is a good remedy
Opium with arsenic, as stimulant is very useful in the aged
Valerian, to relieve flatulence of hypochrondriasis

Hysteria. (*See Vol. I, page 509.*)

Andropogon muricatus is very useful
Anthemis nobilis is useful internally
Annona squamosa, locally to the nostrils
Apomorphine hypodermically to relieve the fits
Asafetida, in hysterical convulsions with flatulence, cough, &c. It removes headache
Atropine, in hysterical aphonia
Avoid alcohol as it leads to excitement
Camphora, to subdue hysterical excitement
Cannabis indica, internally to allay excitement
Chamomile oil, in spasmodic and pseudoneuralgic affections in women
Cimicifuga, in hysterical chorea and fits, also to relieve headache
Conine hydrobromate, internally
Ergot with quinine and iron or with tonics in sub-involution of the uterus with indigestion and anæmia
Galbanum, internally or as plaster
Garlic or onion to smell during the paroxysm
Gynandropsis pentaphylla, decoction, internally
Ignatia, useful to relieve globus hystericus, with hysterical cry, feeling of suffocation, flatulence, &c.
Ipecacuanha, as emetic
Jatamansi like valerian
Lupulin, to procure sleep
Nux vomica, useful in cases with flatulence, flushing, perspiration and weight on the head
Massage
Opium tincture, 1 mn., with nux vomica tincture 2 ms. for the flushes, to relieve depression and weight on the head
Pellitory, to chew
Santonine, if worms exist
Sumbul internally is useful
Valerian fluid extract, or caffein or quinine or zinc valerianate useful in hysterical dyspepsia
Volatile oils to remove flatulence
Wormseed oil is useful

Ichthyosis. (*See Vol. I, page 514.*)

Baths
Camphor with zinc oxide as ointment
Elm bark decoction as a wash
Sumbuca ointment with cupri sulphate locally
Ulmus, decoction, given internally

Impetigo; Impetigo Syphilitica.

Acid chrysophanic, locally in simple form
Grape cure has been very effective
Gutta percha liquor to cover the pustules
Laurel water, to relieve itching
Menthol locally
Picis ointment
Poultices to remove scabs
Quinine and mineral acid when due to imperfect digestion
Tannate of glycerin, locally

Impotence ; Spermatorrhœa ; Emissions.

Aconitum ferox and conium locally to the perineum
Allium sativum (bulb), internally
Atropine in cases of relaxed genitals is useful
Bambusa arundinacea, the silicious concretion is useful when given internally
Batata paniculata (tuberous root), internally is useful
Belladonna, $\frac{1}{8}$ to $\frac{1}{4}$ gr. with zinc sulphate, 1 gr. internally is useful. In atonic state and in extreme cases to check night emissions
Camphor bromide is useful; it excites at first but is soon followed by depression
Cannabis indica, nux vomica and ergot, very useful in functional impotence
Capsicum with cassia absus, internally is useful
Cimicifuga, a nervine tonic is useful in weak and relaxed condition ; it lessens urethral irritation and relieves hypochondriasis
Cocaine, 4 p.c. solution locally upon glans penis
Cubebs, to remove functional impotency
Curculigo orchioides internally
Damiana, a genital stimulant, very useful
Digitalis infusion, very useful in spermatorrhœa with feeble erections, frequent emissions, and cold extremities
Eucalyptus oil locally in sexual exhaustion
Ergotin, hypodermically about the dorsal vein of penis when its enlargement and rapid emptying is the cause of impotence
Fenugreek (seeds) as injection internally
Gelsemium, as an anaphrodisiac given in combination with belladonna or cimicifuga
Hemp, in mild sexual delirium
Hyoscine hydrobromate, by its influence on the spinal centre is useful in seminal emissions
Hydrastis, fluid extract is injected into the prostatic portion of the urethra
Kola, as a general tonic
Lupulin, a good anaphrodisiac ; with camphor, it acts as a genital sedative and thus checks emission
Morphia suppositories, or injected hypodermically into the perineum is of benefit
Mucuna pruriens (seeds) as confection internally is useful
Myristica officinalis, jaipatri (mace)
Nux vomica, with iron, cantharis and phosphoric acid is useful in atonic condition of the genitals with feeble erections and relaxation
Opium, in small doses excites at first, but soon produces depression
Pyrethrum indicum (root), internally
Polygonum hydropiperoides, useful in functional disorder with feeble erection, watery semen, and soft testis
Quinine is sometimes useful
Rhus aromatica, in sexual exhaustion
Sanguinaria, a nice aphrodisiac, only useful in the functional form
Saw palmetto, internally
Serpentaria tincture, in relaxation and feeble erections ; it restores the power
Stramonium and morphia internally
Strychnine in large doses is useful in impotence. It increases general nutrition and exalts reflex excitability of the general centres
Tribulus terrestris (fruit), confection internally
Tinospora cordifolia fecula confection internally
Ternera aphrodisiaca, very useful
Triticum repens, in sexual exhaustion

External remedies—Avoid masturbation, bougies, hard bed, cold douche to the perinium and testicles in atonic cases, cold sponging, electricity (continuous current), use ice bag to the spine, bath warm, and hygienic measures.

Inflammation and Irritability of the Mucous Membranes.

(*See Vol. I, page* 514.)

Aconite tincture, as antiphlogistic, useful in inflammation of the respiratory organs, in eruptive fevers, in inflammatory states with high temperature. Indicated in the early stage of simple inflammatory fevers and in inflammation of serous membrane as pneumonia, tonsillitis, acute rheumatism, and erysipelas
Aleuritis triloba, if alimentry canal is inflamed
Arnica tincture, as antipyretic is useful in inflammation of serous membranes

Inflammation.—(*contd.*)

Belladonna with aconite internally, useful in scarlet fever, erysipelas, and low fevers. Externally in inflammatary sorethroat, inflammation of the eyes, boils, carbuncles, and in inflammation which threatens to end in abscess, in rheumatism, cystitis, pneumonia, &c.
Bryonia in pleurisy, pericarditis, &c.
Capsicum, as poultices
Cannabis, in chronic cases
Cocaine hydrochlorate, locally in acute inflammation of the mucous membranes to constringe the vessels
Colchicum tincture, is useful in bronchitis and conjunctivitis in gouty subjects
Digitalis, locally and internally in pneumonia, bronchitis, rheumatic fever, scarlet fever, inflammation of the joints, breasts, erysipelas, varicocele, &c.
Flax seed, in inflammation of the mucous membranes
Gelseminm, fluid extract, in pneumonia, pleurisy, and acute stage of gonorrhœa
Linium usitatissimum, in inflammation of the genito-urinary and pulmonary organs
Opium, internally and locally in inflammation of the serous membranse as of the peritonium, meninges, and intestines; useful to check it at commencement, and to relieve pain afterwards
Poultices. to check inflammation or formation of pus
Pilocarpine is useful in the exudative stage of pleuritis, keratitis, iritis, &c.
Pulsatilla is useful in acute inflammations with muco-purulent discharges from the eyes, ears, or nose. In epididymitis, it is given with aconite
Quinine, alone or with morphia is useful in peritonitis, to arrest acute inflammation
Ricinus communis if alimentary canal is inflamed
Santalum album, with stramonium locally as a paste
Tectona grandis root, locally to inflamed skin
Veratrum viride tincture with opium in delirium of fever, pneumonia and in arterial excitement

Formula.—Ant. et pot. tart., 2 grs.; magnesia sulphatis, 2 oz.; morphinæ sulphatis, 1 gr.; syrup zingiberis, 2 oz.; acid sulphuric aromat, ½ dr.; tr. veratri veridis, 1 dr,; aqua, 8 oz. Dose, 4 drs. In fever with delirium, in pneumonia, acute rheumatism, &c.

Influenza. (*See Vol. I, page 516.*)

Acid agaric, against sweating
Acid camphoric, on the tongue as a preventive against sweating
Aconite with potassium citrate and spiritus ætheris nitrosi in the early stage
Benzoin tincture compound, with paregoric elixir, as inhalation
Camphor alone in solution, hypodermically or with caffeine and ether internally if nervous prostration
Camphor, monobromate
Cimicifuga, is very useful
Cocaine hydrochlorate, 4 p.c. solution used in the early stage as a spray or as snuff to be blowed up the nostrils
Coca and kola tincture, to be stuffed into the nostrils or internally to relieve nervous depression
Cubeb tincture, with linseed tea subdues subsequent cough
Digitaline, in low state of the system with pneumonia
Ergot, cannabis and bromides, in combination to relieve vertigo
Eserine and cocaine during desquamation stage
Eucalyptus oil, a nice prophylactic; used as inhalation or sprinkled on cotton and placed in a room
Gelsemium extract to relieve headache
Guarana, to relieve pain in the chest
Ipecacuanha as emetic, in cases of biliary derangements
Menthol dissolved in chloroform or with cocaine used as inhalation or as a spray; a nice prophylactic to abort the attack
Opium, to be avoided; with ipecac, nitre and lobelia, useful only for subsequent cough
Quinine hydrobromate, as a prophylactic against fever and to relieve neuralgic pain following the acute stage
Sanguinaria is very useful
Steam medicated inhalations
Strychnine, to relieve weakness and depression following the disease
Turpentine inhalation is useful
Turkish baths

Insanity—Dementia, Mania or Mental Excitement. (*See Vol. I, page 517.*)

Aconite, in high fever and restlessness in early stage
Atropine, hypodermically is useful in acute cases of insainty with delusions of persecution ; useful where bromides have failed
Belladonna is useful in monomania with hallucination and to relieve mental excitement
Cimicifuga, in mania occurring during pregnancy or after confinement
Colchicum in gouty cases
Conium, or its alkaloids, internally or with morphine hypodermically used to soothe muscular excitement and to quiet noisy patients
Croton oil, as a purgative and as revulsive to relieve cerebral congestion
Daturine hypodermically in acute and chronic mania
Digitalis tincture, a useful palliative in acute and chronic mania, complicated with epilepsy ; it should be avoided if the pulse intermits
Duboisine, hypodermically, a good sedative and hypnotic, in acute mania to allay mental excitability of the insane, inducing quiet and refreshing sleep
Ergot, fluid extract, useful in recurrent mania ; it reduces excitement, shortens attacks, widens intervals and prevents exhaustion
Gelsemium tincture, in mania, with great motor excitement and wakefulness
Hyoscine hydrobromate in emergent cases hypodermically, in delirium with hallucination, in hypochondriacal monomania, in violent intermittent noisiness and in abusive restlessness
Morphine, hypodermically to procure sleep ; is dangerous in mania
Opium, with tartar emetic is useful in melancholia, in climacteric cases and in insanity with depression to allay irritation and to induce sleep. It does not produce narcotism
Stramonium tincture, in furious intermittent dilirium, in cerebral excitement with tendency to suicide and in nymphomania. It allays irritaton and induces quiet sleep
Veratrum viride, to allay excitement in acute mania

Insomnia. (*See Vol. I, page 517.*)

Apomorphine, hypodermically given when the patient is ready for bed
Atropine, with morphia injection
Cannabin tannate, as hypnotic is useful
Chamomile tincture, for children is a very useful sedative
Cocaine hydrochlorate is very useful
Coffee in insomnia of chronic alcoholism and from lowering of nervous power
Digitalis, for want of tone in the vessels, a nice soporific in sleeplessness at night, and drowsiness during the day, is useful
Duboisine with morphine, atropine or belladonna hypodermically is hypnotic and very calmative; useful when great mental excitement exists
Gelsemium, a motor depressant in wakefulness of drunkards, in over-excitement, mania or in simple wakefulness
Humulus lupulus tincture, as cerebral sedative is useful
Hyoscyamus tincture, a good substitute for opium in children or hyoscine hydrobromate hypodermically in insomnia of the insane
Ignatia, in nervous erythism to avoid sleeplessness
Narceine and codeine are useful
Opium tincture, with chloral is a useful hypnotic, in insomnia due to pain
Pellotin, an alkaloid from anhalonium lewini (cactus), hypodermically as a hypnotic to be used with care
Scopolamine hydrochlorate is useful
Sumbul tincture, with chloric ether in insomnia due to chronic alcoholism
Tobacco smoking

Intestinal Obstruction ; Intussusception. (*See Vol. I., page 519.*)

Belladonna, internally or as enema to give tone and to relieve painful spasm
Caffeine, to act on muscular tissue and hence useful
Enemata or insufflation often necessary
Opium, internally or morphine hypodermically to prevent inflammation, to relieve pain and other symptoms and to produce painless purgation

Intestinal Obstruction.—(*contd.*)

Strychnine is useful if given with caution in acute cases
Senna infusion is useful as a fine purgative
Tobacco, infusion as enema ; but it often leads to depressing nausea

Formula.—Strychnine, 1 gr.; extract of belladonna, 4 grs.; podophyllin, 4 grs. ; ferri sulphate, 20 grs. ; aloes, 20 grs. ; make a pill mass. Dose, 2 gr s.

Intestinal Ulceration ; Perforation.

Belladonna, to give tone and relieve spasm
Caffeine, acts upon the muscular tissue
Enemata
Hydrastine
Opium or morphine arrests dangerous symptoms and produces a free motion
Senna infusion

Iritis, Syphilitic. (*See Vol. I., page 519.*)

Atropine solution as mydriatic should be used early and perseveringly
Belladonna tincture, or extract internally or as lotion 1 of extract to 25 of water is of great value
Copaiba internally to diminish pain and restore sight
Duboisine, a good substitute for atropine, less irritating to the conjunctivæ; useful to rapidly dilate the pupils
Eserine
Morphine, hypodermically is very useful
Opium as an adjuvant to relieve pain
Quinine and iron if the patient is feeble and anæmic
Santonine
Scopolamine
Turpentine, in small doses is useful in rheumatic iritis
Tropococaine

Itch ; Scabies.

Acid benzoic, as ointment or lotion, very useful
Anthemidis ointment with sulphuric acid and potassii carbonatis very useful
Balsam of peru, with milk of sulphur and vaseline to rub over the body kills itch mite (acarus), disinfects the parts, relieves itching and dermatitis
Cadini oleum with sulphur (1 to 8), with glycerin starch and benzoate of lard
Coal tar naphtha
Cocculus indicus, ointment useful
Kamala
Karanj tel as ointment
Melia superba with sulphur and curd as ointment
Oily inunctions
Staphisagria 1, lard 5, used as friction
Storax 1, to olive oil 2, unirritating, very useful
Tar ointment cures itch quickly
Terminalia chebula with âmlâ fried in castor oil and applied
Walsura piscidia, ointment is useful

Jaundice. (*See Vol. 1, page 520.*)

Acid benzoic
Aloes, in simple jaundice due to atony of the liver
Azadirachta indica, fresh juice
Berberine, in jaundice due to chronic intestinal catarrh
Celandine, given as deobstruent, affects the liver
Delphinium zalil, decoction
Dulcamara, is very useful
Euonymin, as a hepatic stimulant
Gamboge is useful
Hydrastis is useful in malarial jaundice and in that due to catarrh of the bile ducts
Iris, in malarial jaundice and that due to duodenal catarrh
Ipecacuanha
Luffa echinata, infusion internally
Pilocarpine hydrochlorate
Pine apple juice
Podophyllin, in catarrhal or malarial jaundice when stools are clay coloured and exhibit no trace of bile

Jaundice.—(*contd.*)

Quinine when due to malaria or when periodic

Rhubarb, in children with jaundiced skin, and white or clay coloured pasty stools

Stillingea, to relieve torpid liver following intermittent fever and to cure jaundice

Taraxacum

Triticum roots and rhizomes

Turpentine

Compound Powder—Gudashtaka contains—Danti mula, ipomœa turpethum, plumbago root, black pepper, ginger, long pepper and treacle equal parts. Dose, 1 dr. In flatulence, jaundice, anasarca &c.

A compound colocynth pill containing—Colocynth pulp, 4; parakajali, 4; purified sulphur, 4; cardamoms, 4; harde, 4; long pepper, 4; pellitory root, 4; and honey, 8. Dose, 4 to 8 grs. In jaundice, ascites, fever, and rheumatism.

Joint Affections. (*See Vol. 1, page 521.*)

Aconite, locally as liniment in chronic arthritic swellings and internally to relieve pyrexia of polyarthritis and pains in inflamed joints

Digitalis tincture, in water, as fomentation to the joints in acute cases

Gugula, as lep

Rhus toxicodendron, internally and as lotion is useful to relieve itching, and subacute stiffness of joints after acute rheumatic fever

Turpentine liniment, as local application

Vitex negundo leaves as discutient for swollen joints

Labour—Difficult or Tedious Labour. (*See Vol. I, page 522.*)

Althœa decoction as vaginal injection is used in difficult or tedious labour

Aristolochia bractiata, to increase uterine contractions

Atropine with morphia, hypodermically to overcome spasm

Belladonna ointment, locally in long protracted labour to rigid os and cervix

Cannabis indica (flowering tops) tincture, useful in atony of the uterus to stimulate uterine contractions. It is more prompt but less lasting than ergot

Cimicifuga, as an ecbolic, acts like ergot but is less dangerous to life of child and soft parts of mother. It is useful to relieve nervous excitability after labour, and to check or control post partem hæmorrhage and to relieve suppressed lochia

Cinnamon is useful in tedious labour

Cocaine solution, 5 p. c. locally to the os assists dilatation

Cotton root is useful to excite uterine contractions, better than ergot

Ergot is useful in uterine inertia. To accelerate uterine contraction after the head has passed the pelvic brim; it should not be given if there is any obstacle in front. It paralyses the fœtal heart and therefore is dangerous if inadvertently given

Eucalyptus oil, as an antiseptic used locally

Gelsemium fluid extract, is useful to quiet the pains of the first stage; it relaxes spasm, in rigidity of the os

India-rubber bags (Barnes), to dilate the os

Ipecacuanha, is useful after delivery to promote natural functions

Lobelia inflata, to dilate the rigid os.

Morphine, with digitalis and diaphoretics if fever exists

Morphiæ, internally or hypodermically. It is useful in tedious labour. It relieves severe pains due to rigid os, and promotes progress of the child. It also relieves after pains

Opium, internally or as suppository. It promotes dilatation, increases expulsive power of the uterus, lessens hæmorrhage, and stimulates longitudinal and oblique muscular fibres of the os

Ophioxylon serpentinum, useful to increase labour pains

Quinine, in place of ergot to strengthen or promote the uterine contractions

Viscum album (mistletoe), extract or infusion as an oxytoccic very useful

External remedies—Friction over the abdomen, galvanism, hot water douche over the os, incisions to the os.

Laryngismus Stridulus; Spasm of the Glottis. *(See Vol. I, page 523.)*

Aconite, to check spasm and to relieve stridulus breathing
Atropine
Belladonna is of great value
Codeine
Conium is useful
Gelsemium
Ipecacuanha in an emetic dose, to cut short the attack
Lobelia is useful
Quinine, in small doses is given between the attacks with benefit
Morhine hypodermically

Laryngitis, Acute—Catarrhal Laryngitis—Spasmodic Croup. *(See Vol. I, page 523.)*

Aconite given till fever subsides. It is very useful to relieve inflamed state of the respiratory apparatus
Cocaine, 5 p.c. solution locally
Camphorated oil, as embrocation
Cubeb cigarettes, to relieve hoarseness
Morphine, in small doses to allay cough
Mucilaginous drinks
Rumex crispus extract, as a sedative of the laryngeal mucous membrane, relieves cough, catarrh, and a feeling of soreness behind the sternum

Diet—Bland, nutritious, unirritating food.

External remedies.—Inhalation of hot steam or of tincture benzoin comp. or opium, hops, or conium; mustard to the throat. Poultices hot. Abstinence from talking.

Laryngitis, Chronic—Spasmodic Lanryngitis—Catarrhal Croup.

Althæa, as pectoral lozenges to relieve laryngeal irritation
Benzoin on hot coals or inhaled from boiling water
Cocaine, 20 p. c. solution by a brush as paint or by spray is useful
Cubeb berries, to chew in relaxation of the larynx due to cold or long speaking
Croton oil, locally to the skin of the throat
Guaiacum, internally is useful in mucous laryngitis
Tannin olution (1 in 100) by spray or applied by the steam atomizer or used with glycerin as paint in chronic catarrh and ulceration; the solution is useful as gargle

External remedies.—Insufflation of antiseptic powders as starch, and morphine to relieve irritation.

Inhalations.—Balsam of peru or tolu, placed on hot iron, as vapour; benzoin in strumous laryngitis as vapour on hot coal or hot steam; boswelia floribunda as fumigation; diluted hydrocyanic acid as vapour on hot water; fir leaf oil with magnesium carbonate as inhalation; hops with hot steam, tar, tannin, in hot water as vapour by atomizer. Turpentine by steam atomizer.

Laryngeal Tuberculosis; Dysphagia. *(See Vol. I, page 524.)*

Cocaine by insufflation or allowed to melt in the mouth is useful to relieve pain and dysphagia
Menthol, in olive oil used as paint is useful to relieve pain and to destroy local deposits
Tropacocaine is useful

Leprosy. *(See Vol. I, page 525.)*

Atropa belladonna
Aconite in early stage
Anacardium orienlate, cashewnut oil
Bawachi
Chaulmoogra oil with bâwachi, internally or as liniment
Chysarobin, 10 p.c. in lanolin, locally
Crysarobin, salicylic acid and creosote as plaster is useful
Gurjan, balsam or wood oil as ointment and emulsion to alleviate the disease
Gynandropsis pentaphilla, the oil

Leprosy.—(*contd.*)

Gynocardic acid, in early stage
Hoang-nan, in combination with alum and realgar made into pill
Hydnocarpus inebrians oil, locally
Hydrocotyle asiatica, as anæsthetic locally
Ichthyol, internally with chrysarobin, salicylic acid, creasote, and vaseline, as ointment
Pyrogallic acid and lanolin to rub over the arms and legs
Pinus deodara, oil locally
Sero-therapeutic treatment
Sarsaparilla, as tonic and alterative

Leucoderma.

Aplotaxis auricularis locally
Argemone mexicana oil, locally
Azadirachta indica
Bawachi seeds
Cassia tora
Calotropis gigantea
Curcuma aromatica
Gurjan balsam or wood oil
Pterocarpus santalinus
Pangamia glabra oil

Leucorrhœa. (*See Vol. I, page 525.*)

Abies canadensis, fluid extract internally
Acid tannic with iodine and potassium iodide, locally applied round the cervix
Balsams of peru and tolu internally
Belladonna and tannin, as tampon in ulceration of the os; or belladonna tincture, or sodii bicarbonate, and water, as injection, when due to over-secretion of mucous glands about the os
Cascarilla infusion with tincture sabinæ internally
Cimicifuga is very useful
Cocculus indicus tincture, in seropurulent discharge and pain in lumbar region
Gallæ pulv, with decoction of tormentilla internally
Hydrastis fluid extract, applied topically or as an injection in uterine and vaginal leucorrhœa
Myrrh with iron and aloes is very useful
Pulsatilla tincture, internally or as vaginal injection to relieve pain in the loins, depression of spirit, loss of appetite, &c.
Quercus infectoria infusion locally
Sumbul, in atonic cases is very useful
Tannin alone or with salicylic acid and bismuth as tampon locally, or as dusting powder, or as injection of claret, wine or with cocoa butter as suppository if the os is ulcerated
Vinegar, as a wash

Injections.—Acacia bark, cassia auriculata, catechu, dyospyros embryopteris hydrastis, quinine, tar water if the discharge is fœtid. Tea infusion. Tormentilla decoction.

Lithiasis; Lithœmia; Calculi. (*See Vol. I., page 526.*)

Acid benzoic
Biophytum sensitivum
Buchu combined with an alkali is of benefit
Cascara segrada, to promote excretion of uric acid
Chimaphila extract, checks uric acid in the urine
Colchicum wine, or colchicine with oil of winter green is useful
Coffee is an excellent antilithic
Pichi is very useful in lithæmia with cystitis
Piperazine, to promote elimination of uric acid

Locomotor Ataxy. (*See Vol. I, page 527.*)

Belladonna, with turpentine and ergot, to relieve pain
Ergot with sodii bromidi, to relieve pain
Hyoscyamus, to relieve pain
Morphine, in large doses, in the later stage to relieve pain
Physostigma, is very useful
Pilocarpine
Strychnine, with syrup of hypophosphites

Lung Diseases ; Pulmonary Affections. *(See Vol. I., page 528.)*

Aconite, useful in acute congestion and inflammatory state of the respiratory organs
Astragalus verus, to relieve irritation of the respiratory mucous membrane
Belladonna tincture, to retard exudation of serum in pulmonary œdema and to counteract the failure of the heart
Blisters flying to the chest if there is hypostatic congestion
Copaiba, useful in lung diseases generally, when attended with profuse secretions
Cimicifuga extract, is a useful sedative. It relieves irritative cough, promotes expectoration, and improves general condition
Croton oil liniment as counter irritant very useful in chronic cases
Chavica betle, warm leaves locally applied to the chest
Cubeb, useful in old and chronic cases to stimulate the respiratory organs and to check profuse secretion
Dorema ammoniacum, locally
Eucalyptus oil with alcohol as inhalation by a steam atomizer
Ferula galbanifera, as plaster in chronic cases
Glycerrhiza in catarrh of the lungs
Jaborandi, useful in breathlessness complicating lung disease; to be given with care, otherwise collapse ensues
Pinus sylvestris (tar), vapour as inhalation
Storax benzoin, useful as fumigation
Terpin hydrate or terebene, very useful
Turpentine, inhalation or internally in low adynamic pulmonary inflammation
Veratrum viride, in acute parenchymatous pulmonary congestion with high temperature and rapid pulse; to be avoided if there is prostration or collapse

Lymphangitis. *(See Vol. I, page 529.)*

Belladonna with glycerin, as an application, or as poultices to relieve pain
Quinine, with alcohol internally in septic cases

Mastitis ; Mastodynia ; Mammary Abscess. *(See Vol. I, page 530.)*

Aconite tincture, alone or with actæa racemosa tincture internally
Arnica lotion locally
Atropine alone, or with morphine and chloral, locally to relieve pain
Belladonna internally, or with collodion and camphor as paint, or locally as liniment or as ointment to check secretion of milk and thus relieve pain of inflammation
Camphor, saturated solution in glycerin to be applied locally in mammary congestion and threatening abscess
Conium extract, applied locally to the breasts and generative organs; to relieve inflammation and impeuding abscess of breast
Castor oil leaves locally to relieve inflammation
Cimicifuga, to relieve intra-mammary pain of uterine origin in spinsters
Digitalis, infusion of leaves as fomentation to relieve severe inflammation
Hyoscyamus plaster to relieve distress, mammary pain and distension from milk
Morphine with oleate of mercury and iodine applied locally in mammary abscess
Opium and olive oil locally applied with friction to painful breasts after parturition
Phytolacca fluid extract internally and solid extract locally to arrest inflammation of the breast and to prevent suppuration
Plantago plaster, to support and compress mamma
Rosmarini spirit with ammonium chloride as a lotion to remove induration after the abscess has suppurated
Stramonium leaves as poultices or as cataplasm to relieve induration
Tobacco leaves, as poultice

Measles. *(See Vol. I, page 531.)*

Aconite tincture, to arrest bronchial catarrh or pneumonia and to lessen fever
Asclepias infusion or decoction, to promote eruption
Camphor water with liquor ammoniæ acetatis, when cough and catarrh are present
Crocus sativus liquor is useful if there is catarrh or much cough

Measles.—(*contd.*)

Ipecacuanha, to relieve cough and catarrh
Jaborandi, hot bath is a fine diaphoretic to promote eruptions
Mustard foot bath to promote eruptions
Oil or cocao butter is used as inunction to reduce the temperature
Pulsatilla tincture internally or as wash in nasal or intestinal catarrh
Quinine, to relieve hyperpyrexia and in catarrhal pneumonia
Veratrum viride is very useful

Melancholia. (*See Vol. I, page 531.*)

Caffeine citras is useful
Camphor monobromate is very useful
Cannabis indica, to relieve melancholia
Cocaine, as a tonic in nervous affections accompanied by depression
Cimicifuga, in despondency due to uterine derangements or to puerperal state
Ignatia has a very soothing effect in melancholia
Morphine is useful in persons having peculiar idiosyncrasy
Opium tincture, to subdue paroxysms of acute anguish and despair or with suicidal impulse
Valerian, useful in hysterical or suicidal melancholia
Water as wet pack, shower bath, hot and cold douche very serviceable

Meningitis—Cerebral, Spinal and Cerebro-Spinal. (*See Vol. I, page 532.*)

Acid hydrocyanic with sodium carbonate to check vomiting
Aconite with ergot and opium, to reduce the amount of blood in the vessels of the cord
Belladonna, to relieve cerebral excitement, and to lessen hyperæmia of the brain and cord, when due to external violence
Bryonia, useful in serous inflammation with effusion
Croton oil, useful in tubercular meningitis
Digitalis
Ergot fluid extract with potassium bromide to relieve convulsions following meningitis
Flying blisters to the spine and to the nape of the neck to prevent effusion, and to relieve coma
Gelsiemium fluid extract, to check delirium
Hyoscyamus in subacute form, to relieve nervous irritability
Opium with tartar emetic to relieve pain in the head; to be avoided if effusion occurs and stupor and coma supervene
Purgatives at the commencement are useful
Pulsatilla, useful in the acute form
Quinine with belladonna extract or with potassium iodide is useful
Turpentine enema, as a derivative is useful
Veratrum viride

Menses; Vicarious Menstruation.

Aloes
Cimicifuga
Cocculus indicus
Ergot
Hydrastis
Ipomœa digitata
Jasminum grandiflorum
Quinine
Turpentine

Menorrhagia; Metrorrhagia. (*See Vol. I, page 532.*)

Acacia catechu, as vaginal injection
Acid gallic, with acid sulphhuric aromatic is very efficient
Acid tannic, with zinc sulphate as injection
Actœa racemosa
Aloes with iron in anæmic cases
Atropine, with conium pessary or alone hypodermically in hæmorrhage due to abortion
Berberis aristata with gypsum, internally
Bombax malabaricum gum, internally
Cannabis indica, alone or with ergot, as stimulant of the uterine muscular fibres
Cassia auriculata as an astringent injection
Catechu, useful in passive hæmorrhages
Cimicifuga, in passive hæmorrhages, if the coagula are hard and dark and accompanied with headache

Menorrhagia.—(*contd.*)

Cinnamon oil internally is useful to stop oozing from metrorrhagia
Digitalis with morphia and hydrocyanic acid
Digitalis infusion, internally to check menorrhagia when due to disease and in plethoric subjects
Erigeron oil, is very useful
Ergot, internally with ammonium chloride or with sodium bromide, or ergotin with glycerin and water injected hypodermically is very useful
Galls decoction, as injection
Gossypium, extract as uterine hæmostatic, is very useful
Hamamelis, has beneficial effects on the venous system
Hydrastinine hydrochloride, combined with ergot and cannabis and given internally or injected hypodermically; a powerful uterine vaso constrictor
Ipecacuanha
Opium, as a sedative, to reduce uterine circulation
Pomegranate bark decoction as vaginal injection
Quinine sulphas, in cases of subinvolution is next best to ergot
Quercus as local injection in atonic cases
Rue, to lower the vascular tone of the uterus; to be avoided during pregnancy
Savine tincture, is useful as an uterine tonic in relaxed or passively congested uterus
Sclerotic acid as hypodermic injection
Turpentine, internally
Ustilago
Viburnum, internally

Metritis; Endometritis; Parametritis; Peri-Metritis; Uterine Congestion.

Aconite, in the early stage of inflammatory fever is very useful
Aloes, as enema
Belladonna, internally
Camphor monobromate
Ergotine
Heat to the feet and poultices to the abdomen
Hydrastis extract with carbolic acid or with iodine and glycerin as application to cervix
Injections, vaginal, of hot water to abort an attack of cellulitis
Linseed poultices to the hypogastrium to relieve the pain
Leeches in sthenic cases to the hypogastrium
Opium by suppositories or by enema, better borne than when given internally
Turpentine epithem as hot as can be borne
Viburnum prunifolium internally

Myalgia; Pleurodynia; Lumbago. (*See Vol. I, page 533.*)

Aconite tincture internally or as liniment locally
Arnica, useful to relieve contused muscular fibres. Internally the tincture is useful in concussion, or shock
Aqua puncture, useful
Acupuncture, of benefit
Atropine liniment
Belladonna liniment is useful
Burgundy pitch plaster
Cajuput oil liniment
Camphor with chloral, internally or as liniment locally
Capsicum tincture internally or as liniment or infusion locally on lint or as plaster or as oleo resin
Cimicifuga, to relieve general bruised condition. In rheumatic cases and in myalgia due to uterine derangements it is useful
Clove oil, as rubefacient is useful
Colchicum in the gouty state
Gelsemium fluid extract in large doses is useful
Guarana, to remove pain
Massage
Menthol with thymol and eucalyptol locally as plaster
Morphine and atropine hypodermically to relieve pain
Opium liniment to rub in after warm fomentation or internally
Rhus toxicodendron in subacute or tendonous rheumatism
Turpentine is very useful in myalgia if bowels are regular and urine free
Veratrum tincture, internally or as ointment externally
Xanthoxylum, locally and internally

Myalgia ; Pleurodynia.—(*contd.*)

Formula.— Medicated oil, containing—Acorus calamus, ajowan tela, bishop's weed, cinnamon, indian purslane, patchak (aplotaxis auriculata), oleum nigrum, cleome viscosa oil, nutmeg, black pepper, long pepper, catkins, cinnamon, tamala, indian; spikenard and valerian —equal parts, add linseed oil, 1 to 20 and boil ; used as an embrocation in rheumatism, bruises, dislocation, lumbago, &c.

Myelitis (*See Vol. I, page 533.*)

Belladonna locally is very useful when the disease is due to external violence
Ergot, in large doses is very successful
Leeches are useful if there is much localized tenderness
Posture, on one side, or prone is the best
Rest absolute

Nasal Affections. (*See Vol. I, page 534.*)

Camphor
Cocaine, 4 p. c. solution by spray in catarrh to relieve engorged venous sinuse; also in acute catarrh, hay fever, and for rhinoscopy
Eucaine hydrochlorate
Holocaine
Hydrastis externally and internally in chronic catarrh with nasal ulcers
Menthol as snuff
Nasal douche and injections in catarrhal states
Pulsatilla, in nasal inflammations
Sanguinaria
Starch with glycerin locally
Tannin with glycerin in excoriations inside the nose, after measles, or scarlatina, in impetigeneus eruptions inside the nose where hair grows; also in discharge of greenish, black, stinking mucus
Tropacoccaine

Nervous Affections. (*See Vol. I, page 534.*)

Asafetida is useful in nervous affections connected with uterine derangements. In hypochondriasis and nervous gastric dyspepsia it is given with vegetable bitters and aperients
Cocaine, a nerve stimulant; it destroys the sense of fatigue ; as an analgesic it is useful in neuralgia, melancholia, and hypochondriasis.
Lupulin, is useful in nervous affections where opium is intolerable. In hysteria it is very valuable
Nux vomica tincture, is useful in affections of reflex neurotic origin occurring in hysterical subjects as cough, dyspnœa, syncope, palpitation, flatulence, &c.
Opium is useful in insanity, mania, melancholia, and other painful nervous affections; in diabetes it is of great value. It gives repose to body and mind
Physostigma extract, is useful in locomotor ataxia, writer's cramps, and paraplegia
Santonine, in cases of reflex irritation leading to chorea, hysteria, epilepsy, and convulsions
Starch with glycerin or zinc ointment is useful
Sumbul, a nervous stimulant, very useful in neurotic cases as migraine, hysteria, &c.
Valerian and valerianates have special influence in neurotic cases and are very useful

Nervousness or Nervous Debility ; Nervous Irritability or Nervous Excitability. (*See Vol. I, page 537.*)

Aconite tincture in drop doses relieves restlessness
Camphor, is useful in subduing reflex excitability and nervousness
Chamomile tincture, a fine nervous sedative for children to relieve nervine excitability
Caffeine as a stimulant of the nervous system is useful to relieve restlessness due to lowering of nervous power
Coca
Conium, the fluid extract, is useful as a sedative in insomnia with

Nervousness.—(*contd.*)

great restlessness, motor agitation, delirium, &c., resulting from overwork
Gokhru
Hops internally or as pillow
Ignatia, in small doses to relieve mental excitement and nervous erethism
Lupulin, is useful in cases where opium is intolerable
Massage
Morphine valerianate or morphine alone is useful
Opium, to soothe the nervous system and to give repose to mind and body
Piscidia
Quinine preparations are useful
Strychnine, a nervine tonic, useful to assuage restlessness due to functional irritability of the nervous system, to relieve wandering neuralgic pains, and nervousness from over-dose of tobacco
Sumbul tincture, is useful in restlessness of pregnancy
Valerian is a nervine sedative, useful to relieve reflex excitability and to calm the nervous system; useful in fevers with restlessness, anxiety, &c.

Neuralgia. (*See Vol. I, page 535.*)

Aconite, alone internally or with quinine hydrobromate or with morphine as a palliative; useful in congestive or inflammatory affections or aconitine with veratrine as liniment or as ointment locally for headache
Aconitine ointment and aconiti oleas, used for rubbing
Andropogon citratum oil as embrocation locally for neuralgia of the 5th nerve
Atropine, internally or hypodermically in the vicinity of the nerve or as liniment, or as ointment in sciatica or in peri uterine, facial, and intercostal neuralgia.
Belladonna tincture alone, or with chloroform or with gelsemium internally
Caffeine hydrobrom, hypodermically useful in cervico, bronchial neuralgia
Camphor chloral or monobromate internally
Cannabis indica extract, useful in neuralgic headache
Capsicum oleo resin or strong infusion on lint covered with oiled silk locally is useful in facial neuralgia
Chamomile in neuralgia of the 5th nerve is useful
Coccus cacti tincture to relieve pain
Croton seeds and lime juice in orbital neuralgia
Cimicifuga tincture, in ovarian neuralgia and in neuralgia of the 5th nerve when due to cold
Cocaine and its salts, hypodermically along the course of the nerve or in the vicinity of the painful nerve. Given with chloroform internally or used as tampon
Codeine in ovarian neuralgia
Digitalis, useful in sciatica and locally in earache
Ergot alone or with iron chloride in visceral forms as gastralgia
Gelsiemium fluid extract or tincture alone or with pot. iodid. is useful in neuralgia of 5th nerve, especially its dental branches, in supraorbital tic doulereux, trigeminal and ovarian neuralgia,sciatica, &c.
Ichthyol, menthol, thymol as ointment
Ignatia is useful in hysterical and intercostal neuralgia with nervous erethism
Menthol and peppermint campor, locally in facial neuralgia
Morphine, hypodermically in the vicinity of the affected nerve is useful in sciatic, plumbago, tic douloureux, &c.
Nux vomica tincture, with carminatives useful in visceral neuralgia as gastralgia, hepatalgia, &c.
Oil of horse chestnut with camphor and opium as liniment
Oleum cajuputi, externally and internally
Opium, internally and externally
Peppermint oil locally as paint in superficial and facial neuralgia
Physostigmine solution is useful in neuralgia of the eyeball
Piscidia fluid extract, with potas bromidum is very useful in cases due to cold or inflammation
Pyrethrum, root to chew in facial neuralgia
Quinine sulphas, or salicylas, with arsenic just before the attack in periodic neuralgia In small doses in facial, periodic, orbital, and intercostal neuralgia
Sapindus emarginatus, locally in hemicrania
Spigelia anthelmia, in facial neuralgia

Neuralgia.—(*contd.*)

Staphisagria, internally and externally in obstinate facial and cervical neuralgia
Stramonium. To be omitted if any symptoms of narcotism appear. Useful in sciatica, &c.
Strychnine, in all forms of neuralgia
Sumbul extract, in facial, sciatic or ovarian neuralgia in nervous women
Tonga, useful in facial neuralgia
Turpentine oil, with castor oil internally or with liquor ammoniæ and almond oil or with opium and chloroform liniment useful in sciatica tic douloureux, &c.
Theine, with sodium benzoate, sodium chloride, and water hypodermically. A nice analgesic. It improves the nutritive state of the affected nerves
Valerian extract or valerian ammoniated tincture, with guaiacum in facial neuralgia in hysterical subjects
Veratrine oleate or ointment, in facial neuralgia and sciatica, or veratrum viride tincture internally is useful

Diet.—Animal fats, butter cream, &c.

External remedies.—Rest, bathing, shampooing, acupuncture, aquapuncture.

Formula.—Quininæ sulph., 2; morphinæ sulph., $\frac{1}{30}$; aconite extract, $\frac{1}{2}$; strychnine, $\frac{1}{30}$; acid arsenicus, $\frac{1}{30}$. Make one pill. In neuralgia.

(2) Ext. aconite fl., $\frac{1}{2}$; ext. cannabis, $\frac{1}{4}$; extract conii, $\frac{2}{3}$; extract, hyoscyam $\frac{2}{3}$; extract ignatiæ amaræ, $\frac{1}{2}$; extract belladonanæ, $\frac{1}{8}$; extract opii, $\frac{1}{2}$; and extract stramonii $\frac{1}{4}$. Make 1 pill in neuralgia.

Paint—Chloral hydrate, 1 dr.; camphora pulv, 1 dr.; morphiæ sulphatis, 2 grs.; and chloroform, 40 ms. Mix, to be used locally as a paint.

Ointment—Aconite, 4 grs.; veratria, 15 grs.; and cerati, 6 drs. Mix. Ointment.

Elixir—Sodii iodidi, 3 drs.; hydrargyri bichloride 1 gr.; conii extract. fluid, $\frac{1}{2}$ dr. and syrup, 1 oz. Mix. Dose, 1 dr.

Neurasthenia—Brain Weariness or Nervous Exhaustion

(*See Vol. I, page 537.*)

Caffeine, given in nervous breakdown from over-study to relieve brain weariness and nervous exhaustion
Codeine
Cocaine, in nervous exhaustion, is very useful
Coca, in small doses internally
Counter irritation, as cautery along the spine
Kola nut internally useful as it contains caffeine
Rest cure
Strychnine is very useful
Sumbul of benefit

Nipples (Sore, Fissured). (*See Vol. I, page 538.*)

Arnica lotion, locally
Bals of peru and tolu with almond oil or rosewater, a valuable application
Benzoin tincture compound, locally for slight erosions
Catechu locally with honey
Cocaine solution, locally
Gutta percha, solution locally
Quercus infectorius bark infusion locally
Rhatany, as wash or as cerate, locally in fissure
Tannin, with glycerin locally applied to fissured nipples

Nymphomania (*See Vol. I, page 538.*)

Camphor monobromate in large doses, to control inordinate sexual desire
Lupulin, is very useful
Tobacco, given with care, as it is very depressing
Stramonium

Odontalgia. (*See Vol. I, page 539.*)

Acid tannic solution, with ether, a useful application to carious teeth
Aconite tincture, with chloroform, opium and persulphate of iron locally to the gums or aconite ointment or liniment to the face for facial neuralgia due to a caried tooth
Atropine, solution locally
Belladonna extract locally to the face
Camphor rubbed on the gum or with chloral hydrate locally placed into cavities; camphor with chloral as liniment to relieve facial neuralgia, or with morphine and flaxseed as poultices to the cheek
Capsicum, strong infusion, locally on lint is useful
Chamomile oil locally
Cinnamon oil, locally on lint
Cloves, oil as drops into the cavity
Cocaine, solution on cotton applied to a cavity
Cochlearia armoracea, to chew
Conine solution, with alcohol, locally in the hollow of a painful tooth
Delphinium root, to chew
Gelsemium, extract locally to relieve pain
Ginger, as masticatory
Hamamelis tincture, locally on lint and into the cavity
Hyoscyamus, smoke of the seeds applied into the cavity
Mezereon, as masticatory
Morphine, hypodermically for severe toothache
Opium, or tannin or chloroform with creosote placed into the cavity of a caried tooth gives relief
Pilocarpine injection subcutaneously
Plumbago rosea, root to chew
Pyrethrum, as masticatory
Quinine, in full doses
Solanum jaquini, as fumigation into the cavity
Staphisagria, the alcoholic solution, to drop into the caried cavity
Xanthoxylum

Onychia and Paronychia, Inflammation of Nails. (*See Vol. I, page 539.*)

Camphorated spirit, locally
Cocaine, solution used hypodermically as local anæsthetic
Cocaine, locally injected deep into the tissues relieves pain—a nice anæsthetic
Free incision
Firm bandage
Leeches sometimes are of benefit
Morphine powder, locally applied to relieve pain
Poultices hot, very beneficial
Rhubarb powder application
Tar ointment
Turpentine, locally on lint relieves pain

Ophthalmia. (*See Vol. I, page 540.*)

Acid tannic with syrup or glycerin, application to lids in catarrhal or purulent cases
Atropine solution, or belladonna extract in catarrhal or gonorrhœal or purulent cases
Castor oil drops, to allay pain
Cocaine hydrochlorate, solution or the oleate locally, to relieve pain in catarrhal cases
Colchicum, if gouty diathesis exist
Conine, with olive oil locally is useful
Ergot exract, with glycerin and rose-water locally in catarrhal cases and chronic ophthalmia
Hydrastis lotion, in strumous cases
Jequerity infusion as a paint in granular lids and in purulent cases
Myrrh, in asses' milk locally to the eyes
Oil of cade, in persistent cases
Opium wine in drops, to relieve pain
Pulsatilla, as a wash or a lotion ; also useful internally
Physostigma, to contract pupil and shut out the light in catarrhal cases
Spigelia, useful in rheumatic ophthalmia
Staphaisagria, locally

Opium—The Opium Habit. (*See Vol. I, page 541.*)

Atropine relieves the distressing symptoms
Cocaine or coca, the fluid extract is very useful to relieve depression caused by the withdrawal of opium; it restores appetite, induces sleep, promotes digestion, soothes the brain and produces a feeling of contentment and calm
Cannabis tincture in insomnia and restlessness
Codeine alone or with sodium bromide and trional, very useful to relieve nervous agitation
Conium fluid extract, to relieve wandering pains and check motor activity
Capsicum is useful as a gastric stimulant and cerebral sedative
Catechu tincture, if diarrhœa sets in
Duboisine, a nice calmative and hypnotic at the crisis; used as injection to destroy craving for opium
Ergot to relieve headache
Gelsemium, subdues restlessness, and motor excitement
Hyoscyamus internally or hypodermically as a hypnotic to relieve insomnia and motor activity
Lupulin extract with phosphoric acid or with valerian and chloral hydrate acts as a hypnotic, helps to sustain the patient and lessens the force of his suffering
Nux vomica with diluted phosphoric acid and syrup of prunes internally
Physostigmine, a good substitute for opium at the crisis
Piscidia erythrina, a good substitute
Quinine
Reduce the amount of alcohol consumed
Sparteine, hypodermically, to relieve depression
Strychnine, aurum chloride and bromide of arsenic invaluable to complete the cure

Formula.—Anti-opium pill contains—Sodii phosphatis exsic, 1 gr.; extract nux vomica, $\frac{1}{8}$ gr.; pulv. opii, $\frac{1}{12}$ gr.; ipecacuanha, $\frac{1}{4}$ gr.; extract belladonna, $\frac{1}{8}$ gr.; and piperine, 1 gr. Mix. make one pill. Dose, pill 1. To break the opium habit.

Mixture.—Containing bromides of ammonium, potassium, sodium and strontium with a little arsenic and capsicum to which hypophosphites may be added if there is much depression.

Orchitis; Epididymitis. (*See Vol. I, page 482.*)

Aconite tincture, internally in acute epididymitis
Arnica lotion, or tincture with soap liniment as embrocation
Belladonna internally, and as ointment with glycerin or as a paint with iodine locally when inflammation has subsided
Conium leaves alone as poultice, or with opium and mercury as plaster locally
Digitalis leaves locally, very useful
Flax seed poultices
Guaiacol 6 with methyl salicylate 6 and vaseline 8 as a local application to relieve the pain
Morphine with mercury oleate by inunction, or morphine and atropine solution as injection beneath the tunica vaginalis
Pulsatilla with aconite, minute doses to relieve the pain, but not to assuage œdema
Phytolacca decoction internally, or phytolacca extract with belladonna and lanolin as application
Tobacco with linseed meal as poultices

Formula.—Tincture Iodine 1, liq. ammoniæ 1, tinct. opii 1, and ol. olivæ 8, as application.

Otalgia; Earache. (*See Vol. I, page 341.*)

Aconite tincture 1, and opium tincture 1, dropped into the external meatus to relieve pain
Almond oil as drops
Allium cepa, juice as drops
Atropine solution alone or with opium, as drops into the ear to relieve earache of children and to abort otitis
Croton oil liniment behind the ear
Cocaine, 4 p. c. solution as a spray over the tympanum, through the external meatus and then forced into the eustachian tubes by inhaling the spray
Delphinine ointment behind the ear
Garlic with juice of the leaves of ocymum and oleum amygdalæ as drops

Otalgia.—(*contd.*)

Morphia solution, alone or with atropine is used as drops

Olive oil, made hot and locally applied is useful. It sometimes does harm as it often undergoes decomposition and becomes a nidus for the growth of aspergillus or other vegetable fungi

Opium and atropine, solution as drops

Otitis. (*See Vol. I, page 542.*)

Aconite, to relieve the pain, used internally and locally

Atropine solution as drops in acute otitis,

Calendula officinalis, as lotion

Pulsatilla, as lotion, warmed and applied or used as injection in inflammation of external auditory canal

Otorrhœa. (*See Vol. I, page 542.*)

Acid tannic with glycerin locally

Anthemis flowers, with rose petals and sweet oil as drops

Camphor and salol heated together and applied into the middle ear. It causes neither pain nor inflammation

Cleome viscosa, juice as drops

Helicteres isora with castor oil as drops

Opium in sweet oil as drops

Patang powder as insufflation into the middle ear

Quercus infectorius, decoction as injection

Quinine with sulphuric acid in otorrhœa after scarlatina

Ovarian Neuralgia. (*See Vol. I, page 543.*)

Atropine, hypodermically, to relieve pain in the pelvic viscera

Belladonna, combined with stramonium, hyoscyamus and quinine internally

Camphor monobromate with cannabis indica relieves ovarian pain of spasmodic character

Codeine, to relieve ovarian pain either inflammatory or neuralgic

Conium, as vaginal pessary, to relieve ovarian pain either inflammatory or neuralgic

Hydrastis extract with potassium bromide is useful

Opium often relieves the pain of non-inflammatory character

Ovaritis, Oopharitis. (*See Vol. I, page 543.*)

Anemonin

Belladonna

Camphor with opium and cannabis internally to relieve pain

Ergot, with potassium bromide useful in chronic ovaritis

Linseed meal poultice of use

Opium suppository or enema is useful

Salix nigra extract is useful in ovarian hyperæsthesia in nervous women

Turpentine stupes over the ovarian region is useful

Ozæna. (*See Vol. I, page 543.*)

Acid tannic with glycerin by irrigation

Camphor with sugar as snuff

Cubeb, the oleo resin with sugar internally after each meal to lessen the secretion and alter its character

Hydrastis, locally as fluid extract or as lotion or internally as tincture is useful

Krameria decoction with calcium chloride and water used as injection after cleaning the nose with soap and warm water

Menthol, with cosminol as spray

Ocymum sanctum, snuff of leaves

Pix liquida with soda bicarb and water as injection into the nose

Pain. (*See Vol. I, page 544.*)

Aconitine, ointment useful in neuralgia of the 5th nerve in gout and rheumatism

Atropine, hypodermically to relieve local pain, sciatica, glaucoma, &c.

Pain.—(*contd.*)

Belladonna, to relieve every kind of pain in the pelvic viscera with iron for the wandering pains of anæmia where morphine is contra-indicated and bromides fail

Codeine, to relieve abdominal and ovarian pain

Cimicifuga, to relieve pain of neuralgia of dysmen orrhœa, ovarian neuralgia, pain of 5th nerve, rheumatic pain and headache

Cocaine, 4 p.c. solution, locally as anæsthetic to the mucous surfaces in odontalgia, otalgia, &c.; hypodermically for minor operation as extraction of tooth and circumcision

Conium, useful in neuralgia, rheumatism, cancer and ovarian pain; also locomotor ataxia

Duboisine, a good substitute for atropine

Eucaine, to cause anæsthesia of the mucous membranes

Guaiacol, in olive oil or glycerin as anæsthetic, hypodermically injected or locally applied as paint in orchitis, sciatica, rheumatism, and neuralgia

Morphine, hypodermically injected in the vicinity of the nerve is useful when it cannot be borne by the stomach; used as sulphate with atropine, in sciatica and other painful neuralgia. With antipyrin it is more efficient in pain than the use of either drug alone. With chloral it relieves pain of chronic rheumatism, colic, gastralgia and of cancer

Opium, as an analgesic, is used to relieve pain. The liniment is applied with friction in superficial neuralgia; poultices sprinkled with opium, is a useful application to relieve pain of inflammation

Rhatany to relieve pain of ulcerative disease of mucous membranes as pain of burns, blisters, ulcers, &c.

Solanine to relieve gastric pain

Stromoniun ointment is useful

Theine, to relieve neuralgic pains; it affects the nerve if injected

Paralysis and Paresis. (*See Vol. I, page 455.*)

Arnica, in paralysis of the bladder very useful

Belladonna, with ergot internally or as ointment along the spine in paralysis due to chronic inflammation of the cord

Cajuput oil useful in palsy

Cannabis indica, to lessen irritability, for retention of urine in spinal paralysis

Colocynth in cerebral paralysis acts as revulsive or counter irritant

Cocculus indicus tincture, useful in hemiplegia, paraplegia and in paralytic stiffness

Cochlearia armoracia or camphor spirit locally as embrocation

Capsicum, as general stimulant

Ergot, in paralysis of the bladder due to over-distension, in paralytic dysuria, sensation of partial emptying of bladder in paraplegia complicated with menstrual irregularity and in paralysis arising from spinal congestion; useful to relieve constipation in paralysis when other cathartics have failed

Ignatia, in loss of power in the lower extremities

Jatropha oil, as local application

Myristica officinalis, the oil as stimulant locally

Mustard, as an emetic to stimulate the failing heart in certain forms of paralysis

Nux vomica, in hysterical paralysis, or that due to lead poisoning in chronic paralysis, in paraplegia due to softening and wasting of the cord

Oil of bay, is useful

Picrotoxin, is useful in paralysis of the sphinctors, in hemiplegia from cold and in glosso-labio-laryngeal paralysis

Physostigma, in general paralysis of the insane, in progressive muscular atrophy, in long standing hemiplegia, paraplegia, locomotor-ataxia; physostigmine into the eye in ocular paralysis

Rhus toxicodendron, useful in paralysis depending on rheumatism

Senega, in rheumatic paralysis is very useful

Strychnine solution hypodermically into the affected muscles in hemiplegia, paraplegia, local paralysis and mercurial or facial paralysis

Paralysis Agitans. (*See Vol. I, page 545.*)

Cannabis indica, to lower reflex activity

Cocaine, is very beneficial in large and frequent doses

Duboisine

Gelsemium with conium and hyoscyamus, useful to quiet the nervous irritation

Paralysis.—(*cntd.*)

Hyoscyamus tincture or hyoscine hydrobromide as a paliative to control tremors
Hyoscyamine, to relieve trembling
Opium, arsenic, and hyoscyamus are useful
Picrotoxin, very useful

Parasites; Pityriasis; Pediculi; Dandruff. (*See Vol. 1, page 553.*)

Acid chrysophanic
Acorus calamus, rhizome to remove fleas
Anamirta cocculus, powdered fruit to remove lice
Anona squamosa, decoction of seeds to kill pediculi
Aplotaxis auriculata, root
Azadirachta indica, oil of seeds to remove lice
Bawâchee, oil, locally applied with benefit
Cajuput oil, to destroy pediculi
Cleome viscosa, to kill maggots
Cocculus indicus tincture, undiluted as a wash to destroy pediculi
Essential oils, very useful to kill pediculi
Gardinia gummifera, to kill pediculi
Goa powder to kill acarus
Helinium, for mosquitoes
Karanjtel locally to kill lice
Laurel leaves, decoction as a wash against fleas
Melia azadiract, paste of leaves and flowers locally
Picrotoxin against pediculi
Pyrethrum, powdered locally applied kills pediculi
Solamum dulcamara, locally
Sapindus trifoliatus, locally
Stavesacre, as an oil or as an ointment or as tincture locally applied
Tobacco, decoction of the leaf kills lice. The application is to be avoided if the surface is abraded
Vernonia anthelmintica seeds, for pediculi
Vinegar to kill the knits in the hair; it softens the adhesive chitin by which the ova are glued to the hair
Walsura piscida, as a hair wash to kill lice

Pericarditis. (*See Vol. I, page 546.*)

Aconite to relieve violent throbbing and severe pain. If given early, it diminishes vascular excitement or irritability
Bryonia, during the exudation stage is useful
Digitalis with hyoscyamus in the exudation stage when the heart flags, in rapid and feeble heart cyanosis and dropsy
Gautheria oil, internally, or locally with camphor liniment
Opium, is very beneficial
Quinine, with potassium carbonate, a good antipyretic, to suppress an acute attack
Spigelia anthelmia, useful in pericarditis with rheumatism
Turpentine stupes to the chest is useful
Veratrum viride, extract, or succus with calomel, is very valuable

Periostitis. (*See Vol. I, page 465.*)

Free incisions
Mezereon, if complicated, with scrofula or rheumatism
Morphine and mercury oleate, locally
Poultices in the early stage
Staphisagria, if long bones are affected

Peritonitis. (*See Vol. I, page 465.*)

Aconite, to relieve febrile condition in sthenic cases; useful in the early stage in all inflammations of serous membranes
Bryonia, useful in the exudation stage
Cocculus indicus, useful to relieve tympanitis, to remove pain and relieve tension
Morphine, if given early will abort
Opium tincture, to quiet the intestinal peristalsis, with aconite to relieve pain
Poultices, large and hot, and frequently renewed
Quinine is very useful in most inflammation
Turpentine, internally, to relieve tension as turpentine epithem during the early stage locally for tympanitis

Phimosis.

Belladonna, extract in lard as ointment used locally

Cocaine, 4 p. c. solution as an anæsthetic injection before operation to keep the penis at rest

Lupulin, internally after the operation

Surgical removal of the prepuce or circumcision

Phlegmasia Alba; Dolens. (*See Vol. I, page 550*).

Anodyne ointments locally

Belladonna and mercury equal parts as ointment

Hamamelis, is very useful. It has a specific action on the venous system as aconite has on the arterial

Leeches during the acute inflammatory stage

Opium, in large doses internally or locally sprinkled on hot flannel used for fomentation to relieve pain

Phthisis. (*See Vol. I, page 551.*)

Aconite, in small doses, to lessen irritative fever

Acid gynocardic

Agaricin

Acid hydrocyanic to relieve irritative cough

Apomorphine, with morphine relieves dyspnœa and continued cough with thick and tenacious mucus

Atropine, to lessen perspiration

Benzoin as inhalation to lessen cough and expectoration

Burgundy pitch plaster

Camphorated naphthol, in olive oil is used hypodermically

Cannabis indica, relieves cough

Cimicifuga, removes cough, improves digestion and lessens inter-current bronchitis

Cinchona bark, to check hectic and sweats

Clove oil, locally to the chest

Cocaine, locally to the throat before meals relieves irritative cough

Cocos nucifera oil as inunction to the chest

Codeine, as it does not constipate

Croton oil liniment to the chest, as counter-irritant

Eucalyptus oil for inhalation

Grape cure is of benefit

Guaiacol, as a laryngeal spray

Homatropine hydrobromate

Ichthalbin, internally very useful

Ipecacuanha wine as spray to the throat if there is bronchial asthma and emphysema combined with fibroid phthisis

Juglans regia, infusion or extract

Morphia acetas, with sanguinaria, in cough preventing sleep

Morphine, with starch or bismuth, locally to larynx in laryngeal phthisis

Morphia, hypodermically in irritative cough

Myrtol

Opium, with ipecacuanha as lozenges to check sweating and to relieve irritative cough when due to inflamed throat

Picrotoxin, to check prespiration

Pilocarpine, to relieve dyspnœa and to check sweats

Pix liquida, inhalation of tar vapour; also emplastrum to the chest

Prunus virginiana syrup, as a vehicle for cough mixtures useful to relieve cough

Quinine, in large doses, to check sweats, and to lessen temperature

Sanguinaria, promotes expectoration and improves appetite

Terebene with thymol and carbolic acid is very useful as inhalation, to relieve dyspnœa as a spray into the larynx

Verbascum, to facilitate expectoration and to improve health and lessen cough

External remedies—Inhalations—Benzoin inhalation to lessen cough and expectoration ; peppermint oil to the chest ; enemata of starch and opium.

Plague (Bubonic). (*See Vol. I, page 554.*)

Belladonna, with glycerin applied locally to the bubo and poultices

Cocaine, hypodermically, with acid carbolic

Plague.—(*contd.*)

Digitalis, to sustain the heart
Hydrocyanic acid and morphine in the early stage to check vomiting
Hyoscine, with potassium bromide very useful
Morphine, hypodermically, at the onset to induce sleep and to relieve distress and delirium
Olea Europæa, as inunction
Poultices if the buboes are red and inflamed
Sparteine, to support the heart
Strophanthus, to sustain the heart
Strychine, in the early stage alone or with ammonium carbonate in the later stage when the pulse begins to fail

Pleuritis. (*See Vol. 1, page 554.*)

Aconite with tincture opium in the early stage prior to the stage of effusion
Ammoniacum, with mercurial plaster to the chest
Apocynum cannabinum, fluid extract, as hydragogue in pleuritic effusion
Aspiration if effusion is great
Belladonna plaster or liniment to relieve pain due to old adhesions
Bryonia tincture, in the secondary stage, very useful
Burgundy pitch plaster to the chest as a mechanical support
Digitalis, as antipyretic
Guaiacol, locally to promote absorption of the effusion
Jaborandi leaves infusion, to cause absorption of effusion
Morphine, hypodermically or opium internally in the beginning to cut short the attack; also to relieve pain
Pilocarpine nitrate, to absorb fluids, but is too depressing
Pleurisy root is useful
Quinine, with morphine to abort the disease; also as a restorative tonic in low state of the system
Veratrum viride tincture, given till pulse is reduced or nausea occurs
Scilla, with digitalis and mercury internally is useful
Strapping the chest

Pneumonia. (*See Vol. I, page 555.*)

Aconite, useful in catarrhal and fibrinous forms. In the early stage it cuts short the attack; useful to reduce circulation
Apomorphine hydrochlorate is useful
Belladonna, in the first stage as an adjuvant to digitalis to soothe the irritable nervous system and to diminish profuse secretion
Bryonia of service when pleura is affected. It assists absorption and limits effusion
Camphor, morphia hydrochloride and antipyrin, internally to reduce pyrexia better than quinine
Camphor in olive oil hypodermically in fibrinous pneumonia to lower the pulse and to ameliorate general condition
Digitalis, to slow the heart with belladonna as an adjuvant
Ergot, in croupous variety very useful
Ipecacuanha wine, to promote expectoration and to regulate secretion
Muscarine Nux vomica
Opium internally or morphine by hypodermic injection, to relieve pain and arrest delirium
Poultices, jacket encircling the whole chest
Quinine, to reduce the temperature. It acts as a tonic in asthenic cases; very useful if given with aconite and veratrum
Sanguinaria, when fever has abated, to assist improvement
Senega, in later stages, as expectorant when the cough is dry, irritative and painful, with tightness in the chest
Serpentaria with ammonium carbonate, as stimulant about the crisis
Strychnine hypodermically, for impending heart failure, or internally with alcohol if respiration is embarassed or for impending heart failure
Turpentine as stimulant during crisis
Veratrum viride, like aconite to reduce the circulation; useful in the early stage

Polypus (*See Vol. I, page 556.*)

Acid acetic glacial, as injection into the growth, to cause it to shrink
Sanguinaria, as snuff for nasal polypi
Tannin powder, as snuff

Pregnancy, Disorders of, as Albuminuria ; Vomiting ; Ptyalism, &c.

(*See Vol. I, page 556.*)

Aloes, to remove constipation and to cure piles
Berberine, to relieve periodic neuralgic pains ; better than quinine
Calumba, opium, bisumth and antispasmodics to relieve gastrodynia and pyrosis
Camphor liniment, locally to relieve lumbar pains
Castor oil, to clear out the bowels and thus to check diarrhœa
Catechu, tannin or alum as medicated pessaries, to lessen whites
Cocculus indicus, to remove flatulence and lessen frequent desire to micturate which is due to pressure on the bladder
Digitalis infusion, to lessen albuminuria
Galls with opium as ointment to relieve pain of hæmorrhoids
Senna confection, to relieve constipation
Sumbul, as tincture with chloric ether gives sleep at night and relieves restlessness
Tannin pessaries, to lessen leucorrhœa

Prolapsus Ani. (*See Vol. I, page 556.*)

Acacia arabica, decoction in local prolapse
Acid tannic by injection into the rectum
Ergotin or Ergot fluid extract, injected hypodermically into the perinieum gives immediate relief
Excision of the prolapse
Hydrastis, as rectal enema or lotion
Krameria extract, with morphia as suppository
Nut galls as ointment locally
Nux vomica extract or tincture with rhubarb in prolapse in children with constipation
Psidium pyriferum decoction, locally in prolapse
Pad or T. bandage as mechanical support
Punica granatun cortex and leaves locally
Strychnine, hypodermically to be injected into the cellular tissue parallel to the rectum
Soymida febrifuga, locally in prolapse.

Prolapsus Uteri. (*See Vol. I, page 556.*)

Anisomeles malabaricus
Catechu, tannin, kino, rhatany, galls, quercus bark or pomegranate bark as astringent locally
Cimicifuga, to prevent miscarriage in prolapse
Hamamelis
Mechanical support
Peganum harmala
Rhus aromaticus

Prostatitis—Prostate enlarged or hypertrophied. (*See Vol I, page 557.*)

Barosma betulina
Blisters to the perineum
Colchicum, in persons of gouty diathesis if prostate is hypertrophied
Hydrangea
Hydrastis, internally and locally very useful
Prostate dried
Salix nigra
Saw palmetto, acts on the glands of the reproductive organs, used to increase its activity, and to promote secretion
Testicles dried
Triticum repens useful in enlarged prostate of old men
Turpentine oil
Uva ursi

Prostatorrhœa.

Atropine, with potassium bromide
Ergot, to lessen relaxation
Hydrastis is useful locally

Prurigo. (*See Vol. I, page 557.*)

Aconite or conium ointment
Belladonna, is useful in obstinate cases
Cocaine solution, 5 p.c. or oleate locally
Juniper leaves as vapour
Menthol ointment
Quinine, in large doses to control exascerbations
Stavesacre ointment
Tar ointment
Veratria as ointment and internally

Pruritus. (*See Vol. I, page 558.*)

Balsam of peru, locally to relieve itching of pruritus and of scabies
Benzoin compound, tincture as paint on the skin in urticaria and to relieve itching of eczema
Brucine, 20 p.c solution locally applied is useful in chronic pruritus
Camphor with chloral, the liquid so formed is used as an ointment with vaseline as antipruritic or mixed with dusting powders to allay heat and itching of eczema and intertrigo
Cocaine, 5 p.c. solution or oleate, to relieve itching of scrotal eczema, of pruritus ani, or of pruritus pudendi
Gelsemium tincture, internally to relieve itching
Hydrocyanic acid, as lotion alone or with borax or laurel water—useful for pruritus senilis
Menthol, very useful
Piperazine, useful to relieve pruritus of uric acid diathesis
Tar ointment or tar and sulphur as lotion useful for general pruritus
Tobacco, locally is useful, but must be used with care
Tuminol tincture, is used locally with benefit

Psoriasis. (*See Vol. I, page 559.*)

Acid chrysophanic ointment
Acid pyrogallic ointment
Anthrarobin locally
Betula pyroligni oil, locally
Black dammer
Chrysarobin in rose water pomade or with petroleum or vaseline pomade locally applied to each spot. It often irritates
Coptis teeta, very useful
Chaulmoogra oil
Gynocardia oil, made hot and applied locally
Huile de cade, as ointment externally
India-rubber solution to form a coating
Juniperis oleum with olive oil, as application
Lappa major tincture of seeds made in whisky
Mezereon, a useful adjunct
Oils and fats as codliver oil, almond oil, olive oil externally to lubricate the skin in strumous cases
Pongamia glabra oil
Pitch, liquor picis with hydrargyri nitratis locally as ointment
Plantain, locally as poultice
Tar ointment, or as a paint in obstinate cases
Ulmus

Formula.—Chrysarobin, 10; solicylic acid, 10; ether, 15; collodion, 100; Pigment, for application.

(2) Salicylic acid, 25 grs.; pyrogallic acid, 20 grs.; ichthyol, 50 grs.; vaseline, 6 drs., soft soap, 4 drs.; for application.

Ptosis.

Ergot, infusion used as collyrium for the lids
Electricity
Operation of shortening the lid if necessary
Veratrine, with ether, and alcohol to brush over the eye-lids, brows and temples

Ptyalism. (*See Vol. I, page 560.*)

Atropine, hypodermically when ptyalism is the result of some reflex action and not due to any drug poison
Belladonna, useful in ptyalism due to mercury or to pregnancy
Calabar bean
Hyoscine, is very useful
Myrrh
Opium may be used instead of atropine
Pellitory, to stimulate the salivary gland to eliminate the drug poison as mercury, iodine, &c.; to be avoided if the gums are swollen and ulcerated
Santalum album
Tannin or vegetable astringents as gargle in ptyalism from mercury when the gums are swollen and ulcerated

Puerperal Disorders.

Castor oil, or rhubarb to stimulate the bowels after the 4th day
Cimicifuga, in great depression and hypochondriasis
Enema, after the third day
Opium tincture, alone or with alteratives to relieve intestinal irritation, to arrest diarrhœa, and to relieve shock and exahustion

Puerperal Fever. *(See Vol. ', page 561.)*

Aconite, drop doses alone or with castor oil
Arnica tincture, if lochia is excessive
Curette, to remove any membrane or portion of placenta left
Digitalis, hypodermically
Laparotomy
Opium, to relieve wakefulness and delirium, to allay pain and to reduce excitement of the nervous and vascular systems. Laudanum as fomentation or hot poultices
Quinine, in large doses to reduce temperature
Stramonium, to relieve cerebral excitement
Turpentine stupes to the abdomen if there is tympanitis or where the uterine discharge is altogether suspended; also in distension of the abdomen; or given internally when there is depression of the vasomotor nervous system with weak heart and tympanitis
Veratrum viride is very useful
Warberg's tincture, is very useful in puerperal malarial fever

Puerperal Mania and Melancholia. *(See Vol. 1, page 561.)*

Aconite tincture to quiet the puerperal restlessness and mania and to lessen high fever; very useful if given soon after a chill
Cimicifuga, very useful in relieving mania and hypochondriasis
Duboisine, a nice calmative hypnotic; quiets the nervous system in puerperal mania
Hyoscyamus, in milder cases to relieve nervous excitement
Opium, to allay irritation and relieve restlessness
Quinine in cold and sweating-skin with much weakness
Stramonium tincture, to allay cerebral excitement, to soothe the nervous system, to check delirium if mild or furious but intermittent and to remove tendency to suicide or to destroy the child
Weaning is imperative in melancholia

Puerperal Peritonitis.

Aconite, extract, early stage
Apocynum cannabinum, fluid extract
Cimicifuga, in great depression of spirit especially in the rheumatic form
Cocculus indicus, to remove tympanitis and pain
Dover's powder
Morphia hypodermically
Opium, or aconite in cerebral irritation, to prevent exhaustion, to check delirium and to procure sleep; useful in adynamic cases
Quinine alone or with opium, as antipyretic
Stramonium, if there is cerebral excitement
Turpentine, as enema or as hot stupes to the abdomen, or internally in tympanitis as a vasomotor depressant
Veratrum viride with morphia

Pyrosis. *(See Vol. 1, page 562.)*

Almond burned with salt and pepper, to relieve heart burn
Capsicum, in atonic dyspepsia, with heart burn and diarrhœa
Catechu, kino and other astringents and bitter infusions to relieve water brash
Nux vomica tinct, with dilute nitric acid in atonic dyspepsia, heart burn, and hiccough
Podophyllin, in obstinate heart burn with liver derangement
Pulsatilla, to relieve heartburn of dyspepsia
Rhubarb, with ginger, to relieve heart burn

Rectum (Diseases of); Ulceration of Rectum. (*See Vol. I, page 562.*)

Belladonna extract alone or with mercurial ointment locally to fissures, and to irritable ulcers, to relieve burning pain following defœcation
Castor oil, a mild laxative in fissures, and hæmorrhoids
Cocaine (1 in 10) of glycerin and starch, locally applied with a pipe, controls spasm of the rectum
Confectio sennæ, with sulphur as stimulant in fistula, ulcers, and hæmorrhoids
Conium extract, to relieve pain and irritability of cancer of the rectum
Division of the sphinctor in ulcers or fissures and subsequent healing by granulations
Incision through the mucous membrane
Pepper confection, internally a nice stimulant in fistula, ulcers and hæmorrhoids
Podophyllin, internally to relieve prolapse of the rectum
Spigelia anthelmia decoction, internally, the succus is used as an enema
Stramonium ointment, is useful to relieve pain

Retina (Affections of); Retinitis.

Atropine in retinitis due to strain
Dark glasses
Eserine
Physostigmine, locally to contract the pupil and to diminish the amount of light admitted into the eye in optic neuritis
Pilocarpine useful in detached retina and optic neuritis

Rheumatism, Acute and Chronic. (*See Vol. I, page 563.*)

Absinthe
Aconite extract, if there is much heat with dry skin. It relieves pain in inflamed joints and shortens fever. If given from the onset it prevents organic cardiac complication. As a plaster or as liniment it is useful in chronic and subacute rheumatism. It is a valuable adjunct to other remedies
Acupuncture
Acorus calamus, with cashew nut locally
Aletris is useful
Andropogan citratum as embrocation
Anisomeles malabaricus oil from leaves locally
Arnica tincture or infusion, useful to lower the temperature, to relieve articular pain and swelling, and to diminish urea.
Aqua puncture
Atropine, hypodermically as an anodyne or as a prophylactic, in the vicinity of the affected part
Bryonia, to relieve pain and stiffness of joints after the swelling has subsided
Burgundy pitch as plaster, locally
Capsicum oleo resin with lard, 1 to 4, to rub over the joints
Chimaphilla extract, internally useful if lithiasis is present
Cimicifuga, is useful to relieve the pain speedily in rheumatic or neuralgic headaches, and in rheumatism of the uterus; also in lumbago and pleurodynia
Colchicine, with quinine and colocynthidine, is very useful in shortening the duration and alleviating pain in chronic form
Digitalis infusion, 4 drs., or powder, 2grs., with morphine hypodermically and a blister over the prœcordium in cardiac complications with cyanosis and œdema.
Dulcamara, very useful in persons subject to cold or catarrh
Eucalyptus leaves, as local stimulant wrapped up over the joints very useful; but they would cause vesication of the skin if long continued
Euphorbia antiquorum, the juice is used as embrocation
Gaultheria oil, as emulsion, a substitute for salicylic acid
Guaiacum ammoniated tincture, in milk is useful in chronic cases
Ichthalbin internally, very useful. Ichthyol as ointment (1 to 2 of lard), or as liniment with turpentine, or with olive oil and chloroform
Jaborandi, to act on the skin
Jatropha curcas, oil as embrocation or as rubefacient
Lupulin, as an anodyne to relieve pain
Manaca fluid extract, or the root used to shorten the attacks
Menthol, ointment locally to the joints
Mezereon is very useful

Rheumatism.—(contd.)

Mesua ferrea, oil of seeds locally
Morphine acetas, hypodermically if there is cardiac complication
Myristica officinalis, the oil, locally
Nicotiana tabacum, the leaves made hot and applied locally
Ocymum gratissimum for baths or for fumigation
Opium, as anti-rheumatic, very useful in rheumatic cardiac inflammation
Pilocarpine, hypodermically to act on the skin in muscular rheumatism
Plumbago rosea, root with oil as embrocation
Quinine bromide, or quinine salicylas, as antipyretic useful in insomnia
Quinine and iron as tonic, in the later stage
Rhus toxicodendron, externally as liniment, or as lotion, on compresses or as plaster or ointment is very useful in after stage; internally in subacute or chronic muscular or tendinous form when the pain is worse at night
Sassafras officinalis, in chronic cases if circulation is languid
Spigelia anthelmia, to relieve cardiac complication to allay pericarditis and endocarditis; also in rheumatic fever, with pain shifting from joint to joint
Thuja occidentalis, to relieve rheumatic pains
Turpentine, relieves the pain when applied externally as liniment or given internally
Veratrum viride, in small doses alone or with opium, is useful as antipyretic
Vitex negundo, locally to swelled joints or as vapour bath
Xanthoxylum fluid extract, externally in muscular form

External remedies.—Electricity—massage ; hot pack, compresses ; application of ice. of cold, of ice and salt ; baths of steam or vapour or of mineral waters ; pine leaf made hot as fomentation; mustard plaster ; packing splints for fixation of limb ; blisters flying.

Formula—Asafetida, derris uliginosa bark , garlic, plumbago root, and gortel. Medicated oil as application.

Turpentine, camphor, liquor ammonia, capsicum, alcohol and mustard oil as liniment.

Acidi arseniosi, ¼ gr.; pulvis guaiaci, 30 grs. ; pulvis capsici, 10 grs. ; pil aloes et asafetida, 60 grs. Make pills 36. Dose 2 pills. In chronic rheumatism.

Syrup—Pulvis guaiaci resin, 10 grs. ; potas iodid, 10 grs. ; tinct. catechu, 2dr.; tinct. cinnamon, 2 dr.; syrup, 2 drs. Mix. Dose, ½ dr. In chronic rheumatism.

Mixture—Olei gaultheriæ, 30 ms.; acidi salicylici, 30 grs. ; syrup picis liquida, 2 drs.; potassii iodidi, 60 grs.; aquæ menthæ-pip, 6 oz. Dose, 4 drs., three times a day. In acute rheumatism.

Liniment—Olei sinapis, 1 ; ammoniæ liquor, 1; olei terebinthinæ 1; olei origani, 1; ol. hemlock, 1; ol. sassafras, 1 ; spt. camphor, ½; opium, 1 ; cayenne pepper, 1 ; alcohol, 50 ; tinct capsici, 1. Mix ; in chronic cases used as paint.

Rheumatism, Muscular ; Lumbago, Neuritis ; Pleurodynia, Chronic Torticollis, &c., (*See Vol. I, page 565.*)

Cajuput oil, externally and internally
Capsicum powder with lard 1 to 4 locally applied with benefit
Cimicifuga, very useful in lumbago, myalgia, pleurodynia, &c.
Colchicine, solution hypodermically into the muscles affected
Dover's powder as diaphoretic
Jaborandi, hypodermically to act on the skin
Morphine, and atropine hypodermically, of great benefit

Rhinitis ; Cold in the Head.

Camphor in solution alone or with caffeine and ether hypodermically
Cocaine solution, 5 p. c., on cotton to stuff into the nostrils or used as spray into them ; useful in the early stage
Cubeb with linseed tea
Dover's powder, to abort cold
Galvano cautery
Intra-nasal operation
Menthol with chlorlform as inhalation; as a prophylactic it is very useful
Pulsatilla
Quilaja saponaria

Formula—Tinct, aconite, 12 ms. ; tinct. belladonna, 25 ms. ; morphine sulphate, ¼gr. ; pot. bromide, 60 grs.; spt. menthæ piperetæ, 20 ms.; aquæ, 2 oz. Dose, ⅙th.

Cocaine, 2 grs.; ol. pini, 5 ms.; ol. eucalypti, 2 ms. ; menthol, 1 gr. ; thymol 2 grs.; sodæ biboras, 20 grs. A teaspoonful in an ounce of warm water. Used as spray.

Ringworm of the Body ; Tinea Circinata ; Trichophyton Tonsurans.

Butea frondosa, seeds with lime juice for rubbing
Cassia lata tincture of the leaves as paint, or the crushed leaves well rubbed on the part
Chaulmugra oil
Chrysophanic acid, with vaseline
Cocculus indicus, decoction locally applied
Kamala locally
Letœa macrophylla, as a paste
Oil of tar with iodine, locally
Papaya juice, locally applied
Tar, pixliquida ointment
Vista tricolor leaves, well rubbed over the part

Sciatica.

Aconitine, locally as ointment useful in obstinate cases
Acupuncture
Apomorphine, hypodermically is useful to relieve pain in obstinate cases
Aqua puncture
Atropine, hypodermically in the vicinity of nerve
Baths turkish
Belladonna gives relief
Cimicifuga, very useful
Cocaine, 4 p. c. solution, hypodermically along the course of the nerve
Duboisine, a good substitute for atropine, hypodermically very useful
Guaiacol, locally painted over the nerve, acts as a local anæsthetic
Gelsemium, with pot. iodid, very useful
Menthol locally applied
Morphine, hypodermically should be injected deeply into the adjacent muscular tissue
Nerve stretching
Nux vomica, in chronic sciatica very useful
Opium, internally and locally
Pichi extract
Ranunculus bulbosa, fluid extract, internally
Rhus toxicodendron, fluid extract internally useful in rheumatic affections of fibrous tissues
Sarsaparilla with potas iodid, very useful
Stramonium, is useful ; to be avoided if symptoms of narcotism appear
Turpentine sometimes of value
Veratrine, locally as oleate or as ointment, or internally as tincture

Sclerosis ; Atheroma. (*See Vol. I., page 568.*)

Belladonna, useful to retard the progress
Digitoxin
Ergot
Hyoscyamus
Physostigmine
Strychnine

Scrofula. *(See Vol. I, page 568.)*

Berberis aquifolium.
Capsicum infusion, as stimulant, in scrofulous and fistulous ulcerations
Cetraria islandica
Chimaphila umbellata extract.
Conine, in olive oil applied to the conjunctivæ in scrofulous photophobia
Conium maculatum leaves, locally to ulcers
Excision or scraping of gland and packing with iodoform gauze
Fats as inunction
Galium aparine
Gentian, a useful vehicle for chalybeates
Grape cure
Hyoscyamus, leaves bruised as poultice or cataplasm over scrofulous ulcers
McDade's combined fluid extract (succus alterans)
Mezereum, very useful
Prunus virginiana, to check hectic fever
Sarsaparilla extract as tonic and alterative
Stillingia, is very useful

Scurvy. *(See Vol. I, page 569.)*

Acid citric or tartaric, as preventive
Aconite, if there is stomatitis with salivation
Atropine, hypodermically, if profuse salivation
Averrhoa bilimbi, or carumbola internally
Cetraria islandica
Cinchona tincture, with myrrh or with chlorates as gargle
Citrus aurantium, limonis, or medica, as preventive ; the efficacy is due to potassium salts it contains
Ergot, internally to restrain hæmorrhage
Erythroxylon coca
Feronia elephantum
Lemon juice, preventive and curative
Malt
Myrrh tincture, with alum or with potassium chlorate as lotion for ulceration of the gums
Quinine, with mineral acids when much prostration
Tamarindus indicus
Thuja occidentalis tinct
Vegetable charcoal, as tooth powder to remove fœtid odour
Vinegar
Vitis quadrangularis

Septicæmia ; Pyæmia. *(See Vol. I, page 569.)*

Quinine, in large doses, to diminish the temperature
Caryophilli oil, as antiseptic
Gaultheria oil, as antiseptic
Thyme oil, as antiseptic

Shock after Operations. *(See Vol. I, page 570.)*

Atropine and belladonna, hypodermically
Codeine, hypodermically after laparatomy to relieve pain, to prevent intestinal contraction, and to relax tonic spasms of vessels in the first stage of shock as known by small and rapid pulse
Digitalin, with atropine hypodermically is very useful in the second stage of paresis of the vessels
Ergotine
Morphine, a relaxer of spasms of vessels in the first stage of shock
Strychnine, hypodermically in the second or paretic state when the pulse is weak, soft and compressible
Turpentine stupes, internally or rubbing over the limbs

Skin Eruptions : the result of Drugs administered internally or locally applied. *(See Vol. I, page 571.)*

Aconite vesicular exanthemata
Apples, acne about the mouth
Atropine, erythema like the rash of scarlet fever
Belladonna, erythema
Castor oil, urticaria
Cinchona, quinine, like carbolic acid strychnine, erythema, papular eruptions, purpura hæmorrhagica, pemphigus on the face and neck and then on the whole body
Copaiba or cubebs, erythema, urticaria, eczema, pemphigus, rash on ankles and wrists

Skin Eruptions.—*contd.*

Croton oil, locally applied, papules and pustules
Digitalis, erythema
Opium, morphine, codeine :—erythema, itching, papules and marked desquamation
Rhus toxicodendron, and other varietes of senna intolerable itching, vesicles and pustules
Santonine pemphigus and vesicle
Strawberries, urticaria
Tar, acne
Turpentine, like copaiba
Walnuts, inflammation of the buccal mucous membrane

Sore Throat.

Acetum, hot vinegar inhalation
Acid tannic or gallic as spray or dusting powder or gargle, very useful
Aconite tincture when tempnature is high ; useful in ordinary sore throat
Althœa with borax and sodium salicylate
Aristolochia serpentaria, locally as gargle
Belladonna alone or with aconite in high fever to relieve spasm of the pharyngeal muscles
Cochlearia armoracia, as gargle
Capsicum tincture as gargle in relaxed sore throat
Catechu, as astringent gargle
Cimicifuga tincture, in simple sore throat or in malignant sore throat when the pharynx is dry and covered with mucus. Given with opium and syrup of tolu in acute catarrh
Cubeb powder, locally as insufflation
Glycerrhiza glabra
Guaiacum, compound tincture, as gargle in simple sore throat and commencing tonsillitis
Hydrastis fluid extract, as gargle in chronic sore throat and in follicular pharyngitis
Ipecacuanha wine, as spray, very useful in hoaseness and in inflammatory sore throat due to congestion of vocals cords
Kanchan chhal, decoction as gargle
Meriandra strobilifera, infusion of leaves as gargle
Moringa pterygosperma, infusion of bark as gargle
Myrrh, as gargle in ulcerated condition of the throat
Phytolacca, internally and as gargle
Pulsatilla, in acute coryza without gastric irritation
Punica granatum bark, as gargle
Rhus glabra, decoction with potassium chlorate as gargle
Sanguinaria tincture as spray
Soymida febrifuga, the bark as gargle
Tannin, as powder, gargle or spray ; with glycerin it is useful after acute inflammation to relieve aphthous, sore throat with tendency to catarrh
Xanthoxylum, bark decoction, used as gargle or internally in chronic cases

Inhalation of vapours or of pulverized fluid by atomizer.

Formula.—Terminalia belerica, rock salt, piper longum, cloves, liquorice and himaja, equal parts. A linctus to be kept in the mouth ; used in hoarseness, sore throat, cough and catarrh.

Spasmodic Affections.

Aconite, internally or externally as ointment ; useful in mild local spasmodic affections as spasmodic laryngitis, asthma, cough, angina pectoris, &c.
Atropine, hypodermically to relieve local spasm
Belladonna, to relieve spasm of sphincters, especially of pelvic organs
Camphor, to relieve spasm of the bladder causing strangury
Cardamom, to relieve gastric spasm
Chamomile oil, useful in pseudo-angina pectoris and in spasms of hysteria
Hyoscine, very useful in various spasms
Ipecacuanha, useful in spasm of the respiratory organs
Lobelia is useful
Lupulin, in gouty spasms
Mustard poultices, as counter-irritant in spasmodic affections
Opium, useful if given with stimulants as alcohol, chloroform or ether
Strychnine, useful in spasmodic asthma, chorea, epilepsy, tetanus, &c.
Sumbul, to relieve gastric spasms
Tobacco, to relieve muscular spasms, and spasmodic asthma
Veratrine solution, locally applied to the eye lids to relieve spasm of the orbicularis

Spinal Congestion and Concussion. Spinal Irritation. (*See Vol. I, page 572.*)

Aconite, ointment locally in congestion and irritation
Antiphlogistic measures
Arnica, in spinal concussion
Belladonna, locally ; better than aconite to relieve irritation
Bleeding to relieve the heart in concussion
Ergot, in large doses
Leeches to the column
Opium, lead lotion in concussion over the seat of injury
Turpentine stupes or as hot epithem
Vinegar, to restore consciouness
Blisters to spine
Conium, to relieve irritability of the reflex function of the cord
Ignatia, to diminish irritability of cerebro-spinal axis
Strychnine, to stimulate the depressed nerve centres, to relieve wandering pains due to irritability of the nervous system

Spinal Paralysis or Softening; Locomotor Ataxia. (*See Vol. I, page 572.*)

Electricity, to the spine and to nerves and muscles
Ergot, in hyperæmia of the cord, to occlude the spinal arteries and thus starve inflammation
Belladonna, if softening is due to chronic inflammation of the cord
Hyoscyamus, to control tremors
Physostigma, in paraplegia due to myelitis

Spleen Affections. (*See Vol. I, page 572.*)

Carica papaya, the milky juice, given internally
Cinchona and its preparations
Ergot
Luffa amara in enlargement of spleen due to malaria
Quininæ sulphas, in simple malarial enlargement
Quinine fluoride
Salvadora persica
Vitex negundo

Formula.—Confection containing—Nishotar, gulvel, garmâro, kadu, triphla, indrayan, daruhalad, and nimdo equal parts with sugar.

Or Gul-e-banaphsha, hira dakhan, uste-khudus, kâsani, variâlee, dhânâ, and garmâro with sâkar.

Sterility. (*See Vol. I, page 572.*)

Cimicifuga, if due to congestive dysmenorrhœa
Coca extract
Damiana, to cure spermatorrhœa
Electricity, if due to torpor of the uterus
Gossypium radix, if due to dysmenorrhœa
Nux vomica, to relieve spermatorrhœa
Sanguinaria
Stillingia
Dilatation of the os and cervix, when sterility is due to pinhole os or to plugging of the cervix with mucus
Intra-Uterine stem pessary, to stimulate the lining membrane of the uterus

Stomatitis.

Acid tannic with glycerin in ulcerative stomatitis
Acacia catechu, locally applied to ulcerated spongy gum
Balsamodendron myrrha with lime water and honey locally applied
Capsicum tincture with dilute muriatic acid and honey locally
Cascarilla, locally useful for thrush
Cinchona, with creta preperata and acid tannic as dusting powder
Cleansing nipples in breast-fed babies to prevent stomatitis
Cocaine, with soda salicylas and water as tampon or cocaine solution before cauterization to the ulcerated gums
Cydonia, infusion of leaves locally
Eucalyptus decoction of the leaves locally, or the tincture internally

Stomatitis.—*contd.*

Geranium maculatum, as a wash or gargle in aphthæ
Hamamelis tincture, locally
Hydrastis fluid extract, locally in aphthous and mercurial stomatitis
Iris, in dyspeptic mouth ulcers
Krameria, as local astringent
Meriandra strobilifera, as infusion locally applied
Myrrh, borax and potas chlorate topically
Odina wodier, decoction as gargle
Ocymum gratissimum, locally as gargle
Pterocarpus marsupium, locally to relaxed uvula
Rhus glabra (sumach), extract as a mouth wash
Slippery elm, locally to the spongy gums
Starch, locally
Thymol with borax, as a mouth wash
Uncaria gambier, locally to ulcerated gums

Syncope.

Atropine, hypodermically to improve the force and rapidity of heart's action and thus resuscitating the patient
Belladonna, very useful in cardiac syncope
Cinnamon oil, a powerful stimulant
Camphor, as cardiac stimulant
Duboisine, a good substitute for atropine
Lavander, compound tincture very useful
Nux vomica tincture, to restore cardiac action when there is failure of the heart in syncope of a neurotic origin
Digitalis, internally or hypodermically in sudden collapse after hæmorrhage

Synovitis. (*See Vol. I, page 574.*)

Aconite, to relieve pain in inflamed joints
Bandage or strapping to cause absorption of the effused fluid
Blisters flying after the acute stage has passed
Conium, in scrofulous joints very useful
Cupping near the joints
Fomentation, dry heat, or poultices to the joint in the acute stage
Free stimulation in synovitis due to gonorrhœa, acute rheumatism, slight injury occurring in strumous subject
Leeches to the joints
Lotions, evaporating, of arnica, alcohol and water
Morphine and mercury oleate, locally to the affected joints in syphilitic cases
Position straight
Quinine, iron, and potassium iodide internally in syphilitic cases
Splints to keep the limb motionless in synovitis due to injury

Syphilis. (*See Vol. I, page 574.*)

Belladonna and mercury ointment in secondary ulceration of the rectum
Benzoic antiseptic dressing in secondary syphilitic ulcers
Camphor dressing for phagedenic chancres
Calotropis gigantea, useful in secondary syphilis
Guaiacum, as alterative, in secondary and tertiary syphilis as a vehicle for potassium iodide and mercuric chloride
Hemidesmus indicus, internally in constitutional syphilis
Hydrocotyle asiatica, internnlly in secondary form
Kola nuts, useful internally in tertiary form
Manaca, in secondary and tertiary form given internally
Mezereon oil, in secondary cases
Nicotiana tabacum, locally to syphilitic nodes
Papaine, for syphilitic ulcers on the tongue and throat
Plumbago rosea, internally in secondary syphilis
Sassafras oil in secondary cases
Sarsaparilla given with guaiacum and as an adjunct to other alteratives.
Stillingea, in sloughing phagedena and in cachexia due to breaking down by a long course of mercury and iodide of potasium
Sanguinaria, in secondary and tertiary forms, very useful

Formula.—Panch Nimb Churan (a powerful alterative) contains the root, leaves, fruits, flowers and bark of limdo, each 15 parts; loha-bhashm, himaj, tâklâ bij, chitrak, bhilâmo, vâvading, sâkar, âmlâ, halad, trikatu, bâvachi garmaro, gokharu each 1 part. Mix and add the juice of bhângro and decoction of kher chhâl, and make a paste. Dose, 2 to 4 drs. In syphilis.

Ushbo, chobchini, surpunkh, harde, behadânâ, ustekhudus, senna, pastân khubâjee, khatmi, rose buds, gurakhmundi, unâb, gaojabân, and banaphshâ; make decoction for secondary syphilis.

Testicles (Swollen); Tuberculosis of. (*See Vol. I, page 576.*)

Camphorated naphthol, hypodermically used in tuberculosis of the testis
Hyoscyamus
Tectona grandis

Tetanus. (*See Vol. I, page 576.*)

Aconite, very useful to control muscular spasms
Antitetanic serum
Apomorphine, as antagonistic, and motor paralyser
Atropine, injected into muscle to produce mild poisoning
Belladonna extract, internally and locally to wound
Cannabis indica, with chloral, useful in traumatic form
Curare, hypodermically is very useful
Cocaine and morphine, hypodermically injected are very useful in relieving idiopathic cases
Duboisine, like atropine is very useful
Gelsemium, its spinal action is opposed to that of tetanus and hence very useful
Hyoscyamine, in traumatic cases is very useful
Morphine, hypodermically injected deeply into tetanized muscles or to point of entrance of the nerves
Nicotine by rectum, or hypodermically
Physostigma, fluid extract, internally better than nicotine, or by the rectum or hypodermically
Opium, alone or with chloral
Vapour bath, very useful

External remedies.—Acupuncture on each side of the spine. Nerve stretching when a nerve is implicated in the cicatrix. Neurotomy. Baths, warm or vapour. Ice bag to spine.

Thirst.

Bitters with acid drinks quench thirst by promoting secretion of alkoline saliva; but if given in excess, they derange the stomach
Cascarilla or orange peel acidulated with dilute hydrochloric acid quenches thirst in fevers
Cloves
Fruit juices in moderation, very useful
Ice sucking quenches thirst in fevers
Tepid drinks, quenches thirst of diabetic patients

Tic Douloureux. (*See Vol. I, page 576.*)

Aconite with benefit
Atropine, hypodermically and as ointment
Cannabis indica extract, is very useful, next to morphine
Cimicifuga, very useful
Menthol, locally applied
Morphine with atropine, hypodermically is useful
Physostigma extract, solution dropped within the eyelids of the affected side gives relief
Pulsatilla, to relieve tic
Quinine is very useful
Stramonium extract, gives relief; to be omitted if narcotic symptoms set in
Turpentine, when the tic is due to rheumatism or to fœcal accumulations
Veratrine ointment
Valerianate of zinc with hyoscyamus is useful

Tongue (Affections of); Glossitis. (*See Vol. I, page 579*)

Cinnamon oil, a powerful stimulant, useful in paralysis of the tongue
Cloves, as masticatory
Cochlearia as gargle
Conium, is very useful in ulcer of the tongue
Frœnum to be divided in tongue, tie
Ginger, as gargle
Mezereon, as masticatory in paralysis of the tongue
Pyrethrum, as gargle

Tonsillitis. *(See Vol. I, page 579.)*

Aconite tincture, when there are high fever and increased arterial tension, gives relief
Belladonna tincture, internally very beneficial
Capsicum tincture gargle as in severe tonsillitis
Cocaine, 10 p.c. solution locally to remove pain and to promote resolution; it often leads to paralysis of the palate muscles so that liquids regurgitate through the nose, it often when applied as a paint will cut short the attack
Emetics, at the onset to cut short the attack
Guaiacum tincture, with glycerin internally very effective, given as emulsion with mucilage or yolk of egg or as gargle in acute tonsillitis
Morphine and mercury oleate, in obstinate and painful tonsillitis
Opium, as Dover's powder, is very useful
Phytolacca
Quinine
Tannic acid, is useful as gargle

Tonsils (Enlarged.) *(See Vol. I, page 579.)*

Catechu, infusion with tincture of kino is used as gargle
Cimicifuga, decoction of the root as gargle in ulcerated tonsils
Citric acid when rubbed on tonsils removes enlargements
Coptis teeta, the infusion as gargle in ulcerated tonsils
Ergot or ergotin, by injection
Tannin, saturated solution applied locally to the tonsils
Scarification

Torticollis. *(See Vol. I, page 580.)*

Capsicum, infusion locally used
Cimicifuga, is very useful
Conium, when due to spasmodic action of the muscle
Gelsemium, fluid extract, hypodermically administered is useful
Opium liniment or as plaster
Surgical treatment—nerve stretching.
Local pressure

Tremors. *(See Vol. I, page 580.)*

Cocaine, to control tremors due to alcohol or old age
Conine, to control excessive tremor
Gelsemium with conium and hyoscyamus to palliate excessive tremor to quiet the nervous lystem
Hyoscine, useful to relieve tremor, a symptom of disseminated sclerosis or of delirium
Hyoscyamine
Hyoscyamus tincture, to control mercurial tremor
Spartine sulphate
Veratrine, useful in alleviating alcoholic tremor or that due to disseminated sclerosis

Trismus, Lackjaw, in new born Infants. *(See Vol. I, page 580.)*

Belladonna
Cannabis
Conium
Gelsemium
Opium, with castor oil
Warm bath

Tuberculosis—Tuberculous affections. Tabes Mesenterica.

(See Vol. I, page 580.)

Barosma betulina
Camphorated naphthol hypodermically in tuberculosis of the testis, bladder, &c.
Chaulmugra oil, in tabes
Chocolate, or cocoa
Quinine, to subdue the fever, aided by wine, and peptonized food

Tympanitis. (*See Vol. I, page 581.*)

Anisochilus carnosus, in flatulence
Asafetida internally, or as enema in tympanitis, of fever or in hysteria
Capsicum, is very useful
Chamomile oil, internally is ueeful
Cocculus indicus tincture, useful in tympanitis, due to fever or to peritonitis
Ginger, with drastic purgatives relieves tympanitis
Sumbul
Turpentine, useful in tympanitis of typhoid fever with prostration
Vegetable charcoal, in flatulence

Ulcers, Sores. (*See Vol. I, page 583.*)

Acid gallic
Balsam of peru and tolu, very useful
Belladonna, is highly efficient
Benzoin, locally
Camphor dusted over indolent ulcers is useful
Capsicum tincture or infusion is useful locally as a stimulant in scrofulous ulcers and fistulous sores
Catechu powder locally
Charcoal poultice, locally to sloughing sores
Chimaphilla, locally useful
Chinchona bark powder, to be dusted over foul, indolent, sloughing or gangrenous ulcers to clean and stimulate the ulcers and to promote healing
Conium poultices, locally to relieve pain and improve the sore
Hamamelis, is useful in varicose ulcers
Hydrastis, internally and externally in ulcers of the legs, in rectal and rodent ulcers and in uterine ulcers
Ichthyol ointment, useful in ulcers of the leg
Myrrh locally
Opium or morphine with glycerin internally or locally to relieve the pain in phagedenic and indolent ulcers
Papain
Phytolacca, as local application very useful
Pyrogallic acid, useful in venereal sores
Rhatany, locally
Sanguinaria, with glycerin to repress granulations of indolent ulcers
Savine, as an acrid caustic useful to arrest the spread of ulcer
Starch, iodized, dusted locally
Tannin, with glycerin locally as a coating over wounds or discharging sores
Tar water, locally
Turpentine, internally in ulceration of the bowels; locally with olive oil to phagedeinc and indolent ulcers

External remedies.—Bandaging, cleanliness, immersion of the part affected in hot water, recumbent posture, rest, section of exposed nerve filaments in cases of irritable ulcers, support, water dressing, and yeast poultice.

Uræmia; Uræmic Coma, due to Narcotic Poisoning. (*See Vol. I, page 585.*)

Apocynum canabinum is useful
Coffee, useful in diabetic coma
Croton oil, internally as a purgative
Colchicum, an excellent derivative with other purgatives
Digitalis, leaves as infusion, internally or a poultice to the loins and hypogastrium to procure free action of the kidneys
Elaterium, as a free purge. To be avoided if the heart is weak or fatty and œdema of the lungs is present
Jaborandi in uræmic coma is very useful
Mustard poultces to the feet and ankles in coma due to narcotic poisoning
Opium, internally or morphine hypodermically, is very useful in uræmic convulsions and, in acute uræmia; to be avoided in chronic uræmia
Pilocarpine, an active diaphoretic, useful to relieve uræmic symptoms such as headache, drowsiness, and convulsions; to be a voided in weak or fatty heart in œdema of the lungs
Scoparii succus, internally
Turpentine oil, as enema is useful

Urethra, Stricture of. (*See Vol. I, page 585.*)

Aconite, in spasmodic cases
Buchu, in spasmodic form with irritability of the bladder and in gleet
Cocaine, 2 p.c. solution with olive oil locally injected into the urethra
Opium, internally or as suppository or fomentation as in spasmodic stricture

External remedies.—Catheterization under an anæsthetic in spasmodic stricture, and in organic stricture; gradual dilatation, electrolysis, a weak galvanic current, injection of oil before dilatation.

Urethritis. (*See Vol. I, page 585.*)

Acacia, gum arabic, to relieve irrita as an auxiliary to other remedies
Acid tannic, as medicated bougie
Aconite, in urethral stricture (spasmodic); if there is fever after passage of sound. to prevent a chill
Aleuritis triloba, in inflammatory condition
Astragalus verus, to relieve irritation of the mucous membrane of the bladder
Buchu, if the urethra is irritable; also in stricture and gleet
Chimaphilla umbellata, in chronic cases
Cubebs, oleo resin, internally
Mucilaginous drinks
Myrtol, internally in chronic urethritis and chronic cystitis
Opium suppository or fomentation to the bladder
Strophanthus tincture, to prevent chill, after the passage of instruments into the urethra
Tannin bougies for urethritis in females

Uric Acid Diathesis. (*See Vol. I, page 585.*)

Boerhavia diffusa
Ichnocarpus
Piper nigrum
Phyllanthus neruii
Stigmata maidis

Formula:—In brick red deposit. Sodii biboras, 2 drs.; extract uva ursi, 8 drs., spiritus etheris nitrosi, 4 drs.; tinct. opii, 4 drs.; and aquæ, 4 ozs. Dose, 1 dr. internally;

Urinary Disorders. (*See Vol. I, page 587.*)

Acid benzoic, or sodium benzoate to neutralize morbid alkalinity of the urine, to render alkaline urine acid, and to check formation of phosphates
Aconite, useful internally in retention of urine due to chill
Buchu, is very useful in retention or incontinence of urine in cystic catarrh, implicating kidneys or ureters
Cannabis indica, in retention of urine due to spinal diseases
Digitalis leaves, infusion as a diuretic, is very useful in sudden suppression of urine from cold or damp or after scarlatina
Strychnine, useful in retention or incontinence of urine in old people
Triticum infusion to relieve strangury, cystitis, &c.
Turpentine, useful in chronic cystitis, bloody urine, in incontinence of urine due to atony of the bladder

Urticaria. (*See Vol. I, page 527.*)

Benzoic acid solution as lotion or benzoin tincture to paint on the skin to control itching
Colchicum, in gouty persons is very useful
Copaiba, in drop doses, checks urticaria or controls it; although in full doses it produces it
Jaborandi fluid extract, to allay itching; to be avoided if there is much depression or sweating
Menthol, locally applied
Strychnine, with emetics and purgatives is very useful in chronic cases
Tobacco leaves locally
Warm baths, with benefit

Uterine Affections. (*See Vol. I, page 588.*)

Belladonna, with tannin as pessary or as vaginal or rectal injections to relieve neuralgic or inflammatory pains
Caulophyllum thalictroides, a good remedy in prolapse or sub-involution of the uterus
Cannabis indica, to allay neuralgic or inflammatory pains or the pain of cancer
Chiananthus cheiri, to alleviate pain
Cimicifuga, to prevent miscarriage, to relieve irritability and to reduce prolapse
Conium as injection, to relieve pain of uterine cancer
Digitalis is very useful in subinvolution
Ergotin, relieves congestion, lessens chronic inflammation and checks hæmorrhage; as an injection, it diminishes fibroids polypi, &c. In large spongy and sub-involuted uterus its injection into the cervix has been useful

Uterine Affections.—(*Contd.*)

Erigeron canadense, a uterine sedative, useful to relieve pain and irritability
Hydrastis, fluid extract, locally applied in ulceration and erosion of cervix, and also given internally in leucorrhœa and to check uterine hæmorrhages
Ipecacuanha, in subacute metritis during the puerperal state
Opium with starch as rectal injection, to relieve pain and irritation in cancer
Tannin, locally in uterine ulceration

External remedies.—Injections, hot water or hot douche; and rest.

Uvula Relaxed. (*See Vol. I, page 590.*)

Acacia catechu, locally applied to relaxed uvula
Acetum, hot vinegar by inhalation
Anacyclus pyrethrum, to chew in relaxed uvula
Amputation of the elongated uvula after application of cocaine solution, 20 p. c.
Cassia auriculata, decoction as a gargle in relaxed uvula
Capsicum infusion as gargle
Cinchona, decoction as gargle or given internally
Cocaine, with krameria as a local astringent, 20 p. c. solution, useful for enlarged and elongated uvula
Quercus bark, as infusion used as gargle in spongy gums, and relaxed uvula
Rhatany, useful for relaxed uvula
Pyrethrum, to chew in relaxed uvula
Soymida febrifuga, locally applied to relaxed uvula
Tannin, a useful astringent for relaxed uvula
Uncaria gambier, locally applied to relaxed uvula

Vaginismus, Dysparpunia; Vaginal Irritation. (*See Vol. I, page 590.*)

Belladonna extract 1 and lard 8; or belladonna and iodoform as pessary to relieve pain
Cocaine ointment, with morphine and conium to be smeared over the painful spot
Hygiene, fresh air, hot water injection
Ice
Krameria pessaries
Menthol
Morphine
Opium
Sedatives
Tropa cocaine

Formula.—Butter of cocao, 2 grs.: potassii bromidi, 5 grs.; belladonna extract, 3 grs.; acid thymic, ½ gr. Make vaginal suppository. For vaginismus.

Vaginitis. (*See Vol. I, page 590.*)

Acid tannic, with glycerin locally in chronic vaginitis
Caulophyllum thalictroides, very useful locally
Opium with emollients as vaginal injection
Pinus canadensis extract, locally as injection
Vaginal pessaries: Butter of cocoa as excipient with sedative agents as atropine, morphia, opium, and belladonna
Vaginal astringent injections containing alum, iron, catechu, acetate of lead and opium, tannic acid, gallic acid, matico, &c.

Vertigo; Dizziness; Menier's Disease. (*See Vol. I, page 591.*)

Acid hydrocyanic dil
Digitalis with citrate of iron and strychnine, to improve general nutrition
Gastric and hepatic sedatives, as the disease is in some cases symptomatic of stomach and liver disorders
Quinine, useful in aural vertigo

Vomiting; Nausea; Sea Sickness. (*See Vol. I, page 569*)

Acid hydrocyanic dil, useful in nervous vomiting, or in that due to gastric ulcer
Aconite, with bismuth is useful in vomiting of pregnancy
Apomorphine, to empty the stomach of its contents and then to check vomiting
Atropine, hypodermically, or liquor internally gives relief in vomiting or sea-sickness
Bryonia, to relieve bilious vomiting and headache
Calumba, in vomiting due to kidney disease, renal calculi, pregnancy, and dentition
Cinnamon useful
Cloves useful
Cocaine, internally or as spray up the nasal passages to check nausea or locally to the cervix uteri in vomiting of pregnancy
Codeine, useful in vomiting from any cause
Cocculus indicus, in cephalic nausea with ineffectual efforts at vomiting
Ipecacuanha wine, in drop doses is useful in sympathetic nervous vomiting of pregnancy or in vomiting of chronic alcoholism
Iris, in vomiting with supra-orbital pain, hepatic derangements, &c.
Kola nut to chew
Menthol, in olive oil dropped on sugar or with brandy taken internally in obstinate cases
Mustard plaster over the stomach
Morphine, hypodermically or by suppository in severe vomiting
Nutmeg
Nux vomica tincture, or powder alone or with ipecacuanha if the tongue is coated; a good substitute for arsenic in atony of stomach, dyspepsia or in vomiting of pregnancy
Opium as enema or internally in severe vomiting of pregnancy or in that due to biliary or renal calculi, dysmenorrhœa, &c
Pepper, peppermint, or phudino, very useful
Pulsatilla, in vomiting attended with dyspepsia, coated tongue, and headache
Quinine, in sympathetic vomiting
Serpentaria, for bilious vomiting
Staphisagria, in obstinate vomiting of pregnancy
Strychnine, and atropine hypodermically
Tea hot is useful
Veratrum album, in vomiting and purging of summer diarrhœa
Viburnum, in vomiting of pregnancy

Formula.—Cocaine, 2; belladonna, ½; butter of cocoa, 2; make suppository, 1. To relieve nausea of pregnancy.

External remedies.—Blister to the pit of stomach or over 4th and 5th dorsal, vertebræ in sickness of pregnancy, dilatation of the cervix, horizontal posture, absolute rest, ice bag to the spine, ice to suck, iced champagne, nutrient enemata, mustard poultices to the epigastrium, counter irritation.

Whooping Cough; Pertussis.

Acid hydrocyanic dil, in cough from habit or in nervous sympathetic cough
Aconite, useful in acute congestion given with ipecacuanha and cherry laurel water; a good preventive or an abortive remedy
Belladonna tincture, alone or the extract with zinc sulphate is very useful when due to dentition; given in febrile stage, also to relieve spasm and congestion of the air passages, and in determination of blood to the head. It lessens the bronchial secretion when profuse
Camphor monobromide, with syrup of tolu is very useful
Castanea, decoction of chestnut, or the extract, is useful
Chamomile oil in cherry laurel water
Cocaine hydrochlorate, solution, a paint on the tongue, tonsils, fauces, and larynx
Codeine
Conium or hydrobromate of conine, very useful
Drosera is effective
Gelsemium, during the spasmodic stage
Gelaphala internally is useful
Ipecacuanha wine, in bronchitic or pneumonic complication alone or with ammonium bromide

Whooping Cough.—(*contd.*)

Lactucarium syrup as a vehicle for cough mixtures is very useful
Lobelia tincture, internally in spasmodic cases and when the cough is imminent
Myrtol gives great relief
Opium during the paroxysm is useful
Quinine tannas with sodium carbonate, and pulvis acaciæ used as an insufflator
Quinine sulphate in solution locally to the fauces
Quabain
Tar by inhalation
Valerian to control or check the paroxysms

Formula.—Croton chloral, 5 grs.; etheris, 10 ms.; potass bromid, 20 grs.; tr. belladon, 5 ms.; tr. hyoscyam, 30 ms.; and syrup, 4 drs. One dose.

Worms—Anthelmintics; Vermifuges.

Apocynum cannabinum
Areca catechu
Artemisia sieversiana
Atis
Castor oil by the mouth or by injection
Cocoanut
Cyperus pertenuis
Embelia ribes
Gelaphal
Jalap
Jussiæ suffruticosum
Picorrhiza
Punica granatum
Savine oil
Scammony
Spigelia with senna and pimenta
Turpentine oil
Thyme oil
Uva ursi

Vermicides (*a*) Round Worms (Ascaris lumbricoides).

Absinthium
Alstonia
Aristolochia, infusion of leaves
Bawachee
Blumea balsamifera
Brayera anthelmintica
Butea frondosa (seeds)
Callinsonia canadenseis, extract, as rectal injection
Chenopodium anthelminticum
Cleome viscosa
Eucalyptus, for rectal injection
Gloriosa superba
Helleborus niger, fluid extract
Hollarhena antidysenterica (seeds)
Ignatia to check convulsions due to worms
Melia azadirachta, root bark decoction
Myrtol very useful
Mucuna pruriens, hairs as electuary.
Nigella sativa; seeds
Ophioxylon serpentinum root
Papaw juice for lumbrici
Peganum harmala—seeds
Polyporus anthelminticus
Quinine, as a tonic and as a prophylactic, given internally and as injection into the rectum. It prevents the production of abundant' mucus which favours the growth of worms
Santonine and calomel at bed time, and senna draught next morning
Sapindus trifoliatus
Strychnos colubrina (wood)
Vernonia anthelmintica seeds, powdered or infusion
Worm seed oil, 4 ms.
Water-melon seeds

(*b*) Tape Worms; Tænia.

Absinth
Acid embelic
Acid filicic
Ailanthus glandulosa, bark as decoction
Anacardium
Aspidium marginalis (oleo resin)
Cusso fluid extract, or infusion of flowers
Filix mas, extract falicis liquid, upon an empty stomach followed by a purge
Kâlâdanâ
Kamala
Mellotus philippiensis powder
Oleum tigli, with chloroform and glycerin
Pepo
Pelliterine tannate
Polyporus anthelmintica
Quinine as injunction
Turpentine oil with castor oil
Thymol

Formula.—Aspidium, ½ dr.; pomegranate radicis, 4 drs.; pumkin seeds, 8 drs.; ergot, 2 drs.; and aqua, 8 oz. Make decoction, when ready add—croton oil, 6 drops; acaciæ, 2 drs.; and extract of male fern, 8 fluid drs. Dose, ½ oz. internally for tape worms.

(c) Threadworms; Ascaris Vermicularis.

Aloes with potassium carbonate and asafetida as an enema or internally
Eucalyptol, for rectal injection
Gardinia gummifera
Kamal
Musk root
Myrtol
Pharbitis Nil
Picræna excelsa, as enema
Oleum morrhuæ and olive oil in rectal enema
Pepo, as emulsion, against tinea
Papaw juice
Quassia infusion with sodium chloride and simple bitters internally or as an enema
Scammony better than aloes alone or with calomel
Tannin, as injection or as suppository
Valerian
Vegetable, astringents for rectal injection namely, catechu, kino, rhatany, red gum, hæmatoxylon, segat chhal, vinegar vitex negundo and valerian

Wounds; Bedsores.

Aconite in surgical fever
Aloes, as dusting powder locally to favour cicatrization of wounds
Arnica infusion for external bruises, cuts, and for internal injuries
Balsam of peru with carbolic acid to close recent wounds
Benzoin tincture, as a basis for all healing balsams
Bryonia tincture, locally
Camphor carbolate
Charcoal wood
Chaulmugra oil
Cinnamon oil
Cotton wool
Eucalyptus oil locally
Gutta percha, dissolved in tincture or chlorform as a protective to wounds
Hamamelis, locally
Hæmatoxylon with butter of cocao or benzoated lard
Opium camphorated, as tincture locally applied or given internally in abdominal wounds to quiet the intestines
Photoxylon, substitute for collodion
Sesamum indicum, oil as dressing
Tannin with glycerin as protective to wounds
Tar bandage
Thymol with alcohol and glycerin as solution
Tragacanth, as a dusting powder or as a protective agent for granulations
Turpentine oil
Water dressing
Yeast or charcoal poultices in phagedenic sores or ulcers

INDEX.